HEMATOLOGY IN CLINICAL PRACTICE

Notice

A Lange Medical Book

HEMATOLOGY IN CLINICAL PRACTICE

Fifth edition

ROBERT S. HILLMAN, M.D.
Chairman Emeritus, Department of Medicine
Maine Medical Center
Portland, Maine
Professor of Medicine
Maine Medical Center—Tufts University School of Medicine
Boston, Massachusetts

KENNETH A. AULT, M.D.
Director Emeritus
Maine Medical Center Research Institute
Portland, Maine
Associate Professor of Medicine
University of Vermont College of Medicine
Burlington, Vermont

MICHEL LEPORRIER, M.D.
Professor of Hematology
Head, Clinical Hematology Department
Centre Hospitalier & Universitaire
Caen, France

HENRY M. RINDER, M.D.
Director, Hematology Laboratories
Yale-New Haven Hospital
Professor of Laboratory Medicine and
Internal Medicine (Hematology)
Yale University School of Medicine
New Haven, Connecticut

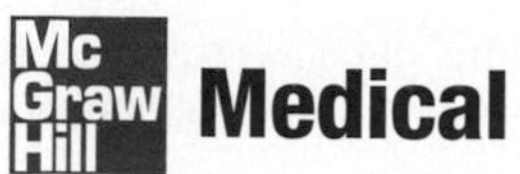

New York Chicago San Francisco Lisbon London Madrid Mexico City
Milan New Delhi San Juan Seoul Singapore Sydney Toronto

The McGraw·Hill Companies

Hematology in Clinical Practice, Fifth Edition

1 2 3 4 5 6 7 8 9 0 CTP/CTP 14 13 12 11 10

ISBN 978-0-07-162699-6
MHID 0-07-162699-9

This book was set in Goudy by Glyph International.
The editors were James Shanahan and Harriet Lebowitz.
The production supervisor was Catherine Saggese.
Project management was provided by Rajni Pisharody at Glyph International.
The text designer was Mary McKeon.
Cover photo: Scanning electron micrograph of red and white blood cells and platelets. Credit: Stem Jems/ Photo Researchers, Inc.
China Translation & Printing Services, Ltd. was printer and binder.

This book is printed on acid-free paper.

Library of Congress Cataloging-in-Publication Data

Hematology in clinical practice / Robert S. Hillman ... [et al.]. —5th ed.
p. ; cm.
Rev. ed. of: Hematology in clinical practice / Robert S. Hillman, Kenneth A. Ault, Henry M. Rinder. 4th ed. c2005.
Includes bibliographical references and index.
ISBN-13: 978-0-07-162699-6 (pbk. : alk. paper)
ISBN-10: 0-07-162699-9 (pbk. : alk. paper) 1. Blood—Diseases. I. Hillman, Robert S., 1934- II. Hillman, Robert S., 1934- Hematology in clinical practice.
[DNLM: 1. Hematologic Diseases—diagnosis. 2. Hematologic Diseases—therapy. 3. Hematologic Diseases—physiopathology. WH 120 H4874 2011]
RC636.H46 2011
616.1′5—dc22 2009053553

McGraw-Hill books are available at special quantity discounts to use as premiums and sales promotions, or for use in corporate training programs. To contact a representative, please e-mail us at bulksales@mcgraw-hill.com

International Edition ISBN 978-0-07-174276-4; MHID 0-07-174276-X.

ill Companies, Inc., for manufacture and export. This book cannot be re-exported from
he International Edition is not available in North America.

CONTENTS

PREFACE

Hematology in Clinical Practice, fifth edition, is written specifically for clinicians—medical students, physicians in training including residents and fellows, primary care internists or family practitioners, and hematologists/oncologists. It is a practical guide to the diagnosis and treatment of disorders of red blood cells, white blood cells, and hemostasis. Each disease state is discussed in terms of the underlying pathophysiology, clinical features that suggest the diagnosis, the use of state-of-the-art laboratory tests in the diagnosis and differential diagnosis of the condition, and current management strategies. For the student or physician in training, chapter sections additionally provide a case-based discussion of the systematic approach to the workup of a patient with hematologic disease, providing a foundation for clinical training.

We would like to thank Dr. Joseph P. Fanning and Dr. James McArthur for photographs from their personal collections, and Catherine Hartung for her artwork.

SECTION I
Red Blood Cell Disorders

NORMAL ERYTHROPOIESIS • 1

The oxygen required by tissues for aerobic metabolism is supplied by the circulating mass of mature **erythrocytes** (red blood cells). The circulating red blood cell population is continually renewed by the erythroid precursor cells in the marrow, under the control of both humoral and cellular growth factors. This cycle of normal erythropoiesis is a carefully regulated process. Oxygen sensors within the kidney detect minute changes in the amount of oxygen available to tissue and by releasing erythropoietin are able to adjust erythropoiesis to match tissue requirements. Thus, **normal erythropoiesis** is best described according to its major components, including red blood cell structure, function, and turnover; the capacity of the erythroid marrow to produce new red blood cells; and growth factor regulation.

STRUCTURE OF THE RED BLOOD CELL

The mature red blood cell is easily recognized because of its unique morphology (Figure 1–1). At rest, the red blood cell takes the shape of a biconcave disc with a mean diameter of 8 μm, a thickness of 2 μm, and a volume of 90 fL. It lacks a nucleus or mitochondria, and 33% of its contents is made up of a single protein, hemoglobin. Intracellular energy requirements are largely supplied by glucose metabolism, which is targeted at maintaining hemoglobin in a soluble, reduced state, providing appropriate amounts of 2,3-diphosphoglycerate (2,3-DPG), and generating adenosine triphosphate (ATP) to support membrane function. Without a nucleus or protein metabolic pathway, the cell has a limited lifespan of 100–120 days. However, the unique structure of the adult red blood cell is perfect for its function, providing maximum flexibility as the cell travels through the microvasculature (Figure 1–2).

Membrane

A. Inner and Outer Layers

The shape, pliability, and resiliency of the red blood cell are largely determined by its membrane. The structure of this membrane is illustrated in Figure 1–3. It is a lipid sheath, just two molecules thick, consisting of closely packed phospholipid molecules. The various surface lipids are in constant motion, forming microdomains or "rafts," which play important physiologic roles. The external surface of the membrane is rich in phosphatidylcholine, sphingomyelin, and glycolipid, whereas the inner layer is largely phosphatidylserine, phosphatidylethanolamine, and phosphatidylinositol. This asymmetry is maintained by **flippase**, an ATP-dependent aminophospholipid translocase that rapidly transports phosphatidylserine and ethanolamine from the outer to the inner membrane. A second calcium-activated transporter, **scramblase**, can disrupt the distribution of membrane phospholipids, leading to a relocation of phosphatidylserine to the cell surface with a resulting increase in the thrombogenic potential of the cell surface. More importantly, accumulation of excess phosphatidylserine on the red cell surface plays a role in red cell senescence and macrophage destruction.

Membrane phospholipids are also vulnerable to oxidation by reactive oxygen species (ROS) resulting in an alteration of the surface organization. This is counteracted by an elaborate antioxidant system, as well as an ATP-dependent regeneration of phospholipids from plasma fatty acids. Approximately 50% of the red blood cell membrane is made up of **cholesterol** that is in equilibrium with the unesterified cholesterol in the plasma. Because of this, the cholesterol content of the membrane is influenced by plasma cholesterol levels, as well as by the activity of the enzyme lecithin cholesterol acyltransferase (LCAT) and bile acids. Patients with liver disease who have impaired

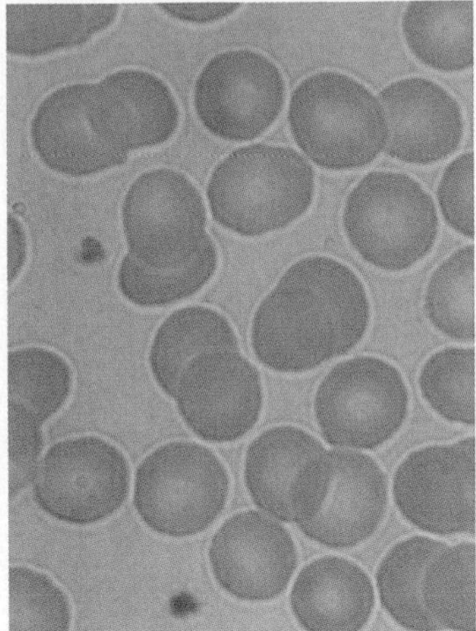

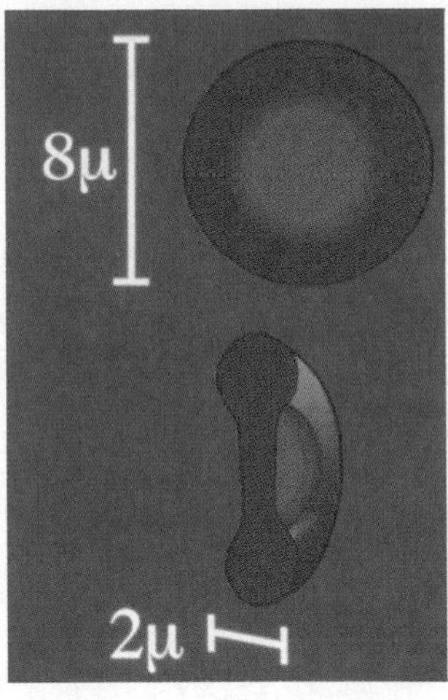

FIGURE I–1. **Red blood cell morphology.** On the stained blood smear, red blood cells appear as a relatively uniform population of anucleate, biconcave cells with a diameter of approximately 8 μm and a width of 2 μm.

LCAT activity accumulate excess cholesterol on the red blood cell membrane, which results in abnormal red blood cell morphology (**targeting**) and at times a shortened survival.

B. Reticular Protein Network

The outer lipid membrane layer is affixed to a reticular protein network consisting of **spectrin** and **actin.** As shown in Figure 1–3, the integral proteins glycophorins (A through C) and band 3, which function as anion exchangers, extend vertically from the spectrin lattice framework through the lipid layer to make contact with the cell surface. Spectrin heterodimers interact horizontally with protein 4.1 and complementary spectrin heterodimers to form a hexagonal lattice framework under the lipid bilayer. Defects in the vertical structure of the membrane (deficiency of spectrin, ankyrin, or band 3, or loss of lipid) result in spherocyte formation. Damage to the horizontal spectrin framework results in severe red cell fragmentation or mild elliptocytosis.

The integral proteins and surface glycosphingolipids are also responsible for the cell's antigenic structure. More than 300 red blood cell antigens have now been classified with the ABO and Rh blood group antigens being of primary importance in typing blood for transfusion (see Chapter 38). Autoantibodies against minor blood group antigens can result in increased red blood cell destruction by the reticuloendothelial cells.

Hemoglobin

The red blood cell is, basically, a container for **hemoglobin**—a 64,500 Da protein made up of 4 polypeptide chains, each containing an active heme group. Each heme group is capable of binding to an oxygen molecule. The **respiratory motion of hemoglobin**, that is, the uptake and release of oxygen to tissues, involves a specific change in molecular structure (Figure 1–4). As hemoglobin shuttles from its deoxyhemoglobin to its oxyhemoglobin form, carbon dioxide (CO_2) and 2,3-DPG are expelled from their position between the β-globin chains, opening the molecule to receive oxygen. Furthermore, oxygen binding by one of the heme groups increases the affinity of the other groups to oxygen loading. This interaction is responsible for the sigmoid shape of the oxygen dissociation curve.

Inherited defects in hemoglobin structure can interfere with this respiratory motion. Most defects are substitutions of a single amino acid in either the α- or β-globin chains. Some interfere with molecular movement, restricting the molecule to either a

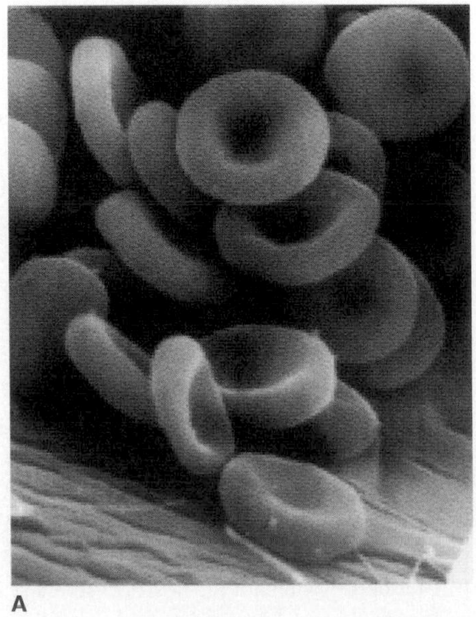
A

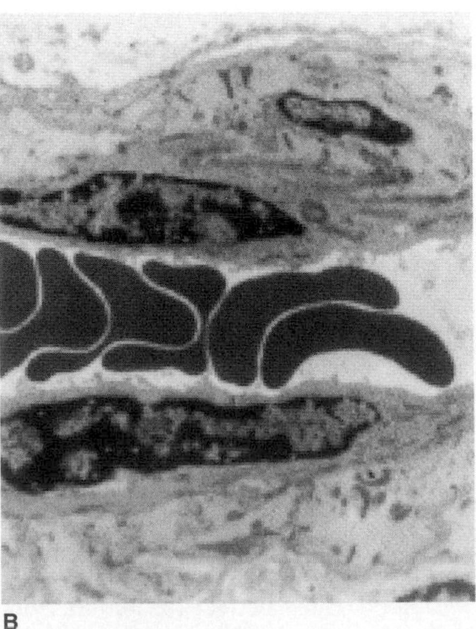
B

FIGURE I–2. **Red blood cell shape and pliability. A:** On scanning EM, the biconcave shape of the red cell at rest is readily apparent. **B:** The exceptional pliability of circulating red cells is shown in this section of a small blood vessel.

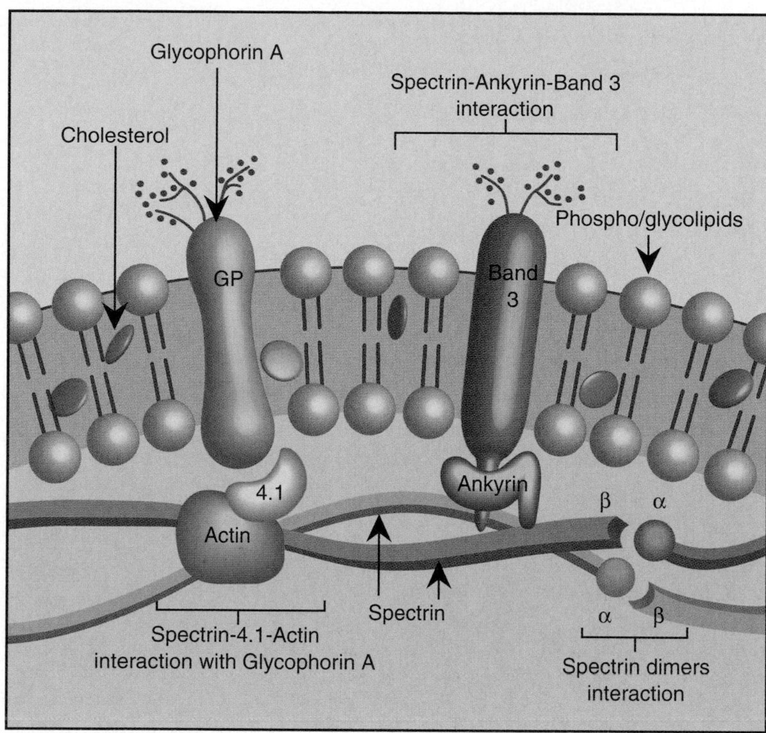

FIGURE 1–3. **Red blood cell membrane structure.** The red blood cell membrane consists of a two-molecule-thick lipid sheath fixed to an intracellular protein network. The outer lipid layer is rich in phosphatidylcholine, sphingomyelin, and glycolipid; the inner layer is made up of the phosphatides of serine, ethanolamine, and inositol. Almost half of the lipid layer is cholesterol. The membrane proteins, glycophorin and band 3, penetrate the lipid sheath and make vertical contact with the reticuloproteins; spectrin; protein 4.1; actin; and in the case of band 3, ankyrin. Spectrin heterodimers provide a horizontal framework by bridging protein 4.1 to complementary spectrin dimers.

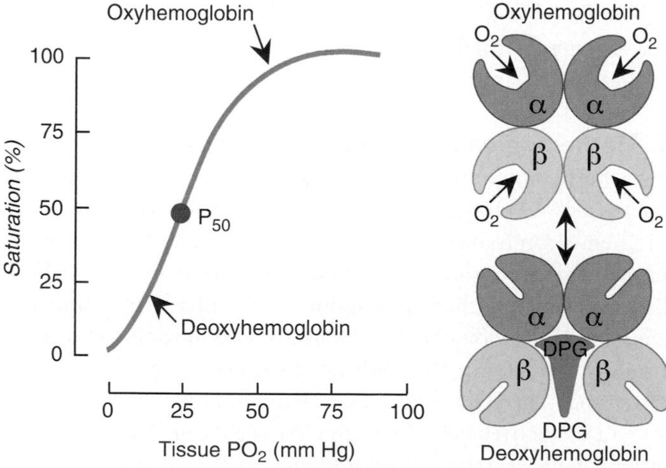

FIGURE 1–4. **Hemoglobin-oxygen dissociation curve.** Hemoglobin is capable of a respiratory motion where oxygen loaded at the lung is unloaded at the tissue level. To accept oxygen, 2,3-DPG and carbon dioxide are expelled, salt bridges are ruptured, and each of the 4 heme groups opens to receive a molecule of oxygen. Oxygen release to tissues reverses the process; salt bridges are reestablished and both 2,3-DPG and carbon dioxide are accepted. The complex interaction of the 4 heme groups is responsible for the sigmoid shape of the hemoglobin-oxygen dissociation curve.

low- or high-affinity state, whereas others either change the valency of heme iron from ferrous to ferric or reduce the solubility of the hemoglobin molecule. Hemoglobin S (sickle cell disease) is an example of a single amino acid substitution that results in a profound effect on solubility.

The normal red blood cell contains approximately 32 pg of hemoglobin (mean cell hemoglobin [MCH] = 32 ± 2 pg). **Normal hemoglobin synthesis** requires an adequate supply of iron and normal production of both protoporphyrin and globin (Figure 1–5). Protoporphyrin synthesis is initiated in the mitochondria with the formation of δ-aminolevulinic acid from glycine and succinyl-CoA. Synthesis then moves to the cell cytoplasm for the formation of porphobilinogen, uroporphyrin, and coproporphyrin. The final assembly of the protoporphyrin ring is carried out by the mitochondria, after which iron is incorporated under the control of the cytoplasmic enzyme, ferrochelatase (heme synthase), to form heme.

Globin chains are assembled by the cytoplasmic ribosomes under the control of two clusters of closely linked genes on chromosomes 11 and 16. The final globin molecule is a tetramer of two α-globin and two non–α-globin chains. In the adult, 96%–97% of the hemoglobin is made up of two α-globin and two β-globin chains (**hemoglobin A**) with minor components of

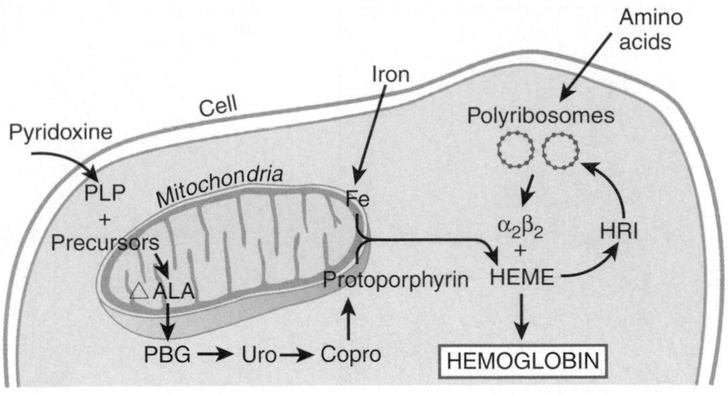

FIGURE 1–5. **Hemoglobin synthesis.** Normal hemoglobin synthesis requires an adequate supply of iron, amino acids, and pyridoxine (vitamin B_6). Porphyrin production is the responsibility of the mitochondria, whereas globin production is controlled by ribosomal RNA. The formation of the complete hemoglobin molecule involves the assembly of heme from protoporphyrin and iron and the union of a heme molecule with the two α- and two β-globin chains that comprise the globin component. Heme regulates globin transcription and translation via HRI (heme-regulated inhibitor [eIF2α] kinase).

hemoglobin F and A_2. The final assembly of the hemoglobin molecule occurs in the cell cytoplasm. Small amounts of iron, protoporphyrin, and free globin chains remain after hemoglobin synthesis is complete. The iron is stored as ferritin, whereas the excess porphyrin is complexed to zinc.

This complex series of reactions is triggered by erythropoietin stimulation of red cell progenitors. With precursor differentiation, there is a coordinated transcriptional induction of heme biosynthesis, globin synthesis, and transferrin receptor expression, which is required for iron transport (see Chapter 5). **The rate of hemoglobin synthesis** is determined by the availability of transferrin iron and level of intracellular heme. Hemoglobin synthesis is maximal in more mature marrow erythroblasts but persists to a lesser degree in the marrow reticulocytes. The cessation of heme synthesis is heralded by a decrease in membrane transferrin receptor expression, followed by a downregulation of heme and globin synthesis. Heme serves both as the essential oxygen-carrying prosthetic group in hemoglobin and as the regulator of the transcription of globin genes, by governing globin translation via HRI (heme-regulated inhibitor [eIF2α] kinase). This is essential to prevent excess globin formation.

Cellular Metabolism

The stability of the red blood cell membrane and the solubility of intracellular hemoglobin depend on four glucose-supported metabolic pathways (Figure 1–6).

A. Embden-Meyerhoff Pathway

The **Embden-Meyerhoff pathway** (**nonoxidative** or **anaerobic pathway**) is responsible for the generation of the ATP necessary for membrane function and the maintenance of cell shape and pliability. Defects in anaerobic glycolysis are associated with

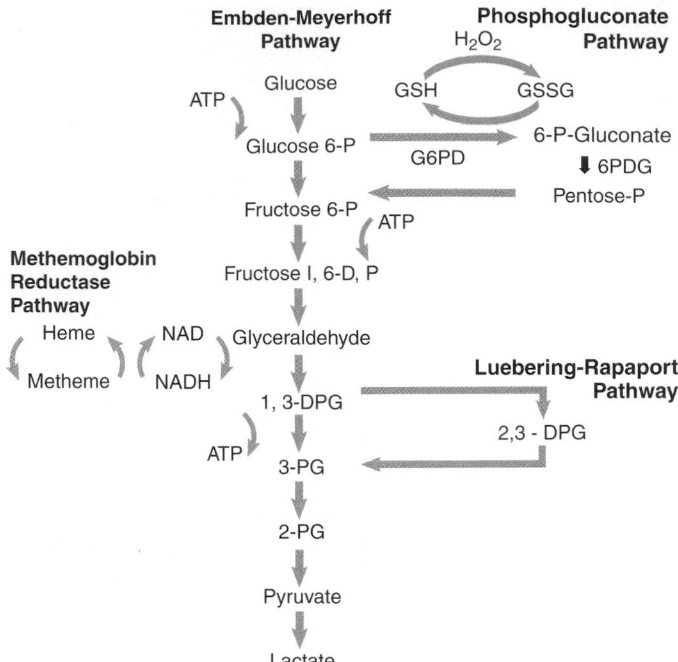

FIGURE 1–6. **Red blood cell metabolic pathways.** The red blood cell depends on 4 metabolic pathways to keep hemoglobin in solution and maintain membrane integrity. The Embden-Meyerhoff pathway is responsible for the generation of high energy phosphate (ATP) for membrane maintenance, whereas the other pathways support hemoglobin function. The methemoglobin reductase (NADH-diaphorase) pathway is required to maintain hemoglobin in a reduced state. The phosphogluconate pathway helps counteract environmental oxidants and the Luebering-Rapaport pathway generates intracellular 2,3-DPG.

increased cell rigidity and decreased survival, which produces a hemolytic anemia.

The Embden-Meyerhoff pathway also plays a role in supporting the methemoglobin reductase, phosphogluconate, and Luebering-Rapaport pathways.

B. Methemoglobin Reductase Pathway

The **methemoglobin reductase pathway** uses the pyridine nucleotide-NADH generated from anaerobic glycolysis to maintain heme iron in its ferrous state. An inherited mutation of the **methemoglobin reductase enzyme** (also referred to as **NADH-diaphorase** or **cytochrome b_5 reductase**) results in an inability to counteract oxidation of hemoglobin to methemoglobin (the ferric form of hemoglobin that will not transport oxygen). Patients with type I NADH-diaphorase deficiency accumulate small amounts of methemoglobin in circulating red cells, whereas type II patients have severe cyanosis and mental retardation.

C. Phosphogluconate Pathway

In a similar fashion, the **phosphogluconate pathway** couples oxidative metabolism with NADP and glutathione reduction. It counteracts environmental oxidants and prevents globin denaturation. When patients lack either of the two key enzymes, **glucose-6-phosphate dehydrogenase (G6PD)** or **glutathione reductase (GSH)**, denatured hemoglobin precipitates on the inner surface of the red blood cell membrane, resulting in membrane damage and hemolysis.

D. Luebering-Rapaport Pathway

The **Luebering-Rapaport pathway** is responsible for the production of 2,3-DPG. It is tied to the rate of anaerobic glycolysis and the action of the pH-sensitive enzyme **phosphofructokinase**. The 2,3-DPG response is also influenced by the supply of phosphate to the cell. Severe phosphate depletion in patients with diabetic ketoacidosis or nutritional deficiency can result in a reduced 2,3-DPG production response.

REGULATION OF OXYGEN TRANSPORT

Red blood cells play a central role in oxygen transport. At the cellular level, oxygen supply is a function of the number of red blood cells perfusing the tissue and their hemoglobin oxygen-carrying capacity. The unique physiology of the hemoglobin-oxygen dissociation curve allows an onsite adjustment of oxygen delivery to match tissue metabolism. At the same time, components such as pulmonary function, cardiac output, blood volume, blood viscosity, and adjustments of regional blood flow are also important contributors to oxygen transport.

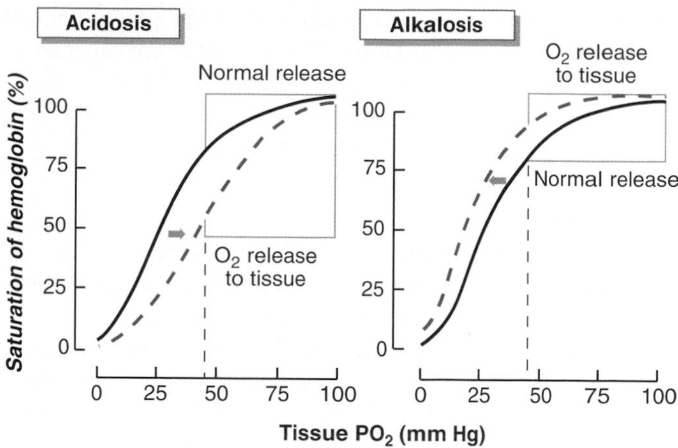

FIGURE 1–7. **pH and hemoglobin-oxygen affinity.** Oxygen delivery responds to tissue metabolism and blood pH—the Bohr effect. When acid products are released at the tissue level, the hemoglobin-oxygen dissociation curve of red blood cells in the vicinity immediately responds with a shift of the curve to the right. This shift has the effect of releasing more oxygen to tissues and opening hemoglobin to receive additional amounts of CO_2. Alkalosis has the opposite effect. It shifts the hemoglobin-oxygen dissociation curve to the left and effectively reduces the amount of oxygen released to tissue.

Hemoglobin-Oxygen Dissociation Curve

Under normal conditions, arterial blood enters tissues with an oxygen tension of 95 mm Hg and hemoglobin saturation greater than 97%. Pooled venous blood returning from tissues has an oxygen tension of 40 mm Hg and a saturation of 75%–80%. Thus, only the top portion of the hemoglobin-oxygen dissociation curve is used in the basal state (Figure 1–7). This provides a considerable excess capacity for increased oxygen delivery to support increased oxygen requirements. The sigmoid shape of the hemoglobin-oxygen dissociation curve also helps in this regard by releasing oxygen more easily as the tissue Po_2 falls below 40 mm Hg.

The affinity of hemoglobin for oxygen is also influenced by temperature, pH, CO_2 concentration, and by the level of red cell 2,3-DPG. As shown in Figure 1–6, the position of the hemoglobin-oxygen dissociation curve is affected by the rate of tissue metabolism, CO_2 production, and blood pH (**the Bohr effect**). When a tissue generates increasing amounts of CO_2 and acid metabolites, the resulting acidosis shifts the dissociation curve to the right. This shift permits the release of more oxygen for the level of tissue Po_2. The reverse is also true. With an increase in pH, such as with an acute respiratory alkalosis, the hemoglobin-oxygen dissociation curve shifts to the left, reducing the amount of oxygen available at any tissue Po_2.

The Bohr effect is instantaneous and can be highly localized to a specific site. For example, the blood perfusing an exercising muscle will be able to deliver 75% or more of its oxygen because of the low tissue Po_2 and the acidosis-induced Bohr effect. Oxygen unloading simultaneously lowers the CO_2 tension in the red cells (**Haldane effect**), thereby facilitating its diffusion from metabolizing tissues. This reciprocal interaction promotes optimal exchange of oxygen and carbon dioxide during exercise.

When the amount of oxygen removed by tissues continues at a high level (**widened arterial-venous difference**), the resulting increase in deoxyhemoglobin in the cell stimulates an increased production of 2,3-DPG. This situation will be true regardless of whether the cause of the hemoglobin desaturation is hypoxia, cardiac failure, or anemia. The rise in intracellular 2,3-DPG sustains the shift of the dissociation curve to the right and provides significant compensation for a chronic anemia or hypoxia.

2,3-DPG metabolism also responds to **systemic acidosis** or **alkalosis**. The initial shift of the curve to the right in a patient with acidosis will be corrected over the next 12–36 hours by a compensatory reduction in the 2,3-DPG level. The Bohr effect is reversed by the lower 2,3-DPG and the curve shifts back to normal. Although this shift readjusts the level of oxygen delivery to match tissue requirements, it can create a problem if the acidosis is suddenly corrected. Because it takes a number of hours to replace the intracellular 2,3-DPG, a sudden return to a normal pH will shift the oxygen dissociation curve to the left owing to the lower than normal 2,3-DPG level. Theoretically, this can be of concern in the treatment of severe diabetic ketoacidosis.

Hemodynamic Factors

The **self-regulating capacity of the oxygen dissociation curve** takes care of most of the variation in tissue oxygen requirements in the basal state. With maximal exercise, the untrained subject will reach a limit determined not by oxygen loading but by a low maximal cardiac output resulting in poor oxygen delivery to tissues. In contrast, highly trained athletes have a greatly increased cardiac output, so that pulmonary loading and peripheral transport determine their limits. The role of the red cell mass in determining exercise capacity has been demonstrated in professional sports, where erythropoietin and blood doping have been used by athletes to improve their performance.

A. Anemia

The oxygen dissociation curve will also compensate for an anemia of moderate severity. However, once the hemoglobin falls below 9–10 g/dL, components such as changes in blood volume, cardiac output, and regional blood flow come into play. Localized vasodilation is a fundamental response to tissue hypoxia. The level of red cell deoxyhemoglobin may be directly linked to this response by acting as a nitrite reductase with the release of nitric oxide and ATP. Both the pulse rate and stroke volume also increase in patients with severe anemia and there is a redirection of blood flow to vital organs. These hemodynamic changes are often appreciated symptomatically by patients. As their anemia worsens, they are increasingly aware of the force of ventricular contraction and often complain of pounding headaches, especially with physical exertion.

B. Oxygen Supply

Impairments in lung function also affect oxygen supply. Although the sigmoid shape of the hemoglobin-oxygen dissociation curve does counterbalance reductions in alveolar PO_2, there is a limit to this compensation. Moreover, desaturation of hemoglobin results whenever unsaturated venous blood is shunted through areas of damaged lung tissue. The physiologic response to a decreased oxygen tension in ambient air, for example, the oxygen tension at moderately high altitudes (3,000–4,000 m), is an increase in 2,3-DPG to raise the P_{50}, that is, shift the oxygen dissociation curve to the right. Moderate exercise will still further elevate the P_{50} via the Bohr effect to maintain oxygen delivery to tissues. Under conditions of more marked hypoxia (altitudes >4,000 m), reflex hyperventilation results in reduced PCO_2 and respiratory alkalosis. The latter shifts the oxygen dissociation curve to the left with a reduction in oxygen delivery to tissues. Still, high hemoglobin affinity for oxygen provides a physiological advantage for acclimatization to high altitudes. Subjects born with high-affinity hemoglobin, such as hemoglobin Andrew-Minneapolis (P_{50} 17 mm Hg), demonstrate normal arterial oxygen saturations at altitudes up to 4,000 m, smaller increases in heart rate, and little or no increases in erythropoietin when compared with normal individuals. Animals that normally live at high altitudes also have high-affinity hemoglobins.

C. Blood Viscosity

Sustained hypoxia usually results in a compensatory rise in the red blood cell mass and hematocrit. Although this increases the oxygen-carrying capacity of blood, it also increases blood viscosity. The interaction of the hematocrit level and blood viscosity is discussed extensively in Chapter 13. Tissue oxygen delivery theoretically is maximal at a hematocrit of 33%–36% (hemoglobin of 11–12 g/dL), assuming no changes in cardiac output or regional blood flow. Above this level, an increase in viscosity will tend to slow blood flow and decrease oxygen delivery. From a physiological standpoint, this effect is relatively minor until the hematocrit exceeds 50%, at which time blood flow to key organs such as the brain can be significantly reduced.

REGULATION OF ERYTHROPOIESIS

Red Blood Cell Production

The **rate of new red blood cell (RBC) production** varies according to the rate of red blood cell destruction and tissue oxygen requirements. Changes in the oxygen delivery to tissue are sensed by peritubular interstitial, fibroblast-like cells in the kidney. A decrease in the oxygen content of hemoglobin (pulmonary dysfunction), the hemoglobin level (anemia), or the hemoglobin affinity for oxygen (shift in the oxygen dissociation curve) will stimulate an increased production of erythropoietin by renal interstitial cells. This is accomplished by recruitment of new cells to initiate transcription of erythropoietin messenger ribonucleic acid (mRNA) by a single gene on chromosome 7. The **mechanism of regulation** involves the sensing of oxygen tension by a flavoheme protein that controls the level of **hypoxia inducible factor (HIF-1)**. The latter interacts with response elements in nuclear DNA to activate erythropoietin gene expression.

Erythropoietin then travels to the marrow, where it binds to a specific receptor (**EPOR**) on the surface of committed erythroid precursors. This receptor is a 508–amino acid glycoprotein coded by a gene on chromosome 19. Within hours, there is a detectable increase in deoxyribonucleic acid (DNA) synthesis. This is followed by proliferation and maturation of committed stem cells to produce an increased number of new red blood cells. Erythroid progenitor apoptosis is also inhibited. The **full marrow response** takes several days. Given a sustained increase in erythropoietin stimulation, a rise in the reticulocyte index will not occur for 4–5 days and a detectable increase in hematocrit will take a week or more.

A. Measuring the Erythropoietin Response

The erythropoietin response to anemia can be directly measured by assaying the serum erythropoietin level (Figure 1–8). Once the hemoglobin level falls below 12 g/dL, there is a logarithmic increase in the serum erythropoietin level. At the same time, it is important to note that with mild anemia (a hemoglobin level greater than 12 g/dL), the erythropoietin level is not increased. This probably reflects the compensation of the 2,3-DPG–induced shift in the hemoglobin-oxygen dissociation curve combined with the sensitivity level of the renal sensor.

B. Other Factors Influencing Erythropoietin Level

Although the erythropoietin response is primarily a function of the severity of anemia or hypoxia, other factors, such as the erythroid marrow mass and levels of inflammatory cytokines, will influence the serum erythropoietin level. Erythropoietin binds avidly to erythroid progenitors and is removed from circulation.

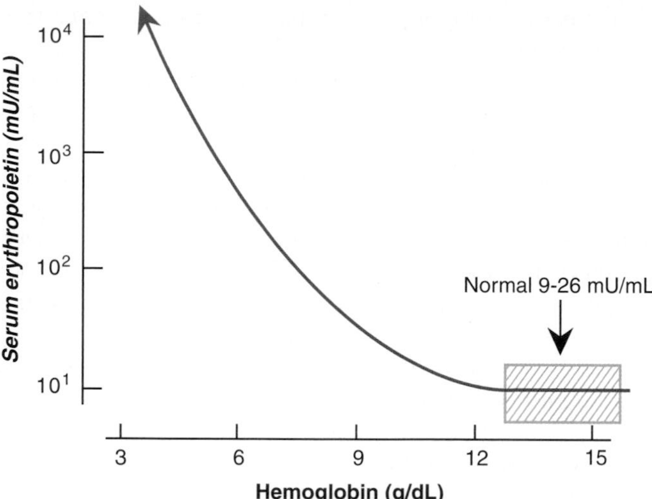

FIGURE 1–8. **Erythropoietin production and anemia.** Once the hemoglobin level falls below 12 g/dL, the plasma erythropoietin level increases logarithmically. Patients with renal disease or the anemia associated with chronic inflammation show a lower than predicted response for their degree of anemia.

Therefore, with **aplastic anemia**, extremely high levels of serum erythropoietin reflect both an increased production and a decreased clearance. In contrast, with **chronic hemolytic anemias**, the expansion of marrow erythroid precursors results in a more rapid clearance of erythropoietin from circulation and, therefore, a lower serum level.

Inflammatory cytokines, including interleukin-1, interleukin-6, tumor necrosis factor (TNF-α), and transforming growth factor β, also play a role in regulating erythropoietin production and erythroid progenitor proliferation. They are responsible for the lower than normal erythroid marrow response in patients with inflammatory disease states (see Chapter 4). Finally, direct suppression of the erythroid marrow response is seen in patients receiving certain drugs (chemotherapeutic agents, cyclosporin A, and theophylline) or who are infected with human immunodeficiency virus (HIV).

Two other factors, **angiotensin II** and **insulin-like growth factor-1 (IGF-1)**, may also play an erythropoietin-like role in certain settings. The erythropoietin-independent growth of erythroid progenitors in polycythemia vera (see Chapter 13) may involve a hypersensitivity to IGF-1, whereas hypoxia has been shown to induce IGF-1 binding protein. Evidence for a role for angiotensin II is indirect. Post–renal transplant erythrocytosis can be reversed by the administration of angiotensin-converting enzyme inhibitors, without affecting the serum erythropoietin level.

ERYTHROID MARROW PRODUCTION

Erythroid marrow production is most often defined for the basal state. When it comes to anemia diagnosis, however, it is more important to recognize the capacity to increase red blood cell production according to the severity of the anemia. Patients who experience acute blood loss or sudden hemolysis of circulating red blood cells can show increases in new red blood cell production of 2–3 times normal; that is, the release of 40–60 mL of new red blood cells per day. With a chronic hemolytic anemia, even higher production levels can be attained. Therefore, the capacity of the erythroid marrow to compensate for an anemia or hypoxia is a key part of the definition of "normal" erythropoiesis.

Measurement

The level of production can be assessed from several measurements of red blood cell production and destruction (Table 1–1). Clinically, the marrow E/G ratio and reticulocyte index are of the greatest value. The **marrow E/G ratio** (the ratio of erythroid to granulocytic precursors) is determined by inspecting a stained smear of aspirated marrow particles. As long as the granulocyte production of the marrow is normal, it is possible to estimate the proliferation of erythroid precursors. In the basal state, there will be approximately 1 erythroid precursor for every 3–4 granulocytic (myelocytic) precursors. With anemia and high levels of erythropoietin stimulation, the number of erythroid precursors increases dramatically to give ratios of 1:1 or greater. The morphology of the precursors is also important. Normal proliferation shows a balanced increase in erythroid precursors at all stages of maturation. If the number is skewed toward a younger population, especially a population with abnormal morphology, this suggests a defect in DNA synthesis or cytoplasmic maturation. These defects can result in a failure of cells to mature and early death in the marrow, so-called **ineffective erythropoiesis**.

Effective red blood cell production is measured clinically by counting the number of **reticulocytes** (new red blood cells containing increased amounts of RNA) entering the circulation. Although both the E/G ratio and reticulocyte count are at best semiquantitative, they do provide sufficient information for clinical diagnosis. A measurement of radioiron incorporation into red blood cells (**erythron iron turnover**) can provide a more accurate measurement of red blood cell production. This technique was used originally to define and classify red blood cell disorders as defects in either marrow proliferation (hypoproliferative anemias), precursor maturation (ineffective erythropoiesis), or red blood cell destruction (hemorrhagic and hemolytic anemias).

TABLE 1–1 • Measurements of red blood cell production and destruction

Production	Destruction
Marrow E/G ratio	Change in hematocrit
Reticulocyte index	Indirect bilirubin
Erythron iron turnover	Lactic dehydrogenase (LDH)
	^{51}Cr—red blood cell survival
	CO excretion/stool urobilinogen

The performance of the erythroid marrow can also be extrapolated from studies of red blood cell destruction. **Clinical indicators of red blood cell destruction** include the serum lactic dehydrogenase level, the indirect bilirubin, and observation of the rate of rise or fall of the hematocrit over time. **Research measurements** that are more accurate in defining levels of red blood cell destruction include carbon monoxide (CO) excretion, stool urobilinogen, and a direct measurement of radiolabeled red blood cell survival (^{51}Cr red blood cell survival). The latter has been used clinically to define both the rate and the site of destruction, whether in spleen or liver. The other measurements are not as practical.

Basal and Stimulated Erythropoiesis

The ability of the erythroid marrow to increase red blood cell production in response to anemia or hypoxia is a basic characteristic of "normal" erythropoiesis. Therefore, when evaluating a patient with an anemia, there is a definable level of response of the marrow (E/G ratio) and the reticulocyte index for acute and chronic anemia (Table 1–2).

A **normal 70-kg adult** has a circulating red blood cell mass of approximately 2,000 mL (300 × 10^9 red blood cells per kg). Since red blood cells have a lifespan of 100–120 days, 1% of the red blood cell mass, approximately 20 mL of red blood cells, is destroyed daily and replaced by new red blood cell production. This steady state is clinically appreciated from the **E/G ratio** of 1:3 and the **reticulocyte index** (the reticulocyte count corrected for hematocrit and reticulocyte shift; see Chapter 2). With an **acute anemia** secondary to hemorrhage or hemolysis, the marrow will respond with a 3-fold increase in cell production within 7–10 days. This can be detected from the increase in the E/G ratio to 1:1 or higher and a rise in the reticulocyte index to 3 times normal. With a **chronic hemolytic anemia**, red blood cell production can increase further, reaching levels of 5–8 times normal. These patients show E/G ratios greater than 1:1 and reticulocyte indices greater than 5 times normal. The highest levels of red blood cell production in patients with hemolytic anemias require an expansion of the erythroid marrow mass to new areas of the marrow cavity. This process takes time and is most prominent in patients who have congenital, lifelong hemolytic anemias.

Several factors play important roles in defining the **marrow's response to anemia or hypoxia**. Obviously, the severity of the anemia or hypoxia and the adequacy of the erythropoietin response are extremely important in setting a level of "expectation." A chronic hypoproliferative anemia develops, for example, when a patient cannot produce increased amounts of erythropoietin because of renal damage.

Other factors that determine the marrow's responsiveness include its anatomical structure, the presence of a normal pool of stem cells, and the supply of essential nutrients. The anatomical structure of the marrow is organized to provide a nurturing environment for cell development. Erythroid precursor cells are maintained in a network of reticular cells and fibers in close proximity to vascular sinusoids. The marrow syncytium is designed to sustain the developing cells in a nutrient-rich environment while they proliferate and mature. Cells lining the sinusoids have the ability to regulate the exit of cells from the marrow into circulation, allowing only those cells that have completed maturation to leave.

The **importance of these marrow characteristics** cannot be overemphasized. An abnormality in marrow structure, as seen with radiation damage or myelofibrosis, significantly impairs new red blood cell production. Overgrowth of other cellular components, as with myeloid leukemias or infiltrating tumors or lymphomas, will decrease red blood cell production by occupying the space required for red blood cell precursor growth.

The **supply of nutrients** to the marrow is also important. The most important nutrient is the iron required for hemoglobin formation. The level of the normal marrow's response to a hemorrhagic or hemolytic anemia is essentially a reflection of iron supply (Figure 1–9). In response to a hemorrhagic anemia, a normal individual with normal iron stores will be able to maintain a

TABLE 1–2 • Normal response to anemia

		Anemia (Hb <8 g/dL)	
	Basal (Hgb >13 g/dL)	Acute	Chronic
Marrow—E/G ratio	1:3	1:1	>1:1
Reticulocyte index	1.0	2–3	3–8

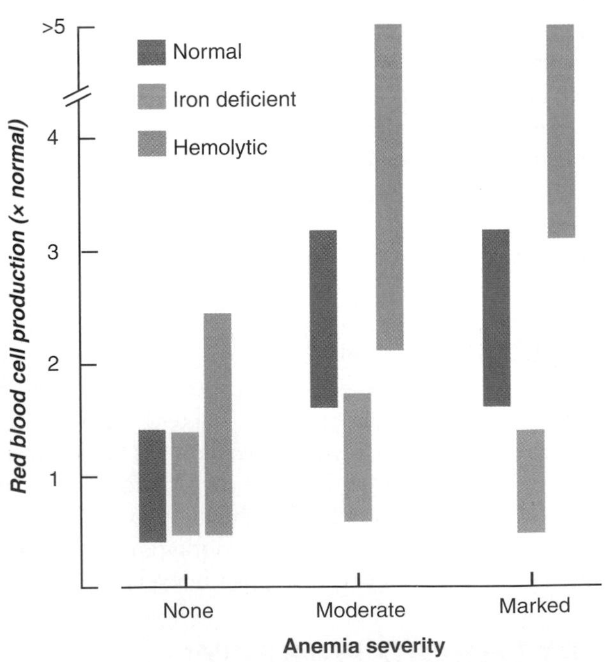

FIGURE 1–9. **Red blood cell production and iron supply.** The ability of the erythroid marrow to increase production is a direct reflection of iron supply. With worsening anemia, a normal individual with 500–1,000 mg of reticuloendothelial iron stores can increase red blood cell production 2- to 3-fold. An individual with iron deficiency will be unable to increase production above basal levels. In contrast, patients with chronic hemolytic anemias show production levels in excess of 3–5 times normal, with moderate to marked anemia.

serum iron level sufficient to support a production increase of up to 3 times normal. As shown in the figure, this level of production is attained as the hematocrit falls to levels between 20% and 30%. More severe anemia with a greater erythropoietin response does not result in a greater marrow production response. The cause of this plateau is the limitation of iron delivery from normal stores.

Figure 1–9 also shows the effect of variations in iron supply. With **iron deficiency**, the erythroid marrow will be unable to respond despite a high level of erythropoietin stimulation. The patient with iron deficiency appears to have a hypoproliferative anemia even though the erythropoietin level is increased and the marrow morphology appears to be normal. In contrast, patients who have **hemolytic anemias**, in which the destruction of adult red cells provides a major source of iron for recycling to the marrow, can have marrow production that increases to levels well above 3 times normal. Chronically, these patients can achieve production levels in excess of 5 times normal.

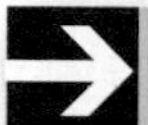

POINTS TO REMEMBER

The circulating red blood cells and the hemoglobin they carry are responsible for oxygen delivery to all organs and tissues.

The mature red blood cell is highly specialized—it lacks a nucleus and is extremely pliable to allow it to squeeze through capillaries and withstand the stress of high velocity blood flow.

The red blood cell's hemoglobin can instantaneously adjust to local tissue oxygen demands by a shift in the hemoglobin-oxygen dissociation curve.

While a sustained shift in the hemoglobin-oxygen dissociation curve can compensate for a mild anemia, changes in cardiac output and regional blood flow come into play with more severe anemia.

An oxygen sensor in the kidney governs the production of erythropoietin, the principal regulator of new red cell production—erythropoiesis.

The capacity to increase erythropoiesis in response to hypoxia or anemia depends on the level of erythropoietin released by the kidney, a normal marrow structure to support red cell precursor growth, and an adequate supply of nutrients, especially the iron needed for hemoglobin synthesis.

An uncompensated anemia can result, therefore, because of a loss of renal function, damage to the marrow structure, nutrient deficiency, poor iron supply, or an excessive loss of circulating red cells from hemorrhage or hemolysis.

Measurements of the level of marrow red cell precursor expansion (the E/G ratio) and new red cell production (reticulocyte index) can be used clinically to determine the adequacy of the erythropoietic response to anemia. As a rule, a normal individual with adequate iron stores can increase red blood cell production 2- to 3-fold (marrow E/G ratio >1:2 and reticulocyte index >2) in response to a fall in the hemoglobin below 9–10 g/dL. Based on these two measurements and changes in mature red blood cell morphology, an anemia can be classified as a hypoproliferative anemia (defect in erythropoietin production, damage to the marrow structure, iron deficiency, or inflammation); a marrow precursor maturation disorder with ineffective erythropoiesis (vitamin deficiency states, myelodysplasia, or preleukemia); or an excessive loss of mature red blood cells (hemorrhage or hemolysis).

BIBLIOGRAPHY

Chen JJ: Regulation of protein synthesis by the heme-regulated eIF2α kinase: relevance to anemias. Blood 2007;109: 2693.

Crawford JH et al: Hypoxia, red blood cells, and nitrite regulate NO-dependent hypoxic vasodilation. Blood 2006; 107:566.

Goodnough LT, Skikne B, Brugnara C: Erythropoietin, iron, and erythropoiesis. Blood 2000;96:823.

Hillman RS, Finch CA: Red Cell Manual, 7th ed. FA Davis, 1997.

Hsia CCW: Respiratory function of hemoglobin. N Engl J Med 1998;338:239.

Lichtman MA et al: Williams Hematology, 7th ed. McGraw-Hill, 2006.

Ponka P: Tissue-specific regulation of iron metabolism and heme synthesis: distinct control mechanisms in erythroid cells. Blood 1997;89:1.

Zwaal RFA, Schroit AJ: Pathophysiologic implications of membrane phospholipid asymmetry in blood cells. Blood 1997;89:1121.

CLINICAL APPROACH TO ANEMIA • 2

CASE HISTORY • *Part I*

A 48-year-old man with poorly controlled type I diabetes is referred for evaluation of a worsening anemia. He reports a long-standing history of general fatigue and poor exercise tolerance, which he feels have worsened of late. Complications of his diabetes include severe retinopathy, peripheral vascular disease with one flight claudication, and worsening neuropathy. On physical examination, he appears chronically ill with a sallow complexion and pale conjunctiva. Findings include bilateral retinal hemorrhages, diminished pulses, and impaired sensation and position sense in both feet.

CBC: Hematocrit/hemoglobin - 29%/9.5 g/dL (IU - 95 g/L)
MCV - 91 fL MCH - 30 pg MCHC - 33 g/dL
RDW-CV - 13.5%
RDW-SD - 48 fL
WBC count - 8,800/μL
Platelet count - 150,000/μL

• SMEAR MORPHOLOGY

Normocytic and normochromic with minimal anisocytosis and no polychromasia. White cell and platelet numbers and morphology appear to be within normal limits.

Reticulocyte count/index - 2.0%/1.2
Sedimentation rate - 30 mm/h (Westergren)

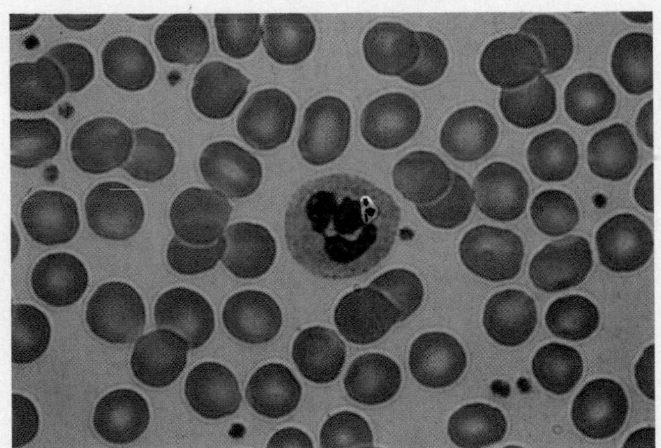

Questions

- How should this anemia be described?
- What physiological factors may be playing a role?
- Are there other tests that can be ordered to find the cause?

The presence and nature of an anemia may be apparent from the clinical presentation. Acute blood loss, when severe, can be expected to produce a hemorrhagic anemia; chronic blood loss will generally result in an iron deficiency anemia. More often, however, a routine measurement of the complete blood count (CBC) provides the most sensitive method for both detection and diagnosis. Thus, the clinical approach to an anemia involves both a bedside evaluation and the skilled use of the laboratory.

CLINICAL PRESENTATION

The signs and symptoms of an anemia are a function of its severity, its rapidity of onset, and the age of the patient. Mild anemias produce little in the way of symptoms other than a loss in stamina and an increase in heart rate and dyspnea with exercise. This reflects the ability of the hemoglobin-oxygen dissociation curve to compensate for modest reductions in the hemoglobin level in the basal state. It also shows the loss of the capacity of the hemoglobin-oxygen dissociation curve to respond to situations of increased demand once it is used to compensate for the anemia.

With more pronounced anemia, the patient's exercise capacity can be markedly reduced. Any exertion is accompanied by palpitations, dyspnea, a pounding headache, and rapid exhaustion. In younger individuals, these symptoms and signs do not appear until the hemoglobin has fallen below 7–8 g/dL (hematocrit of less than 20%–25%). However, older individuals, especially those with atherosclerotic cardiovascular disease, can become symptomatic with more modest anemia (a hemoglobin of 10–12 g/dL). This can include worsening of ischemic manifestations, including angina and claudication. Moreover, anemia can precipitate heart failure in the older patient with underlying heart disease.

The rapidity of onset of the anemia is also important. Although the hemoglobin-oxygen dissociation curve can rapidly compensate for modest falls in the hemoglobin level, cardiovascular compensation for more severe anemia takes time. This situation is worsened if the anemia is the result of **acute blood loss** (a deficit in both red blood cells and plasma volume). The reduction in total blood volume jeopardizes the cardiovascular response. Patients with acute hemorrhagic anemias are at risk for signs and symptoms of both tissue hypoxia and acute vascular collapse. In contrast, patients with long-standing anemias are able to expand their total blood volume over time and compensate with an increase in cardiac stroke volume and changes in regional blood flow.

CLINICAL EVALUATION

The cause of anemia may be suggested from the history and physical examination. Ongoing blood loss is an obvious and dramatic clue to the cause of the patient's anemia. The history can be equally revealing in diagnosing other types of anemia. A documented history of anemia that reaches back to childhood is highly suggestive of a hereditary disorder, especially a congenital hemolytic anemia. The sudden onset of pancytopenia in an otherwise healthy individual may be explained from the patient's history of occupational or environmental exposure to toxic chemicals or the introduction of a new medication just prior to development of the cytopenia. A more gradual onset of anemia or a pancytopenia may herald myelodysplasia or other marrow disorder. Race can also be an important clue, because many of the hemoglobinopathies and enzyme deficiency states follow ethnic lines.

History

The patient should be questioned extensively regarding the timing of the onset of symptoms, transfusion history, past blood count measurements, nutritional habits, alcohol intake, and any associated symptoms of acute or chronic illness such as weight loss, fever, or night sweats. A few complaints are unique to specific types of anemia. For example, the adult iron-deficient patient may report craving ice, whereas children may be observed eating dirt or clay (picophagia). Complaints of a sore mouth and difficulty swallowing are expressed by patients with vitamin B_{12} and iron deficiency. The sickle cell anemia patient will have a lifelong history of episodic bone and joint pains.

Physical Examination

The physical signs of an anemia depend very much on the acuity of onset. The patient with acute blood loss will show signs of hypovolemia and hypoxia. A loss of more than 30% of the blood volume in less than 12 hours cannot be compensated by the normal mechanisms of venospasm and redirection of regional blood flow. Such patients will show signs of hypovolemia, including postural hypotension and tachycardia with exertion. Once the acute volume loss exceeds 40% of the total blood volume, the patient will exhibit all the symptoms and signs of hypovolemic shock, including anxiety, confusion, air hunger, diaphoresis, rest tachycardia, and hypotension even while supine. The appearance of symptoms and signs of hypoxia in such patients is as much a result of inadequate perfusion of vital organs because of a decreased blood volume as a reflection of their anemia.

When an anemia develops gradually so that the plasma volume has time to increase, compensation is accomplished by a combination of the shift in the hemoglobin-oxygen dissociation curve, an increase in cardiac output, and a redistribution of blood flow (Figure 2–1). By physical examination, it is possible for one to detect the changes in cardiac output and blood flow. The patient demonstrates a more forceful apical impulse, a wide pulse pressure, and tachycardia with exertion. Flow murmurs secondary to increased blood turbulence are frequently heard as midsystolic or holosystolic murmurs at the apex or along the sternal border with radiation to the neck.

An anemia may also be suggested from the patient's general appearance. In fair-skinned patients, skin and mucous membrane pallor are relatively good indicators of anemia. However, skin color is a less reliable measure of the hemoglobin level in heavily pigmented patients, or in those with marked vasoconstriction or dilatation. Marked edema, as seen in patients with nephrotic syndrome or myxedema, can also interfere with

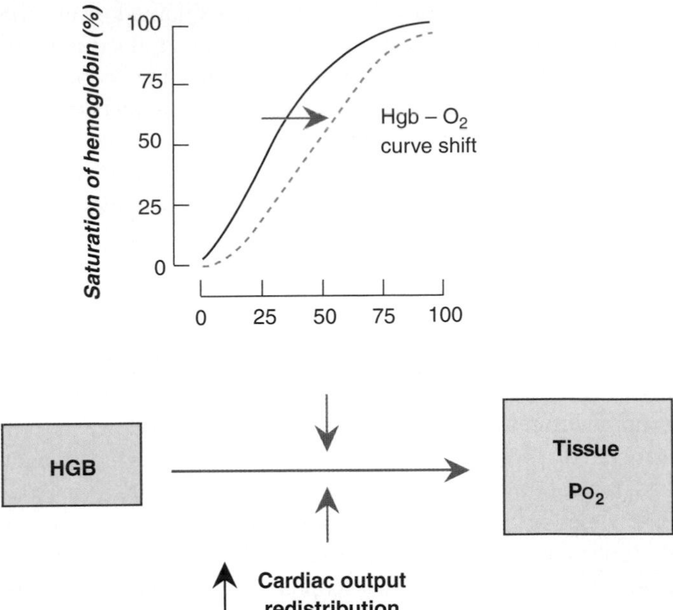

FIGURE 2–1. **Tissue oxygen supply.** Delivery of oxygen to tissues is a function of the hemoglobin level, the hemoglobin-oxygen dissociation curve, and the characteristics of tissue blood flow. With anemia, the hemoglobin-oxygen dissociation curve shifts to the right so as to deliver additional oxygen for a level of tissue Po_2. As the anemia worsens, cardiac output increases and there is a redistribution of blood flow to critical organs.

TABLE 2–1 • Routine laboratory tests in anemia diagnosis

Complete blood count
Red blood cell number—Red blood cell count, hemoglobin, hematocrit
Red blood cell indices—Mean cell volume (MCV), mean cell hemoglobin (MCH), mean cell hemoglobin concentration (MCHC), red blood cell distribution width (RDW)
Reticulocyte count, immature reticulocyte fraction—Reticulocyte production index
White blood cell count—White blood cell differential
Platelet count
Blood film morphology—Cell size, hemoglobinization, anisocytosis, poikilocytosis, polychromasia
Marrow examination
Marrow aspirate—E/G ratio, cell morphology, iron stain
Marrow biopsy—Cellularity, morphology
Iron studies
Iron transport—Serum iron, total iron-binding capacity
Iron stores—Serum ferritin, marrow iron stain

anemia detection. To avoid these confounding variables, it is best for one to look at the conjunctiva, mucous membranes, nail beds, and palmar creases of the hand when assessing the hemoglobin level.

Laboratory Evaluation

Although the history and physical examination may point the way to the presence of anemia and suggest its cause, a thorough laboratory evaluation is essential to the definitive diagnosis and treatment of any anemia. The routine hematology laboratory offers several tests relevant to anemia diagnosis: the more routine tests such as the CBC and reticulocyte count as well as studies of iron supply that serve both as screening tests and a jumping-off point to diagnosis (Table 2–1). A larger number of more specific tests come into play when one is confirming the diagnosis of specific anemic conditions.

A. Complete Blood Count

The CBC includes determinations of the hemoglobin, hematocrit, red blood cell count, red blood cell volume; and hemoglobin content, platelet count, and white blood cell count. These measurements are provided by any of the common automated counters, including instruments manufactured by Abbott, Bayer, Beckman-Coulter, Sysmex, and Technicon Instruments vary somewhat in their technology, with most using either a combination of a highly focused light source, an electric field, laser-based flow cytometry, or a radiofrequency wave to discriminate between cells. Newer instruments that incorporate technologies such as flow cytometry not only measure the white blood cell count, but also perform a 3- or 5-part automated white blood cell differential that also flags bands, immature and atypical cells, and blasts.

Automated instruments are not only fast but extremely accurate. The coefficient of variation (measurement error) of an automated counter is usually less than 2%, and each of the major measurements, including the hemoglobin level, red blood cell count, and mean cell volume, can be standardized independently with commercial red blood cell and hemoglobin standards. A printout of an automated blood count is shown in Figure 2–2. A range of normal values with 95% confidence limits is provided as a part of the report.

B. Hemoglobin/Hematocrit

The hematocrit and hemoglobin levels are used interchangeably in identifying the presence of an anemia. Many counters directly measure the hemoglobin and then calculate the hematocrit from measurements of the red blood cell count and mean cell volume (MCV). Other counters measure the hematocrit from the red blood cell size-distribution curve. This can make the hemoglobin measurement somewhat more accurate, because artifacts introduced by cell agglutination can increase the MCV and falsely elevate the hematocrit. This is usually flagged by the automated counters because of the simultaneous marked increase in the mean corpuscular hemoglobin concentration (MCHC).

To diagnose an anemia, any patient value must be compared with a "normal" reference range. Table 2–2 summarizes the mean normal values for hemoglobin and hematocrit according to age and sex. At birth, the hemoglobin averages 17 g/dL, with a hematocrit of 52%. These values then decrease during childhood only to recover during adolescence until a mean

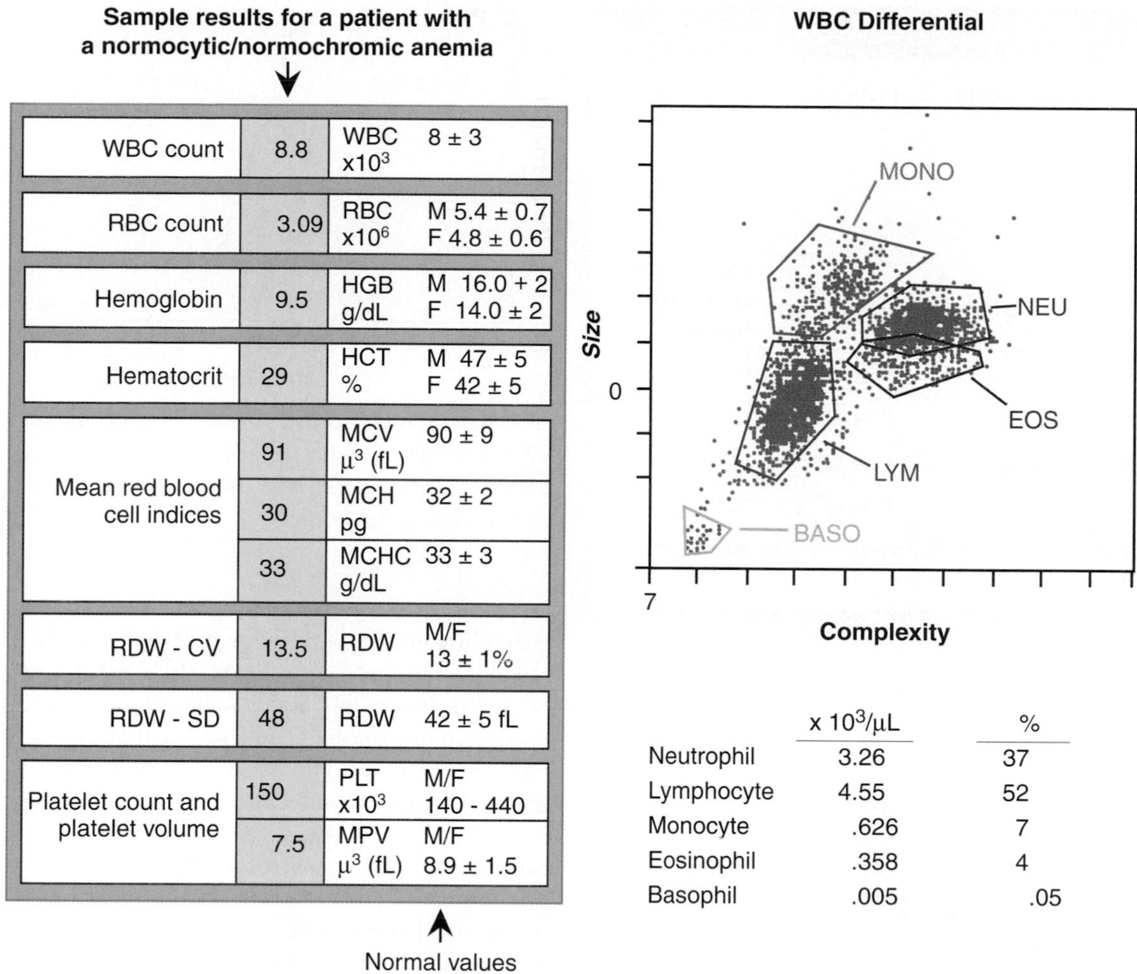

FIGURE 2–2. **CBC results.** Direct measurements on an automated counter include the white blood cell count, red blood cell count, hemoglobin, MCV, platelet count, and the mean platelet volume. Calculated values include the hematocrit, MCH, MCHC, and RDW. A 3- or 5-part white blood cell differential also is provided by many of the automated counters. As shown in the right-hand data plot, white blood cells can be separated and counted based on their light scatter characteristics. Abnormal white blood cells (blasts, promyelocytes, and metamyelocytes) also can be identified and counted.

hemoglobin level of 16 g/dL (hematocrit of 47%) is reached in adult men and 14 g/dL (hematocrit of 42%) in adult women.

These are mean values, however, and any normal population of men or women will vary around the mean in a Gaussian distribution (Figure 2–3). Therefore, it is common practice to state 95% confidence limits (2 standard deviations [SD]) for the mean normal value. For the purpose of clinical decision making, it is best to focus on a set of lower limit of normal values that best separates normal from anemic individuals. As shown in Table 2–2, data from Scripps-Kaiser and NHANES studies have been used to derive a set of lower limits of normal for adults living at sea level, which should exclude all but 5% of normal individuals (95% confidence limit). At the same time, the lower limits of normal for apparently healthy American black men and women are approximately 1 g/dL lower (12.9 g/dL for black men and 11.5 g/dL for black women).

The probability that a patient's hemoglobin is normal will also depend on the incidence of disease in any population, as illustrated in Figure 2–3. When the prevalence of a hematological abnormality is high, for example, as in the inheritance of a hemoglobinopathy, the overlap of abnormal and normal populations will increase, thereby reducing both the sensitivity and specificity of the hemoglobin and hematocrit measurements. This effect may well play a role in determining the lower limits of normal for black men and women. A higher incidence of iron deficiency and α-thalassemia has been detected in the Scripps-Kaiser population studies, which, at least in part, explains the difference between white and black values. Normal values for the hemoglobin and hematocrit are also influenced by several environmental and physiologic factors. Populations living at higher altitudes have predictable increases in their hemoglobin levels of approximately 1 g/dL of hemoglobin for each 3%–4% decrease in arterial oxygen saturation. The same effect is produced by cigarette smoking because carbon monoxide decreases the hemoglobin-oxygen saturation. A patient who smokes more than one pack of cigarettes per day will show an increased

TABLE 2–2 • Normal hemoglobin/hematocrit values

Age/Sex	Hgb (g/dL)	Hct (%)	
At birth	17	52	
Childhood	12	36	
Adolescence	13	40	
			Lower Limit of Normal (Hgb)[a]
Adult man <60	16 (± 2)	47 (± 6)	13.7
Adult woman <60	14 (± 2)	42 (± 6)	12.2
Adult man >60	15 (± 2)	45 (± 6)	13.2
Adult woman >60	14 (± 2)	42 (± 6)	12.2

[a]*Based on Scripps-Kaiser and NHANES data—Beutler E, Waalen J: Blood 2006;107:1747.*

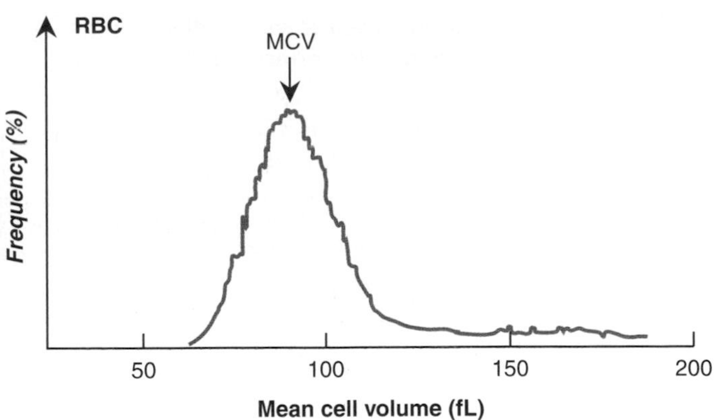

FIGURE 2–4. **A red blood cell size-distribution curve.** Automated counters display a distribution curve for the red blood cell volume. Direct inspection of the curve offers a sensitive method for detecting small populations of macrocytic or microcytic red blood cells.

hemoglobin level of between 0.5 and 1 g/dL. During normal pregnancy, there is a steady decline in the hemoglobin level to 11–12 g/dL during the second and third trimesters. This decline is caused by an expansion of plasma volume and does not represent a true anemia. In fact, a pregnant woman's red blood cell mass is actually increased late in pregnancy.

C. Mean Cell Volume

Automated counters produce a size-distribution curve for the red blood cell population (Figure 2–4), which is then used to calculate the mean MCV. The normal MCV ± 2 SD is 90 ± 9 fL and generally coincides with the peak of the Gaussian distribution of red blood cell size. The "normal" MCV in black populations can be 1–2 fL lower (88.5 ± 7). Again, this in part represents the incidence of iron deficiency and α-thalassemia in American black populations. The MCV accurately detects any general increase **(macrocytosis)** or decrease **(microcytosis)** in red blood cell volume. It is less sensitive to the presence of small populations of microcytes or macrocytes, because they have little impact on the mean. To detect small numbers of abnormal cells, the clinician should look at the calculated red cell distribution width and the shape of the size-distribution curve, or, even better, inspect the stained blood smear. Figure 2–5 shows the effect on the distribution curve of blood transfusions in a patient with thalassemia. The broad two-peak distribution curve can be

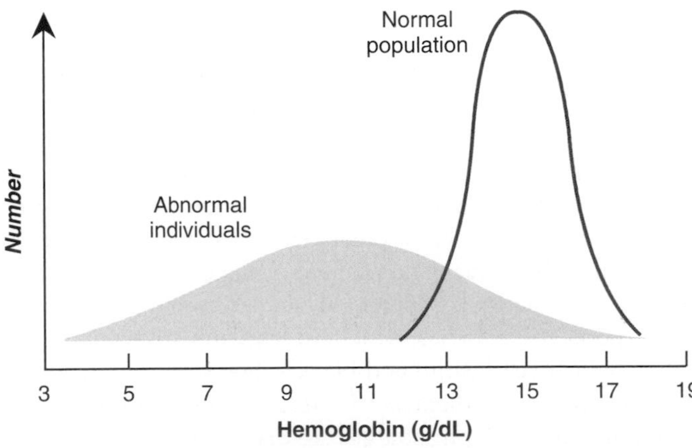

FIGURE 2–3. **Distributions of normal and abnormal hemoglobin values.** The unshaded area shows the expected distribution for a normal population of adult males. Patients with red blood cell disorders may or may not fall outside this normal distribution (shaded area). Very anemic patients will have hemoglobin values well below the normal distribution, whereas those with less severe disease may fall within the normal range.

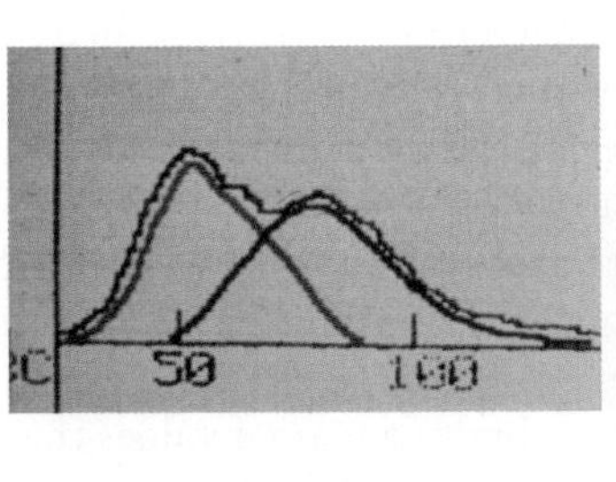

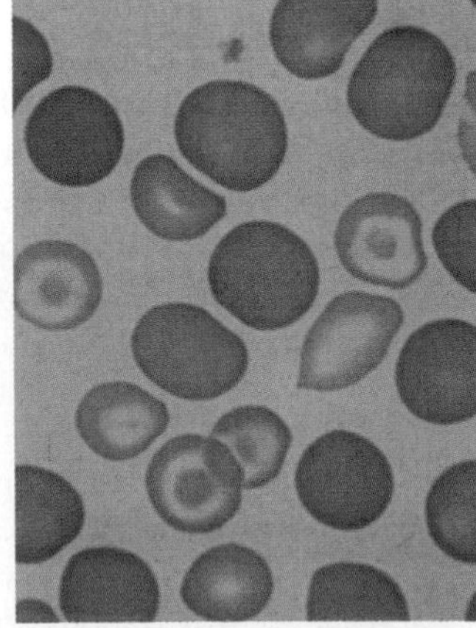

FIGURE 2–5. **Mixed populations of red blood cells.** As seen in this thalassemic patient with marked microcytosis and targeting, blood transfusions will distort the MCV size-distribution curve (shown on the left as a superimposition of 2 distinct distribution curves) and result in a greater-than-normal RDW value. Examination of the smear clearly shows the differences between the two populations: microcytic/hypochromic/targeted cells versus normocytic, normochromic cells.

explained by the coexistence of a microcytic population (red curve) and a normocytic population (blue curve).

Although the MCV is both accurate and highly reproducible, errors may be introduced by red blood cell agglutination, distortions in cell shape, the presence of very high numbers of white blood cells, and sudden osmotic swelling. The latter is seen in patients with very high blood glucose levels or, rarely, with hypernatremia, when the red blood cell sample is diluted for counting. Since the diluent is isotonic, cells containing excess glucose or sodium will act as tiny osmometers and swell.

D. Mean Cell Hemoglobin

The automated counter provides a calculated mean cell hemoglobin (MCH; ie, the hemoglobin level divided by the red blood cell count). The normal MCH is 32 ± 2 pg. This is an excellent measure of the amount of hemoglobin in each individual red blood cell. Patients with iron deficiency or thalassemia who are unable to synthesize normal amounts of hemoglobin show significant reductions in the MCH.

E. Mean Corpuscular Hemoglobin Concentration

The counter also provides a calculated mean corpuscular hemoglobin concentration (MCHC). The normal value of the MCHC is 33 ± 3 g/dL. This is the least revealing value provided by the counter. Although it should provide a measurement of the relative concentration of intracellular hemoglobin, it is not very sensitive to disease states where hemoglobin production is defective. This is in part due to counter error, but primarily reflects the fact that defects in hemoglobin production are accompanied by a simultaneous reduction in cell size. Thus, empty cells are also small cells. The principal value of the MCHC is to detect patients with hereditary spherocytosis who have very small, dense spherocytes in circulation. These spherocytes represent cells that have lost considerable intracellular fluid because of a membrane defect. When present in significant numbers, they will cause the MCHC to increase to levels in excess of 36 g/dL.

F. Red Blood Cell Distribution Width

In addition to the MCV, MCH, and MCHC, automated counters provide an index of the distribution of red blood cell volumes, termed the red blood cell distribution width (RDW). Counters may use 2 methods to calculate this value. The first is referred to as the RDW-CV. As shown in Figure 2–6, the **RDW-CV** is the ratio of the width of the red blood cell distribution curve at 1 SD divided by the MCV (normal RDW-CV = 13 ± 1%). Since it is a ratio, changes in either the width of the curve or the MCV will influence the result. Microcytosis will tend to magnify any change in the RDW-CV simply by reducing the denominator of the ratio. Conversely, macrocytosis will tend to counterbalance the change in the width of the curve and thereby minimize the change in the RDW-CV. A second method of measuring the RDW, the RDW-SD, is independent of the MCV. The **RDW-SD** is a direct measurement of the red blood cell distribution width taken at the 20% frequency level (normal RDW-SD = 42 ± 5 fL).

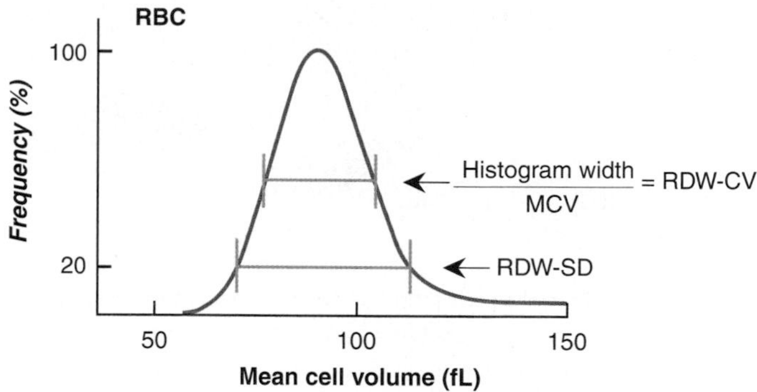

FIGURE 2–6. **Red blood cell distribution width (RDW).** Automated counters provide measurements of the width of the red blood cell distribution curve. The RDW-CV is calculated from the width of the histogram at 1 SD from the mean divided by the MCV. The normal RDW-CV is 13 ± 1%. The RDW-SD is the arithmetic width of the distribution curve measured at the 20% frequency level. The normal RDW-SD is 42 ± 5 fL.

Both measurements of the RDW are essentially mathematical representations of anisocytosis (ie, variations in red blood cell size). Increases in the RDW suggest the presence of a mixed population of cells. Double populations, whether microcytic cells mixed with normal cells or macrocytic cells mixed with normal cells, will widen the curve and increase the RDW. The RDW-SD is more sensitive to the appearance of minor populations of macrocytes or microcytes since it is measured lower on the red cell volume-distribution curve (Figure 2–6). At the same time, it is overly sensitive to the impact of increased numbers of reticulocytes, which, because of their larger MCV, will broaden the base of the distribution curve. The RDW-CV is less sensitive to the appearance of small populations of microcytes, true macrocytes, or reticulocytes, but better reflects the overall change in size distribution seen with well-established macrocytic or microcytic anemias.

G. Stained Blood Film

Although automated instruments provide accurate red blood cell counts and indices and white blood cell counts and differentials in both healthy and diseased individuals, red blood cell morphology can provide important additional information as to the nature of the anemia. Blood films are easily prepared by hand using glass slides (Figure 2–7) or by using automated slide preparation technology coupled to the cell counter. The well-dried blood film is then stained with Wright stain to bring out cytoplasmic and nuclear detail. On inspection, red blood cells should form a single cell layer with most of the cells appearing biconcave, that is, having the distinctive doughnut shape associated with biconcavity (Figure 2–8). If the film is too thick, cells will overlay each other and appear overly dense. When the film is too thin, as, for example, at the feathered edge of a hand-prepared blood smear, cells will lose both their biconcavity and round shape. Therefore, it is extremely important that any interpretation of red blood cell morphology be based on inspection of the best area of a

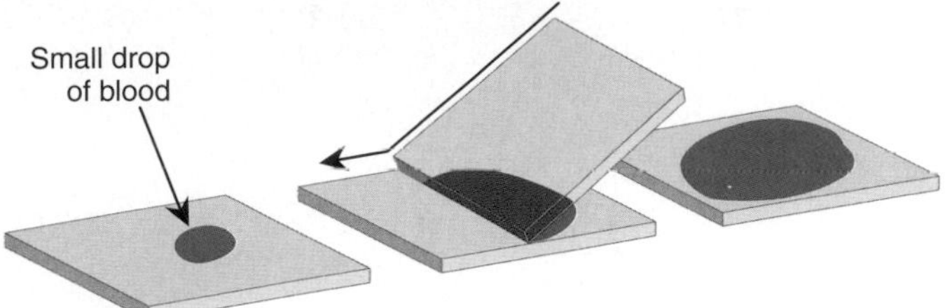

FIGURE 2–7. **Blood film preparation.** Blood films can be prepared by hand or as part of an automated cell count. Using 2 glass slides and a small drop of anticoagulated blood, it is easy to draw the blood along the length of the slide with a single smooth motion. Once the film is completely dry, the slide is stained with Wright stain. The slide is first flooded with stain for 2–3 minutes and then a buffer solution is added until a green sheen appears on the surface. After another 3–5 minutes, the slide is rinsed with tap water and air-dried. To interpret red blood cell morphology, one should select an area on the film where the red blood cells show the typical biconcave, doughnut shape.

well-prepared film. This is usually close to but not at the feathered end of the film.

The blood film complements the automated counter measurements of MCV and MCH. Visible changes in cell diameter, shape, and hemoglobin content can be used to distinguish both microcytic and macrocytic cells from normocytic/normochromic red blood cells (Figure 2–9). It should be emphasized, however, that the diagnosis of microcytosis or macrocytosis on a blood film involves extrapolation from an observed change in cell diameter to a volume estimate. This is not as sensitive or accurate as the direct measurement of cell volume by an automated counter. Therefore, the counter MCV should be used as the gold standard measurement for average changes in cell volume. At the same time, the stained film provides a more sensitive way to detect small populations of microcytic or macrocytic cells that are missed in the mean cell volume measurement.

The blood film is also used to detect and describe variations in red blood cell size **(anisocytosis)** and shape **(poikilocytosis)** (Figure 2–10). The former complements the automated counter measurement of the RDW. Film morphology provides more information than the RDW, however. It is possible to not only grade the degree of anisocytosis on a scale of 0–4+ but also comment on the population mix, whether microcytic, macrocytic, or another distinctive red blood cell shape (spherocytes, sickle cells, etc). Poikilocytosis can only be appreciated from the blood film. It is an important finding, because increasing poikilocytosis is associated with defects in red blood cell precursor maturation and certain types of red blood cell destruction. Like anisocytosis, it is graded on a scale of 0–4+.

The presence of **polychromatic macrocytes (polychromasia)**—cells that are slightly larger than the normal red cell by 1–2 μm (cell volume >100 fL), are of bluish-grayish color, and often lack the normal biconcave shape—is an important finding (Figure 2–10B). These cells represent young reticulocytes (immature marrow reticulocytes) that still contain large amounts of RNA and ribosomes. Their presence, even in small numbers, indicates a "shift" of marrow reticulocytes into circulation in response to an increased level of erythropoietin stimulation. Polychromasia can be used, therefore, to assess the adequacy of the erythropoietin response to anemia. It is also a key finding when it comes to calculating the reticulocyte index.

Other distinctive changes in red blood cell morphology, such as red cells that contain small inclusions (nuclear remnants, Howell-Jolly bodies, Pappenheimer bodies, siderocytes), sickle cells, spherocytes, target cells, and elliptocytes are seen in patients with various hemoglobinopathies, marrow damage, and loss of normal splenic function. The morphologic appearance of each of these abnormalities is illustrated and discussed extensively in the chapters and sections dealing with individual anemic states.

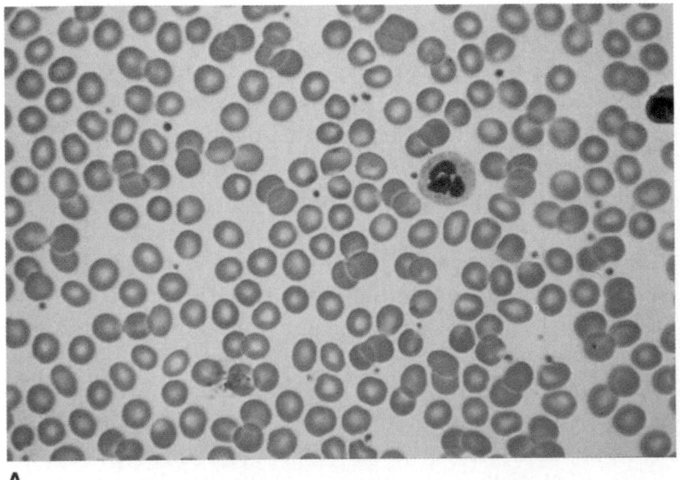
A

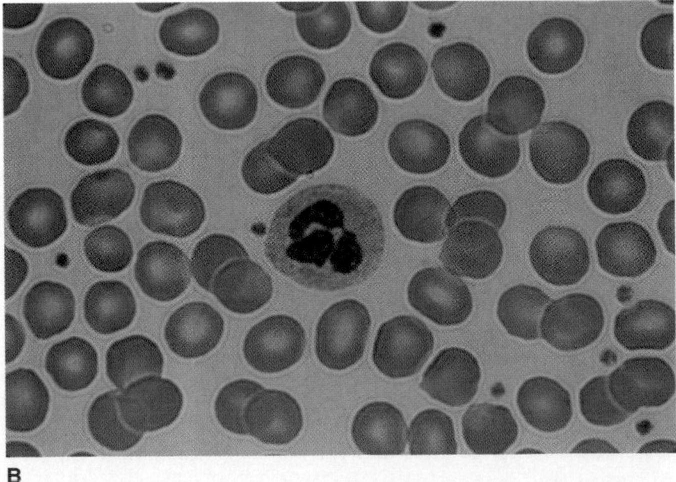
B

FIGURE 2–8. **Normal red cell morphology.** The red blood cells on a normal blood smear (low power—**A**, high power—**B**) typically are uniform in size and shape and show a clear center area because of their biconcave shape. Their diameter (compared to the single leukocyte in the center of this photograph) is roughly one-half the diameter of a leukocyte or only slightly smaller than a mature lymphocyte.

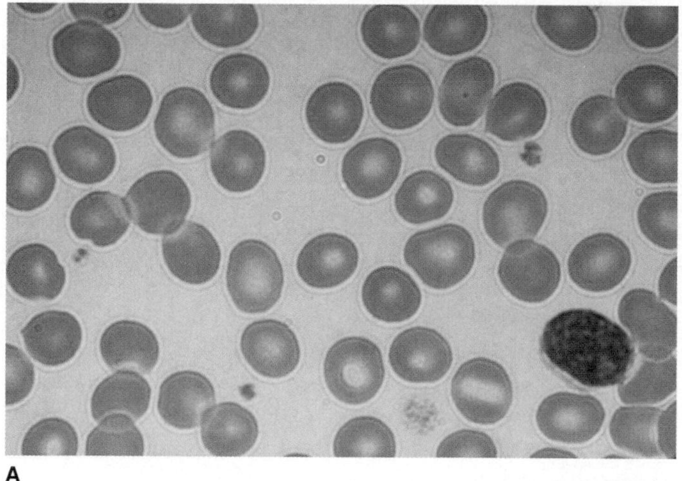
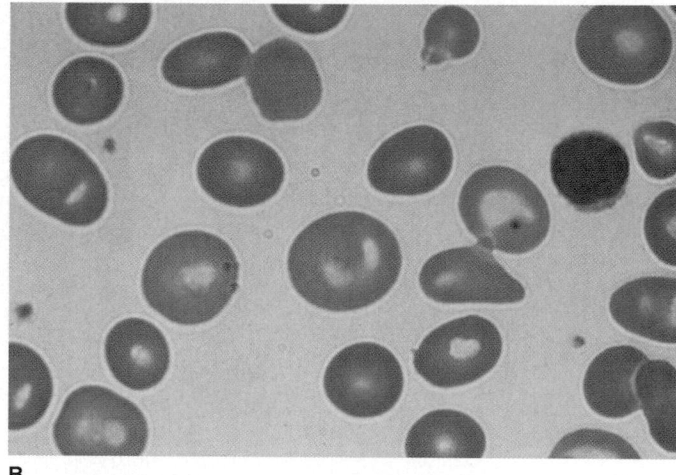

A B

FIGURE 2–9. **Microcytosis versus macrocytosis.** Example of a slightly microcytic **(A)** versus a macrocytic **(B)** smear. The lymphocyte on each smear can be used as a reference point; normocytic red cells are only slightly smaller than a mature lymphocyte.

H. Reticulocyte Count

The reticulocyte count is an essential component of the CBC and plays a prominent role in initially classifying any anemia. The reticulocyte is a young red blood cell containing residual ribosomal RNA that can be stained with a supravital dye such as acridine orange or new methylene blue. In the manual method, a drop of fresh blood is incubated with a few drops of new methylene blue solution and a blood smear is then prepared. The dye precipitates and stains the RNA, marking the cell as a reticulocyte and permitting a technician to count the number of reticulocytes versus the number of adult red blood cells (Figure 2–11). For accuracy, at least 1,000 red blood cells should be counted to determine the reticulocyte percentage. The relative intensity of RNA staining can also provide a clue to the presence of marrow reticulocytes in circulation.

Most automated counters now incorporate technologies that allow direct instrument measurement of the reticulocyte count. As one example, the Abbott Cell-Dyne instrument uses a proprietary dye that binds to reticulocyte RNA and emits fluorescence that is detected using an Argon-ion laser. The presence of marrow reticulocytes can also be measured as an immature reticulocyte fraction, that is, macrocytic cells containing larger amounts of RNA.

The normal reticulocyte count for both the automated and new methylene blue methods is 1% with a range of 0.6%–2.0%. Even though the standard error for the manual method is quite high because it is based on a limited count, the accuracy is generally good enough for clinical purposes. In response to anemia, the reticulocyte count will increase several-fold in patients with normal renal (erythropoietin production) and bone marrow function. In addition, high levels of erythropoietin stimulation

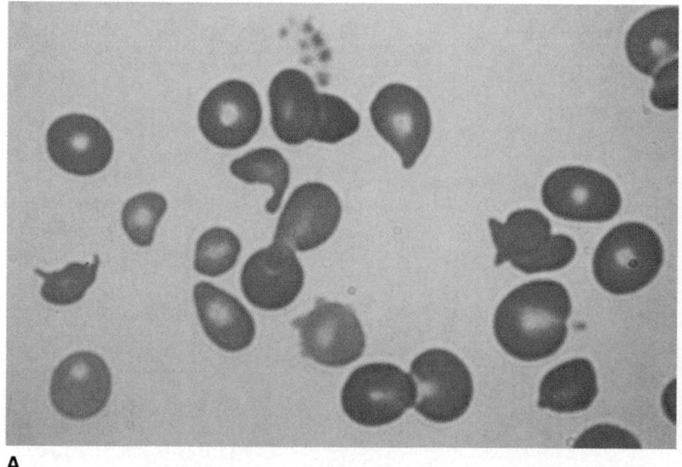
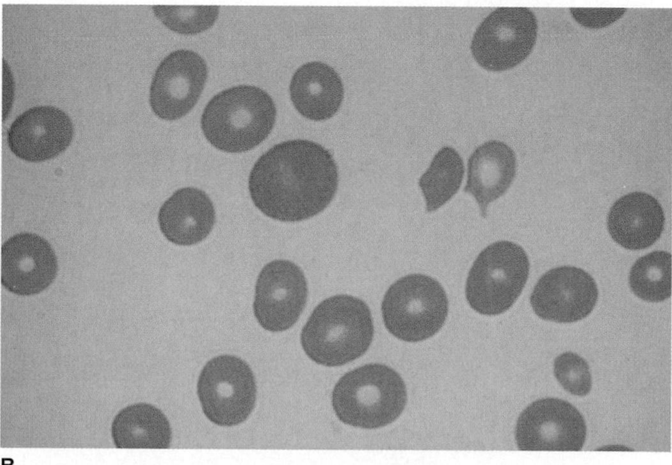

A B

FIGURE 2–10. **Abnormalites of size and shape.** The blood smear is also invaluable for the detection of anisocytosis (variations in cell size) and poikilocytosis (variations in cell shape) **(A)**, and polychromasia (polychromatophilic macrocytes or shift cells) in circulation **(B)**.

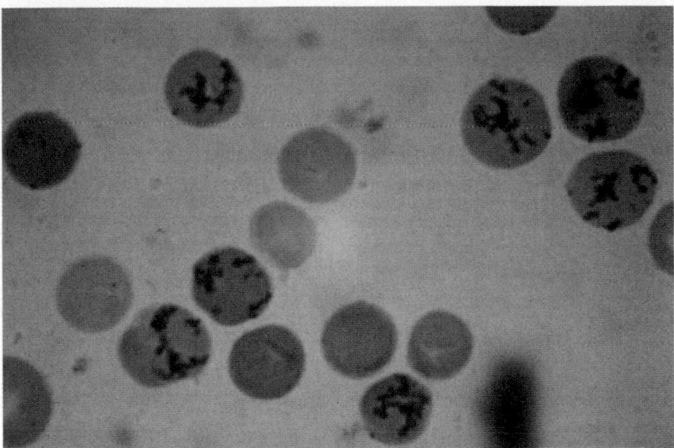

FIGURE 2–11. **Reticulocyte stain.** The new methylene blue stain allows ready identification of reticulocytes—cells containing deep blue precipitates. The amount of precipitate correlates with the age of the reticulocyte—marrow reticulocytes (shift cells) contain more blue staining material than the reticulocytes released into circulation in the basal state.

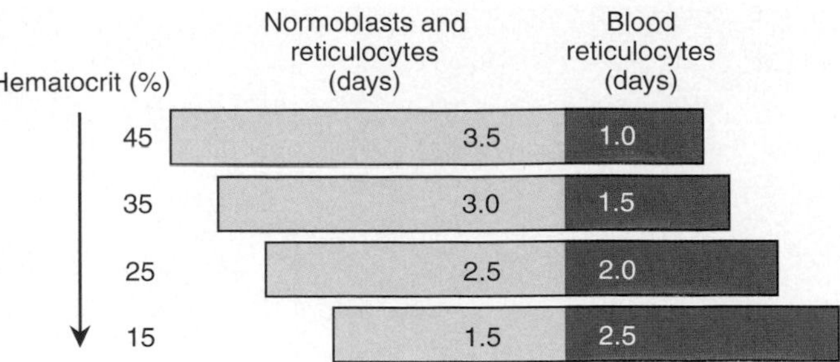

FIGURE 2–12. **Reticulocyte shift.** As anemia worsens and the level of erythropoietin stimulation increases, marrow reticulocytes leave the marrow at an earlier point in their maturation. This prolongs their maturation time in circulation. Whereas the normal reticulocyte matures in less than a day, reticulocytes in anemic patients take from 1.5–2.5 days. This must be taken into account when calculating the reticulocyte production index.

seen with certain anemias result in the release of large numbers of immature marrow reticulocytes (shift cells or polychromasia) into circulation.

For one to use the reticulocyte count as a measure of red blood cell production, the count needs to be corrected for both changes in hematocrit (red blood cell count) and the effect of erythropoietin on reticulocyte release from the marrow. Most laboratories automatically convert the reticulocyte percent count to an absolute number either by multiplying it against the red blood cell count (normal absolute count = ~50,000 reticulocytes/μL) or multiplying it by the fraction of the patient's hematocrit (Hct) over the normal hematocrit as illustrated in the following formula:

$$\%\text{ Reticulocytes} \times \frac{\text{Patient Hct}}{45}$$

$$= \text{Absolute Reticulocyte Percentage}$$

or

$$\%\text{ Reticulocytes} \times \text{Red Blood Cell Count}$$

$$= \text{Absolute Reticulocyte Count}$$

An example for a patient with a reticulocyte count of 6% and a hematocrit of 22% (red cell count of 2.6×10^6) would provide the following results:

$$6\% \times \frac{22}{45} = 3\%$$

or

$$6\% \times 2.6 \times 10^6 = 156{,}000 \text{ Reticulocytes}/\mu\text{L}$$

To obtain the true index of marrow production in a severely anemic patient, a second correction must be made if marrow reticulocytes have entered circulation in response to high levels of erythropoietin. As shown in Figure 2–12, marrow reticulocytes are shifted out of the marrow and into circulation at an earlier stage with increasingly severe anemia. This process has the effect of lengthening the maturation time of reticulocytes in circulation. Whereas normal reticulocytes lose their RNA within 24 hours, a severely anemic patient with a full erythropoietin response will release reticulocytes that take from 2–3 days to lose their RNA. This has the effect of raising the reticulocyte count simply because reticulocytes produced on any single day will spend more than 1 day in circulation as reticulocytes and, therefore, will be counted for 2 or more days. The simplest method for correcting the reticulocyte count, to obtain a more accurate daily production index, is to divide the absolute count by a factor of 2 whenever polychromasia (the presence of immature marrow reticulocytes or shift cells) is observed on the smear or the immature fraction on the automated counter is increased, as follows:

$$\frac{\text{Absolute Reticulocyte Percentage (or number)}}{2}$$

$$= \text{Production Index}$$

When applied to the prior example, results in a patient with an initial reticulocyte count of 6% would be corrected as follows:

$$6\% \times \frac{22}{45} \times \frac{1}{2} = 1.5 \text{ (Production Index)}$$

or

$$6\% \times 2.6 \times 10^6 \times \frac{1}{2} = \frac{78{,}000}{50{,}000} = 1.5 \text{ (Production Index)}$$

As a practical matter, the correction for the reticulocyte shift phenomenon should be applied to any patient with a severe anemia and/or a very high reticulocyte count, because erythropoietin levels are predictably high. In patients with more modest anemia or a poor reticulocyte response, it is very important to document whether there has been a release of marrow reticulocytes (polychromasia). Not only will this help characterize the mechanism behind the anemia, but also the second correction should not be applied in the absence of polychromasia. For example, polychromasia is not seen in most patients with inflammatory anemias (the anemia of chronic disease) where the erythropoietin response is suppressed. In contrast, a patient with a marrow damage anemia will have a poor reticulocyte response but readily recognized polychromasia on smear because of the high level of erythropoietin release.

The principal application of the reticulocyte count (corrected to obtain a production index) is to distinguish between patients with a functionally normal marrow response to anemia/hypoxia and those with a failed marrow response. Whenever the reticulocyte production index increases to levels greater than 3 times normal in response to an anemia (hematocrit <30%), it can be assumed that the patient has normal renal function with an appropriate erythropoietin response and a normal erythroid marrow with an adequate supply of key nutrients (iron, folic acid, and vitamin B_{12}). Moreover, it strongly suggests that the anemia is the result of an increased destruction of circulating red blood cells, either because of hemorrhage or hemolysis. Diseases that interfere with the erythropoietin response, nutrient supply, or erythroid precursor proliferation/maturation are characterized by a low reticulocyte production index indicative of a low level of effective red blood cell production.

Other routine laboratory measurements can also help define the physiologic defect responsible for the anemia. Elevations in the serum bilirubin (indirect fraction) and lactic dehydrogenase (LDH) are seen in patients with increased hemolysis and disorders of marrow precursor maturation with high levels of ineffective erythropoiesis (death of immature red cell precursors within the marrow). The indirect (unconjugated) serum bilirubin concentration correlates with the rate of red blood cell turnover. Normally, serum bilirubin is between 0.4 and 1 mg/dL, most of which is indirect bilirubin (70%–80%). With hemolysis or severe ineffective erythropoiesis, indirect bilirubin increases to 0.8–3 mg/dL. The direct or conjugated bilirubin level shows little change, as long as the patient's liver function is normal.

The serum LDH is extremely sensitive to increased rates of red blood cell destruction, because red blood cells are rich in LDH, especially LDH 1. Patients with hemolytic anemias show rises in their serum LDH concentrations in excess of 1,000 IU/L (normal 300–600 IU/L), without abnormalities in other liver enzymes. With severe hemolysis or marked ineffective erythropoiesis, the LDH level can reach several thousand units.

I. Marrow Examination

A sample of marrow can easily be obtained by needle aspirate or biopsy to evaluate overall cellularity, the ratio of erythroid to granulocytic precursors **(E/G ratio)**, and cellular morphology. The marrow examination is of greatest value in patients who fail to show an appropriate increase in the reticulocyte production index in response to anemia. In these patients defects in erythroid precursor proliferation or maturation play a major role.

In adults, the marrow aspirate or biopsy is best obtained from the posterior iliac crest (Figure 2–13). The **iliac crest** is identifiable as a palpable bony ridge, approximately 2 cm from the midline at the level of the sacrum. The cortex of the crest is quite thin and easily punctured with a standard aspiration or

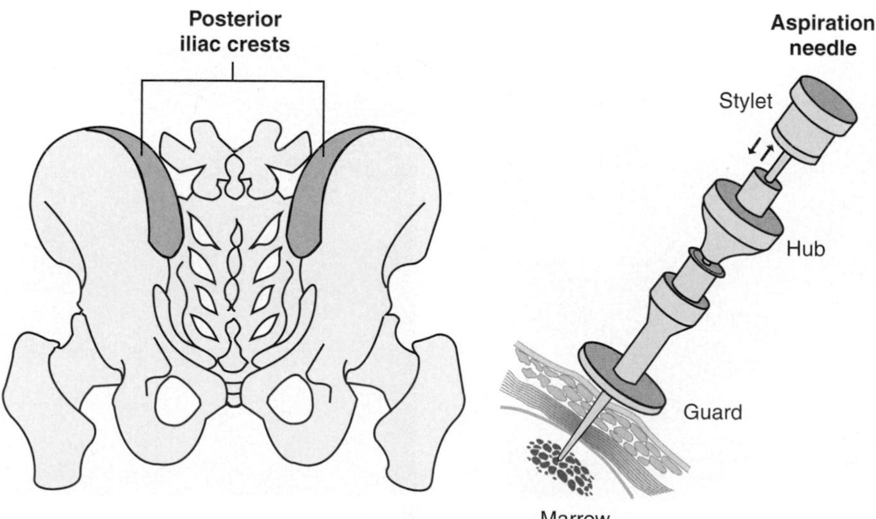

FIGURE 2–13. **Marrow aspiration technique.** A marrow aspirate is most easily obtained from the posterior iliac crest, a bony ridge that is usually easily palpable 2 cm from the midline at the level of the sacrum. An aspiration needle with stylet in place is easily pushed through the external cortex of the crest using a slight twisting motion. Once the needle is firmly in the marrow cavity, the stylet is withdrawn and a small (1–2 mL) syringe is used to aspirate a few drops of marrow. The marrow is then expelled on a watch-glass and particles are harvested to make marrow smears.

biopsy needle, using a small amount of local anesthetic to numb the skin and periosteal membrane. The marrow aspirate specimen is used for evaluating cell morphology, whereas needle biopsy is best suited for evaluating overall cellularity and the relationship of marrow structure to hematopoietic cells.

1. Marrow aspirate—The quality of the marrow aspirate specimen is extremely important. Very small amounts of marrow should be aspirated using a 1- to 2-mL syringe and immediately expressed onto a watch-glass. Marrow particles can then be harvested with a capillary tube and spread on slides or coverslips. Once air-dried, smears are stained with a Wright-Giemsa stain to bring out the details of nuclear and cytoplasmic structure. The best aspirate specimens show stromal particles surrounded by a field of hematopoietic cells of all types (Figure 2–14). It should also be possible under oil immersion to identify and classify each cell as myeloid or erythroid and as a mature or immature precursor. If cells are sparse or severely distorted, the preparation is not interpretable. Inspection of a marrow aspirate starts with a low power scan for particle cellularity, and distribution and frequency of megakaryocytes, which because of their large size and multiple nuclei are easily identified. There is no exact way of enumerating megakaryocytes. It should not be difficult, however, to find them in a normal marrow specimen. Inspection of the other cell types is then carried out under oil immersion (100×).

Several high-power fields adjacent to a stroma particle should be scanned to estimate the E/G ratio (Figure 2–15). As long as the patient's white blood cell production is normal, the E/G ratio provides a rough index of red blood cell production. Figure 2–15 shows an example of a shift in the E/G ratio to greater than 1:1 (Figure 2–15A) in a patient responding normally to a severe anemia, while a patient with a severe hypoproliferative anemia will show an E/G ratio of 1:3 or lower (Figure 2–15B).

The normal marrow red blood cell precursor population is characterized by a predictable progression from primitive blasts

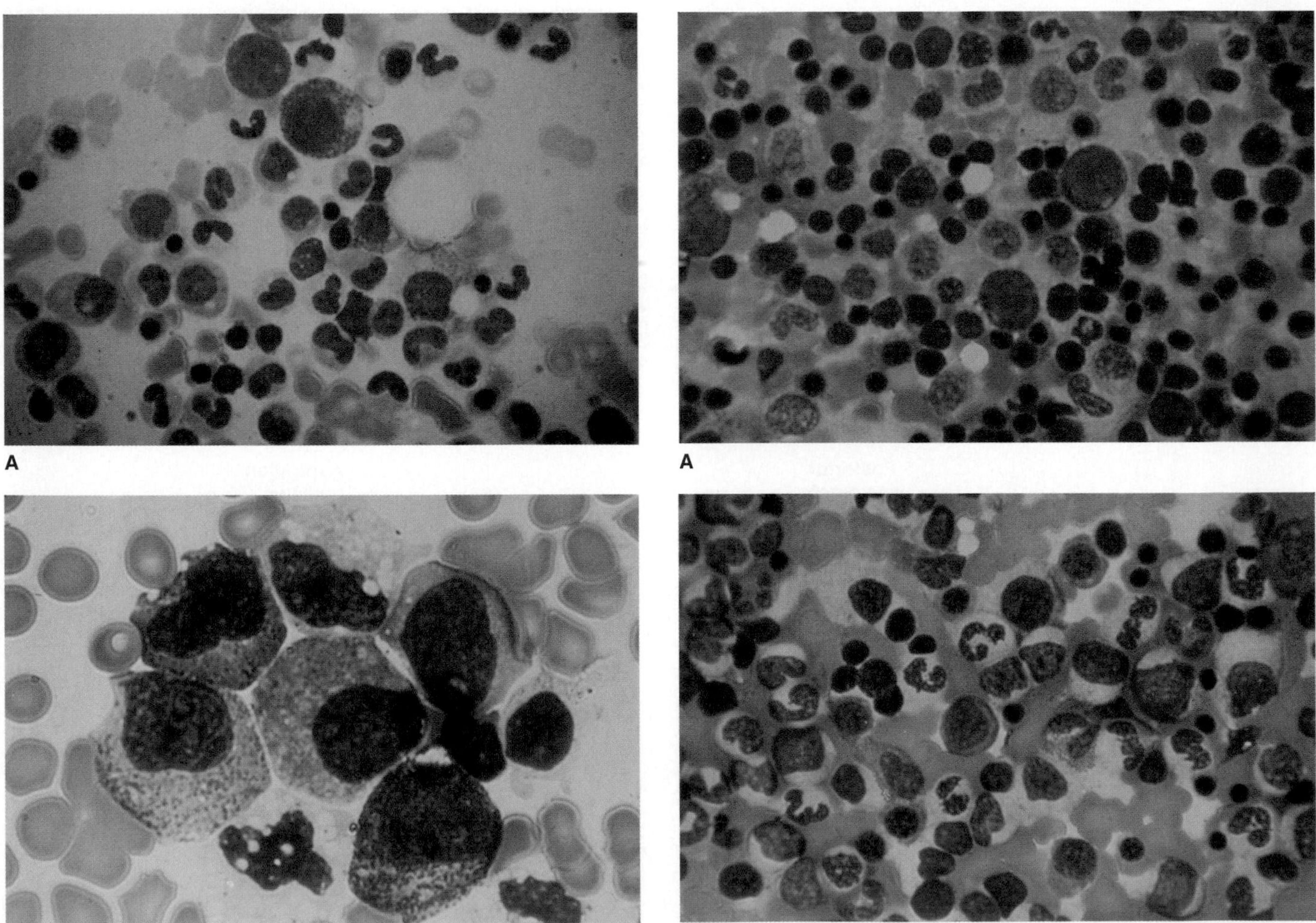

FIGURE 2–14. **Bone marrow aspirate.** Normal marrow aspirate particles provide information as to cellularity, cell types, and the ratio of erythroid precursors to white cell precursors (E/G ratio). This example of a marrow aspirate shows a mix of cell types from early precursors to mature granulocytes **(A)**. Under very high power it is possible to identify the minute structures of early white cell precursors **(B)**.

FIGURE 2–15. **Examples of abnormal E/G ratios.** The estimation of the marrow E/G ratio (normally 1:3) is key to the functional classification of anemias. This composite photograph shows examples of 2 abnormal ratios: **(A)** increased red cell production (E/G ratio >1:1) and **(B)** decreased red cell production (E/G ratio < 1:3).

(committed stem cells) through a morphologically distinct maturation sequence—pronormoblast; basophilic, polychromatic, and orthochromatic normoblasts; and, finally, marrow reticulocytes (Figure 2–16). Morphologically, this maturation sequence is characterized by a progressive reduction in cell size, shrinkage and disappearance of the cell's nucleus, loss of cellular mitochondria and RNA, and a steady increase in hemoglobin content. The final product of this maturation sequence is the anucleate, fully hemoglobinized adult red blood cell.

Examination of any marrow aspirate should include a careful assessment for evidence of a red cell maturation abnormality, especially changes in cell size, nuclear morphology, and hemoglobin development. A number of anemias are characterized by distinct abnormalities in the maturation sequence and the morphology at each stage of maturation. For example, patients with a megaloblastic marrow (defect in DNA metabolism) show a preponderance of young, large erythroblasts with nuclei containing lacy, poorly staining chromatin (see Chapter 8). Older precursors show a discrepancy between nuclear maturation and hemoglobin synthesis, where the nucleus appears less mature than it should for the amount of hemoglobin synthesized. In contrast, patients with defects in hemoglobin synthesis, iron deficiency, or thalassemia show normal nuclear maturation but poor cytoplasmic maturation.

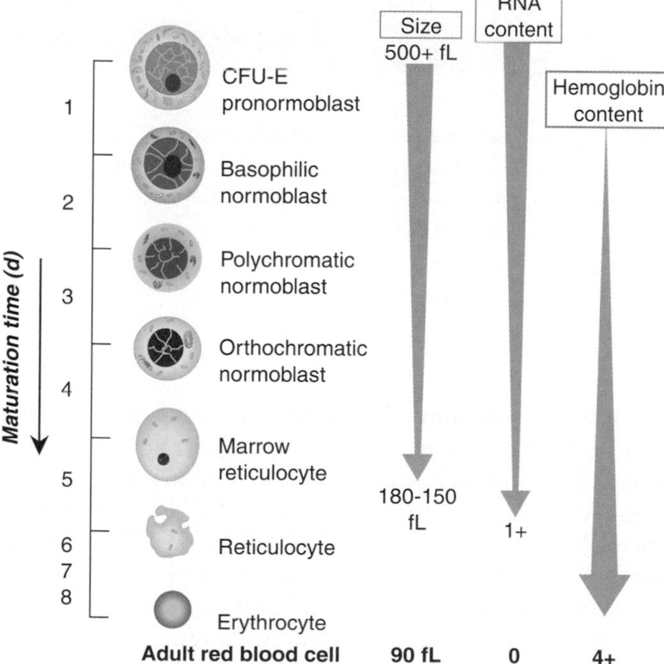

FIGURE 2–16. **Erythroid marrow maturation.** Red blood cell precursor maturation proceeds through a series of morphologically distinct stages over 6–7 days. Identifiable populations in this maturation sequence include pronormoblasts; basophilic, polychromatic, and orthochromatic normoblasts; and the marrow reticulocytes. With development, there is progressive reduction in cell size, shrinkage of the cell's nucleus, loss of cellular mitochondria and RNA, and a dramatic increase in hemoglobin. Specific red blood cell disorders can be identified from disruptions in this normal maturation sequence.

Marrow aspirate particles should also be routinely stained with Prussian blue to evaluate reticuloendothelial cell iron stores and iron deposits in individual red blood cell precursors. Hemosiderin particles within the reticuloendothelial cells of the marrow stroma stain a deep blue color. The greater the amount of iron stores, the more dramatic the staining. Iron stores can be estimated using a scale of 0–4+, where the normal adult male with 1,000 mg of iron stores will be 2–3+ and a normal adult female with 200–300 mg of iron stores will be 1+. Transfusion iron overload is associated with 4+ iron stores, while 0 stores indicate iron deficiency (Figure 2–17).

Close inspection of individual red blood cell precursors will also reveal a few dustlike iron (ferritin) granules in maturing normoblasts. Up to one-third of red blood cell precursors will contain blue-staining ferritin granules. These cells are referred to as **sideroblasts**, whereas marrow reticulocytes containing iron granules are **siderocytes**. A decrease in the number of sideroblasts and siderocytes is a morphologic indication of iron-deficient erythropoiesis. In contrast, an increase in the number and size increase in iron granules in erythroid precursors suggests a defect in hemoglobin synthesis. Patients with specific disorders of mitochondrial function can exhibit **ringed sideroblasts**, which are distinctive cells with several large granules distributed in a ring around the nucleus (see Chapter 9). This condition results from iron loading of the mitochondria that surround the nucleus.

2. Marrow biopsy—A marrow needle biopsy should also be obtained if an adequate specimen cannot be obtained by aspiration and, as a routine, whenever a patient is being evaluated for tumor infiltration of the marrow, fibrosis, or aplasia. The biopsy specimen permits a better evaluation of the marrow's structural elements and the relationship of stroma to hematopoietic cells. Independent of the type of needle used, it is important to obtain a good core of marrow (Figure 2–18). The core specimen is fixed, decalcified, and stained with

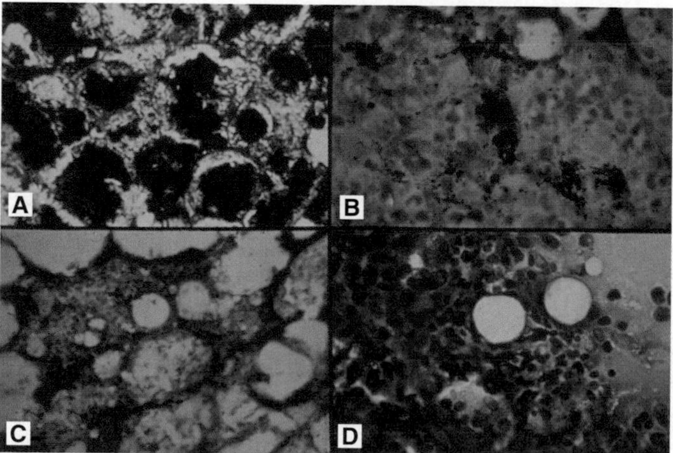

FIGURE 2–17. **Iron stain.** A marrow aspirate slide stained with Prussian blue can be used to estimate iron stores. As shown in this composite photograph, iron stores can be roughly graded as **(A)** increased (4+); **(B)** normal (2–3+); **(C)** reduced (1+); or **(D)** absent (0).

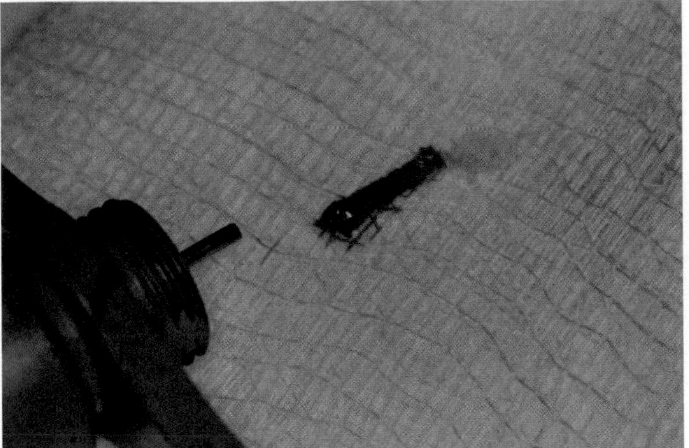

FIGURE 2–18. **Core needle biopsy.** On needle biopsy, it is important to obtain an adequate core specimen for a successful evaluation of marrow structure and cellularity.

periodic acid–Schiff, and hematoxylin and eosin stains. Other special stains, such as a silver stain for reticulin fibers or a trichrome stain for collagen, can help in diagnosing specific disorders of marrow structure.

As with the aspirate, initial inspection of a biopsy specimen should be carried out under both low power and high power to evaluate adequacy of the specimen, general architecture, and overall cellularity (Figure 2–19). The cellularity of hematopoietic tissue in the central skeleton decreases with age. Two-thirds or more of the marrow space in a young adult is taken up by hematopoietic tissue and one-third is filled with fat cells. This ratio reverses over the next several decades; older individuals have one-half to two-thirds of their marrow space filled with fat cells. The biopsy specimen is also good for evaluating the presence of megakaryocytes. As with the aspirate, the megakaryocytes are easily identified because of their large size and multinuclearity. Finally, needle biopsy is clearly preferred for the detection of structural abnormalities such as myelofibrosis and infiltration of the marrow by malignant cells, especially lymphomas and carcinomas.

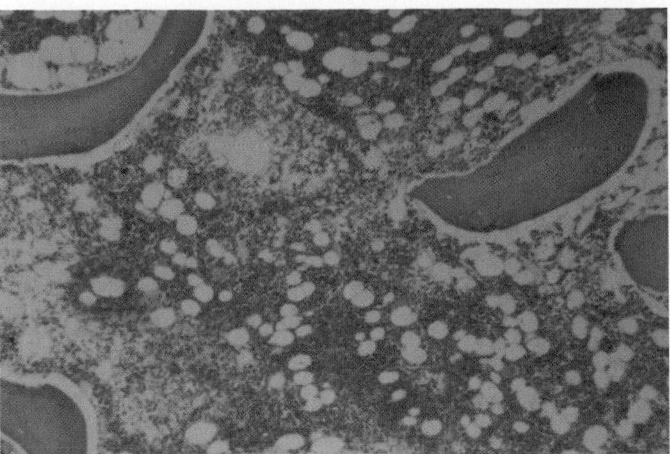

A

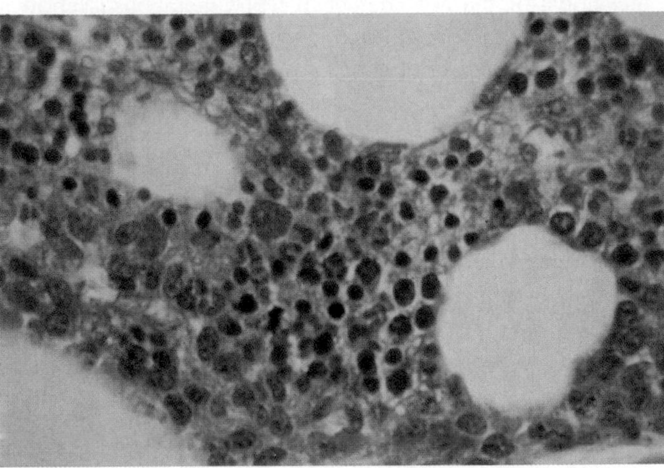

B

FIGURE 2–19. **Fixed and stained marrow biopsy.** A marrow biopsy specimen, shown here under low **(A)** and high **(B)** power, shows the relationship of marrow precursor elements to fat cells and the bony trabecular structure of the marrow cavity. The biopsy offers the best measure of overall cellularity and the relative number of megakaryocytes. It also is invaluable in diagnosing structural abnormalities, such as tumor infiltration, fibrosis, and marked aplasia.

J. Tests of Iron Supply

Studies of iron supply, including measurements of serum iron, transferrin iron binding capacity, and serum ferritin level, play an important role in the initial differential diagnosis of an anemia. They are essential companions to the marrow iron stain whenever a marrow aspirate is performed.

1. Serum iron level—The serum iron (SI) is a measure of the amount of iron bound to transferrin. A normal individual has an SI of 50–150 μg/dL. The proliferative capacity of the erythroid marrow and its ability to synthesize hemoglobin are functions of the serum iron level. When the SI falls to levels below 50 μg/dL, the erythroid marrow cannot increase production above basal levels and new red blood cells will be poorly hemoglobinized. Levels of marrow production that are 3 times the basal level or greater require a serum iron in excess of 100 μg/dL.

2. Total iron-binding capacity—The **total iron-binding capacity (TIBC)** is a measure of the amount of iron that can be bound by transferrin. In effect, it is equivalent to measuring the level of transferrin protein. The normal TIBC is 300–360 μg/dL. The importance of the TIBC is 2-fold. First, the TIBC changes independently of the serum iron in situations of iron deficiency. Although TIBC declines in patients with the anemia of chronic disease (inflammation), it typically increases in excess of 360 μg/dL in patients with severe iron deficiency. The TIBC is also used to calculate a percent saturation of transferrin:

$$\frac{\text{SI}}{\text{TIBC}} = \%\ \text{Saturation}$$

A normal individual has a percent saturation of between 20% and 50%. When the percent saturation falls below 10%, the patient usually has absolute iron deficiency. With values between 10% and 20%, it is more likely that the decrease in iron supply is the result of an inflammatory state. Iron overload, especially hereditary hemachromatosis, is associated with an increased percent saturation, which exceeds 50% and often approaches 90%–100%.

3. Serum ferritin level—Ferritin is a spherical protein made up of 24 subunits: L (light), H (heavy), and G (glycosylated). **Serum ferritin** contains mostly L and G subunits, whereas tissue ferritins are largely L and H subunit types. Since the serum ferritin level generally parallels total body storage iron, it is used clinically to evaluate body iron stores. A normal adult male will have a serum ferritin level of between 50 and 150 μg/L, reflecting iron stores of 600–1,000 mg. When iron stores are depleted, the serum ferritin falls. Levels below 10–15 μg/L indicate store exhaustion and iron deficiency. With iron overload, the serum ferritin level will exceed 300 μg/L and may reach several thousand micrograms per liter. Liver disease and inflammation disproportionately elevate the serum ferritin, perhaps by the release of tissue ferritins.

4. Serum transferrin receptor level—Erythroid precursor cells express transferrin receptors (TfR) on their surface according to their level of maturation and the adequacy of iron supply (see Chapter 5). Measurements of the serum TfR level (normal level = 4–9 μg/L) generally reflect the level of expression of receptors on the cell surface as well as the absolute number of erythroid precursors. Therefore, the serum TfR increases with both iron deficiency **(iron store exhaustion)** and erythroid precursor proliferation. It can be useful in the differential diagnosis of absolute iron deficiency versus the anemia of chronic disease **(inflammatory anemia)**, where iron stores are maintained and the anemia is hypoproliferative (see Chapters 4 and 5).

K. Other Laboratory Measurements

Several other laboratory tests are used in the diagnosis of specific hematopoietic disorders. A partial list of these assays grouped according to category of disease is provided in Table 2–3. Detailed descriptions of assay methods and test interpretations are provided as a part of the discussion of individual disorders.

TABLE 2–3 • Laboratory assays in the diagnosis of specific red cell disorders

Hypoproliferative anemias
Cytometric assay of CD59/CD55 levels (paroxysmal nocturnal hemoglobinuria)
Chromosomal analysis (leukemias)
Marrow aspirate/biopsy special stains
Trichrome stain (myelofibrosis)
Silver stain for reticulin (myelofibrosis)
Peroxidase, esterase, and PAS stains (acute leukemia)
Maturation disorders
Serum vitamin B_{12} level (vitamin B_{12} deficiency)
Serum/red blood cell folate levels (folic acid deficiency)
Urine/serum methylmalonic acid level (B_{12} and folate deficiency)
dU suppression test (B_{12} deficiency)
Hemoglobin electrophoresis (thalassemia)
Hemoglobin A_2 level–HPLC (β-thalassemia)
Hemoglobin F level—HPLC (β-thalassemia)
Cytometric assay for hemoglobin F (thalassemia versus hereditary persistence of hemoglobin F)
Brilliant cresyl blue stain/isopropanol stability (hemoglobin H)
Red blood cell protoporphyrin level (iron deficiency—lead poisoning)
Hemolytic anemias
Hemoglobin electrophoresis and HPLC (hemoglobinopathies)
Coombs test (autoimmune hemolytic anemia)
Cold agglutinin titer (autoimmune hemolytic anemia)
Haptoglobin level (hemolysis)
Serum/urine hemosiderin (intravascular hemolysis)
Osmotic fragility (hereditary spherocytosis)
Incubated autohemolysis test (congenital nonspherocytic hemolytic anemias)
G6PD screen (G6PD deficiency)
Heat/isopropanol denaturation tests (unstable hemoglobins)

APPROACH TO THE PATIENT

The key to any anemia evaluation is the clinician's skill in applying and interpreting the results of these laboratory tests according to the clinical presentation. Often, the workup of the anemia is carried out as a part of the evaluation and management of another illness. This process requires knowledge and understanding of the impact of disease states on red blood cell production and survival. It is also important to complete the basic workup as quickly as possible, since delay can lead to confusion. For example, a patient with a maturation defect secondary to drug effect or vitamin deficiency can show dramatic changes in the CBC, serum iron studies, and marrow morphology within a few days of changes in medication and diet, or the treatment of a second illness.

Therefore, the battery of routine laboratory tests and marrow aspirate or biopsy (or both) should be performed on the same day whenever possible. This approach will help avoid any misinterpretation of a test result simply because it was drawn at a time when the patient's clinical picture had changed. For example, because the reticulocyte count measures red blood cell production on a daily basis, it will change much more quickly than red blood cell morphology, which takes 2–3 months to correct completely, based on the lifespan of red blood cells in circulation.

Another important rule is never to merely assume a diagnostic relationship. Even though the nature of the anemia may be suggested by the clinical presentation, the true cause can only be diagnosed based on a full laboratory evaluation. Moreover, the anemia is often the product of several contributing factors. For example, the patient with small-bowel disease and malabsorption can present with a combination of deficiencies in iron, folic acid, and vitamin B_{12}, as well as an anemia typical of a chronic inflammatory disease state. Therefore, the diagnostic challenge is to not just assume the causal basis of the anemia but identify each pathophysiologic component.

Classification of Anemia

Anemia diagnosis can be organized as a 3-branch algorithm based on routine laboratory test results. The first step is to categorize the erythropoietic abnormality as one of 3 functional defects: (1) a failure in red blood cell production, (2) an abnormality in cell maturation, or (3) an increase in red blood cell destruction. This first step relies on the CBC and reticulocyte index. As shown in Figure 2–20, defects in production (hypoproliferative anemias) are characterized by a low reticulocyte production index coupled with little or no change in red blood cell morphology. Maturation disorders demonstrate a low reticulocyte production index together with either macrocytic or microcytic red blood cell morphology. In contrast, patients with increased red blood cell destruction owing to hemolysis show a compensatory increase in the reticulocyte index to levels greater than 3 times normal and red blood cell morphology that may or may not be distinctive for the disease process.

This first step in classifying an anemia is important for both diagnosis and management. From the diagnostic viewpoint, each category encompasses a limited number of possibilities (Figure 2–21). This situation makes it possible to organize the rest of the laboratory evaluation around those tests that best discriminate among several diagnostic choices. Management of the patient will also vary according to the functional defect. For example, the need to provide a transfusion for a patient early in the course of the workup will depend on the expected ability of the patient to respond to a specific therapy.

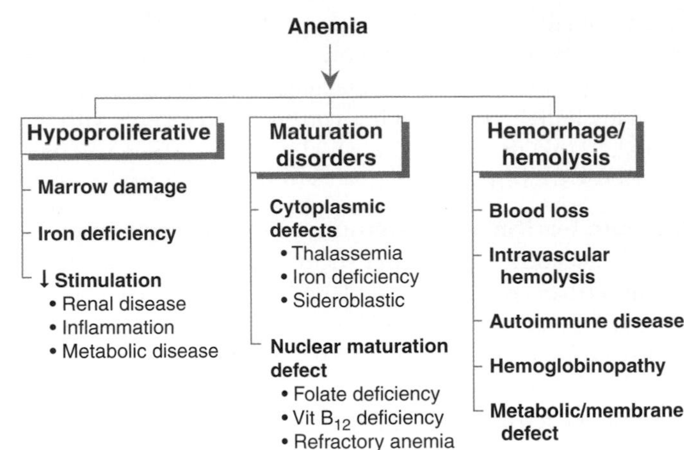

FIGURE 2–21. **Functional classification of anemia.** Each of the major categories of anemia (hypoproliferative, maturation disorders, and hemorrhage/hemolysis) can be further subclassified according to the functional defect in the several components of normal erythropoiesis.

Hypoproliferative Anemias

A **hypoproliferative anemia** (ie, an anemia resulting from a failure in the erythroid marrow production response) can result from damage to the marrow structure or precursor stem cell pool, a lack of stimulation by erythropoietin, or iron deficiency. Patients with these conditions usually present with a normocytic, normochromic anemia of moderate severity. The reticulocyte production index is less than 2 and the marrow E/G ratio is less than 1:2. Measurements of red blood cell destruction such as the bilirubin and LDH are normal or decreased. In essence, this is the profile of a marrow that has not responded appropriately (increased red cell production) to the patient's anemia.

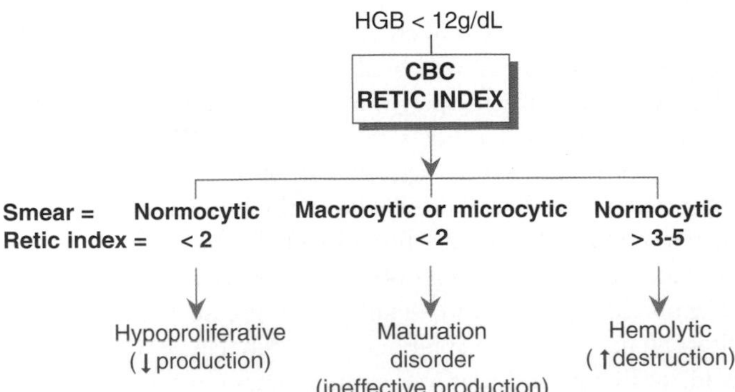

FIGURE 2–20. **Initial classification of anemia.** The CBC and reticulocyte index is used to classify an anemia as hypoproliferative, a maturation disorder, or a hemorrhagic/hemolytic anemia.

Most anemias encountered in clinical practice are hypoproliferative. They are generally associated with a chronic illness, especially disorders with a significant inflammatory component. Iron deficiency is another prominent cause of hypoproliferative anemia. Therefore, a careful clinical evaluation is required to understand the cause of the anemia (the nature of the inflammatory illness or site of blood loss producing iron deficiency) and plan management. A full discussion of marrow damage anemias is covered in Chapter 3, whereas anemias associated with chronic disease are discussed in Chapter 4.

Maturation Defects

Disruption of the erythroid precursor maturation sequence can result from deficiencies in vitamins such as folic acid and vitamin B_{12}, exposure to chemotherapeutic agents, or a myelodysplastic or preleukemic state. Since these are all defects in nuclear maturation, patients present with macrocytic anemias, megaloblastic bone marrow morphology, and varying degrees of ineffective erythropoiesis. By contrast, defects in hemoglobinization, including severe iron deficiency and inherited defects in globin chain synthesis, the thalassemias, produce a microcytic, hypochromic anemia and ineffective erythropoiesis. An extensive discussion of maturation disorders is provided in Chapter 5 ("Iron-Deficiency Anemia"), Chapter 6 ("Thalassemia"), and Chapter 8 ("Macrocytic Anemias").

Increased Red Blood Cell Destruction

Blood loss or hemolysis will stimulate a compensatory red blood cell production response. Thus, the increased cell destruction category of anemia is characterized by an increase in the reticulocyte production index to greater than 3 times normal and a similar increase in the E/G ratio to levels greater than 1:1. The impact of high levels of erythropoietin stimulation in the marrow is also apparent from the appearance of large numbers

CASE HISTORY • *Part 2*

From a morphologic perspective, the patient has a normocytic/normochromic anemia of moderate severity without changes in white blood cell or platelet levels. This is confirmed by the normal red blood cell indices (MCV, MCH, MCHC, and RDW) and blood smear morphology. His reticulocyte count (2%) and calculated reticulocyte index (1.2—*after correction for anemia but without correction for "shift" since no polychromasia on smear*) suggest a **hypoproliferative anemia**, that is, an anemia secondary to a failure of the erythroid marrow response to a worsening anemia.

The most likely physiological mechanisms in this case are an inflammatory condition and/or renal failure with decreased erythropoietin production. To address these questions, the patient had iron (serum iron, iron-binding capacity, and serum ferritin) and renal function studies (BUN and creatinine/creatinine clearance). The results of these tests were:

Serum iron - 70 μg/dL
Iron-binding capacity - 320 μg/dL
% Saturation - 21%
Serum ferritin - 240 μg/dL
BUN - 85 mg/dL
Serum creatinine - 4.5 mg/dL

The normal iron studies rule out an inflammatory process of any significant importance. The elevated BUN and serum creatinine suggest a loss of renal function, a common complication of poorly controlled type I diabetes. This would correlate with a fall in erythropoietin stimulation of the marrow, a recognized mechanism responsible for the "anemia of renal disease" (see Chapter 4).

of polychromatic macrocytes (marrow reticulocytes) on the peripheral blood smear. Other changes in morphology may provide a specific clue as to the cause of a hemolytic anemia. A full discussion of both diagnosis and management of blood loss anemia is provided in Chapter 10. The approach to diagnosis and management of the various hemolytic anemias is discussed in Chapters 7 and 11.

MANAGEMENT GUIDELINES

The management of any anemia must be based on the diagnosis. Therefore, the sooner the workup is complete and the diagnosis confirmed, the better. Shotgun therapy, where several therapeutic agents are given simultaneously, can make accurate diagnosis nearly impossible and can lead to inappropriate maintenance therapy with one or more hematinics. Thus, the clinician should withhold therapy at least until all of the necessary laboratory tests have been obtained.

Therapy should not be delayed, however, if the patient is physiologically unstable. Severe anemia in the elderly patient can lead to confusion, obtundation, heart failure, and organ ischemia. This condition needs to be treated immediately with transfusion of packed red blood cells to stabilize the patient while the anemia workup proceeds. As long as the volume of blood transfused is limited, it will not interfere with the diagnostic workup. However, massive transfusion will obscure the results of key laboratory tests, including the CBC, reticulocyte count, serum iron studies, and marrow morphology.

A wide range of therapies is available for treating various anemias, ranging from red blood cell transfusion and vitamin replacement therapy to bone marrow transplantation. With the availability of recombinant erythropoietin, the anemias associated with renal damage and chronic disease can be effectively treated. The details of specific treatments are covered in the individual chapters on these topics.

POINTS TO REMEMBER

The routine CBC (complete blood count) is the most sensitive measure of the presence and severity of an anemia.

The worst thing a clinician can do is merely assume the patient's anemia is the result of another illness. Skill in ordering and interpreting a basic set of laboratory tests/results (CBC, reticulocyte count, blood smear morphology changes, iron balance studies, bone marrow morphology reports) is essential for anemia evaluation.

These tests should always be performed as a battery to avoid confusion due to rapid changes over time.

The severity of the hematocrit/hemoglobin depression and changes in red blood cell volume (MCV), the distribution width (RDW), and blood smear morphology are the first results to consider. These help define the anemia as either normocytic, microcytic, or macrocytic.

The reticulocyte index (ie, corrected reticulocyte count) and the presence or absence of polychromasia (marrow "shift" reticulocytes) serve to define the adequacy of the erythropoietin and red cell production response.

Examination of the bone marrow can also provide information as to the proliferative response (cellularity and E/G ratio) and the presence of a visible defect in precursor maturation.

Based on these studies, anemias can be broadly classified physiologically as either hypoproliferative, a maturation disorder, or a hemorrhagic/hemolytic anemia.

Each of these "functional" categories has a well-defined set of underlying etiologies that can be elucidated using additional laboratory tests, especially the measurements of the serum iron, iron-binding capacity of transferrin (TIBC), and serum ferritin. For this reason, iron studies should always be included in the initial anemia workup "battery."

BIBLIOGRAPHY

Bain BJ: Diagnosis from the blood smear. N Eng J Med 2005;353:498.

Beutler E, Waalen J: The definition of anemia: what is the lower limit of normal of the blood haemoglobin concentration? Blood 2006;107:1747.

Beutler E, West C: Hematologic differences between African-Americans and whites: roles of iron deficiency and α-thalassemia on haemoglobin levels and mean corpuscular volume. Blood 2005;106:740.

Buttarello M, Plebani M: Automated blood cell counts. Am J Clin Pathol 2008;130:104.

Fauci AS et al: Harrison's Principles of Internal Medicine, 17th ed. McGraw-Hill, 2008.

Hillman RS, Finch CA: Red Cell Manual, 7th ed. FA Davis, 1997.

McPherson RA, Pincus MR: Henry's Clinical Diagnosis and Management by Laboratory Methods, 21st ed. Saunders Elsevier, 2007.

MARROW-DAMAGE ANEMIA · 3

CASE HISTORY • *Part 1*

A 27-year-old auto mechanic presents with a 1-month history of increasing fatigue, shortness of breath with strenuous exertion, easy bruising, and gum bleeding. His past history is negative, except for hepatitis A as a teenager. His occupation does involve the use of cleaning solvents on auto parts. Examination reveals a well-muscled male with pale conjunctiva, petechiae limited to the ankle areas, and hand and forearm bruises. No lymphadenopathy or hepatosplenomegaly.

CBC: Hematocrit/hemoglobin - 20%/6 g/dL
MCV - 91 fL MCH - 32 pg MCHC - 33 g/dL
RDW-CV - 13%

• SMEAR MORPHOLOGY

Normochromic/normocytic red cells with ± anisocytosis and the rare polychromatic macrocyte. Platelets and neutrophils markedly decreased without blast cells. Lymphocytes appear normal.

Reticulocyte count/index - <1%/<0.5
White blood cell count - 1,600/μL
Absolute differential: Neutrophils - <200/μL
Lymphocytes - 1,200/μL
Monocytes - 320/μL
Platelet count - 9,000/μL

Questions

- How should the anemia be classified?
- What tests should be ordered?

Disruption of the erythroid precursor pool or the structure of the marrow can produce a marrow-damage anemia. The severity of the anemia depends on the nature of the disorder. **Relatively mild marrow-damage anemias** are seen in association with drug toxicity and tumor infiltration. **More severe anemias** are typically seen in patients with acute leukemia and aplastic anemia.

The **prevalence** of marrow-damage anemias in any population is a function of the incidence of various disease states and environmental challenges. Impairment of red blood cell production is anticipated in most patients receiving tumor chemotherapy. In contrast, aplastic anemia characterized by a marked reduction in all hematopoietic precursors is a relatively rare event. Higher rates of aplastic anemia in the developing world are usually a result of the level of exposure to toxic drugs and chemicals in the workplace and environment.

MARROW STRUCTURE

Anatomical Distribution

The capacity of the erythroid marrow to compensate for anemia or hypoxia requires a normal pool of committed stem cells and a nurturing environment. The anatomical distribution of the marrow is illustrated in Figure 3–1. In normal adults, marrow is concentrated in the axial skeleton and proximal portions of the long bones. It can, however, extend out into more peripheral sites in

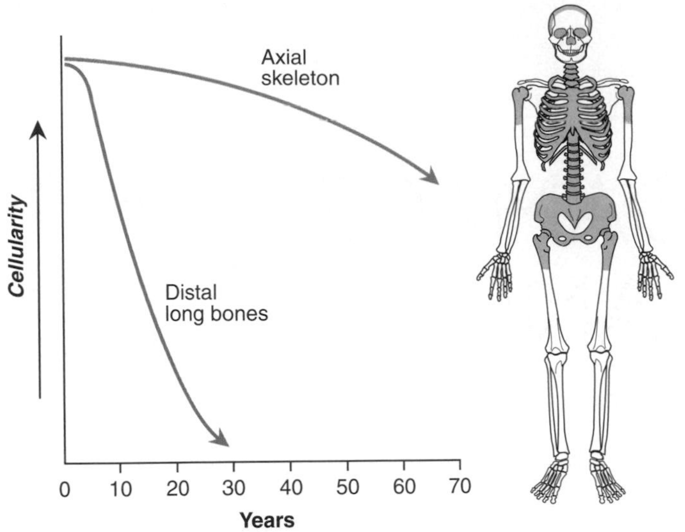

FIGURE 3–1. **Anatomical distribution of the marrow in the adult.** At birth, the marrow is widely distributed throughout the skeleton. During childhood and early adult life, marrow in the more distal portions of the long bones is replaced by fat. Active marrow is limited to the axial skeleton and proximal ends of the long bones, as indicated by the shading of the skeleton.

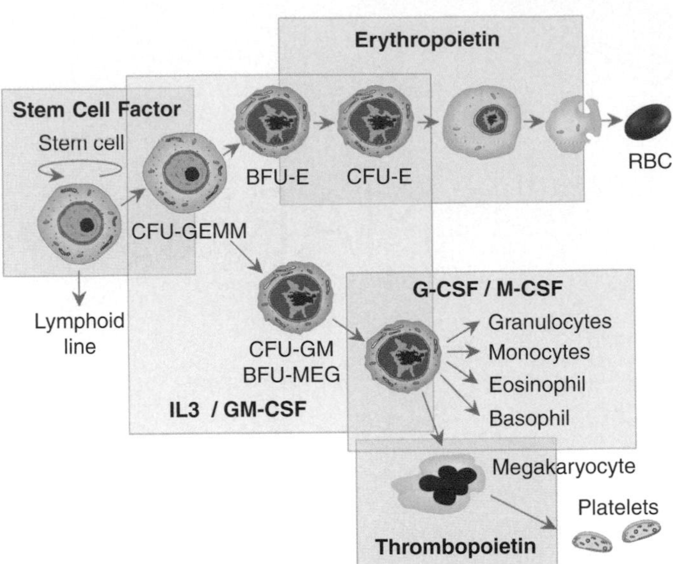

FIGURE 3–2. **Marrow cell differentiation and proliferation.** A pool of replicating pluripotent stem cells differentiates into the several cell lineages required for erythropoiesis, myelopoiesis, and platelet formation. The most primitive cell in the red blood cell lineage is the blast-forming unit–erythroid (BFU-E). Under the influence of erythropoietin, the BFU-E differentiates to the colony-forming unit–erythroid (CFU-E) and the more mature normoblast series. This process involves both the series of cell divisions and the progressive formation of hemoglobin in the cytoplasm. Growth factors such as IL-3, GM-CSF, G-CSF, and M-CSF are important first steps in cell differentiation and the proliferation and maturation of myelopoietic cell lines. Thrombopoietin governs the proliferation and maturation of the megakaryocyte cell line.

response to long-standing anemia or as a result of myeloproliferative disease. Patients with thalassemia major can show extension of marrow even into the small bones of the hand.

Red Blood Cell Growth

On a microscopic level, erythroid progenitors grow in clusters within a matrix of stromal cells, reticular fibers, and a network of vascular sinusoids. Long-term hematopoietic stem cells (LT-HSC) are found in close approximation to osteoblasts lining the marrow cavity. More mature progenitors tend to cluster around marrow macrophages, suggesting a nurse cell role for these structural cells. There is evidence for direct reticuloendothelial cell transfer of iron to red blood cell precursors to support hemoglobin synthesis. Other structural cells play an equally important role in providing growth factors (interleukin-3 [IL-3], granulocyte macrophage colony-stimulating factor [GM-CSF], and stem cell growth factor [SCF]), which are essential to the first steps in cell differentiation and proliferation (Figure 3–2). T cells also influence early stem cell growth. Erythropoietin has its principal effect on committed red blood cell precursors such as the burst-forming unit–erythroid (BFU-E) and colony-forming unit–erythroid (CFU-E).

Aging Process

Humans are born with a self-replicating stem cell pool that supports all hematopoietic cell lines throughout the natural lifespan. There is no evidence for a stem cell–based failure of red blood cell production as a part of the aging process (see Chapter 12). The ratio of hematopoietic tissue to fat cells in younger patients favors hematopoietic tissue, whereas older patients show a relative decrease in marrow cellularity because of an increased number of fat cells. This is not a sign of marrow damage or a failed capacity to respond to anemia or hypoxia. With a sustained stimulus, marrow cellularity, at any age, can increase to the point of displacing all visible adipose tissue.

Damaging Factors

Both the stem cell pool and marrow structure can be damaged by external factors. Ionizing radiation can result in a loss of HSC and irreversible damage to the blood supply and suspensary structures of the marrow. Several chemicals and drugs will also cause irreversible loss of replicating HSC, such that the extent of recovery is dependent on the number of LT-HSC remaining. Finally, the nurturing environment of the marrow can be impaired by overexpansion of a single line of hematopoietic cells, as with leukemia, or invasion by metastatic tumor. These cells compete for both the space and nutrients required for normal red blood cell growth. Immune-mediated aplasia is a common cause of severe aplastic anemia. Some 30%–80% of patients presenting with severe aplastic anemia without an obvious external factor respond to immunosuppressive therapy.

CLINICAL FEATURES

Many of the marrow-damage anemias can be anticipated from the clinical presentation. **Patients undergoing high-dose multidrug chemotherapy** are expected to develop a temporary marrow-damage anemia. The more strenuous the treatment protocol, the more severe the anemia and the more likely there will be an associated leukopenia and thrombocytopenia. If one anticipates both the course and severity of this type of marrow-damage anemia, a workup is usually unnecessary and management, whether red blood cell transfusion or treatment with erythropoietin and/or other growth factors, is easily planned.

In a similar fashion, **marrow-damage anemias associated with hematopoietic malignancies, myelodysplasia, myeloproliferative disease, or widespread invasion of the marrow by tumor** are usually obvious from the patient's clinical picture and the presence of marked abnormalities in other hematopoietic cell lines. The onset is most often very gradual but can be as rapid as that seen with acute leukemia. However, even though the anemia may be severe, it usually is overshadowed by defects in the myelocyte and megakaryocyte cell lines. Patients with marked pancytopenia usually present with varying combinations of severe bleeding, acute infection, and symptomatic anemia.

The most characteristic clinical features of a patient with a so-called **idiopathic "aplastic anemia"** are the suddenness of onset and the apparent absence of other illness or other predisposing factors. Once again, the associated pancytopenia can produce a mixed picture of bleeding, infection, and anemia. However, many patients have variable depressions in their white blood cell and platelet counts, so the presenting symptoms of anemia may predominate. There is even the rare patient who presents with solitary red blood cell aplasia.

Laboratory Studies

The **complete blood count (CBC), reticulocyte count, serum iron studies, and a well-performed marrow aspirate and biopsy** should make it possible to quickly diagnose a marrow-damage anemia. Typical erythropoietic profiles of moderate and severe marrow damage are illustrated in Table 3–1. The CBC and reticulocyte count are characteristic of a hypoproliferative anemia. Red blood cell morphology is normocytic and normochromic, and the reticulocyte index is inappropriately low for the severity of the patient's anemia. A careful inspection of the blood smear may reveal important clues to the presence of marrow structural damage, including the appearance of nucleated red blood cells and abnormal white blood cell precursors.

TABLE 3–1 • Marrow-damage anemia erythropoietic profile

	Moderate	Severe
Red blood cell morphology	Normocytic/normochromic	
Polychromasia	Present	Rare/absent
Nucleated red blood cells	Present with structural damage	
Reticulocyte index	<2	<1
Marrow E/G ratio[a]	<1:3	<1:3
Marrow morphology	Can be diagnostic of disease process	
Serum iron	Normal or slightly increased	Increased
TIBC	Normal	Normal
Percent saturation	30–50	50–100

[a]*May be impossible to assess due to severe aplasia.*

A. Iron Studies

Iron studies, including the serum iron, total iron-binding capacity (TIBC), and serum ferritin level, provide an indirect measure of erythroid marrow cellularity. With severe damage and a marked reduction in red blood cell precursors, iron destined for hemoglobin synthesis accumulates in the plasma and iron storage sites. This situation results in an increase in the serum iron level even to the point of full saturation of the TIBC. The serum ferritin level also increases, reflecting a rise in reticuloendothelial cell iron stores. Although the serum ferritin level may only be modestly elevated when the patient first presents, it increases to very high levels (>1,000 μg/L) when the patient is repeatedly transfused.

B. Marrow Aspirate and Biopsy

A well-performed marrow aspirate and biopsy is essential for diagnosis. In patients with severe aplastic anemia, advanced myelofibrosis, or marked infiltration of the marrow with tumor, the aspirate can be difficult or impossible to obtain (a "dry tap"). In this circumstance, a **marrow core biopsy** should be performed using a standard marrow biopsy needle. The core sample is used to make touch preparations for cell morphology and, after fixation and sectioning, for study of overall structure and cellularity. In addition to the standard **hematoxylin and eosin** and **periodic acid–Schiff stains** for cell characteristics, special stains such as a **trichrome stain** for collagen tissue and a **silver stain** for reticulin fibers are used to identify marrow structural abnormalities. Patients with myelofibrosis or tumor metastases to marrow can show increasing amounts of collagen and reticulin fibers, even to the point of obliterating the space available for hematopoietic cells (Figure 3–3).

A **Prussian blue stain** of marrow aspirate and biopsy material is also important. In addition to permitting evaluation of the level of iron stores, it also allows the detection of red blood cell precursors with abnormal amounts of intracellular iron (see Chapter 9). A marrow-damage anemia pattern is seen in some patients with sideroblastic anemias. Likewise, occasional ringed sideroblasts are seen in patients with secondary marrow-damage anemias. The amount of iron stored in reticuloendothelial cells is dramatically increased in patients with severe marrow-damage anemias who have received many transfusions.

Although marrow biopsy provides an excellent measure of the structure and cellularity of a small area of marrow, it does not provide a sense of total marrow mass and distribution.

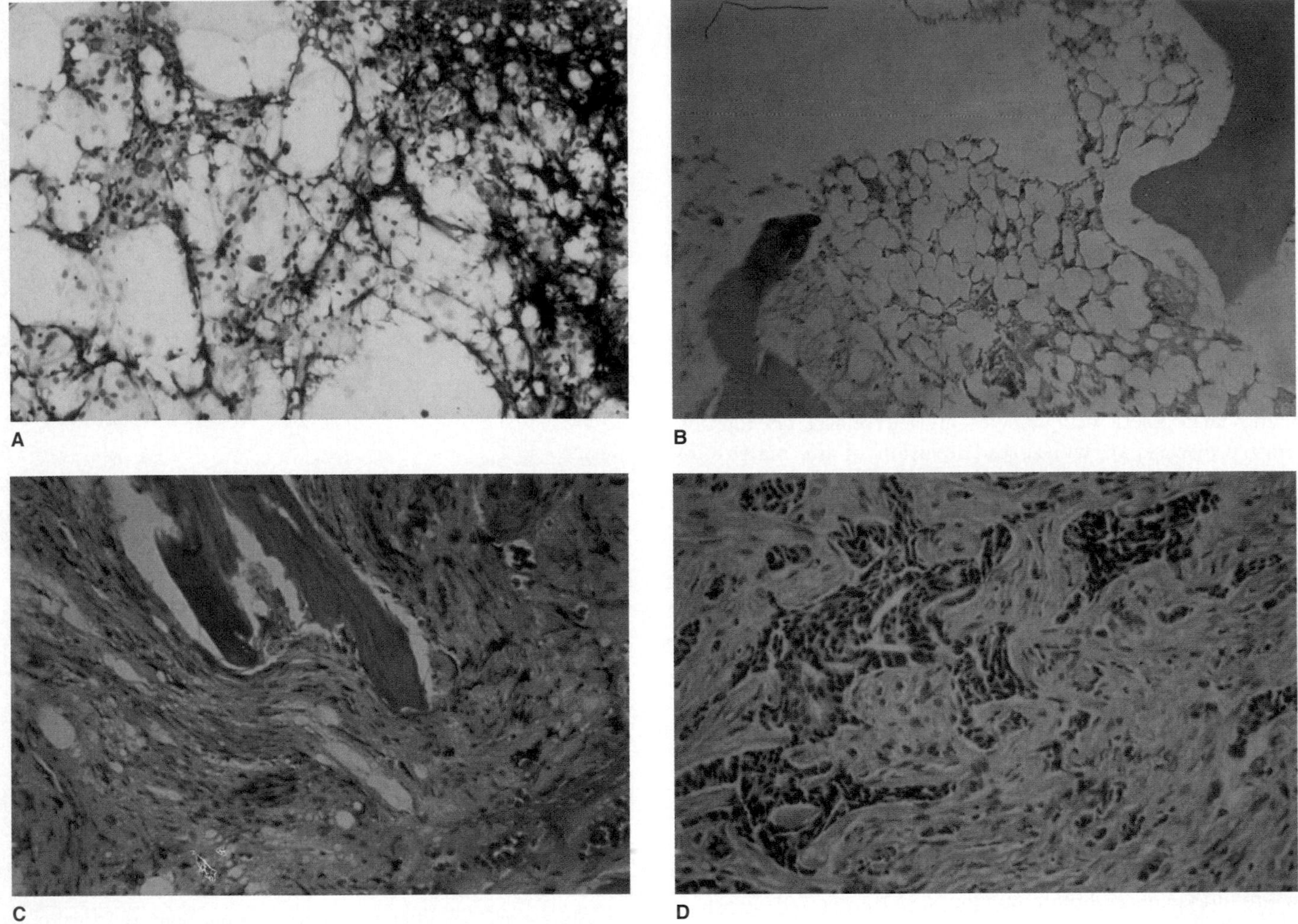

FIGURE 3–3. **Marrow-damage specimens.** A well-performed marrow aspirate and biopsy will often reveal the cause of a severe pancytopenia. **A:** Marrow aspirate specimen showing empty stroma in a patient with severe aplastic anemia. **B:** Biopsy specimen showing widespread marrow loss. **C:** Dense collagenous fibrosis of the marrow space. **D:** Solid tumor infiltration with fibrosis.

Radiologic techniques can be used to measure marrow distribution. The **technetium sulfa colloid scan** measures the integrity of the vascular and structural elements of the marrow. In patients with severe fibrosis or widespread invasion of marrow by tumor, the technetium scan will be abnormal, showing either total loss of uptake or a patchy distribution. The presence and distribution of red blood cell precursors can also be imaged using ^{111}In. Indium, like iron, is avidly absorbed by red blood cell precursors.

Magnetic resonance imaging (MRI) of the vertebral spine provides qualitative information as to the cellularity of the marrow by discriminating between marrows that are largely replaced by fat cells and those where hematopoietic or tumor tissue is present. In patients with an aplastic or hypoplastic anemia, the characteristic fatty appearance may not be observed when there are excessive marrow iron deposits **(hemosiderosis)** secondary to iron loading. MRI is the preferred imaging technique in the evaluation of patients with myeloma, lymphoma, or tumor metastases—diseases where marrow involvement is focal and patchy. It also allows a better assessment of complications of marrow disease, such as compression/pathological fractures, epidural disease with cord compression, and soft-tissue/node extension. Finally, serial MRI studies are much more useful in monitoring responses to therapy and/or disease progression.

C. Miscellaneous Studies

Other studies for evaluating patients with marrow-damage anemia include **cytogenetic and phenotypic studies** of cells in circulation and in the marrow. Both techniques are helpful in detecting a malignant cell line and providing supporting evidence for diagnoses such as myelodysplasia, myelofibrosis, and leukemic states. Conversion from a normal to an abnormal karyotype is seen in 15%–20% of patients during the first 5 years after diagnosis of a marrow-damage anemia. Chromosome 7 abnormalities are the most common (approximately 40% of cases) and carry the worst prognosis. Other findings include trisomy of chromosome 8 or 6, deletion of Y, abnormalities of chromosome 13, and complex abnormalities. Unlike the

CASE HISTORY • Part 2

This patient has a marked pancytopenia with normocytic, normochromic red cell morphology, and a reticulocyte production index far below basal levels. His neutrophil and platelet counts are also severely depressed. Given the rapidity of onset and the severity of the pancytopenia, the most likely diagnosis is "severe aplastic anemia".

An immediate **marrow aspirate and biopsy**, to evaluate overall cellularity and to look for abnormalities in progenitor morphology, will usually confirm the diagnosis and provide another measure of severity. Aplastic marrows with less than 20% cellularity indicate a poor prognosis. Infiltration by tumor, fibrosis, or hematological malignancy should be readily evident.

Iron studies provide another measure of the severity of damage to red cell progenitors. With severe aplasia, the serum iron will rise to the point of full saturation of transferrin (TIBC), while patients with less severe damage will have relatively normal percent saturations.

In this case, the marrow biopsy revealed an overall cellularity of less than 10% of normal without evidence of tumor, fibrosis, or a leukemic infiltrate. Serum iron - 280 mg/dL, TIBC - 300 mg/dL for a saturation of 93%.

Questions

- What etiologies and additional testing need to be considered in the differential diagnosis?
- How should this patient be managed?

myelodysplastic anemias (see Chapter 9), abnormalities of chromosomes 5 and 20 are much less common.

A change in the red cell surface glycosylphosphatidylinositol (GPI) anchor protein (appearance of GPI$^-$ cells) may also be seen and can predict response to immunosuppressive therapy. Minor clones of GPI$^-$ red blood cells (CD59/CD55 negative cells) can be detected by flow cytometric analysis. A measurement of red cell levels of hemoglobin F has been used in screening for Fanconi anemia patients; F levels are usually increased.

DIAGNOSIS

The approach to diagnosis of any marrow-damage anemia depends on the clinical setting. As summarized in Table 3–2, marrow-damage anemias predictably result from diseases that have a destructive impact on the marrow, or as a side effect of chemotherapy or radiotherapy. When the primary disease diagnosis is obvious, the workup of the anemia can be truncated. CBC, reticulocyte count, iron studies, and marrow examination are usually all that is required, and even this workup is unnecessary when patients are undergoing high-dose chemotherapy.

In contrast, the diagnostic workup needs to be pursued aggressively when a patient presents with a **sudden onset of severe anemia or pancytopenia** without clear evidence of other disease. While the basic diagnosis of marrow damage may be obvious, successful management of a patient with an **idiopathic aplastic anemia** depends on rapid and accurate diagnosis of the underlying cause. In some patients, clues to the cause may be provided by the CBC and marrow studies, especially the marrow biopsy, while in others, more elaborate studies of marrow precursor cytogenetics and growth characteristics may be necessary. In many cases, the nature of the disorder may only become clear with the patient's response to therapy.

Drug and Radiation Damage Anemia

A. Drug Toxicity

Marrow-damage anemia is a predictable side effect of chemotherapy. When a single chemotherapeutic drug is given, the resulting

TABLE 3–2 • Causes of marrow-damage anemias

Stem cell/marrow structural damage
Chemo-/radiotherapy
Radiation
Gaucher disease
Myelofibrosis
Autoimmune disease
Rheumatologic disorders
Viral infections
Graft-versus-host disease
"Idiopathic" aplastic anemia
Pure red cell aplasia
Congenital disorders
Fanconi anemia
Diamond-Blackfan anemia
Shwachman-Diamond syndrome
Dyskeratosis congenita

TABLE 3–3 • Classes of drugs associated with marrow damage

Antibiotics (**chloramphenicol**, penicillin, cephalosporins, sulfonamides, amphotericin B, flucytosine, dapsone, streptomycin)
Antidepressants (**lithium**, **tricyclics**)
Antiepileptics (**dilantin, carbamazepine, felbamate**, phenacemide, primidone, ethosuximide, valproic acid)
Anti-inflammatory drugs (**phenylbutazone**, **gold salts**, nonsteroidals, salicylates, penicillamine)
Antiarrhythmics (lidocaine, quinidine, procainamide)
Antithyroid drugs (propylthiouracil)
Diuretics (**acetazolamide**, thiazides, pyrimethamine, furosemide)
Antihypertensives (captopril)
Antiuricemics (allopurinol, colchicine)
Antimalarials (**quinacrine**, chloroquine, pyrimethamine)
Hypoglycemics (tolbutamide, chlorpropamide)
Tranquilizers (prochlorperazine, meprobamate)
Platelet inhibitors (ticlopidine)

anemia is usually mild. However, patients with marrow damage secondary to malignancy can have a significant worsening of an already existing anemia, even to the point of becoming transfusion dependent. **High-dose, multidrug chemotherapy** results in severe pancytopenia that requires both red blood cell and platelet transfusion support. However, the drug effect falls short of irreversibly damaging the marrow stem cells, thereby allowing recovery once the drugs are discontinued. Moreover, growth factors can be used therapeutically to counteract the drug effect and speed recovery.

A number of drugs have been associated with the development of severe, often irreversible, **aplastic anemia**. Table 3–3 lists the more common classes of drugs associated with marrow damage. At the same time, the clinician must suspect any drug as a possible cause of marrow damage when a patient lacks other obvious reasons for having pancytopenia. Several drugs can be highlighted for their common association with **severe aplasia**, including chloramphenicol, phenylbutazone, propylthiouracil, and tricyclic antidepressants. Obviously, the frequency of the association of marrow damage with these drugs will reflect the relative frequency of their use. More important, the marrow damage that results is hard to predict, and can be both severe and irreversible. This situation is especially true with chloramphenicol because irreversible aplastic anemia can appear without warning after only a few doses of the drug. Therefore, even though the actual incidence of fatal aplastic anemia in patients treated with chloramphenicol is less than 1 in 20,000, routine use of the drug is strongly discouraged. The pancytopenia experienced with phenylbutazone, propylthiouracil, and the tricyclic antidepressants has a more gradual onset and is reversible if the drug is immediately withdrawn.

The development of **pancytopenia** secondary to any of the drugs listed in Table 3–3 is best detected with a routine CBC and not the symptoms or signs of anemia, leukopenia, or thrombocytopenia. This is important both diagnostically and therapeutically. Periodic measurements of blood counts during hospitalization or as a part of long-term drug therapy are necessary. Moreover, careful attention needs to be paid to the results in order to detect any early trends to anemia, leukopenia, and/or thrombocytopenia. As a rule, drug-induced cytopenias will rapidly reverse if the inciting drug or drugs are quickly removed at the first sign of marrow damage.

B. Radiation

High-energy radiation can also produce a **marrow-damage anemia and pancytopenia**. The effect can be predicted according to the type of radiation, the dose, and the extent of marrow exposure. High-energy radiation can be used therapeutically at high doses without the appearance of marrow damage as long as the treatment fields spare major marrow sites. In patients who receive **whole body irradiation**, the effect on the marrow is dose dependent. At doses less than 1 Sv (equivalent to 1 Gy or 100 rad for x- and γ-rays), there will be little effect on the marrow. A reversible fall in the blood counts is seen between 1 and 2.5 Sv (100 and 250 rad). Irreversible loss of stem cells is seen at higher doses. With doses of 5–10 Sv, patients will die of marrow failure if they do not receive a bone marrow transplant. Long-term exposure to low levels of external radiation or ingested radioisotopes can also produce **aplastic anemia**, although the dose relationship is much less predictable.

C. Other Chemicals

Several chemicals have also been implicated in causing severe aplastic anemia. **Benzene and chemicals containing benzene derivatives** have been associated both with aplastic anemia and acute myelocytic leukemia. These findings have led to very strict federal regulations limiting occupational exposure to organic solvents containing benzene derivatives. Many other chemicals, insecticides, and heavy metals have also been associated with marrow-damage anemia and pancytopenia. It is essential, therefore, to question a patient with marrow-damage anemia at length regarding occupational chemical exposure.

Marrow-Damage Anemia Related to Infection

Marrow-damage anemia can result from direct invasion of the marrow structure by an infectious agent or immunosuppression of stem cell growth. **Miliary tuberculosis** is perhaps the best example of the first mechanism. Extensive involvement of the marrow as evidenced by widespread granuloma formation and marrow fibrosis can produce a marrow-damage anemia and in some cases pancytopenia. Early on, the clinician's index of suspicion must be high to successfully make this diagnosis. The patient can present with little evidence of widespread tuberculosis, and on hematologic evaluation may appear to have idiopathic myelofibrosis or a myelodysplastic syndrome. Therefore, a careful search for granulomas in the marrow biopsy specimen, using an acid-fast stain to help identify the organism, is essential.

Aplastic anemia is also seen following viral illnesses such as viral hepatitis, Epstein-Barr virus infection, HIV, and rubella. Parvovirus B19 infection can cause an acute, reversible pure red blood cell aplasia in patients with congenital hemolytic anemias (sickle cell anemia, hereditary spherocytosis, etc). In immunocompromised patients who fail to produce neutralizing antibody to parvovirus, a chronic form of red cell aplasia can develop. The most dramatic relationship of viral infection to severe pancytopenia is the fatal aplastic anemia seen during recovery from viral hepatitis. Generally, this occurs in young males who have had an uncomplicated episode of hepatitis, and is most common in poorer socioeconomic populations in Asian countries. Although this anemia was originally associated with non-A and non-B hepatitis, recent studies would appear to exclude hepatitis C as the putative agent. Thus, the responsible agent and the nature of the subsequent immune process that results in marrow stem cell suppression are still unknown.

Malignancy and Marrow Damage

Marrow-damage anemias can result from an infiltration of the marrow by nonhematopoietic tumors or a malignant transformation of marrow stem cells. **Metastatic malignancies** such as prostate and breast carcinoma generally produce a relatively mild anemia without changes in other cell lines. The mechanism involved is a progressive interference with the support structure of the marrow. The tumor occupies the space needed for marrow precursors, stimulates collagen growth, and cuts off normal blood supply. The resultant disorganization is frequently detectable simply by inspecting the blood smear. The appearance of nucleated red blood cells in the circulation in a patient with a mild, normocytic, normochromic anemia can be a tip-off to the presence of metastatic tumor within the marrow (Figure 3–4).

Malignant transformations of hematopoietic stem cells produce severe marrow-damage anemias. This process involves a loss of stem cells committed to differentiation along the erythroid line. The same is true for the other cell lines, which makes the diagnosis relatively easy. Patients presenting with leukemia have characteristic changes both in the number of cells in circulation and in cellular morphology. The examination of the marrow also reveals the nature of the malignant cell line. Although the diagnosis of an acute leukemia is relatively easy, patients with myelodysplasia, myelofibrosis, paroxysmal nocturnal hemoglobinuria, or a sideroblastic anemia can be more of a diagnostic challenge (see Chapter 9).

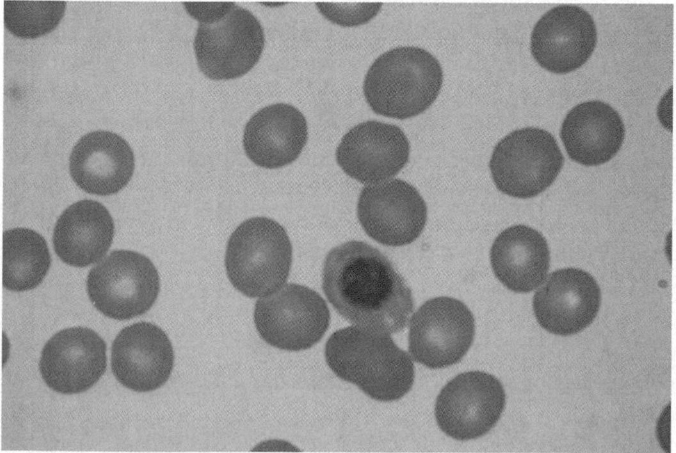

FIGURE 3–4. **Nucleated red blood cells in circulation.** The presence of nucleated red blood cells in circulation suggests either severe damage to the structure of the marrow as seen with tumor infiltration or splenic dysfunction (hyposplenism, extramedullary hematopoiesis, or tumor infiltration).

Aplastic Anemia of Unknown Etiology ("Idiopathic")

An otherwise healthy patient who presents with the sudden onset of pancytopenia and a markedly hypoplastic or aplastic ("empty") marrow, most likely has an idiopathic or acquired aplastic anemia. In some instances, the bone marrow shows a persistence of a small population of early precursors, raising the question of damage from a drug or chemical agent. Therefore, all drugs should be discontinued immediately, and any further contact with a toxic chemical avoided. If a drug or chemical is involved and the injury is reversible, the marrow will repopulate and blood counts will improve. However, the presence of a few precursor cells in the marrow aspirate or biopsy does not guarantee recovery. It is much more likely that the aplasia is permanent. This is almost always true when the pancytopenia is severe, leukocyte counts are less than 200/μL, and the marrow cellularity is below 20% of normal.

The most likely cause of a sudden severe aplastic anemia (pancytopenia) is an autoimmune process. This is especially true if the patient has had an episode of seronegative hepatitis, a recent pregnancy, eosinophilic fasciitis, or a T-cell non-Hodgkin lymphoma, but an autoimmune etiology should be considered even without a history of preceding illness. Typically, these patients are found to have a polyclonal expansion of CD8+CD28– T cells, expressing the Th1 cytokines—γ-interferon and tumor necrosis factor-α, which induce apoptosis in LT-HSC. The fact that the T-cell response is polyclonal would further suggest a viral antigen or chromosomal abnormality as the initiating factor leading to a change in the LT-HSC. Yet, despite a major research effort, it is unclear as to exactly what factors can initiate the autoimmune process. From a research viewpoint, T-cell depletion of cultured marrow will demonstrate an increase in the BFU-E and CFU-E colonies in many of these patients. Of course, this will depend on the presence of a few viable HSC. From a clinical viewpoint, the patient's response to immunosuppressive therapy provides the best indicator of autoimmune disease.

Aplastic anemia may also present as or evolve to resemble other hematologic disorders, especially paroxysmal hemoglobinuria (PNH) and myelodysplasia (MDS). Up to 50% of patients present with detectable clones of GPI^- cells (somatic *PIG-A* mutations leading to an absence of GPI membrane proteins) in circulation. One explanation for this is that these GPI^- cells (CD55/CD59 negative red cells and leukocytes or CD16/CD66b negative leukocytes) are normally present in small numbers and somehow escape the immune destruction. This finding has been used as a predictor of responsiveness to immunosuppressive therapy.

As for the association with MDS, chromosomal abnormalities, monosomy 7 and trisomy 8, can appear in aplastic anemia patients over time. Moreover, MDS patients with trisomy 8 can show immune abnormalities similar to aplastic anemia (oligoclonal expansion of cytotoxic T cells) and will respond to immunosuppressive therapy. Monosomy 7, the more frequent cytogenetic abnormality, has been associated with refractoriness to therapy and a poor outcome. Overall, severe aplastic anemia patients run a significant risk of developing a clonal malignancy within 10 years of the diagnosis. This is true regardless of the mode of therapy, whether bone marrow transplantation or immunosuppression.

Any patient with **severe "idiopathic" aplastic anemia** needs to be quickly and fully evaluated as a guide to management. When there is no obvious reversible cause for the marrow damage, early bone marrow transplantation or immunosuppressive therapy should be considered. The patient's age and availability of a histocompatible sibling will determine the choice of therapy. Younger patients with a matched donor should receive transplants without delay since the risk of graft-versus-host disease (GVHD) is low and the opportunity for a sustained recovery is high. Older patients and patients who have received multiple blood transfusions are better managed with immunosuppressive therapy.

Fanconi Anemia

Fanconi anemia (FA) is an autosomal recessive disorder that presents as severe pancytopenia during the first 2 decades of life, although more than a third of FA patients present with cancer at an early age and anemia as a secondary finding. In Western societies, the frequency of the heterozygous state is about 1 in 200 persons, though it may be as high as 1 in 80 in white South Africans. When fully expressed (1 per 100,000 live births), the disorder is characterized by progressive marrow failure, multiple physical defects (short stature, microcephaly, microopthalmia, hypoplastic radii, abnormal thumbs, and abnormal pigmentation, including café au lait spots), chromosomal abnormalities (particularly partial trisomies or tetrasomies of 3q), and a pronounced predisposition to cancer. However, patients can present without the typical physical defects, such that the diagnosis should be considered in a child or young adult presenting with AML or a solid tumor. The risk of developing marrow failure, hematologic cancers, and nonhematologic cancers, as reported by the International Fanconi Anemia Registry, increases dramatically with age, reaching 90%, 33%, and 28%, respectively, by age 40–50. In patients who are successfully transplanted, the probability of developing a solid tumor is not affected—if anything, it continues to steadily increase with age.

The **diagnosis** of FA can be confirmed by testing for DNA hypersensitivity to crosslinking agents. The traditional test uses mitomycin C or diepoxybutane as provocative agents in lymphocyte culture to bring out chromosomal abnormalities. FA patients demonstrate an increased number of cells with chromosomal breaks and an increase in breaks per cell. Definitive proof of FA requires the isolation of a characteristic FA gene mutation. Thirteen FA genes have now been cloned. Of these, *FANCA*, *FANCC*, *FANCE*, and *FANCG* are the most common, while *FANCC*, *FANCD1* and *2*, and *FANCN* mutations are associated with especially severe disease.

Dyskeratosis Congenita

Aplastic anemia is seen in at least 50% of patients with dyskeratosis congenita (DC), an inherited X-linked, autosomal dominant or recessive disorder characterized by lacy-reticulated skin pigmentation, leukoplakia, and dysplastic nails. The mucocutaneous abnormalities generally appear well before puberty, whereas the aplastic anemia occurs late in the second or third decades. Since the clinical presentation can be quite variable, even within the same family, DC should be considered in the differential diagnosis of adult aplastic anemia. Four putative genes, the X-linked genes *DKC1*, *TERT*, and *TERC*, and the autosomal recessive gene *NOP10*, have been identified in up to 40% of DC patients. These genes are involved in telomere maintenance, and abnormal telomere shortening may be the root cause of the marrow failure. However, much more needs to be learned about the 60% of DC patients who lack one of these gene mutations.

Pure Red Blood Cell Aplasia

Isolated aplasia of erythroid progenitors (producing anemia without leukopenia or thrombocytopenia) can present as a self-limited "aplastic crisis" or as severe irreversible marrow-damage anemia. As with pancytopenia, pure red blood cell aplasia can result from exposure to a number of drugs and infections. Short periods of pure red blood cell aplasia have been reported in patients with mycoplasma and parvovirus (HPV B19) infections, mumps, and viral hepatitis. Patients with congenital hemolytic anemias, especially hereditary spherocytosis and sickle cell anemia, are especially sensitive to parvovirus infection. Patients with immunosuppression, especially those infected with HIV-1, may be unable to resolve an HPV B19 infection, resulting in severe, persistent red cell aplasia. In all of these situations, the patient presents with the sudden appearance of anemia without pancytopenia. Inspection of a marrow aspirate shows essentially normal cellularity and morphology except for the red cell progenitor component. Normal red cell precursors are virtually absent and may be replaced by giant pronormoblasts containing viral inclusions in the nucleus.

Prolonged red blood cell aplasia has been associated with several other diseases including lupus erythematosus, rheumatoid arthritis, chronic active hepatitis, parvovirus infection, lymphoid malignancies, myelodysplasia, and thymoma. It also occurs without apparent cause, although studies of BFU-E and CFU-E growth characteristics suggest that most patients with pure red cell aplasia have a T-cell or antibody-mediated inhibition of erythropoiesis. This has been reflected clinically in the success of immunosuppressive therapies. Pure red cell aplasia unresponsive to immunosuppressive therapy is most often the initial presentation of a dysplastic/sideroblastic anemia (see Chapter 9).

The **workup** for a patient with a pure red cell aplasia should include, in addition to a detailed history, physical examination, and routine CBC and blood chemistries, a bone marrow examination, cytogenetics, lymphocyte immunophenotyping or T-cell gene rearrangement studies (or both), and serum analysis for HPV B19 (both antibodies and polymerase chain reaction [PCR]). A search should be made for thymic enlargement, which may play an etiologic role in up to 15% of patients. Typically, the thymomas associated with pure red blood cell aplasia remain encapsulated and can be easily resected. Histologically, they are comprised of spindle cells with loss of germinal centers and infiltration by small polyclonal lymphocytes, with no evidence of lymphoma.

Diamond-Blackfan Anemia

Diamond and Blackfan described a congenital form of pure red blood cell aplasia that appears early in childhood. By 6 months of age, 80% of Diamond-Blackfan anemia (DBA) children are anemic; by 9 months, 90% are affected. Mildly affected familial cases may not be diagnosed until later in childhood. The typical erythropoietic profile shows a somewhat macrocytic, normochromic anemia; reticulocytopenia; and an absence of red blood cell progenitors in a marrow with normal white blood cells and platelet production. Serum levels of erythropoietin are increased. Many children have minor physical defects including growth retardation, strabismus, and bony abnormalities of fingers and ribs. Similar to FA, 50% of DBA patients will develop leukemia or a solid tumor by the end of the third decade.

Disruption of the **ribosomal protein genes**, *RPS19* and *RPSA24*, leading to a failure in ribosomal function, has been implicated in a quarter or more of cases of DBA. The impact of *RPS19* deficiency is greatest in the maturing erythroid precursors where the demand for ribosome biogenesis is especially high. This leads to increased apoptosis of erythroid precursors. Although the presence of a humoral or cellular inhibitor has not been detected, 70% or more of patients with DBA will respond clinically to relatively low doses of **prednisone**. Allogeneic bone marrow transplantation has also proved effective in patients with matched donors. **Transfusion** is the mainstay for all other DBA patients. Overall, life expectancy has improved significantly; patients now live cancer-free into their third or fourth decade.

Shwachman-Diamond Syndrome

Shwachman-Diamond syndrome (SDS) is an autosomal recessive disorder that usually presents in childhood with pancreatic insufficiency and malabsorption. Fifty percent of SDS patients also have bony abnormalities and/or learning disabilities. Neutropenia progressing to pancytopenia, aplastic anemia, myelodyplasia, and leukemia is seen in more than 70% of SDS patients during the second and third decades. Chromosomal abnormalities, particularly of chromosome 7, with progression to myelodysplasia are common. Virtually all SDS patients have mutations in a single gene, *SBDS*, which, similar to DBA, is involved in ribosome formation and function. However, the exact mechanism of action is still unclear, although abnormal telomere shortening may be involved.

DIFFERENTIAL DIAGNOSIS

Severe aplastic anemia is readily detected and easily distinguished from most other forms of hypoproliferative anemia. The one exception is **myelodysplasia** with a severely hypoplastic marrow (see Chapter 9). With this exception, the involvement of all cell lines in the marrow both confirms the diagnosis and often explains the reason for the marrow failure. Iron studies provide another indicator of severe marrow damage. Patients with **aplastic anemia** show an elevation in the serum iron level to full saturation of the TIBC (see Table 3–1). Similarly, the diagnosis of **pure red blood cell aplasia** is relatively straightforward. The striking reticulocytopenia, the virtual absence of red blood cell precursors in an otherwise normal marrow, and the increase in serum iron level are unique and are not mimicked by other forms of anemia.

Less severe marrow-damage anemia is not as easily distinguished from other hypoproliferative anemias such as early iron deficiency, the anemias of renal failure and hypothyroidism, and the anemia that develops as a part of an inflammatory disease process. As long as the patient's hemoglobin level is greater than 11 g/dL, changes in red blood cell and marrow morphology may not be diagnostic. The only distinguishing feature is the pattern of iron studies (Table 3–4). Patients with **iron deficiency** or **an inflammatory anemia** can usually be identified on the basis of changes in serum iron, TIBC, and serum ferritin levels.

The differential diagnosis of a **hypoproliferative anemia characterized by normal iron studies** is more difficult. Studies of renal function and thyroid function should be performed. In addition, careful examination of the peripheral blood smear and both the marrow aspirate and biopsy specimen are recommended. The appearance in circulation of even a few nucleated red blood cells in a patient with a hypoproliferative anemia can

TABLE 3–4 • Iron studies in hypoproliferative anemias

	Iron Deficiency	Inflammation	Renal/Endocrine Disease	Marrow Damage	
				Mild	Severe
Serum iron (μg/dL)	<30	<40	Normal	50–150	>150
TIBC (μg/dL)	>350	<300	Normal	Normal	Normal
Percent saturation (%)	<10	10–20	Normal	30–60	>60
Ferritin (μg/L)	<12	30–300	Normal	30–600	>1,000
Marrow iron stores	Absent	Increased	Normal	Increased	Increased

TABLE 3–5 • Marrow-damage anemias associated with abnormal marrows

Disease State	Marrow Morphology
Myelofibrosis	Increased collagen and reticulin fibers
Lymphoid malignancies (CLL, lymphomas, Hodgkin disease)	Increased numbers of lymphocytes, paratrabecular lymphoid nodules, granulomas, Reed-Sternberg cells
Metastatic malignancies (breast, prostate, lung, etc)	Clusters of tumor cells, fibrosis
Myeloma	Increased plasma cells (>20% of cells)
Drug/radiation damage	Decreased hematopoietic cells, relative increase in plasma cells, mast cells, and structural cells
Marrow infections (tuberculosis, sarcoidosis, etc)	Granulomas, fibrosis, increased plasma cells

be an early clue to involvement of the marrow with a malignancy. A close examination of the marrow specimens may also reveal the cause of an early marrow-damage anemia. Table 3–5 lists several disease states that are associated with marrow-damage anemia and that can be detected by inspecting the marrow.

THERAPY

The management of a marrow-damage anemia will vary considerably according to the cause of the anemia or pancytopenia, the severity of the damage, and both the patient's age and transfusion history. The importance of the cause as a predictor of final outcome is obvious. In the patient with a hematologic malignancy, return to normal marrow function will depend on responsiveness of the tumor to chemotherapy. The same is true with marrow-damage anemias secondary to a metastatic malignancy. It is **essential to consider drug exposure** as a potential cause of marrow damage, even in patients who have other disease. Although some drugs are known for their propensity to cause damage, virtually every drug must be considered as a possible etiologic agent and, if possible, withdrawn.

Patients who present with a **severe aplastic anemia** need special attention. They should be quickly evaluated to identify any possible reversible cause of the aplasia and to rule out malignant disease. When the marrow is severely hypo- or aplastic, the chance of spontaneous recovery is very low. Younger patients should be considered immediately for marrow transplantation. They also need to be protected from exposure to blood-component transfusions if transplantation is to be successful. If possible, transfusions should be withheld until immunosuppressive therapy is begun in preparation for the transplant to avoid alloimmunization. Finally, both patients with severe aplastic anemia and patients who are at risk for severe marrow damage should be human leukocyte antigen (HLA) typed. This is not only required for marrow donor selection but is also important in planning transfusion support. Patients not eligible for transplantation can show a high rate of response to immunosuppressive therapy alone. Unfortunately, up to 40% of patients treated with immunosuppression who survive 10 years or longer are at subsequent risk for developing a clonal malignancy, paroxysmal nocturnal hemoglobinuria, or myelodysplasia progressing to acute myeloid leukemia.

The identification of patients with an inherited defect, whether FA, DC, DBA, or SDS, is essential to planning appropriate therapy. FA and DC patients should be considered for a marrow transplant once their hemoglobin falls below 8 g/dL, platelet count less than 30,000/μL, or an absolute neutrophil count below 500/μL. For those patients who can't be matched to an appropriate donor, androgens and colony-stimulating factors may improve their blood counts. However, caution should be exercised in DC patients, where the combination of granulocyte colony-stimulating factor (G-CSF) and androgens has been reported to cause splenic rupture.

The management of DBA patients is quite different. The majority of DBA patients respond to steroids. Oral prednisone should be given, initially at a high dose, and then tapered to maintain the hemoglobin at a level greater than 8–10 g/dL. A quarter of treated patients will experience a sustained remission, allowing discontinuation of the steroid therapy, although they may relapse in later years. Those who respond poorly should be considered for marrow transplantation. Regardless of the inherited defect, chronic transfusion may be necessary, especially during periods of rapid physical growth when prednisone therapy may be a detriment. Chronic transfusion also runs the risk of progressive iron overload and may therefore require iron chelation therapy.

Transfusion Support

A **relatively mild anemia or pancytopenia** can be observed or, if necessary, treated with 1 or more hematopoietic growth factors. **More severe marrow damage** will generally require supportive therapy with red blood cell and platelet transfusions to maintain oxygen delivery and prevent bleeding. In the adult patient with little or no red blood cell production and a relatively normal rate of destruction, a hemoglobin level of 7–8 g/dL can be achieved with the transfusion of 1 unit of packed red blood cells every other week. Older patients and patients with cardiovascular disease may require transfusion to a higher hemoglobin level.

Patients with aplastic anemia who require long-term transfusion are at high risk of becoming alloimmunized. Prestorage leukoreduction of blood products (both packed red cells and platelets) can significantly reduce the rate of alloimmunization. Clinically, **alloimmunization** may be suspected when the patient repeatedly has fever and chills during or immediately following a red blood cell or platelet transfusion. Another possible sign of alloimmunization is failure to achieve a significant increase in the platelet count following platelet transfusion. The severity of the febrile reaction often correlates with the number of white blood cells contaminating the unit of red blood cells and can be reduced by transfusing only leukopoor red blood cells (see Chapter 38).

Another predictable side effect of repeated transfusion is the **accumulation of excessive tissue iron stores**. Patients who have severe marrow damage and an elevated serum iron are at risk for iron toxicity and damage to the anterior pituitary, heart, and liver. Tissue damage correlates with the total body iron burden and is likely once 100 units or more of red blood cells have been transfused. These patients should be considered for iron chelation therapy using oral deferasirox and/or subcutaneous or intravenous deferoxamine (see Chapters 6 and 15).

Leukopenia to levels as low as 300–500 neutrophils/μL is usually well tolerated. Below this level, patients are at risk for **bacterial infections and sepsis**. Localized infections should be treated with the appropriate antibiotic, whereas septic patients should receive broad-spectrum antibiotic coverage, usually a semisynthetic penicillin or a later-generation cephalosporin in combination with an aminoglycoside. Recovery from transient neutropenia can be accelerated by treatment with G-CSF.

Bleeding complications in patients with aplastic anemia are usually the result of the patient's thrombocytopenia. However, in the septic patient, disseminated intravascular coagulation with decreased levels of coagulation factors must also be considered. Any bleeding episode in a patient with aplastic anemia should be initially treated with platelet transfusions, either random donor or single pheresis donor platelets. A transfusion of 6 units of random platelets or the platelets from a single pheresis donor should raise the 1-hour posttransfusion platelet count by 50,000/μL unless the patient is alloimmunized or actively septic (see Chapter 38).

Patients receiving repeated platelet transfusions who develop anti-HLA antibodies will, in addition to experiencing fever and chills with transfusion, show poor platelet increments and shortened survivals. When a sensitized patient is experiencing a life-threatening hemorrhage, repeated platelet transfusions (2–3 or more times per day) or a continuous infusion may be required to attain hemostasis. The use of HLA-matched platelets may also be required. Unrelated HLA-matched donors can be provided as part of a community donor pool. At the same time, it is important to know the patient's HLA type and to have surveyed the patient's family and siblings for HLA-compatible donors.

Prophylactic transfusion of platelets may be necessary in patients with severely impaired platelet production. In leukemic patients who are not bleeding and do not have an active infection or fever, a platelet count transfusion trigger of 10,000/μL will generally be adequate to maintain hemostasis. In the presence of spontaneous bleeding or signs of infection, the platelet count should be maintained above 20,000/μL. To maintain hemostasis during a minor surgical procedure, platelet counts in excess of 50,000/μL are usually required. Finally, thrombocytopenic patients should avoid antiplatelet drugs, especially aspirin.

Hematopoietic Growth Factors

Erythropoietin, G-CSF, and GM-CSF can be used for treating reversible marrow-damage anemias and pancytopenia. Patients receiving high-dose multidrug chemotherapy can be treated with erythropoietin to reduce the severity of the anemia and avoid transfusion. Several randomized clinical trials have shown an improvement in quality-of-life measures such as energy and activity levels, depression/anxiety, and treatment regimen tolerance in patients receiving erythropoietin who had a greater than 2 g/dL rise in hemoglobin or achieved a hemoglobin level greater than 12 g/dL. At the same time, routine use of erythropoietin in patients undergoing treatment for a solid tumor malignancy is both expensive and, according to some reports, associated with a worse prognosis.

G-CSF and GM-CSF will speed the recovery of the neutrophil count in patients receiving ablative chemotherapy for treatment of a hematopoietic malignancy. This application has been of greatest value in patients receiving allogeneic and autologous bone marrow transplants. GM-CSF or G-CSF (given in a dose of 10 μg/kg/d beginning 2–4 days after the reinfusion of the marrow stem cells) has been shown to significantly speed recovery following transplantation, thereby decreasing the incidence of infection and the need for broad-spectrum antibiotic coverage. In the case of high-dose chemotherapy, G-CSF is now used routinely to shorten the period of marked neutropenia, especially when the patient has previously experienced a period of febrile neutropenia associated with a neutrophil count below 100/μL. Not only does this serve to prevent complicating infections, but it also helps keep the patient on schedule for successive chemotherapy treatments and allow the use of more intensive drug regimens.

The usefulness of growth factors in the treatment of **severe aplastic anemia** is less certain. Patients with severe marrow-damage anemias usually have very high serum erythropoietin levels. Administration of additional exogenous erythropoietin would appear to add little to this natural stimulus, and therefore cannot be expected to increase red blood cell production. Limited trials of erythropoietin in the treatment of patients with myelodysplasia have reported the occasional response; trials with very high levels of recombinant erythropoietin have not been carried out.

GM-CSF and G-CSF therapy may hold greater promise for treating the **leukopenia associated with aplastic anemia**. However, the effectiveness depends on the severity of the marrow damage. Patients with absolute granulocyte counts of less than 200/μL generally fail to respond to either growth factor, whereas 60%–70% of patients with counts of 200–1,500/μL show excellent responses. Growth factors have also been given in varying combinations to patients undergoing immunosuppressive therapy. While the hematological response rate is more rapid, the incidence of infections and febrile episodes is unchanged and overall survival is no different. The effectiveness of growth factors that act at earlier stages in cell development (IL-3 and SCF) still needs to be studied. Limited trials of IL-3 as a single agent suggest that a few patients may experience increases in leukocytes, red blood cells, and platelets. The true test will require studies of a larger number of patients and using combinations of IL-3 and SCF with erythropoietin, GM-CSF, and G-CSF.

The role of growth factors in the treatment of FA and DBA is limited. Trials involving small numbers of patients with FA have shown that the leukopenia and anemia can improve transiently with growth factor therapy. At the same time, there is the concurrent risk of speeding evolution to acute leukemia. The bottom line is there still is no role for growth factors in the long-term treatment of FA, DBA, or SDS.

The use of growth factors in the treatment of **"idiopathic" aplastic anemia** is also hampered by a lack of knowledge regarding the most appropriate dose and schedule of administration. Studies of erythropoietin in patients with marrow-damage anemia have evaluated doses ranging from 100–300 U/kg given subcutaneously 2–3 times each week. Very-high-dose regimens have not been attempted. Therefore, it is likely that only those patients with an anemia associated with a failed erythropoietin response will have a chance of responding. The best dosages and dose schedules for G-CSF and GM-CSF alone and in combination with IL-3, IL-6, IL-11, and SCF are also unclear.

Marrow Transplantation

The recommended treatment for the younger patient with a severe aplastic anemia is marrow transplantation. Of course, this therapy requires the availability of a histocompatible family member, either a parent or sibling with a 4-locus HLA match or an identical twin. Transplants with nonidentical or unrelated donors are less successful and should only be considered in patients who fail immunosuppressive therapy.

The success of a marrow transplant depends on the patient's age, transfusion history, clinical status at the time of transplant, and the cause of the marrow damage (Figure 3–5). A younger patient has a greater chance of success, largely because the incidence of GVHD (the major cause of graft failure) increases with age. Although children, teenagers, and young adults can expect a better than 80% chance of long-term survival with good return of marrow function, patients over age 20 will experience significant complications from **GVHD**. Graft rejection is more frequent, and the incidence of posttransplant infections, including interstitial pneumonitis, is much higher. This will be true even if the patient is immunosuppressed both prior to and following transplant.

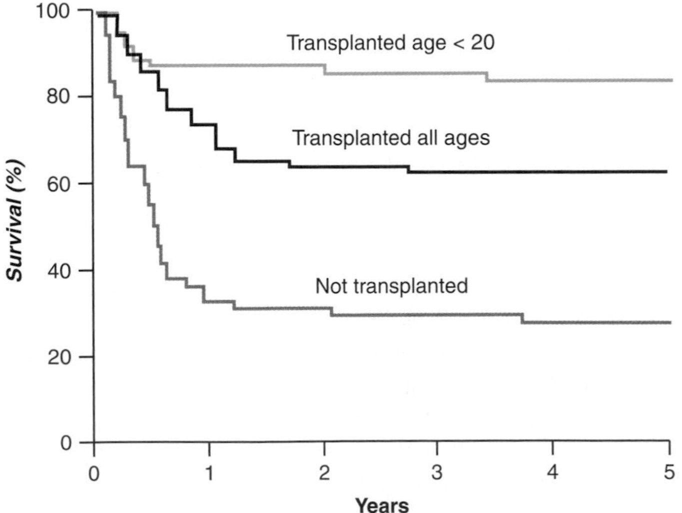

FIGURE 3–5. **Marrow transplantation in aplastic anemia.** The success of an allogeneic marrow transplant in patients with aplastic anemia depends on the availability of a related or unrelated matched donor, the age of the patient, and the nature of the disease. Young patients who receive transplants early with a well-matched donor have sustained remissions up to 90% of the time. Overall survival for patients of all ages is better than 60%. This rate is in dramatic contrast to patients who do not receive transplants and who did not receive effective immunosuppressive therapy. Their survival over a 5-year period is less than 40%.

Transfusions prior to preconditioning immunosuppression can increase the chance of graft rejection and GVHD. It is important, therefore, to try to avoid multiple transfusions for the few weeks it takes to search the family for a suitable donor and, when transfusion is required, to use only leukocyte depleted, irradiated red blood cell and platelet products. However, a conditioning regimen of cyclophosphamide and fludarabine has been reported to achieve a high rate of graft acceptance and survival even in heavily transfused patients. The cause of the disease and the medical condition of the patient at the time of the transplant also make a big difference, and patients whose transplant course is complicated by infection do less well. Children or teenagers with severe aplasia of unknown cause who receive a transplant early in their course have the best prognosis. Older patients and patients with less severe hypoplasia are best treated with immunosuppressive therapy initially and should only receive transplants if the response is inadequate.

Patients with **aplastic anemia of unknown cause** must have immunosuppressive therapy prior to transplant, not only to guarantee engraftment of the marrow (prevent rejection), but also to treat any underlying autoimmune disease process. Even in identical twins, a simple infusion of marrow without immunosuppression will not be successful. With the current use of combinations of high-dose cyclophosphamide, antithymocyte globulin (ATG), and cyclosporine as pretransplant conditioning therapy, and both methotrexate and cyclosporine to manage the patient's GVHD, long-term survivals are 70%–80% for patients under the age of 40 and 30%–50% for those over age 40. Patients under age 16 conditioned with 200 mg/kg cyclophosphamide have been reported to show survivals of 91% with a matched sibling transplant, making this the preferred therapy by far for this age group. Total body irradiation (TBI) has fallen out of favor because of the high incidence of secondary cancers, greater than 20% at 8 years. In addition, TBI in children is also associated with impairment of endocrine functions and growth retardation.

Although there is less experience with unrelated marrow transplants, small series of patients transplanted between 1993 and 2000 using a conditioning regimen of cyclophosphomide, ATG, and TBI have reported graft rejection rates of 2%–11%, chronic GVHD in 20%, and survivals of 40%–60%. In a more recent multicenter trial, 62 severely aplastic anemic patients who failed immunosuppressive therapy and then received an unrelated transplant demonstrated a graft rejection rate of 2%, chronic GVHD of 52%, and survivals of 60%. Changes in conditioning regimens (addition of fludarabine and/or cytosine arabinoside, CD34 purification, T-cell depletion, and monoclonal antibodies) and improvements in donor-recipient matching have all been reported to improve outcome in small studies of children without matched sibling donors, even to the point of rivaling matched donor results. In light of this, children and young adults who lack a sibling donor should still be considered for an unrelated donor transplant. As for the use of umbilical cord stem cell transplants, results to date have not been encouraging.

Immunosuppression

Immunosuppression alone with combinations of steroids, antithymocyte globulin, and cyclosporine is highly effective when the aplasia is caused by an autoimmune disease process. The decision to use an immunosuppressive regimen rather than marrow transplantation will depend on the suspected etiology, the patient's age, the overall clinical condition, and the availability of a marrow donor. An algorithm for selecting therapy is shown in Figure 3–6. Young patients with severe aplastic anemia should receive transplants immediately if a matched donor is available. Patients who lack a donor, patients over age 40 years, and patients with less severe marrow aplasia/hypoplasia are **candidates for immunosuppressive therapy**. With modern regimens that include cyclosporine, overall long-term survival rates are probably comparable to those achievable with transplantation.

Corticosteroids given alone can occasionally result in improved marrow function. This is especially true for patients with pure red cell aplasia. However, **horse-derived antithymocyte globulin (ATG) or the equivalent rabbit preparation of antilymphocyte globulin (ALG)** in combination with cyclosporine are considered to be more effective immunosuppressive agents. Response rates range from 25%–85% of patients with moderate to severe aplastic anemia, and survival of responders can reach 90% at 5 years. Improvement in peripheral blood counts is typically slow, requiring several months of therapy, and is generally less complete than that seen with marrow transplantation. Patients with very severe aplastic anemia may not survive long enough to benefit from the therapy unless supportive care is excellent. Partial responses are not uncommon (less than half of patients achieve normal blood counts) and as many as 40% of patients relapse a few months to years after successful treatment. However, 50% or more of patients who relapse will respond to additional courses of immunosuppression or, in some cases, maintenance therapy with cyclosporine. The addition of G-CSF to the initial regimen may result in fewer relapses. **Long-term cyclosporine therapy** must be carefully monitored since it is associated with significant adverse effects, including hypertension, hypertrichosis, and nephrotoxicity.

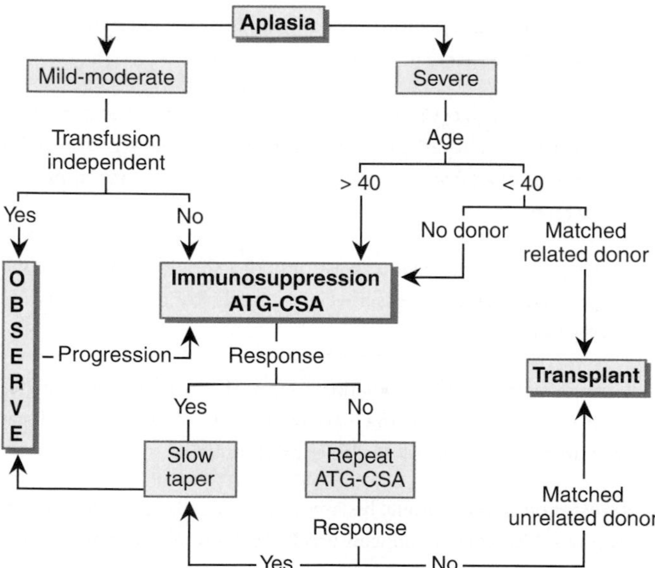

FIGURE 3–6. **Therapy selection in patients with aplastic anemia.** Management of a patient with aplastic anemia will depend on the patient's age, the severity of the aplasia, and the availability of a matched related or unrelated donor for transplantation. Patients with mild to moderately severe disease may be observed or treated with immunosuppressive therapy if they show progression. The young patient with severe aplasia should receive a transplant without delay if a matched sibling donor or twin is available. Immunosuppressive therapy in older patients and patients who do not have donors can provide a partial or complete remission in a majority of patients. Those who do not respond can be considered for an unrelated matched transplant.

ATG administration is not without its problems. Patients are at risk for an **anaphylactic reaction** to the horse or rabbit proteins in the preparation, and **serum sickness–like reaction** to the ATG/ALG is very common. Patients experience fever, chills, and urticaria with the first infusions and later a flu-like illness with fever, arthralgias, myalgia, a maculopapular rash, and diarrhea. Liver and renal function abnormalities are also common. The severity of these side effects can be in part controlled by the administration of 60–80 mg of methylprednisolone per day in divided doses.

The **mechanism of action of ATG** is not well understood. Although it may decrease subsets of lymphocytes responsible for immune suppression of marrow precursors, it may also stimulate a proliferation of T lymphocytes that produce growth factors such as GM-CSF and IL-3. Clinical trials of ATG and ALG have also reported varied success rates for different lots of material. This has raised questions as to the actual active component of the preparations. It is not simply a matter of decreasing the number of T–suppressor cells, since monoclonal preparations of antihuman T-cell antibodies have had little therapeutic effect.

Cyclosporine alone or in combination with ALG and methylprednisolone has also been found to be therapeutically effective. Patients with aplastic anemia treated with the combination of drugs have now been reported to have a 92% survival at 3 years. However, although the early response is better when cyclosporine is used, long-term survival may be no different, and the frequency of the subsequent appearance of a clonal malignancy (eg, acute leukemia, sideroblastic anemia, or paroxysmal nocturnal hemoglobinuria) may be increased. Patients who receive cyclosporine therapy to treat their aplastic anemia are also at greater risk for the development of ***Pneumocystis carinii*** pneumonia.

The choice of therapy for patients with **pure red cell aplasia** will depend on the diagnosis. Patients with thymomas can respond with a complete remission after successful surgical resection of the tumor. Patients with chronic parvovirus respond to

CASE HISTORY • Part 3

Given the fact that the patient is 27 years of age and has no physical deformities, the likelihood of an inherited defect (FA, DBA, SDS, or DCA) is extremely low. Tumor or leukemic infiltration was ruled out by the marrow examination, and the pancytopenia excludes pure red cell aplasia as a diagnosis. His occupation does raise the issue of chemical exposure and this deserves further exploration, especially if he doesn't respond to immunosuppressive therapy.

The most likely diagnosis is an **autoimmune severe aplastic anemia/pancytopenia**, underlying etiology unknown. One test that may help confirm this diagnosis is the detection of GPI^- (CD55/CD59 negative) clones in circulation by flow cytometry. They can be detected in 50% or more of autoimmune aplastic anemia cases and predict a response to immunosuppression.

Depending on the availability of a matched sibling marrow donor, the management of the patient will involve making a choice between immediate bone marrow transplantation after conditioning therapy versus immunosuppressive therapy with ATG and cyclosporine (Figure 3–4). Both therapies can produce a partial to complete response in 60%–80% of patients under the age of 40 years, and even higher rates in children.

intravenous immune globulin or ATG. Corticosteroids alone can be effective in many of the patients who have an immune component to their disease, whereas most will respond to some combination of prednisone, with ATG, cyclosporine, or cyclophosphamide. Patients with myelodysplasia (see Chapter 9) are generally refractory to immunosuppressive therapy.

Androgen Therapy

Androgen therapy was used extensively to treat aplastic anemia prior to the advent of marrow transplantation and immunosuppressive therapy. Although most patients do not benefit, an occasional patient will show a response, usually limited to the red blood cell line. To achieve even a modest therapeutic response, androgens must be given for 4–6 months or longer. Side effects with prolonged therapy include acne, virilization, and hyperlipidemia.

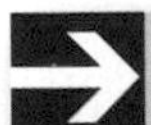

POINTS TO REMEMBER

Marrow-damage anemias and pancytopenias are routinely seen in patients receiving chemotherapy or radiation therapy and as a complication of diseases that cause structural damage to the marrow—leukemia, solid tumor metastases, and granulomatous infections.

Aplastic anemia, that is, severe hypo-/aplasia of all marrow elements, is seen in association with certain drugs, toxic chemicals, viral diseases, or without apparent etiology, although most of the latter are likely to be autoimmune disorders.

The workup of a patient with a severe aplastic anemia, especially the younger patient, must be aggressive. Effective management with bone marrow transplantation and/or immunosuppressive therapy depends on early diagnosis and early treatment.

Four genetic abnormalities need to be considered in the workup of children and young adults, especially those with skeletal defects—Fanconi anemia, dyskeratosis congenita, Blackfan-Diamond syndrome, and Shwachman-Diamond syndrome.

Patients under age 16 with severe aplastic anemia and a matched sibling donor should be transplanted immediately. If a sibling donor is unavailable, a search for an unrelated donor should be undertaken.

Older patients with severe aplastic anemia should receive immunosuppressive therapy, unless a well-matched sibling donor or twin is readily available.

Growth factors (erythropoietin and G-CSF) have limited usefulness in aplastic anemia, unless the marrow damage is less severe and marrow progenitors are still available for stimulation.

Transfusion therapy should be limited or avoided, if possible, and only irradiated leukocyte reduced products used in order to diminish alloimmunization and avoid both graft rejection and GVHD.

Immunosuppressive therapy with ATG, cyclosporine, and G-CSF can induce a complete or partial remission in up to 85% of patients, depending on the underlying cause and the patient's physical condition.

BIBLIOGRAPHY

Clinical Features and Diagnosis

Bacigalupo A et al: Antilymphocyte globulin, cyclosporine, prednisolone, and granulocyte-stimulating factor for severe aplastic anemia: an update of the GITMO/EBMT study of 100 patients. Blood 2000;95:1931.

Barrett J, Saunthararajah Y, Molldrem J: Myelodysplastic syndrome and aplastic anemia: distinct entities or diseases linked by a common pathophysiology? Semin Hematol 2000;37:15.

Blank U et al: Signaling pathways governing stem-cell fate. Blood 2008;111:492.

Brown KE et al: Hepatitis-associated aplastic anemia. *N Engl J Med* 1997;336:1059.

Calado RT et al: Mutations in the *SDRS* gene in acquired aplastic anemia. Blood 2007;110:1141.

Flygare J, Karlsson S: Diamond-Blackfan anemia: erythropoiesis lost in translation. Blood 2007;109:3152.

Kutler DI et al: A 20-year perspective on the International Fanconi Anemia Registry (IFAR). Blood 2003;101:1249.

Moulopoulus LA, Dimopoulus MA: Magnetic resonance imaging of the bone marrow in hematologic malignancies. Blood 1997;90:2127.

Taniguchi T, D'Andrea AD: Molecular pathogenesis of Fanconi anemia: recent progress. Blood 2006;107:4223.

Young NS: Hematopoietic cell destruction by immune mechanisms in acquired aplastic anemia. Semin Hematol 2000;37:3.

Young NS, Calado RT, Scheinberg P: Current concepts in the pathophysiology and treatment of aplastic anemia. Blood 2006; 108:2509.

Therapy

Charles RJ et al: The pathophysiology of pure red cell aplasia: implications for therapy. Blood 1996;87:4831.

Crump M et al: Treatment of adults with severe aplastic anemia: primary therapy with antithymocyte globulin (ATG) and rescue of ATG failures with bone marrow transplantation. Am J Med 1992;92:596.

Deeg HJ et al: Optimization of conditioning for marrow transplantation from unrelated donors for patients with aplastic anemia after failure of immunosuppressive therapy. Blood 2006; 108:1485.

Doney K et al: Immunosuppressive therapy of aplastic anemia: results of a prospective, randomized trial of thymocyte globulin (ATG), methylprednisolone, and oxymetholone to ATG, very high-dose methylprednisolone and oxymetholone. Blood 1992; 79:2566.

Doney K et al: Primary treatment of acquired aplastic anemia: outcomes with bone marrow transplantation and immunosuppressive therapy. Ann Intern Med 1997;126:107.

Frickhofen N, Rosenfeld SJ: Immunosuppressive treatment of aplastic anemia with antithymocyte globulin and cyclosporine. Semin Hematol 2000;37:56.

Lieschke GJ, Burgess AW: Granulocyte colony-stimulating factor and granulocyte-macrophage colony-stimulating factor. N Engl J Med 1992;327:28, 99.

Marsh J, Ganser A, Stadler M: Hematopoietic growth factors in the treatment of acquired bone marrow failure states. Semin Hematol 2007;44:138.

Rackoff WR et al: Prolonged administration of granulocyte colony-stimulating factor (filgastrim) to patients with Fanconi anemia: a pilot study. Blood 1996;88:1588.

Rizzo JD et al: Use of epoietin in patients with cancer: evidence-based clinical practice guidelines of the American Society of Clinical Oncology and the American Society of Hematology. Blood 2002;100:2303.

Sugimori et al: Minor populations of CD55$^-$CD59$^-$ blood cells predicts the response to immunosuppressive therapy and prognosis in patients with aplastic anemia. Blood 2006;107:1308.

Teramura M et al: Treatment of severe aplastic anemia with antithymocyte globulin and cyclosporine A with and without G-CSF in adults: a multicenter randomized study in Japan. Blood 2007;110:1756.

Welte K et al: Filgrastim (r-metHuG-CSF): the first 10 years. Blood 1996;88:1907.

Zeidler C, Welte: Hematopoietic growth factors for the treatment of inherited cytopenias. Semin Hematol 2007;44:133.

ANEMIAS ASSOCIATED WITH A REDUCED ERYTHROPOIETIN RESPONSE · 4

CASE HISTORY • *Part I*

A 66-year-old woman presents with more than 6 months of pain and stiffness of the muscles of the neck, shoulders, and lower back. Within the past 2 weeks, she has also suffered from recurrent headaches, unresponsive to aspirin, acetaminophen, and nonsteroidals. Review of systems is negative for collagen vascular disease or vasculitis, but she has had a 10–15 lb weight loss, and is a heavy smoker. Examination is notable for sallow complexion and depressed mood. Neck and shoulder muscles are tender to palpation but no arthritic changes or temporal artery nodularity or tenderness are noted.

CBC: Hematocrit/hemoglobin - 29%/9 g/dL
MCV - 84 fL MCH - 30 pg MCHC - 30 g/dL
RDW-CV - 14%
WBC count - 9,500/μL
Platelet count - 210,000/μL

• SMEAR MORPHOLOGY

Normocytic/normochromic, with minimal anisocytosis, no poikilocytosis, and no polychromasia.
Reticulocyte count/index - 1.3%/<1
Sedimentation rate - 115 mm/h (Westergren)
C-reactive protein - 37 mg/L

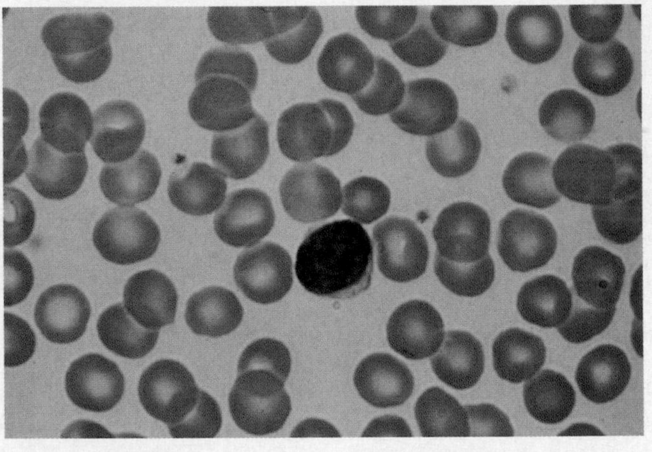

Questions

- How should the anemia be described and classified, given the above data?
- What additional tests should be ordered?

Anemia is common in patients with acute and chronic inflammatory diseases, renal insufficiency, and hypothyroidism. In each situation, there is an apparent failure in the erythropoietin stimulation of the marrow. Serum erythropoietin levels, although not decreased below basal levels, are not appropriately increased for the severity of the anemia. Marrow cellularity and reticulocyte response are typically hypoproliferative.

The importance of this class of anemias cannot be overemphasized. The clinical incidence of hypoproliferative anemias associated with acute infection or chronic inflammatory disease (the anemia of chronic disease) is far greater than that of all other types of anemia. In some cases, appearance of a typical hypoproliferative anemia is the first sign of underlying disease. The pattern of the anemia can also be of considerable value in the diagnosis of the etiology and severity of the disease process. It is important, therefore, that clinicians be skilled in evaluating the patient with a hypoproliferative anemia, even when the anemia is mild.

NORMAL MARROW PROLIFERATION

The **normal proliferative response** of the erythroid marrow to anemia requires an appropriate erythropoietin response, an intact erythroid marrow, and an adequate supply of iron (Figure 4–1). Dedicated peritubular interstitial cells in the kidney are capable of sensing changes in oxygen delivery. A **decrease in hemoglobin level to values less than 12 g/dL** stimulates an increased production of erythropoietin. This process involves recruitment of additional peritubular interstitial cells rather than an upregulation of existing cellular production. The role of the kidney in regulating erythropoietin production is well maintained even with significant renal damage. However, end-stage renal disease is uniformly associated with a failure in the erythropoietin response. Since hepatocytes also produce some erythropoietin, anephric patients have measurable serum erythropoietin levels but markedly reduced red blood cell production.

The erythropoietin produced by the kidney travels to the marrow, where it binds to specific receptors (EPOR) on the surface of the burst-forming unit–erythroid (BFU-E) and colony-forming unit–erythroid (CFU-E) precursors (Figure 4–2). This process initiates a sequence of proliferation and maturation of these committed stem cells to produce new adult red blood cells. The magnitude of the erythropoietin response correlates with the severity of the anemia, and the higher the serum erythropoietin level, the greater the marrow proliferative response. This response can be assessed clinically both from changes in the marrow ratio of erythroid to granulocytic precursors (E/G ratio) and the reticulocyte response. The normal production response to anemia of increasing severity is discussed in Chapter 2.

The proliferative response also requires an adequate supply of **iron**. The iron recycled from red cell breakdown and reticuloendothelial iron stores largely provides iron required for erythropoiesis. Only a small amount is derived through absorption of food iron. It is transported through the plasma bound to transferrin. The transferrin-iron complex then binds to transferrin receptors on the surface of erythroid precursors. The expression of transferrin receptors and rate of transport of iron into the cell appear to be governed by erythropoietin and a genetically controlled transmembrane protein—HFE (see Chapters 5 and 15).

Red blood cells

O_2

Erythroid marrow

Erythropoietin

Iron

Gut

RE cells

FIGURE 4–1. **Components of the normal marrow proliferative response.** A full response to an anemia requires an appropriate excretion of erythropoietin by the kidney, an adequate supply of iron, and a fully responsive marrow.

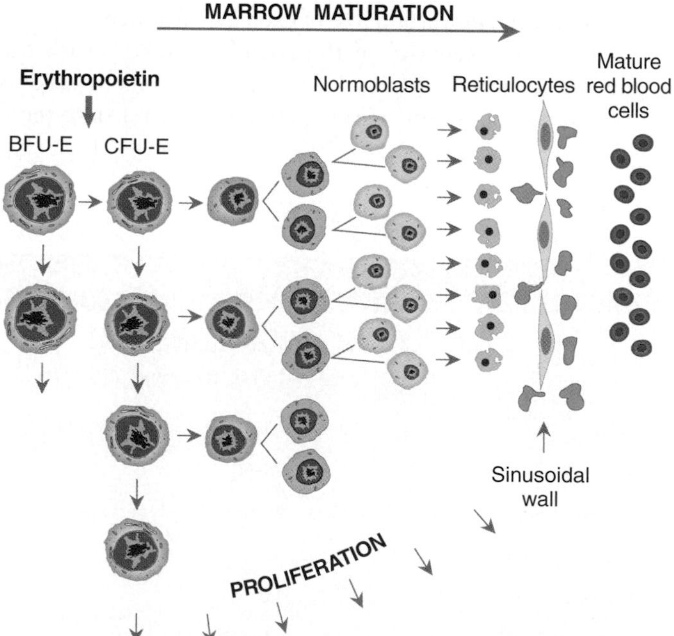

FIGURE 4–2. **Erythroid marrow proliferation and maturation.** Erythropoietin stimulates marrow BFU-E and CFU-E to proliferate and differentiate to produce an increasing number of maturing red blood cell precursors. Each committed precursor undergoes 4 cell divisions, producing 14–16 adult red blood cells. Increased levels of erythropoietin also accelerate normoblast maturation and the release of marrow reticulocytes into circulation.

When the amount of iron on transferrin is reduced (a lower than normal serum iron level), both hemoglobin synthesis and the proliferative response of erythroid precursors to erythropoietin are inhibited. Erythropoietin production, iron supply, and erythroid precursor proliferation are also influenced by cytokines produced during inflammation (tumor necrosis factor α [TNF-α], interleukin-1 and -6 [IL-1, IL-6], and γ and α interferon [IFN-γ, IFN-α]). Direct T-cell suppression of stem cells has also been postulated in some cases of hypoplastic anemia.

Hepcidin, a liver-produced peptide, plays a central role in the regulation of dietary iron absorption and the storage and release of iron from reticuloendothelial cell stores. Inflammatory cytokines, especially IL-6, induce the overexpression of hepcidin, resulting in elevated levels in circulation and reductions in both iron absorption and release from stores. As stated above, the resulting fall in serum iron is a major inhibitor of erythroid marrow proliferation.

CLINICAL FEATURES

Hypoproliferative anemias are most often detected as a result of the workup of the patient's primary condition. For example, when a patient is admitted for an acute inflammatory illness such as lobar pneumonia, the complete blood count (CBC) reveals a mild to moderate anemia. The same is true for a patient who is being followed up for progressive **renal failure;** routine CBCs typically show a worsening anemia. Unless the anemia is severe, the patient can be asymptomatic. This situation is not true for **older patients,** in whom even a moderate anemia can exacerbate the symptoms and signs of cardiovascular disease, or at least result in fatigue and loss of exercise tolerance.

As a rule, the **severity of the anemia** correlates with the severity of the primary illness. Symptomatic anemia in patients with renal disease is only seen in patients with end-stage renal disease. An exception to this observation is in patients with diabetic nephropathy where anemia of moderate severity can occur before significant increases in the blood urea nitrogen (BUN) and creatinine. The anemia that accompanies chronic inflammatory disease, either collagen vascular disease or chronic infections, will correlate with the activity of the inflammatory process. This relationship between illness severity and anemia severity is demonstrated when the patient's primary illness is treated. When a patient with rheumatoid arthritis or polymyalgia rheumatica responds to anti-inflammatory drug therapy, the anemia also improves. Finally, the hypoproliferative anemia seen in patients with hypothyroidism or panhypopituitarism will also correlate best with the severity and duration of the hypometabolic state.

Laboratory Studies

The **CBC, reticulocyte count**, and **serum iron studies**, including a measurement of serum ferritin, should be enough to diagnose this type of anemia. **Typical erythropoietic profiles of anemias** associated with acute and chronic inflammatory disease, renal failure, and hypometabolic states are illustrated in Table 4–1. The CBC and reticulocyte count are characteristic of a hypoproliferative anemia. Red blood cell morphology is normocytic and normochromic, and the reticulocyte index is inappropriately low for the severity of the patient's anemia. In patients with severe, chronic inflammatory disorders, a mild microcytic/hypochromic anemia may develop. However, microcytosis is not as marked as that seen in patients with an iron-deficiency anemia of comparable severity.

A. Iron Studies

Iron studies, including **measurements of serum iron, total iron-binding capacity (TIBC), serum ferritin, and serum transferrin receptor,** provide important diagnostic information. As illustrated

TABLE 4–1 • Erythropoietic profiles of reduced erythropoietin anemias

	Acute and Chronic Inflammatory	Renal Disease	Hypometabolic States
Anemia	Mild	Minor to severe	Mild
MCV (fL)	75–90	90	80–100
Film morphology	Normocytic → microcytic	Normocytic	Variable
Reticulocyte index	<2	<2	<2
Marrow E/G ratio	1:3	1:3	1:3
Serum iron/TIBC	<50/<300	Normal	Normal
% Saturation	10–20	Normal	Normal
Marrow iron stores	Increased	Normal	Normal
Serum ferritin	Increased	Normal	Normal
Bilirubin/LDH	Normal	Normal	Normal

in Table 4–1, patients with renal disease or a hypometabolic state demonstrate essentially normal iron studies. Serum iron, total iron-binding capacity (TIBC), and serum ferritin levels are all normal. This may not be true, however, for patients with renal disease on chronic dialysis or predialysis patients receiving multiple transfusions. In the former case, repeated hemodialysis can result in a negative iron balance and iron-deficient erythropoiesis, especially in those patients receiving recombinant erythropoietin (see Therapy section). On the other hand, patients with end-stage renal disease who receive chronic transfusions are at risk for iron overload and can show elevated serum ferritin levels.

Most patients with anemia associated with **acute or chronic inflammatory disease** (the anemia of chronic disease) demonstrate a characteristic pattern of low serum iron and low TIBC with percent saturations between 10% and 20%, coupled with a rising serum ferritin level. This pattern is distinctly different from a true iron-deficiency anemia, where a very low serum iron level accompanies a rising TIBC and a very low serum ferritin level (<12 μg/L). The relationship of illness severity to anemia is mirrored in the iron studies. The more pronounced the inflammatory component of the patient's illness, the lower the serum iron and TIBC and the higher the serum ferritin level. The level of reticuloendothelial iron stores also influences the latter measurement. Women, with smaller stores, show smaller increases (ferritin levels of 20–200 μg/L), whereas men show a greater rise (ferritin levels of 100–500 μg/L). As an even more simplistic rule of thumb, any patient with a hypoproliferative anemia, together with an elevated C-reactive protein and a normal to increased serum ferritin level, will have an inflammatory anemia (anemia of chronic disease), whereas a patient with a normal C-reactive protein and low ferritin level will be iron deficient.

The **serum transferrin receptor (sTfR)** measurement has been popularized as another way to discriminate the anemia of chronic disease from that of iron deficiency. The sTfR increases once the serum ferritin falls to less than 40 μg/L, as a result of *HFE-IRE* induction of increased numbers of receptors on the surface of individual erythroid precursors. At the same time, the sTfR also rises in response to the proliferation of red cell precursors for whatever reason, reflecting an increased shedding of receptors from an increased number of precursors. Therefore, elevated sTfR values cannot be interpreted as indicative of iron deficiency unless proliferation of erythroid precursors is ruled out.

Recognizing this point of possible confusion, the sTfR, together with the serum ferritin level, can help distinguish uncomplicated iron deficiency from the anemia of chronic disease. Using the calculated log (serum TfR/ferritin) ratio, **patients with iron-deficiency anemia** typically have values greater than 2.5 (reflecting a rising sTfR together with a marked fall in the ferritin level), whereas **patients with the anemia of chronic disease** have values less than 2.5 (reflecting a lower sTfR together with a rising ferritin level). The latter pattern also reflects the hypoproliferative nature of the anemia. **Patients with severe iron-deficiency anemia** exhibit not only a very low serum ferritin level (<12 μg/L) but also erythroid marrow expansion and ineffective erythropoiesis, causing a further rise in the sTfR level to even higher ratios (>4).

B. Marrow and Erythropoietin Studies

The diagnosis of a hypoproliferative anemia that is clearly associated with a known inflammatory disorder, renal disease, or an abnormality in thyroid or pituitary function usually does not require a marrow aspirate or biopsy. The combination of normocytic, normochromic morphology, and a lower than predicted reticulocyte response without polychromasia is enough to confirm the hypoproliferative nature of the anemia. Performance of a marrow aspirate merely to assess the E/G ratio is unproductive. Moreover, as long as the patient demonstrates normal leukocyte and platelet counts, it is unlikely that a marrow biopsy specimen will identify a defect in marrow morphology or cellularity.

When a serum ferritin level is unavailable or is in a range that does not support the diagnosis, a marrow aspirate stained with Prussian blue can be used to distinguish true iron deficiency from the anemia of chronic disease. Patients with absolute iron deficiency should have no visible iron stores in reticuloendothelial cells once the percent saturation of transferrin is below 15%. Patients with a low serum iron secondary to inflammatory disease will have normal to increased iron stores on the Prussian blue stain. In patients with chronic inflammatory disease, iron stores often appear increased, with extra large hemosiderin granules in the marrow reticuloendothelial cells.

Direct measurements of the serum erythropoietin level are not helpful in either identifying this class of anemias or in separating individual abnormalities. Although a reduced erythropoietin response is an inherent component of the anemia, the observed range of measured values is quite large. Patients can demonstrate erythropoietin levels that are above basal, although they fall short of the levels achieved by the normal individual responding to a blood loss anemia. This phenomenon is best illustrated by the observed pattern of serum erythropoietin measurements in patients with renal disease (Figure 4–3).

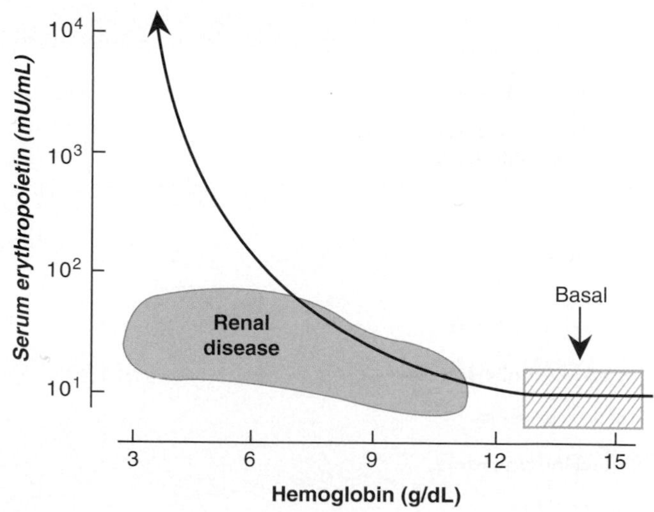

FIGURE 4–3. **Serum erythropoietin levels in renal disease.** Serum erythropoietin levels in patients with the anemia of end-stage renal disease fall well below the levels observed in normal individuals responding to a hemorrhagic event.

CASE HISTORY • *Part 2*

Based on smear morphology and the red blood cell indices (MCV, MCH, MCHC), the patient has a normocytic, normochromic anemia of mild to moderate severity. From a physiological perspective, it is a hypoproliferative anemia, that is, an anemia resulting from a failure of the marrow to respond to and compensate for the anemia. This is apparent from the reticulocyte index of less than 1. Furthermore, the absence of polychromasia suggests a failure to increase erythropoietin production.

Additional studies of immediate importance include serum iron, iron-binding capacity, serum ferritin, renal function studies (BUN and creatinine/creatinine clearance), and thyroid function studies (T4 and TSH). The following results were obtained:

Serum iron - 30 μg/dL
Iron-binding capacity - 230 μg/dL % Saturation - 13%
Serum ferritin - 180 μg/L BUN - 15 mg/dL
Serum creatinine - 0.6 mg/dL
T4 and TSH - Within normal limits

Questions

- What does this pattern of iron studies suggest?
- Are there other studies that will confirm your diagnosis?
- What treatment is indicated?

DIAGNOSIS

The approach to diagnosis of a hypoproliferative anemia in a patient with an acute or chronic inflammatory disease, renal damage, or a hypometabolic state depends on the nature and severity of the primary illness and the severity of the anemia (Table 4–2). Since mild to moderate anemia in a patient with progressive renal failure is predictable, there is less need to repeatedly assess the patient for other possible causes of anemia. **For patients with acute or chronic inflammatory disease**, definition of the anemia can be helpful in diagnosing the disorder and assessing its severity. In this case, even a mild anemia should be evaluated with a full panel of studies—CBC, reticulocyte count, sedimentation rate/C-reactive protein, and serum iron studies, including a serum ferritin level.

TABLE 4–2 • Diseases associated with reduced erythropoietin response

Inflammatory states	Acute and chronic bacterial infections
	Collagen vascular disorders
	AIDS
	Malignancies
Renal disease	Nephritis
	End-stage renal disease
Hypometabolic states	Protein deprivation
Endocrine disorders	Hypothyroidism
	Hypopituitarism
	Hyperparathyroidism

Acute Inflammatory States

Anemia is a common component of acute inflammatory states, especially bacterial infections and collagen vascular disorders. Viral diseases are less likely to produce anemia, or if they do, the anemia is secondary to an autoimmune process or a general failure of stem cells that results in pancytopenia. Parvovirus infection in patients with congenital hemolytic anemias produces a reversible suppression of marrow erythroid precursors without affecting other cell lines (see Chapters 3 and 11).

Anemia appears rapidly with the onset of an acute bacterial infection. It is not unusual to see the patient's hemoglobin fall to levels of 10–12 g/dL (hematocrit of 30%–36%) within 1 or 2 days after the onset of a bacterial infection, such as acute lobar pneumonia. This initial fall in the hemoglobin level results from a loss of older red blood cells, which are nearing the end of their natural lifespan in circulation, demonstrating the sensitivity of older cells to changes in the external environment. The release of various cytokines, fever, and local changes in the infected tissue may all play a role in stressing the older red blood cell beyond its metabolic capacity to maintain hemoglobin solubility and cell membrane continuity.

Even though the first step in the evolution of an acute inflammatory anemia is a self-limited hemolytic event, the principal defects are a failure in the erythropoietin response and a limitation in iron supply, both of which inhibit the erythroid marrow response. Therefore, the **erythropoietic profile is typically hypoproliferative**. Red blood cell morphology is normocytic and normochromic, the reticulocyte count remains low (a reticulocyte index <2), and there is little or no polychromasia apparent on the blood film. **Iron studies confirm the nature of the anemia.** Within a matter of hours of the onset of an inflammatory condition, serum iron and TIBC fall and the ferritin level begins to rise. Serum transferrin receptor levels remain low, resulting in a low (<2.5) serum TfR/ferritin ratio. This pattern is so distinctive that it is used diagnostically to confirm the presence of an inflammatory component to the patient's illness, even when there is some question as to the primary diagnosis (see Table 4–1).

The subpar erythropoietin response and a fall in iron supply are responsible for the inhibition of erythroid precursor proliferation. Several cytokines are involved, including TNF-α, IL-1, IL-6, IFN-α and IFN-γ, and neopterin. Increased TNF-α may suppress erythroid progenitor proliferation directly and via the induction of IFN-γ from marrow stromal cells. IL-1, in the presence of both T cells and interferon, also may play a role in the inhibition of erythroid progenitor proliferation. **Hepcidin**, a liver-produced cysteine-rich peptide with antimicrobial properties, appears to be the principal mediator in restricting iron supply to the marrow in patients with infection or inflammation. As illustrated in Figure 4–4, hepcidin regulates iron absorption and reticuloendothelial cell release of iron to transferrin in response to iron balance, oxygen supply, and erythropoiesis. With acute infection and acute or chronic inflammation, hepcidin levels rise rapidly and strongly inhibit iron absorption and the release of iron from reticuloendothelial stores, by binding to and degrading the export protein ferroportin. The inflammatory cytokine IL-6 appears to play a key role in the regulation of hepcidin synthesis via STAT3-mediated mRNA expression.

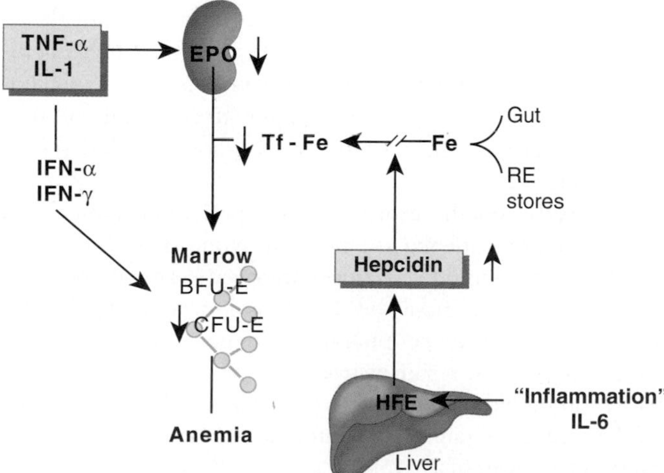

FIGURE 4–4. **Suppression of erythropoiesis by inflammation.** Inflammatory conditions, acute infections, and certain neoplasms are associated with increased blood levels of TNF-α and IL-1, which can suppress erythropoietin production and marrow BFU-E/CFU-E proliferation. Hepcidin, a peptide produced by the liver in response to IL-6 and other inflammatory signals, also plays a major role by suppressing iron absorption and recirculation from reticuloendothelial cells.

Chronic Inflammatory States: The Anemia of Chronic Disease

Any disease state with a major inflammatory component will be accompanied by a hypoproliferative anemia. Moreover, the erythropoietic profile of that anemia will be typical of an inflammatory cytokine–induced defect (see Table 4–1). However, when an inflammatory state is present for a long period, the **anemia of chronic disease can take on some of the manifestations of iron deficiency.** The smear becomes mildly microcytic (mean cell volume [MCV] 75–85 fL) and hypochromic as the hemoglobin falls to levels below 10 g/dL. At the same time, the reticulocyte response continues to be well below that expected for the severity of the anemia, the E/G ratio does not increase, and the serum iron studies show the typical pattern of low serum iron, low TIBC, and elevated serum ferritin level. Moreover, patients with severe, chronic inflammatory states often show an apparent increase in the stainable amounts of iron in a marrow aspirate (Figure 4–5).

The patient with **active rheumatoid arthritis** is a prime example of a disease state that can lead to a severe inflammatory anemia (anemia of chronic disease) with hemoglobin levels below 8–10 g/dL, MCVs in the low-normal to microcytic range, and iron studies typical of a marked inflammatory block in iron supply (low serum iron and low TIBC). TNF-α may play a major role in the pathogenesis of the anemia of rheumatoid arthritis. TNF-α–mediated apoptotic depletion of $CD34^+$ precursors is apparent in marrow cultures from active rheumatoid patients and is reversed by the addition of anti–TNF-α antibody. At the same time, interference with iron supply (increased hepcidin levels) and decreased erythropoietin stimulation of erythroid precursors appears to play the most critical role clinically. Patients with the anemia of chronic disease generally have suboptimal levels of erythropoietin in circulation and, despite their defects in precursor growth and iron supply, can respond to treatment with recombinant erythropoietin.

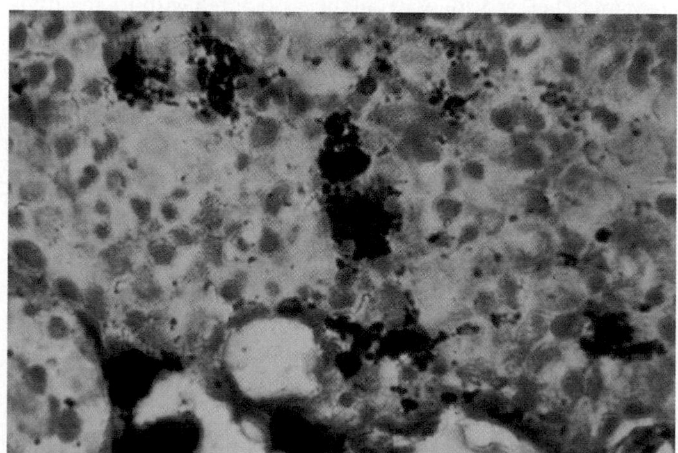

FIGURE 4–5. Increased levels of hepcidin in inflammatory anemias reduce the export of iron from reticuloendothelial cells to the circulation, resulting in an increase in hemosiderin iron as readily seen on Prussian blue stain of a marrow aspirate particle.

Unlike adult rheumatoid arthritis, **juvenile rheumatoid arthritis** patients present with a severe microcytic anemia, low serum iron, and elevated ferritin levels associated with elevated serum erythropoietin and sTfR levels, and respond well to intravenous iron. The explanation for this appears to be an excessive production of IL-6 resulting in enhanced ferritin synthesis and liver iron uptake, and a severe block in reticuloendothelial iron release without the other components of an inflammatory anemia (anemia of chronic disease).

Patients with AIDS demonstrate a hypoproliferative anemia in association with progression of their disease and complicating bacterial infections. Early on, the characteristics of the anemia are those of the anemia of chronic disease, although the severity of the anemia is often made worse by zidovudine therapy, so that the patient becomes transfusion dependent. Later in the course of the disease, HIV involvement of marrow precursor cells can produce a severe marrow damage picture. This process may be recognized from the appearance of a marked pancytopenia. Measurement of the serum erythropoietin level may also help distinguish between the 2 types of anemia and has been used as a guide to therapy. Patients with AIDS who have low serum erythropoietin levels typical of a chronic inflammatory anemia (<500 IU/L) can be expected to respond to treatment with recombinant erythropoietin.

The Anemia of Renal Disease

Severe renal disease is almost always accompanied by a **failure of the normal erythropoietin response**. As with other hypoproliferative anemias, the **erythropoietic profile** is characterized by normocytic, normochromic morphology; a normal MCV; a low reticulocyte count; and an absence of polychromasia on the peripheral blood smear. The severity of the anemia correlates with the severity of the renal failure. Acute loss of renal function as with acute tubular necrosis is associated with the rapid development of a moderately severe anemia, with hemoglobin levels of 7–9 g/dL. Progressive renal failure with a BUN in excess of 50 mg/dL, serum creatinine above 3 mg/dL, and creatinine clearances below 30% of normal is associated with increasingly severe anemia (hemoglobin levels below 7 g/dL). This situation reflects the added impact of marked nitrogen retention on red blood cell survival; patients with end-stage renal disease and untreated uremia also show significant reductions in red blood cell lifespan.

There are clinical situations where the erythropoietin response and the loss of renal function do not correlate. One example is the patient with diabetes mellitus, where the severity of the anemia can be greater than that predicted by measurements of the BUN and creatinine. Patients with diabetes have a moderately severe hypoproliferative anemia relatively early in the evolution of their renal disease. An even more striking dissociation of erythropoietin production from renal function is seen in patients with **hemolytic-uremic syndrome.** They present with severe uremia requiring dialysis but are able to respond to an increased rate of red blood cell destruction with an increase in red blood cell production typical of a hemolytic anemia (see Chapter 11). This situation is one where, despite glomerular-tubular damage, peritubular interstitial cells are preserved.

Iron studies are important both in the diagnosis and management of a patient with renal disease anemia. Early in the evolution of the anemia, the serum iron, TIBC, and serum ferritin levels should all be normal (see Table 4–1). This is of value in the differential diagnosis of the renal disease anemia by helping to rule out iron-deficiency anemia or an inflammatory state. Repeated studies are important to patient management. Patients can develop iron deficiency at any time secondary to blood loss, especially if they are receiving chronic hemodialysis. At the same time, if repeated transfusions are required, they are at risk for progressive iron overload. It is especially important to monitor the patient's iron status whenever recombinant erythropoietin therapy is used to correct the anemia of renal disease. The appearance of iron deficiency during the course of erythropoietin therapy is a primary cause of therapeutic failure.

Hypometabolic States

Modest falls in the hemoglobin level are seen with protein starvation and endocrine deficiency states. In both situations, the anemia appears to be secondary to a reduced erythropoietin response that is appropriate for the reduction in tissue metabolism. **Kidney sensor cells,** which measure oxygen delivery according to their metabolic rate, appear to downregulate erythropoietin production because of their lower oxygen requirement.

A. Protein Deprivation

The **hypoproliferative anemia of protein deprivation is mild**, a 1–3 g/dL reduction in the hemoglobin level. However, in the markedly marasmic individual, the severity of the anemia may be masked by a simultaneous reduction in the patient's plasma volume and total blood volume. This situation is revealed when the patient is fed. As the production of albumin recovers, the plasma volume expands, which results in a further drop in the hemoglobin level. Poor protein nutrition without calorie deprivation has been considered as a possible cause of mild hypoproliferative anemias in the elderly. However, it is more likely that the patient is suffering from an inflammatory anemia, iron or vitamin deficiency, renal failure, or early-onset myelodysplasia (see Chapter 12).

The **erythropoietic profile** of these patients is typical of a hypoproliferative anemia secondary to reduced erythropoietin stimulation. Cell indices and morphology are normal, the reticulocyte count is not increased above basal levels, and polychromasia is absent on the peripheral blood smear. Since prolonged starvation can also result in iron or vitamin deficiencies, the evaluation should include both **iron studies and measurements of folic acid and vitamin B_{12}**. Rarely, deficiencies in vitamin B_6 and riboflavin can play a role.

B. Endocrine Disorders

Testosterone, thyroid hormone, and parathormone all play roles in the regulation of red blood cell production. Testosterone is responsible for the 1–3 g/dL difference in the hemoglobin level between men and women. Anabolic steroids in general are capable of enhancing the erythropoietin stimulation of erythroid precursors. Estrogen administration or castration results in a fall in the hemoglobin level by as much as 2 g/dL.

Hypothyroidism and pituitary deficiency are associated with a modest anemia (hemoglobin levels of 10–12 g/dL). The anemia has all the characteristics of a hypoproliferative anemia secondary to reduced erythropoietin stimulation. The severity of the anemia is usually a good reflection of the severity of the hypometabolic state; the more myxedematous the patient, the lower the hemoglobin level. Iron and folate deficiency can also be present, since patients with markedly hypothyroid conditions demonstrate malabsorption of iron and folic acid as well as a reduced dietary intake. On occasion, one or another of these deficiencies can result in an erythropoietic profile more typical of a nutritional anemia. However, iron and folate therapy will usually not resolve the anemia unless thyroid replacement is also provided.

In patients with **severe pituitary or adrenal insufficiency (Addison disease),** the severity of the anemia may initially be hidden. This is especially true for patients presenting in addisonian crisis, when the total blood volume and plasma volume are significantly reduced. This obscures the severity of the anemia until the patient receives volume replacement. The patient with severe addisonian features may also demonstrate decreased white blood cell counts (3,000–5,000/μL) and have difficulty mounting a granulocyte response to acute infection.

Patients with **hyperparathyroidism,** often in association with renal disease, may exhibit a mild hypoproliferative anemia. The mechanism involved is not well defined. It has been suggested that parathormone may directly inhibit erythroid progenitor proliferation or cause sclerosis of the marrow cavity. More likely, it relates to the development of renal calcification with interference in erythropoietin production. The anemia does respond to parathyroidectomy.

DIFFERENTIAL DIAGNOSIS

Differential diagnosis of a hypoproliferative anemia secondary to a poor erythropoietin response can be difficult. The milder the anemia is, the harder the task. This can be even more difficult in women where the range of "normal" hemoglobin values extends to levels as low as 11 g/dL. Therefore, as often as not, the nature of the anemia is attributed to the clinical setting. For example, patients with progressive renal disease who present with a mild to moderate anemia are assumed to have the anemia of renal failure, that is, failure of the kidneys' ability to increase erythropoietin production. This can result in a major diagnostic error. Other factors may be playing a role, for example, concurrent iron deficiency, inflammation, an endocrine disorder, or marrow damage. Therefore, a diagnosis can only be reached by excluding other possible etiologies.

Iron studies can be invaluable in detecting even the mildest anemia associated with infection or inflammation and also discriminating between inflammatory anemias (anemia of chronic disease) and iron deficiency. There is, however, an opportunity for confusion when both inflammation and iron deficiency are present in the same patient. This has the potential of preventing the typical fall in serum ferritin seen with iron deficiency or the predicted rise associated with inflammation. Simultaneous measurements of the serum ferritin, sTfR, C-reactive protein, and hemoglobin level should solve this dilemma (Table 4–3). The patient with a pure iron-deficiency anemia will have a ferritin well below 30 μg/L, a normal C-reactive protein, and an elevated log (serum TfR/ferritin) ratio (>2.5). Patients with inflammatory anemias typically have ferritins greater than 100 μg/L, an increased C-reactive protein, and serum TfR/ferritin ratios less than 2.5.

TABLE 4–3 • Iron studies in patients with iron deficiency and/or inflammation

	Iron Deficiency	Both	Inflammation
Serum ferritin (μg/L)	<30	30–100	>100
C-reactive protein	Normal	Increased	Increased
Log (sTfR/ferritin) ratio	>2.5	<2.5	<2.5

When both inflammation and iron deficiency are present, the serum ferritin will generally fall between 30 and 100 μg/L with an elevated C-reactive protein and a serum TfR/ferritin ratio less than 2.5, rising quickly to greater than 2.5 once the inflammation is successfully treated. This is an important point, because undetected iron deficiency or iron store depletion can prevent the resolution of an anemia after treatment of an inflammatory condition. Therefore, it is good practice to repeat the measurements of iron status during the treatment of any patient who may have a dual abnormality.

Pregnancy

Pregnancy can make the diagnosis of a hypoproliferative anemia much more difficult. Although the red blood cell mass increases during the second and third trimesters of pregnancy, the plasma volume expands to an even greater extent, which results in a fall in the hemoglobin level. This situation has been referred to as the "physiologic anemia" of pregnancy, even though it is not a true anemia. The pregnant woman's oxygen delivery capabilities are actually supernormal.

The physiologic reduction in hemoglobin during pregnancy can mask other types of anemia. Iron and folic acid deficiency are common during pregnancy and can result in hemoglobin falls of 1–3 g/dL without changes in cell morphology. Mild inflammatory conditions and renal damage also can be responsible for a reduced hemoglobin level. As a general rule, a **hemoglobin level below 10 g/dL during pregnancy should be carefully evaluated** for a treatable cause for the anemia. When the hemoglobin level is between 10 and 13 g/dL, it is hard to distinguish true anemia from a physiologic change in the hemoglobin level. Therefore, routine prophylaxis with oral iron and folic acid is recommended as a preventive measure during pregnancy.

CASE HISTORY • *Part 3*

The pattern of the iron studies (low serum iron; low iron-binding capacity, % saturation below 15%; and normal to slightly elevated serum ferritin) is characteristic of an inflammatory anemia. Given the right history, additional studies, including bone marrow aspiration, are not necessary. In this case, the patient's history and physical examination suggest a diagnosis of polymyalgia rheumatica or temporal arteritis and a temporal artery biopsy may help confirm the latter diagnosis.

If there is the possibility of confusion between an inflammatory anemia diagnosis and iron deficiency, a measurement of the serum transferrin receptor and a bone marrow aspirate to assess iron stores can help with the differential. The patient with inflammatory anemia will show a normal or only slightly elevated serum transferrin receptor, a serum TfR to ferritin ratio of less than 2.5, and prominent iron stores, while iron deficiency dramatically increases the transferrin receptor level, resulting in a serum TfR/ferritin ratio well above 3–4. The ferritin level with iron-deficiency anemia is very low and marrow stores are absent.

The treatment of an inflammatory anemia is basically the treatment of the underlying inflammatory disease. An acute inflammatory anemia associated with a bacterial infection will resolve with effective antibiotic therapy. In a patient with polymyalgia rheumatica, treatment with prednisone and/or immunosuppressive therapy will rapidly correct the anemia. In fact, the hematocrit/hemoglobin response has been used to measure overall improvement from corticosteroids.

THERAPY

The management of a hypoproliferative anemia will obviously vary according to the patient's primary disorder. There is also the issue of severity. Patients with mild to moderate anemia (hemoglobin levels greater than 9–10 g/dL) tolerate it quite well. Unless they are elderly or have significant cardiovascular disease, they maintain good exercise tolerance and a general sense of well-being. Although effective, **transfusion therapy** carries a finite risk of complications, including transmission of infections, alloimmunization, and iron overload. **Erythropoietin therapy,** although effective in selected situations, is expensive.

When **hypoproliferative anemia is severe,** accurate diagnosis is very important. Even when the anemia is clearly related to a primary disorder such as end-stage renal disease, **iron studies** still need to be performed to rule out combination anemias and plan therapy. The presence of iron deficiency in a patient with renal anemia will effectively prevent a response to recombinant erythropoietin. In the case of the anemia of inflammatory disease, the best cure is the effective treatment of the inflammatory condition. With acute bacterial infections, the anemia will resolve spontaneously with effective antibiotic therapy. In the case of chronic inflammatory disorders such as rheumatoid arthritis, treatment with anti-inflammatory drugs will often result in an increase in the hemoglobin level. Recombinant erythropoietin therapy has been approved for use in the treatment of patients with HIV and as an adjunct to chemotherapy in patients with cancer to reduce transfusion requirements.

Transfusion Support

Severe hypoproliferative anemias that are not expected to respond to either disease-specific therapy or erythropoietin administration will need to be transfused. Amounts of blood required and frequency of transfusion must be determined by carefully following the patient's response to each transfusion. **Younger patients** will usually tolerate hemoglobin levels of 7–8 g/dL, even though their exercise tolerance is somewhat reduced. **Older patients** will need to be transfused to hemoglobin levels of 10–11 g/dL. Each unit of packed red blood cells should increase the hemoglobin by approximately 1 g/dL (hematocrit by 3%–4%). The frequency of transfusion will depend on the patient's own level of red blood cell production. Transfusions can usually be scheduled at intervals of weeks or even months.

When patients receive **multiple transfusions,** they are at risk for alloimmunization and iron overload. However, in contrast to patients with aplastic anemia who have much higher transfusion requirements, sufficient iron overload to produce tissue damage is rarely seen. To avoid the severe fever and chills associated with cytokine release by white cells or an alloimmune reaction or both, patients requiring multiple units of red blood cells over a prolonged period should receive **leukocyte-reduced red blood cells** (see Chapter 38).

Erythropoietin Therapy

Recombinant erythropoietin therapy has become the standard treatment in patients with end-stage renal disease with severe anemia. It has proved effective in both predialysis and dialysis patients. Three recombinant erythropoietins are currently approved by the US Food and Drug Administration (FDA): **epoetin alfa** (Procrit, Epogen); **epoetin beta** (Recormon); and **darbepoetin alfa** (Aranesp). Their principle difference is their half-lives following injection—20.5, 24, and 48 hours, respectively.

A number of newer erythropoiesis-stimulating agents (ESAs) are under development and are currently being tested. **Epoetin**

delta (Dynepo) is the first human cell line–derived erythropoietin and is approved for use in renal patients in Europe but not the United States. **Continuous erythropoietin activator** (CERA) is a modified EPO molecule with different binding characteristics to the EPO receptor and a greatly prolonged half-life of approximately 130 hours. It can be given at intervals of 2–4 weeks. **Hematide** (Affymax) is a mimetic peptide (a short-chain amino acid peptide that has EPO-like activity) with a very long half-life. Early studies have shown sustained increases in the hemoglobin levels in both renal disease and cancer patients when Hematide was administered subcutaneously once every 3 weeks.

An interesting class of ESAs is the hypoxia-inducible factor (HIF) prolyl hydroxylase inhibitors that increase the levels of HIF-1. These agents appear to act to increase EPO synthesis, even in patients with little or no renal function, by way of preventing HIF-α degradation. This suggests that disturbed oxygen sensing, not outright destruction of EPO-producing cells of the kidney, plays a significant role in the anemia of renal disease. A number of such agents are under development. They have a potential advantage of being orally administered.

A. Anemia of Renal Disease

Recombinant erythropoietin, epoetin alpha (Epogen, Procrit), can be administered either intravenously or subcutaneously in doses of 10–300 U/kg 3 times per week. **A typical starting dose** is 50–150 U/kg given 3 times each week. The drug is supplied in single-use vials of 2,000, 4,000, and 10,000 U of erythropoietin, and dosages should be adjusted to use the entire vial and avoid wastage. The comparable dosage of darbepoetin alfa is 0.45 μg/kg, given once a week.

At the beginning of therapy, a **CBC must be performed at least once each week** to determine the rate of rise of the hemoglobin (hematocrit). The rise should not exceed 1 g/dL (4% hematocrit rise) over 2 weeks. This will help prevent complications such as exacerbation of the patient's hypertension or induction of seizures. At the same time, an adjustment in coexistent hypertensive medications is usually needed during the early treatment phase with erythropoietin.

Once the hemoglobin level approaches 10 g/dL, the dose of erythropoietin must be reduced to avoid a rise to levels in excess of 12 g/dL (hematocrit 35%). This will involve frequent follow-up visits with measurements of CBC and serum iron and ferritin levels. The **final maintenance dose for renal patients can vary from as little as 10 U/kg to more than 300 U/kg.** The average maintenance dose is close to 75 U/kg 3 times per week. If a patient does not respond, the dose of erythropoietin should be increased by increments of 25–50 U/kg at monthly intervals up to a level of 300 U/kg. Some patients will require both the higher dose and several months of treatment before they will respond.

Iron deficiency, even a relatively poor supply of iron, can block the response. Therefore, **all patients must be evaluated prior to therapy to determine iron store status and then monitored repeatedly** during therapy to detect exhaustion of iron stores. Patients with serum ferritin levels below 200 μg/L (or below 400 μg/L when the percent saturation is less than 20%) should be considered for iron loading prior to therapy with 1 or more injections of intravenous iron dextran (INFeD) (see Chapter 5). Maintenance iron dextran therapy in patients receiving dialysis can reduce the amount of erythropoietin needed by up to 46%, demonstrating the close relationship between iron supply levels and the erythropoietic response. As a general guideline, parenteral iron should be administered to maintain the serum ferritin above 100 μg/L as long as the C-reactive protein is normal and above 200–300 μg/L when C-reactive protein is elevated.

Sodium ferric gluconate (Ferrlecit) and iron sucrose (Venofer) given in approximately 100-mg doses by intravenous push at the time of dialysis are reasonable alternatives to iron dextran therapy and carry less risk of acute or delayed reactions (see Chapter 5). Oral iron therapy with 1 tablet of oral iron 3–4 times per day can be used, although this will usually not provide sufficient iron to match the requirements generated by higher-dose erythropoietin therapy.

The National Kidney Foundation has published guidelines for the treatment of the anemia of chronic renal failure. Recommendations regarding iron therapy include the following:

- To achieve target hematocrit levels of 33%–36%, **sufficient iron** should be administered to maintain a transferrin saturation greater than 20% and a ferritin greater than 200 μg/L.
- **In patients who have a poor response to erythropoietin**, it may be necessary to maintain higher transferrin saturation and ferritin levels (saturations of up to 50% and ferritin levels as high as 400–800 μg/L).
- **Patients receiving hemodialysis** will almost certainly require intravenous iron therapy on a regular basis (50–100 mg once or twice per week) to avoid functional iron deficiency; oral iron will not be sufficient.

Infection with the release of inflammatory cytokines will inhibit red blood cell production, necessitating higher erythropoietin doses to overcome both the inhibition of erythropoietin and the block in iron supply. To help control the high costs of replacement therapy, it may make sense to discontinue erythropoietin during periods of acute inflammatory illness. Often, the patient's anemia will worsen despite erythropoietin treatment, requiring a reinstitution of periodic red blood cell transfusions. Other factors that may affect the response to erythropoietin in the patient receiving hemodialysis include aluminum toxicity, secondary hyperparathyroidism with marrow fibrosis, carnitine deficiency, and the use of angiotensin enzyme inhibitors.

B. AIDS

Erythropoietin therapy has been approved for treatment of patients with AIDS, especially those receiving zidovudine (AZT) therapy. Erythropoietin therapy will help counteract the erythroid marrow defect induced by AZT. Responses are also observed in patients who exhibit inflammatory-type anemias with low serum erythropoietin levels. However, patients with high serum erythropoietin levels (>500 IU/L) or advanced marrow damage do less well.

C. Cancer-Related Anemia

Erythropoietin therapy can also reduce transfusion requirements in patients with cancer-related anemia and improve quality-of-life measures such as energy and activity levels. Up to 50% of patients with myeloma will demonstrate a poor erythropoietin response before chemotherapy or with the onset of advanced disease. Most of these respond to epoetin alpha given in doses of 150–250 IU/kg 3 times a week, or once a week in larger doses of 40,000–60,000 U. Darbepoetin, an erythropoietin analog with 2 additional N-linked carbohydrate side chains with additional sialic acid residues, has a prolonged half-life of more than 40 hours after subcutaneous injection. It can be given in doses of 1–4.5 μg/kg every 2 weeks with equivalent results. The same may be true for patients with Hodgkin and non-Hodgkin lymphomas. Patients with solid tumors receiving chemotherapy can show a statistically significant change in hematocrit, a decrease in transfusion requirement, and an improved quality of life when treated weekly with epoetin or every 2 weeks with darbepoetin. There is a question, however, whether long-term survival is negatively impacted in certain cancer patients. Also, the expense of overuse in patients with less severe anemia is considerable, resulting in more stringent guidelines.

D. Allogeneic Bone Marrow Transplantation

Erythropoietin has also been used to speed the recovery of red blood cell production after allogeneic bone marrow transplantation.

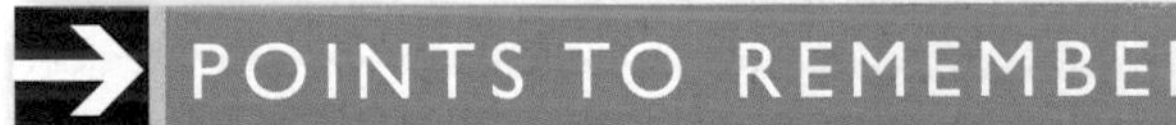

Anemias associated with a "reduced erythropoietin response" are routinely seen in patients with inflammatory illnesses, renal disease, and hypometabolic states. They are physiologically classified as hypoproliferative anemias with normal red blood cell morphology and indices, a below normal reticulocyte response for the severity of the anemia, and an absence of polychromasia on smear (suggestive of a failed erythropoietin response).

Acute and chronic inflammatory (anemia of chronic disease) anemias are the most common anemias seen in clinical practice.

The physiological mechanisms behind the anemia of inflammation are several, including direct suppression of erythroid progenitor growth, a failure of the erythropoietin response by the kidney, and IL-6 stimulation of hepcidin production resulting in a reduced iron supply to the marrow.

Renal disease and progressive renal failure are associated with a loss of erythropoietin-producing cells and a moderate to severe hypoproliferative anemia according to the degree of renal failure.

Hypothyroidism, pituitary/adrenal failure, and protein starvation are associated with a mild hypoproliferative anemia, which appears to be appropriate for the severity of the hypometabolic state (reduced oxygen demand).

Distinctive patterns of serum iron studies can usually distinguish between the anemia of inflammation, the anemia associated with renal or thyroid disease, and absolute iron deficiency.

The anemia of inflammation will resolve once the underlying inflammatory illness is effectively treated. The anemia of severe renal disease, especially in patients on chronic dialysis, involves long-term maintenance on erythropoietin and iron supplementation. A hypoproliferative anemia secondary to hypothyroidism will respond to thyroid replacement therapy.

When a patient fails to fully correct an anemia associated with inflammation or thyroid disease, a repeat evaluation is needed to rule out a previously undetected iron or vitamin deficiency.

BIBLIOGRAPHY

Cazzola M et al: Defective iron supply for erythropoiesis and adequate endogenous erythropoietin production in the anemia associated with systemic-onset juvenile chronic arthritis. Blood 1996;87:4824.

Cook JD et al: The quantitative assessment of body iron. Blood 2003;101:3359.

Drueke TB et al: Management of iron deficiency in renal anemia: guidelines for the optimal therapeutic approach in erythropoietin-treated patients. Clin Nephrol 1997;48:1.

Ganz T: Hepcidin, a key regulator of iron metabolism and mediator of anemia of inflammation. Blood 2003;102:783.

Krantz SB: Erythropoietin. Blood 1991;77:419.

Lee GR: The anemia of chronic disease. Semin Hematol 1983;20:61.

Malope BI et al: The ratio of serum transferrin receptor and serum ferritin in the diagnosis of iron status. Br J Haematol 2001;115:84.

Means RT, Krantz SB: Progress in understanding the pathogenesis of the anemia of chronic disease. Blood 1992;80:1639.

Nemeth E et al: Hepcidin, a putative mediator of anemia of inflammation, is a type II acute-phase protein. Blood 2003; 101:2461.

Nissenson AR, Miner SD, Wolcott DL: Recombinant human erythropoietin and renal anemia: molecular biology, clinical efficacy, and nervous system effects. Ann Intern Med 1991;114:402.

Weinstein DA et al: Inappropriate expression of hepcidin is associated with iron refractory anemia: implications for the anemia of chronic disease. Blood 2002;100:3776.

Wrighting DM, Andrews NC: Interleukin-6 induces hepcidin expression through STAT3. Blood 2006;108:3204.

IRON-DEFICIENCY ANEMIA · 5

CASE HISTORY • *Part I*

A 43-year-old woman presents with complaints of increasing fatigue, exercise intolerance, and difficulty swallowing. She also reports palpitations and shortness of breath when climbing stairs. She has a past history of fibromyalgia for more than a decade, managed with liberal doses of aspirin and nonsteroidal preparations. She also reports prolonged and irregular menstrual periods for the last 6 months. Examination is notable for pallor of the conjunctiva and mucous membranes; a beefy, red, smooth tongue; and flattened nails. She has considerable tenderness to palpation of the muscles of the neck and shoulders and restricted motion of both shoulders.

CBC: Hematocrit/hemoglobin - 21%/6 g/dL
MCV - 67 fL MCH - 24 pg/cell MCHC - 28 g/dL
Reticulocyte count/index - 3.0%/<1
White blood cell count - Normal
Platelet count - 720,000/μL
Sedimentation rate - 42 mm/h
(Westergren) Stool hemoccult - Brown
stool/4+ heme positive

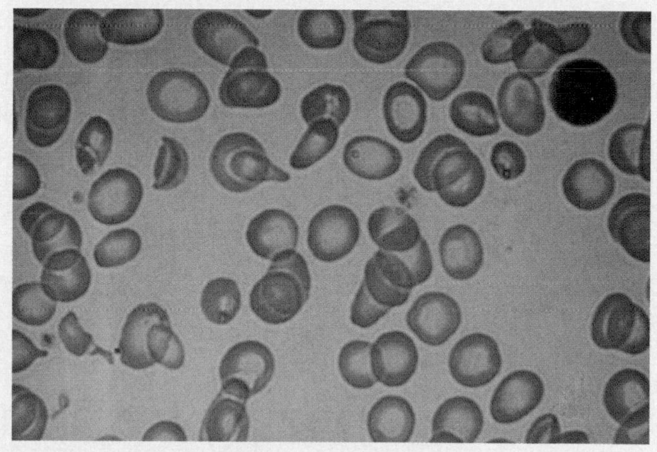

Questions

- How should this anemia be described?
- What is the differential diagnosis?
- What other tests should be ordered?

Iron deficiency is a leading cause of microcytic anemia in children and adults. When iron supply to the erythroid marrow is deficient, red blood cell production is impaired and new cells released into circulation are poorly hemoglobinized. The severity of the anemia and the degree of microcytosis and hypochromia generally reflect the severity and chronicity of the iron-deficiency state.

The prevalence of iron deficiency in a population depends on the interaction of several factors, including the adequacy of dietary iron supply and the incidence of disease states, which are accompanied by malabsorption or chronic blood loss. In developing countries, inadequate nutrition is a major factor and iron deficiency is the principal cause of nutritional anemia. In Europe and the United States, by contrast, chronic blood loss is more frequently responsible for an iron-deficiency anemia.

NORMAL IRON METABOLISM

Iron is an essential component in the synthesis of hemoglobin, myoglobin, and several heme and metalloflavoprotein enzymes. It also plays a direct role in governing erythropoiesis by influencing the cell cycle of proliferating red blood cell precursors. A fall in iron supply to the marrow is associated with a fall in cyclin D1 protein and an arrest of erythroid precursors in the G_1/S phase, thereby decreasing the proliferative response to erythropoietin.

Iron Loss

Iron is highly conserved in humans. Still, enough is lost to require absorption of between 1 and 4 mg of elemental iron from the diet each day to maintain normal iron balance. The intestine responds to negative iron balance by increasing the efficiency of transport. At the same time, the intestine can virtually shut off transport once stores of iron exceed metabolic requirements.

Iron Transport

Once absorbed, iron binds to a specific plasma protein, transferrin, which transports it to tissues (Figure 5–1). At any moment, about 3 mg of iron is in circulation bound to transferrin. This pool turns over 10 times each day, with a predominant portion of the iron (ie, 25–30 mg) going to the erythroid marrow. Maturing erythroid precursors express transferrin receptors (TfR) on the cell surface, which bind diferric iron-laden transferrin. Aggregate iron-TfR complexes are then incorporated into the erythroid cell in intracytoplasmic endosomes. The iron is released and the transferrin-TfR complex returns to the cell surface, where the transferrin molecule reenters the plasma. The free iron within the endosomes is then reduced by a ferrireductase (STEAP3) to Fe^{2+} and exported into the cytosol via DMT1, a key transmembrane transporter, for incorporation into heme or storage as ferritin. Heme synthesis also requires transport of the free iron into the mitochondria via a second transporter, mitoferrin.

The end result of this pathway is incorporation of 80%–90% of the iron into the hemoglobin of new erythrocytes that then have a lifespan of 100–120 days. The process of new red cell production is not perfect; 10%–20% of precursor red blood cells are destroyed by marrow reticuloendothelial cells prior to release. In addition, about 1% of the red blood cells in circulation are destroyed each day as they reach the end of their lifespan. Together, these 2 processes result in the recovery of 25–30 mg of iron each day by the reticuloendothelial cells of the marrow and spleen. This iron can then be transported back to the marrow by transferrin for new cell production.

Hepcidin, a liver-produced peptide, plays a major role in regulating the release of iron from reticuloendothelial cells by inducing the degradation of ferroportin, the sole transport protein on both duodenal and reticuloendothelial cells. Hepcidin gene expression is in part regulated by erythropoietin. Therefore, with anemia or hypoxia and the resulting rise in erythropoietin levels, hepcidin production is downregulated, allowing an increase in iron absorption and release from reticuloendothelial cells. The resulting increase in iron supply to the marrow is essential for a normal proliferative response.

An iron-transport pathway to parenchymal tissues is also shown in Figure 5–1. Approximately 6 mg of iron is delivered to other tissues each day, especially the liver, where it is incorporated into ferritin stores or used in iron-containing enzymes. At least 1 mg each day is required to replace the iron lost in cells desquamated from the skin, and both the gastrointestinal and urinary tracts.

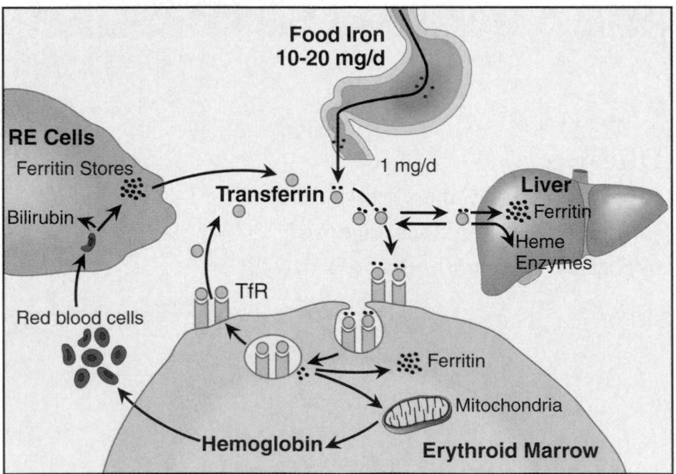

FIGURE 5–1. **Iron transport pathways.** Iron absorbed from food and iron recovered from senescent red blood cells is transported by transferrin to the marrow and tissues. The iron-laden transferrin binds to transferrin receptors (TfR) on the surface of erythroid precursors. It is then internalized, at which time the iron is released for use in hemoglobin production. The transferrin-TfR complex is then returned to the surface of the cell and the transferrin is released to complete the cycle. Hepcidin, a small peptide produced by the liver in response to oxygen supply, iron balance, and the level of erythropoiesis, regulates iron absorption and the return of iron from the reticuloendothelial cells to transferrin.

Body Iron Content

The impact of these variables on body iron content is summarized in Table 5–1. Normal adult males have a total body iron content of close to 4,000 mg, including 500–1,000 mg of hepatic and reticuloendothelial iron stores. Because of menstrual blood loss and a lower dietary iron intake, adolescents and adult women have significantly lower amounts of storage iron (usually <200 mg).

Ferritin and Transferrin Receptor Levels

The intracellular balance of iron needed for heme production is controlled by 2 highly regulated iron-regulated proteins

TABLE 5–1 • Body iron content

	Adult—Male (80 kg) (mg)	Adult—Female (60 kg) (mg)
Hemoglobin	2,500	1,700
Myoglobin and enzymes	500	300
Serum iron	3	3
Iron stores	500–1,000	0–200

(IRP-1 and -2) and an mRNA, noncoding iron-responsive element (IRE). The IRE/IRP regulatory system controls ferritin production and TfR expression. When iron is scarce, IRP-1 binds to the mRNA IRE and inhibits ferritin synthesis. When abundant, IRP binding is inhibited and ferritin production increases. The opposite is true for TfR; low iron induces receptor expression, whereas high iron allows more rapid mRNA degradation and reduced levels of TfR. Together, this guarantees the delivery of optimal amounts of iron for heme production and immediate storage of any excess as ferritin.

Serum Transferrin Receptor

Transferrin receptor is shed from the membrane of red blood cell precursors and other cells during development and circulates as a monomeric fragment bound to transferrin. A measurement of the serum transferrin receptor (sTfR) level will reflect the patient's iron status. Patients with iron deficiency show serum sTfR levels of 2–4 times normal. This reflects both an increased expression of TfR on the surface of red cell precursors and, as the anemia worsens, a proliferation of red cell precursors.

Serum Ferritin Level

While most ferritin is stored in reticuloendothelial cells, a small, but proportional, amount is glycosylated and released into circulation. Why this occurs is unclear, but the serum level has been used clinically to assess iron stores (Figure 5–2). Each microgram per liter of serum ferritin roughly correlates to 8–10 mg of tissue stores. Children, adolescents, and menstruating women typically have ferritin levels of 20–50 μg/L (200–500 mg of iron stores), whereas adult men and postmenopausal women have levels of 50–200 μg/L (500–2,000 mg of iron stores), depending on their age and level of dietary iron. With iron deficiency leading to exhaustion of body iron stores, the serum ferritin level falls to levels below 15 μg/L. Iron overload can produce ferritin levels of 300 μg/L to more than 1,000 μg/L. The ratio of the sTfR to the serum ferritin—log (serum TfR/ferritin ratio)—has been advanced as a more quantitative method for estimating total body iron stores in populations at risk for iron deficiency. However, just as with the serum ferritin level, the serum TfR/ ferritin ratio can be distorted by inflammation or liver disease.

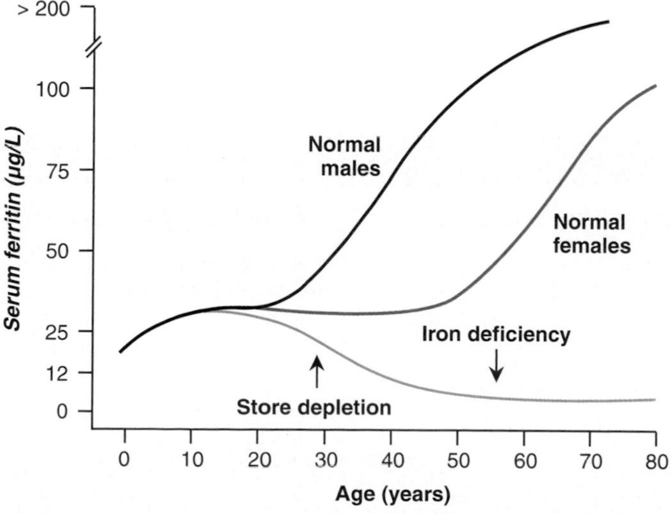

FIGURE 5–2. **Serum ferritin levels.** The serum ferritin level correlates with the level of iron stores. Ferritin levels in both sexes are less than 50 μg/L throughout childhood. Adult males and females demonstrate different normal ranges of values based on their levels of iron intake and loss. Iron store depletion and iron deficiency are accompanied by a fall in the serum ferritin level to below 15–20 μg/L.

Hepcidin

Hepcidin (HAMP) is a cysteine-rich antimicrobial peptide produced by the liver in response to iron balance, oxygen supply, and the level of erythropoiesis (erythropoietin). It plays a key role in governing iron absorption and the recirculation of iron from reticuloendothelial cells. Elevated levels of hepcidin are seen in patients with inflammatory anemias, resulting in a block in both iron absorption and iron release from reticuloendothelial stores. Iron deficiency suppresses hepcidin production, and thereby increases both iron absorption and recirculation of storage iron.

IRON NUTRITION

Iron content of the diet depends on the types of foods eaten and the total daily caloric intake. Meat-derived heme iron is much more available for absorption. Although making up the greater proportion of the daily intake, nonheme vegetable iron is far less bioavailable. Compounds within vegetables, especially phosphates and phytates, inhibit iron absorption to a significant degree. In developed countries, a diet consisting of a balance of meat and vegetable products contains approximately 6 mg of iron per thousand calories. Thus, an adult male ingests between 15 and 20 mg of iron each day, whereas the adult female takes in 10–15 mg.

Adult males and nonmenstruating females with normal dietary habits have little difficulty maintaining normal iron balance. Menstruating females, rapidly growing infants, children, adolescents, and frequent blood donors are at some risk of iron store depletion and may require supplementation to maintain an adequate iron balance. Iron supplementation is almost always required during pregnancy. During the last 2 trimesters, the daily requirement for iron increases to 5–6 mg, a level that cannot be easily attained by diet alone unless it is especially rich in heme iron.

CLINICAL FEATURES

Clinical states of iron deficiency can be classified as iron store depletion, iron-deficient erythropoiesis, or iron-deficiency anemia (Table 5–2). In its mildest form, iron store depletion results simply from an imbalance between normal physiologic demands, such as rapid growth and menstrual blood loss versus dietary iron intake. More severe iron deficiency with limitation of red blood cell production is usually the result of protracted blood loss from

TABLE 5–2 • Causes of iron deficiency

Iron Store Depletion	Iron-Deficient Erythropoiesis	Iron-Deficiency Anemia
Inadequate diet	Excessive menses	Chronic blood loss
Rapid growth	Pregnancy	Varices
Infancy	Acute hemorrhage	Peptic ulcer disease
Adolescence	Malabsorption	Large-bowel tumors
Normal menses	Gastrectomy	Diverticulitis
Blood donation	Regional enteritis	Angiodysplasia
	Inflammation	Intravascular hemolysis
	Acute infections	Hookworm infestation
	Chronic inflammatory states	Severe malabsorption
	Polycythemia vera treated with phlebotomy	Postgastrectomy
		Sprue
		Regional enteritis

the gastrointestinal tract or uterus. Less frequently, the cause is malabsorption secondary to small intestinal disease or gastric surgery. Iron deficiency with marked anemia and microcytosis is seen in patients with severe malabsorption or chronic blood loss.

Iron store depletion and iron-deficient erythropoiesis are not associated with any distinctive clinical findings. The symptoms and signs of severe iron deficiency are primarily those of severe anemia. Patients complain of fatigue and exercise intolerance, and may show signs of cardiac decompensation. When patients are iron deficient for a prolonged period, they may complain of a sore mouth, difficulty swallowing, or a tendency for their nails to soften and curl, at times producing a characteristic spooning of the nails (koilonychia). In children, iron deficiency has been associated with learning and behavioral problems.

Laboratory Studies

Accurate diagnosis of an iron-deficiency state requires several laboratory tests (Table 5–3). Measurements of the serum iron, transferrin iron-binding capacity, and the serum ferritin level are of greatest importance and often are enough to make the diagnosis. Other measurements used include direct inspection of marrow reticuloendothelial iron stores using a marrow aspirate, and measurements of the red cell protoporphyrin level and the sTfR to ferritin ratio.

A. Serum Iron Studies

The **serum iron (SI)** is a direct measure of the amount of iron bound to transferrin. A normal individual has an SI of 50–150 μg/dL. The total iron-binding capacity (TIBC) is a measure of the amount of iron that can be bound by transferrin and, therefore, is a surrogate measure of the serum transferrin level. The normal TIBC is 300–360 μg/dL. Together, the SI and TIBC (transferrin level) are used to calculate the percent saturation of transferrin with iron (SI/TIBC = percent saturation). In states of normal iron balance, the percent saturation is between 20% and 50%. When it falls below 20%, the erythroid marrow has difficulty obtaining sufficient iron to support increased levels of erythropoiesis. When the percent saturation exceeds 50%–60%, iron delivery to parenchymal tissues increases, resulting in iron loading of hepatocytes, heart muscle, skin, and pituitary gland.

B. Serum Ferritin

The **serum ferritin** is used to evaluate total body iron stores. Normal adult males have serum ferritin levels of 50–200 μg/L. This correlates with the 800–1,000 mg or more of tissue iron stores seen in men. As iron stores are depleted, the serum ferritin

TABLE 5–3 • Laboratory studies in iron deficiency

	Iron Store Depletion	Iron-Deficient Erythropoiesis	Iron-Deficiency Anemia
Hemoglobin	Normal	Slight decrease	Marked decrease (microcytic/hypochromic)
Iron stores (mg)	<100 (0–1+)	0	0
Serum iron (μg/dL)	Normal	<60	<40
TIBC (μg/dL)	360–390	>390	>410
% Saturation	20–30	<15	<10
Ferritin (μg/L)	<40	<20	<15
% Sideroblasts	40–60	<10	<10
Red blood cell protoporphyrin (μg/dL RBC)	30	>100	>200

TABLE 5–4 • Measurements of iron stores

Iron Stores	Serum Ferritin (μg/L)	Marrow Iron Stain (0–4+)
0	<15	0
1–300 mg	15–20	1+
300–800 mg	20–50	2+
800–1,000 mg	50–150	3+
>1–2 g	150–300	4+
Iron overload	>500	4+ or more

falls, eventually reaching levels below 15 μg/L once stores are exhausted and iron-deficient erythropoiesis appears. In iron overload states, serum ferritin can reach levels of several thousand micrograms (Table 5–4).

C. Serum Transferrin-Receptor

An enzyme-linked immunosorbent assay (ELISA) for **serum transferrin receptor (sTfR)** can be used in conjunction with the serum ferritin measurement in diagnosing iron store depletion and defects in iron delivery to the marrow, that is, iron deficiency and the block in iron release from stores seen with inflammation. Levels of sTfR (normal = 5–9 μg/L) increase rapidly as iron stores are exhausted (serum ferritin <40 μg/L). Iron-deficiency anemia is accompanied, therefore, by an elevation of sTfR proportional to the severity of the anemia. However, sTfR levels also increase in association with erythroid precursor proliferation, whether effective or ineffective erythropoiesis, as well as in some patients with myeloproliferative and lymphoproliferative disease. Therefore, a high sTfR level must be interpreted in light of a full evaluation of the underlying marrow abnormality. Patients with inflammatory anemias (the anemia of chronic disease) show near normal serum TfR levels, reflecting their normal to increased reticuloendothelial iron stores and hypoproliferative erythroid marrows. The log (serum TfR/ferritin) ratio is the best discriminator between iron deficiency and inflammation. Low values (<2.5) are typical of an inflammatory anemia (anemia of chronic disease); values greater than 2.5 suggest iron-deficiency anemia.

D. Marrow Iron Stores

The presence of **iron stores** in reticuloendothelial cells can be determined by inspection of a Prussian blue stain of marrow aspirate particles (Figure 5–3). A simple scale of 0–4+ stores has been used to estimate the amount of storage iron (see Figure 2–17). This grading system correlates fairly well with the amount of iron available for erythropoiesis (see Table 5–4 and the discussion of iron store measurements in Chapter 2). It is very reliable for determining the total absence of reticuloendothelial iron stores in patients with iron-deficiency anemia. At the same time, it does not provide as good a measure of total tissue loading as the serum ferritin level. Patients with hereditary hemochromatosis will demonstrate near normal reticuloendothelial stores in the face of marked liver parenchymal cell loading.

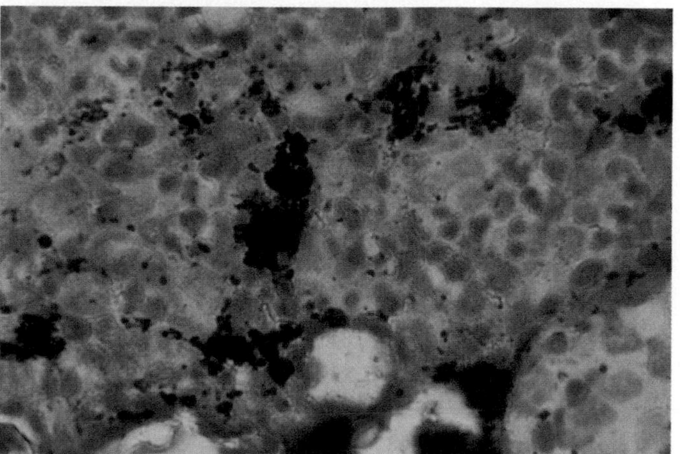

A

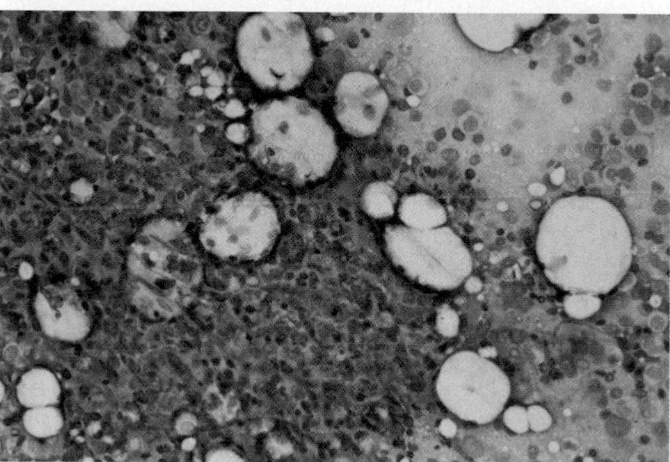

B

FIGURE 5–3. **Reticuloendothelial cell iron storage.** In a patient with abundant iron stores, blue staining particles are visible throughout the reticuloendothelial cells on a Prussian blue stain **(A)**. Iron-deficient patients show no stainable stores **(B)**.

The marrow iron stain has also been used to evaluate delivery of iron to erythroid precursors. Normally, 40%–60% of developing red blood cell precursors has visible, dust-like, iron granules in their cytoplasm, which represents the excess iron not used for hemoglobin production. These cells are referred to as **sideroblasts**. The number of sideroblasts in marrow decreases rapidly when iron supply to the marrow falls, which provides a sensitive but highly qualitative measure of iron-deficient erythropoiesis.

E. Erythrocyte Zinc Protoporphyrin

A measurement of **erythrocyte zinc protoporphyrin** can also be used to detect early iron-deficient erythropoiesis. Intracellular levels of protoporphyrin will increase even before anemia is present. This process is a result of the imbalance between iron supply and the production of protoporphyrin by mitochondria. It is especially useful for detection of iron-deficient erythropoiesis in children since the assay requires extremely small amounts of blood, and the ratio of zinc protoporphyrin to heme can be measured quickly on a portable hematofluorimeter. The average normal red blood cell protoporphyrin is 30 μg/dL of red blood cells. The level rises quickly to values in excess of 100 μg/dL with iron-deficiency anemia. Increased protoporphyrin levels are also seen in children exposed to lead, which inhibits heme synthetase, the enzyme necessary for the final assembly of iron and the protoporphyrin ring required to form heme. Falsely elevated values can also be seen in patients with increased bilirubin levels or on hemodialysis.

F. Reticulocyte Hemoglobin Content

Whereas the mean cell volume (MCV) and mean cell hemoglobin (MCH) are insensitive parameters to iron deficiency because of the slow turnover of circulating red blood cells, the hemoglobin content of reticulocytes (CHr) declines within a few days of the onset of iron-deficient erythropoiesis. However, the CHr has a poor specificity when used as a screening test and only 1 automated counter (Bayer Advia) is currently equipped to make that measurement.

DIAGNOSIS

The diagnosis of an iron-deficiency state is largely a laboratory exercise. As summarized in Table 5–3, iron store depletion, iron-deficient erythropoiesis, and iron-deficiency anemia can be distinguished from one another by a combination of measurements of the hemoglobin, red blood cell morphology, SI, TIBC, serum ferritin, serum TfR, and marrow iron stores.

Iron Store Depletion

Depletion of iron stores is best assessed using the serum ferritin level or a Prussian blue iron stain of aspirated marrow particles. A serum ferritin of less than 40 μg/L or visible iron stores of 1+ or less (<200–300 mg) (or both) suggests iron store depletion. The sTfR/ferritin ratio is an even more sensitive indicator of total body iron and has been used in the evaluation of populations at risk for iron deficiency. In the absence of complicating inflammatory illness, the sTfR/ferritin ratio will begin to rise once the serum ferritin falls below 40 μg/L. In contrast, as long as some iron stores are still present, the SI, TIBC, and hemoglobin level should be normal.

Iron-Deficient Erythropoiesis

Iron-deficient erythropoiesis is also readily diagnosed from the pattern of SI, TIBC, and serum ferritin. The serum ferritin is less than 15 μg/L and the SI falls to levels below 60 μg/dL. This situation is most often accompanied by a rise in the TIBC, which results in a percent saturation of less than 15%. If a marrow aspirate is performed, stainable reticuloendothelial cell iron stores are absent and the number of sideroblasts is markedly reduced.

In the earliest stages of iron-deficient erythropoiesis, the decrease in iron supply impairs the proliferative capacity of the erythroid marrow. Clinically, this situation is expressed as a modest fall in the hemoglobin level to as low as 11–12 g/dL. At the same time, there is little or no change in red blood cell morphology and the MCV and MCH remain normal. It is important that the clinician recognize this fact. With iron-deficient erythropoiesis and early iron-deficiency anemia, red cell morphology/indices are normocytic, normochromic. Microcytosis and hypochromia only appear when the anemia is more severe and has been present for weeks or months.

Iron-Deficiency Anemia

Full-blown **iron-deficiency anemia** is easy to diagnose. The SI is very low and the TIBC high, producing a percent saturation of less than 10% (see Table 5–3). The serum ferritin level is always less than 15 μg/L, the sTfR level is elevated (as is the serum TfR/ferritin ratio), and inspection of marrow aspirate particles reveals absent iron stores and no sideroblasts. Patients with severe iron deficiency also present with a moderate to severe anemia and distinctive changes in red blood cell morphology. Once the hemoglobin falls to below 10–11 g/dL, erythropoietin stimulation of the marrow forces the production of cells that are morphologically abnormal. Initially, the cells are microcytic without abnormalities in cell shape or hemoglobin content. However, as the anemia worsens, new red blood cells become increasingly microcytic and hypochromic (Figure 5–4).

The relationship of cell morphology to the severity of the anemia is illustrated in Figure 5–5. While the hemoglobin level is in the range of 9–11 g/dL, the reduction in cell size is roughly equivalent to the loss of cell hemoglobin, so that cells tend to be uniformly microcytic with little or no hypochromia. There are also modest variations in cell size (anisocytosis) and cell shape (poikilocytosis). As the hemoglobin falls below 9 g/dL, cell morphology becomes increasingly bizarre, with the appearance of many misshapen cells (poikilocytes). This situation is a sign of increasing ineffective erythropoiesis in response to high levels of erythropoietin stimulation. Finally, the presence or absence of cigar- or pencil-shaped red blood cells and target cells (Figure 5–6) can help in the differential diagnosis of iron deficiency from thalassemia. Cigar-shaped cells are typically seen with iron-deficiency anemia, whereas target cells are associated with thalassemia, not iron deficiency.

Determination of the cause of the iron loss is essential to the diagnosis of any iron-deficiency anemia. Because the cause is most often chronic blood loss, symptoms and signs of abnormal bleeding should be sought. If no obvious site of external loss is present, a full evaluation of the gastrointestinal tract for the bleeding site is required. Any prolonged delay in working up the patient can result in a missed opportunity to detect a malignancy while it is still at a treatable stage.

The depth of the evaluation of less severe degrees of iron deficiency depends on the setting. The tenuous nature of iron balance in infants, rapidly growing adolescents, and pregnant women usually makes an exhaustive workup unnecessary. In these situations, a therapeutic trial of iron supplementation is appropriate.

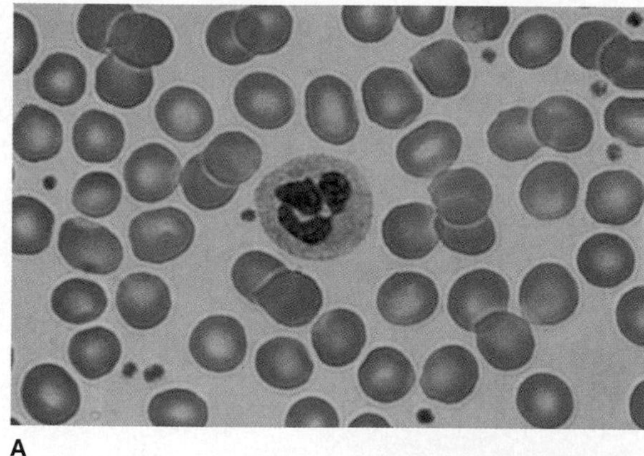
A

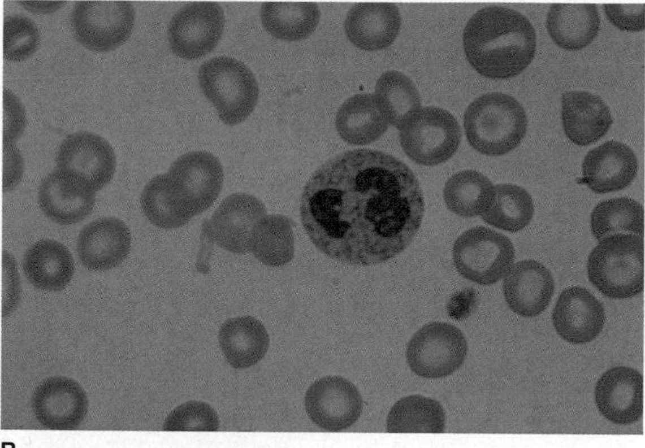
B

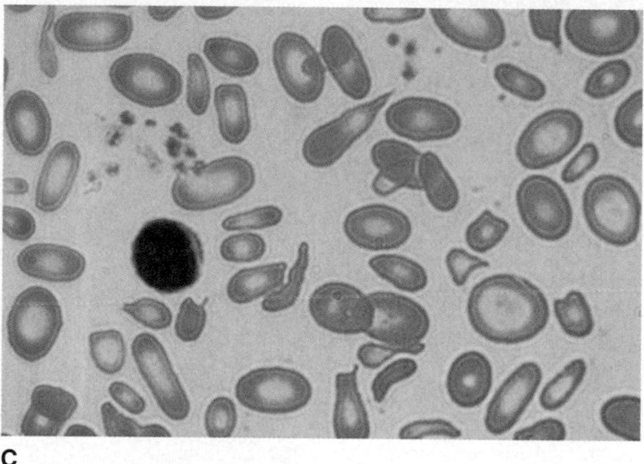
C

FIGURE 5–4. **Smear morphology with iron deficiency.** Depending on the severity and duration of the anemia, the smear in a patient with iron-deficiency anemia can appear to be normocytic and normochromic **(A)**, slightly microcytic with minimal hypochromia and anisocytosis **(B)**, or severely microcytic and hypochromic, with marked aniso- and poikilocytosis **(C)**. In the latter case, the diameter of some red cells may appear to be increased due to the marked deficiency of intracellular hemoglobin, which results in flattening of the cells on smear.

CASE HISTORY • *Part 2*

The patient has a severe microcytic, hypochromic anemia—a hematopoietic profile that fits the class of disorders characterized as defects in cytoplasmic maturation. This class of disorders includes iron deficiency, severe inflammatory anemia, the thalassemias (genetic defects in globin formation), and the inherited form of sideroblastic anemia.

As for the most likely diagnosis, the presence of a smooth, beefy, red tongue; the nail changes; difficulty swallowing; and a positive test for blood in the stools would strongly suggest iron deficiency. Moreover, the absence of target cells on the smear rules against β-thalassemia, and inflammatory anemias rarely get this severe or have MCV levels much below 80 fL.

Tests needed to confirm the diagnosis include, at a minimum, measurements of the serum iron, iron-binding capacity, and serum ferritin. In cases where thalassemia or sideroblastic anemia are likely possibilities, a bone marrow aspirate with Prussian blue staining for cellular storage patterns, and globin analysis (hemoglobin electrophoresis/HPLC to quantitate hemoglobins A_2 and F) are required. In this case the studies showed:

Serum iron - 13 μg/dL	TIBC - 420 μg/dL
% Saturation - 3%	Serum ferritin - 10 μg/L

This pattern is diagnostic for severe iron deficiency.

Questions

- How should the patient be evaluated and treated?
- What factors may interfere with the response?

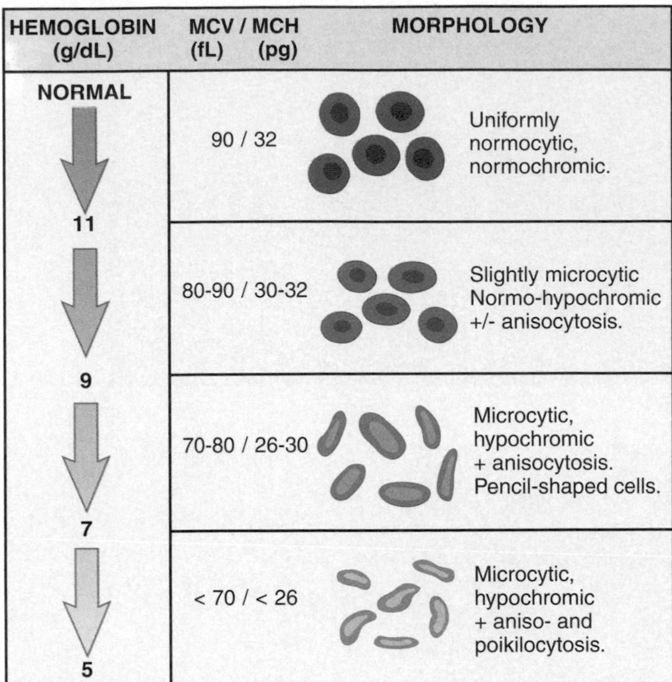

FIGURE 5–5. **Anemia severity and red blood cell morphology.** The appearance of microcytosis and hypochromia in patients with iron deficiency depends on the severity of the anemia. As long as the hemoglobin is above 11–13 g/dL, red blood cells will be normocytic and normochromic. With more severe anemia, new red blood cells will be increasingly microcytic and hypochromic with marked poikilocytosis.

A

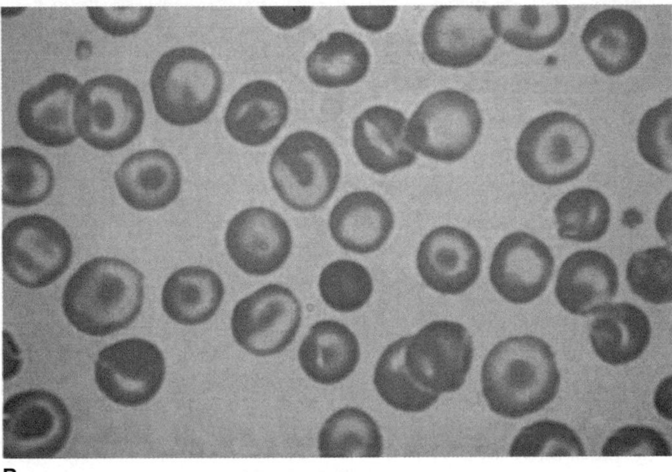

B

FIGURE 5–6. **Cigar-shaped and target cells.** Cigar- or pencil-shaped red cells **(A)** are typically seen with severe iron-deficiency anemia, while targeting **(B)** is commonly seen with thalassemia but not uncomplicated iron deficiency.

However, even the mildest iron deficiency in a male or postmenopausal female should never be dismissed as simple iron imbalance and treated with iron supplements. These patients should always be evaluated for abnormal sites of bleeding.

DIFFERENTIAL DIAGNOSIS

Only a few diseases need to be considered in the differential diagnosis of a microcytic, hypochromic anemia. Congenital defects in globin production (the thalassemias) typically have moderate to severe microcytosis with varying degrees of anemia. An approach to diagnosis of these conditions is discussed in Chapter 6. Unless both conditions are present simultaneously, iron studies and red cell morphology (uniformity of red cell shape, the presence of target or pencil-shaped cells) will clearly separate the 2 entities.

A more common diagnostic dilemma is separating iron-deficient erythropoiesis secondary to iron loss from iron loss that accompanies acute and chronic inflammation. As a part of the inflammatory process, the normal recirculation of iron from reticuloendothelial cells to erythroid precursors is disrupted. When the serum iron falls to less than 50 μg/dL, the number of sideroblasts in the marrow declines, and red blood cell production is suppressed. With an acute inflammatory illness such as a pneumonia or cellulitis, the anemia that results is mild (hemoglobin >10 g/dL) and red blood cell morphology is unaffected. With long-standing, chronic inflammatory illnesses such as rheumatoid arthritis, the defect in iron supply can result in a moderately severe, microcytic/hypochromic anemia.

Iron studies will usually distinguish between true iron deficiency, an inflammatory block in iron delivery (the anemia of chronic disease), and thalassemia (Table 5–5). The pattern of a low serum iron, high TIBC (percent saturation <10%), low ferritin level, increased serum TfR/ferritin ratio, and absent iron stores is unique for true iron deficiency. Although patients with inflammatory anemia also have low serum irons and low percent saturations of transferrin, iron stores will still be visible in the marrow and their serum ferritins will be normal or increased (see Chapter 4). Moreover, the sTfR/ferritin ratio will be less than 2.5, not the increase seen with true iron deficiency or the ineffective erythropoiesis of thalassemia. Finally, patients with thalassemia minor will have an essentially normal iron profile.

Several rare genetic defects can result in iron-deficient erythropoiesis, including mutations in genes regulating DMT1, ferroportin, ceruloplasmin, hepcidin, transferrin production, and

TABLE 5–5 • Differential diagnosis of microcytic anemia

	Thalassemia	Iron Deficiency	Chronic Inflammation
SI	Normal/increased	Low	Low
TIBC	Normal	High	Low
% Saturation	>20	<10	10–20
Serum transferrin receptor (sTfR)	Increased	Increased	Normal
Ferritin (μg/L)	>50	<15	30–200
Log (sTfR/ferritin) ratio	>2.5	>2.5	<2.5
Iron stores	3–4+	0	1–4+

ferroxidase activity needed for iron store mobilization. Microcytosis can also occur in patients with congenital or acquired defects in mitochondrial function, the so-called sideroblastic anemias. These are uncommon, however, and rarely result in the degree of microcytosis and hypochromia that are typical of severe iron-deficiency anemia. The characteristics of the sideroblastic anemias are discussed in Chapter 9.

THERAPY

Management of the patient with iron deficiency will depend on the severity of the anemia, the cause of the iron deficiency, and the ability of the patient to tolerate medicinal iron preparations. With a severe anemia, immediate red blood cell transfusion may be advisable. This suggestion is especially true for patients who require surgery or are in cardiac failure. The guidelines for transfusion are no different for iron-deficiency states than other types of anemia.

Cause of Iron-Deficient State

It is always important to know the cause of the iron-deficient state. Chronic blood loss needs to be controlled if iron therapy is to be effective. If significant gastrointestinal malabsorption is present, the route of iron administration must be modified. The patient should also be questioned regarding any complicating inflammatory illness or a previous history of gastric intolerance to oral iron preparations. Complicating inflammatory illnesses will inhibit both iron absorption and the release of iron from reticuloendothelial iron stores. This situation will have the effect of dampening the response to treatment.

Gastrointestinal Intolerance to Oral Iron Preparations

Gastrointestinal intolerance to oral iron preparations can interfere with patient compliance. For maximum effect, patients must maintain a constant oral intake of iron. The response of the erythroid marrow correlates with the severity of the anemia (level of erythropoietin stimulation), the structural integrity of the marrow, and the continuous level of serum iron. Erythropoiesis will be suppressed whenever the SI is less than 50 μg/dL. When the SI concentration is kept between 50 and 150 μg/dL, production will increase 2- to 3-fold, resulting in a hemoglobin rise of 0.2–0.5 g/dL/d. In the patient with iron deficiency with a moderately severe anemia, this should result in a 2–3 g/dL rise in hemoglobin within 3–4 weeks. When the anemia is less severe, hemoglobin greater than 10 g/dL, the response will be slower because of the lower level of erythropoietin stimulation.

Lack of Response to Oral Iron

When the response to oral iron seems to be inadequate, the patient's ability to comply with the regimen should be reviewed and the clinical diagnosis reevaluated. If patient compliance appears to be good, sources of continued bleeding should be looked for and studies performed to detect the presence of inflammatory disease. Oral iron therapy should not be continued beyond 3–4 weeks without evidence of a response. In addition, medicinal iron supplementation should not be routinely prescribed beyond 6 months without a definite reason. There is a small but finite risk of iron overload if the patient has inherited the trait for hemochromatosis.

Oral Iron Preparations

Several oral preparations of iron are available in tablet, capsule, and elixir forms (Table 5–6). Ferrous sulfate tablets and elixir are the least expensive and, therefore, the preferable iron preparations. Ferrous fumarate, ferrous gluconate, and polysaccharide-iron complex tablets are equivalent preparations, even though the actual iron contents are somewhat different. Carbonyl iron is about 70% as efficacious as ferrous sulfate. However, because of its slower intestinal release of iron, patients with gastrointestinal side effects may better tolerate carbonyl iron. Generally, when any of these preparations are given 3–4 times a day before meals, between 40 and 60 mg of iron will be absorbed and delivered to the erythroid marrow. This process will support marrow production levels of up to 3 times normal in patients with moderate to severe anemia.

TABLE 5–6 • Oral iron preparations

	Tablet (Iron Content) (mg)	Elixir (Iron Content) (mg)
Ferrous sulfate	325 (65)	300/5 mL (60)
Ferrous gluconate	325 (38)	300/5 mL (35)
Ferrous fumarate	300 (99)	100/5 mL (33)
Carbonyl iron	50 (50)	—
Polysaccharide—iron	150 (150)	100/5 mL (100)

Several other compoundings of iron are available. Enteric-coated and delayed-release preparations hold no great advantage and may actually result in decreased absorption. Some preparations also contain "absorption-enhancing substances," including other vitamins, amino acids, and a range of other ingredients. Ascorbic acid is one of the more popular additives. Iron absorption is increased when ascorbic acid is present in amounts of 200 mg or more. At the same time, increased uptake is accompanied by an increase in gastrointestinal side effects. All of these preparations are more expensive than ferrous sulfate, while not providing much of an advantage to the patient.

Dosage Guidelines

Moderate to severe iron-deficiency anemia in an adult should be treated with 150–200 mg of elemental iron per day (2–3 mg/kg)—1 tablet of ferrous sulphate (or equivalent iron preparation), 3–4 times a day, between meals and at bedtime. Children and infants can tolerate doses of iron of up to 5 mg/kg, somewhat larger than the adult dose by weight. At the same time, children are at special risk of a life-threatening overdose if they ingest several pills or a large amount of elixir at one time.

The patient's compliance is the key to an effective marrow response to oral iron therapy. The best oral iron regimen requires multiple doses during the day since absorption following each dose is limited to a few hours (Figure 5–7). To achieve a maximum effect, it is also important to ingest the iron medications between meals. This procedure will avoid the inhibiting effect of food substances on iron transport. At the same time, it will tend to increase the gastrointestinal intolerance to the medication. A typical oral iron regimen is 1 tablet of iron 3 or 4 times a day taken prior to meals and at bedtime. The final dose can be very important to maintain an elevated SI during the late evening and night hours. Without it, the SI will fall to levels below 50 μg/dL during the night.

As the hemoglobin level responds to iron therapy, the rate of increase will slow, reflecting a decrease in erythropoietin stimulation as the anemia disappears. Once the hemoglobin rises above 10–12 g/dL, the recovery rate is much slower, regardless of the level of oral iron intake, and a reduction in the dose can help maintain patient compliance. Finally, at least 6 months of dietary iron supplementation is required in the normal adult to rebuild reticuloendothelial iron stores from an iron-deficient state.

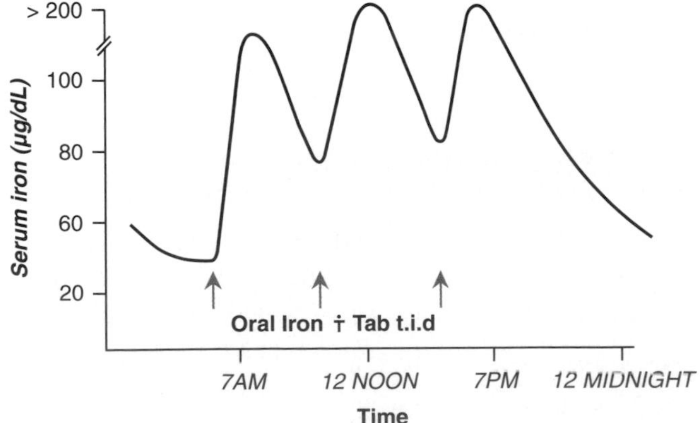

FIGURE 5–7. **Oral iron absorption.** When medicinal iron is given 3 times a day, each dose raises the SI for several hours. A fourth dose at bedtime can help sustain the SI during nighttime hours; however, this later dose may be poorly tolerated.

A. Adjusting Dose for Patient Tolerance

In all situations, the dose must be adjusted according to patient tolerance. With a full treatment dose of 150–200 mg of elemental iron per day (1 iron tablet, 3 or 4 times a day), up to 25% of individuals will complain of gastrointestinal side effects. If a patient experiences significant gastrointestinal distress, especially nausea and epigastric discomfort, the dose will need to be reduced. Carbonyl iron may be better tolerated because it is more slowly absorbed, but at the same time it is less bioavailable. Generally, tolerance to oral iron will improve over several days with continued treatment. Constipation and diarrhea, also common complaints of patients taking oral iron, are not dose related and should be managed symptomatically. When iron is given over a long period, using a lower dose can increase patient compliance. Moreover, higher doses do not carry any advantage in patients with mild anemia or where iron is being given to rebuild iron stores, since iron absorption is limited.

B. Iron Absorption

Absorption of iron given in tablet form requires the acid milieu of the stomach to remove the tablet coat. In patients who have had gastric surgery, tablet iron may be poorly absorbed or not absorbed at all. In this situation, therapy with iron elixir should be tried. It may also be necessary to administer the iron with meals to prevent gastric intolerance.

Parenteral Iron Therapy

For those situations where gastrointestinal malabsorption or severe intolerance prevents effective oral iron therapy, parenteral iron can be administered. Two iron dextran preparations are available for use in the United States: INFeD (Schein) and DexFerrum (USP/American Regent Laboratories). Two other parenteral preparations, sodium ferric gluconate (Ferrlecit) and iron sucrose (Venofer), also approved by the US Food and Drug Administration (FDA), offer an alternative to the use of a iron dextran compound.

A. Iron Dextran

Iron dextran for injection is a ferric hydroxide-dextran compound, average molecular weight of 165,000, packaged as a viscous solution containing 50 mg/mL of iron. The preferred method of administration is by bolus intravenous injection of 500–2,000 mg. However, it can also be administered in smaller amounts either intravenously or intramuscularly. When given as a single intravenous dose, the total amount of iron needed by the patient can be calculated as follows:

$$\text{Body Weight (kg)} \times 2.3 \times (15 - \text{Patient's Hgb in g/dL}) + 500 \text{ mg (for Stores)} = \text{Total Dose (mg)}$$

An alternative calculation, recommended by the manufacturer, is as follows:

[0.476 × Lean Body Weight (kg) × Hemoglobin Deficit]
+ 1 mL per 5 kg Body Weight to a Maximum of 14 mL
(to Reconstitute Iron Stores) = Total Dose
(mL of Iron Dextran Solution)

1. Clearance—Iron dextran given intravenously is rapidly cleared by reticuloendothelial cells. The iron is then released from the dextran over a period of days or weeks and transported by transferrin to the erythroid marrow. The rate of release is in part a function of the particle size of the iron dextran; larger particles are sequestered in reticuloendothelial cells and are slow to dissolve. Over time, when patients receive repeated injections, this can result in the accumulation of considerable unused iron dextran particles in the reticuloendothelial cells. Moreover, the sequestered iron dextran can be so unavailable that the serum iron can fall to iron-deficient levels even while visible iron stores (iron dextran) are abundant.

2. Administration and complications—When administering intravenous iron dextran, great care must be taken to anticipate and avoid a life-threatening anaphylactic reaction. A careful history should be taken to identify those patients who have had a prior reaction to iron dextran. In addition, regardless of the patient's history, a small test dose (less than 0.5 mg given over several minutes followed by a period of observation) should be administered before intravenous infusion of the drug. If the initial test dose is well tolerated, the remainder of the dose can be administered slowly. When 500–1,000 mg is used on a single occasion, it is best diluted in 250 mL of 0.9% sodium chloride solution and administered over 30–60 minutes. The infusion should be stopped immediately if the patient complains of itching, shortness of breath, chest pain, or back pain. The blood pressure should also be monitored over the first hour of administration to detect sudden hypotension.

Iron dextran can also be administered by intramuscular injection but this is generally not recommended. Five milliliters (250 mg) of iron dextran can be given each time with half of the dose injected in each buttock area. Significant skin staining can occur. It is also possible to produce sterile abscesses at the site of injections that will take considerable time to resolve. The rate of release of iron from intramuscular iron dextran injection can be slower and less reliable, and the risk of acute anaphylaxis is not avoided. Late reactions to intramuscular or intravenous iron dextran include a serum sickness–like reaction with malaise, fever, arthralgias, skin rash, and lymphadenopathy.

B. Iron Sucrose

Iron sucrose (Venofer) is packaged in 5-mL vials containing 100 mg of elemental iron. It can be infused directly or after dilution in 100 mL of saline over 15 minutes to avoid hypotension. The risk of a severe "anaphylactic-type" reaction is negligible when compared to iron dextran preparations. At the same time, the maximum dose of iron administered at one time is limited to 100 mg.

C. Sodium Ferric Gluconate

Sodium ferric gluconate (Ferrlecit) is packaged in 5-mL vials containing 62.5 mg of elemental iron. The recommended dose is 5–10 mL (62.5–125 mg) given by intravenous push over 10 minutes. Unlike the slow release of iron from iron dextran, up to 80% of the dose is available for transport by transferrin within 24 hours. Like iron sucrose, the risk of an "anaphylactic-type" reaction is negligible, as are delayed immune reactions. However, just as with iron sucrose, the maximum dose of iron administered at any one time is limited to 125 mg. This makes sodium ferric gluconate (and iron sucrose) ideal for the maintenance of iron supply in hemodialysis patients where iron infusions can be timed to dialysis treatments. It makes it less useful in situations where a single, large-dose iron infusion is appropriate.

CASE HISTORY • *Part 3*

The treatment of any patient with iron-deficiency anemia must begin by defining the etiology of the blood loss. In this case, there were two possible leads—the positive stool hemoccult test and the history of excessive menses. Both issues were fully explored—workup of the bowel failed to reveal a cause and repeat hemoccult tests were negative. She was then referred to a gynecologist to deal with her menstrual abnormality.

To treat the anemia, she was started on oral iron—ferrous sulphate, 1 tablet TID between meals—which she tolerated with minimal gastric distress. Follow-up CBC at 4 weeks showed a hematocrit/hemoglobin of 30%/10 g/dL, an MCV of 79 fL, and a mixed population of normocytic and microcytic cells on smear. By 2 months her hematocrit had reached 35% with an MCV of 88 fL. She was then advised to continue her iron regimen for another 3–4 months to rebuild iron stores.

POINTS TO REMEMBER

Iron deficiency due to a nutritional imbalance, malabsorption, or excessive blood loss is a leading cause of anemia worldwide.

The iron content of the Western diet is largely a function of the caloric intake and the types of foods eaten. Children, adolescents, frequent blood donors, and women with heavy menses may not ingest sufficient iron and require supplementation.

Iron supplementation is always in order during pregnancy.

Iron deficiency may present as asymptomatic iron store depletion, iron-deficient erythropoiesis, or, when severe, an iron-deficiency anemia.

Iron store depletion can only be detected by a fall in the serum ferritin level and a reduction in iron stores on a marrow aspirate or biopsy. Store depletion decreases the ability of the marrow to respond to sudden blood loss.

Iron-deficient erythropoiesis is characterized by a reduced marrow response to erythropoietin stimulation, often resulting in a modest fall in the hematocrit without accompanying changes in red cell morphology (cells remain normocytic and normochromic).

Iron-deficiency anemia is notable for the appearance of microcytic/hypochromic red blood cells in circulation, and characteristic changes in the serum iron, iron-binding capacity, percent saturation, and serum ferritin level.

Other causes of microcytic/hypochromic red cell morphology, including severe inflammatory anemia, thalassemia, and sideroblastic anemia, may need to be ruled out.

You can't treat iron deficiency effectively without diagnosing and, if at all possible, correcting the cause—chronic blood loss, malabsorption, malnutrition.

An oral iron preparation is the recommended first-line therapy, unless the patient is elderly with cardiopulmonary disease or needs immediate surgery, when red blood cell transfusions are indicated. Parenteral iron therapy is available for patients who cannot tolerate oral iron preparations or have severe malabsorption.

Correction of an iron-deficiency anemia will take 1–2 months, while full replacement of iron stores can take another 3–4 months on an oral iron regimen.

Correction of an iron-deficiency anemia may be dampened by the continued presence of an inflammatory disease, blood loss, renal failure, or marrow damage. An iron-deficient thalassemia patient may show an improvement in hematocrit but little change in MCV or smear microcytosis.

BIBLIOGRAPHY

Andrews NC: Forging a field: the golden age of iron biology. Blood 2008;112:219.

Cook JD, Flowers CH, Skikne BS: The quantitative assessment of body iron. Blood 2003;101:3359.

Cook JD, Skikne BS: Iron deficiency: definition and diagnosis. J Intern Med 1989;226:349.

Cook JD, Skikne BS, Boynes RD: Serum transferrin receptor. Annu Rev Med 1993;44:63.

Finch CA, Huebers H: Perspectives in iron metabolism. N Engl J Med 1982;306:1520.

Guyatt GH et al: Laboratory diagnosis of iron-deficiency anemia: an overview. J Gen Intern Med 1992;7:145.

Malope BI et al: The ratio of serum transferrin receptor and serum ferritin in the diagnosis of iron status. Br J Haematol 2001;115:84.

Massey AC: Microcytic anemia: differential diagnosis and management of iron deficiency anemia. Med Clin North Am 1992;76:549.

Mast AE et al: Clinical utility of the reticulocyte hemoglobin content in the diagnosis of iron deficiency. Blood 2002;99:1489.

Michael B et al: Sodium ferric gluconate complex in hemodialysis patients: adverse reactions compared to placebo and iron dextran. Kidney Int 2002;61:1830.

Oski FA: Iron deficiency in infancy and childhood. N Engl J Med 1993;329:190.

THALASSEMIA • 6

CASE HISTORY • *Part I*

As a part of a routine physical examination for college sports, an 18-year-old college freshman with a completely negative past medical history has a routine CBC. The results are as follows:

CBC: Hematocrit/hemoglobin - 39%/13 g/dL
MCV - 74 fL MCH - 29 pg MCHC - 30 g/dL
RDW-CV - 18%
WBC count - 7,500/µL
Platelet count - 180,000/µL
Reticulocyte count/index - 2.0%/1.7

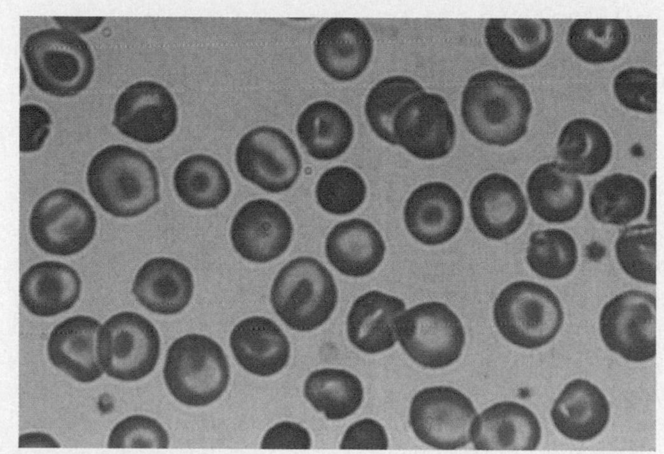

Questions

- How should this anemia be described/categorized?
- What is the most likely diagnosis based on the history and CBC?

In addition to iron deficiency, an inherited defect in globin chain synthesis is the other leading cause of microcytic anemia worldwide in children and adults. The frequency and severity of the several types of thalassemia depend on the **racial or ethnic background** of the population. For example, β-thalassemia is commonly seen in individuals from Africa and the Mediterranean area, whereas α-thalassemia and hemoglobin E disease are common in Southeast Asian populations. For certain subpopulations, the incidence of a microcytic, hypochromic anemia secondary to thalassemia can exceed that due to iron-deficiency anemia.

The diagnosis of thalassemia requires an understanding of normal globin chain synthesis, familiarity with the laboratory tests used to identify chain deficiencies, and a careful clinical evaluation of the patient. Because it is easy to confuse the microcytosis of iron deficiency with that of thalassemia, **iron studies** need to be performed on all microcytic patients. Moreover, both conditions can coexist. **Accurate diagnosis of the chain synthesis abnormality** is also very important for genetic counselling.

NORMAL GLOBIN CHAIN SYNTHESIS

Types of Globin

Globin, the protein portion of the hemoglobin molecule, is a tetramer of 2 α and 2 non–α-globin chains (Figure 6–1). The α-globin chains are encoded by 2 closely linked genes (α_2 and α_1) on chromosome 16. The non-α genes, β, γ, and δ, are encoded by a cluster of genes on chromosome 11. The pairing of these

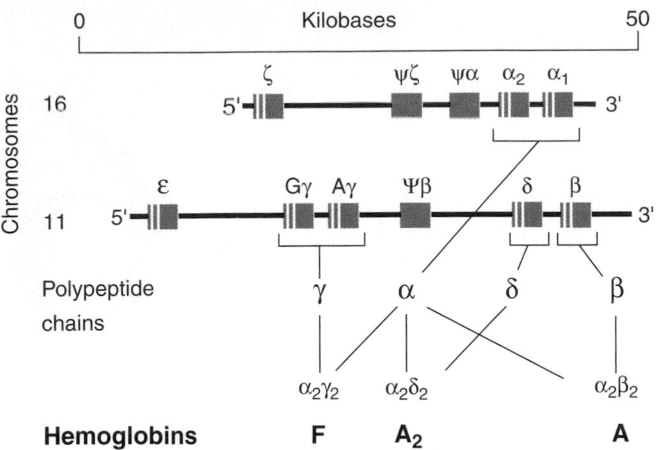

FIGURE 6–1. **Globin genes.** Specific genes on chromosomes 16 and 11 control the production of the α-, β-, γ-, and δ-globin chains.

several globin chains produces 3 **types of hemoglobin**: hemoglobin F ($\alpha_2\gamma_2$), hemoglobin A ($\alpha_2\beta_2$), and hemoglobin A_2 ($\alpha_2\delta_2$). A failure in α-globin chain synthesis can result in hemoglobin H, a tetramer of β-globin chains.

Quantity of Hemoglobin and Diagnosis

Globin gene expression varies with the patient's age. **Throughout fetal life**, red blood cells contain only hemoglobin F (Figure 6–2). During the first several months of life, γ-globin gene expression is gradually suppressed and both β-globin and δ-globin syntheses are activated. In adults, red blood cells contain primarily hemoglobin A (96%–97% of the cell's hemoglobin) and only small amounts of hemoglobin A_2 (<3.5%) and F (<1%). The quantity of each hemoglobin type is important in the diagnosis of thalassemia. Because gene mutations are associated with a quantitative failure in chain production, diagnosis is based on changes in intracellular levels of the major hemoglobin types.

Globin gene expression in adults can also vary according to the level of erythropoietin stimulation and availability of iron. One example is the upregulation of hemoglobin F production in sickle cell anemia patients who are treated with hydroxyurea. The increased synthesis of hemoglobin A_2, typically seen in β-thalassemia minor patients, is inhibited by concomitant iron deficiency. This factor needs to be taken into account when one is analyzing any abnormal hemoglobin electrophoretic pattern.

CLINICAL FEATURES

Depending on the genetic mutation, thalassemia can present as an incidental laboratory finding in an otherwise asymptomatic patient or as a moderate to severe anemia. One unifying feature is the presence of microcytosis and hypochromia, which reflects the decreased synthesis of globin chains.

Racial Background/Family History

Although the morphologic abnormality is very much the same for the various thalassemias, racial and ethnic background and family history can help in diagnosis. Patients with the **most severe forms of either α- or β-thalassemia** have parents who are heterozygotes for the globin chain defect and are generally members of high-prevalence population groups (Figure 6–3). Geographic distribution of the major thalassemias appears to reflect the survival advantage of the mutation in regions with a high incidence of malaria. α-Thalassemia is most common in Southeast Asia and Africa, whereas β-thalassemia has a more worldwide distribution. Various combinations of globin chain defects can be seen with intermarriage among distinct racial/ethnic backgrounds.

Classification

Thalassemia patients are classified as having thalassemia major, thalassemia intermedia, or thalassemia minor, depending on the

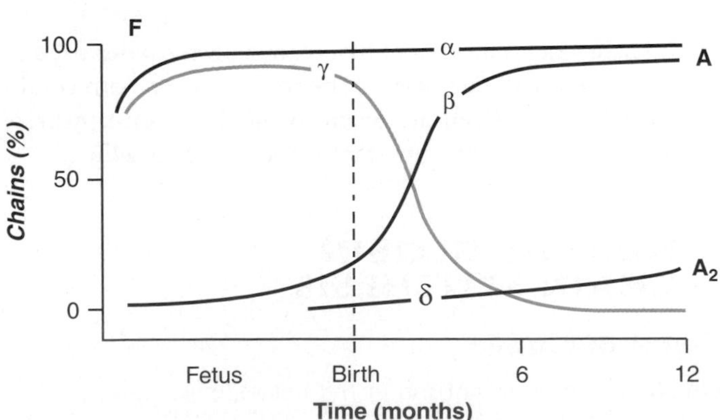

FIGURE 6–2. **Globin chain production and development.** Fetal red blood cells contain primarily hemoglobin F ($\alpha_2\gamma_2$). Soon after birth, γ-globin chain synthesis is suppressed and β-globin and δ-globin chain production increase, which results in the appearance of hemoglobins A and A_2.

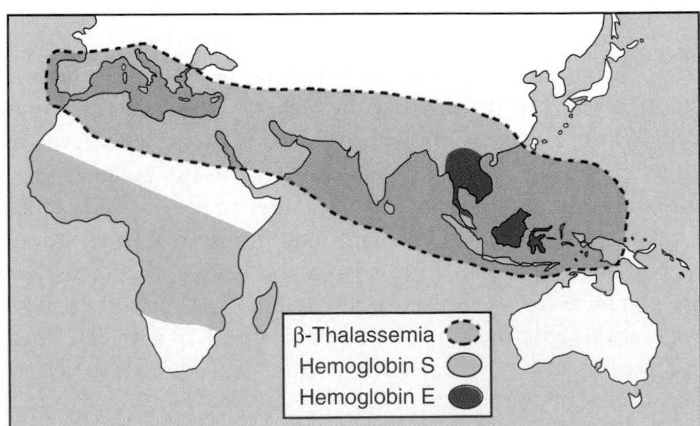

FIGURE 6–3. **Geographic distribution of hemoglobinopathies.** β-Thalassemia has a near worldwide distribution, as indicated by the dotted line. Hemoglobin S (sickle cell trait and sickle cell anemia) is concentrated in Africa, whereas hemoglobin E and α-thalassemia are most prevalent in Southeast Asia.

TABLE 6–1 • Clinical classification of thalassemia

Clinical Class	Genotype	Severity
Thalassemia minor		
β-Thalassemia trait	β/β^0	
α^0-Thalassemia trait	$—/\alpha\alpha$	Microcytosis, hypochromia, mild anemia
Hemoglobin Constant Spring	$\alpha\alpha^{CS}/\alpha\alpha^{CS}$	(Hemoglobin 10–14 g/dL)
α^+-Thalassemia trait	$-\alpha/-\alpha$	
Lepore trait	$\beta/(\delta\beta)^{+Lepore}$	
δβ-Thalassemia trait	$\beta/(\delta\beta)^{0\text{ or }+}$	
$(\delta\beta)^0$ HPFH homozygotes	$(\delta\beta)^0HPFH\beta/(\delta\beta)^0HPFH$	
Thalassemia intermedia		
$\beta^{+Africa}$-Thalassemia	$\beta^{+Africa}/\beta^{+Africa}$	
α^+ and β^0-Thalassemia double heterozygote	$-\alpha/-\alpha/\beta/\beta^0$	Microcytosis, hypochromia, moderate anemia
β^0-Thalassemia major with high hemoglobin F	β^0/β^0 with increased F production	
$(\delta\beta)^{0\text{ or }+/Lepore}$ Homozygotes	$(\delta\beta)^{0\text{ or }+Lepore}/(\delta\beta)^{0\text{ or }+Lepore}$	
Thalassemia major		
β^0-Thalassemia major	β^0/β^0	Severe microcytosis, hypochromia, and severe anemia
β^0/Hemoglobin E disease	β^0/β^E	(Hemoglobin 3–6 g/dL)
Hemoglobin H disease		
α^+ and α^0 double heterozygote	$—/-\alpha$	Microcytosis, hypochromia, moderate anemia with reticulocytosis
α^0 and Constant Spring double heterozygote	$—/\alpha\alpha^{CS}$	

severity of their anemia (Table 6–1). Worldwide, there are nearly 200 million individuals with thalassemia.

A. Thalassemia Minor

Most individuals with thalassemia are thalassemia minor patients who are heterozygotes for either an α-globin or β-globin gene mutation and have a very mild, asymptomatic anemia. α-Thalassemia trait patients with deletion of 2 genes, heterozygous β-thalassemia patients, and patients with partial but heterozygous deletions of both the δ- and β-genes, such as hemoglobin Lepore [$(\delta\beta)^+$ thalassemia] and hereditary persistence of fetal hemoglobin [$(\delta\beta)^0$ HPFH], demonstrate microcytosis and hypochromia, which is usually out of proportion to the severity of their anemia. Patients with α-thalassemia (deletion of a single gene), hemoglobin Constant Spring [(α^{CS}), a non-deletion form of α-thalassemia], and certain subtypes of β-thalassemia have little or no hematologic disease. They deserve the title of "silent" carrier state.

B. Thalassemia Intermedia

Thalassemia intermedia patients present with more severe anemia and prominent microcytosis and hypochromia. Not only do they complain of symptoms secondary to their anemia, but they also have related physical abnormalities such as hepatosplenomegaly, cardiomegaly, and on occasion skeletal changes secondary to marrow expansion. These patients have either a milder form of homozygous β^+-thalassemia, a combined α- and β-thalassemia defect, β-thalassemia with high levels of hemoglobin F, or $(\delta\beta)^0$-thalassemia.

C. Thalassemia Major

Thalassemia major (Cooley anemia) patients develop a severe, life-threatening anemia during their first year or two of life. To survive childhood, they require chronic transfusion therapy to correct their anemia and suppress their high level of ineffective erythropoiesis. Otherwise, they either die during childhood or have marked skeletal changes, growth retardation, and failure to reach sexual maturity. The anemia of β-thalassemia major is also associated with a high serum iron (SI) level, saturation of the total iron-binding capacity (TIBC), and a marked tendency for tissue iron loading. Most patients are homozygous for a β-globin gene deletion, although some are double heterozygotes for β-thalassemia minor and an abnormal hemoglobin such as hemoglobin E (β^E).

D. Hemoglobin H Disease

Patients who are double heterozygotes for α^0 and α^+ or α^{CS} are classified clinically as having hemoglobin H disease. Because of the involvement of 3 of the 4 β genes, these patients produce an excess of β-globin chains that combine to form β_4 hemoglobin **(hemoglobin H)**. Clinically, patients with hemoglobin H disease have characteristics of both thalassemia and a hemolytic anemia. Red blood cell production is not as ineffective as with other forms of thalassemia, but hemoglobin H is highly unstable, resulting in increased destruction of circulating red blood cells.

E. Hydrops Fetalis

When both parents are α^0-thalassemia heterozygotes, there is a chance of producing a fetus with deletion of all 4 α-globin genes. This condition, hydrops fetalis, is a lethal defect. The complete absence of α-globin production results in the formation of **hemoglobin Bart**, which is a poorly functioning hemoglobin made up of 4 γ-globin chains. The involved fetus has a profound anemia with marked extramedullary hematopoiesis, hepatosplenomegaly, and anasarca. These children die in utero or soon after birth.

Laboratory Studies

The **routine complete blood count (CBC)** and **peripheral blood film** provide the first clues to the presence of a thalassemia (Table 6–2). **Thalassemia minor** patients demonstrate microcytosis (MCV <75 fL) and hypochromia with little or no anemia (Figure 6–4). Because the microcytosis is quite uniform, the red blood cell distribution width (RDW) is not increased. The peripheral blood film is microcytic and hypochromic but shows little in the way of anisocytosis, poikilocytosis, or polychromasia. Many red blood cells have a target shape as a result of a reduction in intracellular hemoglobin content that is not matched by an equal reduction in cell membrane. Excess membrane tends to accumulate in the center of the cell, resulting in the target shape.

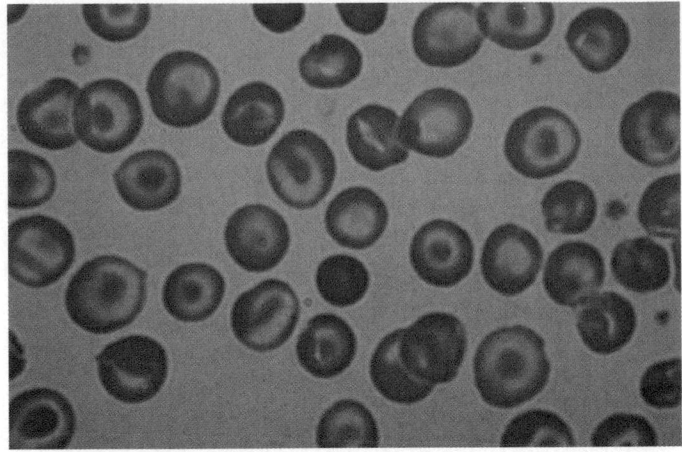
A

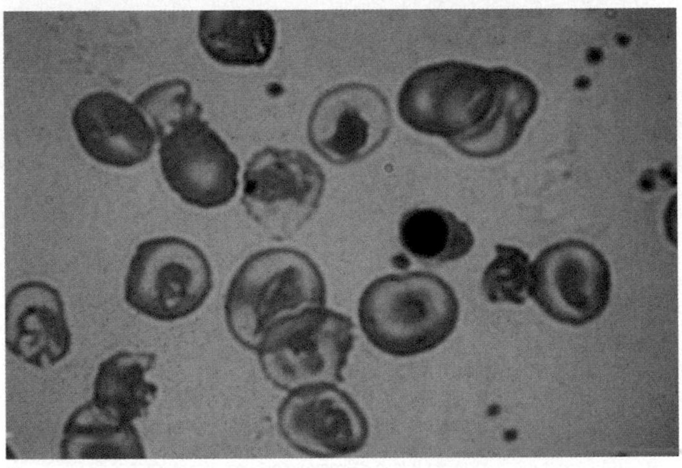
B

FIGURE 6–4. **Red blood cell morphology in thalassemic patients.** The blood smear in patients with β-thalassemia minor typically shows microcytosis and hypochromia with frequent target cells **(A)**; β-thalassemia major smears show much more dramatic microcytosis, hypochromia, poikilocytosis, and targeting **(B)**. With thalassemia major, the diameter of the red blood cells on the dried smear appears greater than expected for the marked microcytosis. This reflects the fact that severely hypochromic (major reduction in the MCH) cells tend to flatten out on the glass surface.

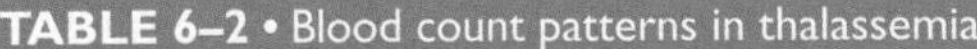
TABLE 6–2 • Blood count patterns in thalassemia

	Minor	Intermedia	Major
Hemoglobin (g/dL)	10–14	6–10	<6
MCV (fL)	60–80	50–70	50–60
MCH (pg)	28–32	22–28	16–22
RDW-CV	Normal	Slightly increased	Increased
Microcytosis, hypochromia	Mild	Moderate	Severe
Polychromasia	Very little	Moderate	Marked
Anisocytosis	None	Moderate	Marked
Poikilocytosis	None	Moderate	Marked
Targeting	Present	Present	Present

Thalassemia intermedia and thalassemia major patients present with a much more dramatic picture. Their anemia is more severe and the microcytosis and hypochromia are much more pronounced (Figure 6–4). There is a greater amount of anisocytosis and poikilocytosis on the peripheral film with a concomitant increase in the RDW. Polychromasia and targeting are also much more pronounced.

A. Marrow and Iron Studies

Although examination of the marrow is usually not required to detect or diagnose thalassemia in individual patients, it does provide information regarding the level of ineffective erythropoiesis and complications such as folic acid or iron deficiency. In some populations, the incidence of iron deficiency can compete with that of thalassemia minor, or both defects can be present simultaneously. **Accurate diagnosis of thalassemia minor** in this situation requires measurements of the SI, TIBC, and serum ferritin level, and at times, a careful inspection of a marrow specimen stained with Prussian blue.

Patients with thalassemia intermedia and thalassemia major have high levels of **ineffective erythropoiesis**. This situation results in an erythropoietic profile that is quite distinctive from that of iron deficiency (Table 6–3). The **marrow of the patient with severe thalassemia** is very hyperplastic, with the ratio of erythroid to granulocytic precursors (E/G ratio) easily exceeding 1:1 or 2:1. Since most of the proliferating erythroid cells fail to complete maturation and die within the marrow, the reticulocyte index is lower than expected for the degree of erythroid hyperplasia. In addition, measurements of cell turnover including the lactic dehydrogenase (LDH) level and serum indirect bilirubin are both elevated.

Although severe iron deficiency can cause a degree of ineffective erythropoiesis, the **severely iron-deficient marrow** is never as hyperplastic, the E/G ratio does not exceed 1:1, and even though the reticulocyte index is usually low, the serum bilirubin and LDH levels are never increased. The most obvious difference, however, is that patients with thalassemia intermedia and major show a marked tendency to iron loading. They exhibit high SI levels even to full saturation of the TIBC, very high serum ferritin levels, and increased reticuloendothelial stores on the marrow aspirate. In contrast, iron-deficient patients show low SI levels, low ferritin levels, and absent stores (see Chapter 5 for further discussion).

B. Hemoglobin Analysis and Quantitation

Definitive diagnosis and classification of thalassemia requires quantitative measurement of cellular hemoglobins, including hemoglobins A, A_2, F, and H. In populations with a high incidence of double heterozygotes for other hemoglobinopathies, tests must be performed to identify other abnormal hemoglobins, including S, C, D, E, Lepore, and Constant Spring. Clinical laboratories routinely perform hemoglobin electrophoresis to identify these common hemoglobinopathies. Quantitative measurements, such as high-pressure liquid chromatography (HPLC), of both hemoglobin A_2 and F are of special value in the diagnosis of β-thalassemia minor. A qualitative measure of red blood cell hemoglobin H is possible using the supravital stain, **brilliant cresyl blue** and quantitation is possible by **starch gel electrophoresis**. As part of genetic counselling, DNA-based diagnosis is now the optimal method for precisely defining the genetic mutations.

1. Screening for and measuring the amount of different hemoglobins—Reference laboratories screen for abnormal hemoglobins using automated HPLC testing (eg, BioRad instrumentation). Software programs that accompany the HPLC instrumentation can be set for both β-thalassemia detection (A_2 level) and variant hemoglobin screening. HPLC analysis provides accurate measurement of the levels of hemoglobins A, A_2, and F, and any abnormal variant. At the same time, the identity of an abnormal hemoglobin (Lepore, S, C, D, and E) requires electrophoretic analysis for confirmation. HPLC results coupled with the CBC can diagnose β-thalassemia minor based solely on the A_2 level and the MCV. Besides HPLC, hemoglobin F can be measured using the alkaline denaturation technique. This test takes advantage of the greater resistance of hemoglobin F to denaturation by strong alkali. The same principle has been used to assess amounts of hemoglobin F in individual red blood cells. The acid elution slide test for hemoglobin F (**Kleihauer-Betke acid elution test**) uses a citric acid–phosphate buffer to elute the hemoglobin A from the cells. The hemoglobin F remains behind and can then be stained with hematoxylin and eosin. Normal quantities of these hemoglobins and the most common patterns for both the β- and α-thalassemias are summarized in Tables 6–4 and 6–5.

2. Electrophoresis techniques—Electrophoresis techniques commonly used in diagnosing hemoglobinopathies are cellulose acetate, starch, and agar gel with either an alkaline or acid buffer. **Cellulose acetate electrophoresis** with an alkaline buffer is used to initially screen blood samples for common hemoglobinopathies such as S and C. **Citrate agar electrophoresis** with an acid buffer is used to confirm the results of a cellulose acetate study. It is especially valuable in separating hemoglobin C from hemoglobins A and S in infants. More complex electrophoresis of globin chains after separation from their heme groups using both **citrate agar and cellulose acetate** makes it possible to identify many of the hemoglobin subtypes without expensive structural analysis.

3. β-Thalassemia minor—Patients with β-thalassemia minor due to either a gene deletion (β^0) or mutation (β^+) can be identified from the slight elevation in fetal hemoglobin and an increase in the hemoglobin A_2 level to between 4% and 7%. Confusion can arise if the patient is simultaneously iron deficient

TABLE 6–3 • Erythropoietic profiles of thalassemia and iron deficiency

	Thalassemia	Iron Deficiency
Anemia	Minor to severe	Minor to severe
MCV (fL)	<70	<80
Film morphology	Microcytic, hypochromic with prominent targeting	Normal to microcytic, hypochromic with pencil forms, no targeting
Reticulocyte index	<2	<2
Marrow E/G ratio	>2:1	1:1–1:3
Serum iron/TIBC	Increased/normal	Very low/increased
% Saturation	>50	<10
Marrow iron stores	Increased	Absent
Serum ferritin (μg/L)	>100	<15
Bilirubin/LDH	Increased	Normal

TABLE 6–4 • Hemoglobin patterns in β-thalassemia variants

	Hemoglobin (%)				
	A	*F*	*A₂*	*Lepore*	*S*
Normal	97	<1	2–3	0	0
β-Thalassemia minor					
Trait $\beta/\beta^{0 \text{ or } +}$	90–95	1–5	4–7[a]	—	—
Lepore trait $\beta/(\delta\beta)^{+\text{Lepore}}$	80–85	1–5	2–3	10–15	—
β-Thalassemia intermedia					
$\beta^{+\text{Africa}}/\beta^{+\text{Africa}}$	30–50	50–70	0–5	—	—
β-Thalassemia major					
β^0/β^0	0	95–100	0–5	—	—
$(\delta\beta)^{+\text{Lepore}}/(\delta\beta)^{+\text{Lepore}}$	0	80	0	20	—

[a]*Iron deficiency can lower the hemoglobin A_2 level to normal.*

because this will lower the hemoglobin A_2 level to normal. It is essential, therefore, that iron studies be run simultaneously to exclude this possibility.

4. β-Thalassemia intermedia or β-thalassemia major— Patients with β-thalassemia intermedia or β-thalassemia major are easily identified from their severe microcytosis and hypochromia and greatly increased levels of hemoglobin F with markedly decreased or absent hemoglobin A on electrophoresis. Hemoglobin A_2 levels are variable and can be reduced, normal, or slightly increased. β-Thalassemia can present as a double heterozygote with α-thalassemia or another β-hemoglobinopathy gene, such as hemoglobin S, C, or E. From a clinical standpoint, the most important of these is the sickle/thalassemia combination. The patient with hemoglobin S/β^0-thalassemia presents with the typical symptoms and signs of homozygous (S/S) sickle cell disease (see Chapter 11). However, the presence of the β^0-thalassemia mutation (gene deletion and total absence of normal β chain production) results in a major deficit in hemoglobin production and pronounced microcytosis, hypochromia, and targeting. If the patient has a mutational defect (β^+), the presentation is much more like sickle trait (see Chapter 11), since β-chain production, though reduced, is still present. These patients are readily identified from the relative quantities of hemoglobins S and A on HPLC or electrophoresis. The quantity of hemoglobin S will typically be greater than hemoglobin A. This is distinctly different from the pattern seen with hemoglobin S trait where the quantity of hemoglobin A (60%–70%) always exceeds hemoglobin S (30%–40%) (Table 6–6).

5. α-Thalassemia—The most common hemoglobin patterns for α-thalassemia are summarized in Table 6–5. When only 1 of the 4 α-globin chain genes is defective, the patient has little clinical disease and this silent condition can only be detected at birth from the presence of a small amount of Bart hemoglobin, a hemoglobin made up of 4 γ-globin chains. Current HPLC techniques are relatively insensitive to the very low level of Bart hemoglobin with a single chain defect and are, therefore, not useful for the diagnosis of α-thalassemia carriers. Heterozygous α^0 and homozygous α^+ patients show microcytosis, hypochromia, and a mild anemia, suggesting thalassemia minor. In contrast to those with β-thalassemia minor, however, they have normal hemoglobin F and A_2 levels. Hemoglobin H is not

TABLE 6–5 • Hemoglobin patterns in α-thalassemia variants

	Hemoglobin (%)			
	A	*H(β₄)*	*Bart (γ₄) (at Birth Only)*	*Constant Spring*
Normal	97	0	0	0
α⁺-Thalassemia silent –α/αα	98–100	0	(0–2)	0
α⁰-thalassemia trait				
–α/–α(homozygous α^+)	85–95	Red blood cell inclusions	(5–15)	0
or —/αα (heterozygous α^0) $\alpha\alpha^{CS}/\alpha\alpha^{CS}$	85–95	0	(5–15)	5
Hemoglobin H disease				
—/–α(α^0/α^+)	70–95	5–30	Trace	Trace
—/$\alpha\alpha^{CS}$ (α^0/α^{CS})	60–90	5–30	Trace	5–10
Hydrops fetalis				
—/—(α^0/α^0)	0	5–10	90–95	0

TABLE 6–6 • Hemoglobin patterns in combined hemoglobinopathies

	Hemoglobin (%)			
	A	*F*	*A_2*	*E/S/C*
Normal	97	<1	2–3	0
Hemoglobin E				E
Trait β/β^E	60–65	1–2	2–3	30–35
Homozygous β^E/β^E	0	0	5	95
E/β Thal β^E/β^0	0	45	1–5	40–50
E/α Thal	70	0	2–3	30
Hemoglobin S				S
Trait β/β^S	60–70	1–2	2–3	30–40
Homozygous β^S/β^S	0	5–10	—	90–95
S/β Thal β^S/β^0	0	5–10	4–7	80–90
β^S/β^+	20–30	5–10	4–7	50–70
Hemoglobin C				C
Trait β/β^C	55–65		3–5	30–40
Homozygous β^C/β^C	0	5–10	—	90–95
C/B Thal β^C/β^0	0	5–10	—	90–95
β^C/β^+	20–30	5–10	—	60–75

detected on routine electrophoresis, but H inclusions can be demonstrated in occasional red blood cells using brilliant cresyl blue stain. Definitive diagnosis of α-thalassemia minor requires electrophoresis at birth when from 5%–15% Bart hemoglobin is present, or later in life with extensive gene sequencing. Patients who are double heterozygotes for hemoglobin Constant Spring also have up to 15% Bart hemoglobin at birth and approximately 5% hemoglobin Constant Spring as adults.

6. Hemoglobin H disease and hydrops fetalis—Hemoglobin H disease is produced when a patient is a double heterozygote for α^0 and α^+, or α^0 and hemoglobin Constant Spring. In both situations, only 1 gene is truly operating. In the adult, hemoglobin H disease is detected using HPLC and starch gel electrophoresis where from 5%–30% of hemoglobin H is present with small amounts of both Bart hemoglobin and hemoglobin Constant Spring. Finally, a deletion of all 4 α-globin chain genes results in the condition called **hydrops fetalis**, where only Bart and hemoglobin H are produced. This condition is not compatible with life and results either in fetal wastage or death soon after delivery.

7. Hemoglobin E—Hemoglobin E (β^E) is an important mutation especially in Southeast Asia. Hemoglobin E can be detected using combined acid and alkaline hemoglobin electrophoresis (hemoglobin E migrates with A_2 at an acid pH and C, O^{Arab}, and A_2 at an alkaline pH). Patients carrying the trait are asymptomatic but have a red cell profile similar to that of β-thalassemia minor, with microcytosis and targeting. However, they have normal hemoglobin A_2 levels. Even homozygous patients with hemoglobin E levels exceeding 90% are relatively asymptomatic with little more than a mild microcytic/hypochromic anemia. Double heterozygotes—β^E/β^+; β^E/β^0; $\beta^E/\delta\beta^{+Lepore}$; $\beta^E/\delta\beta^0$; and β^E/α-thalassemia—present with highly variable clinical pictures from a mild asymptomatic anemia to full blown thalassemia major. The clinical variability may, in part, be related to the level of hemoglobin F; the higher the F level the less severe the disease. Sequencing studies are required to accurately classify these heterozygotes.

CASE HISTORY • *Part 2*

The presentation—a mild microcytic anemia identified on routine screening in a young individual with a negative medical history—is supportive of a diagnosis of an inherited defect in globin production. A family history of anemia and racial heritage would be further evidence of a thalassemia and can even help in the differential diagnosis of the specific globin defect.

The combination of little or no anemia and an impressive microcytosis and hypochromia is highly suggestive of thalassemia minor. The presence of target cells on smear further supports the diagnosis—targeting is seen with globin production defects where the failure of hemoglobin production is not matched by a decrease in cell membrane. With iron deficiency, reductions in cell size and membrane generally parallel the fall in hemoglobin content; red cell morphology is normocytic or only slightly microcytic/normochromic, without targeting.

Questions

- Given the fact that the young man almost certainly has a form of thalassemia, are additional tests needed?
- Are there health issues associated with this diagnosis and should he be restricted from sports?

C. Molecular Diagnosis

Detection of the actual mutation responsible for a thalassemia is now possible using either sequencing or polymerase chain reaction (PCR) together with primer-specific probes complementary to the most common mutations. More than 200 different mutations have been described in patients with β-thalassemia, but fewer than 10 mutations are responsible for the majority of cases. When one of these common mutations is not detected the gene defect can be determined by direct sequencing of the area of interest.

Most β-thalassemias are due to a point mutation involving 1 or several nucleotides that then interferes with the coding of the gene; rarely is there gross deletion of the β-gene. Other mutations result in abnormal splicing or a defect in RNA processing. The location of the gene mutation determines hematologic phenotype, whether β^0, β^+, or a complex thalassemia such as $\delta\beta^0$ or $^+$-thalassemia, where there is a partial deletion of both the δ-and β-genes. Mutations in or near to the promoter sequences and in the 5′ untranslated regions of the gene interfere with transcription and usually result in mild (β^+)-thalassemia. Mutations that interfere with translation of the globin chain tend to produce more severe (β^0)-thalassemia. Molecular diagnosis has also helped identify compound heterozygotes with more severe disease.

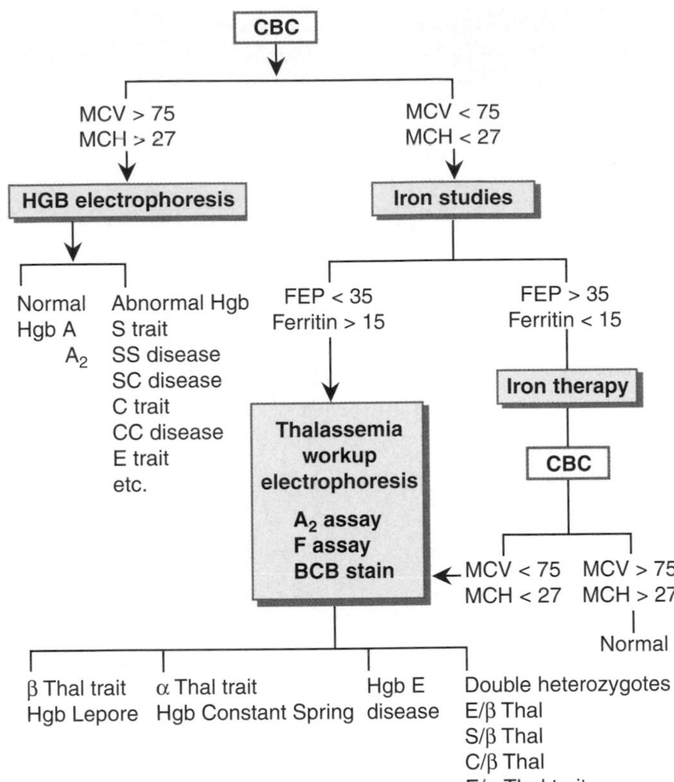

FIGURE 6–5. **Stepwise approach to the diagnosis of the thalassemias.** The CBC, free erythrocyte protoporphyrin (FEP), hemoglobin electrophoresis, and measurements of iron supply can be used to separate patients with iron deficiency anemia from those with hemoglobinopathies.

DIAGNOSIS

Initial detection and diagnosis of a thalassemia depends to a large extent on the severity of the gene defect. **Silent carrier states,** by definition, cause no clinical illness and can only be picked up by screening programs that use the combination of HPLC, MCV quantitation, and red cell supravital staining, often as a part of a family analysis. **Thalassemia minor patients** will be identified during screening programs, as a part of routine health maintenance, or, less frequently, because of a clinical symptom or sign relating to their hematologic defect. In contrast, **patients with thalassemia intermedia or thalassemia major** require medical attention because of their symptomatic anemia. β-Thalassemia major is often identified early in childhood because of the severe anemia, if not at birth, as a result of prenatal screening of the parents.

Initial Detection

National screening programs have developed **stepwise diagnostic strategies** for detecting and diagnosing thalassemias. Figure 6–5 gives an example of one such algorithm. Another entry point to the diagnosis of thalassemia is the **detection of some combination of anemia, microcytosis, and hypochromia on the routine CBC**. Since these patients are at equal or greater risk for an iron-deficiency state, testing for iron deficiency with measurements of SI, TIBC, serum ferritin, and red blood cell protoporphyrin can be highly productive. At the same time, laboratory testing is expensive. As an alternative, young patients who are at little or no risk for pathologic blood loss can be treated with oral iron therapy for 2–3 months followed by a repeat CBC. Correction of the anemia and microcytosis will rule against, but not necessarily rule out, thalassemia.

A. Thalassemia Minor Versus Iron Deficiency

Some simple hematologic observations can help discriminate between thalassemia minor and iron deficiency. The first is the **degree of microcytosis versus the severity of the anemia**. As a rule, **thalassemia minor patients** have more severe microcytosis (MCV below 75 fL), at a time when there is little or no anemia. In addition, they usually have a normal RDW, which indicates a uniform population of microcytic cells. The **iron-deficient patient** is just the opposite. Microcytosis is not seen until the hemoglobin falls below 10–11 g/dL for some period of time. An exception is the **patient with iron deficiency and polycythemia vera** where the increased drive for red blood cell production will result in prominent microcytosis even while the hemoglobin/hematocrit is normal or increased. In addition, the RDW in iron-deficient patients is usually increased, indicating a mixed population of microcytic and normocytic cells.

Inspection of the blood smear provides additional clues. **Patients with α- or β-thalassemia minor** show a uniform population of microcytic, hypochromic cells with frequent target cells. In contrast, **iron deficiency anemia patients** show a mixed population of small and normal-sized cells (**anisocytosis**) with variable hypochromia. More important, targeting is not a common feature of iron deficiency; instead, these patients will show occasional pencil-shaped red blood cells.

B. Combination Anemias

Since populations at risk for thalassemia are also at risk for iron deficiency, combination anemias are clearly possible. The patient who presents with a hematocrit below 35%, an MCV less than 70 fL, an RDW that is above normal, and a film showing anisocytosis, poikilocytosis, and target cells must be considered for a combined abnormality. The situation can be made more complicated by the presence of other diseases. For example, a **vitamin deficiency state or liver disease**, both of which are common in populations at risk for thalassemia, can affect all elements of the CBC, including the severity of the anemia, the MCV, RDW, and film morphology.

Prenatal Diagnosis

For high-risk populations, **prospective screening programs** have been established to identify young individuals at risk for transmitting a thalassemia gene to their children. The more frequent the expression of an abnormal gene(s), the more likely that couples will be at risk of producing a child with double heterozygous or homozygous thalassemia. A well-organized, skilled professional group that not only can accurately diagnose the genetic defect but also has experience in counselling affected individuals/couples should provide screening.

Another approach is to screen mothers at the time of their **first prenatal visit**. If the mother is a thalassemia carrier, the father should also be evaluated. When there is a risk of the child being a homozygote or double heterozygote (ie, having thalassemia major or intermedia), prenatal diagnosis is possible using the techniques of fetal blood sampling or chorionic villus biopsy. The latter can be performed as early as the ninth week of gestation with the diagnosis made by direct analysis of fetal DNA. Prenatal diagnosis is essential for the pregnant woman who has already had an affected child, especially a child with β-thalassemia intermedia or major, or homozygous α^0 (hydrops fetalis). When both parents are carriers of a severe form of thalassemia (β^0 or α^0), accurate prenatal diagnosis makes it possible to offer the option of a therapeutic abortion during the first trimester.

DIFFERENTIAL DIAGNOSIS

The differential diagnosis of the various thalassemias can appear to be a daunting task. Despite the large number of genetic defects and their combinations, however, individual thalassemias present as one of only a half dozen clinical vignettes. This fact is of great value not only in selecting and interpreting the necessary laboratory tests, but also in organizing the differential diagnosis and treatment plan.

Silent Carrier States

Thalassemia in these patients is rarely detected since they have no hematologic disease; their CBC and blood film are usually normal. A slightly low MCV coupled with a slight increase in the hemoglobin A_2 level by HPLC may be the only clue. The existence of thalassemia can also be discovered during a family study initiated because of disease in a sibling or offspring. The most common silent carrier states are β^+-thalassemia minor, α^0 and $^+$-thalassemia single-gene defects, and heterozygous hemoglobin Constant Spring.

Microcytosis with Little or No Anemia

These patients present with a normal to slightly reduced hemoglobin level, a definite microcytosis (MCV below 75 fL), and hypochromia. They are not clinically symptomatic and not at risk for iron overload. In fact, such patients actually run a greater risk of iron deficiency, which can make diagnosis difficult. Therefore, patients who present with what appears to be thalassemia minor should be tested for iron deficiency with an SI, TIBC, and serum ferritin level.

A. Most Common Genotypes

The most common genotypes responsible for thalassemia minor include heterozygous β^0-thalassemia, $\delta\beta^0$ and $\delta\beta^{+Lepore}$-thalassemia, $\delta\beta^0$ HPFH, homozygous α^+-thalassemia, heterozygous α^0-thalassemia, hemoglobin E, and β^E/α-thalassemia (see Table 6–1). As long as the patient is not iron deficient, patients with β-thalassemia minor will show an increased level of hemoglobin A_2 (4%–7%), with a slight increase in hemoglobin F. Patients with $\delta\beta^0$-thalassemia and hemoglobin Lepore trait will show normal hemoglobin A_2 and F levels. Patients with $\delta\beta^0$ HPFH show levels of hemoglobin F that approach 100%. Patients with α^0- and α^+-thalassemia demonstrate small amounts of Bart hemoglobin at birth and occasional hemoglobin H red blood cell inclusions on blood films stained with crystal violet. Finally, patients with homozygous hemoglobin Constant Spring show small amounts of Bart hemoglobin at birth and up to 5% hemoglobin Constant Spring as adults. The latter can easily be diagnosed by HPLC and gel electrophoresis.

B. α-Thalassemias

α-Thalassemias, both α^0 and α^+, are most common in Asian populations. This situation sets the stage for the inheritance of a multiple gene defect to produce a more severe form of α-thalassemia in Asian patients, either hemoglobin H disease or hydrops fetalis. In Africa, the α^0 (—/αα) genotype is very rare. Only single gene (–α/αα) and double gene (–α/–α) (homozygous) forms of α^+ thalassemia are observed in blacks. The first of these is a silent carrier state, whereas the homozygotes show clinical manifestations of thalassemia minor. Hemoglobin H disease and hydrops fetalis are less common in blacks. They do occur in Mediterranean and Arabian populations secondary to nondeletion mutations of the α-globin gene.

Moderate Anemia with Marked Microcytosis

These patients present with a definite anemia and marked microcytosis (MCV less than 70 fL) and hypochromia on the blood film. They commonly seek medical attention because of symptoms and signs related to their anemia. Splenomegaly, skeletal changes secondary to marrow expansion, and cardiomegaly are usually present, and patients are at risk for iron overload. This situation can worsen if the patient requires chronic blood transfusions.

This hematologic picture is typical of patients with thalassemia intermedia (see Table 6–1). Principal causes genetically are homozygous β-thalassemia of the $\beta^{+Africa}$ subtype, coinheritance of α- and β-thalassemia, compound heterozygosity for 2 mild β-globin gene mutations, or homozygous β-thalassemia with variably increased hemoglobin F production. Rarely, a mutation at the third exon of the β-globin gene will result in an intermedia phenotype despite a β-trait genotype.

Severe Anemia and Microcytosis

During the first year or two of life, these patients present with a severe, life-threatening anemia, marked microcytosis (MCV less than 60 fL), and hypochromia with pronounced targeting on the blood film. Symptoms and signs of anemia are striking. Children require long-term transfusion to grow and develop. They can also manifest marked splenomegaly, skeletal changes secondary to marrow expansion, growth and sexual retardation, and aggressive iron loading even without transfusion. Without treatment, affected children will die of heart failure during the first 2 decades of life.

This presentation is typical of patients with thalassemia major. Principal genetic mutations responsible are homozygous deletion (β^0) and nondeletion (β^+) forms of β-thalassemia, and the compound heterozygote for β-thalassemia and hemoglobin E (β^E). Hemoglobin electrophoresis patterns show mostly hemoglobin F with little or no hemoglobin A in all of these genotypes.

Hemolytic Anemia and Microcytosis

These patients present with mild to moderate anemia (hemoglobin 7–10 g/dL), an elevated reticulocyte count, and microcytosis and hypochromia with targeting on the blood film. Their erythropoietic profile is more typical of a hemolytic anemia than the ineffective erythropoiesis seen with thalassemia intermedia or major. Moreover, their clinical course is characteristic of hemolysis. Most patients have splenomegaly and exhibit reticulocytopenic crises in response to infections or exposure to oxidant drugs.

This clinical pattern is typical of patients with hemoglobin H disease secondary to deletion of 3 α-globin genes—the double heterozygote for α^0 and α^+-globin gene or the compound heterozygote α^0 and hemoglobin Constant Spring. The **definitive test for hemoglobin H disease** is demonstration of excess hemoglobin H by starch gel electrophoresis, HPLC, or supravital stain of blood with brilliant crystal blue. Depending on the severity of the illness and whether the patient has had a splenectomy, 5%–30% of the hemoglobin on electrophoresis will be hemoglobin H (β_4). If blood is tested at birth, red blood cells will contain up to 40% Bart hemoglobin. Patients with α^0/hemoglobin Constant Spring show 5%–10% hemoglobin Constant Spring on electrophoresis in addition to the hemoglobin H.

The **supravital stain film** shows a mix of heavily stained reticulocytes and cells with a fine, lightly stained, granular inclusion pattern. The latter are the cells that contain hemoglobin H. If the patient has a functional spleen, only a small number of circulating cells will have hemoglobin H inclusions. After splenectomy, virtually all cells will be filled with inclusions, reflecting the loss of the pitting function of the spleen.

Lethal Defect

Asian couples who are carriers for α^0 (—/αα) are at risk for producing a fetus that is homozygous for α^0 resulting in complete failure of α-chain production. This lethal defect results in death in utero or shortly after birth. The fetuses have a characteristic appearance with marked anasarca, hepatosplenomegaly, and extramedullary hematopoiesis. On hemoglobin electrophoresis, only Bart hemoglobin can be detected.

Compound Hemoglobinopathies

Both α- and β-thalassemia can present as a double heterozygote with another β-globin hemoglobinopathy gene. The most common combinations are with hemoglobin S, C, and E. The clinical presentation combines aspects of both gene defects. The incidence of the various combinations is geographically quite different. Combinations of hemoglobin E with thalassemia, as well as homozygous E disease, which clinically resembles thalassemia minor, are limited to Southeast Asia. Hemoglobin S and C/thalassemia have a more worldwide distribution.

A. Hemoglobin E/β-Thalassemia

Hemoglobin E results from a **β-globin chain defect** (substitution of lysine for glutamic acid at position 26), which interferes with mRNA processing and the synthesis of β^E-globin chains. Moreover, the β^E hemoglobin is unstable, which further contributes to the production of microcytosis and hypochromia. Both heterozygous and homozygous forms of hemoglobin E disease show microcytosis (MCV less than 75 fL) and hypochromia with prominent targeting on the blood film. Heterozygotes are not anemic and the homozygous state is associated with a mild anemia similar to that observed with β-thalassemia minor. The **incidence** of hemoglobin E/β-thalassemia in Southeast Asian populations is extremely high; more than a million people are affected. A gene frequency for hemoglobin E of up to 60% for certain groups of immigrants from Laos, Cambodia, and Thailand has translated into a hemoglobin E incidence of 1 in 4 Cambodian and 1 in 9 Thai/Laotian children born in the United States. Moreover, E/β-thalassemia is now more common in US Asian populations than β-thalassemia.

Patients with hemoglobin E/β-thalassemia can have **clinical features** of severe β-thalassemia major or much milder disease, resembling thalassemia minor or intermedia. In part, this reflects genetic factors such as the nature of the β-thalassemia mutation, the level of hemoglobin F, and coinheritance of α-thalassemia. The latter can result in a much milder phenotype when the β^+ mutation is present. Environmental factors, such as exposure to infections, may also play a role in disease severity. **Children with severe disease** usually require chronic transfusion and are at risk for iron loading. The severity of the clinical condition clearly separates hemoglobin E/β-thalassemia from homozygous hemoglobin E disease. Hemoglobin electrophoresis, a hemoglobin A_2 level, and the appearance of the smear will also help separate the conditions (see Table 6–6).

B. Hemoglobin S/β-Thalassemia

The double heterozygote, hemoglobin S(β^S)- and β-thalassemia, is most commonly seen in African and Mediterranean populations. These patients present with the symptoms and signs of sickle cell disease including a severe anemia and painful vasoocclusive crises. In contrast to those with homozygous S sickle cell anemia, most patients have splenomegaly. Otherwise, their symptoms, signs, and clinical course are the same.

The **erythropoietic profile** shows features of both gene defects. Patients are moderately to severely anemic, microcytic (MCV less than 65 fL), and hypochromic with prominent poikilocytosis and targeting. Sickle cells may be seen, but are rare in patients with intact spleens. Following splenectomy, sickle cell forms are common. The **hemoglobin electrophoresis pattern** also reflects the double gene defect (see Table 6–6). Patients with a β-globin chain deletion defect (β^0) can have a pattern identical to that of homozygous SS disease, although the microcytosis and increased A_2 levels are clues to the diagnosis. Patients with hemoglobin β^S/β^+-thalassemia typically show small amounts of hemoglobin A (20%–30%), increased amounts of hemoglobin F, and up to 7% hemoglobin A_2.

Hemoglobin S can also be inherited together with $(\delta\beta)^0$-thalassemia or hemoglobin Lepore $(\delta\beta)^{+Lepore}$-thalassemia, resulting in a moderately severe hemolytic anemia with splenomegaly. The patient's CBC is microcytic and hypochromic with prominent targeting on the blood film. These patients tend to have milder disease with few if any painful vasoocclusive events, perhaps because of increased amounts of hemoglobins Lepore and F. **Patients with hemoglobin $\beta^S/(\delta\beta)$-thalassemia** present with a much milder disease. They are not anemic and do not have vasoocclusive events. Their CBCs do show microcytosis, hypochromia, targeting, and occasional sickle cells. Here again, concentrations of hemoglobin F from 20%–40% appear to be protective.

C. Hemoglobin C/Thalassemia

In Mediterranean and African populations, hemoglobin C can be inherited as a double heterozygote with β-thalassemia. Hemoglobin β^C/β^0-thalassemia is associated with a moderately severe hemolytic anemia, splenomegaly, and a microcytic, hypochromic red blood cell population. In blacks, hemoglobin C is often associated with the β^+-thalassemia gene producing a milder disease. In both situations, the peripheral blood film shows close to 100% targeting of red blood cells.

THERAPY

Management of the patient with thalassemia varies according to the severity of the anemia. **Heterozygote patients with α- and β-thalassemia** are not clinically symptomatic, have only a mild anemia, and are not at risk for iron overload. They should be reassured of the benign nature of the inherited defect and, when appropriate, counselled regarding the risks of transmitting the defect with childbearing. Thalassemia minor patients should not receive long-term iron therapy and do not require folic acid supplementation.

Patients with thalassemia intermedia or major who are homozygotes or double heterozygotes for α- or β-thalassemia will require almost continuous medical attention beginning early in childhood. Principal management issues include transfusion support, prevention of iron overload, and management of hypersplenism. Thalassemia major patients represent the greatest challenge. Children with the homozygous, deletional form of β-thalassemia (β^0/β^0) present during the first year of life with severe, life-threatening anemia. Their survival depends on a carefully orchestrated program of transfusion support and iron chelation therapy to prevent iron overload and tissue toxicity.

Transfusion Therapy

The decision to initiate a program of chronic transfusion will depend on the type of gene defect and the severity of the anemia. In general, **children with β-thalassemia major and hemoglobins of less than 6–7 g/dL** should receive chronic transfusions. It is

CASE HISTORY • *Part 3*

The presentation, CBC, and family history strongly support the diagnosis is β-thalassemia minor. However, iron deficiency still needs to be ruled out. This is especially important if a hemoglobin electrophoresis is ordered, since iron deficiency will mask the increase in hemoglobin A_2 needed for the definitive diagnosis of β-thalassemia minor.

There are no health risks associated with β-thalassemia minor and no contraindication to sports activities. Moreover, unlike thalassemia intermedia and major, there is no risk of iron overload. If appropriate, the patient should be counselled as to the implications of passing the genetic trait to his progeny, especially if he marries a woman who also carries the β-thalassemia trait. In this case, there is a 1 in 4 chance of giving birth to a child with thalassemia major.

important to start early before the child has a chance to develop splenomegaly and hypersplenism, and before skeletal changes and growth retardation. It is also important to establish a reliable, routine transfusion schedule that maintains hemoglobin levels of 9–10 g/dL. Below this level, the marrow will be stimulated to maintain a high level of ineffective erythropoiesis. This will lead to expansion of the marrow cavity, causing skeletal changes and increasing the splenomegaly and hypersplenism. Metabolic requirements of the expanded marrow will also result in growth retardation. Erythropoiesis will be suppressed when the hemoglobin is kept close to 10 g/dL. However, transfusion to levels higher than 10 g/dL increases the risk of organ damage from iron loading.

A. Reducing Risks of Transfusion

Care should always be taken to reduce the potential risks of transfusion. Early in life, children should be immunized for hepatitis B. They should also be monitored for the development of minor blood group antibodies and should receive only leukocyte-reduced packed red blood cells. If, over time, a patient does develop HLA alloantibodies and exhibits febrile reactions with transfusion, the patient can be premedicated with acetaminophen (Tylenol) and diphenhydramine (Benadryl).

B. Transfusion Requirements

Transfusion requirements will obviously vary according to the patient's age and physical size. As a general rule, it should be possible to maintain hemoglobin levels of 10 g/dL with a transfusion of 12–15 mL/kg of packed red blood cells every 3–4 weeks. This requirement can increase if the patient develops significant red blood cell antibodies or hypersplenism. The latter is signaled by the development of increasing splenomegaly, splenic discomfort, and, on occasion, infarction. When the yearly red blood cell transfusion requirement exceeds 250–300 mL/kg, hypersplenism is almost certainly present and a therapeutic splenectomy should be considered. If performed, both **pneumococcal** and ***Haemophilus influenzae* type B vaccine** should be given prior to surgery.

Iron Chelation Therapy

Severe iron overload leading to cardiac arrhythmias and heart failure is a major threat to the survival of the thalassemia major patient. Iron absorption is increased in all thalassemic patients with high levels of ineffective erythropoiesis, to the extent that they are at risk for iron overload even without transfusion. Abnormal iron absorption can increase body iron by 2–5 g each year, depending on the severity of the anemia and ineffective erythropoiesis. This represents a failure in the level of hepcidin production needed to suppress iron absorption; hepcidin levels are inappropriately low in thalassemia patients with marked ineffective erythropoiesis. In part, this may represent a suppression of hepcidin mRNA by growth factor 15, a member of the transforming growth factor superfamily, which is released in increased levels from apoptotic erythroblasts. Chronic transfusion therapy only worsens the situation. Therefore, such patients must be considered as early candidates for iron chelation therapy with deferoxamine or deferasirox. They are also candidates for antioxidant therapy in the form of daily vitamin E supplementation, since vitamin E levels are uniformly low in iron overload patients, setting the stage for increased lipid peroxidation.

A. Therapy in Children

Children with thalassemia major should begin therapy at the earliest possible age and certainly by the time they have accumulated more than 7 g of excess iron. In young children, a serum ferritin level much greater than 1,000 μg/L or 1 year of regular transfusions (or both) can be used as surrogate indicators to initiate chelation therapy.

B. Monitoring Iron Concentration

Correlation of ferritin levels with tissue iron loading is less than precise and, in fact, can be totally unreliable. Severe ineffective erythropoiesis, hepatic damage, ascorbate deficiency, and inflammation can all interfere with the serum ferritin–iron overload relationship. Therefore, liver biopsy with quantitative measurement of hepatic iron concentration is the gold standard. Normal individuals have hepatic iron concentrations of approximately 1–2 mg/g dry weight tissue. Concentrations exceeding 15 mg/g dry weight tissue are associated with progressive organ damage and early death.

C. Treatment with Deferasirox/Deferoxamine

Iron overload can be reduced (and when treated from childhood on, largely prevented) by the administration of an iron chelator, either deferasirox or deferoxamine. Deferasirox is a relatively new oral tridentate iron chelator now approved by the US Food and Drug Administration (FDA). Given as a single oral dose of 20–30 mg/kg/d, it can prevent iron overload in all but the most heavily transfused patients. Side effects include abdominal pain, nausea and vomiting, diarrhea, rash, and a slight elevation in the serum creatinine, most prominent at the start of therapy.

A more long-standing therapy for the control of iron overload is the subcutaneous or intravenous administration of the hexadentate iron chelator deferoxamine. It can be administered at the time of red blood cell transfusions and subcutaneously during sleep hours using a syringe pump. A dose of 25–50 mg/kg of deferoxamine infused over 12 hours each day should maintain a negative iron balance despite the high level of iron absorption and ongoing red blood cell transfusions. In adults with severe iron overload and life-threatening cardiac disease, deferoxamine can be administered as a continuous intravenous infusion through a central venous catheter in doses of 40–100 mg/kg/d. This will more rapidly unload iron from tissues and improve cardiac function. A third chelator, deferiprone, has shown a special ability to unload iron from the myocardium. It potentially could be used in combination with deferasirox or deferoxamine to treat patients with severe cardiac disease but has yet to be approved by the FDA.

Deferoxamine therapy is not without its **complications**. Some patients may be unable to tolerate the drug because of local skin reactions. Others are at risk for the development of neurotoxic side effects, including changes in visual acuity with central scotomata and impaired color vision, as well as the appearance of a high-frequency auditory sensory deficit. These abnormalities are dose related, most often seen in patients receiving more than 50 mg/kg/d of deferoxamine, and can be reversed by reducing the dose. Since the toxicity increases as the iron burden falls, a useful rule of thumb is to **keep the ratio of the daily (in milligrams per kilogram) dose to the serum ferritin level (in micrograms per liter) below 0.025**. It is also important to monitor the patient very closely with **periodic audiometry and eye examinations**. Deferasirox is rarely associated with changes in visual acuity or deafness.

Survival can be correlated with the hepatic iron concentration or the patient's mean ferritin level. If periodic ferritin levels fall below 2,500 μg/L, children can expect a better than 90% survival at 15 years. When most values fall above 2,500 μg/L, only 20% of children will survive 15 years without cardiac disease. Repeated liver biopsy can be used to give a definitive measure of iron control. Follow-up liver biopsy can be important in children who receive treatment at an early age with a lower dose of deferoxamine, 25 mg/kg/d, to guarantee effective therapy as they grow. The therapeutic goal is to keep the hepatic iron concentration between 3 and 7 mg/g dry weight tissue.

Augmentation of Fetal Hemoglobin Production

It is well recognized that coinheritance of hereditary persistence of fetal hemoglobin with homozygous β-thalassemia results in milder disease. This has led to studies of several agents that have been used to increase hemoglobin F in the treatment of sickle cell anemia, including 5-azacytidine, hydroxyurea, erythropoietin, and butyric acid compounds. In clinical trials involving small numbers of patients with thalassemia intermedia or major, each of these agents, or combination of agents, has demonstrated a modest increase in hemoglobin, with or without a concomitant increase in hemoglobin F. Certainly, any increase in hemoglobin level will help reduce the transfusion requirement, especially in milder thalassemias. However, the "best" therapy still needs to be defined in large clinical trials.

Bone Marrow Transplantation

More than 1,000 children and adults with thalassemia major have now received bone marrow transplants from HLA-identical siblings that have led to reversal of the genetic disorder. To succeed, patients must be treated with both busulfan to eradicate hematopioesis and cyclophosphamide to suppress their immune system. Azathioprine, hydroxyurea, and fludarabine have also been added to treatment regimens with a reported improvement in the incidence of graft rejection. Graft-versus-host disease (GVHD) can usually be ameliorated by the use of prophylactic cyclosporine. Children who undergo the procedure at an early age before iron overload and organ damage become problems do the best, with disease-free survivals of better than 80%. Overall survival falls to 60%–70% and disease-free survival falls to 50% in older patients with disease-related complications, especially chronic active hepatitis. Marrow rejection and nonrejection mortality are both increased in these patients. Although ablation of the patient's own marrow is required for a successful long-term transplant, the procedure can result in stable mixed chimerism in a small number of patients. However, persistence of recipient marrow cells post-transplant usually predicts a subsequent failure of the graft. The experience with unrelated donor transplants is limited to date and the success rate with cord blood transplants has been limited by the need for relatively large numbers of stem cells for engraftment. Cord blood may become the treatment of choice if and when ex vivo expansion of stem cells becomes possible.

GENE THERAPY

Induction of β-globin production or correction of the mutant splicing defect holds the greatest promise for lifelong correction of thalassemia major. Recent studies of gene implantation using lentiviral vectors have shown sufficient induction of β-chain production to correct the anemia of β-thalassemia intermedia in a mouse model and in an in vitro model of human β-thalassemia major stem cells. Correction of the splicing defect responsible for the failure in β-chain production has also been demonstrated using antisense oligonucleotides in the laboratory. Clinical trials for either approach are still a way off.

CLINICAL COURSE

Without long-term transfusion and iron chelation therapy, **children with thalassemia major** will not survive much past the second decade of life. In addition, they will exhibit major growth and sexual retardation. Complications from iron overloading include cardiac, hepatic, and endocrine abnormalities. Iron loading of myocardial muscle cells results first in diastolic and then systolic dysfunction, and life-threatening atrial and ventricular arrhythmias. Often arrhythmias are preceded by an episode of pericarditis. **When patients with less severe thalassemia develop heart failure** during middle age, they should be aggressively treated with iron chelation therapy at a maximum dose. This procedure can result in an improvement in cardiac function.

As with hereditary hemochromatosis, iron overload in thalassemia can result in **cirrhosis and diabetes** (see Chapter 15). This situation can be prevented by effective iron chelation therapy during childhood. **Other endocrine abnormalities** include a marked failure of sexual development secondary to iron damage to the anterior pituitary. Children will fail to enter puberty and will have low levels of luteinizing and follicle-stimulating hormones. Once this occurs, it is irreversible by chelation therapy, and either testosterone or estrogen supplementation will be required to achieve sexual maturation. Osteopenia/osteoporosis can result from the combination of expansion of bone marrow, endocrine dysfunction, and overly vigorous chelation therapy. Finally, a few patients may present with **hypoparathyroidism**, characterized by tetany, hypocalcemia, and hyperphosphatemia.

The **survival potential** of well-treated thalassemic individuals is quite good. Patients should be followed up in a clinic experienced in the rigors of both transfusion and iron chelation therapy. Successful treatment and survival will depend on the patient's ability to comply with the rigors of the treatment schedule. A few thalassemia major patients have been treated definitively by **allogeneic marrow transplantation**. There is, however, a significant risk of death as a part of the transplantation procedure, and patients are at risk for both acute and chronic GVHD.

POINTS TO REMEMBER

Inherited defects in α- or β-globin chain production are common in selected populations and are leading causes of microcytic/hypochromic anemias, worldwide.

Individuals with ancestral roots in Africa and the Mediterranean region are especially at risk for inheriting a β-chain defect, either the trait (β-thalassemia minor) or the homozygous defect (β-thalassemia major).

Southeast Asian populations are at the added risk for inheriting α-chain defects and hemoglobin E, which can appear by itself or in combination with either α- or β-chain abnormalities to produce severe disease.

Patients presenting with β-thalassemia minor are generally asymptomatic with a mild microcytic/hypochromic anemia, often first detected on a routine screening CBC. They need to be distinguished from early iron deficiency anemia, which can also be asymptomatic. They are not at risk for associated disease or iron loading.

β-Thalassemia major and intermedia patients usually present in childhood with a severe microcytic/hypochromic anemia, growth retardation, and a marked tendency to develop iron overload, made worse by their transfusion dependency.

α-Thalassemia can present as a silent trait (single gene defect), with a thalassemia minor profile (double gene defect), more severe hemoglobin H disease (triple gene defect), or, in the case of deletion of all 4 genes, in utero death (hydrops fetalis).

Both α- and β-gene defects can be inherited in combination with other hemoglobinopathies, including hemoglobins S, C, and E, resulting in more severe disease with combined characteristics of the individual hemoglobinopathies.

Accurate diagnosis, especially the detection of double heterozygotes, requires a reference laboratory expert in the application of hemoglobin electrophoresis, HPLC, supravital stains, and DNA analysis.

Thalassemia major patients with marked ineffective erythropoiesis are at risk for progressive iron overload, cardiac toxicity, and early death if not aggressively treated with iron chelating drugs (deferasirox and deferoxamine).

BIBLIOGRAPHY

Cao A et al: Molecular diagnosis and carrier screening for β-thalassemia. JAMA 1997;278:1273.

Cazzola M et al: Relationship between transfusion regimen and suppression of erythropoiesis in β-thalassemia major. Br J Haematol 1995;89:473.

Cohen A, Glimm E, Porter J: Effect of transfusional iron intake on response to chelation therapy in β-thalassemia major. Blood 2008;111:583.

Davis BA, Porter JB: Long-term outcome of continuous 24-h DFO infusion via indwelling intravenous catheters in high-risk β-thalassemia. Blood 2000;95:1229.

Glickstein H et al: Action of chelators in iron-loaded cardiac cells: accessibility to intracellular labile iron and functional consequences. Blood 2006;108:3195.

Lucarelli G et al: Bone marrow transplantation in adult thalassemic patients. Blood 1999;93:1164.

Neufeld E: Oral chelators deferasirox and deferiprone for transfusional iron overload in thalassemia major: new data, new questions. Blood 2006;107:3436.

Rund D, Rachmilewitz E: β-Thalassemia. N Eng J Med 2005;353:1135.

Sodani P et al: New approach for bone marrow transplantation in patients with class 3 thalassemia aged younger than 17 years. Blood 2004;104:1201.

HEMOGLOBINOPATHIES • 7

CASE HISTORY • *Part 1*

A 22-year-old African American woman presents to her obstetrician for prenatal care. She reports that she has been anemic since childhood but is unclear as to what kind of anemia. Past medical history is positive for splenectomy following blunt trauma to the abdomen in a car accident at age 16. Otherwise review of systems negative. A routine CBC shows the following results:

CBC: Hematocrit/hemoglobin - 33%/11 g/dL (IU - 110 g/L)
MCV - 75 fL MCH - 28 pg MCHC - 30 g/dL
RDW-CV - 16%
WBC count - 7,400/μL
Platelet count - 245,000/μL

• SMEAR MORPHOLOGY

Findings on the blood smear include microcytosis, targeting, sickle cell forms, and both the occasional nucleated red blood cell (not shown) and red cells with Howell-Jolly bodies (also not shown).
Reticulocyte count - 4.5%/3.0 Index - 1.5–2

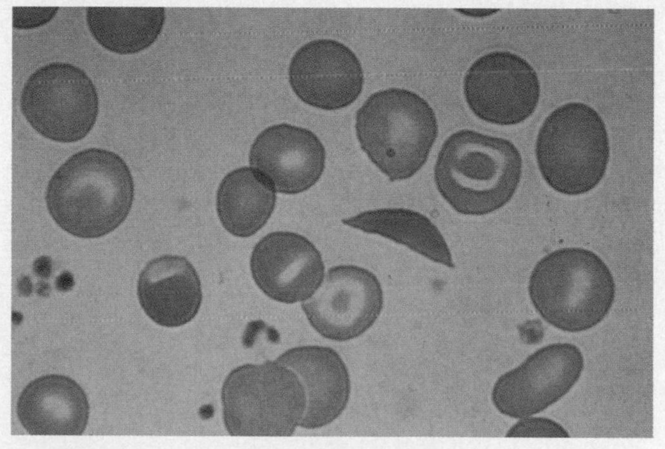

Questions

- How should this anemia be described/categorized?
- Do the smear abnormalities indicate a specific abnormality?
- What additional tests should be ordered?

Inherited defects in globin structure are common in individuals of African, Indian, Asian, and Mediterranean descent. Most of these involve a single amino acid substitution in one of the globin chains. The resulting structural defect can be clinically silent or produce a significant anemia. Sickle cell disease, secondary to the substitution of valine for glutamic acid in position 6 of the β-globin chain, is the paradigm of the hemoglobinopathies. It has a worldwide distribution with a very high frequency, and it was the first hemoglobinopathy to be defined at a molecular level.

Management of a patient with a hemoglobinopathy depends not only on an accurate diagnosis of the disorder but also on an understanding of the clinical expression of the defect. In addition, there is an obligation for screening and genetic counseling of populations with any increased prevalence of a hemoglobinopathy.

NORMAL GLOBIN CHEMISTRY

The globin portion of the hemoglobin molecule can be defined according to combinations of α-globin and β-, γ-, or δ-globin chains; the amino acid sequence of the individual chains; and the 3-dimensional structure of the folded molecule. As discussed in Chapter 6, genetic defects resulting in **impaired globin chain**

synthesis produce microcytic, hypochromic anemias and distinctive changes in pairing of the several globin chains. In contrast, **amino acid substitutions** in either the α-globin or β-globin chains can disrupt the molecular structure and function of hemoglobin.

Normal globin is made up of 2 α-globin chains, each with 141 amino acids, and 2 β-globin chains, each with 146 amino acids. The 4 polypeptide chains form a helical structure with hydrophobic pockets holding 4 heme groups. A central cavity between the two β-globin chains houses 2,3-diphosphoglycerate (2,3-DPG) (Figure 7–1). This complex structure is essential to hemoglobin function.

Even a single amino acid substitution can interfere with the helical structure and make the globin unstable. The most common clinical example of this is sickle cell disease (hemoglobin S-β^S). Replacement of glutamic acid with valine at position 6 on the β-globin chain results in a dramatic change in its solubility. Deoxygenated hemoglobin S polymerizes to form twisted rope-like fibers that align and deform the red blood cell, producing the characteristic sickle shape. Substitutions at other sites can disrupt the respiratory motion of the hemoglobin molecule and either increase or decrease hemoglobin-oxygen affinity.

More than **400 hemoglobin variants** have now been defined. Nearly half of these variants are clinically silent and most of the others are structural defects that produce either a change in hemoglobin-oxygen affinity or a physically unstable molecule. The latter is most often associated with a mild hemolytic anemia. Changes in hemoglobin-oxygen affinity can produce either anemia or polycythemia. Only a handful of amino acid substitutions are associated with unique structural changes that can be defined morphologically. The most clinically important of these are hemoglobins S and C.

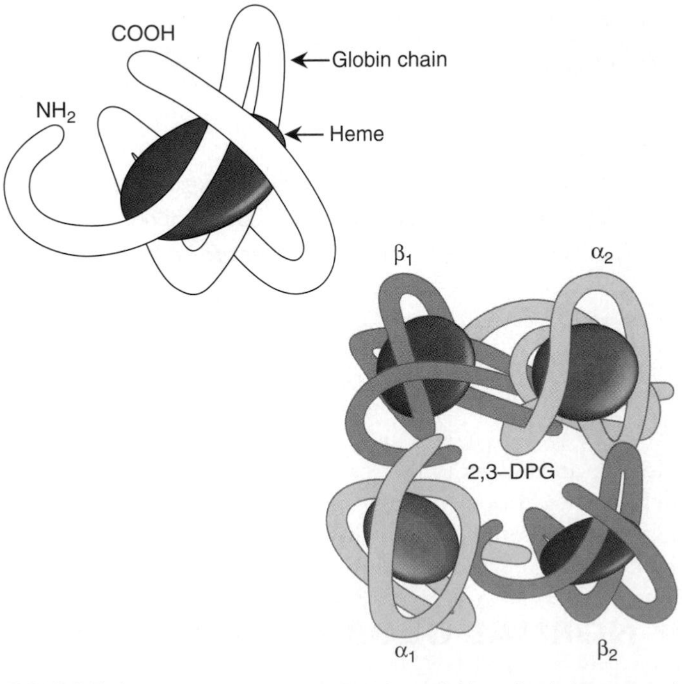

COOH
Globin chain
NH_2
Heme
β_1
α_2
2,3–DPG
α_1
β_2

FIGURE 7–1. **Hemoglobin structure.** Each hemoglobin molecule is composed of 2 α globin (light shading) and 2 β-globin chains (dark shading), each of which contains a single heme group in a hydrophobic pocket. A central cavity between the 2 β-globin chains houses a molecule of 2,3-DPG. This is important for the respiratory function of hemoglobin.

CLINICAL FEATURES

The clinical presentation of a hemoglobinopathy is a function of the severity of the genetic defect and its impact on hemoglobin structure and function. Heterozygote patients tend to have little or no clinical disease and are most often identified by routine screening. In contrast, some heterozygote and most homozygote patients present with a moderate to severe hemolytic anemia, or, in the case of high oxygen–affinity hemoglobins, erythrocytosis (see Chapter 13). The most common of the hemoglobinopathies (hemoglobins S, C, D, and E), when present in their homozygote form or as a compound heterozygote, generally result in severe disease (Table 7–1).

Sickle Cell Anemia

Sickle cell anemia, the homozygous form of hemoglobin S disease ($\beta^S\beta^S$), presents early in life with a severe hemolytic anemia and vasoocclusive disease involving the marrow, spleen, kidney, and central nervous system (CNS). **Involved children** first complain of recurrent painful crises characterized as deep-seated bone and joint pain that may or may not be associated with other intercurrent illness. When frequent, these painful episodes are devastating, and over time, patients can become disabled and dependent on pain medications. Organ damage starts early in childhood. **Splenic infarction** with eventual complete loss of splenic function occurs in the first decade of life. The renal medulla is another prime target. The concentrating ability of the kidney is invariably lost, and patients can experience episodes of gross hematuria. Sickle cell anemia patients are also

TABLE 7–1 • Common hemoglobinopathies

Severe anemia/disease
Hemoglobin S/S (sickle cell anemia)
Hemoglobin S/C
S/β^0-thalassemia
Hemoglobin S/E
Mild anemia/disease
S/β^+-thalassemia
Hemoglobin C/C
Hemoglobin S/Lepore
Hemoglobin S/D
Hemoglobin S/$O^{\text{-Arab}}$
Minimal anemia/no disease
Hemoglobin S trait
Hemoglobin C trait
Hemoglobin D trait

at risk for death from cerebrovascular thrombosis or overwhelming sepsis. Loss of splenic function and the recurrent infarction of marrow and bone set the stage for infections with organisms such as ***Streptococcus pneumoniae***, ***Haemophilus influenzae***, and salmonella species.

Adult sickle cell anemia patients who have recurrent vasoocclusive crises can develop significant bone and joint disease, including **aseptic necrosis** of the femur and humerus heads, muscle wasting, and flexion contractures of major joints. During the second and third decades of life, damage to the pulmonary vasculature can result in pulmonary hypertension, cardiac failure, and death. When patients receive long-term transfusion therapy, crises can be prevented but only at the risk of progressive **iron overload**.

Compound Hemoglobinopathies

Compound hemoglobinopathies, such as combinations of hemoglobin S with hemoglobin C (SC disease) or hemoglobin S with either α- or β-thalassemia, vary in their presentation. **Hemoglobin SC disease patients** tend to have less difficulty with painful crises and do not have infarction of their spleens. At the same time, they do have problems with gross hematuria, aseptic necrosis, retinopathy, and, in women, increased risk of maternal or fetal death with pregnancy. **Hemoglobin S/β^+-thalassemia patients** usually present with a variable anemia and can experience vasoocclusive crises, but often have milder forms of vascular disease. The severity of the clinical picture in these patients in large part depends on the level of hemoglobin F in red blood cells.

Hemoglobin C Disease and the Unstable Hemoglobinopathies

Homozygous hemoglobin C disease and hemoglobinopathies associated with an unstable hemoglobin molecule generally present with a well-compensated hemolytic anemia. Although they do not have vasoocclusive disease, patients are subject to hemolytic crises where an increased rate of red blood cell destruction, secondary to intercurrent illness or drug ingestion, produces a sudden worsening of their anemia. They also exhibit the symptoms and signs associated with continuous high levels of red blood cell turnover, including jaundice, splenomegaly, and an increased risk of gallstone formation.

Several amino acid substitutions of the globin chain result in a change in **hemoglobin-oxygen affinity**. When the oxygen affinity is reduced, patients generally have a well-compensated hemolytic anemia. The shift in the hemoglobin-oxygen dissociation curve maintains tissue oxygen delivery despite the hemoglobin level. In contrast, patients with high oxygen–affinity hemoglobinopathies present with erythrocytosis (see Chapter 13).

Laboratory Studies

The complete blood count (CBC), high-performance liquid chromatography (HPLC), and hemoglobin electrophoresis are the key tests for detecting and diagnosing common hemoglobinopathies. The characteristic erythropoietic profile for these patients is shown in Table 7–2. Most hemoglobinopathies are associated with a lifelong hemolytic anemia. This situation is readily apparent when the reticulocyte index increases to greater than 3–5 times normal when patients are otherwise healthy and in a well-compensated state. Other signs of increased hemoglobin turnover include high lactic acid dehydrogenase (LDH) and indirect bilirubin levels. Patients with moderately severe hemolytic anemias will demonstrate a reticulocyte index greater than 3 times normal, LDH levels of greater than 1,000 IU, and indirect bilirubins of 1–3 mg/dL.

TABLE 7–2 • Hemoglobinopathy erythropoietic profile

Red blood cell morphology	Normocytic, normochromic to slightly microcytic (MCV 70–80 fL), abnormal cell shapes (sickle cells, target cells, etc)
Polychromasia	Present to prominent
Nucleated red blood cells	Present after splenic infarction
Reticulocyte index	>3–5
Marrow E/G ratio	>1:1
Bilirubin and LDH	Increased
Serum iron	Normal to increased
TIBC	Normal
Serum ferritin	>100 μg/L

A. Red Blood Cell Indices and Morphology

Red blood cell indices and film morphology can provide important clues to the cause of the anemia. Although most hemoglobinopathies present with a normocytic, normochromic anemia, sickle cell anemia patients with large numbers of sickle cells in circulation can show a slight reduction in the mean cell volume (MCV). Combinations of hemoglobin S or C with α- or β-thalassemia or hemoglobin E will have more marked microcytosis with concomitant reductions of the MCV to levels below 70 fL (see Chapter 6). To complicate the situation, all hemolytic anemia patients are at risk for development of folic acid deficiency, since their folate requirements are increased in line with their increased level of erythropoiesis. Folate deficiency results in megaloblastic erythropoiesis and the production of macrocytic red blood cells and, over time, can normalize or increase the MCV. An early measure of complicating folate deficiency is the detection of occasional macroovalocytes or multilobed polymorphonuclear leukocytes on the peripheral film.

Cell **morphology** can make the diagnosis. With homozygous hemoglobin S disease, sickle forms are usually present on a Wright stained film, although in small numbers (Figure 7–2). The classic sickle cell looks like a crescent moon or banana. This is dramatically magnified on a phase microscopy wet preparation. Other shapes include fragments of cells and partially distorted cells with sharp, pointed extensions. The distinctive sickle shape is the result of the tendency for hemoglobin S to

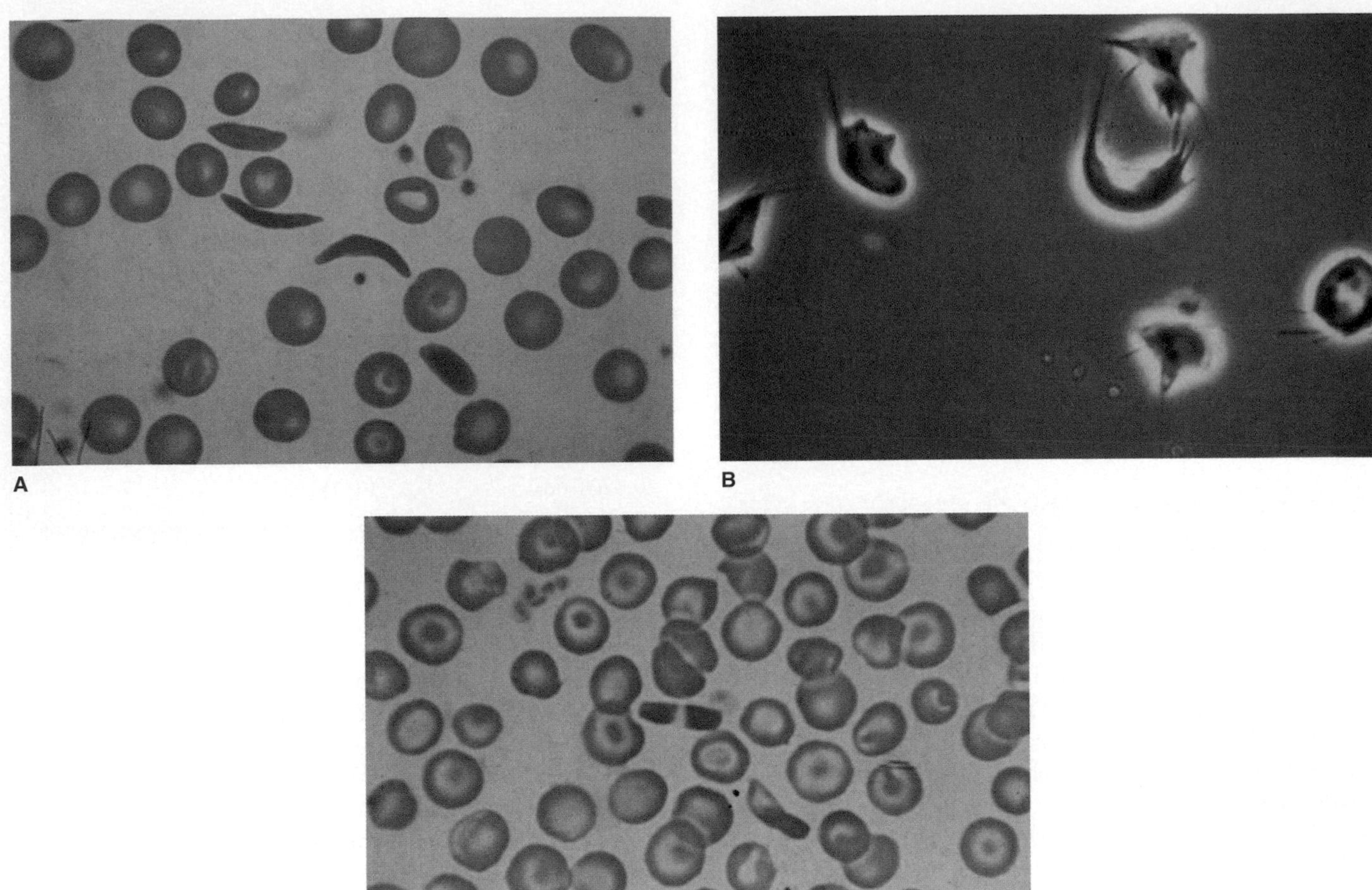

FIGURE 7–2. **Abnormalities in cell morphology.** On a Wright stained blood film, sickle cells appear as crescent moon or banana-shaped red cells **(A)**; phase microscopy of a sickle-prep specimen shows the same sickle-shape distortion but in a more dramatic way **(B)**; hemoglobin C crystals appear as dense block or bricklike formations in red cells **(C)**.

form rigid, crystal-like structures within the cell. Since sickle cell anemia patients generally have infarcted spleens at an early age, nuclear remnants (Howell-Jolly bodies and nucleated orthochromatic normoblasts) may also be detected on the blood smear (Figure 7–3).

Morphologic features of other hemoglobinopathies include targeting, the presence of intracellular inclusions of precipitated hemoglobin (**Heinz bodies**), and, in homozygous hemoglobin C disease, the formation of a blocklike crystal in the center of the red blood cell (Figure 7–2). Prominent targeting is most common in patients with hemoglobin C or SC disease and those with hemoglobin S or C/β-thalassemia.

B. Hemoglobin Electrophoresis

Screening for hemoglobinopathies is best accomplished by HPLC analysis, which can rapidly detect and quantify any abnormal hemoglobin(s). Although certain HPLC programs can distinguish among hemoglobins S, C, and D, confirmation generally requires further testing by cellulose acetate and citrate agar hemoglobin electrophoresis. When performed at an alkaline pH, hemoglobin S migrates more slowly than hemoglobins A and F (Figure 7–4). Moreover, hemoglobin C migrates even more slowly, permitting the separation of the more common hemoglobinopathies including hemoglobin S, hemoglobin C, and combinations of hemoglobins S and C with β^+-thalassemia. Sickle cell anemia can be detected at birth using both HPLC and electrophoresis to separate small amounts of hemoglobin S from the predominant hemoglobin F of the fetal red blood cell. Prenatal diagnosis in families where both parents carry sickle cell trait is possible using the technique of **chorionic villus biopsy** with restriction fragment length polymorphism/Southern blot analysis or polymerase chain reaction amplification of genomic DNA. The more rare hemoglobinopathies may require identification by the technique of isoelectric focusing.

Genetic **defects resulting in unstable hemoglobins** generally present with evidence of increased hemolysis, including an

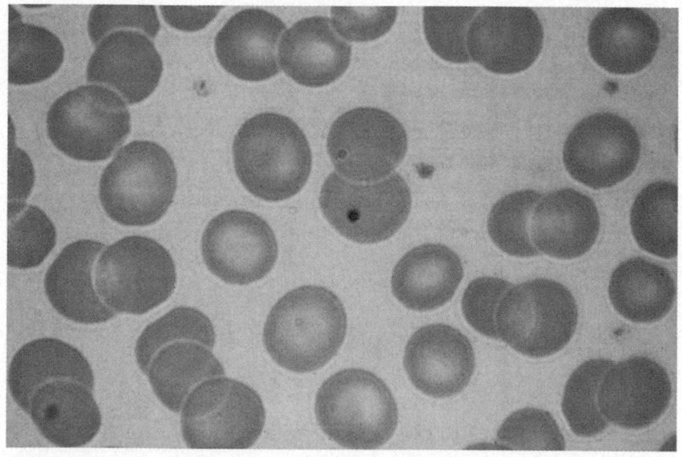

A

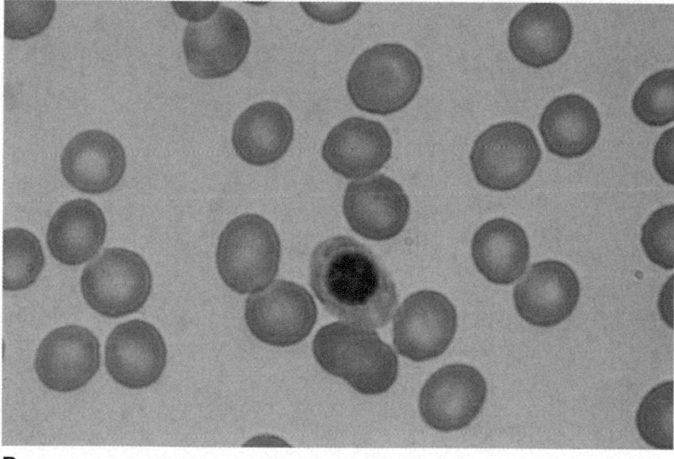

B

FIGURE 7–3. **Morphological abnormalities with hyposplenism.** A red blood cell containing a tiny nuclear remnant—Howell-Jolly body **(A)** and a single nucleated red cell–orthochromatic normoblast **(B)**. Both findings are commonly seen on the blood smear in patients with a loss of splenic function.

Hemoglobinopathy	Origin ↓	Hemoglobin electrophoresis A_2	C	S	F	A	Ratio S/A
Normal	▌	▌				█	—
Sickle cell anemia	▌	▌		█	█		100/0
Sickle cell trait	▌	▌		█	▏	█	40/60
Hemoglobin S/C	▌	▌	█	█	▏		—
S/B^{+} thalassemia	▏	▏		█		█	60/40
S/B$^{°}$ thalassemia	▏	▌		█	▌		100/0
B$^{°}$ thalassemia trait	▏	█			▏	█	—
Hemoglobin C trait	▏	▌	█		▏	█	—
Hemoglobin C/C	▏	▌	█		▏		—

FIGURE 7–4. **Cellulose acetate hemoglobin electrophoresis at an alkaline pH.** Cellulose acetate electrophoresis is used clinically to separate the more common hemoglobinopathies. Top: The normal hemoglobin pattern. More than 97% of the hemoglobin in normal individuals is hemoglobin A, with very small amounts of hemoglobin A_2 (2%–3%) and F (trace). Hemoglobins S and C migrate more slowly than hemoglobin A and are clearly separated by this technique. Patients with β-thalassemia trait show an increase in hemoglobin A_2; double heterozygotes for hemoglobin S and β-thalassemia show variable amounts of hemoglobin F. The ratio of hemoglobin S/A is important in distinguishing sickle cell trait from hemoglobin S/β^{+}-thalassemia.

elevated reticulocyte index, high LDH level, and an increase in the indirect bilirubin level with clinical jaundice. Hemoglobin levels may be decreased, normal, or increased according to the oxygen affinity characteristics of the abnormal hemoglobin. Red blood cell morphology can be either normocytic and normochromic or show slight hypochromia with aniso- and poikilocytosis, secondary to intracellular hemoglobin denaturation and pitting of red blood cell inclusion bodies by the spleen. Diagnosis depends on demonstrating hemoglobin instability and defining its oxygen carrying characteristics.

C. Isopropanol Stability Test

The **isopropanol stability test** is performed by adding fresh red blood cell hemolysate to a 17% buffered solution of isopropanol kept at 37°C. The mixture is then observed at frequent intervals for the appearance of a flocculent precipitate. Unstable hemoglobins will usually precipitate within the first 5–20 minutes, whereas normal hemoglobin is stable for 40–60 minutes.

D. Heat Stability Test

The **heat stability test** is performed by mixing 3 mL of a fresh hemolysate of washed red blood cells with 3 mL of tris buffer, followed by heating in a water bath at 50°C for 2 hours. Normal hemoglobin is stable at this temperature, whereas unstable hemoglobins will precipitate. Centrifuging the sample after 2 hours and measuring the hemoglobin level in the supernatant can detect this result.

E. Detection of Intracellular Inclusion Bodies

Two stains, brilliant cresyl blue and methyl violet, can be used to identify intracellular inclusions of denatured hemoglobin. When fresh whole blood is incubated with **brilliant cresyl blue**, unstable hemoglobins are induced to precipitate, resulting in a diffuse cobblestone-type stippling of red blood cells. The **methyl violet stain** does not by itself denature hemoglobin. It can be used, however, to detect free-form hemoglobin inclusions (Heinz bodies) in circulating red blood cells. This test works best in patients who lack splenic function, in whom Heinz bodies appear as from a few to many small, violet-colored inclusions in red blood cells. Heinz bodies are seen not only with unstable hemoglobins but also in patients with α- and β-thalassemia and glucose-6-phosphate dehydrogenase (G6PD) deficiency.

DIAGNOSIS

Diagnosis of a hemoglobinopathy involves both accurate identification of a specific gene defect and assessment of the patient's clinical status. The first step may be possible simply from the

CASE HISTORY • Part 2

Based on the CBC, the patient has a microcytic/hypochromic anemia of modest severity, which could indicate a diagnosis of iron deficiency, thalassemia minor, or a combination of the two. At the same time, the blood shows the presence of sickle-shaped cells, target cells, Howell-Jolly bodies, and the rare nucleated red cell.

This morphology raises the immediate question of a compound hemoglobinopathy. While the presence of sickle cells is diagnostic for hemoglobin S disease, targeting is seen with thalassemia, hemoglobin C disease, liver disease, or a loss of splenic function (hyposplenia). The appearance in circulation of Howell-Jolly bodies and the occasional nucleated red blood cell (see Figure 7–3) are typically seen with hyposplenia (patient had a splenectomy).

To look for the presence of a hemoglobinopathy, a hemoglobin electrophoresis was performed with the following result:

Hgb A - 25% Hgb F - 10% Hgb A_2 - 5% Hgb S - 60%

Questions

- Does this result indicate a specific diagnosis?
- If so, what are the health implications?
- Does the patient run the risk of iron overload?

clinical presentation, as with sickle cell anemia. However, other hemoglobinopathies may only be diagnosed after a careful laboratory evaluation. As for assessment of the patient's overall clinical status, this involves a broader evaluation of both the erythropoietic profile and the functional status of various organ systems.

Hemoglobin S Diseases

Diagnosis of homozygous sickle cell disease (hemoglobin SS) is usually not difficult. Detection and diagnosis of the hemoglobin S heterozygote and the patient with a compound hemoglobinopathy are greater challenges.

A. Sickle Cell Trait

Sickle cell trait, the heterozygous form of hemoglobin S ($\beta\beta^S$), is not associated with anemia or clinical disease. It is, however, a very common genetic abnormality; some 7%–8% of American blacks carry the trait. The frequency of sickle cell trait in certain African countries can be even higher, and the chance of forming a compound heterozygote with thalassemia is greatly increased. This situation is thought to reflect a survival advantage that sickle hemoglobin imparts in those regions where there is a high incidence of malaria. The protective role of hemoglobin S is further demonstrated by the observation that the same β-globin chain position 6 Glu to Val mutation has originated in 4 different locations in Africa.

Overall clinical health of the individual is not affected by the inheritance of a single sickle gene (Table 7–3). Lifespan is normal and these individuals do not have painful crises or organ damage. The **only abnormality that has been associated with sickle cell trait** is the occurrence of self-limited episodes of painless hematuria in up to 3% of patients. There have also been a few case reports of sickle crisis and sudden death with severe exertion and dehydration, or from exposure to very low oxygen tensions.

The routine CBC is normal and sickle cells are not observed in the peripheral blood film. Furthermore, the lifespan of the red blood cells is not significantly shortened, so there is no evidence of a hemolytic anemia, and the reticulocyte index, LDH, and indirect bilirubin levels all are normal. The hemoglobin electrophoresis pattern is diagnostic; 35%–45% of the hemoglobin in red blood cells migrates as hemoglobin S (see Figure 7–2 and Table 7–3). The disparity between the levels of hemoglobin

TABLE 7–3 • Clinical features of sickle hemoglobinopathies

	Clinical Abnormalities	CBC/Hgb Electrophoresis
Sickle trait	None, rare painless hematuria	Hgb: 11–14 g/dL Hgb S/A 40/60
Sickle cell anemia	Vasoocclusive crises with infarction of spleen, marrow, kidney, etc Aseptic necrosis of bone Gallstones Priapism Ankle ulcers	Hgb: 7–10 g/dL MCV: 80–100 fL Hgb S/A: 100/0 Hgb F: 2%–25%
S/β^0-Thalassemia	Vasoocclusive crises Aseptic necrosis of bone	Hgb: 7–10 g/dL MCV: 60–80 fL Hgb S/A: 100/0 Hgb F: 1%–10%
S/β^+-Thalassemia	Rare vasoocclusive disease or aseptic necrosis	Hgb: 10–14 g/dL MCV: 70–80 fL Hgb S/A: 60/40
Hemoglobin S/C	Rare vasoocclusive disease or aseptic necrosis; painless hematuria more common	Hgb: 10–14 g/dL MCV: 80–100 fL Hgb S: 50% Hgb C: 50%

A (60%) and S (40%) reflect the different production efficiencies for the 2 globin (β and β^S) chains.

B. Sickle Cell Anemia

Sickle cell anemia, the homozygous form of hemoglobin S disease ($\beta^S\beta^S$), is easier to diagnose. It is largely limited to black populations and occurs in families where both parents are heterozygotes for hemoglobin S. It almost always causes clinical disease once the affected infant approaches 6 months of age, because for the first 6–12 weeks of life, high levels of fetal hemoglobin prevent severe intravascular sickling.

1. Classic symptoms and signs—As described in the section on clinical presentation, classic symptoms and signs of sickle cell anemia include recurrent, painful crises secondary to intravascular sickling, small-vessel occlusion, and tissue infarction. The organs that are at greatest risk for infarction include marrow, kidney, spleen, lung, and brain. **Young children** can present with acute dactylitis secondary to marrow necrosis in the small bones of the hands and feet. **Older children** complain of recurrent episodes of joint or bone pain, and abdominal pain secondary to splenic infarction. Pneumococcal sepsis is a leading cause of death in children with sickle cell anemia, because of the loss of spleen function. Damage to vital organs including lung, heart, and brain increases as the child grows older. In **untreated patients**, there is a constant risk of vascular occlusion, with death occurring from either a stroke or major cardiopulmonary damage before the fourth decade. Risk of stroke in untreated children is on the order of 10% per year. This can be reduced to less than 1% by chronic transfusion therapy. This observation has led to the recommendation that all children with homozygous sickle cell disease, between 2 and 16 years of age, be screened every 6 months by **transcranial doppler**, with the clinician looking for elevated blood flow velocity in the middle cerebral or internal carotid arteries. From 5%–30% of adult sickle cell anemia patients develop pulmonary hypertension secondary to repeated vascular occlusion (acute chest syndrome) and pulmonary fibrosis. The median survival after the development of pulmonary hypertension is about 2 years.

2. Severity—The severity of the sickle process is a function of several variables including the concentration of hemoglobin S, the degree of hemoglobin deoxygenation, the intracellular hemoglobin concentration, and the level of hemoglobin F. Homozygous $\beta^S\beta^S$ cells also show a **tendency to become dehydrated** secondary to an increased rate of potassium-chloride cotransport out of the cell and an activation of the calcium-dependent **(Gardos) potassium export channel** when the red cell membrane is distorted. This hastens the polymerization process, and plays a similar role in the formation of target cells in patients with SC and CC disease.

Interference **with blood flow through the tissue microcirculation (viscosity)** correlates with the degree of deoxygenation and formation of irreversibly sickled cells. Oxygenated sickle blood has a viscosity of 1.5 times normal, rising to 10 times normal with deoxygenation. In part, the increase in viscosity is compensated for by the patient's anemia. However, with deoxygenation, blood flow is strikingly diminished, especially at the level of the small arterioles. Any rise in the patient's hematocrit, as with marked dehydration, will further increase viscosity and contribute to the severity of the disease.

The **frequency and severity of vasoocclusive events** also reflects the tendency of sickle cells to adhere to dysfunctional endothelial cells. Endothelial dysfunction in sickle cell disease, as well as with other hemolytic anemias, has been correlated with hemolysis-driven low arginine and nitric oxide (NO) bioavailability. Free-radical and plasma hemoglobin levels produce a dramatic resistance to NO, resulting in upregulation of endothelin-1, a potent vasoconstrictor, as well as platelet activation and thrombogenesis.

Sickle cells express several adhesion receptors including CD36, CD44, B-CAM/LU, ICAM-4, $\alpha_4\beta_1$ integrin, and increased phosphatidylserine exposure. The latter appears to correlate with repeated cycles of sickling and unsickling and is a potential driver of a persistent hypercoagulable state. Cytokine-induced endothelial vascular adhesion molecule-1 (VCAM-1) and $\alpha_v\beta_3$ integrin that binds von Willebrand factor and thrombospondin also help mediate sickle cell adherence. Red cell binding to endothelial cells, together with platelet adhesion and white cell activation/adhesion, contributes to the severity of any occlusive event.

The rate of hemolysis would appear to play a major role in the clinical expression of these abnormalities. Two overlapping thrombogenic phenotypes have been proposed: a viscosity-vasoocclusion subtype and a hemolysis-driven endothelial dysfunction subtype. Patients with lower levels of hemolysis are less anemic and suffer primarily from recurrent vasoocclusive pain crises, osteonecrosis, and acute chest syndrome. In contrast, patients with more severe hemolysis (LDH >500 IU) are more anemic and have a greater incidence of pulmonary hypertension, priapism, leg ulceration, and stroke. The appearance of pulmonary hypertension (echo-detected tricuspid regurgitant jet velocity [TRV] >2.5 m/sec) is perhaps the strongest predictor of early death. Fifty percent of patients with elevated TRVs (mean pulmonary artery pressures >30 mm Hg) will die within 2–3 years.

Sickle cell anemia patients are also at risk for sudden and repeated aplastic crises where a self-limited failure of stem cells precipitates a major worsening of their anemia. Parvovirus infection (HPV B19) can be one cause of aplastic crisis; another is major damage to the kidney with loss of erythropoietin stimulation. From 30%–50% of children with sickle cell disease will show serologic evidence of HPV B19 infection and half of these will present with an episode of transient red cell aplasia. The impact of erythroid marrow expansion on bone structure can be impressive. Active marrow can be detected in distal bones, at times accompanied by thinning of the bony cortex and remodeling of the bone, especially in the skull where frontal bossing is a sign of severe disease.

3. Complications—Slight to moderate **growth retardation** with delayed puberty may be observed. This condition may be related to zinc deficiency. However, sickle cell anemia patients will attain normal physical size and sexual maturation by age 18–21. Women have no difficulty bearing children, although the number and severity of **crises can increase during pregnancy**. With puberty, young men often have recurrent episodes of **priapism**.

Other complications of sickle cell anemia include proliferative retinopathy (especially with SC disease), gallstones, aseptic necrosis of the femoral and humeral heads, leg ulcers, renal insufficiency, and acute chest syndrome. A **proliferative retinopathy** usually appears later in life, whereas most sickle cell anemia patients will develop bilirubin pigment **gallstones** by the second or third decade. Poorly healing **leg ulcers** secondary to infarction of the subcutaneous fat and skin over the malleoli appear in the second and third decades.

Aseptic **necrosis of the femoral or humeral heads** can produce a crippling arthritis requiring prosthetic surgery. Furthermore, aseptic necrosis is associated with pulmonary fat embolism and is a risk factor for the development of a ***Salmonella*** or ***Staphylococcus aureus*** osteomyelitis. **Renal insufficiency**, which leads to renal failure, may be seen later in life. **Acute chest syndrome** is a life-threatening complication in adult sickle cell patients. It presents with symptoms of fever, cough, hypoxemia, and chest pain, usually without evidence of a viral or bacterial infection. Chest x-ray shows multilobar infiltrates that reflect widespread thrombosis/fat embolism on autopsy. This can lead to marked hypoxia, respiratory failure, and death. **Multiorgan damage** and **"watershed" strokes**, often associated with sudden increases in hematocrit and whole blood viscosity, are also life-threatening complications.

4. Overall course of the disease—The frequency of vasoocclusive events, the severity of the hemolytic anemia, and the presence of other abnormal hemoglobins mark the overall course of the patient's disease (Figure 7–5). High levels of intracellular

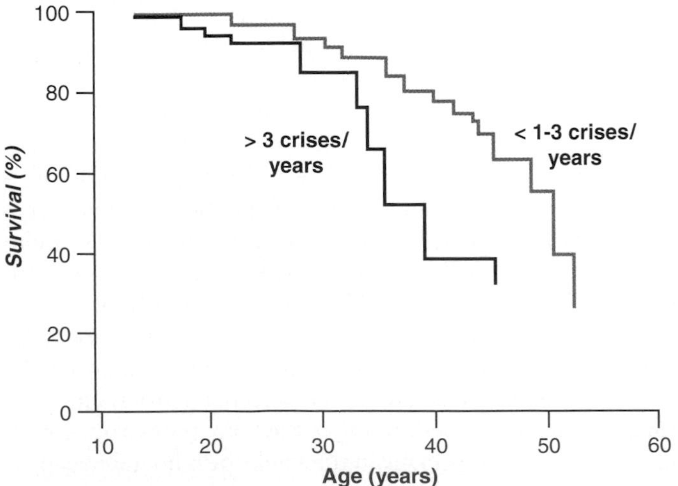

FIGURE 7–5. **Survival of sickle cell anemia patients.** The overall survival of patients with sickle cell anemia correlates with the severity of their disease state, especially the number of crises per year. Patients who experience between 1 and 3 crises per year have a median survival of nearly 50 years, whereas patients with more than 3 crises per year will experience fatal complications during the fourth and fifth decades of life.

hemoglobin F are associated with milder disease. Sickle cell patients from the Middle East and West Africa who have a strong predilection for hereditary persistence of hemoglobin F production have very mild disease. A decrease in the hemoglobin concentration in the red blood cell secondary to iron deficiency or combined inheritance of α-thalassemia can also significantly reduce the sickling tendency and the frequency of vasoocclusive crises.

The likelihood of death at an early age correlates best with the number and severity of vasoocclusive events, especially episodes of acute chest syndrome, the severity of the hemolytic anemia, and the appearance of pulmonary hypertension. The patient's LDH level, an easily measured marker of hemolysis severity, may correlate best with the frequency of painful crises, priapism, leg ulcerations, and life-threatening pulmonary hypertension.

C. Hemoglobin SC Disease

Hemoglobin SC disease ($\beta^S\beta^C$) is less common than SS disease. Clinically, it can present with the same manifestations as sickle cell anemia, although frequency and severity of the vasoocclusive manifestations are somewhat less. In contrast to sickle cell anemia, splenic infarction is uncommon and most adult patients with SC disease have an easily palpable, enlarged spleen. Damage to other organs, including renal medullary infarction, CNS thrombosis, and cardiopulmonary thrombosis, is also less common. Hemoglobin SC patients present more frequently with gross hematuria, and the rate of spontaneous abortion in women with SC disease is very high.

The **laboratory diagnosis** of SC disease is straightforward. Patients show a mild to moderate hemolytic anemia, prominent red blood cell targeting on the peripheral blood film, hemoglobin C crystal formation in some red blood cells, a tendency to form spherocytes with a slight rise in the mean corpuscular hemoglobin concentration (MCHC), but an absence of true sickle cells. HPLC will rapidly quantitate both hemoglobins, whereas the hemoglobin electrophoresis pattern is diagnostic (see Figure 7–2 and Table 7–3).

D. Hemoglobin S/β-Thalassemia

The combined inheritance of hemoglobin S and β-thalassemia is another common disorder in black and Mediterranean populations. **When S hemoglobin is combined with β^+-thalassemia,** the patient's disease is mild and more closely resembles sickle cell trait. Patients can demonstrate a mild to moderate hemolytic anemia and splenomegaly. On hemoglobin electrophoresis, they show a reduction in hemoglobin A production, which results in a hemoglobin S to A ratio of 60%/40% or higher depending on the level of production of hemoglobins F and A_2. The preponderance of S hemoglobin clearly distinguishes patients with S/β^+-thalassemia from those with heterozygous S (sickle cell trait) (see Figure 7–4 and Table 7–3).

The combination of hemoglobin S with β^0-thalassemia in Mediterranean populations results in more severe disease. These patients present with most or all of the symptoms of sickle cell anemia, although their spleens do not infarct. The severity of the vasoocclusive manifestations of hemoglobin S/β^0-thalassemia depends on the level of hemoglobin F in red blood cells. When hemoglobin F levels are greater than 10%–15% and are evenly distributed throughout the red blood cell population, the patient manifests much less severe disease. When hemoglobin F production is low, the clinical picture, blood film findings, and hemoglobin electrophoresis pattern mimic SS disease.

E. Other Double Heterozygotes

Hemoglobins D, O^{-Arab}, and Lepore are other β-globin chain defects that may be inherited together with hemoglobin S. Hemoglobin SD disease and S/O^{-Arab} disease produce clinical manifestations similar to but milder than those of sickle cell anemia. Hemoglobin S/Lepore also results in milder disease.

Hemoglobin C Disease

Hemoglobin C production results from the substitution of lysine for glutamic acid at the sixth position of the β-globin chain. Hemoglobin C tends to form intracellular blocklike crystals, which increase the rigidity of the red blood cell, shorten its lifespan, and cause fragmentation and formation of spherocytes in circulation.

Patients **with homozygous hemoglobin C disease** ($\beta^C\beta^C$) have a mild to moderate hemolytic anemia, hemoglobin levels of 8–12 g/dL, and obvious splenomegaly. They do not have the vasoocclusive problems of the sickle cell anemia patient. The diagnosis may be apparent from the blood film based on the prominent targeting that accompanies both homozygous (80%–90% of red blood cells) and heterozygous (20%–50% of red blood cells) C disease and the presence of blocklike crystals of hemoglobin C (see Figure 7–2). **Patients with C trait** ($\beta\beta^C$) demonstrate a normal erythropoietic profile other than the presence of targeting on the blood film.

Hemoglobin D Disease

Hemoglobin D (β^D) production results from the substitution of glutamine for lysine at position 121 on the β-globin chain. Hemoglobin D disease is most prevalent in India. Heterozygotes are not anemic, whereas homozygotes demonstrate a mild hemolytic anemia. Laboratory diagnosis requires electrophoresis on acid citrate agar, since hemoglobin D comigrates with S on cellulose acetate electrophoresis at an alkaline pH.

The Unstable Hemoglobins

Mutations in the amino acid sequence of the globin chains can also produce unstable hemoglobins that tend to denature and form insoluble precipitates in the cell, so-called **Heinz bodies**. Other unstable hemoglobins have an increased tendency to form methemoglobin. In both situations, the loss of soluble, functional hemoglobin results in a chronic hemolytic anemia. Often, the mutation also changes the oxygen affinity of the abnormal hemoglobin. When the oxygen affinity is decreased, the patient's anemia is compensated for by increased delivery of oxygen to tissues. When affinity is increased, the patient can present with an abnormally high hemoglobin level (see Chapter 13).

Although many unstable hemoglobins have now been described, the clinical frequency of patients with disease is very low. Most of the unstable hemoglobins represent **defects of the α-globin chain** and are inherited as autosomal dominant traits. Two relatively prevalent β-globin chain mutants are hemoglobins Zurich and Koln. Those patients that do come to medical attention usually have a well-compensated hemolytic anemia, characterized by a normal or slightly decreased hemoglobin level and a high reticulocyte index. The mean cell hemoglobin (MCH) may be decreased, and inspection of the film may show hypochromia, and mild anisocytosis and poikilocytosis. Basophilic stippling and occasional Heinz bodies may be observed, but generally they are not impressive unless the patient has had a splenectomy. Episodes of increased hemolysis can occur with exposure to oxidant drugs or illness, similar to those seen with G6PD deficiency and other hemolytic anemias.

Laboratory confirmation of an unstable hemoglobinopathy involves using both the isopropanol and heat stability tests and the brilliant cresyl blue and methyl violet stains. Although these

CASE HISTORY • *Part 3*

This patient's hemoglobin pattern (A - 25%; F - 10%; A_2 - 5%; S - 60%) is characteristic of S/β^+-thalassemia. Heterozygous β^+ thalassemia (β/β^+) is a clinically silent mutation, unless combined with another β-chain abnormality such as hemoglobin S. This results in a clinical picture quite similar to sickle trait (β/β^S). However, the 60/40 ratio of hemoglobin S to A (plus A_2 and F) is quite different from the 40/60 ratio typical for sickle cell trait (β/β^S). This reflects the different levels of β^+-globin and β^S-globin production in the 2 entities and is a useful clue to the diagnosis.

S/β^+-thalassemia patients typically have only a modest anemia, little or no ineffective erythropoiesis or tendency to iron overload, rare if any vasoocclusive episodes and, in this case, no increased risk of complications with pregnancy. As with any pregnancy, however, the patient should receive iron and folic acid supplements, and during the third trimester iron studies may be in order to exclude a complicating iron deficiency anemia. Because the patient is also asplenic (surgical removal after trauma), she should also be immunized with *H. influenzae*, meningococcal, and polyvalent pneumococcal vaccines.

tests have the ability to uncover an unstable hemoglobin, they do not define the specific genetic defect. This process requires hemoglobin electrophoresis, globin chain purification, peptide analysis, and gene sequencing.

THERAPY

The management of a patient with a hemoglobinopathy varies greatly according to the genetic defect. Patients with **homozygous S disease or one of the combinations** of hemoglobin S and another β-globin chain defect present the greatest challenge. The patients who are **heterozygous for one of the hemoglobinopathies** generally do not have significant clinical disease. Effective screening and accurate diagnosis of the heterozygous individual is essential, however, for appropriate counseling and prenatal diagnosis. **Patients at risk because of racial or ethnic background** should be routinely screened with a CBC and HPLC. This battery of tests will detect most high-risk hemoglobinopathies. Furthermore, if a heterozygous individual plans to bear children, it is essential that the mate be screened both for counseling and to guide the use of prenatal diagnostic techniques.

Prenatal diagnosis makes it possible to anticipate the birth of homozygous and compound heterozygous children, thereby permitting parents to make an early decision regarding abortion. Accurate diagnosis of fetal hemoglobin SS disease is now possible using fetal DNA from amniotic fluid or chorionic villus biopsy and a specific restriction enzyme that recognizes the A to T base switch responsible for the Glu to Val substitution.

Sickle Cell Anemia

Management of the sickle cell anemia patient begins in the first year of life. Continuous, unbroken medical follow-up is essential, and a full range of health care and social support services needs to be provided. Several medical issues will need to be addressed during the lifespan of the patient. These issues include the recurrent, painful sickle crises, the severe hemolytic anemia, organ damage from vasoocclusive disease, priapism in teenage males, the tendency to form pigment gallstones, the poorly healing leg ulcers, the danger of overwhelming sepsis due to hyposplenism, and the tendency for patients to become disabled and narcotic dependent.

A. Painful Sickle Crises

The pain and painful crises experienced by sickle cell patients can vary considerably. Children are at risk for vasoocclusive infarction of marrow, spleen, and renal medullary tissue. They present with recurrent episodes of extremity and abdominal pain that may or may not be precipitated by other illness. Unless very severe, **crises can usually be managed at home** with varying combinations of pain medications such as nonsteroidal analgesics, acetaminophen, and, if necessary, oral narcotics. A high level of **fluid intake must be maintained and the CBC monitored** for evidence of acute infection or sudden worsening of the patient's anemia. As the child grows older and splenic function is lost, there is an **increased risk of life-threatening sepsis** with organisms such as ***S. pneumoniae*** and ***H. influenzae***, and osteomyelitis secondary to infection with ***Salmonella.***

The **severely ill child may need to be admitted to the hospital** to receive parenteral fluid therapy, higher-dose narcotic analgesia, and, if necessary, red blood cell transfusion to correct a worsening anemia. Although a vasoocclusive crisis that is well established cannot be reversed, red blood cell transfusions will decrease the tendency to further vessel occlusion by diluting the number of sickle cells in circulation. Long-term prophylactic cell transfusion can be used to decrease the frequency of painful crises in patients who have frequent crises or life-threatening vasoocclusive episodes, but the concomitant risks of iron overload must then be anticipated.

Teenage and adult patients develop their own characteristic pattern of recurrent painful crises. One-third or more patients report relatively infrequent episodes of slight to moderate aching pain in bones and joints, requiring nothing more than a few days of nonnarcotic analgesia. Others have frequent, severe crises presenting as incapacitating pain of large joints, especially the wrists, ankles, knees, hips, and shoulder joints. These crises are only occasionally associated with other illness. The inciting event can be completely unknown or may relate to small changes in routine activity, diet, or fluid intake. Survival correlates with the frequency of crises (see Figure 7–3). Patients who have 3 or more crises each year have a significantly shortened lifespan.

A **severe crisis in the adult** is a devastating illness. It can be difficult to control pain despite the use of large amounts of narcotics, and patients will generally require hospitalization for fluid management. Because sickle cell anemia patients are unable to adequately concentrate their urine owing to renal medullary damage, they need to be aggressively hydrated with a mix of dextrose 5% in water (D5W) and one-half normal saline (NS). An adequate regimen of pain medication is also essential. Patients should have a **fixed-schedule narcotic regimen** using opioids such as morphine, hydromorphone, and fentanyl (meperidine is not recommended by some—see below) at dosages that will relieve their pain. From 5%–10% of sickle patients lack the enzyme CYP2D6 needed for conversion of codeine, hydromorphone, and oxycodone to the active metabolite. This makes morphine the most reliable narcotic. Morphine is, however, associated with histamine release from mast cells, which may require concomitant antihistamine therapy with hydroxyzine or diphenhydramine. Younger patients often require higher doses. Continuous intravenous morphine or patient-controlled analgesia is the preferred route of administration as long as limits are set for total narcotic dosage.

The total dose of narcotic needed to control the pain can be quite high. It is important, therefore, to **closely monitor the patient for side effects**. In the case of meperidine, the accumulation of the toxic metabolite nor-meperidine, which has a half-life of 18 hours, can produce marked anxiety, tremors, myoclonus, and seizures. Accumulation of the morphine-6-glucuronide metabolite in patients receiving high-dose morphine therapy is associated with marked sedation and respiratory depression. Serotonin syndrome, characterized early on by tremors and diarrhea, which can progress to marked delirium and life-threatening hyperthermia, can also be seen in critically ill patients receiving high-dose opioid therapy, especially if they are also receiving serotonergic drugs.

There is **little risk for narcotic abuse when patients are managed well**. Poor control of pain during a crisis, inadequate follow-up, and overuse of emergency rooms by the sickle cell patient can lead to addictive behavior. When painful crises occur at frequent intervals, sickle cell anemia is a debilitating illness that interferes with every aspect of normal living. Patients are chronically ill, unable to work or go to school, and in need of long-term support. The sickle cell anemia patient has every reason to be angry and depressed and to feel poorly served by the medical system. This situation needs to be recognized in the long-term care of the patient. Painful episodes, and even mild ones, must be taken seriously. The patient needs to be educated on how to use pain medications, emphasizing dosing at frequent, fixed intervals rather than as needed. In addition, the tendency to become depressed should be recognized and treated with appropriate use of antidepressants and social support.

B. Prevention of Painful Crises

It has been well recognized that **decreasing the relative amount of sickle hemoglobin** in circulation can reduce the frequency and severity of painful crises. This process is possible either by diluting the number of sickle cells in circulation by transfusion of normal red blood cells or reducing the amount of intracellular sickle cell hemoglobin by increasing hemoglobin F production. Iron deficiency may also reduce the frequency of sickle crises by reducing intracellular hemoglobin S concentration. It is difficult, however, to induce iron deficiency in a sickle cell anemia patient. Attempts at phlebotomy are frustrated by the severity of the patient's anemia.

1. Transfusion therapy—When transfused with normal red blood cells sufficient to reduce the number of sickle cells by one-third or more, most patients will experience a reduction in the frequency of painful crises. At least 2 U of packed red blood cells must be transfused every 2–4 weeks in the adult patient. If larger amounts of red blood cells are given to increase the hemoglobin to levels greater than 10–11 g/dL, the patient's erythropoietin response will be suppressed, and new sickle cell production will decrease, as illustrated by the reticulocyte index.

It is possible to hypertransfuse a patient and virtually shut off hemoglobin S production. This approach, however, increases the exposure of the patient to transfused blood with its associated complications. Therefore, **hypertransfusion** is only indicated for the severely ill patient who does not respond to smaller amounts of blood. For **patients undergoing general anesthesia**, transfusion to a hematocrit of 30% is sufficient to prevent perioperative complications. Recent clinical trials have demonstrated the efficacy of repeated transfusion in reducing the risk of recurrent stroke in children with sickle cell anemia. **Prophylactic transfusion is now recommended in children** with transcranial doppler blood flow velocities of greater than 200 cm/s in the middle cerebral or internal carotid arteries. Sufficient red cell transfusions need to be given to reduce the S hemoglobin to 30% of the total hemoglobin concentration. **Other indications for acute and long-term transfusion** are listed in Table 7–4.

TABLE 7–4 • Indications for transfusion

Acute Transfusion	Long-Term Transfusion
Acute, increasingly severe anemia Aplastic crisis Inflammatory illness Hemolytic event	Recurrent acute chest syndrome Pulmonary hypertension Congestive heart failure Chronic lung disease with hypoxia
Acute chest syndrome	Recurrent stroke
Acute stroke/TIA	Abnormal transcranial doppler
Multiorgan failure	Severe, recurrent pain crises
General anesthesia	
Severe, prolonged pain crisis	

Exchange transfusion, entailing a volume-for-volume replacement of the patient's blood with transfused red cells either manually or by apheresis, is used to treat critically ill patients presenting with stroke, acute chest syndrome, or multiorgan failure. The goal of an exchange transfusion is to reduce the hemoglobin S level to 30% and increase the hematocrit to 30% but no higher to avoid viscosity problems. When used in stroke patients, it should be performed as the first step in management, even before confirmatory studies, such as computed tomography (CT)-scan or magnetic resonance imaging (MRI). Exchange transfusion has also been used to prepare hemoglobin SC patients with hematocrits less than 30% for surgery or delivery.

Complications of transfusion therapy include formation of alloantibodies to minor blood group antigens, acute or delayed hemolytic transfusion reactions, and, with chronic transfusion, iron overload. **Alloantibody formation** to red blood cell antigens is a difficult problem. For unclear reasons, up to 30% of sickle cell anemia patients will form alloantibodies, making cross-matching of future transfusions increasingly difficult. Therefore, it is important that all transfused units be matched for minor blood groups such as C, c, E, e, and Kell. Moreover, if the pool of donors used for transfusion is kept relatively small, it can help avoid antibody formation.

Hemolytic transfusion reactions can be acute or delayed and are of particular concern. With acute hemolysis, patients will complain of back, flank, or chest pain (or all of these) and will develop fever and malaise. Transfusion-induced hemolysis may also precipitate a typical vasoocclusive crisis. At the same time, reticulocytopenia and a fall in the hematocrit to levels below that present prior to transfusion may be the first and only clue to an acute or delayed hemolytic reaction. While formation of alloantibodies often explains the reaction, the mechanism behind some of these events remains unclear.

Iron overload is the major downside of chronic transfusion therapy. Although sickle cell patients can demonstrate an increased tendency to iron absorption even before transfusion, every transfused unit of red blood cells adds 200 mg of iron to the patient's total body iron pool. Even a minimum transfusion regimen of 1 U every 2 weeks contributes an excess load of iron of nearly 5 g each year. This places the patient at significant **risk for tissue iron overload** and damage, especially cardiac damage. The risk of iron overload must be anticipated by keeping careful records of the patient's transfusion history. Measurements of serum ferritin as an indicator of total body iron and liver iron load in sickle cell patients are notoriously unreliable. Patients can have liver iron loads of greater than 15 mg/g dry weight tissue when the serum ferritin is still below 1,000 μg/L.

If **long-term transfusion therapy is used in a sickle patient**, it is essential that the patient be considered for long-term maintenance therapy using the new oral chelator, deferasirox, or deferoxamine. As long as the patient can comply with the rigors of chelation therapy, the risk of iron overload can be greatly diminished, if not completely mitigated. Vitamin E supplementation is also important to counteract the increased tendency to lipid peroxidation seen with iron overload.

2. Induction of hemoglobin F—The observation that high levels of intracellular hemoglobin F in sickle cell anemia patients are associated with milder disease has led to attempts to induce hemoglobin F production with drugs. At least 4 drugs—5-azacytidine, the deoxy form of the drug decitabine, hydroxyurea, and arginine butyrate—have been shown to increase γ-globin gene expression. Hydroxyurea was the first to be approved for long-term use in sickle patients. It is an oral agent with a good safety profile and has a demonstrated ability to increase hemoglobin F levels from 1.5- to 16-fold (2%–20%). Both the number of F cells and the intracellular level of F are increased. The latter can be easily monitored by quantitative HPLC. The response correlates both with the patient's initial hemoglobin F level and the maximally tolerated hydroxyurea dosage. Even patients who realize relatively small increases in hemoglobin F (5%–10%) appear to benefit from therapy. In fact, correlation of the frequency of vasoocclusive crises with the rise in hemoglobin F has only been documented during the first few months of therapy. Sustained improvement with hydroxyurea correlates better with reductions in the neutrophil, monocyte, and reticulocyte counts, and expression of sickle cell and endothelial adhesion receptors.

In **adult patients**, therapy should begin with a daily dose of 500 mg of hydroxyurea (10–15 mg/kg/d). After 6–8 weeks of therapy, the dose can be increased to 1,000 mg/d if the patient's blood counts are stable. Most patients will tolerate hydroxyurea doses of 1,000–2,000 mg/d (20–30 mg/kg/d), although up to 10% will not tolerate a dose of even 10 mg/d. Blood counts need to be checked frequently, every 2 weeks until the dose is stabilized, and then every 6–8 weeks for the duration of therapy. Up to 30% of patients will fail to respond to even high doses of hydroxyurea.

Hydroxyurea can be given without apparent toxicity for relatively long periods. However, depending on the dose, patients will develop a significant macrocytosis, usually without becoming more anemic, and a slight to moderate leukopenia, thrombocytopenia, or both. Small numbers of **patients have now received hydroxyurea for 5 or more years** without evidence of increased risk for secondary malignancy, myelodysplasia, or marrow chromosomal abnormalities. Much longer-term experience with chronic hydroxyurea therapy is necessary, however, before its effectiveness can be compared with possible long-term complications. There is still no firm evidence that hydroxyurea will prevent or reverse organ damage over time.

The 5-azacytidine analogue, decitabine, now approved by the US Food and Drug Administration (FDA), will also increase hemoglobin F levels (10%–25%) and the percentage of F cells (30%–40%) in nearly all patients, making it the drug of choice in hydroxyurea-resistant patients. It also raises the hemoglobin level by up to 2 g/dL with a concomitant fall in the reticulocyte index and hemolysis parameters. The drug can be administered either intravenously or by subcutaneous injection. The major side effect is reversible neutropenia. The long-term risks of decitabine therapy, especially the potential for tumor induction, are still unknown. However, in studies in animal models decitabine actually appears to be a potential chemopreventive agent for certain tumors.

Arginine butyrate is also capable of inducing fetal hemoglobin production. In fact, when given in intermittent doses intravenously every 2–3 weeks, the increase in fetal hemoglobin was immediate (within 1–2 days) and even more dramatic than that seen with hydroxyurea. A rise in the total hemoglobin levels was also observed. Combination therapy with hydroxyurea and butyrate may well be synergistic based on their different mechanisms of action. Moreover, the use of combination therapy may make it possible to achieve hemoglobin F levels of 30%–45%, which would completely inhibit polymerization of hemoglobin SS. The major disadvantage is that the drug must be given as a continuous infusion over several days. Since clinical improvement is best correlated with the level of induced hemoglobin F, combination therapies using all 3 agents may hold promise.

3. Reduction in intracellular hemoglobin concentration—Hemoglobin SS polymerization is highly dependent on the intracellular hemoglobin concentration. Therefore, a sustained reduction in MCHC will, theoretically, decrease the chance of a sickle crisis. Currently, clinical trials are studying the ability of clotrimazole, an antifungal drug, to inhibit calcium-dependent (Gardos channel) potassium efflux and prevent cell water losses. Another trial involves oral magnesium (Mg) supplementation with Mg picolate, which, by increasing intracellular red cell Mg, appears to inhibit the K-Cl cotransport system. Future therapies may well combine hydroxyurea with clotrimazole, Mg, or both.

4. Bone marrow (stem cell) transplantation—A number of children and adolescents (under age 20) with severe sickle cell disease and an increased risk for stroke have successfully received **transplants with allografts from human leukocyte antigen (HLA)-identical siblings** (A/A or A/S hemoglobin patterns). The patients were initially treated with a combination of busulfan, cytoxan, and antithymocyte globulin. Overall survivals exceed 90% with stable engraftment and little or no graft-versus host disease (GVHD) or recurrent sickle complications. Event-free survival has been reported to be better than 85%. Since the availability of a normal HLA-matched related donor is low, future trials may look at the use of unrelated matched donors and cord-blood stem cells.

Future therapeutic strategies will involve altering the interaction between sickle cells and endothelial cells. Possible points of interruption include decreasing the activation of sickle cell adhesion receptors, downregulating inflammatory mediators, and improving endothelial function. Endothelin receptor blockade in patients with pulmonary hypertension using the ET_A blocker, bosenton, is currently being used in clinical trials. Inhaled NO has appeared to reduce the severity of vasoocclusive crises in a small series of sickle cell anemia children. Amplification of endogenous NO using sidenafil has also shown some promise in patients with pulmonary hypertension. The hypercoagulable state associated with hemolysis will also need to be addressed. To date, however, many small clinical trials of anticoagulation, usually during crisis episodes, have failed to provide clear evidence for a therapeutic role for anticoagulants or antiplatelet agents.

Management of Other Complications

Most sickle cell anemia patients form **pigment gallstones** and are at **risk for cholecystitis and cholangitis**. Cholecystectomy is indicated at an early age in patients who are symptomatic. To prevent a sickle crisis in the perioperative period, patients should be transfused to a hemoglobin of 10–11 g/dL and a hemoglobin S/A ratio of 60/40 or lower. In addition, laparoscopic cholecystectomy is associated with less postoperative morbidity and a shorter length of stay. **Aseptic necrosis of the femoral and humeral heads** is another common complication. It can usually be managed conservatively with pain medications, although severe bony destruction can require the placement of an orthopedic prosthesis.

Acute chest syndrome in adults can rapidly proceed to respiratory failure and death in up to 5% of patients. Therefore, it should be aggressively treated with red blood cell exchange transfusion, fluid resuscitation, oxygen, and antibiotics. The latter is important because about one-third of adults dying of acute chest syndrome are bacteremic. Anticoagulation therapy also may be considered in patients with signs of **marked pulmonary thrombosis/fat embolism**. Recent studies of acute chest syndrome have shown a pathologic expression of **VCAM-1**, suggesting a possible therapeutic role for inhibitors of VCAM-1 such as dexamethasone and nitric oxide gas. However, the mainstay of acute chest syndrome therapy is rapid and complete red cell exchange. With adequate venous access, a complete red cell exchange using hemapheresis instrumentation can be accomplished within 2–3 hours, reducing the percent of sickle cells from greater than 90% to less than 30%.

Priapism in teenaged males can usually be managed with pain medications alone or in combination with nifedipine, given in repeated dosages of 10 mg. Priapism that lasts for more than a day can be treated by penile aspiration and epinephrine irrigation of the corpora cavernosa and, finally, red cell exchange. **Leg ulcers**, which usually appear in the third or fourth decades, are very difficult to treat. Meticulous local care to prevent superinfection and the application of an Unna boot (zinc oxide, impregnated bandage) can provide protection and encourage healing. Patients will also need to decrease their activity level and keep their legs elevated. Blood transfusion, even hypertransfusion, usually will not speed healing.

Women with sickle cell anemia can undergo **pregnancy** without an increase in the frequency of crises or complications. Spontaneous abortion is rare. However, women of SS phenotype tend to have low-birth-weight infants. An increase in number and severity of crises during the third trimester and the induction of premature labor put both mother and child at risk. **Transfusion therapy can be quite effective in the third trimester** to prevent painful crises and life-threatening vasoocclusive events during labor.

Similarly, **prophylactic red blood cell transfusion** can be used when patients undergo **major surgery** to prevent a perioperative crisis. As a rule, reducing the hemoglobin S level to less than 30% will prevent a perioperative vasoocclusive event. The decision to transfuse prophylactically is a clinical one. There is no protocol regarding which surgical procedures or which patients will require this level of therapy.

Sickle cell anemia patients are at risk for overwhelming **sepsis** with organisms such as ***S. pneumoniae*** and ***H. influenzae***. They should receive both Haemophilis influenzae Type B (Hib) and meningococcal vaccines and a pneumococcal vaccine (PCV7 – Prevnar in infants or PPSV – Pneumovax after age 2) and should be carefully instructed regarding their response to sudden fever. Young children should also receive prophylactic oral penicillin at 125 mg twice a day. Adult sickle cell anemia patients who have repeated infarctions of marrow and demonstrate aseptic necrosis of the femoral or humeral heads are at risk for developing **salmonella osteomyelitis**. This needs to be considered in any patient who complains of chronic, localized bone pain or manifests a fever of unknown origin.

Routine Health Maintenance

Sickle cell anemia patients should be routinely monitored for progression of their disease. **Periodic CBCs** are very important. Patients will demonstrate an erythropoietic profile that is normal for their compensated state. Severity of their anemia can vary according to the **level of intracellular hemoglobin F**. The higher the hemoglobin F level, the less severe the anemia based on the reduced tendency to form irreversibly sickled cells that are rapidly destroyed. The likelihood of the patient experiencing painful crises also correlates with the hemoglobin F level.

Any **sudden change in the patient's hemoglobin level**, whether a decrease or increase, can trigger a major vasoocclusive event. A fall in the hemoglobin level can result from a sudden increase in the rate of hemolysis, a decrease in erythropoietin production, or appearance of a maturation defect secondary to folic acid deficiency. The latter should be anticipated and the diet of a sickle cell anemia patient should always be supplemented with 1–2 mg of folic acid taken orally daily. Increased rates of red blood cell destruction are seen with any intercurrent illness and as a part of organ infarction, whereas falls in red blood cell production occur with inflammatory diseases and renal damage. Sickle cell anemia patients are also at risk for self-limited failure of stem cell proliferation secondary to parvovirus infection.

A full **evaluation of the erythropoietic profile** should be performed whenever a patient presents with a vasoocclusive crisis and a fall in hemoglobin level or reticulocyte index. Renal function studies are important to look for a failure in erythropoietin stimulation. A marrow aspirate and measurements of parvovirus serology, and both iron and folic acid supply will uncover reversible defects in red blood cell progenitor proliferation and maturation. A worsening anemia secondary to chronic inflammatory disease or renal damage will increase the risk for severe vasoocclusive crises. This situation is also true for patients who develop severe cardiopulmonary disease and hypoxia. In these situations, long-term transfusion therapy may be the only way to maintain a patient's functional status.

Compound Hemoglobinopathies

Management of a patient with a compound hemoglobinopathy will depend largely on the incidence of vasoocclusive disease. **Patients with hemoglobin S/β^0-thalassemia** follow a clinical course similar to that of patients with sickle cell anemia. They have frequent painful crises and have a very high incidence of aseptic necrosis. In contrast, **patients with S/β^+-thalassemia** have much milder disease (see Table 7–3). **Patients with hemoglobin S/C disease** tend to have fewer vasoocclusive crises and a milder hemolytic anemia. At the same time, they should be followed up closely for complications such as retinopathy, gross hematuria, and, in women with S/C disease, spontaneous abortion and complications with delivery.

The Unstable Hemoglobins

Patients with unstable hemoglobins tend to have well-compensated hemolytic anemias or tendency to erythrocytosis. Those patients with hemolytic anemia should **receive 1–2 mg oral folic acid daily**. Otherwise, they require little in the way of therapy unless they present with a sudden fall in their hemoglobin level. As with other compensated hemolytic anemias, they are at risk for increased hemolysis secondary to intercurrent illness or drug ingestion and reversible red blood cell aplasia secondary to parvovirus infection.

POINTS TO REMEMBER

The principle hemoglobinopathies (hemoglobins S and C) involve a single amino acid substitution in the β-globin chain, resulting in a structural/functional abnormality.

Hemoglobin S or C can present as a heterozygous (β/β^S or β/β^C), homozygous ($\beta^S\beta^S$ or β^C/β^C), or a compound hemoglobinopathy (SC [β^S/β^C] disease, S/β^+- or S/β^0-thalassemia).

Some 7%–8% of African Americans are heterozygous for hemoglobin S–sickle cell trait. Their overall health is not affected, but they carry the potential for having a child with a severe sickle cell anemia if their spouse carries either hemoglobin S or β^0-thalassemia.

Sickle cell anemia is a severe hemolytic anemia with major complications related to intravascular sickling and repeated vasoocclusive events, leading to permanent organ damage. It generally presents in the first year of life with recurrent painful episodes of joint and abdominal pain (splenic infarction). Untreated children and young adults are at high risk for stroke and pulmonary complications (acute chest syndrome).

The severity of sickle cell anemia is significantly less in patients who have high levels of hemoglobin F, especially patients from West Africa and the Middle East with hereditary persistence of fetal hemoglobin production.

The prompt treatment of painful crises is essential and involves aggressive hydration, blood transfusion, and liberal use of narcotics and antibiotics. Acute chest syndrome can rapidly progress to respiratory failure and death and should be treated with exchange transfusion and maximum pulmonary support.

Long-term management of the sickle cell anemia patient involves stem cell/bone marrow transplantation for severely affected children with a matched sibling donor (limited applicability), chronic transfusion therapy, and induction of hemoglobin F with hydroxyurea, arginine butyrate, or 5-azacytadine.

Late complications of sickle cell anemia include pigment gallstones, aseptic necrosis of the hip, recurrent priapism, proliferative retinopathy, and recurrent episodes of acute chest syndrome leading to pulmonary hypertension. Patients on chronic transfusion therapy will require aggressive chelation therapy to prevent iron overload and cardiac disease.

Compound hemoglobinopathies can display a wide range of disease severity with different sets of complications. Hemoglobin S/C patients have few if any vasoocclusive problems, but painless hematuria and aseptic necrosis of the hip are a problem. Pregnant S/C patients have a very high spontaneous abortion rate. Hemoglobin S/β^+-thalassemia present with a picture similar to sickle trait with little or no anemia and rare vasoocclusive episodes, while S/β^0-thalassemia patients are clinically indistinguishable from homozygous S patients.

Sickle cell anemia patients are at special risk of overwhelming sepsis secondary to their loss of splenic function in childhood. They should be immunized with *H. influenzae*, meningococcal, and polyvalent pneumococcal vaccines and treated immediately with antibiotics upon the onset of a high fever.

BIBLIOGRAPHY

Hemoglobin Structure and Function

Steinberg ME et al: Disorders of Hemoglobin. Cambridge University Press, 2001.

Clinical Features

Castro O et al: Pulmonary hypertension in sickle cell disease: cardiac catheterization results and survival. Blood 2003; 101:1257.

Gladwin MT, Vichinsky E: Pulmonary complications of sickle cell disease. N Eng J Med 2008;359:2254.

Kato GJ et al: Lactic dehydrogenase as a biomarker of hemolysis-associated nitric oxide resistance, pripism, leg ulceration, pulmonary hypertension, and death in patients with sickle cell disease. Blood 2006;107:2279.

Petz LD et al: The sickle cell hemolytic transfusion reaction syndrome. Transfusion 1997;37:382.

Reed W et al: Acute anemic events in sickle cell disease. Transfusion 2000;40:267.

Smith-Whitley K et al: Epidemiology of human parvovirus B19 in children with sickle cell disease. Blood 2004;103:422.

Vichinsky EP et al: Acute chest syndrome in sickle cell disease: clinical presentation and course. Blood 1997;89:1787.

Therapy

Adams RJ et al: Prevention of a first stroke by transfusion in children with sickle cell anemia and abnormal results on transcranial doppler ultrasonography. N Engl J Med 1998;339:5.

Atweh GF et al: Sustained induction of fetal hemoglobin by pulse butyrate therapy in sickle cell disease. Blood 1999;93:1790.

Bernaudin F et al: Long-term results of myeloablative stem-cell transplantation to cure sickle cell disease. Blood 2007; 110:2749.

Brugnara C et al: Therapy with clotrimazole induces inhibition of the Gardos channel and reduction of erythrocyte dehydration in patients with sickle cell disease. J Clin Invest 1996;97:1227.

Charache S et al: Effect of hydroxyurea on the frequency of painful crises in sickle cell anemia. N Engl J Med 1995;332: 1317.

DeSimone J et al: Maintenance of elevated fetal hemoglobin levels by decitabine during dose interval treatment of sickle cell anemia. Blood 2002;99:3905.

Ferster A et al: Hydroxyurea for treatment of severe sickle cell anemia: a pediatric clinical trial. Blood 1996;88:1960.

Haberken CM et al: Cholecystectomy in sickle cell anemia patients: perioperative outcome of 364 cases from the National Preoperative Transfusion Study. Blood 1997;89:1533.

Kato GJ et al: Lactic dehydrogenase as a biomarker of hemolysis-associated nitric oxide resistance, pripism, leg ulceration, pulmonary hypertension, and death in patients with sickle cell disease. Blood 2006;107:2279.

Kinney TR et al: Safety of hydroxyurea in children with sickle cell anemia: results of the HUG-KIDS study, a phase I/II trial. Blood 1999;94:1550.

Koshy M et al: 2-Deoxy 5-azacytidine and fetal hemoglobin induction in sickle cell anemia. Blood 2000;96:2379.

Lee MT et al: Stroke prevention trial in sickle cell anemia (STOP): extended follow-up and results. Blood 2006;108:847.

Ohene-Frempong K: Indications for red cell transfusion in sickle cell disease. Semin Hematol 2001;38:5.

Saunthararajah Y et al: Effects of 5-aza-2′-deoxycytidine on fetal hemoglobin levels, red cell adhesion, and hematopoietic differentiation in patients with sickle cell disease. Blood 2003;102:3865.

Sickle Cell Disease: Screening, Diagnosis, Management, and Counseling in Newborns and Infants. Agency for Health Care Policy and Research, Public #93-0562, 93-0563, and 93-0564.

Steinberg MH: Management of sickle cell disease. N Engl J Med 1999;340:1021.

Steinberg MH et al: Effect of hydroxyurea on morbidity and mortality in adult sickle cell anemia. JAMA 2003;289:1645.

Walters MC et al: Impact of bone marrow transplantation for symptomatic sickle cell disease: an interim report. Blood 2000;95:1918.

Zimmerman SA et al: Sustained long-term hematologic efficacy of hydroxyurea at maximum tolerated dose in children with sickle cell disease. Blood 2004;103:2039.

MACROCYTIC ANEMIAS • 8

CASE HISTORY • *Part I*

A 42-year-old male presents to the emergency room confused and combative with alcohol on his breath. He has a history of chronic alcoholism, alcoholic liver disease, and dementia. He had been "dry" for almost a year before resuming drinking a month ago. On examination he has normal vital signs, a sallow complexion, and multiple bruises over both shins and forearms. Liver and spleen are both palpable. Neurological examination is notable for stocking glove anesthesia and poor position sense. Routine labs are ordered:

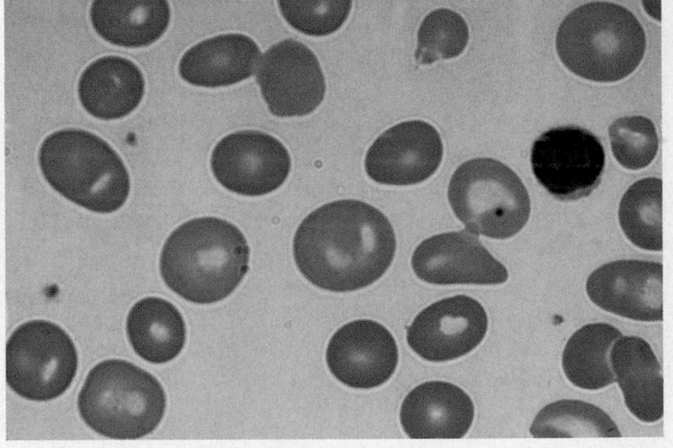

CBC: Hematocrit/hemoglobin - 29%/9 g/dL
MCV - 107 fL MCH - 34 pg MCHC - 32 g/dL
RDW-CV - 15%
RDW-SD - 55 fL
Reticulocyte count/index - 1.5%/<1
White cell count - 5,300/μL
Platelet count - 65,000/μL

• BLOOD SMEAR MORPHOLOGY

Mixed population of normocytic and macrocytic red cells with moderate aniso- and poikilocytosis, polychromasia, and the occasional target cell.

A bone marrow aspirate is also obtained and on preliminary reading shows a relatively hypercellular marrow with a ratio of erythroid to granulocytic precursors (E/G ratio) of 1:1, megaloblastic maturation of both the erythroid and granulocyte progenitors, and normal megakaryocyte numbers.

Questions

- How should this anemia be described?
- What is the differential diagnosis?
- What additional tests are in order?

Folic acid and vitamin B_{12} deficiency are primary causes of macrocytic anemia in adults. Both vitamins are essential for normal DNA synthesis, and high turnover tissues such as marrow are especially sensitive to any deficiency state. With either deficiency, the marrow becomes megaloblastic; marrow precursors appear much larger than normal and are unable to complete cell division. This results in ineffective erythropoiesis, release of macrocytic red blood cells into circulation, and worsening anemia. The severity of the anemia and the degree of macrocytosis depend on the severity and duration of the deficient state.

The **prevalence of folic acid deficiency** depends on the frequency of diseases associated with a decreased dietary intake of folic acid, malabsorption, or an increased metabolic requirement. Alcoholism is a common cause of folic acid deficiency in Western societies because of the poor dietary habits of the alcoholic and alcohol's interference with folate metabolism. In developing countries, tropical and nontropical sprue are more common etiologies. **Vitamin B_{12} deficiency** can result from a dietary deficiency, an autoimmune process directed at intrinsic factor (IF), or any one of a number of gastrointestinal disorders that lead to vitamin B_{12} malabsorption.

NORMAL FOLIC ACID AND VITAMIN B_{12} METABOLISM

Major metabolic pathways of folic acid and vitamin B_{12} are illustrated in Figure 8–1. These 2 vitamins are closely linked in the support of DNA synthesis. Within the cell, vitamin B_{12} is present in 2 forms. As deoxyadenosyl B_{12}, it supports conversion of l-methylmalonyl-CoA to succinyl-CoA. It also accepts a methyl group from methyltetrahydrofolate to support synthesis of methionine. The transfer of a methyl group from methyltetrahydrofolate provides the tetrahydrofolate necessary for synthesis of various folate coenzymes needed for purine and glycine synthesis and for conversion of deoxyuridylate to thymidylate for DNA synthesis.

A lack of either vitamin interferes with **DNA synthesis**. When methyltetrahydrofolate is in short supply, tetrahydrofolate cannot be generated to support other folate coenzymes. When vitamin B_{12} is lacking, there is no acceptor for the methyl group from methyltetrahydrofolate. This situation creates a "methylfolate trap" and reduced availability of tetrahydrofolate to support DNA synthesis.

Absorption and Distribution of Vitamin B_{12}

Pathways of absorption and distribution of vitamin B_{12} to tissues are shown in Figure 8–2. Food B_{12} is initially bound to a salivary binding protein (an R-protein) until it reaches the small bowel, where pancreatic proteases release the vitamin for subsequent binding to the glycoprotein, intrinsic factor. The **B_{12}-intrinsic factor (cobalamin-IF) complex** then binds to a receptor on ileal mucosal cells and is transported across the gut wall to the circulation. In the absence of IF, vitamin B_{12} absorption virtually ceases. Several transcobalamin proteins in circulation are capable of binding free B_{12}. However, **transcobalamin** II is the principal transport protein for delivery of B_{12} to tissues and liver. Daily turnover of vitamin B_{12} reflects tissue requirements and the size of body stores and can range from as little as 0.5 to as much as 8 μg per day. From 1–10 mg of vitamin B_{12} accumulate in liver stores in a normal adult on an adequate diet.

Absorption and Distribution of Folic Acid

Dietary folic acid follows a similar metabolic pathway (Figure 8–3). An essential step in absorption is hydrolysis of folate

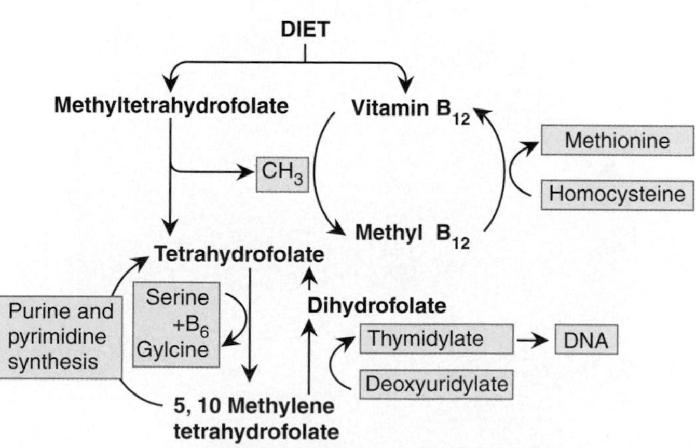

FIGURE 8–1. **Metabolic pathways of folic acid and vitamin B_{12}.** An adequate supply of both methyltetrahydrofolate and vitamin B_{12} are required for normal DNA synthesis. Methyltetrahydrofolate donates a methyl group to vitamin B_{12} in support of methionine metabolism. This generates the tetrahydrofolate needed for purine and pyrimidine synthesis and the production of thymidylate for DNA synthesis.

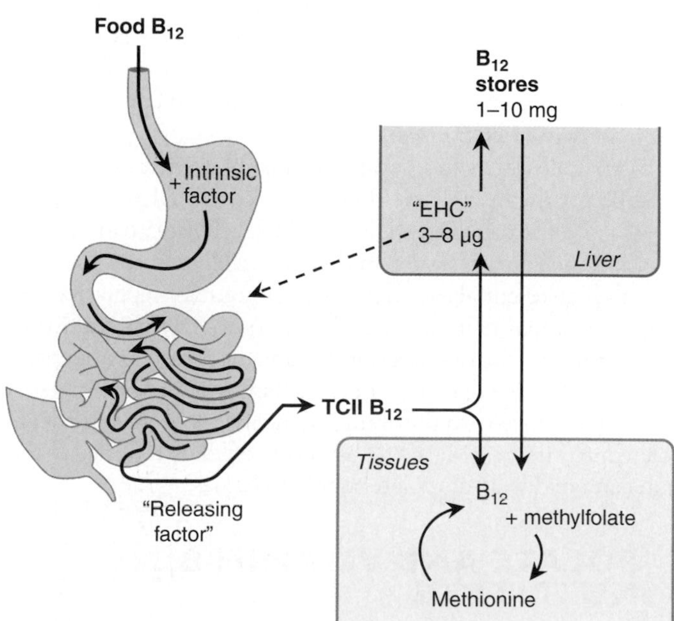

FIGURE 8–2. **Vitamin B_{12} absorption and transport to tissues.** Dietary vitamin B_{12} is sequentially bound to R-protein and intrinsic factor in preparation for binding to receptors on ileal mucosal cells. It is then transported on TC II to liver and tissues.

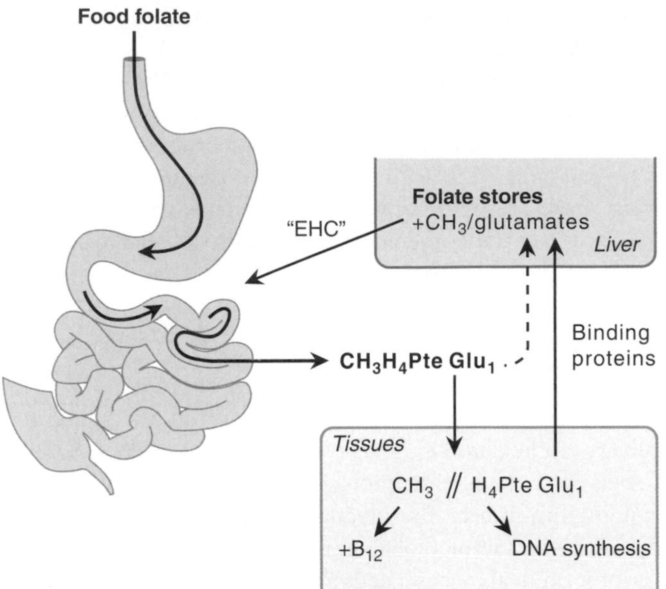

FIGURE 8–3. **Folic acid absorption and transport.** Folate polyglutamates in food are hydrolyzed, reduced, and methylated to form methyltetrahydrofolate monoglutamate. This is then transported to tissues where it participates actively as a methyl donor and as substrate for both purine and pyrimidine metabolism and DNA synthesis. Liver folate stores play an important role in providing a constant supply of folate through the enterohepatic cycle for reabsorption.

polyglutamates present in food to methyltetrahydrofolate monoglutamate. This process depends on a carboxypeptidase located on the mucosal cell membrane and a dihydrofolate reductase enzyme in mucosal cells. Most absorption occurs in the proximal portion of the small intestine. The methyltetrahydrofolate is then rapidly transported to tissues to enter the intracellular metabolic cycle required for purine and pyrimidine metabolism and DNA synthesis. Although there are proteins in plasma that bind folate, their primary affinity appears to be for nonmethylated congeners that are not essential for transport to tissues.

Both methylated and nonmethylated congeners of folate are absorbed by the liver, where they are stored as methyltetrahydrofolate polyglutamate. Depending on the level of folate in the diet, the liver can contain several milligrams of folate stores. The liver also plays an essential role in providing a constant supply of folate to tissues. It maintains an active transport of methyltetrahydrofolate into bile for reabsorption by the gut. This enterohepatic cycle of folate is important for maintaining folate homeostasis. Any interference with the ability of the liver to store and release folate into bile, or with the reabsorption of folate returned to the gut, can rapidly disrupt folate supply to tissues.

FOLATE AND VITAMIN B_{12} NUTRITION

Most foods, especially leafy vegetables, are rich in folate. However, excessive cooking and food processing significantly reduce folate content, so that an unfortified Western diet may provide as little as 50–100 μg per day. This amount barely meets the minimum daily requirement of an adult and may be insufficient during pregnancy or for patients with high rates of cell turnover (hemolytic anemias). Chronic alcoholics, whose principal source of calories is derived from their alcohol intake, are at great risk of developing folate deficiency.

Dietary supply of vitamin B_{12} is derived largely from meat and meat by-products; vegetables are essentially free of the vitamin. Usually, the daily requirement of 3–5 μg is easily supplied by a Western diet. Only strict vegetarians are at risk for a true dietary deficiency state.

CLINICAL FEATURES

Symptoms and signs of a **severe vitamin B_{12} deficiency** include those of **marked anemia** and **neuropathy**. Most often, patients complain of the gradual onset of fatigue, exercise intolerance, and progressive cardiac decompensation. The latter is associated with a severe anemia (hematocrit <15%–20%). Vitamin B_{12} deficiency also has an impact on the central nervous system. Patients develop a demyelinating lesion of the neurons of the spinal column and cerebral cortex. This condition results in paresthesias of the hands and feet, unsteadiness of gait, and eventually memory loss and personality changes. The most distinctive characteristics of the neuropathy are the focal dorsal column and corticospinal tract lesions (Figure 8–4), which result in a loss of vibration and position sense and the development of an unsteady gait and a positive Romberg test. Neuropathy may be present without anemia. It is important, therefore, to consider vitamin B_{12} deficiency in the differential diagnosis of a peripheral neuropathy, dementia, or a psychiatric disorder.

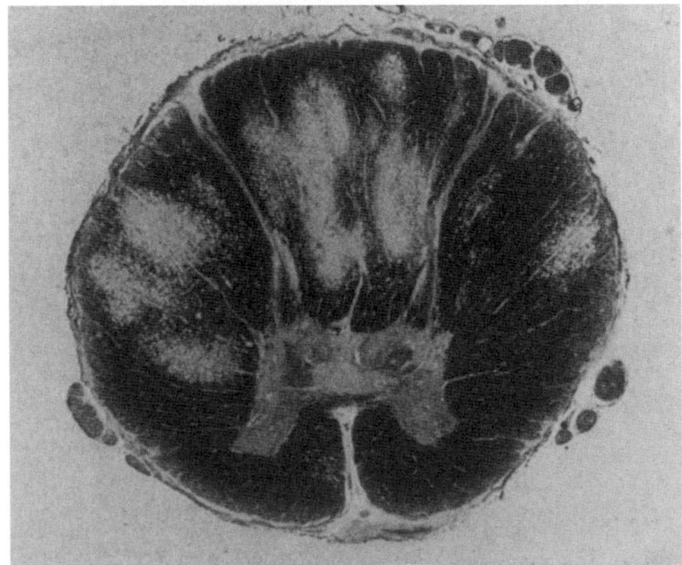

FIGURE 8–4. **Spinal cord section from a pernicious anemia patient.** The characteristic neuropathological lesion of vitamin B_{12} deficiency is localized to the dorsal column and corticospinal tracts as shown in this cross section of the spinal column.

Other symptoms and signs of vitamin B_{12} deficiency include complaints of a **sore mouth and loss of taste**, in addition to **atrophy of the mucosa of the tongue**. The tongue appears smooth, red, and shiny on physical examination. In addition, patients who develop pernicious anemia often have **vitiligo** and are prematurely gray. Several **disorders of the gastrointestinal tract** can result in vitamin B_{12} deficiency. The most common causes in the United States include pernicious anemia associated with antibodies to parietal cells, IF, or the cobalamin-IF complex; gastrectomy, gastric bypass, or bowel resection; bacterial overgrowth of the small intestine; and pancreatic insufficiency.

Patients with folic acid deficiency anemia often go undiagnosed, especially alcoholics who have a very poor diet and maintain blood alcohol levels above 100 mg/dL for extended periods. At this level of alcohol intake, the enterohepatic cycle of folate supply to the intestine and tissues is impaired, setting the stage for the rapid onset of a folate-deficiency anemia. However, unless anemia is severe, the patient is relatively insensitive to its symptoms when compared to the other problems associated with alcoholism. Diagnosis is also made difficult by the rapid return of intracellular folate metabolism to normal once alcohol ingestion ceases. Within hours of alcohol withdrawal and resumption of a normal diet, the serum folate returns to normal and the megaloblastic defect begins to resolve. Therefore, clinicians must be highly suspicious of the possibility of folate deficiency in alcoholics and perform the workup while the patient is still inebriated and prior to institution of a healthy diet.

Folate deficiency during pregnancy is associated with a high incidence of fetal developmental abnormalities, especially neural tube defects. **Peripheral neuropathies** and **neuropsychiatric disorders** (dementia, psychosis, and depression) in adult patients who are folate deficient and have normal vitamin B_{12} levels may also be observed. **Subacute degeneration of the cord**, usually associated with vitamin B_{12} deficiency, has been reported in the occasional patient with folate deficiency. The difference in incidence may have more to do with the duration of the deficiency state than the vitamin involved.

Laboratory Studies

Accurate diagnosis of folic acid or vitamin B_{12} deficiency requires several laboratory studies (Table 8–1). **Serum folate and serum cobalamin levels** provide the most sensitive measure of ongoing supply of these vitamins to tissues and enjoy the greatest popularity as screening tests to identify clinically important deficiency states. **Other tests**, including serum methylmalonic acid and homocysteine levels, and measurements of plasma transcobalamin protein and transcobalamin saturation can help when the diagnosis is unclear. Measurements of anti-IF antibodies and the absorption of radiolabeled vitamin B_{12} (Schilling test) are used to determine the pathophysiology of a malabsorption defect.

TABLE 8–1 • Laboratory studies in the diagnosis of macrocytic anemias

Screening tests
Complete blood count/reticulocyte index
Marrow aspirate
Iron studies—SI, TIBC, serum ferritin level
Multilobed polymorphonuclear leukocyte count
Serum/urine methylmalonic acid and homocysteine levels
Vitamin B_{12} deficiency
Serum cobalamin (vitamin B_{12}) level
Transcobalamin protein levels
Serum antiparietal cell and anti-intrinsic factor antibody assays
Schilling test
DU suppression test
Folic acid deficiency
Serum and red blood cell folate levels

A. Serum and Red Blood Cell Folate Levels

The serum folate level is exquisitely sensitive to the intake of dietary folate. Normal serum folate levels range from 5–30 ng/mL, but can be even higher with the intake of folate-rich foods. A minimal level of at least 4 ng/mL is required to sustain normal DNA synthesis. As a rule, stores of folate in the liver will, via the enterohepatic cycle, sustain the serum folate level during periods of poor folate intake. Stores are limited, however, and can be depleted within a few weeks of dietary restriction, malabsorption, or chronic alcohol ingestion. The serum folate level will also quickly return to normal when alcohol is withdrawn and/or food intake resumes, or when a folate supplement is provided. In this circumstance, it is still possible to detect a folate-deficient state by assaying **red blood cell folate**, which reflects the state of folate supply at the time the cells were first produced. However, intracellular folate is stored as folate polyglutamate, which must first be hydrolyzed to monoglutamate prior to assay. This preparation step is difficult to standardize, making the red cell measurement less reliable. In addition, the red blood cell folate level will only be abnormal if the patient has been folate deficient for some period and has not received a transfusion. A falsely low level is also seen in 50%–60% of patients with primary vitamin B_{12} deficiency.

B. Serum Cobalamin (Vitamin B_{12}) Level

The normal range for serum cobalamin levels is most often stated to be from 200–500 pg/mL (ng/L). The traditional lower limit of normal, 200 pg/mL, has been challenged, however, based on the ability to detect subclinical cobalamin deficiency with the methylmalonic acid and homocysteine assays. It is more accurate to state the probability of a metabolic abnormality according to the serum cobalamin level, as follows:

- Patients presenting with hematological findings typical of a vitamin B_{12}-deficient macrocytic/megaloblastic anemia have serum cobalamin levels below 200 pg/mL 95%–97% of the time. In addition, the more severe and protracted the anemia the more likely the serum cobalamin level will fall below 100 pg/mL. However, 10%–30% of patients present with little or no anemia, a hypoproliferative anemia secondary to complicating illness or iron deficiency, or nothing more than a neuropathy.

- From the opposing viewpoint, 60%–80% of individuals with serum cobalamin levels less than 200 pg/mL will have anemia or metabolic evidence of vitamin B_{12} deficiency (abnormal methylmalonic acid and homocysteine levels).
- When the serum cobalamin level is between 200 and 350 pg/mL, there is still a considerable chance of a metabolic abnormality suggestive of a subclinical deficiency state. From 30%–35% of apparently normal individuals with cobalamin levels in this range will have an abnormal methylmalonic acid level without hematologic abnormalities.
- The negative predictive value of a single cobalamin level is a major issue. In a retrospective study of a group of ambulatory patients who showed an improvement in hematological/neurological findings when given pharmacological doses of vitamin B_{12}, more than 50% had cobalamin levels greater than 300 pg/mL. Moreover, measurements of methylmalonic acid and homocysteine failed to identify apparently deficient patients 30%–45% of the time. This raises a major concern as to the accuracy of the commercially available tests or suggests a significant fluctuation of cobalamin and metabolite levels over time, making it difficult to get a consistent and therefore diagnostic value.

Misleading cobalamin levels are also seen in certain clinical settings. Falsely low measurements have been reported with normal pregnancy, oral contraceptive use, multiple myeloma, and transcobalamin I deficiency. Patients who are folic acid deficient or are taking large doses of ascorbic acid can have low serum cobalamin levels because of interference with vitamin B_{12} absorption and metabolism. Conversely, normal or elevated cobalamin levels are seen in patients with inborn errors of cobalamin metabolism, isolated transcobalamin II deficiency, and high levels of plasma transcobalamin I and III secondary to severe liver disease or a myeloproliferative disorder.

C. Methylmalonic Acid and Homocysteine Levels

Methylmalonyl-CoA mutase and methionine synthase are both cobalamin-dependent enzymes (Figure 8–5). Methyltetrahydrofolate is required as a methyl donor to cobalamin in the methionine synthase conversion of homocysteine to methionine. Therefore, low cobalamin levels result in elevations of both methylmalonic acid and homocysteine, whereas folate deficiency is accompanied only by an increase in serum homocysteine. The **normal range for serum methylmalonic acid** is 73–271 nM/L (19–76 ng/mL), whereas the **normal serum homocysteine** ranges from 5.4–12.1 μM/L. Serum methylmalonic acid and total homocysteine levels are elevated in 95%–97% of vitamin B_{12}–deficient megaloblastic anemia patients (the same sensitivity as the serum cobalamin measurement). Methylmalonic acid levels are increased 2–100 times the upper limit of normal, and homocysteine elevations are 2–20 times normal. Although homocysteine elevations occur with both cobalamin and folic acid deficiency, less than 2% of folate-deficient patients will have an elevation of serum methylmalonic

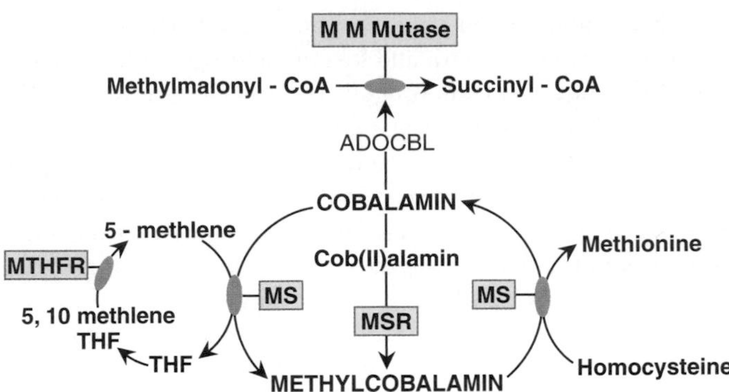

FIGURE 8–5. **Key enzymes in the cobalamin metabolic pathways.** Methionine synthase (MS) catalyzes the synthesis of methionine from homocysteine using the methyl group transferred from methyltetrahydrofolate via methylcobalamin. Methylenetetrahydrofolate reductase (MTHFR) catalyzes the reduction of methylenetetrahydrofolate methyltetrahydrofolate, the obligate methyl donor in the formation of methylcobalamin. The methionine synthase reductase (MSR) enzyme maintains cobalamin in its active form. Methylmalonyl-CoA mutase (MM Mutase) with adenosylcobalamin (ADOCBL) as cofactor catalyzes the conversion of methylmalonyl-CoA to succinyl-CoA.

acid. Folate-deficient patients typically have elevations of homocysteine of 2–10 times normal.

The assay for serum methylmalonic acid is complex and expensive, requiring gas chromatography/mass spectroscopy. Moreover, it is not available in most routine clinical laboratories, making it less valuable in the immediate diagnosis of a deficiency state. Elevated values also are seen in patients with renal insufficiency and severe methylmalonyl mutase deficiency. Homocysteine levels are easier to measure (immunoassay), rise early in and correlate with the severity of the cobalamin deficiency state, and only normalize with cobalamin therapy. However, they are far less specific. Folate and vitamin B_6 deficiency are both associated with increases in serum homocysteine levels. In fact, slight elevations in serum homocysteine are common in otherwise normal populations and appear to respond to dietary folate supplementation. Other causes of serum homocysteine elevation include renal insufficiency, folate enzyme polymorphisms, alcohol abuse, certain drugs (eg, folate and vitamin B_6 inhibitors, such as methotrexate and isoniazid), hypothyroidism, and inborn errors of homocysteine metabolism. Delays in sample processing also can falsely elevate levels. Anticoagulated plasma should be used for assay and the blood sample must be centrifuged within 1 hour of collection.

D. Serum Vitamin B_{12} Binding Proteins

Transcobalamin II (TC II) is the primary plasma-binding protein responsible for the transport of vitamin B_{12} to tissues. Cobalamin absorbed from food or given parenterally is avidly bound to TC II in gastrointestinal mucosal cells and serum. The cobalamin-TC II complex gains access to cells by binding to a specific membrane receptor that is then internalized and delivered to a lysozyme for digestion and release of free cobalamin.

The turnover of cobalamin-TC II complex (holoTC II) in plasma is very rapid, in contrast to the slower turnover of cobalamin and cobalamin analogues bound to transcobalamin I and III.

The level of **holoTC II** may be a more sensitive measure of early negative vitamin B_{12} balance, although this is far from proven and there is the question as to whether it adds anything clinically to the usual serum cobalamin measurement. A commercial immunoassay (AxSYM Holo-TC assay) is available. The "normal level" of holoTC is said to be greater than 50 pmol/L (range 50–300 pmol/L), which best correlates with cobalamin levels greater than 350 pg/mL. The range of values for patients with cobalamin levels between 0 and 100 pg/mL is 0–40 pmol/L, and for cobalamin levels of 150–350 pg/mL it is 0–100 pmol/L. Therefore, there is an indeterminate range of values which, while suggesting store depletion, does not necessarily correlate with a metabolic deficiency state.

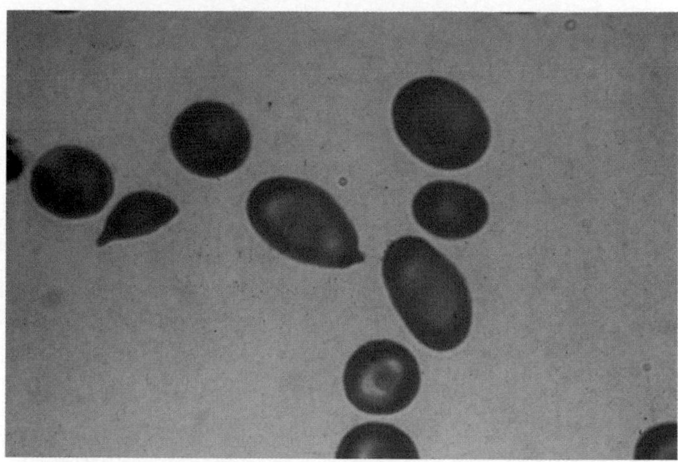

FIGURE 8–7. **Macroovalocytes.** The appearance of macroovalocytes in circulation is an early and reliable sign of an evolving macrocytic/megaloblastic anemia.

E. Tests of Vitamin-Deficient Erythropoiesis

From a morphologic standpoint, the earliest sign of vitamin B_{12} or folic acid deficiency is the appearance in circulation of **hypersegmented (multilobed) polymorphonuclear leukocytes (leukocytes with 5 or more lobes) and giant band forms (Figure 8–6)**. In part, sensitivity of the leukocyte to vitamin deficiency reflects the more rapid turnover of this cellular population. However, unlike the appearance of macrocytosis, this leukocyte response is not easily quantitated. It is either present or not present on examination of the smear. In addition, multilobed leukocytes may also be observed in the occasional patient with severe iron deficiency, myelodysplasia, or simply as an inherited characteristic, making it a somewhat less-specific finding.

Red blood cell morphology changes come on more slowly. At first, a few macroovalocytes (Figure 8–7) can be detected on the peripheral film; later on, as the anemia worsens, the mean cell volume (MCV) becomes elevated.

Patients with severe anemia, macrocytosis (MCV >110), and a megaloblastic marrow are easier to diagnose. Morphologically, megaloblastic changes are characterized by an increase in the size of the earliest progenitor cells (blast forms) and a failure of cell division and maturation. The marrow E/G ratio is generally increased, 1:1 or higher, with depletion of the marrow mature leukocyte pool and expansion of early erythroid precursors. The morphology of the megaloblastic erythroid precursors is distinctive. The earliest blast forms are very large with lacey nuclear chromatin and obvious nucleoli. More mature erythroid precursors typically display prominent nuclear remnants (misshapen or fragmented pieces of nuclei) in what appear to be fully hemoglobinized macrocytes, so-called nuclear-cytoplasmic asynchrony (Figure 8–8).

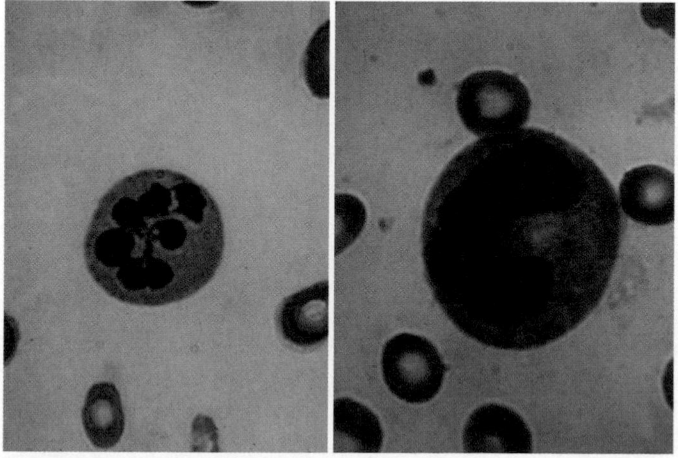

FIGURE 8–6. **Hypersegmented leukocytes.** A hypersegmented (multilobed) polymorphonuclear leukocyte is shown on the left and a giant band (metamyelocyte) on the right.

Full-blown megaloblastosis is associated with **severe ineffective erythropoiesis** (Table 8–2). This is reflected in the disparity between the marrow erythroid hyperplasia (E/G ratio >1:1) and the output of new red blood cells (reticulocyte index <1). Ineffective erythropoiesis represents a death of red cell progenitors prior to leaving the marrow due to defects in cell division and maturation. Additional signs of ineffective erythropoiesis include marked poikilocytosis on the peripheral blood film, an increase in the serum lactic dehydrogenase (LDH) level, and an increase in the serum iron level to the point of full saturation of the total iron-binding capacity (TIBC).

In the research setting, the **deoxyuridine (DU) suppression test** can be used to directly test the DNA synthesis of marrow precursors. This method measures the ability of the cells to convert radiolabeled deoxyuridine monophosphate to thymidylate. Because this reaction requires adequate levels of both vitamin B_{12} and folic acid, the DU suppression test can be made even more specific by testing the effect of adding each vitamin to the reaction mixture. An abnormal DU suppression test that is corrected by the addition of cobalamin, but not methyltetrahydrofolate, is a sensitive measure of early vitamin B_{12} deficiency. However, this sophisticated radioisotope technique is not available in most clinical laboratories.

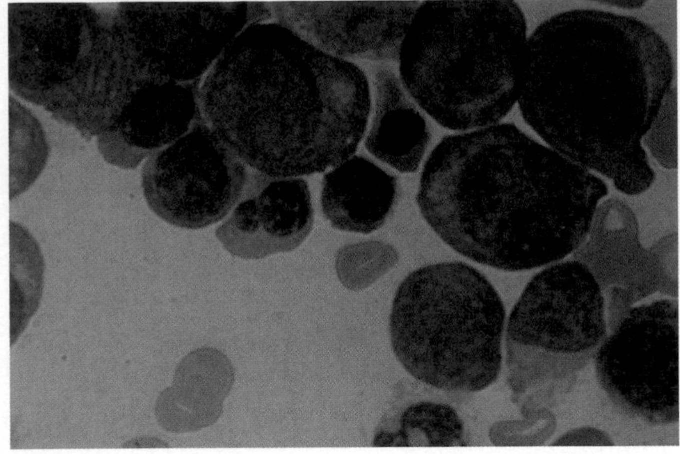

A

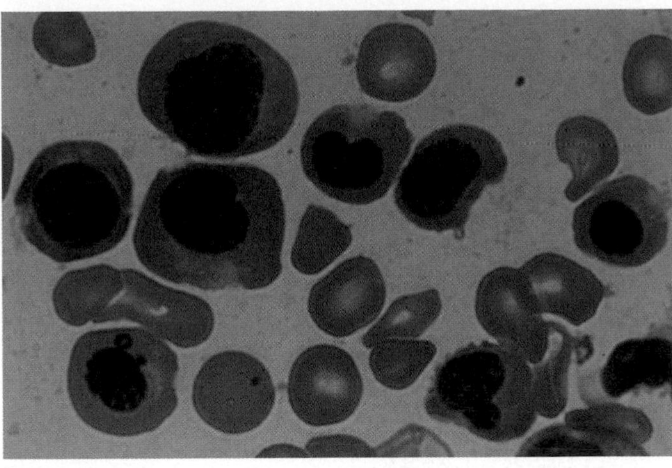

B

FIGURE 8–8. **Megaloblastic marrow morphology.** Primitive erythroid "megaloblasts" with distinctive lacey nuclear chromatin **(A)**. Note that some of these very early blast forms are already forming small lakes of hemoglobin in their cytoplasm. More mature erythroid progenitors showing the delay in nuclear maturation and a tendency for distorted nuclear remnants in otherwise fully hemoglobinized cells **(B)**.

F. Anti–Intrinsic Factor Antibody and Serum Gastrin

Autoantibodies against parietal cells, IF, and cobalamin-IF complex can be detected in the sera of most patients with so-called "pernicious anemia," the most common clinical form of vitamin B_{12}-deficient megaloblastic anemia. **Antiparietal cell antibody** appears to be the most sensitive for atrophic gastritis leading to vitamin B_{12} malabsorption but is not as specific or reliable. **Antibodies against IF and cobalamin-IF complex** are seen in 60%–70% of pernicious anemia patients and have a specificity of close to 100%. Serum gastrin levels, at the same time, should be normal; a lack of serum gastrin casts doubt on the diagnosis.

TABLE 8–2 • Erythropoietic profile of severe macrocytic anemia

Anemia	Severe (Hgb <8–10 g/dL)
MCV (fL)	110–140
Film morphology	Macrocytic, normochromic
Reticulocyte index	<1
Marrow	
E/G ratio	>1:1
Morphology	Megaloblastic
Serum iron/TIBC	Increased/normal
% Saturation	>50
Marrow iron stores	Increased
Serum ferritin	Increased
Bilirubin/LDH	Increased/increased

G. Schilling Test

The **Schilling test** can be used to help define the nature of a vitamin B_{12} malabsorption defect. Unfortunately, the test is a difficult one and has fallen out of favor. Many hospitals no longer offer the test, which involves the use of a tracer isotope, radiolabeled cyanocobalamin. The test involves oral administration of 0.5 μc (0.5–2.0 μg) of radiolabeled cyanocobalamin while the patient is fasting, followed by measurements of the appearance of radioactivity in serum and urine. For the urine test of absorption, 1 mg of nonradioactive cyanocobalamin must be given intramuscularly (IM) 2 hours after the ingestion of the isotope to saturate the serum-binding proteins and flush the radioactive cobalamin into the urine. A 24-hour complete urine collection is essential. Normal subjects should excrete 7% or more of the ingested isotope in the first 24 hours after the flushing dose.

To determine whether vitamin B_{12} malabsorption is related to a lack of IF or an interference with intestinal absorption of the cobalamin-IF complex, the Schilling test is repeated with the simultaneous ingestion of 60 mg of purified, hog-derived IF. This should correct malabsorption secondary to IF deficiency but not the malabsorption owing to small-bowel disease. To avoid a false-positive result because of a vitamin deficiency–induced malabsorption, the Schilling test should be performed some days or weeks after vitamin therapy is initiated.

Accuracy of the Schilling test requires cooperation by the patient. Inadequate flushing with nonradioactive vitamin B_{12} or an incomplete urine collection will lead to false-positive results. In addition, if the IF preparation used in the second part of the Schilling test is not fully active, confusion can arise as to the cause of the vitamin B_{12} malabsorption. Finally, use of crystalline cyanocobalamin in the test will not detect those patients who malabsorb food cobalamin secondary to hypochlorhydria or achlorhydria. Acid gastric juice containing pepsin is essential to normal absorption of food cobalamin.

DIAGNOSIS

As with iron deficiency, the diagnosis of vitamin B_{12} or folic acid deficiency relies heavily on laboratory tests. The concept of stages of deficiency including store depletion, abnormal DNA synthesis without anemia (subclinical deficiency), and a fully developed deficiency state with a macrocytic anemia also applies to vitamin B_{12} and folic acid deficiency. However, unlike iron deficiency, available laboratory methods do not provide as clear-cut a definition of each state.

Vitamin B_{12} and Folic Acid Store Depletion

Accurate measurement of liver stores of either vitamin B_{12} or folic acid would require a direct assay of liver tissue. There are no indirect measures of the quantity of stores of these vitamins similar to the serum ferritin level in iron metabolism. An exception to this statement may be the use of the holoTC II level (the amount of cobalamin bound to TC II) as a more sensitive indicator of negative vitamin B_{12} balance. When vitamin B_{12} intake is inadequate and stores are progressively depleted, the **holoTC II level** could be expected to fall first because of its primary role in delivery of cobalamin to tissues and its rapid turnover as compared to transcobalamins I and III. However, this correlation is not fully proven and, even if true, still does not provide a quantitative measure of total body store depletion.

Once vitamin stores are exhausted, serum cobalamin and folic acid levels measured in the fasting state will indicate inadequate tissue supply. **Serum cobalamin** falls to levels below 200 pg/mL and the **serum folate** to less than 4 ng/mL. This decrease reflects the fact that liver stores must be present to support normal serum vitamin levels in the fasting state. To make this interpretation with any certainty, however, other causes of false elevations or depressions of the vitamin levels must be excluded.

Subclinical Cobalamin Deficiency

The observation that otherwise normal individuals can have elevated methylmalonic acid and homocysteine levels, which return to normal with vitamin B_{12} therapy, has led to the concept of "subclinical cobalamin deficiency." The clinical implications of this finding have not been well defined. Some patients with subclinical deficiency may go on to develop a neuropathy without hematologic changes, suggesting a significant metabolic defect. However, this is a small fraction of the large number of such individuals who can be identified in screening programs. Up to 35% of individuals with serum cobalamin levels between 200 and 350 pg/mL can be shown to have elevated methylmalonic acid and homocysteine levels without anemia or neuropathy. Moreover, in studies of elderly populations, up to 15% of subjects can have evidence of a metabolic defect, even while cobalamin levels are greater than 350 pg/mL.

The implications of classifying individuals with serum cobalamins between 200 and 350 pg/mL, and elevations of serum methylmalonic acid as clinically abnormal and, therefore, in need of a full diagnostic evaluation for vitamin B_{12} malabsorption, are staggering. Because one-third or more elderly Americans have serum cobalamin levels less than 350 pg/mL and a third of these also have minor elevations of their serum methylmalonic acid, several million elderly persons would be eligible for evaluation. Not only is this beyond available resources, but it also ignores the fact that the clinical benefit of finding, evaluating, and treating subclinical cobalamin deficiency has yet to be shown.

To make matters worse, a retrospective study of patients treated with pharmacological doses of vitamin B_{12} for suspicious hematological or neurological findings reported a significant incidence of clinical improvement (predominantly neurological) in patients with apparently normal cobalamin, methylmalonic acid, and/or homocysteine levels. It is unknown whether this is a result of inaccurate measurements using existing commercial assays, an in vivo fluctuation of metabolite levels, or actual subclinical cobalamin deficiency. It does raise the issue, however, of blindly treating patients with vitamin B_{12}, a practice that has been common in the past. Vitamin B_{12} has a long-standing reputation as a "health tonic," which may help and certainly can't hurt.

Vitamin B_{12} and Folic Acid–Deficiency Anemia

A full-blown macrocytic anemia secondary to vitamin B_{12} or folate deficiency is relatively easy to diagnose (see Table 8–2). With **moderate to severe anemia**, the MCV increases to values in excess of 110 fL and the peripheral blood film shows a marked distortion of morphology with macroovalocytes, aniso- and poikilocytosis, and multilobed polymorphonuclear leukocytes. As the anemia worsens, the hematocrit can fall to levels below 15%–20% (hemoglobin 6 g/dL or less), and both leukopenia and thrombocytopenia can develop.

Distortions of marrow morphology are equally impressive. The marrow is strikingly megaloblastic with a shift in the E/G ratio to 1:1 or greater. Most of the erythroid marrow proliferation is limited to the earliest precursors (ie, the basophilic and polychromatophilic normoblasts). This is, in fact, a demonstration of the ineffective erythropoiesis that accompanies megaloblastosis. Erythroid precursors are arrested in S phase, cannot go through cell division, and die within the marrow. This is reflected by a mismatch between the E/G ratio of 1:1 (>3 times normal) and a reticulocyte production index of less than 1. Other laboratory signs of the ineffectiveness of erythropoiesis include elevations in serum LDH level and an increase in the serum iron that approaches full saturation of the TIBC. There may also be a modest increase in the indirect bilirubin level.

Serum cobalamin levels should confirm the diagnosis (Table 8–3). The patient with a pure vitamin B_{12} deficiency and a well-developed macrocytic anemia will almost certainly have a serum cobalamin level less than 200 pg/mL, with more severe anemia patients falling below 100 pg/mL. At the same time, the serum folate level will be normal or increased. If the cobalamin level is low, measurements of serum methylmalonic

TABLE 8–3 • Testing for vitamin B_{12} and folic acid deficiency

	Vitamin B_{12} Deficiency	Folic Acid Deficiency
Serum B_{12} (normal >200 pg/mL)	<100	>200
Serum folate level (normal >4 ng/mL)	>4	<4
Serum methylmalonic acid (normal <270 nM/L)	2–100 × normal	Normal
Serum homocysteine (normal <16 nM/L)	2–20 × normal	2–10 × normal

acid and homocysteine are not needed; they only add expense. Patients with severe liver disease or myeloproliferative disorders who have very high levels of transcobalamin I/III are exceptions to this rule.

The **diagnosis of a macrocytic anemia secondary to folic acid deficiency** can be more difficult. This diagnosis is especially true for the alcoholic patient where there is a close relationship between the patient's diet, level of alcohol ingestion, and serum folate level. Alcohol has a dramatic and rapid effect on the serum folate level. At blood alcohol levels of 100 mg/dL or higher, release of folate from hepatic stores to recycle through the enterohepatic pathway for tissue supply is impaired. In the patient who has little or no dietary intake of folate, this results in a rapid and sustained fall in the serum folate level to values below 4 ng/mL. Thus, an acute alcoholic can show low serum folate levels within a matter of a few days of a drinking binge, even though liver folate stores are not exhausted.

This phenomenon is easily detected if a serum folate level is drawn while the patient is still inebriated. However, any delay following withdrawal of alcohol and/or resumption of a normal diet will result in a rise in the serum folate to normal levels. Delays of several days or a week can result in an even more confusing picture. By this time, the patient's abnormal marrow morphology will have disappeared. Moreover, the anemic patient will mount a reticulocyte response suggesting either a hemolytic anemia or a recovery from a bleeding episode. In this situation, the only clue to a prior deficiency in folic acid will be the occasional macroovalocyte on the peripheral blood film and a lower than normal red blood cell folate level.

The approach to diagnosis is also influenced by the **severity of the anemia**. If the patient requires immediate treatment, it is essential that all necessary laboratory studies be drawn prior to transfusion or vitamin administration. The tests should include a complete blood count (CBC), reticulocyte count, marrow aspirate for morphology and assessment of iron stores, serum

CASE HISTORY • *Part 2*

The CBC shows a moderately severe pancytopenia with red cell morphology and cell indices notable for a mixed population of normocytic and macrocytic cells with some aniso- and poikilocytosis and polychromasia. The increase in the red blood cell distribution width (RDW)-SD greater than the RDW-CV is another indicator of a subpopulation of very macrocytic cells on a background of otherwise normocytic red cells, suggesting that the appearance of macrocytosis is a relatively recent event. A more balanced increase in both the RDW-CV and -SD would suggest a shift in the overall MCV curve and, therefore, a more long-standing anemia.

As a rule, the presence of even a few macroovalocytes indicates the presence of a macrocytic anemia—a "nuclear maturation disorder." The "megaloblastic" bone marrow morphology and E/G ratio of 1:1 support this diagnosis. The imbalance between the erythroid hyperplasia in the marrow and the low reticulocyte index suggests ineffective erythropoiesis—another characteristic of the megaloblastic anemias.

The diagnostic differential includes vitamin B_{12} deficiency, folic acid deficiency, a combination of the 2, drug toxicity (folate antagonists, nitrous oxide exposure), or a myelodysplastic nuclear maturation defect. To confirm the diagnosis, the patient should have measures of serum vitamin B_{12} and folate levels, as well as a battery of iron studies to exclude iron deficiency as a complicating factor. In this case, these tests should be drawn immediately before any of the acute effects of alcohol ingestion and dietary folate deficiency are corrected. Even a delay of 24 hours can make the interpretation of the study results inconclusive.

These studies are drawn with the following results:

Serum vitamin B_{12} level - 580 pg/mL
Serum folate level - 3 ng/mL
Serum iron - 85 μg/dL TIBC - 270 μg/dL
Serum ferritin - 460 μg/L

Questions

- What diagnosis is supported by these results?
- What possible underlying etiologies must be considered?
- How should the patient be managed given the various blood abnormalities?

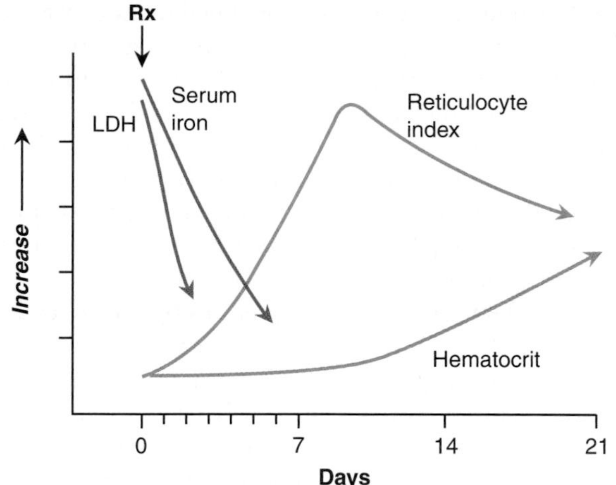

FIGURE 8–9. **Therapeutic response to vitamin B_{12} or folic acid.** The first sign of an effective response to one or the other vitamin is a fall in serum iron and LDH levels. This reflects a correction of the patient's ineffective erythropoiesis. On or about day 3, the reticulocyte index increases, peaking by the eighth day. The subsequent level of red blood cell production and rate of hematocrit rise will reflect the severity of the patient's anemia, adequacy of iron supply, and the presence of other complicating illness.

cobalamin and folate levels, and serum iron, TIBC, and ferritin levels. This battery of tests should make it possible to confirm any defect in cell maturation, distinguish vitamin B_{12} from folic acid deficiency, and provide an assessment of iron stores. The latter is especially important in planning therapy. Patients with small bowel malabsorption can present with a single deficiency of vitamin B_{12}, folic acid, or iron, or any combination of the 3. Moreover, it is not uncommon that therapy with vitamin B_{12} and folic acid, alone or in combination, will uncover an iron deficiency state.

In patients with less-marked anemias, **vitamin B_{12} and folic acid therapy can be used diagnostically**. This therapy is most applicable for patients with vitamin B_{12} deficiency owing to an autoimmune process (pernicious anemia), where folic acid and iron deficiency are unlikely. To perform a therapeutic trial, the patient is given 1–10 μg vitamin B_{12} parenterally each day for 10–14 days. The response to therapy can be measured in several ways. As shown in Figure 8–9, the LDH level and elevated serum iron level fall rapidly over the first 2–3 days as the patient's erythropoiesis becomes effective. This decrease is followed on days 3–5 with an increase in the reticulocyte count. Recovery of the hematocrit is much slower and takes several weeks. Although a response to small amounts of vitamin B_{12} strongly suggests a vitamin B_{12} deficiency state, it is not absolute proof; serum vitamin levels are still important to confirm the diagnosis.

DIFFERENTIAL DIAGNOSIS

The differential diagnosis of a vitamin deficiency state involves not just identifying whether it is vitamin B_{12} or folic acid deficiency but also the cause of the vitamin deficiency. There is also the task of distinguishing the macrocytic anemia associated with vitamin B_{12} and folic acid deficiency from the macrocytosis observed in patients with dysplastic anemias, liver disease, hemolysis, and exposure to chemotherapeutic agents.

Macrocytosis

Macrocytosis, an MCV greater than 100 fL, is seen in several clinical settings (Table 8–4). In patients with a hemorrhagic or hemolytic anemia, where there is a high level of stimulation of the marrow by erythropoietin, the release of marrow reticulocytes with an MCV in excess of 140 fL will increase the MCV. The higher the reticulocyte count, the greater the increase in MCV. Patients with reticulocyte counts greater than 20% can have MCVs in excess of 110–120 fL, and the red blood cell–volume histogram will clearly show the double population of very large reticulocytes and normal mature red blood cells. In that situation, the RDW-SD will be increased out of proportion to the RDW-CV. Much less dramatic, uniform **macrocytosis, MCVs of 95–105 fL**, is observed in patients with hypothyroidism and liver disease. In the latter case, it may represent an accumulation of excess membrane secondary to disturbed cholesterol metabolism and is usually accompanied by the appearance of target cells in circulation.

More severe macrocytosis with red cell poikilocytosis and megaloblastic marrow morphology is seen not only in vitamin-deficient patients but also with myelodysplasia and in patients receiving chemotherapeutic agents such as **hydroxyurea and methotrexate**. Just as with the vitamin deficiency states, these patients have a true nuclear maturation defect. Their marrow morphology is abnormal and they exhibit varying degrees of ineffective erythropoiesis. Abnormalities in white blood cell and platelet components of the blood count are also common.

Macrocytosis can also be an **artifact of the automated cell counter technique**. Patients with cold agglutinins or marked elevations of their white blood cell count may be reported to have an MCV in excess of 110 fL. In the first case, it is related to clumping of red blood cells in the counter, whereas with marked leukocytosis, white blood cells are being counted as red blood cells. Modest increases in the MCV can be seen in

TABLE 8–4 • Causes of macrocytosis

	MCV (fL)	Morphology
Normal	90	Normocytic
Reticulocytosis	90–110	Polychromasia (shift reticulocytes)
Liver disease	95–110	Uniform macrocytosis, targeting
Megaloblastic anemia	100–130	Macroovalocytosis, marked poikilocytosis
Cell counter artifact	100–130	Red blood cell agglutination or marked leukocytosis

patients with hyperglycemia. This condition is an artifact of the dilution step when the cells are prepared for counting. Because of the high intracellular glucose content, cells swell rapidly when they are placed in the isosmotic diluent. Hematology laboratories are aware of such artifacts and take steps to confirm that the MCV is accurate.

Causes of Vitamin B_{12} Deficiency

Evaluation of a patient with a vitamin B_{12} deficiency anemia demands consideration of several possible causes (Table 8–5). Dietary history may suggest **poor intake of vitamin B_{12}**. However, only the strictest of vegetarians and breast fed infants born to vegetarian mothers are at risk for developing a deficiency state. In the case of the adult patient with anemia, impaired **vitamin B_{12} absorption**, either IF deficiency or a defect in small-bowel absorption, is almost certainly present. In children, congenital defects in transport and intracellular metabolism must be considered. Transport defects include defective IF synthesis, impaired intestinal transport (Imerslund-Gräsbeck syndrome) and TC II deficiency. Except for the TC II–deficient patients where normal levels of TC I are present, these conditions will have low serum cobalamin levels. Diagnosis of TC II deficiency requires assay of TC II total protein. Inborn errors of intracellular metabolism include abnormalities of the methionine synthase, methionine synthase reductase, and methylmalonyl mutase enzymes (see Figure 8–5). Patients with an impaired methionine synthase reaction present with megaloblastic anemia, a normal serum cobalamin level, and an elevated serum homocysteine.

TABLE 8–5 • Causes of vitamin B_{12} deficiency

Congenital defects
Intrinsic factor deficiency
TC II deficiency
Imerslund-Gräsbeck disease
Juvenile pernicious anemia
Poor vitamin B_{12} intake (vegans)
Malabsorption
Intrinsic factor deficiency
Autoimmune—antiparietal cell/anti-intrinsic factor antibody (pernicious anemia)
Gastric surgery
Pancreatic insufficiency
Small intestine absorption defect
Crohn disease
Sprue
Lymphoma
Diverticulosis or blind loop with bacterial overgrowth
Fish tapeworm
Ileal resection
Zollinger-Ellison syndrome
HIV infection
Vitamin B_{12} destruction
Nitrous oxide exposure

The impairment of vitamin B_{12} metabolism by nitrous oxide oxidation of the cobalt atom of the vitamin and inhibition of methionine synthase is also suggested by the patient's clinical history. The resulting defect in methionine and S-adenosylmethionine synthesis can have a major impact on both hematopoiesis and the central nervous system. It occurs following exposure to high levels of nitrous oxide anesthesia for several hours or with repeated low-level exposures over a long time in at-risk individuals, such as dentists.

A **full evaluation of vitamin B_{12} absorption** includes a careful review of the clinical history and an evaluation of small-bowel anatomy and function. Patients with ileitis, ileal resection, small-bowel dysfunction secondary to diverticulitis and bacterial overgrowth, fistula formation, or sprue may be recognized from the clinical presentation with the help of radiologic and endoscopic studies. Patients with nontropical sprue may be diagnosed by biopsy of the small bowel. The presence of any one of these conditions obviously sets the stage for vitamin B_{12} malabsorption. To confirm this, a Schilling test first without and then with IF can be performed. Any of the defects in vitamin B_{12} transport or absorption secondary to small-bowel disease will show abnormal absorption of crystalline B_{12} in both parts of the study. The addition of IF does not correct the absorption defect.

The patient with IF deficiency can be diagnosed using a combination of laboratory studies and the Schilling test. The patient presenting with a macrocytic anemia, a serum cobalamin level less than 200 pg/mL, and a positive anti-IF antibody is almost certainly an example of vitamin B_{12} deficiency secondary to an IF defect. This is a relatively common diagnosis that is most frequently detected in adult patients in their later years (classic pernicious anemia). IF deficiency is seen in children who are born with an IF production defect. Adults who have gastrectomies, where a major portion of the fundus of the stomach is removed, or a gastric bypass operation will predictably develop vitamin B_{12} deficiency secondary to a lack of IF, usually within 2–4 years if they do not receive parenteral vitamin B_{12} on a regular basis. Some patients with low serum cobalamin levels can be shown to have abnormal food-B_{12} absorption.

Causes of Folic Acid Deficiency

The causes of folic acid deficiency are listed in Table 8–6. **Poor dietary intake coupled with alcohol ingestion** is a major cause of folic acid deficiency in the adult population. Obviously, the history and physical examination are important in identifying the alcoholism and the level of dietary intake. Still, it is even more important to fully evaluate the patient at presentation. Accurate diagnosis requires an immediate workup, including measurements of serum cobalamin and folate, at a time when the impact of alcohol on folate metabolism is still operative.

There are clinical settings where even a normal diet will not maintain folate requirements. **Patients with high levels of cell turnover** (eg, hemolytic anemias, psoriasis, and exfoliative dermatitis) can develop folic acid deficiency even while on a normal diet. Sickle cell anemia patients are at considerable risk due to their increased requirement and irregular dietary intake,

TABLE 8–6 • Causes of folic acid deficiency

Poor folic acid intake	Increased requirement
Dietary lack/alcoholism Goat's milk anemia Parenteral nutrition	Hemolytic anemias Exfoliative dermatitis/psoriasis Pregnancy
Malabsorption	**Metabolic inhibition**
Sprue (nontropical and tropical) Lymphoma Small-bowel resection Crohn disease Anticonvulsant drugs	Dihydrofolate reductase inhibitors (methotrexate, trimethoprim, etc) Alcohol Vitamin C deficiency
Loss/destruction	
Hemodialysis Tropical sprue	

especially with frequent crises. Inadequate folate intake is a major issue during normal pregnancy. It has been associated with a high incidence of neural tube defects. Therefore, folic acid supplementation is required for each of these situations.

As with vitamin B_{12} deficiency, **disease of the small intestines** can result in folic acid malabsorption. Patients with sprue (especially tropical sprue), bacterial overgrowth, and short-bowel syndrome are at risk for developing a macrocytic anemia due to folic acid deficiency. In the case of tropical sprue, folate deficiency is thought to play an integral role in the small-bowel mucosal transport defect, since treatment with folic acid is actually therapeutic.

Several **drugs have an antifolate action**. Methotrexate, triamterene, and sulfamethoxazole with trimethoprim (Bactrim) are competitive inhibitors of methyl folate and DNA metabolism. Methotrexate given in therapeutic amounts is the strongest of these agents and with long-term therapy can be expected to produce macrocytosis and pancytopenia. Anticonvulsants (phenytoin, primidone, and phenobarbital) appear to be weak inhibitors of folic acid absorption. These drugs can cause macrocytosis and anemia when given in high doses to children.

As regards congenital defects, severe methylenetetrahydrofolate reductase and cystathione beta-synthetase deficiencies are the most common of the inborn errors of folate metabolism. Patients present as children or adults with neurologic abnormalities, developmental delay, and thrombotic disease, probably secondary to their high levels of homocysteine. Because thymidylate synthesis remains unaffected, they do not have a megaloblastic anemia. Methylenetetrahydrofolate reductase polymorphisms resulting in 30%–60% reductions in enzyme activity are also quite common. They are cited as a primary cause of mild hyperhomocysteinemia in population studies and, therefore, as risk factors for cardiovascular disease, neural tube defects, and colon cancer. Because serum homocysteine levels in these individuals can be normalized with folate supplementation, this has led to even more enthusiasm for dietary fortification. At the same time, supplementation trials have not conclusively shown a beneficial effect.

THERAPY

General Guidelines

Folic acid and vitamin B_{12} are available in their purified forms for oral and parenteral use and are incorporated in several multivitamin preparations sold as nutritional supplements. The selection of preparation, dose, and treatment schedule must be appropriate to the clinical setting. Misdiagnosis can result in a treatment failure and worsening of the patient's clinical condition. This fact is of special importance in the patient with vitamin

CASE HISTORY • *Part 3*

The serum vitamin B_{12} level is normal to high, while the folate level is below 4 ng/mL, suggesting folic acid deficiency. Folic acid deficiency can result from poor dietary intake, malabsorption (sprue), drug toxicity (folate antagonists), and acute and chronic alcoholism. The latter involves both an absence of folate in the alcoholic's diet and interference by alcohol in the normal enterohepatic recirculation of active folate metabolites. Even short exposures to intoxicating levels of alcohol (days to weeks), together with a lack of dietary folate, will produce a macrocytic anemia.

The treatment of this patient is a simple matter of alcohol withdrawal and folate replacement by diet, oral folic acid supplements, or both. The reduced levels of leukocytes and platelets should also respond, although the pancytopenia may well be multifactorial—a combination of direct alcohol toxicity, folate deficiency, and hypersplenism (the patient has a palpable spleen). The role of each will become clearer after alcohol withdrawal and folic acid replacement. If the anemia fails to resolve after a month or more, a full evaluation will be necessary to rule out chronic blood loss, iron deficiency, or an inflammatory anemia (alcoholic patients may have chronic active hepatitis).

B_{12} deficiency because a delay in therapy or mistreatment with folic acid alone may result in irreversible neurologic damage. Therefore, both the nature and cause of the deficiency state must be well defined as a foundation for planning management.

A. Severe, Life-Threatening Anemia

The treatment of a patient with a severe macrocytic anemia will need to **proceed prior to completing the diagnostic workup**. Once appropriate laboratory studies including serum cobalamin, folate, and iron studies are drawn, the patient should receive full therapeutic doses of both vitamin B_{12} and folic acid, using the parenteral route to avoid the issue of malabsorption. Furthermore, this treatment should be continued with daily administration of both vitamins until a response is evident or the diagnosis is clear. If the patient is unstable from a cardiovascular standpoint, the patient should receive a transfusion with red blood cells. This must be done with caution, however, since patients with vitamin B_{12} deficiency are usually older and have marginal cardiovascular compensation. Any sudden increase in blood volume as with a rapid red blood cell transfusion can induce a fatal arrhythmia or acute congestive heart failure. Therefore, red blood cells should be infused slowly and carefully with concomitant use of a diuretic or simultaneous phlebotomy to avoid increasing the blood volume.

Treatment with both vitamin B_{12} and folic acid does not interfere with the subsequent evaluation of the patient for malabsorption. Radiologic and functional studies of the small bowel can still be performed once the anemia is corrected. This includes the use of the Schilling test to distinguish IF deficiency from an abnormality in small intestinal absorption.

B. Less Symptomatic Deficiency States

Whenever possible, therapy should be targeted to the specific deficiency state. In the patient with a **mild to moderate macrocytic anemia**, this will mean a delay until a full hematologic workup can be performed and the serum cobalamin and folate levels are measured. If the patient presents with **neurologic disease and no anemia**, measurements of serum methylmalonic acid and homocysteine can suggest the diagnosis. It is these settings where a therapeutic trial with a specific vitamin can also help confirm the deficiency state. For the **vitamin B_{12}–deficient patient**, a therapeutic trial can be performed using 1–10 μg of vitamin B_{12} given IM daily for 10 days while monitoring changes in the methylmalonic acid level, or when anemia is present, the serum iron, LDH, reticulocyte count, and over several weeks, the hematocrit and MCV. Similarly, a therapeutic trial can be performed using 50–100 μg of folic acid given parenterally on a daily schedule for 10–14 days to confirm an isolated **folic acid–deficiency** state. This low level of folic acid will not run the risk of either inducing a hematologic response or worsening the neurologic signs in a vitamin B_{12}–deficient patient. Also, it will not correct the high serum methylmalonic acid level of vitamin B_{12} deficiency.

As a practical point, therapeutic trials with small amounts of either vitamin B_{12} or folic acid are difficult to perform and often hard to interpret because other disease states can interfere with the response. If the patient is iron deficient or has an inflammatory illness, the lack of iron substrate and suppression of erythropoietin will dampen the reticulocyte and hematocrit responses. In addition, a therapeutic trial with low doses of vitamin B_{12} will delay the performance of a Schilling test since the latter includes administering a flushing dose of 1,000 mg of nonisotopic vitamin B_{12}. In effect, the flushing dose is therapeutic.

The issue of "subclinical deficiency," where there are no hematological or neurological findings typical of a deficiency of vitamin B_{12}, is a clinical conundrum. If you believe patients benefit from pharmacological doses of vitamin B_{12} even though their levels of cobalamin, methylmalonic acid, and homocysteine are within normal limits, then it is easy to defend a therapeutic trial of high doses of vitamin B_{12} in patients with dementia or other neurological findings. It also gives life to an old issue of clinical practice—the administration of B_{12} injections to elderly patients as a "tonic." In either case there is no downside and some patients may improve, or at least feel better.

C. Vitamin Prophylaxis

There are clinical situations where vitamin B_{12} or folic acid therapy should be given prophylactically. These situations include conditions where the rate of use of either vitamin exceeds the dietary supply, and disease states where malabsorption can be anticipated. For example, patients who have had a gastrectomy will exhibit vitamin B_{12} malabsorption and should, therefore, receive long-term vitamin prophylaxis. Normal pregnancy is an example of an imbalance between folate needs for fetal growth and folate supply in the diet. All pregnant women should receive supplementation with a multivitamin that contains folic acid.

Vitamin B_{12} Preparations

Vitamin B_{12} is available in its pure form, **cyanocobalamin**, in concentrations of 30, 100, and 1,000 mg/mL for IM or deep subcutaneous injection. The dose administered will depend on the management plan. A dose of 1–10 μg IM daily is typically used in therapeutic trials where the purpose is to confirm vitamin B_{12} deficiency or distinguish vitamin B_{12} deficiency from folic acid deficiency. When a diagnosis of vitamin B_{12} is established, the patient with a **severe macrocytic anemia** should be treated with at least 100 μg of cyanocobalamin daily for at least 2 weeks. This regimen will guarantee a maximum therapeutic response and encourage rebuilding of liver vitamin B_{12} stores. Subsequently, patients should receive 100–1,000 μg of cyanocobalamin once a month for the rest of their lives. This situation will maintain their balance unless there is a high level of cell turnover, in which case twice-monthly injections are advised. Patients with a **vitamin B_{12}** deficient neuropathy should be treated more aggressively with weekly or biweekly injections for several months to encourage maximum recovery.

Administration of more than 100 μg of cyanocobalamin in any single injection exceeds the binding capacity of TC II and results in a rapid clearance of most of the excess vitamin B_{12} into urine. Therefore, there is no advantage to using a dose of 1,000 μg of cyanocobalamin. At the same time, cyanocobalamin is very inexpensive and the higher dose is harmless.

Several vitamin preparations that contain vitamin B_{12} are marketed as **nutritional supplements**. Some of these contain not only cyanocobalamin but also IF concentrate prepared from animal stomachs. Theoretically, the latter should provide an effective oral medication for the treatment of patients with poor absorption secondary to IF deficiency, especially those with some residual IF activity. However, its effectiveness cannot be assumed. Patients can develop refractoriness to these preparations possibly because of the development of an antibody against the animal protein. Oral maintenance therapy is possible using very high doses of vitamin B_{12} (1,000 μg daily) on the rationale that a small amount of it will leak across the intestine. Although this does work, patients will need to be monitored closely for any clinical evidence of recurrence of their deficiency. The cost of this increased level of observation can cancel any advantage of oral over parenteral therapy.

Multivitamin preparations containing small amounts of vitamin B_{12} are marketed as **over-the-counter medications**. Some of these contain as much as 80 μg of cyanocobalamin combined with 500–1,000 μg of folic acid, ascorbic acid, and iron. They are very useful as nutritional supplements in patients who are on an inadequate diet or have an increased requirement.

Folic Acid Preparations

Pharmaceutical preparations of folic acid include **pteroylglutamic acid folate congener** (folic acid, folvite), and **5-formyltetrahydrofolate congener** (folinic acid, leucovorin, citrovorum factor). Both are formulated for either oral or parenteral administration. Folic acid tablets **(folvite)** contain 0.1, 0.4, 0.8, or 1 mg of pteroylglutamic acid, whereas folic acid for injection contains 5 mg/mL. Pteroylglutamic acid must first be reduced and methylated by either intestinal mucosal cells or hepatocytes before it participates in cellular DNA metabolism.

Folinic acid tablets (leucovorin) contain 5, 10, 15, or 25 mg of 5-formyltetrahydrofolate. The principal application of folinic acid is to circumvent the inhibition of dihydrofolate reductase by the chemotherapeutic agent, methotrexate. Leucovorin will also correct the defect in thymidylate production both in patients who lack methyltetrahydrofolate and those who are vitamin B_{12} deficient. It should be avoided when treating vitamin B_{12}–deficient patients because it can correct the hematologic abnormality while allowing the neurologic findings to progress.

The approach to folic acid therapy will vary according to the management plan. If a **therapeutic trial** is attempted, the patient should be given a daily parenteral injection of 50–100 μg of folic acid (folvite). This treatment will require a meticulous dilution of the 5-mg/mL commercial preparation in order to avoid a high dose that might give a partial response in the vitamin B_{12}–deficient patient. It is also important to recognize the difficulties associated with a therapeutic trial of folic acid. Patients with alcohol-induced defects in folate metabolism often demonstrate a spontaneous recovery of their hematologic abnormality with alcohol abstention. This reflects the reversal of the alcohol-induced defect in liver folate store metabolism. Patients with folic acid deficiency can also demonstrate a combined defect in vitamin B_{12} and iron metabolism. In this situation, a therapeutic trial with a single vitamin will not give an interpretable response.

Patients with **severe macrocytic anemias** are best treated with a combination of 100 μg of cyanocobalamin IM and either oral or parenteral doses of 1–5 mg of folic acid. Generally, oral doses of folic acid are adequately absorbed, even in patients with known defects in small intestinal absorption. It is a water-soluble vitamin that can cross the mucosal barrier by passive diffusion when given in large doses. Therefore, it is common practice to treat patients with oral folic acid in daily doses of 1–5 mg regardless of the cause of the deficiency state.

Prophylactic administration of folic acid in patients with poor diets or high levels of cell turnover will vary according to the individual clinical situation. Multivitamin preparations containing as much as 1 mg of folic acid are used in pregnancy and as a supplement for nursing mothers because as much as 50 μg of folate is secreted each day in breast milk. Patients with hemolytic anemias or exfoliative dermatitis are usually given a higher dose (1 or 2 mg of folic acid orally each day). Like vitamin B_{12}, the safety range of folic acid is very large and no side effects are seen even with doses exceeding 20 mg per day. However, there have been reports of an increase in the frequency of seizures in children who receive large amounts of folic acid to prevent the antimetabolite effect of antiepileptic medications.

The **long-term management** of any patient with vitamin B_{12} or folic acid deficiency requires periodic reevaluation to guarantee therapeutic effectiveness. Since the deficiencies are most often the result of an underlying defect in absorption, patients may need to maintain their vitamin therapy for the rest of their lives or at least until the absorption defect has been cured. There is also a constant risk that multiple vitamin and mineral deficiencies will occur. This risk is most typical of the patient with sprue or widespread intestinal disease from other causes where the patient is at risk for folic acid, vitamin B_{12}, and iron deficiency. Less commonly, vitamin C deficiency can play a role. The patient with scurvy can exhibit a macrocytic/megaloblastic anemia secondary to a defect in intracellular folate metabolism resulting from low cellular vitamin C levels.

Periodic evaluations of patients receiving maintenance vitamin therapy should include a careful history and physical to look for the reappearance or progression of the patient's neuropathy, a complete blood count, iron studies, and measurements of serum cobalamin and folate levels. Additional studies may be needed to evaluate and monitor the underlying disease process responsible for the vitamin deficiency.

POINTS TO REMEMBER

Folic acid and vitamin B_{12} deficiency are the primary causes of macrocytic anemia in adults. Patients with myelodysplasia and erythroleukemia may also present with a modest to severe macrocytic anemia, and macrocytosis with targeting may be seen in patients with advanced liver disease.

Vitamin B_{12} and folic acid are key nutrients in the diet. Deficiency states can develop in the absence of an adequate intake, an interference with absorption, an abnormality in metabolism, or an increased requirement.

Most patients with vitamin B_{12} deficiency represent either a dietary deficiency (vegans) or more likely a defect in absorption. The etiologies behind malabsorption are multiple, ranging from intrinsic factor abnormalities to competition for vitamin B_{12} by parasites/bacteria to disorders of small bowel function.

Folic acid deficiency is common in patients with severe malabsorption (sprue) and in alcoholics, where both poor dietary intake and interference with the normal folate metabolism contribute.

The differential diagnosis of the cause of macrocytic anemia depends on a timely evaluation using studies of bone marrow morphology and measurements of serum cobalamin and folic acid levels. Iron studies are also important and may need repeating to rule out the emergence of iron deficiency once the vitamin deficiency is treated.

The evaluation of an alcoholic patient with a macrocytic anemia must be done promptly, preferably while the patient's blood alcohol level is still elevated and before any dietary folate replacement. Otherwise, the impact of alcohol on the serum folate level will be missed.

The measurement and interpretation of the serum cobalamin level can present problems, including potential false results from commercially available assays, a broad indeterminate range (100–350 pg/mL) where deficiency may go undetected, abnormalities in the transcobalamin proteins, concomitant folate deficiency, and inborn errors of cobalamin metabolism. There is also evidence that "subclinical" deficiency may exist even with levels greater than 350 pg/mL.

Methylmalonic acid and homocysteine levels can be used to identify metabolic signs of vitamin B_{12} and folate deficiency. However, they are expensive, and while identifying some patients with "subclinical" deficiency, they still miss a third or more of patients who appear to respond hematologically and neurologically to pharmaceutical levels of vitamin B_{12}.

The full evaluation of a patient with suspected vitamin B_{12} malabsorption involves radiographic studies of the stomach and small bowel, measurements of intrinsic factor antibodies and serum gastrin, and, in some cases, the performance of a Schilling test.

When the etiology is not clear, a therapeutic trial with folic acid or vitamin B_{12} in small amounts may be useful. However, in the presence of a life-threatening anemia, serum cobalamin and folate levels should be drawn and both vitamins given in pharmacologic doses. Elderly patients in heart failure should also be judiciously transfused.

Once initiated, vitamin B_{12} therapy in a deficient patient secondary to an uncorrectable defect in absorption must be continued for life, preferably with monthly injections of the vitamin.

A missed diagnosis or inappropriate therapy (high doses of folic acid given to a vitamin B_{12} anemia patient) runs the risk of progressive and irreversible neurological abnormalities (combined systems disease).

BIBLIOGRAPHY

Carmel R: Current concepts in cobalamin deficiency. Annu Rev Med 2000;51:357.

Carmel R: How I treat cobalamin (vitamin B_{12}) deficiency. Blood 2008;112:2214.

Carmel R: Prevalence of undiagnosed pernicious anemia in the elderly. Arch Intern Med 1996;156:1097.

Carmel R, James SJ: Alcohol abuse: an important cause of hyper-homocysteinemia. Nutr Rev 2002;60:215.

Chanarin I et al: Cobalamin and folate: recent developments. J Clin Pathol 1992;45:277.

Clarke R et al: Screening for vitamin B_{12} and folic acid deficiency in older persons. Am J Clin Nutr 2003;66:750.

Cooper BA, Rosenblatt DS: Inherited defects of vitamin B_{12} metabolism. Ann Rev Nutr 1987;7:291.

Green R, Miller JW: Folate deficiency beyond megaloblastic anemia: hyperhomocysteinemia and other manifestations of dysfunctional folate status. Semin Hematol 1999;36:47.

Hillman RS: Hematopoietic agents: growth factors, minerals and vitamins. In: The Pharmacological Basis of Therapeutics, 10th ed. McGraw-Hill, 2001.

Lederle FA: Oral cobalamin for pernicious anemia: medicine's best kept secret? JAMA 1991;265:94.

Lindenbaum J et al: Diagnosis of cobalamin deficiency: II. Relative sensitivities of serum cobalamin, methylmalonic acid and homocysteine concentrations. Am J Hematol 1990;34:99.

Rosenblatt D, Fenton W: Inherited disorders of folate and cobalamin transport and metabolism. In: Scriver CR et al: The Metabolic Bases of Inherited Disease, 8th ed. McGraw-Hill, 2001.

Solomon L: Cobalamin-responsive disorders in the ambulatory care setting: unreliability of cobalamin, methylmalonic acid, and homocysteine testing. Blood 2005;105:978.

Stabler SP et al: Clinical spectrum and diagnosis of cobalamin deficiency. Blood 1990;76:871.

Toh BH, vanDriel IR, Gleeson PA: Mechanisms of disease: pernicious anemia. N Engl J Med 1997;337:1441.

Wald DS et al: Homocysteine and cardiovascular disease: evidence on causality from a meta-analysis. BMJ 2002;325:1.

THE DYSPLASTIC AND SIDEROBLASTIC ANEMIAS • 9

CASE HISTORY • *Part I*

A 65-year-old woman seen for a routine checkup reports a decrease in exercise tolerance, especially during routine workouts at the gym. She denies other recent illness. Review of systems is positive, however, for a history of Hodgkin lymphoma, stage IA, diagnosed at age 25 and treated successfully with mantle radiation. Physical examination reveals a well-developed white female looking younger than her stated age. Conjunctiva may be somewhat pale. No evidence of lymphadenopathy or hepatosplenomegaly. No recent weight loss.

CBC: Hemoglobin/hematocrit - 10 g/dL/30%
MCV - 99 fL MCH - 32 pg MCHC - 33 g/dL
RDW-CV - 16%
White blood cell count – 4,900/μL
Absolute differential: Neutrophils - 2,600/μL
Lymphocytes - 2,100/μL
Monocytes - 200/μL
Platelet count - 180,000/μL

• SMEAR MORPHOLOGY

Slightly macrocytic, normochromic with 1+ aniso- and poikilocytosis. Few if any polychromatic macrocytes observed. Leukocytes are normal except for occasional bilobed cells (Pelger-Huët anomaly). Platelets appear somewhat pale—poorly granulated.

Reticulocyte count/index - 1.2%/<1.0

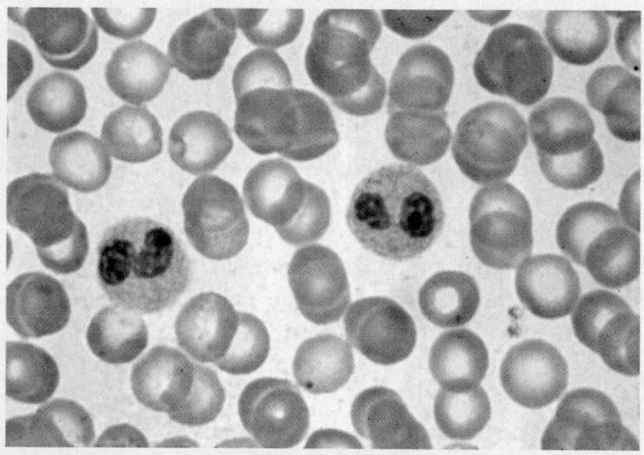

Questions

- How should the CBC findings be described?
- What additional studies should be ordered?

The dysplastic and sideroblastic anemias are primary stem cell disorders, many of which eventually result in progressive bone marrow failure or evolve to acute leukemia. Clinical recognition and differential diagnosis of these disorders revolves around characteristic changes in blood film and marrow morphology. The **dysplastic anemias (myelodysplasia)** present with varying combinations of anemia, leukopenia, and thrombocytopenia together with macrocytosis, distorted marrow precursor maturation, and ineffective erythropoiesis. **Sideroblastic anemias** are defined by the distinctive appearance of ringed sideroblasts on the Prussian blue stain of the marrow. The overall incidence of these disorders is said to be low, only 1–3:100,000 population. However, the incidence increases with age, rising to 15–50: 100,000 in older populations.

The **pathophysiology of myelodysplasia** is complex. There is evidence for impairments in stem cell growth, progenitor maturation, and both growth factor production and progenitor responsiveness. The presence of ineffective hematopoiesis (increased apoptosis of maturing marrow precursors) is a hallmark of myelodysplasia. It appears to correlate in part with CD95 expression and persistent high levels of Fas receptor, resulting in increased fas-ligand apoptosis. Upregulation of the cytokines tumor necrosis factor α (TNF-α) and interleukin 1β (IL-1β) also may play a role in promoting apoptosis of long-term hematopoietic stem cells (LT-HSC) and committed precursors in myelodysplastic marrows. Vascular endothelial growth factor (VEGF) overproduction is thought to be involved in the promotion of myeloblastic elements, and perhaps the evolution to acute myeloid leukemia (AML).

The level of apoptotic activity varies with the stage and progression of the dysplastic disorder. Lower-risk patients (refractory anemias with few if any blasts) generally have higher levels of apoptosis (ineffective hematopoiesis). With evolution to more advanced disease, the apoptotic index decreases and the number of myeloblasts in the marrow increases. Possible reasons for this include an upregulation of *BCL2/BCLX$_L$*, loss of the *p15* protooncogene, and downregulation of Fas receptor.

The variable presentations make the diagnosis of a dysplastic or sideroblastic anemia difficult, requiring a high level of suspicion and skill in identifying distortions in blood and marrow morphology. This is especially true in older populations where the presenting anemia/pancytopenia is often relatively mild (see Chapter 12). At the same time, management of a patient with myelodysplasia is very dependent on accurate classification of the dysplastic subtype.

NORMAL BLOOD FILM AND MARROW MORPHOLOGY

Morphology of the marrow aspirate and peripheral film provides a sensitive measure of precursor proliferation, maturation, and adult blood cell production. **Marrow biopsy** is used to estimate overall cellularity. Normal aging is associated with a gradual increase in the marrow's ratio of fat cells to hematopoietic cells. Although less than one-third of the biopsy is comprised of fat cells in a young adult, 50% or more of the marrow in an elderly patient will be fat. Reversal of this ratio suggests hematopoietic cell hyperplasia.

Marrow cellularity and distribution can also be assessed using a technetium Tc 99 or indium In 111 scan or magnetic resonance imaging. Indium, like iron, is preferentially taken up by erythroid precursors, whereas **technetium** measures the reticuloendothelial portion of the marrow. In normal adults, activity is limited to the axial skeleton and proximal portions of the long bones. In patients with dysplastic syndromes, marrow can expand into shafts of long bones, skull, and, on occasion, extramedullary sites.

A **marrow aspirate stained with Wright-Giemsa** provides a vivid display of the proliferation and maturation of each cell line. The **E/G ratio** is an estimate of the relative numbers of erythroid to myeloid precursors (see Chapter 2). It is very useful for detecting a marked decrease or increase in the proliferation of 1 cell line as long as other lines are relatively normal. The E/G ratio is less useful when a disorder of the marrow involves all cell lines.

Individual cell morphology is equally important. Distribution of cells in a marrow aspirate is not random. By scanning a number of fields using high power, however, it is possible to estimate the numbers of the most distinctive cell types (Table 9–1). For example, about 25% of all the cells in a normal marrow are **mature granulocytes** that comprise the marrow granulocyte reserve pool. Another 25% or more are **developing myelocytes** and monocytes that may be distinguished by their size, nuclear shape, and cytoplasmic granulation. Maturing myelocytes can be subdivided into promyelocytes, myelocytes, and metamyelocytes (bands) according to their nucleus and content of primary and secondary granules. **Erythroid progenitors** are readily identified from their progressive condensation of the nucleus and a cytoplasm that contains increasing amounts of hemoglobin, not enzymatic granules. Together, these 3 components make up 80% or more of the cells observed in a normal marrow.

Several minor cell populations may also be identified, including megakaryocytes, lymphocytes, plasma cells, undifferentiated blasts, and mast cells. The **number and morphologic characteristics of megakaryocytes** are best evaluated using

TABLE 9–1 • Normal marrow cell types

Type	Percentage (%)
Erythroid progenitors	20–25
Myeloblasts	<2
Promyelocytes	5
Myelocytes	10–15
Metamyelocytes (bands)	10–20
Mature granulocytes	20–30
Lymphocytes	5–15
Plasma cells	5

low-power magnification. In a cellular marrow, it should not be difficult to identify megakaryocytes based on their large size and multinuclearity. Because they make up less than 1% of a normal marrow, it is difficult to accurately estimate their level of proliferation. Still, increases in the number of megakaryocytes in patients with immune thrombocytopenia can usually be appreciated, as can decreases in number after marrow injury or chemotherapy. Moreover, distortions in individual megakaryocyte morphology, as in, for example, a decrease in nuclear ploidy or diminution in megakaryocyte size, both typical of a dysplastic marrow, are easily appreciated.

The **number of lymphocytes** in a marrow aspirate can vary. Normal marrow contains focal areas of lymphocyte hyperplasia, and when one of these areas is sampled, 20% or more of the cells in an aspirate can be lymphocytes. Moreover, they may appear in an irregular distribution; some high-power fields will show mostly lymphocytes, whereas others very few. This normal characteristic must be kept in mind when examining a bone marrow for lymphoma. Each of the other cell lines including primitive blasts, plasma cells, and mast cells should not exceed 5% of the total population in normal marrow. **Mast cells** are also integral to the structure of the marrow stroma. Because of this fact, they are best viewed by low-power inspection of stromal particles.

Individual cell morphology provides important information regarding **defects in cell maturation** such as size of the cell; size and shape of the nucleus; ratio of the nucleus to the cytoplasm; presence, number, and size of nucleoli; and presence of cytoplasmic granules. **Leukemias** can be recognized morphologically by proliferation of either primitive, poorly differentiated cells or the presence of a monomorphic cell population, regardless of the level of differentiation. Increases in cell and nuclear size, presence of one or several large nucleoli in the nucleus, and proliferation without maturation are all **signs of leukemia**. By contrast, **dysplastic and sideroblastic anemias** are identified based on unique distortions in precursor maturation. Cells appear megaloblastic with a predominance of younger forms **(maturation arrest)**, failure of the nucleus to mature in conjunction with the cytoplasm (nuclear:cytoplasmic dysynchrony), and the presence of mature cells containing distorted (lobulated) nuclei. **Sideroblastic anemias** are distinguished by the characteristic appearance of excess cytoplasmic iron granules in a perinuclear distribution (mitochondrial iron encrustation).

CLINICAL FEATURES

The initial presentation of the dysplastic and sideroblastic anemias follows a bimodal age distribution. The rare infant or child who presents with a refractory anemia may be found to have marked erythroid precursor multinuclearity **(congenital dyserythropoietic anemia)** or prominent ringed sideroblasts on iron stain **(hereditary sideroblastic anemia)**. Most often, however, the dysplastic and sideroblastic anemias are disorders of the elderly, usually men or women in the fifth, sixth, or seventh decade of life. The incidence of secondary myelodysplasia leading to AML has been reported to be as high as 3%–7% in lymphoma patients exposed to multiple courses of chemotherapy and autologous bone marrow/stem cell transplantation. The use of alkylating agents in patients with multiple myeloma and breast, ovarian, or lung cancer is also associated with a higher incidence of myelodysplasia.

Presenting symptoms and signs of these disorders are a function of the severity of the anemia or pancytopenia. The patient may complain of nothing more than weakness or easy fatigability. **Severe anemia** can provoke congestive heart failure. A **tendency to easy bruising** may signal thrombocytopenia, and **recurrent infections** may reflect significant leukopenia. If the patient is asymptomatic, the disorder is first detected from a routine complete blood count (CBC). Patients typically show varying combinations of pancytopenia and abnormal cell morphology.

The onset is usually so gradual that patients will have difficulty identifying a starting point for the illness. A few patients will present with an immune-mediated disease such as skin vasculitis, temporal arteritis, or polymyalgia rheumatica. Since the **initial symptoms and signs are nonspecific**, a broad search should be made for an inciting cause or clues that suggest another type of anemia or pancytopenia. Dysplastic refractory anemias can be seen in younger patients as a result of exposure to radiation, cytotoxic drugs, or toxic chemicals. Patients exposed to alcohol, lead, and certain antibiotics such as chloramphenicol and isoniazid can present with a sideroblastic anemia. It is important not to miss these reversible conditions.

Laboratory Studies

Routine CBC, blood film, and marrow aspirate and biopsy are the key studies used in diagnosing and classifying the various dysplastic syndromes. Most patients are anemic on presentation. With time, most patients also develop leukopenia and thrombocytopenia. The severity of the anemia can vary from very mild to so severe that the patient becomes transfusion dependent.

A. Peripheral Blood Film Morphology

Peripheral blood film morphology may be helpful. Patients can present with a macrocytic, normocytic, or slightly microcytic anemia with varying degrees of anisocytosis and poikilocytosis. Teardrop forms and nucleated red blood cells may be present, especially if the patient has a severely dysplastic or fibrotic marrow with extramedullary hematopoiesis. Both granulocytes and platelets can be morphologically abnormal. Leukocytes with bilobed nuclei **(Pelger-Huët anomaly—see case problem smear)** may be observed and platelets can be pale and poorly granulated. With progression of the disease to acute leukemia, the number of leukocytes and platelets falls even farther and blasts appear in the circulation.

B. Marrow Aspirate and Biopsy

A good marrow aspirate and biopsy are essential. **Marrow cellularity** is usually increased, although it can be irregularly distributed in the medullary cavity and separated by areas of excess fat or fibrous tissue. Often this situation is associated with expansion of actively proliferating marrow into the shafts of long bones or extramedullary sites. Some patients will present with a

TABLE 9–2 • Dysplastic/sideroblastic anemia profiles

	Dysplastic	Sideroblastic
Red blood cell morphology	Mixed macro-, normo-, microcytic; moderate aniso- and poikilocytosis	
Reticulocyte index	<2	
Marrow E/G ratio	>1:1 to hypoplastic	
Marrow morphology	Megaloblastic to normoblastic	
		Ringed sideroblasts
Serum iron/TIBC	Normal/normal	Increased/normal
Serum ferritin	Normal	

normocellular or even hypocellular marrow. This can present a diagnostic dilemma if the hypoplasia is severe enough to suggest aplastic anemia. Inspection of the blood smear may help distinguish the 2 conditions; the presence of agranular neutrophils or the Pelger-Huët anomaly is suggestive of a dysplastic anemia.

Marrow aspirate morphology will reveal disturbances in **cell proliferation and maturation**. If the patient has a macrocytic anemia, the erythroid marrow is usually hyperplastic and megaloblastic with ineffective erythropoiesis (Table 9–2). Moreover, megakaryocyte and white cell morphology are generally abnormal. The number of megakaryocytes tends to be increased, with individual cells that are smaller than normal, exhibit decreased ploidy, and may have three separate nuclei **(pawn-ball nuclei)**. Similarly, myelocytic maturation may be abnormal, with an apparent maturation arrest and poor granulation of mature granulocytes.

The percentage of "blasts" (myeloblasts, monoblasts, and megakaryoblasts) is important in determining prognosis (Figure 9–1). Patients with more than 10%–20% blasts have a distinctively worse prognosis. Flow cytometric analysis of the number of CD34$^+$ cells in the marrow has been advanced as a better way to estimate the number of blasts. It may also help distinguish myelodysplastic from aplastic anemia patients, where the CD34$^+$ population is dramatically reduced. Immunophenotyping can also reveal evidence supportive of myelodysplasia, specifically myeloid precursor aberrant expression of surface markers such as CD56, CD13, CD16, and CD10, with a loss of CD71. Finally, an iron stain of the marrow aspirate is important to look for abnormal sideroblasts, especially ringed sideroblasts.

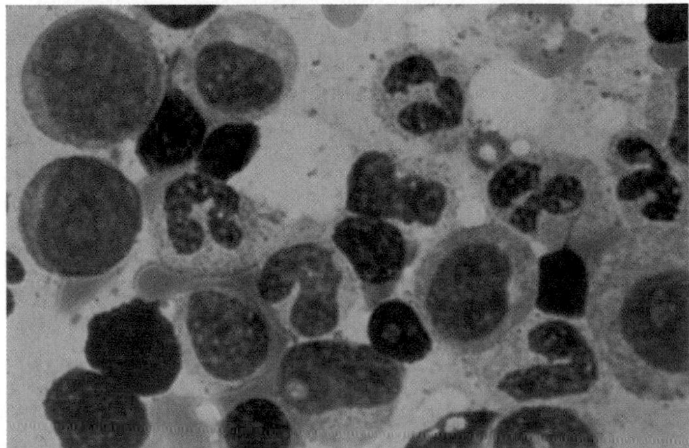

FIGURE 9–1. **Blast percentage in myelodysplasia.** The percentage of blast forms—typically relatively large cells with small amounts of agranular cytoplasm and large nuclei with prominent nucleoli—is key to the classification of the dysplastic anemias.

C. Chromosomal Analysis

While a single genetic marker that reliably identifies myelodysplastic patients has not been identified, chromosomal analysis can help both in diagnosis and prognosis. Early on, most patients with evolving myelodysplasia have normal karyotypes, while up to 80% of patients with more advanced myelodysplasia demonstrate a chromosomal abnormality (Table 9–3). Deletions of chromosomes 5, 7, 11, 13, and 20, and trisomies of 8 and 21, are the most common abnormalities (60%–70% of patients) and are strong indicators of myelodysplasia. Complex karyotypes (more than 3 chromosomal aberrations) are seen in 30% of de novo myelodysplasia cases and up to 50% of chemotherapy-related myelodysplasias.

Patients with a deletion of the long arm of chromosome 5 (5q minus syndrome—usually a deletion of band 5q31–32), seen in 15% of de novo myelodysplasias and 50% of secondary dysplasias, represent a subgroup with a relatively good prognosis. Several genes are lost in 5q minus syndrome, including those responsible for IL-3, -4, -5, and -9; granulocyte macrophage colony stimulating factor; c-fms; platelet-derived growth factor (PDGF)-receptor; interferon regulatory factor 1 (IRF-1); epidermal growth factor 1 (EGR-1); Flt-4; and CD14. In contrast, point mutations that activate the *RAS* and *AML1* genes and/or multiple chromosome abnormalities, involving chromosomes 5 and 7, predict a worse outcome. Mutations of mitochondrial DNA have also been observed and may underlie the ultrastructural deformities and abnormal iron loading of mitochondria in patients with ringed sideroblasts. A number of patients will also have a positive sugar water or Ham-acid hemolysis test or, preferably, a flow cytometric assay showing glycosylphosphatidylinisotol (GPI) anchored protein deficiencies (CD59/CD55 negative

TABLE 9–3 • Chromosomal abnormalities in dysplastic anemias

Partial or Full Deletions	Numeric Abnormalities
Chromosome 5:5q minus syndrome	Monosomy 5, 7
	Trisomy 8, 21
Chromosome 7, 11, 13, and 20	**Structural defects**
Loss of Y chromosome	Nonspecific defects, 6, 9, 11, 12, 13, and 17

CASE HISTORY • *Part 2*

The patient has a moderately severe, slightly macrocytic anemia (mean cell volume [MCV] - 99 fL) and leukopenia. The reticulocyte index is compatible with either hypoproliferative or ineffective erythropoiesis. Platelet count is in the low normal range. The finding of bilobed leukocytes (Pelger-Huët anomaly) on the smear suggests a myelodysplastic process.

To evaluate the possibility of a myelodysplastic anemia, the patient should have a bone marrow aspirate and biopsy and marrow cytogenetic analysis. Iron studies, folic acid and vitamin B_{12} levels, and flow cytometric analysis for surface antigen abnormalities, especially the CD55/CD59 phenotype of paroxysmal nocturnal hemoglobinuria (PNH), should be performed. The results of these studies are as follows:

Bone marrow—Hyperplastic marrow with an E/G ratio of 1:2, a decreased number of mature leukocytes, and increased numbers of myelocytic and monocytic precursors with 5% blasts (type I myeloblasts). Megakaryocyte numbers are increased with micro- and hypolobated forms. Biopsy shows a patchy marrow distribution without evidence of metastatic tumor or fibrosis. Iron stain—normal iron stores with few ringed sideroblasts (<5%).

Cytogenetic analysis is remarkable for a 5q deletion. Iron, vitamin, and flow cytometry studies of surface markers are all normal.

Questions

- Based on these studies can you categorize the patient according to the French-American-British (FAB) classification of myelodysplasia?
- What implications does this category have for management and prognosis?

red cells or CD16/CD66b negative granulocytes) indicative of paroxysmal nocturnal hemoglobinuria.

D. Hemoglobin Analysis

Dysplastic syndromes may also be associated with abnormal laboratory findings in the character of red cell hemoglobin. Many, if not most, patients show slightly increased levels of hemoglobin F and, less commonly, an altered globin chain synthetic rate that results in **production of hemoglobin H**.

DIAGNOSIS

Classifications of dysplastic and sideroblastic anemias have been developed based on marrow and peripheral blood morphology, the number of cytopenias, percentage of marrow blasts, and marrow cytogenetics. **The WHO/FAB (World Health Organization/French-American-British) classification of myelodysplasia** is based primarily on morphological abnormalities—the predominant cell line involved, the number of blasts, the number of cell lineages involved, and the presence or absence of ringed sideroblasts. Major categories include refractory anemia (RA), refractory anemia with ringed sideroblasts (RARS), refractory cytopenias with multilineage dysplasia (RCMD and RCMD-RS), refractory anemia with excess blasts (RAEB-1 and -2), myelodysplasia with a 5q deletion, and undifferentiated myelodysplastic syndrome (MDS-U) (Table 9–4). The older RAEB-T subclassification (refractory anemia with excess blasts in transformation) has been dropped; patients with more than 20% blasts are now considered to have MDS-related AML (see Chapter 18). In addition, the **International Prognostic Scoring System (IPSS)** for predicting outcome in myelodysplasia has been introduced, which focuses on age and gender, marrow blast percentages, the number of cytopenias, and cytogenetics. It can help identify higher-risk individuals in each of the WHO/FAB subgroups. It does not change the fact that all of these conditions are clonal malignancies with varying potential for evolution to acute leukemia.

TABLE 9–4 • WHO/FAB classification of the dysplastic syndromes

Disease Category	Blood/Marrow Morphology
Refractory anemia (RA)	Anemia/erythroid hypo/dysplasia with <5% blasts, <15% ringed sideroblasts
RA with ringed sideroblasts (RARS)	Anemia/erythroid dysplasia with <5% blasts, >15% ringed sideroblasts
RA with multilineage dysplasia (RCMD)	Bi- or pancytopenia/dysplasia in 2 or more myeloid lineages, <5% blasts. If >15% ringed sideroblasts, RCMD-RS
RA with excess blasts (RAEB-1 and -2)	Anemia or multiple cytopenias/dysplasia in 1 or more lineages RAEB-1, 5%–9% blasts/RAEB-2, 10%–19% blasts
Myelodysplasia with isolated del (5q) "5q minus syndrome"	Anemia/normal to increased megakaryocytes with hypolobation, <5% blasts; isolated deletion of 5q
Myelodysplasia, unclassified (MDS-U)	Cytopenia(s)/myeloid or megakaryocyte dysplasia, <5% blasts
Myelomonocytic leukemia (CMML)	Cytopenias with monocytosis/increased monocyte precursors, <20% blasts

When typical morphologic clues and/or chromosomal abnormalities are not present, the diagnosis can be much more difficult, if not impossible. This situation often applies to the older patient with a refractory anemia or mild pancytopenia and a "megaloblastoid" marrow. Such patients tend to progress very slowly and are hard to distinguish from patients with a marrow-damage anemia (see Chapter 3). They should be followed with repeated CBCs.

Refractory Anemia

Refractory anemia (RA) patients present with a mild to moderately severe anemia, variable macrocytosis, mild to moderate anisocytosis and poikilocytosis, and a hypoplastic, normal, or hyperplastic erythroid marrow. Many of the features of other dysplastic and sideroblastic disorders are not present. Less than 5% of the marrow cells are blasts and there are fewer than 15% ringed sideroblasts. Cytogenetic studies generally do not reveal a specific chromosomal defect. Research studies of mutations of the *N-ras* oncogene have shown point mutations in fewer than 10% of RA patients, in contrast to the higher incidence in RAEB and chronic myelomonocytic leukemia (CMML).

Since distinctive clinical and laboratory findings are less prominent in RA, **it is important to exclude reversible marrow damage causing anemia or pancytopenia**. Any history of exposure to radiation, drugs, or toxic chemicals is important. If the patient is young, has a significant exposure history, and demonstrates a somewhat hypoplastic marrow without morphologic or cytogenetic abnormalities, marrow damage is a good possibility (see Chapter 3). Of course, these same exposures can incite a preleukemic condition, presenting as RA or myelodysplasia. Similar to idiopathic aplastic anemia, there is now evidence that T cell–mediated suppression of marrow progenitors is 1 important component in the clinical picture of RA. However, $CD8^+$ T-cell expansion is usually a secondary polyclonal response to 1 or more progenitor cell mutations and not a primary autoimmune disorder.

Refractory Anemia with Ringed Sideroblasts

Refractory anemia with ringed sideroblasts (RARS) is most often seen in older males. It usually appears in the fifth or sixth decade of life and follows a long, indolent course. Since the initial anemia is mild and the clinical findings are nonspecific, diagnosis is frequently delayed. Many patients will give a history of several years of treatment with various hematinic agents, including vitamin B_{12}, folic acid, vitamin B_6, and even iron, without noticeable effect. Over time, RARS patients demonstrate a worsening anemia, increasing macrocytosis, aniso- and poikilocytosis, and both leukopenia and thrombocytopenia. Other morphologic clues include appearance on the blood film of small numbers of hypochromic cells and, on occasion, heavily stippled red blood cells. The stippling tends to be coarser than that seen with lead poisoning and represents fragments of iron-encrusted mitochondria (Figure 9–2).

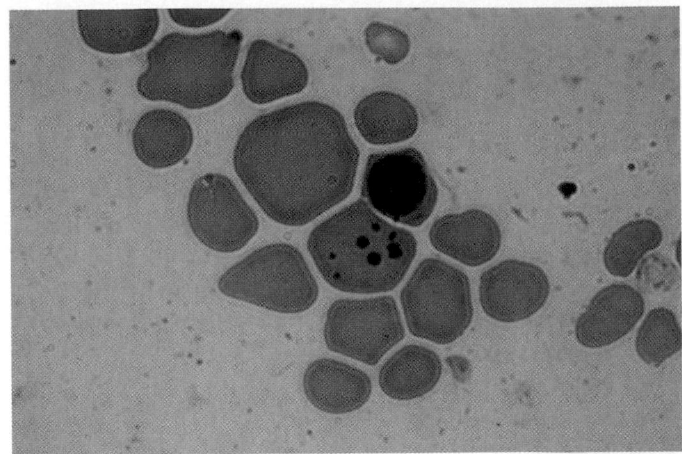

FIGURE 9–2. **RARS red cell stippling.** Heavily stippled cells indicate retention of nuclear fragments and are a clue to the presence of ringed sideroblastic anemia. In comparison, lead poisoning is associated with much finer stippling.

Definitive diagnosis is made from the marrow morphology, in particular the appearance of large numbers of ringed sideroblasts (>15% of maturing erythroblasts). Typically, RARS patients have hyperplastic erythroid marrows that can be slightly megaloblastic with ineffective erythropoiesis. Often, many late erythroid marrow precursors show distorted, lobated nuclei with heavy stippling of the cytoplasm. The more hyperplastic the marrow, the easier it is to find abnormal late forms **(orthochromatic normoblasts)**. These patients also show larger numbers of **ringed sideroblasts** on the Prussian blue stain, that is, erythroid precursors that show a ring or collar of large, blue-staining granules immediately surrounding the nucleus (Figure 9–3). These "granules" can be demonstrated by electron microscopy to be iron-encrusted mitochondria and fragments of mitochondria. By light microscopy, their size and position readily distinguish them from the much finer cytoplasmic ferritin granules.

The frequency of ringed sideroblasts and the severity of the erythroid hyperplasia can vary widely. In some patients, virtually all of the late erythroid precursors contain excess iron granules. More often, however, ringed sideroblasts represent a smaller proportion of the developing erythroblasts. The latter is more typical of patients who demonstrate less erythroid hyperplasia or appear to have a relatively hypoplastic marrow. Whether this represents a difference in mechanism of disease or simply reflects a stage in the evolution of RARS is unclear. Patients with less proliferative marrows, few blasts, and fewer ringed sideroblasts generally demonstrate a more prolonged, indolent clinical course. Five-year survivals exceed 50% with RARS, and the potential for conversion to AML is very low. Patients with extreme erythroid hyperplasia or added dysplasia in 2 or more myeloid lineages have a worse prognosis with less than 40% surviving after 5 years and a greater conversion rate to AML. The latter patients are better categorized as **RCMD-RS (refractory cytopenia with multilineage dysplasia and ringed sideroblasts).**

A subset of RARS patients may also present with an elevated platelet count (>450,000/μL). These patients have provisionally been classified at RARS-T. They share characteristics with the myeloproliferative disorder thrombocytosis, including

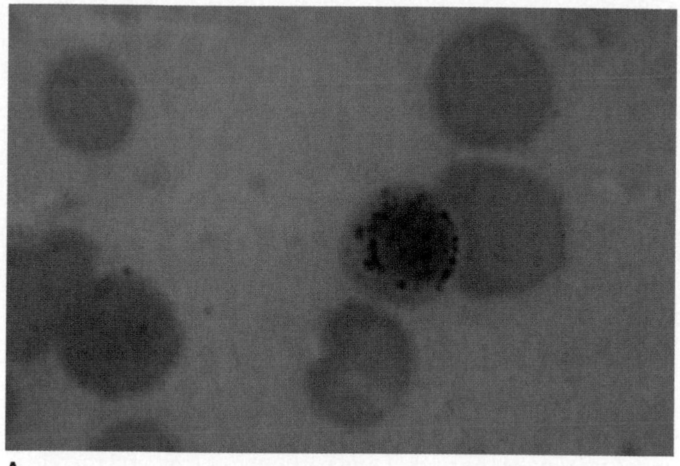

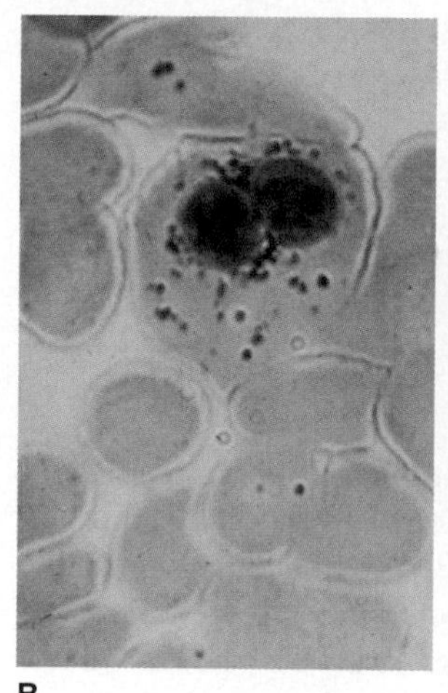

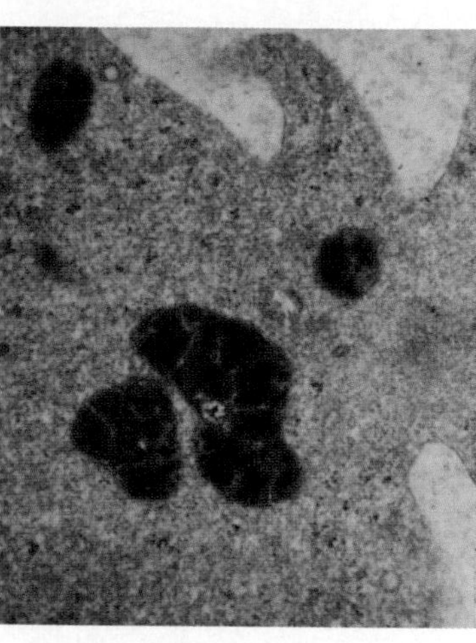

FIGURE 9–3. **Ringed sideroblasts.** The ringed sideroblast **(A)** is a red blood cell precursor, which on iron stain has a collar of blue staining particles just around the nucleus. On electron microscopy these particles are, in fact, iron-laden fragments of mitochondria **(B)**. When ringed sideroblasts are present in the marrow aspirate in sufficient numbers, they are diagnostic for RARS.

abnormal megakaryocyte morphology and the presence of the *JAK2* gene mutation in more than 50% of patients.

Patients with RARS with marked erythroid hyperplasia and **severe ineffective erythropoiesis** typically have high serum iron and serum ferritin levels. They are at the added risk for tissue iron loading with potential damage to the liver and myocardium. Iron loading is also an issue when RARS patients require long-term transfusion therapy.

RARS must always be distinguished from other "environmental" causes of sideroblastic anemia (Table 9–5). Several antibiotics and heavy metals can impair mitochondrial function (Figure 9–4). Isoniazid, pyrazinamide, cycloserine, azathioprine, D-penicillamine, and alcohol impair the vitamin B_6–dependent initial step in porphyrin production. Lead has a wider inhibitory effect. Patients with neoplasms or inflammatory disorders can occasionally present with a hypoproliferative anemia and occasional ringed sideroblasts. These appear to relate to the primary disease process and cannot be explained by drug effect or the appearance of true RARS. The potential interaction of heterozygosity for idiopathic hemachromatosis as a cofactor in mitochondrial iron loading has not been well defined.

Refractory Cytopenia with Multilineage Dysplasia

When there is multilineage dysplasia involving more than 10% of 2 or more cell lineages with fewer than 5% blasts and no Auer rods, the patient meets the criteria for the **refractory cytopenia with multilineage dysplasia (RCMD)** category. If more than 15% ringed sideroblasts are also present, the patient may be designated as having RCMD-RS. The original FAB classification of RA and RARS included patients with varying amounts of multilineage dysplasia, making it difficult to compare outcomes.

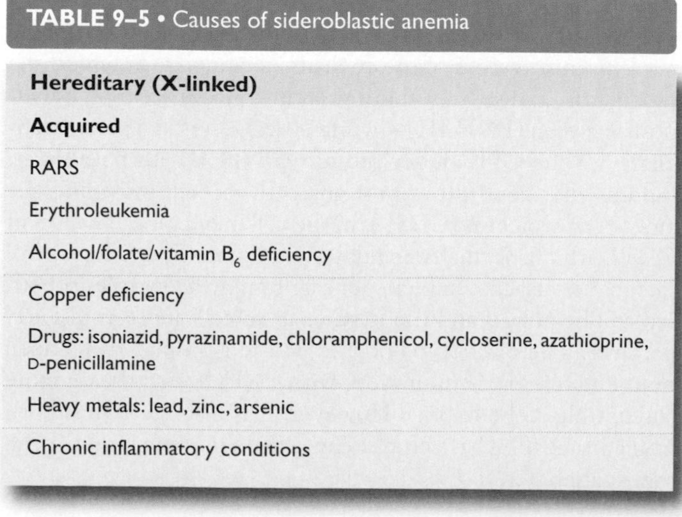

TABLE 9–5 • Causes of sideroblastic anemia

Hereditary (X-linked)
Acquired
RARS
Erythroleukemia
Alcohol/folate/vitamin B_6 deficiency
Copper deficiency
Drugs: isoniazid, pyrazinamide, chloramphenicol, cycloserine, azathioprine, D-penicillamine
Heavy metals: lead, zinc, arsenic
Chronic inflammatory conditions

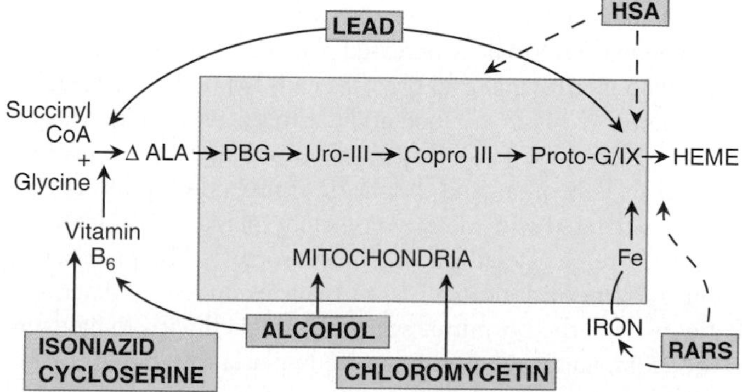

FIGURE 9–4. **Impairment of mitochondrial function and porphyrin synthesis.** Several drugs and heavy metals can interfere with several steps in porphyrin metabolism necessary to produce ringed sideroblasts. RARS and hereditary sideroblastic anemia (HSA) appear to interfere with the final heme synthetase step, possibly in conjunction with an inherited tendency to iron overload.

The separation of patients with RCMD from patients with RA and RARS better predicts the course and propensity for developing AML. In 1 retrospective study, the response rate to granulocyte colony-stimulating factor (G-CSF) and erythropoietin (EPO) of patients with RARS as compared with RCMD-RS patients was striking, 75% versus 9%, with median survivals of 67 versus 29 months, respectively.

Refractory Anemia with Excess Blasts

Patients with **refractory anemia with excess blasts (RAEB)-1 or -2** generally present with pancytopenia or severe anemia and granulocytopenia. Unlike RA and RARS, the blood film shows small numbers (usually <5%) of myeloblasts and, in some cases, bilobed granulocytes **(Pelger-Huët anomaly)**. Diagnosis is made from marrow morphology. Cellularity of the marrow can vary from hyperplastic to hypoplastic with a patchy distribution on biopsy. On examination of the marrow aspirate, fewer than 20% of the cells are blasts, either undifferentiated **(type I myeloblasts)** or containing azurophilic granules **(type II myeloblasts)**. In addition, the number of monocytes and monocyte precursors may be increased, especially in patients with granulocytopenia. Finally, many of these patients show an increased number of small megakaryocytes with reduced ploidy and abnormal morphology.

The original classification of dysplastic anemias recognized a subset of patients with **RAEB-T (refractory anemia with excess blasts in transformation)**. These patients were defined as having similar morphologic abnormalities, but the number of blasts in peripheral blood was greater than 5% and the number of types I and II myeloblasts in marrow greater than 20%. For prognostic and management decisions RAEB-T has been replaced by the subclassifications RAEB-1 and RAEB-2 according to the number of marrow myeloblasts (5%–9% and 10%–19%, respectively). RAEB-2 patients are also more likely to have multiple chromosomal abnormalities. Patients with higher marrow blast counts (>20%) are best classified as myelodysplasia-related AML and should be treated as such (see Chapter 18).

Myelodysplasia with Deletion of 5q

Patients with **myelodysplasia and deletion 5q (5q minus syndrome)** are typically elderly women who present with a macrocytic anemia, a normal to increased platelet count, and increased numbers of marrow megakaryocytes with hypolobulated nuclei. The number of blasts in blood and marrow is fewer than 5% and Auer rods are absent. Although deletions of 5q are seen in a number of leukemias and dysplastic states, the 5q minus syndrome associated with de novo myelodysplasia is characterized by q31–32 region deletions on chromosome 5. The presence of other cytogenetic abnormalities virtually excludes this diagnosis. Patients with the 5q minus syndrome do well with longer survivals, compared to the other myelodysplasia categories.

Chronic Myelomonocytic Leukemia

Chronic myelomonocytic leukemia (CMML) can arise de novo or evolve from preexisting myelodysplasia, most often a blood picture that resembles RAEB-1 or -2. One distinguishing feature of CMML is an increase in the monocyte count to levels greater than 1,000/μL, and a marrow that shows an increased number of monocytic precursors. The marrow blast count is less than 20%, and megakaryocyte maturation usually is normal. Cytogenetic abnormalities are seen in up to 50% of CMML patients, but no specific chromosomal defect has been identified that could serve as a diagnostic marker. With time, CMML patients can exhibit a progressive increase in white cell and blast counts, more typical of acute myelomonocytic leukemia (M4). While CMML patients presenting with white cell counts greater than 13,000/μL have been classified at times as having a myeloproliferative disorder, they generally lack the *JAK2* and/or *BCR-ABL* markers typically seen with this class of disorders (see Chapter 19). This clearly is a situation where the understanding of the underlying pathophysiology, and therefore the appropriate place in the classification, is unsatisfactory.

Both leukocyte and platelet function defects may be detected, leading to an increased susceptibility to infection and abnormal bleeding. In CMML patients, the blood and urinary lysozyme levels are usually increased, and the leukocyte alkaline phosphatase can be decreased in up to 20% of cases. Finally, some patients with RAEB and CMML will show progressive fibrosis on marrow biopsy, together with hepatosplenomegaly secondary to extramedullary hematopoiesis.

DIFFERENTIAL DIAGNOSIS

With the diversity of clinical and laboratory findings in dysplastic and sideroblastic anemias, it is not surprising that other disorders share features with these conditions. Paroxysmal nocturnal hemoglobinuria, primary myelofibrosis, DeGuglielmo anemia/erythroleukemia, and rare benign conditions such as congenital dyserythropoietic anemia (CDA) and hereditary sideroblastic anemia (HSA) all need to be considered in the differential diagnosis.

Paroxysmal Nocturnal Hemoglobinuria

Paroxysmal nocturnal hemoglobinuria (PNH) is a clonal disorder of hematopoietic cells caused by a somatic mutation of the ***pig-A*** gene on the short arm of the X chromosome. More than 170 mutations in the ***pig-A*** gene have been reported. Some result in inactivation of the gene and a complete failure in the production of the GPI anchor protein—glycosylphosphatidylinositol glycan **(PNH III)**—while others result in a partial deficiency of the GPI anchor protein **(PNH II)**. In both cases, binding of several other proteins is disturbed, including the amount of **protectin (CD59)** on the cell membrane. The loss of CD59, which normally regulates the assembly of the C5b-9 membrane attack complex, appears to play a key role in both red cell hemolysis and the hypercoagulable state seen in PNH patients. The phenotype of the disease is in part influenced by the nature of the mutation, with PNH III cells being more susceptible to hemolysis. However, it is also clear that both PNH II and PNH III clones can exist simultaneously in the same patient.

A. Presentation and Complications

Patients with PNH present either with a **hemolytic anemia** with intravascular hemolysis and episodes of nocturnal hemoglobinuria, or with **pancytopenia** with a dysplastic or aplastic marrow morphology. Hemolytic disease is more often associated with a large, dominant clone of PNH cells, while aplastic and dysplastic individuals usually have fewer GPI-negative cells in circulation. One conclusion drawn from this observation is that marrow damage (bone marrow failure) somehow induces the PNH somatic mutation as a secondary manifestation of the disease, such that the mutation is not the primary cause of the dysplastic or aplastic anemia.

Patients with PNH are also at **increased risk for venous thrombosis,** owing to complement-driven activation of platelets lacking CD59 and also, perhaps, impaired fibrinolysis. Thrombosis of hepatic veins **(Budd-Chiari syndrome)** or the portal, splenic, or mesenteric veins is a common manifestation of the hypercoagulable state and can lead to severe morbidity and a clinical picture similar to that of disseminated intravascular coagulation. Patients with chronic hemolysis are at risk for developing **iron deficiency secondary to urine iron loss.** Finally, severe thrombocytopenia and granulocytopenia can lead to **major bleeding or infection.**

PNH can present any time from the second to the eighth decade of life. The diagnosis should be considered as a part of the differential diagnosis of an anemia when accompanied by other cytopenias (myelodysplasia or aplastic anemia), a history of passing dark urine, iron deficiency without an obvious cause, or signs or symptoms suggesting venous thrombosis. **Recurrent attacks of abdominal pain** may indicate intra-abdominal thrombotic disease. PNH tends to be a chronic disorder; the median survival in uncomplicated patients can easily exceed 10 or even 20 years. Up to 15% of patients will demonstrate a spontaneous remission, but many patients die of either uncontrolled hemorrhage or thrombosis. Patients presenting with a marrow picture of aplasia or dysplasia frequently go undiagnosed if no one thinks to order a flow cytometric assay of cell surface CD59/CD55 and CD16/CD66b levels.

B. Diagnostic Tests

Historically, the **sugar water test** was used as a convenient screen for PNH. It is performed by adding a small amount of the patient's red blood cells to an isotonic sucrose solution laced with fresh complement. A somewhat more definitive test is the **Ham-acid hemolysis test,** which detects sensitivity of the PNH red blood cells to fresh complement and acidification. However, the current **cytometric assay of red cell CD59/CD55 levels** is clearly preferred. It is more sensitive and specific and can identify small subpopulations of abnormal cells. Two other GPI-anchored proteins, **CD16 and CD66b, can also be measured** on granulocytes in patients with equivocal red cell results to further increase the sensitivity of the test to small clones in patients presenting with aplasia.

All cell lines, including granulocytes and platelets, are involved in PNH and are susceptible to lysis. Although this may be responsible in part for the pancytopenia, many patients present with a hypocellular, even aplastic, marrow. In these patients, **marrow culture studies** have demonstrated a reduced number of all progenitor lines, similar to the findings in marrow damage/aplastic anemia. The presence of GPI-negative cells is most often seen with T cell–mediated marrow failure. It has now been reported that 15%–50% of patients with idiopathic aplasia or myelodysplasia will demonstrate a PNH clone. In contrast, patients with marrow failure after chemotherapy, transplantation, immunotherapy, or secondary to large granular lymphocytosis (T-cell lymphoma) rarely have GPI-negative cells detected.

Primary Myelofibrosis (Myeloid Metaplasia)

Myelofibrosis is another clonal malignancy that, while classified as a myeloproliferative disorder (see Chapter 19), can share many of the features of the dysplastic anemias. Patients usually present later in life with a gradual onset of anemia, pancytopenia, and impressive splenomegaly. The dominant feature of the disorder is **progressive fibrosis of the marrow cavity** that results in dramatic expansion of extramedullary hemopoiesis in the spleen and liver. The basis for this severe marrow fibrosis appears to be release of fibroblastic growth factors from an abnormal megakaryocyte line. Fibroblasts themselves do not share the chromosomal abnormalities observed in the hematopoietic cells.

Several **clinical features help distinguish myelofibrosis** from other dysplastic anemias. The blood film typically shows a combination of teardrop-shaped red blood cells and nucleated red blood cells (Figure 9–5). When extramedullary hematopoiesis is advanced, normal and abnormal myelocytes, blasts, and Pelger-Huët cells may be observed in the circulation. The platelet count may be decreased, normal, or increased. In the latter case, it can reach levels in excess of 1 million/μL with the appearance in the circulation of giant platelets and fragments of megakaryocytes.

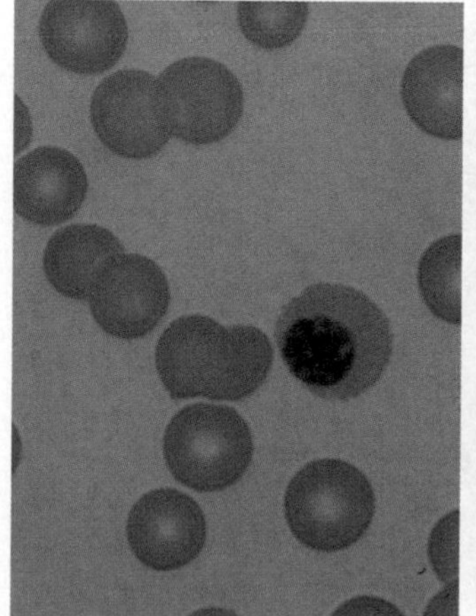
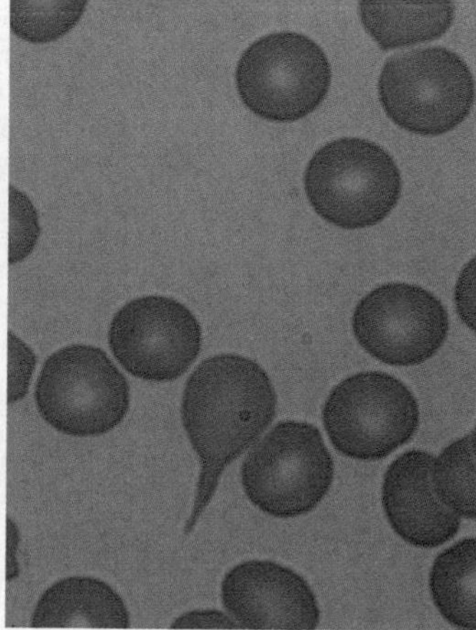

FIGURE 9–5. **Nucleated and teardrop red blood cells in myelofibrosis.** Nucleated red blood cells and "teardrop" red cells are typically seen on the blood smear of patients with primary myelofibrosis, especially in the presence of extramedullary hematopoiesis. They are also seen with splenic hypoplasia and in asplenic patients.

A. Diagnostic Tests

Definitive diagnosis is made from the **marrow examination**. Often as not, attempts to aspirate marrow are unsuccessful and a biopsy is needed to demonstrate the fibrotic lesion. The marrow cavity can be virtually obliterated by dense collagenous tissue or demonstrate a patchy involvement with alternating areas of hyperplastic marrow (Figure 9–6A). A **reticulin or silver stain of the marrow biopsy** will highlight the fibrotic abnormality (Figure 9–6B). Typically, myelofibrosis patients show a marked increase in reticulin fibers throughout the marrow. Granulocyte and megakaryocyte hyperplasia, with abnormal maturation of the latter, may also be observed.

B. Causes of Myelofibrosis

The more abnormal the appearance of the hematopoietic cells, the more likely the patient will demonstrate a **chromosomal abnormality**. This abnormality includes deletions and translocations of chromosomes 1, 5, 7, 8, 9, and 20. Myelofibrosis can also occur secondary to infiltration of the marrow by **metastatic carcinoma** or as a result of **infections with mycobacteria**. The latter should always be considered in the differential diagnosis of myelofibrosis especially, because it is a reversible cause of myelofibrosis.

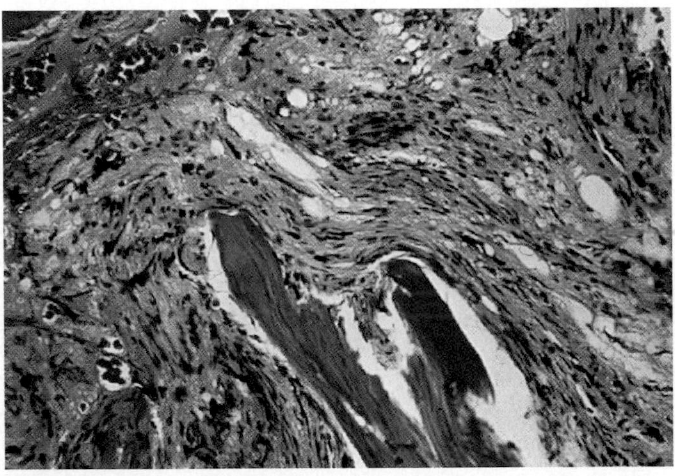

A

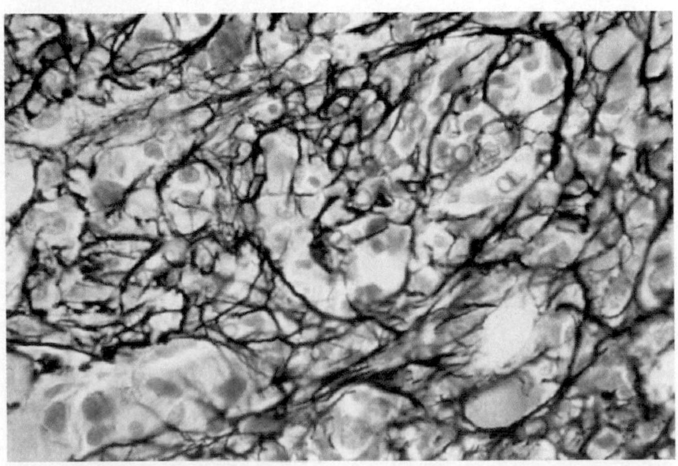

B

FIGURE 9–6. **Myelofibrosis.** Marrow biopsy (H&E stain) will typically show a dense infiltrate of collagenous tissue, virtually obliterating the marrow space **(A)**. A reticulin stain (silver stain) of the same marrow shows a marked increase in reticulin fibers (black-staining threads) **(B)**.

DeGuglielmo Anemia/Erythroleukemia

DeGuglielmo anemia has been described in the past as a **clonal malignancy that rapidly progresses to erythroleukemia**. At the same time, it shares features with RARS and RAEB. Some patients will present with a slightly macrocytic anemia, pancytopenia, and a hyperplastic marrow. With time, the pancytopenia worsens and the patient takes on characteristics of an acute leukemia of the erythroid line.

Common features of DeGuglielmo anemia include red blood cell macrocytosis, marked aniso- and poikilocytosis, siderocytes and nucleated red blood cells on the peripheral blood film, and the appearance of ringed sideroblasts in the marrow of some patients. **Distinguishing features** for the condition include late erythroid precursors with multiple nuclei, nuclear budding, and cloverleaf-shaped nuclei. Some of the late precursors also show heavy cytoplasmic stippling, reminiscent of RARS. A unique finding, however, is the dramatic appearance of the periodic acid–Schiff (PAS) stain. The cytoplasm of mature red blood cell precursors is filled with large PAS-positive granules. Finally, close examination of the reticuloendothelial portion of the marrow aspirate may reveal erythrophagocytosis.

Congenital Dysplastic and Sideroblastic Anemias

Inherited defects in precursor maturation can result in a lifelong anemia with features similar to those of acquired dysplastic and sideroblastic anemia. Congenital dyserythropoietic anemias are a group of disorders **characterized by the striking multinuclearity of erythroid precursors. Hereditary sideroblastic anemia** is defined by the presence of ringed sideroblasts in marrow and a defect in hemoglobin production.

A. Congenital Dyserythropoietic Anemia

Patients with congenital dyserythropoietic anemia (CDA) are usually diagnosed during childhood, although when anemia is mild they may escape detection until well into adult life. They present with a slightly macrocytic anemia with aniso- and poikilocytosis, a low reticulocyte index, and an otherwise normal CBC. The finding that leads to the diagnosis is **marked dysmorphology of the erythroid marrow** (Table 9–6).

CDA is classified according to unique distortions of the nuclei of erythroid precursors. **CDA type I** is a rare autosomal recessive disorder characterized by a macrocytic anemia, megaloblastic erythroid hyperplasia with ineffective erythropoiesis, binucleate erythroblasts, and prominent intranuclear chromatin bridging. **CDA type II** is characterized by more prominent binuclearity, karyorrhexis, and lobulation of the nuclei of the late erythroid precursors (Figure 9–7). In addition, these patients have a positive Ham-acid hemolysis test. Because of the latter

TABLE 9–6 • Profiles of congenital dyserythropoietic anemias

Type	MCV (fL)	Marrow Morphology
CDA I	95–110	Megaloblastic with binucleate erythroblasts and chromatin bridging
CDA II HEMPAS	90	Normoblastic with marked binucleate erythroblasts; positive acid hemolysis test
CDA III	90–100	Giant, multinucleate erythroblasts
CDA IV	80–90	Normoblastic with marked bi- or multinucleate erythroblasts; negative acid hemolysis test

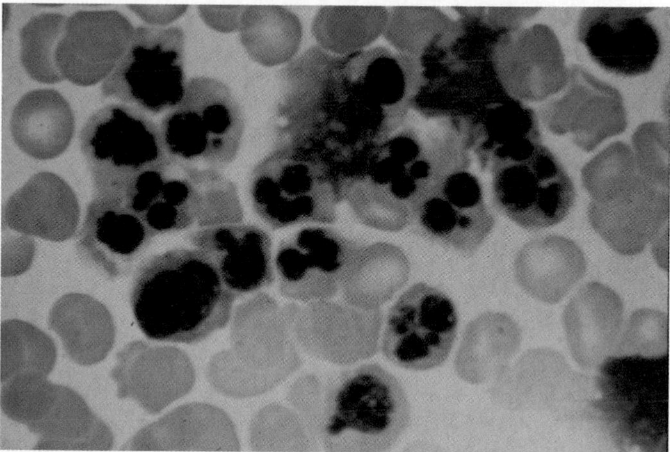

FIGURE 9–7. **HEMPAS.** Marrow aspirate from a patient with HEMPAS (CDA type II). Note the marked lobulation and nuclear bridging in the late erythroid precursors.

finding, type II CDA is also referred to as **HEMPAS (hereditary erythroblastic multinuclearity associated with a positive acidified serum test). CDA type III** is distinguished by the appearance of extremely large late erythroid precursors with up to 12 nuclei per cell. **CDA type IV** has morphologic characteristics of type II CDA but a negative acid hemolysis test.

Chromosome studies have shown the presence of a number of codanin-1 gene (*CDAN1* on chromosome 15) mutations in CDA type I patients. These conditions do not evolve into leukemia and, depending on the severity of the anemia, the prognosis is quite good. As with other conditions characterized by abnormal precursor maturation with ineffective erythropoiesis, **iron overload** can be a significant complication. This situation is worsened if the patient requires long-term transfusion.

B. Hereditary Sideroblastic Anemia

Patients with hereditary sideroblastic anemia (HAS) usually present during infancy or childhood with a severe microcytic, hypochromic anemia. The defect is usually X-linked, so males present with the most severe form of the disease. It is most commonly caused by a mutation of the erythroid-specific δ-aminolevulinic acid synthase gene (*ALAS2*). This leads to inadequate protoporphyrin IX synthesis, mitochondrial iron loading, and ineffective erythropoiesis. Carrier females may be identified because of a dimorphic blood film with even proportions of microcytic, hypochromic, and normal red blood cells. The **diagnostic finding** is the presence of classic ringed sideroblasts on Prussian blue stain.

X-linked sideroblastic anemia with ataxia (progressive truncal ataxia with cerebellar hypoplasia), a rare form of hereditary sideroblastic anemia, is the result of partial loss of function mutations in the mitochondrial iron transporter gene, *ABCB7*. ABCB7 protein enables the transport of excess mitochondrial iron back to the cytoplasm.

THERAPY

The most important principles in managing the dysplastic and sideroblastic anemias are to **provide maximum support and encouragement** to patients over the prolonged course of their disease and to **avoid potentially harmful treatments in early stages** of the disease. As a general principle, patients with mild anemias and other cytopenias should be simply monitored for progression of their disease. With progession, they will require supportive therapy, including periodic red blood cell and platelet transfusion and/or hematopoietic growth factor therapy. Patients presenting with RAEB or CMML almost always deserve more aggressive therapy, for example, allogeneic bone marrow transplantation

CASE HISTORY • *Part 3*

The patient has a myelodysplastic anemia with leukopenia, an isolated 5q deletion, and fewer than 5% marrow blasts. This is diagnostic for 5q minus syndrome, a category of dysplastic anemias that generally carry a better prognosis. Management will include judicious transfusion, growth factor administration, and treatment with the immunomodulatory drug lenalidomide. The latter is highly effective with up to 80% of 5q minus syndrome patients experiencing a sustained improvement, including a reduction in the number of deletion 5q clonal cells in the marrow.

when possible, or both growth factor therapy and chemotherapy. The **classification of dysplastic anemias** provides guidance as to the patient's prognosis and therapy (Figure 9–7).

Prognosis and Survival

Patients with RA and RARS have a less severe anemia that is slow to evolve to more refractory disease or to acute leukemia. Patients with RA and RARS have median survivals in excess of 36–72 months, and less than 10% become leukemic, whereas **patients with RAEB** have median survivals of 5–15 months with a better than 50% chance of transformation to acute myelogenous leukemia or, less commonly, CMML (Figure 9–8).

The **International Prognostic Scoring System (IPSS)** classifies myelodysplastic anemias into 1 low-risk, 2 intermediate-risk (INT-1 and INT-2), and 1 high-risk categories. By weighting the impact of cytopenias, blast percentage, and chromosomal abnormalities, it is somewhat more accurate in its prediction of survival (Table 9–7).

Overall, **low-risk** patients (score of 0) have median survivals of almost 6 years, as compared with 3.5 years for those with **INT-1** (score of 0.5–1), 1 year for those with **INT-2** (score of 1.5–2), and less than 6 months for **high-risk** patients (score >2).

Blood Component Therapy

As patients become more severely anemic or pancytopenic, they need to be supported with red blood cell and platelet transfusions. Red blood cell transfusions should not be initiated until the patient is symptomatic. In an otherwise healthy individual, this will often translate into a hemoglobin level of 8 g/dL or less. Elderly patients with cardiovascular disease may need to receive transfusions at an earlier stage, however. With time, patients usually become very good judges of their own transfusion needs, decreasing the need for frequent hemoglobin measurements.

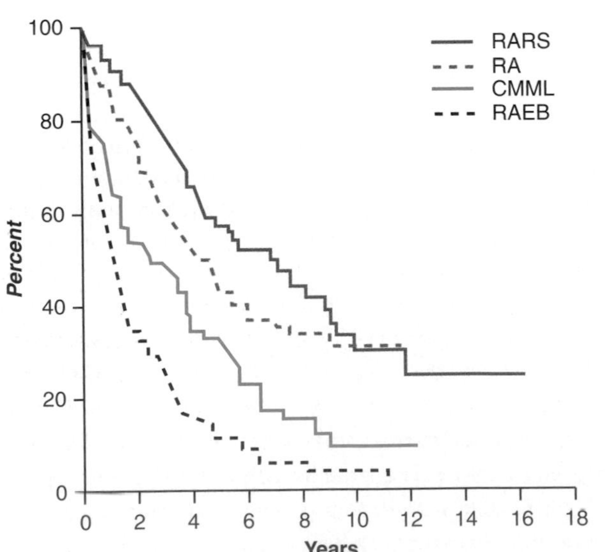

FIGURE 9–8. **Patient survival according to the classification of the dysplastic anemias.** Patients with RARS or RA have significantly better survivals when compared with patients with RAEB or CMML.

TABLE 9–7 • International prognostic scoring system (IPSS)

Variable	Score 0	0.5	1	1.5	2
Cytopenias	0/1	2/3			
Chromosomal abnormalities[a]	NL/1+	2+	3+		
Blast (%)	<5	5–10		11–20	>20

[a]*Patients with normal karyotypes (NL) or deletions of only 20q, 5q, or the Y chromosome (1+) do much better than those with* ***multiple abnormalities*** *involving chromosomes 5 and 7 (3+). Other abnormalities are graded as 2+.*

An increased transfusion requirement is associated with a decrease in survival and a greater likelihood of evolution to leukemia.

Once transfusion therapy is initiated, it is likely that patients will eventually become **transfusion dependent**. Moreover, it can be anticipated that the transfusion requirement will gradually increase. This tendency is accelerated in patients who develop red blood cell antibodies or splenomegaly **(hypersplenism)**. Long-term transfusion therapy also runs the risk of stimulating human leukocyte antigen (HLA) alloantibodies. It is advisable, therefore, to **use leukocyte-reduced red blood cells** for transfusion. Certainly, any patient who experiences chills and fever with transfusions should only receive leukocyte-reduced red blood cells.

A. Iron Overload

Patients with sideroblastic or dysplastic anemias with marked ineffective erythropoiesis and a high transfusion requirement are at great risk for iron overload. This needs to be considered early in the course of their management and they need to be followed up closely over time. Repeated iron studies are an essential component of patient management. Treatment with deferasirox or deferoxamine can prevent organ damage, and on occasion, by reducing the patient's iron load, improve hematopoiesis (see Chapters 6 and 15).

B. Platelet Transfusion

Prophylactic platelet transfusions should not be used routinely because of the increased risk of HLA alloimmunization, leading to platelet refractoriness. If possible, platelet transfusions should only be used to prepare a patient for a surgical procedure or treat an acute hemorrhage. Usually, myelodysplasia patients can tolerate platelet counts as low as 5–10,000/μL without spontaneous bleeding. They should be advised, however, to avoid aspirin and nonsteroidal anti-inflammatory agents that can inhibit platelet function.

C. Infections

Life-threatening infections are uncommon in dysplastic and sideroblastic anemia patients unless the absolute granulocyte count falls below 300–500/μL. Localized infections should be treated promptly with the appropriate antibiotic, since these patients often lack granulocyte reserves and can develop worsening leukopenia with uncontrolled infections. Dysplastic anemia patients do appear to be at greater risk for reactivation of mycobacterial infections. Any patient who presents with sustained fever, malaise, a worsening pancytopenia, and abnormal liver chemistries should be evaluated for a systemic mycobacterial or fungal infection.

Hematopoietic Growth Factors

Most patients with dysplastic and sideroblastic anemias can be expected to have very high levels of endogenous erythropoietin and, therefore, be unresponsive to therapeutic levels of recombinant erythropoietin. This assumption can be confirmed by **measurements of plasma erythropoietin**. However, selected patients with a favorable response profile (endogenous erythropoietin level <500 mU/mL; transfusion requirement of <2 U per month; bone marrow blasts below 10%) have a 40%–70% chance of a response to standard doses of 150–300 U/kg of recombinant erythropoietin given subcutaneously 3 times a week or an equivalent dose of darbepoietin given every 1–3 weeks. Routine therapeutic trials with erythropoietin in unselected patients are to be discouraged, simply on the basis of cost-effectiveness.

Granulocyte colony-stimulating factors (both G-CSF and GM-CSF) are effective in stimulating granulocyte production. When given in dosages of 1–3 μg/kg/d, G-CSF will increase the granulocyte count in 40%–50% of patients. Similarly, GM-CSF given in dosages of 3 μg/kg/d will increase the granulocyte count to a level of 5–10,000/μL in most leukopenic patients. This increase can be useful in managing pancytopenic patients with acute infection. Combination therapy with erythropoietin may also augment the erythroid response in up to 40% of apparently nonresponsive patients.

Long-term administration of growth factors has raised concern that they may actually speed progression to acute leukemia. In fact, the opposite appears to be true. Responding patients have an improved survival and a lower rate of evolution to leukemia when compared to case-based controls treated with supportive care alone. Patients with 5q deletions may be an exception; they appear to have a significantly shorter duration of response to growth factors.

Immunosuppressive and Immunomodulatory Therapy

T cell–mediated suppression of marrow progenitor cells has been implicated as a mechanism contributing to pancytopenia in dysplastic anemias. A limited number of trials of anti-thymocyte globulin (ATG) and cyclosporine have shown responses in a third or more of patients, with the highest response rate in RA and low/intermediate risk (INT-1) patients. Variables predictive of response include age less than 60 years, reduced marrow cellularity, presence of a PNH clone, HLA-DR15 phenotype, and low transfusion requirement of short duration. In some responders, a clonal $CD8^+$ T-cell suppression of colony-forming unit–granulocyte, monocyte (CFU-GM) progenitors has been identified as an underlying mechanism, raising the question of whether they represent a form of autoimmune aplastic anemia (see Chapter 3).

Immunomodulatory drugs that suppress proinflammatory cytokines, TNF-α, VEGF, basic fibroblast growth factor (bFGF), and neoangiogenesis also have a role in the treatment of selected patients with myelodysplasia. **Lenalidomide**, a derivative of thalidomide, has shown remarkable activity in patients with deletions of 5q (5q minus syndrome). In several trials, up to 80% of patients with this karyotype have shown a robust response with the majority achieving transfusion independence. Moreover, an observed cytogenetic response with suppression of the deletion 5q clonal cells is further indicative of the cytotoxic action of the drug. Patients with major reductions in deletion 5q clonal cells appear to have more durable responses and a lower rate of evolution to leukemia. The principle complication of prolonged lenalidomide therapy is myelosuppression, requiring intermittent dosing.

Chemotherapy and Bone Marrow Transplantation

Cytotoxic chemotherapy has been used in younger patients with RAEB with approximately the same response as seen in AML (excluding acute promyelocytic leukemia). Therefore, as the patient takes on more features of acute leukemia, it makes sense to attempt a regimen similar to that used in treating AML, a 2- or 3-drug regimen containing a cell cycle–specific agent. **Elderly patients** do not do well with these regimens. They tolerate less drug, develop marked marrow hypoplasia, and fail to enter a sustained remission. **Patients with complex chromosomal abnormalities or monosomy 7** also do less well; fewer than 50% will achieve a complete remission. Even with the best candidates, event-free survival at 2–3 years is less than 30%.

Epigenetic therapy, using drugs that impact DNA methylation and histone code alterations, would also appear to have a significant role in the management of myelodysplastic patients. Two hypomethylating agents: 5-azacytadine and 5-aza-2′-deoxycitidine have been approved by the US Food and Drug Administration (FDA), and a number of ongoing trials are studying dose schedules and combination regimens with valproic acid, a histone deacetylase inhibitor. The response rate with combination therapy may approach 50%. The retinoid, 13-cis-retinoid acid, can also induce cell differentiation, and may therefore be useful in combination regimens.

Allogeneic bone marrow transplantation can be "curative" in patients with RAEB. The largest series of some 66 patients reported a 24% 5-year disease-free survival rate regardless of their pretransplant chemotherapy history. A recent report of allogeneic and syngeneic transplantation in older patients (aged 55–66) with RA and RAEB showed even better success rates—30%–60% estimated 3-year survivals according to the extent of cytogenetic abnormalities. It would also appear that marrow transplantation can be carried out successfully even when the patient's marrow is quite fibrotic.

Vitamin Therapy

Although many of the dysplastic anemias present with a macrocytic anemia and megaloblastic marrow, treatment with vitamin B_{12} and folic acid is always ineffective. Patients with hereditary, X-linked, sideroblastic anemia often respond to **pyridoxine**

therapy and should be tried on a regimen of pyridoxine 50 mg/d orally for 2–3 months to document response. Rarely, patients with RARS may also respond to pyridoxine given in doses of 50 mg or more per day by mouth. Parenterally administered **pyridoxal-5-phosphate** has been reported to partially correct the anemia in some patients with acquired ringed sideroblastic anemia (RARS). This has not been accepted as standard therapy, however. Other hematinics are not indicated. Certainly, iron should not be administered to patients with a sideroblastic anemia or ineffective erythropoiesis where there is a tendency to iron overload. Androgens, steroids, and immunosuppressive therapy have also been of little value.

Patients with Paroxysmal Nocturnal Hemoglobinuria

Management of patients with PNH will vary according to the nature of the clinical presentation. When hemolysis is the dominant feature (PNH III patients), folic acid and iron supplementation are needed to sustain red blood cell production levels. Iron therapy can worsen episodes of PNH by increasing the daily production of PNH cells. This should not, however, be taken as a reason to stop iron therapy. Long-term anticoagulation should be considered in all PNH patients, especially those with a history of thrombotic disease, unless there is a major contraindication such as severe thrombocytopenia. Platelet and red blood cell transfusions will be necessary in patients with marked marrow dysplasia or aplasia.

A monoclonal antibody (eculizumab) that binds to complement component 5 (C5) and blocks complement-mediated lysis is now available for the treatment of PNH III patients. Given in a dose of 900 mg every 12–14 days, eculizumab dramatically decreases the number and severity of episodes of paroxysmal hemoglobinuria. It also reduces transfusion requirements, normalizes the lactic dehydrogenase (LDH), and improves quality of life. At the same time, the number of PNH type III red blood cells increases and patients continue to exhibit a moderately severe extravascular hemolytic anemia. This is the result of continued binding of activated C3 on the red cell membrane (eculizumab does not block C3 activation).

Eculizumab therapy is well tolerated with little or no side effects. All patients should be vaccinated against *Neisseria meningiditis* prior to initiating therapy. Even so, vaccination is not fully protective; a few episodes of meningococcal meningitis have been reported. It is anticipated that the frequency and severity of thrombotic events will be significantly decreased with long-term therapy. However, until this is well proven, anticoagulation therapy should be continued.

Prior to the availability of eculizumab, young patients with PNH and severe disease, especially life-threatening thrombotic disease or evolving myelodysplasia, were considered to be candidates for allogeneic stem cell transplantation, especially if a matched sibling donor was available. While a successful transplant can result in a "cure," the overall survival after 10 years ranges from 50%–60%. The future role of transplantation in the management of PNH will depend on the experience with long-term eculizumab therapy.

POINTS TO REMEMBER

The dysplastic (myelodysplasia) and sideroblastic anemias are generally diagnosed on the basis of changes in blood counts, blood smear and marrow morphology, and cytogenetics.

The WHO/FAB classification recognizes 6 different conditions: refractory anemia (RA); RA with ringed sideroblasts (RARS); RA (cytopenias) with multilineage dysplasia (RCMD); RA with excess blasts (RAEB-1 and -2); 5q minus syndrome; and myelodysplasia unclassified (MDS-U).

RA patients typically present with a moderately severe anemia, without other cytopenias, ringed sideroblasts, or cytogenetic changes. T cell–mediated suppression of erythroid progenitors may play a significant pathophysiologic role.

RARS is distinguished by the presence in the marrow of large numbers of ringed sideroblasts (erythroid progenitors containing iron-encrusted mitochondria in a ring around the nucleus) in the marrow. RARS patients tend to have an indolent course, although those with marked ineffective erythropoiesis are at risk for tissue iron overload.

RCMD is characterized by dysplasia in 2 or more cell lineages, fewer than 5% blasts, and varying numbers of ringed sideroblasts (RCMD-RS). Both types (RCMD and RCMD-RS) have a worse prognosis.

RAEB patients present with a pancytopenia or severe anemia with neutropenia. The number of myeloblasts in the marrow is increased from 5%–19% and blasts may be seen on the blood smear. Cytogenetics is very helpful in making this diagnosis; most patients have 1 or more chromosomal defects.

Patients with deletion of 5q (5q minus syndrome) are a unique subset of RAEB. They respond dramatically to treatment with immunodulatory agents (lenalidomide) and have an improved prognosis.

The differential diagnosis of myelodysplasia requires excluding disorders with similar presentations, including CMML, paroxysmal nocturnal hemoglobinuria (PNH), myelofibrosis, erythroleukemia, congenital dyserythopoietic anemias (CDA I–IV), and hereditary sideroblastic anemia.

The management and prognosis of a patient with myelodysplasia depends on the classification and severity of the patient's cytopenias, blast percentage, and chromosomal abnormalities (IPSS score). RA, RARS, and RCMD (IPSS low-risk) patients have the best prognosis and are generally managed with judicious use of red cell transfusions and growth factors.

The prognosis of RAEB (IPSS intermediate- to high-risk) patients is least favorable, but varies according to the severity of their pancytopenia, the number of blasts in the marrow, and their karyotype. Younger patients are candidates for immunosuppressive therapy, chemotherapy, and transplantation if a matched sibling donor is available.

BIBLIOGRAPHY

Dysplastic and Sideroblastic Syndromes

Bottomley SS: The spectrum and role of iron overload in sideroblastic anemia. Ann NY Acad Sci 1988;526:331.

Greenberg P et al: International scoring system for evaluating prognosis in myelodysplastic syndromes. Blood 1997; 89:2079.

Heimpel H et al: Congenital dyserythropoietic anemia type I (CDA I): molecular genetics, clinical appearance, and prognosis based on long-term observation. Blood 2006;107:334.

Nimer SD: Myelodysplastic syndromes. Blood 2008;111: 4841.

Rollison DE et al: Epidemiology of myelodysplastic syndromes and chronic myeloproliferative disorders in the United States, 2001–2004, using data from the NAACCR and SEER programs. Blood 2008;112:45.

Wang SA et al: Chronic myelomonocytic leukemia evolving from preexisting myelodysplasia shares many features with de novo disease. Amer J Clin Pathol 2006;126:789.

Paroxysmal Nocturnal Hemoglobinuria

Dunn DE et al: Paroxysmal nocturnal hemoglobinuria cells in patients with bone marrow failure syndromes. Ann Intern Med 1999;131:401.

Hill A et al: Sustained response and long-term safety of eculizumab in paroxysmal nocturnal hemoglobinuria. Blood 2005;106:2559.

Hillmen P et al: Natural history of paroxysmal nocturnal hemoglobinuria. N Engl J Med 1995;333:1253.

Parker C et al: Diagnosis and management of paroxysmal nocturnal hemoglobinuria. Blood 2005;106:3699.

Peffault de Latour R et al: Paroxysmal nocturnal hemoglobinuria: natural history of disease subcategories. Blood 2008; 112:3099.

Rosse WF, Ware RE: The molecular basis of paroxysmal nocturnal hemoglobinuria. Blood 1995;86:3277.

Therapy

Chang C et al: Hematopoietic cell transplantation in patients with myelodysplastic syndrome or acute myeloid leukemia arising from myelodysplastic syndrome: similar outcomes in patients with de novo disease and disease following prior therapy or antecedent hematologic disorders. Blood 2007; 110:1379.

Deeg HJ et al: Allogeneic and syngeneic transplantation for myelodysplastic syndrome in patients 55 to 66 years of age. Blood 2000;95:1188.

Howe RB et al: The WHO classification of MDS does make a difference. Blood 2004;103:3265.

Vardiman JW, Harris NL, Brunning RD: The World Health Organization (WHO) classification of the myeloid neoplasms. Blood 2002;100:2292.

BLOOD LOSS ANEMIA • 10

CASE HISTORY • *Part I*

A 27-year-old man is brought to the emergency room by the rescue service after suffering significant blood loss from a chain saw laceration of the right thigh. The EMTs have applied a pressure dressing to the wound and initiated an intravenous saline drip at a rapid rate. Vital signs in the field were BP - 110/60 mm Hg, P - 120 bpm, R - 22 bpm.

On examination, the patient is pale, anxious, and breathing rapidly but is alert and able to answer questions. He denies other illness or injuries besides the thigh wound. Supine vital signs are BP - 100/55 mm Hg, P - 130 bpm, R - 24 bpm. On sitting his blood pressure falls to 60/40 mm Hg and he feels faint.

A second intravenous line is placed and blood is drawn for a complete blood count (CBC), coagulation profile, and STAT type and crossmatch for 4 U of red blood cells. Ringer lactate is infused at a maximum rate and vital signs are continuously monitored. Surgical consultation is requested.

Questions

- Based on the patient's appearance and vital signs, how much blood would you estimate he has lost?
- In order to correct for this loss, what volume of Ringer lactate/electrolyte solution should be infused and how rapidly?
- Is he a candidate for an immediate type O-negative blood transfusion?

Acute blood loss has a direct impact on the integrity of the blood volume and oxygen supply to tissues. Sudden, severe hemorrhage can induce hypovolemic shock, cardiovascular failure, and death. When blood loss is more gradual, the hemoglobin level can fall to a point where oxygen delivery to vital organs is compromised. Chronic blood loss will deplete iron stores and produce an iron-deficiency anemia. Therefore, diagnosis and management of a blood loss anemia must take into account the reason behind the loss, the rate and amount of blood loss, and the capacity of the patient to compensate for both volume losses and anemia.

NORMAL RESPONSE TO BLOOD LOSS

Compensation for acute hemorrhage involves both a well-defined cardiovascular response to hypovolemia and the erythropoietic response to a reduction in red blood cell mass.

Cardiovascular Response

A normal individual readily tolerates blood volume **losses of up to 20% of the total blood volume** (Table 10–1). This is accomplished by redistribution of blood flow, principally a contraction of the venous blood pool by reflex venospasm. Pain, fever, or a vasovagal response can interfere with this normal compensatory mechanism. An obvious example of this is the vasovagal syncope reaction to a painful injury or the anxiety initiated by acute blood loss.

When acute blood loss exceeds 20% of the total blood volume (more than 1,000 mL in a 70-kg adult with an estimated blood volume of 5,000 mL), venospasm alone will not compensate for the reduction in blood volume. These individuals will want to remain supine and may demonstrate a postural drop in blood pressure on sitting or standing. They will also become tachycardic with exercise. Once blood loss **exceeds 30% of the blood volume (1,500 mL)**, postural hypotension is clearly

TABLE 10–1 • Symptoms and signs of blood volume losses in the adult

Percent Lost (%)	Volume Lost (mL)[a]	Symptoms	Signs
<20	<1,000	+/– Anxiety	+/– Vasovagal reaction
20–30	1,000–1,500	Anxiety, exercise intolerance, may faint on standing	Orthostatic hypotension, exertional tachycardia
30–40	1,500–2,000	Syncope when sits or stands	Orthostatic, anxious, tachycardic at rest
>40	>2,000	Anxious, restless, often confused, may be short of breath	Hypovolemic shock, fall in supine blood pressure, tachycardic with cool, clammy skin

[a]*Calculated for a 70-kg adult with a blood volume of 5,000 mL.*

present and patients may faint if they stand up. **Hypovolemic shock** starts once blood loss exceeds 40% of the total blood volume (2,000 mL).

When blood loss is gradual, compensation is provided by expansion of plasma volume. The ability to acutely mobilize **albumin**, the principal oncotic protein of plasma, from extravascular sites is limited, however. New production of albumin is a relatively slow process, so full restoration of an acute volume loss of 1,000–1,500 mL can take 20–60 hours. At the same time, healthy individuals easily tolerate chronic blood losses of 1,000 mL or more per week, producing sufficient albumin to replace their plasma losses. Albumin production is well maintained even when nutrition intake is temporarily restricted.

Erythroid Marrow Response

As discussed in Chapter 1, the normal erythroid marrow rapidly increases red blood cell production in response to anemia or hypoxia. The **capacity of the marrow to respond** depends on the level of erythropoietin stimulation, the presence of a normal complement of erythroid precursors in a normal marrow structure, and an adequate supply of iron. The erythropoietin response is a function of anemia severity. Once the hemoglobin falls to levels below 11 g/dL, the normal kidney secretes increasing amounts of erythropoietin. This response occurs within a matter of hours. At the same time, marrow expansion, which leads to an increase in the reticulocyte count and a rise in the total number of circulating red blood cells, takes days to weeks.

The **pattern of response to a sudden reduction in hematocrit** is summarized in Table 10–2. During the first 2 days, initial evidence of an increased level of erythropoietin stimulation is the appearance in circulation of **polychromatic macrocytes (shift cells)**. These are marrow reticulocytes that are released 1–2 days early under the stimulation of a high level of erythropoietin. Although appearance of these young reticulocytes will raise the percent reticulocyte count, the actual **index of production** (absolute reticulocyte count corrected for the early release of marrow reticulocytes) will not have increased (see Chapter 2). Furthermore, if the marrow is examined, the ratio of erythroid to granulocytic precursors (E/G ratio) is still 1:3. Overall, the erythropoietic profile during the first 1–2 days after an acute hemorrhage fits the description of a hypoproliferative anemia.

TABLE 10–2 • Erythropoietic response to acute hemorrhage

Days After Bleed	1–2	3–6	7–10
Marrow reticulocyte shift (polychromasia)	+	++	+++
Reticulocyte production index (times normal)	1	1–2	>2–3
E/G ratio	1:3	1:1	>1:1

A definite **increase in erythroid marrow response** should be detectable during the next several days. Initially, by days 3–6 the marrow E/G ratio increases to levels of 1:1 (a 3-fold expansion of erythroid precursors), followed by an increase in the reticulocyte index. An **apparent imbalance** between the level of proliferation of the marrow and the reticulocyte response should not be interpreted as ineffective erythropoiesis. Rather, it reflects the fact that the erythropoietic response has not yet reached steady state. By days 7–10, the reticulocyte production response should reach a level of at least 3 times basal. At this point, the marrow E/G ratio of 1:1 and the reticulocyte production index of 3 times normal are in balance. This process depends, however, on the level of iron supply. When reticuloendothelial iron stores are depleted, red blood cell production may never reach 3 times basal and certainly cannot be sustained at that level without iron supplementation.

Red Blood Cell Oxygen Delivery

Although the marrow response to a blood loss anemia is slow, circulating red blood cells are able to quickly compensate by increasing their transfer of oxygen to tissues. This is a 2-step process. When acute hemorrhage reduces the number of red blood cells or the blood flow to tissue (or both), the red blood cells perfusing the tissue respond to the more acidic environment with an instantaneous shift in the hemoglobin-oxygen dissociation curve to the right, which is known as the **Bohr effect**. In effect, it facilitates transfer of oxygen to tissues. Over the next several hours, this phenomenon leads to an **increased production of 2,3-diphosphoglycerate** in the red blood cell. This process maintains the higher level of oxygen delivery. Together, these mechanisms can maintain relatively normal levels of oxygen delivery to key organs with only half the normal number of circulating red blood cells.

CLINICAL FEATURES

Clinical presentation of a blood loss anemia will vary according to the site and severity of blood loss. Massive hemorrhage from the gastrointestinal tract or an external trauma site will be immediately obvious. The rate and magnitude of the blood loss may also be apparent. Slower bleeding internally can be harder to diagnose. In the case of gastrointestinal blood loss, patients may only present once they have developed an iron-deficiency anemia. With bleeding into tissues or a closed cavity (especially the peritoneal space), the presenting anemia may mimic acute hemolysis. Therefore, severity of the bleed, rate and site of the bleed, and capacity of the patient to respond are each integral in defining the clinical presentation.

Large Volume Blood Loss

Sudden loss of a large volume of blood has an immediate impact on the patient's cardiovascular status. Relatively healthy, young to middle-aged individuals can tolerate acute volume **losses of up to 30% of their blood volume** with few symptoms other than mild postural hypotension (see Table 10–1). This situation may not be true, however, for elderly individuals or patients with complicating illness. Fever, severe pain, and exposure can all interfere with the reflex mechanisms that compensate for modest volume losses. Once an acute loss of blood **exceeds 30% of the patient's blood volume**, postural hypotension worsens and symptoms and signs of hypovolemic shock appear, including a rapid, thready pulse; cool, clammy skin; air hunger; and confusion. **When blood loss approaches 50% of blood volume**, heart failure and death are imminent unless volume expanders are administered immediately.

The impact on the blood volume overshadows the effect of acute blood loss on red blood cell mass. Even as a patient approaches death from hypovolemia and cardiovascular shock, **depletion of red blood cell mass** is still less than 50%. This level of red blood cell loss would not be life threatening in a normal individual with a normal blood volume and cardiovascular system. Oxygen delivery to tissues will remain close to normal because of the shift in the hemoglobin-oxygen dissociation curve. When red blood cell loss is combined with blood volume loss, however, tissue perfusion fails and severe tissue hypoxia appears as a major component of hypovolemic shock.

Important features in the clinical presentation include the cause, location, magnitude, and duration of the blood loss. External trauma can result in either arterial or venous hemorrhage and produce hypovolemic shock within a matter of minutes. Large-volume bleeding from the gastrointestinal tract is seen with esophageal varices, esophageal tears, or ulcer-induced arterial bleeds. A less obvious presentation is a major bleed into a closed cavity or tissue. Patients who fracture their hip or pelvis can lose 1–2 L of blood into the thigh and pelvic area. Bleeds into the pleural and peritoneal cavities can easily exceed 30% of the patient's blood volume and result in the rapid onset of hypovolemic shock.

Lower Volume, Slower Blood Loss

When the amount of blood loss is less and the rate slower, the **plasma volume expands to maintain a relatively normal total blood volume**. A normal individual can usually keep up with rates of 200–300 mL of whole blood loss per day without experiencing symptoms or signs of hypovolemia. This level may not suffice for patients with liver disease or a chronic debilitating illness that interferes with their ability to produce new oncotic protein. These patients will exhibit a combination of postural hypotension and congestive heart failure. Severe right heart failure with marked edema and ascites can be anticipated in these patients if their albumin production is significantly impaired.

In the absence of hypovolemia, patients with ongoing, gradual losses of blood will present with the **symptoms and signs of anemia**. These signs will vary depending on the rate of onset, the severity of the anemia, and the patient's age. Younger, healthy individuals will tolerate moderately severe anemias with little complications other than a loss in stamina and some increase in heart rate and dyspnea with exercise. Older individuals become symptomatic with even mild anemias (hemoglobins of 10–11 g/dL). They are also at risk for the early onset of heart failure if they have coexisting cardiovascular disease.

Once the hemoglobin level falls below 8–9 g/dL, most patients will report palpitations, shortness of breath, and easy fatigability with exertion. They may also report difficulty with concentration, sleep disturbance, and pounding headaches. Clinical signs of a **worsening anemia** include tachycardia, signs of an increased cardiac stroke volume, and a loss of skin and mucous membrane color. On physical examination of the heart, the apical impulse is more forceful, and flow murmurs secondary to increased blood turbulence can be heard as mid- or holosystolic ejection murmurs at the apex and along the left sternal border.

Small Volume, Chronic Blood Loss

Loss of small volumes of blood (<100 mL/d) is **easily compensated by albumin production and plasma volume restoration**. In addition, anemia develops over weeks, permitting maximum compensation by the shift of the oxygen dissociation curve, production of new red blood cells by the erythroid marrow, and, when anemia is severe, changes in cardiac output and blood flow. Because of this, patients may not be symptomatic enough to seek medical attention. This will delay the diagnosis and lead to the appearance of an iron-deficiency anemia.

The slower and more protracted the bleeding, the more likely the patient will **present with symptoms and signs of iron deficiency**, which include a general loss of stamina and well-being, cardiovascular symptoms and signs of severe anemia, sore mouth and difficulty swallowing, and a softening and spooning of the fingernails. Children often develop **pica**, an unusual appetite for ice or dirt.

Chronic blood loss leading to iron deficiency is usually caused by gastrointestinal blood loss. However, some patients may present with a defect in iron absorption, secondary to small-bowel disease, such as non-tropical sprue or extensive Crohn disease. Patients who have had a Billroth II operation with vagotomy for ulcer disease can also exhibit food iron malabsorption. In developing countries, hookworm infestation is a frequent cause of chronic blood loss leading to severe iron deficiency. Less frequently, patients can present with a blood loss anemia secondary to hemoglobinuria (paroxysmal nocturnal hemoglobinuria, see Chapter 9), pulmonary hemosiderosis, or self-induced blood loss.

Perisurgical Blood Loss

Blood losses can usually be predicted according to the surgical procedure. Unanticipated excessive bleeding can, however, result in a large-volume loss picture, requiring both **plasma volume and red cell mass support**. With massive blood losses, **platelet and coagulation factor replacement** will be necessary to guarantee hemostasis. In order to minimize the patient's exposure to blood products, patients should not be overtransfused. It is preferable to leave the physiologically stable patient with a significant postoperative anemia, hematocrit in the 25%–30% range. This will not interfere with recovery and wound healing.

In the case of a significant preoperative anemia (hematocrit <30%), small body size predicting a small blood volume, or an expected blood loss of more than 1,000 mL, consideration should be given to **autologous blood storage, perioperative erythropoietin therapy, or both**. Given the appropriate candidate and procedure, acute normovolemic hemodilution and intraoperative blood salvage can also be used to reduce the transfusion requirement. When these therapies are used in combination, it is possible to avoid homologous blood transfusion in many patients undergoing elective noncardiac procedures with predictable major blood losses.

Laboratory Studies

Laboratory findings will also vary according to the size and rate of blood loss. The behavior of the CBC is a good example. Although it would seem to make sense that the hemoglobin level (hematocrit) would provide a good measure of red blood cell loss, it is not necessarily the case. Hemoglobin and hematocrit measurements are volume ratios where the quantity of red blood cells depends on the volume of diluent plasma. Immediately after an acute, severe hemorrhage, there will be little change in the hemoglobin (hematocrit) until the plasma volume has time to expand (Figure 10–1). Without fluid administration, this process takes more than 24 hours. If a volume expander is given, the change in hemoglobin level correlates as much with the volume transfused as with the volume of blood lost.

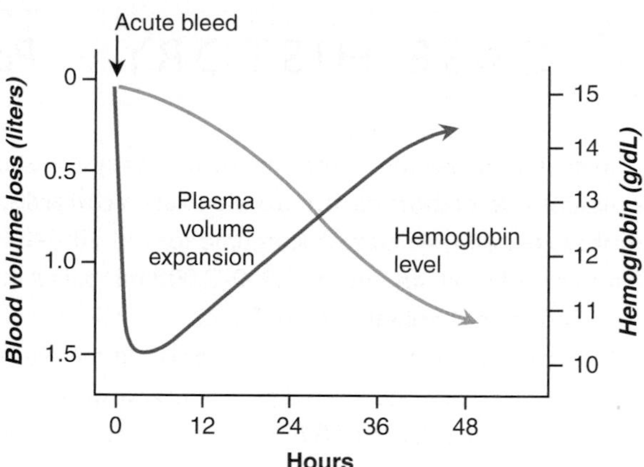

FIGURE 10–1. **Changes in blood volume and hemoglobin level after an acute bleed.** The compensatory expansion of the plasma volume following an acute bleed can take more than 48 hours if a volume expander is not administered. The hemoglobin level will reflect this delay in volume expansion. It will not reach its lowest point until full plasma volume expansion has occurred.

Severe hemorrhage may be accompanied by other changes in the CBC. The granulocyte count can increase dramatically to levels of 20,000/μL or higher, and immature white cell forms can appear in circulation. This situation reflects a demargination of granulocytes secondary to the patient's catecholamine response and a release of granulocytes from the marrow storage pool. With **hypovolemic shock and hypoxia**, very immature cells, including metamyelocytes, myelocytes, and nucleated red blood cells, can also appear in circulation. A rise in the platelet count to levels exceeding 1 million/μL can also occur in the days after a severe hemorrhage. The explanation for this rise in platelet count is unclear.

A. Findings in the Days After Blood Loss

In the days following a significant blood loss, laboratory studies will demonstrate a normal erythroid marrow compensatory response to anemia. The first surge of erythropoietin will, within a matter of hours, cause marrow reticulocytes to enter circulation. This shift phenomenon can be appreciated from the appearance of polychromatic macrocytes on the peripheral film. Changes in the marrow E/G ratio and reticulocyte index will then follow the predictable, normal response pattern to anemia (see Table 10–2). Laboratory studies during the first week after hemorrhage must be interpreted against this template of the "normal" erythropoietic response.

B. Findings After the First Week

After the first 7–10 days, the **reticulocyte count** should provide a good measure of effective red blood cell production. This

CASE HISTORY • *Part 2*

The patient's appearance and vital signs (low systolic blood pressure with orthostatic hypotension, rest tachycardia, and modest tachypnea) suggest a volume loss of 30%–40% of his normal blood volume or 1,500–2,000 mL based on an assumed normal volume of 5,000 mL.

In order to stabilize his vital signs, he should receive 3–4 L of Ringers lactate or normal saline at a maximum rate, which should provide at least 1,000 mL of blood volume support (electrolyte solutions immediately equilibrate with the extravascular space). This should also provide enough time to access red blood cells and plasma if necessary. Type O-negative blood should only be given if he fails to show a rapid response to the fluid infusion and then, only if type-specific blood is unavailable on an emergency basis.

In his case, he does respond to the electrolyte infusion. His blood pressure rises to 120/75 mm Hg, P - 94 bpm, R - 16 bpm. Inspection of the wound reveals considerable soft-tissue and muscle damage with bits of cloth and wood chips in the wound and continued rapid bleeding. CBC is reported as normal, hematocrit of 42%, platelet count - 380,000/μL.

Questions

- Anticipating he will need to go the operating room for debridement, possible vessel repair, and wound closure, how do you manage his transfusion requirements, including his need for red cell replacement, platelets, and coagulation factors?

count requires calculating the **reticulocyte index**, which is the percent count corrected for anemia and shift (see Chapter 2). With an acute, self-limited blood loss, recovery of the **hemoglobin (hematocrit)** over the next several weeks can also be used to estimate effective red blood cell production. The change in the hemoglobin level is much slower than the reticulocyte production index, however, and full recovery can take many weeks.

Laboratory testing is of greatest value during **recovery. Serial measurements of reticulocyte count** in the weeks following a hemorrhage provide an important indicator of the effectiveness of the marrow's response. Given an adequate supply of reticuloendothelial iron stores, normal adults should increase their reticulocyte production index to 2–3 times basal after 7–10 days and sustain this production level over the next several weeks. If the reticulocyte index falls back toward the basal level, iron studies should be performed to look for the emergence of iron deficiency or an inflammatory suppression of both the erythropoietin response and iron supply.

DIAGNOSIS

Types of Bleeding

When patients present with **severe, ongoing hemorrhage**, the diagnosis can be made at the bedside, and the location and rate of the bleeding can help predict the magnitude of the red blood cell loss. If symptoms and signs of hypovolemia are present, the patient will almost certainly develop a relatively severe blood loss anemia. Patients presenting with **less severe, slower bleeding** are a greater diagnostic challenge. Most of these patients will have a gastrointestinal abnormality and will follow a clinical course typical for their disease. The timing and location of the bleed will determine the patient's presenting symptoms, physical signs, and laboratory findings. For example, patients with advanced cirrhosis have episodic, large-volume bleeds from varices, accompanied by sudden, dramatic hematemesis and melena. Patients with gastritis or peptic ulcer disease present in a similar fashion or with melena alone.

Bleeding from the small or large intestine may only be evidenced by routine hemoccult screening. When the amount of blood lost exceeds 50–100 mL per day, patients will report black, often foul-smelling stools. If the loss into the small intestine is greater than 200 mL per day, the blood will act as a laxative, resulting in multiple black- to maroon-colored, loose stools. The more rapid the bleeding, the greater chance the patient will exhibit symptoms and signs of hypovolemia.

Physical examination and laboratory findings in **patients with slower bleeds** will depend on the clinical course of the illness. Many patients will bleed for some period before seeking medical attention and will have had time to respond with an expansion of their plasma volume. It should be possible, therefore, to detect many symptoms and signs of anemia. Laboratory studies such as the hemoglobin (hematocrit) should provide a fair measure of anemia severity, whereas the reticulocyte count and red blood cell indices provide a sense of the level of effective red blood cell production and adequacy of iron supply.

Timing of the Bleeding Episode

Interpretation of any set of laboratory studies depends on the timing of the bleeding episode. If a patient presents soon after the bleeding begins, laboratory studies must be interpreted according to the template of the normal erythropoietic response to acute anemia or hypoxia. In contrast, when patients present with a more protracted course of bleeding, it may be assumed that the erythroid marrow has had an opportunity to respond.

In this latter situation, studies of red blood cell production and iron supply are important to look for the appearance of iron deficiency.

Chronic, low-grade blood loss can go undetected for long periods, until the patient presents with symptoms and signs of anemia and/or iron deficiency. The more severe the anemia, the easier the laboratory diagnosis of iron deficiency. Normal adult males will exhaust their iron stores when more than 1,000 mL of red blood cells are lost. The young to middle-aged adult female can become iron deficient with losses of as little as 200–300 mL of red blood cells. Once stores are exhausted, the serum iron falls to below 30 μg/dL and the serum ferritin to below 20 μg/L. In addition, the erythroid marrow begins to produce microcytic, hypochromic red blood cells.

Iron Deficiency

As described in Chapter 5, the pattern of laboratory findings in **iron deficiency** varies according to the severity and duration of the anemia. As long as the hemoglobin level is greater than 10 g/dL, patients will exhibit a normocytic or slightly microcytic anemia with a low reticulocyte production index. At lower hemoglobin levels, microcytosis and hypochromia become more pronounced. Initially, the red cell distribution curve and blood film show a mixed population of microcytic and normocytic cells while the mean cell volume (MCV) is still normal. This situation reflects the initial mixing of newly produced microcytic cells with existing normocytic cells. After some weeks or months, the entire circulating population becomes microcytic with a fall in the MCV and mean cell hemoglobin. The red blood cell distribution width (RDW) can also give a sense of the evolution of the film morphology from normocytic to microcytic. Both RDW-CV and RDW-SD will increase as greater numbers of small cells are mixed with the normal population.

THERAPY

Management of a patient with a blood loss anemia requires not only good clinical decision making but also appropriate use of volume expanders, blood components, and iron supplements. The **first steps in stabilizing a severely hemorrhaging patient** are the essential components of first aid. Most important, any obvious bleeding sites should be controlled. If available, **military antishock trousers (MAST)** can be applied to redistribute intravascular volume and maintain the patient's blood pressure until adequate fluids are administered. The MAST suit can provide an autotransfusion of 600–1,500 mL of blood by compressing the lower extremities and abdomen. It can also tamponade arterial or venous bleeders in the lower extremities of a trauma victim.

The next important step is to establish reliable intravenous access and begin an aggressive program of **fluid and volume expander administration**. The choice of volume expanders will depend on the type and severity of the bleeding, symptoms and signs of hypovolemia, and patient age. There is also the issue of what products are readily accessible. Electrolyte solutions and purified colloid preparations are immediately available, whereas the administration of red blood cells, platelets, and fresh frozen plasma will involve some delay, unless the patient is brought to a major trauma center.

Electrolyte Solutions

Two standard electrolyte solutions, **Ringer's lactate** and **normal saline**, can be used as volume expanders. Although they lack oncotic protein, they will expand the intravascular volume if given in sufficient quantities. To attain an intravascular volume expansion of 1 L, 3–4 L must be infused at a rapid rate, since electrolyte solutions immediately equilibrate with the extravascular space, which is about twice the size of the intravascular space. In a life-threatening situation, volumes of 8 L or more of electrolyte can be safely administered to younger patients. However, older patients and patients with cardiovascular disease can have difficulty tolerating this much fluid. They almost certainly will develop subcutaneous edema and may experience pulmonary edema or, even worse, acute respiratory distress syndrome (ARDS). The latter is most commonly seen in patients who are also septic or have experienced a severe crush injury.

There are **limits to how long a patient can be sustained solely on electrolyte solutions**. When 6 or more liters of fluid are required in the first 1–2 hours, it is unlikely the patient can be maintained without the infusion of a colloid solution and red blood cells. Older patients should be considered for colloid and red blood cells at an even earlier stage to prevent cardiovascular decompensation.

Colloid Solutions

Several colloid solutions are available that provide reliable volume expansion for volume infused. These include 5% albumin solution, purified plasma protein fraction, and hydroxyethyl starch solution (Table 10–3). For management of an acute, severe hemorrhage, these products are interchangeable. When large volumes are required, protein-containing products are preferred.

TABLE 10–3 • Volume expanders

Product	Advantages	Disadvantages
Electrolyte solution (saline, Ringer's lactate)	Readily available, inexpensive	Need to give large volumes; can induce congestive failure
Protein solutions (PPF, Albumisol)	Volume-for-volume expansion, no side reactions	Expensive; may be in short supply, hyponatremia
Hydroxyethyl starch solution	Volume-for-volume expansion, less expensive	Can inhibit platelet function
Fresh frozen plasma	Contains coagulation factors	Allergic reactions; expensive

A. Protein Solutions

Albusimol, a purified preparation of 5% albumin in isotonic saline, is a hepatitis-free, HIV-free, extremely reliable volume expander. It can be stored at room temperature for long periods and infused at rapid rates without allergic reactions. In a hypovolemic patient, it gives volume-for-volume expansion. Moreover, because human albumin is the primary oncotic protein in plasma, volume expansion is sustained for several days until the patient's own albumin production can compensate. This product is also quite safe if excess volumes are given. As long as cardiac and renal functions are relatively normal, patients will compensate with a salt and water diuresis, even raising serum albumin concentrations to supernormal levels.

Plasma protein fraction (PPF) (Plasmanate) is a popular alternative to 5% albumin solution. PPF contains a mixture of albumin (4 g/dL) and other globulins (1 g/dL). The protein fraction is prepared as a sodium acetate precipitate of human plasma proteins. Because of this, the protein is resuspended in a solution that may vary from isotonic to hypotonic with sodium levels of 140–110 mEq/L and very low chloride levels. Because of this, the patient should be followed up for hyponatremia if large volumes are administered (more than 2–3 L). Otherwise, PPF is also hepatitis- and HIV-free and gives predictable volume expansion.

B. Hydroxyethyl Starch Solution (Hetastarch, Hespan)

Hydroxyethyl starch solution is another popular alternative. It is made up as a 6% solution in isotonic saline, which will give volume-for-volume intravascular expansion. It is much less expensive than either 5% albumin solution or PPF, and it has a stable shelf life. Its **use is limited**, however, by its more rapid removal from circulation and its tendency to inhibit platelet function, even resulting in an acquired form of von Willebrand disease. It is usually recommended that infusions of hydroxyethyl starch solution be limited to 1–2 L.

When massive transfusion is needed to save an exsanguinating patient, volume expanders will need to be accompanied by transfusions of red blood cells, platelets, and fresh frozen plasma. Hypovolemic shock and hypoxia, which lead to lactic acidosis, ARDS, and brain damage, are still the principal issues. They need to be dealt with by very aggressive administration of volume expanders and red blood cells. It is also important to anticipate the diluting effect of electrolyte and colloid solutions on the levels of plasma coagulation factors and platelets. Hydroxyethyl starch may directly lower factor VIII and von Willebrand factor (vWF) levels. When the volume of blood lost exceeds the patient's blood volume (more than 5 L), a mix of colloid expander, fresh frozen plasma, red blood cells, and platelets must be administered. The patient's bleeding can be worsened if this therapy is not implemented.

C. Fresh Frozen Plasma

Fresh frozen plasma (FFP) is essentially frozen normal human plasma, prepared as a part of routine fractionation of whole blood. Each unit of FFP contains approximately 200 mL of plasma with levels of coagulation factors, including fibrinogen, prothrombin, and factors XI, IX, VIII, X, V, and VII, which approach those found in fresh plasma. When administered to a patient with a plasma volume of approximately 3 L, each unit will increase individual factor levels by only 5%–7%. In order to make a significant impact on the coagulation profile of a massively bleeding patient, at least 4–6 U of FFP must be given. This infusion will temporarily provide a level of 30% or more of the coagulation factors needed for normal hemostasis.

FFP is also a protein-containing volume expander, similar to 5% albumin solution or PPF. However, it is not as trouble-free as the other 2 solutions. **FFP can induce an IgE immune-mediated allergic reaction** in sensitive patients. In addition, when large volumes of FFP are administered, there is a significant risk in up to 10% of patients of inducing an **acute sensitivity reaction** characterized by widespread urticaria, generalized subcutaneous edema, and acute bronchospasm. On occasion, an allergic reaction is severe enough to actually reduce the plasma volume at a time when the need for volume expansion is critical. It is essential, therefore, that patients receiving FFP be watched for symptoms and signs of a hypersensitivity reaction, including a worsening of the patient's hypotension.

Red Blood Cell Transfusion

A major loss of red blood cells with severe hemorrhage needs to be treated by transfusion of red blood cells. A unit of red blood cells contains approximately 200 mL of red blood cells suspended in 50–75 mL of plasma and preservative solution. Depending on the method of preparation, a unit can also contain nonviable platelets and granulocytes and viable lymphocytes.

A. Filtration of Red Blood Cells

In some blood centers, red blood cell units are filtered prior to storage. This filtration removes most but not all of the granulocytes and platelets. When available, leukofiltered red blood cells do have an advantage of reducing the frequency of acute febrile reactions secondary to cytokines, or alloantibodies to white blood cell human leukocyte antigens (HLAs), or both (see Chapter 38).

B. Severity and Rate of Blood Loss

The need to transfuse red blood cells will depend on the severity and rate of blood loss. Usually, it is not as urgent as the need to treat the patient's hypovolemia. As long as adequate amounts of volume expanders are administered, the patient will tolerate up to 50% loss of circulating red blood cells. This may not be true, however, for elderly patients or patients with cardiovascular disease. The decision to transfuse should be based on the bedside evaluation of the patient's clinical status with emphasis on cardiovascular compensation, mentation, age, and complicating illness.

When blood loss is massive, red blood cell transfusion should be initiated as soon as possible as a part of blood volume support. Hypovolemic shock can result in metabolic acidosis, a situation which possibly may be made worse by the transfusion of blood older than 14 days. Some centers, therefore, elect to use fresh blood in massively transfused patients to avoid complications of worsening acidosis, hypocalcemia, and hyperkalemia. It is also essential to transfuse either type-specific fresh whole blood (blood that contains red blood cells, coagulation factors, and platelets in normal amounts) or a combination of red cells, fresh frozen plasma, and stored platelets to, in effect, reconstitute fresh whole blood.

C. Blood Typing

If red blood cell transfusion can be delayed for 30 minutes or more, the patient's ABO blood type should be determined and the patient's plasma screened for anti–red blood cell antibodies. ABO typing takes only a few moments. With this information, type-specific red blood cells can be transfused with little or no risk of a transfusion reaction. The only faster way of providing a relatively safe and compatible red blood cell transfusion is to administer type O (Rh-negative) red blood cells. **Type O red blood cells** lack both A and B antigens and are therefore universally accepted by patients regardless of blood type. At the same time, the supply of O-negative blood is quite limited; only 7% of donors are O Rh-negative. Therefore, even major trauma centers are unable to supply enough of this product to manage every patient with a massive hemorrhage.

When using type-specific blood to manage a life-threatening hemorrhage, the **patient's Rh status may have to be ignored**. For men and women who have passed the childbearing age, a transfusion of Rh-positive red blood cells to an Rh-negative recipient is of little consequence. If the patient is free of Rh antibody, there is less than a 1 in 5 chance of sensitizing a patient, and even then this will not result in a significant hematologic abnormality. If necessary, the chance of immunization can be eliminated by the administration of **anti-D antibody (RhoGAM)** for up to 3 days following small red blood cell transfusions. This has the effect of suppressing the anti-D immune response. When a young Rh-negative woman receives an entire unit of Rh-positive red blood cells, she should be treated with RhoGAM. The amount required is considerable, however—20 mg of anti-D per milliliter of transfused red blood cells. Since this option may not be effective, especially when several units of blood are transfused, Rh-compatible blood should be used in females of childbearing age.

D. Volume Expanders

Each unit of red blood cells should increase the hemoglobin level by approximately 1 g/dL (hematocrit increase of 3%–4%). Although very little plasma is infused with each unit, there can be a significant volume expansion effect when several units of red blood cells are transfused. This should be recognized when calculating the amount of volume expander administered so as not to induce congestive heart failure. If a patient has received a large amount of volume expander, especially electrolyte solution, and is stable, the rate of red blood cell transfusion should be slowed and the patient treated with a diuretic.

E. Allergic Reactions

Like FFP, rapid transfusion of several units of red blood cells can induce an immune-mediated allergic reaction. Appearance of urticaria, bronchospasm, or a sudden fall in blood pressure suggests an IgE-related reaction, whereas chills, fever, or both are usually caused by cytokines that accumulate during storage or, rarely, bacterial contamination. Prestorage leukoreduction of red cell units is effective in reducing the level of leukocyte-derived cytokines and the incidence and severity of febrile reactions to transfusion. Transfusions of red blood cells also run the risk of transmitting blood-borne infections.

Platelet Transfusions

Thrombocytopenia is a problem in patients who receive massive transfusions of volume expanders and red blood cells. It is good practice, therefore, to closely monitor the platelet count and to prophylactically administer platelets in severely hemorrhaging patients. As a simple rule, a 6-pack of platelets (the platelets from 6 random donors) should be administered with every 5–6 U of red blood cells. This treatment should prevent thrombocytopenia and avoid the question of whether the patient has sufficient platelets to guarantee hemostasis. If a complicating illness that might contribute to platelet consumption is present, frequent platelet counts should be obtained to confirm the adequacy of platelet transfusion support.

Iron Therapy

Iron plays a key role in the erythroid marrow response to a blood loss anemia. A normal adult male with 1,000 mg of reticuloendothelial stores can acutely increase red blood cell production to 2–3 times normal. This production level cannot be sustained, however, if the blood loss exceeds the amount of stored iron. At this point, the patient must receive iron therapy.

A. Dosage Guidelines

Detailed guidelines of oral and parenteral iron therapy are presented in Chapter 5. As a rule, oral iron therapy should be used whenever possible. Adult patients with an acute, self-limited hemorrhage can be treated with 1 tablet of a standard oral iron preparation 3–4 times each day, preferably given between meals to increase absorption. Iron therapy should be initiated as soon as possible after the patient is stabilized and should be maintained for 3–6 months. This treatment plan will give time both to repair the anemia and to rebuild reticuloendothelial iron stores.

B. Response to Oral Iron Therapy

Response to oral iron therapy will be influenced by such factors as the severity of the anemia, patient compliance, intestinal absorption, and any complicating illnesses that suppress the erythropoietin response. Red blood cell production levels as high as 3 times normal can be observed in patients with significant anemia (a hemoglobin level <10 g/dL) who faithfully take their oral iron and do not have a complicating illness. Renal disease or an inflammatory illness can dampen the erythropoietin response to anemia. Breaks in the oral iron regimen will also interfere with the marrow's response. To maintain a constant supply of iron to erythroid precursors, the doses of oral iron must be taken at even intervals throughout the day.

If the patient has a **less severe anemia** (a hemoglobin level >10 g/dL) because of a more modest bleeding episode or as a result of transfusion, oral iron therapy should be modified to encourage gastrointestinal tolerance and patient compliance. Otherwise, the patient will not cooperate with the prolonged course of iron therapy, which is required for the reconstitution of iron stores.

C. Iron Dextran Therapy

Patients with malabsorption or a marked intolerance to oral iron will not be amenable to oral iron therapy. Their anemia can obviously be corrected with red blood cell transfusions. They will need to receive parenteral iron, however, to correct their iron balance and rebuild stores. Iron can be given intravenously or intramuscularly as **iron dextran complex**. Detailed instructions for the administration of iron dextran are presented in Chapter 5. When iron dextran is used to treat a patient who is recovering from a blood loss anemia, it is best given as a single, total dose infused intravenously.

Iron dextran can also be of value in treating patients with **chronic blood loss**. Hereditary hemorrhagic telangiectasia is perhaps the best example of a clinical condition where a relentless, daily loss of blood from the gastrointestinal tract can overwhelm the normal routes of iron supply. Reticuloendothelial stores are quickly exhausted, and even maximum iron absorption on a full oral regimen cannot match cell losses of 50 mL or more of red blood cells each day. As these patients become severely anemic, they develop a severe iron-deficiency anemia with marked microcytosis and hypochromia. They can also exhibit signs of **tissue iron deficiency**.

Acute, severe episodes of bleeding in patients with **hereditary hemorrhagic telangiectasia** should be treated with red blood cell transfusions, just like any acute blood loss anemia. To counteract the slower, daily loss of blood in these individuals, attempts should be made to provide maximum iron therapy (see Chapter 30). Not only should the patients receive a constant regimen of oral iron but they should also receive periodic intravenous injections of iron dextran, according to the rate of blood loss. The combination of oral iron and iron dextran can be quite effective (Figure 10–2). In severely anemic patients with hereditary telangiectasia, red blood cell production levels of up to 5–6 times normal may be achieved for several weeks following an intravenous injection of 500–1,000 mg of iron dextran.

To maintain erythroid marrow production at its maximum level over a prolonged period, the iron dextran **injections must be given every 3–4 weeks**. Otherwise, the level of red blood cell production will fall gradually back to basal level as the release of iron from the iron dextran complex slows. Larger complex particles in the preparation are only slowly dissolved by the reticuloendothelial cell. In fact, the release from some particles can fall behind the rate of the patient's blood loss, so that microcytosis and hypochromia will appear despite the presence of visible iron dextran particles within marrow reticuloendothelial cells. This phenomenon needs to be recognized in the laboratory evaluation of anemia in patients with hereditary hemorrhagic telangiectasia who receive long-term iron dextran therapy. They may present with characteristic findings of an iron-deficiency anemia but have easily visible or even increased iron stores of their marrows on the Prussian blue stain.

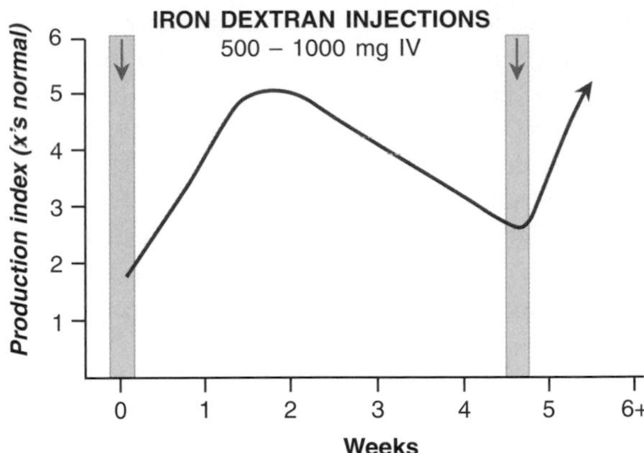

FIGURE 10–2. **Marrow production levels following iron dextran injection.** Patients with severe anemia and chronic blood loss can be treated with a combination of oral iron and intermittent intravenous injections of iron dextran. Each bolus of intravenous iron will increase red blood cell production to as high as 5–6 times normal for several weeks.

Perisurgical Blood Loss Management

Elective surgery patients undergoing major noncardiac procedures are candidates for autologous blood storage, perisurgical recombinant erythropoietin therapy, acute normovolemic hemodilution, and blood salvage, alone or in combination. Patients who are moderately anemic (hemoglobins between 10 and 13 g/dL) or of small body size can also benefit, even when the anticipated surgical blood loss is not above 1,000 mL.

Together, these several techniques should make it possible to avoid, if not significantly reduce, exposure to homologous blood transfusion. Benefits are considerable. Allogeneic blood transfusion is associated with a demonstrable decrease in cellular immunity, and the postoperative infection rate in patients receiving transfusions has been reported to increase 7- to 10-fold. Furthermore, the postoperative length of stay and hospital charges can be correlated with the number of homologous units transfused, a relationship that is not seen in a comparable group of patients given autologous blood or erythropoietin.

A. Autologous Blood Storage

The amount of blood that can be deposited for subsequent transfusion (autologous donation) will depend on the patient's initial hematocrit and marrow production response. As long as the hemoglobin is above 13 g/dL, the **average-sized patient should be able to donate 3–4 U of red cells**. Smaller patients with hemoglobins below 13 g/dL will require simultaneous erythropoietin therapy to donate more than 2 U without causing the hematocrit to fall below 33%.

Autologous blood storage is notoriously **expensive**. When blood is stored for surgical procedures with a low risk of major hemorrhage (hysterectomy, transurethral prostatectomy, normal vaginal delivery, etc), up to 90% of the units collected will be discarded. Even with higher-risk procedures, 50% or more of the units will go unused.

There is also the issue of **postoperative anemia**, which can be made worse by autologous donation. Together these drawbacks tend to discourage its use.

The **marrow response to erythropoietin** correlates with the dose and the duration of treatment. When given in a dose of 100–150 IU/kg (approximately 10,000 U) subcutaneously twice a week for 3 weeks, patients will produce 300–400 mL of red blood cells, the equivalent of 1.5–2 U of red cells. This will usually guarantee storage of up to 4 autologous units. In addition, they will enter surgery with a higher than normal reticulocyte count. Much higher erythropoietin doses will result in greater production but at considerable financial cost.

An adequate **iron supply** is very important. Patients must be maintained on oral iron, 1 tablet of Feosol 3 times per day (200 mg of elemental iron per day), or receive intravenous iron as iron dextran (1,000 mg single infusion) or iron saccharate (200 mg at the time of each autologous donation).

B. Perisurgical Recombinant Erythropoietin Therapy

Perisurgical erythropoietin therapy without autologous donation can also help decrease homologous (allogeneic) blood exposure. Dosing studies have looked at a number of regimens, including daily 100–300 IU/kg injections for 10 days preoperatively to 4 days postoperatively to once or twice per week injections of 600 IU/kg subcutaneously. Aggressive iron supplementation is again key to the patient's response. This therapy will generally produce a 1–2 g/dL rise in the hemoglobin level (3%–6% rise in hematocrit), the equivalent of a 1–2 U red cell transfusion. When continued postoperatively, erythropoietin therapy will also accelerate the rate of recovery of the hemoglobin level.

C. Acute Normovolemic Hemodilution

In selected settings, acute normovolemic hemodilution can help decrease the need for homologous blood. Normovolemic hemodilution follows the same principle as autologous blood storage. Whole blood is removed using standard blood storage bags just prior to surgery and replaced with crystalloid/colloid to maintain normovolemia. It can then be reinfused during or after the procedure to treat major blood losses. Advantages include the elimination of testing requirements, less preoperative planning, and a lower cost. Candidates for this approach include patients without symptomatic cardiovascular disease who are expected to experience a blood volume loss in excess of 20% of their blood volume. Acute normovolemic hemodilution can be combined with erythropoietin therapy, autologous blood storage, and intraoperative blood salvage to further reduce the need for homologous transfusion.

D. Blood Salvage

Intraoperative blood salvage provides another method for reducing exposure to homologous blood. It is most effective in orthopedic and vascular surgery patients where blood can be scavenged from a relatively sterile field. Cell-washing devices can handle blood losses equivalent to 10 U/h of stored blood. This can be lifesaving in patients with massive blood losses associated with vascular procedures. Blood can also be recovered postoperatively from surgical drains and reinfused. The blood collected is, however, partially hemolyzed and contains activated platelets as well as cytokines released from fragmented cells. Devices such as the Haemonetics Cell Saver incorporate a saline wash and centrifugation to remove white blood cells, platelets, plasma, and anticoagulants prior to reinfusion.

E. Coagulopathy Management

Depending on the condition of the patient prior to surgery, every attempt should be made to promote normal hemostasis. Thrombocytopenic patients are at great risk for uncontrollable capillary bleeding if the platelet count at the time of operation is less than 50,000/μL (see Chapter 31). They should, therefore, be transfused perioperatively to maintain the platelet count as close to 100,000/μL as possible. DDAVP can be used immediately before and for several days after an operation to improve platelet function in patients with a prolongation of the bleeding time secondary to von Willebrand disease, aspirin ingestion, mild hemophilia A, or uremia (see Chapter 31). Coagulation factor replacement with purified or recombinant factor preparations is essential in patients with severe hemophilia A or B (see Chapter 32). Patients with consumptive coagulopathies must be aggressively supported with platelet transfusions and factor replacement (see Chapter 33).

For certain clinical situations where activation of the fibrinolytic system is an issue (cardiac, prostate, or orthopedic surgery; liver transplantation; and following a subarachnoid hemorrhage), ε-aminocaproic acid (EACA) or tranexamic acid can be used to inhibit plasminogen activation to plasmin. EACA is given as a loading dose of 100–150 mg/kg intravenously followed by a constant infusion of 10–15 mg/kg/h. Tranexamic acid, a more potent inhibitor, is given as a loading dose of 10 mg/kg followed by a constant infusion of 1 mg/kg/h.

Recombinant factor VIIa (rFVIIa) may play an important role in patients with uncontrollable diffuse hemorrhage. A number of anecdotal studies of the use of rFVIIa in perioperative and postoperative patients have reported improvement in the coagulopathy and a significant decrease in subsequent transfusion requirements. Dosages have ranged from 40–120 μg/kg administered intravenously over 2–5 minutes, sometimes with repeated doses as needed. However, most studies report a good result after a single dose.

F. Controlled Hypotension

A deliberate reduction in systolic blood pressure to 80–90 mm Hg (~30% reduction in baseline mean arterial pressure) may be used to reduce intraoperative blood loss. This can be attained with anesthetic techniques or by the administration of a vasodilator

CASE HISTORY • *Part 3*

The patient's need for red blood cell replacement depends on his physiological status, the continued rate of blood loss, and the need to keep his hematocrit at a level appropriate for general anesthesia. His initial CBC (as well as repeat hematocrits during the first several hours) is of little value in as much as the hematocrit/hemoglobin will not reflect the magnitude of his blood loss until the plasma volume loss has been fully corrected. As for his platelet count and coagulation profile, they need to be monitored closely, especially if blood loss during surgery is inordinate and the patient requires massive transfusion, at which time platelet and coagulation factor replacement are essential.

(eg, sodium nitroprusside, nitroglycerin, calcium channel blockers, prostaglandin E1). Proper patient selection and experience with this technique are essential. It has been used in elective orthopedic surgery with positive results.

Massive Blood Transfusion

The experience in the acute resuscitation of the severely wounded in the Iraq and Afghanistan conflicts has emphasized the need for the immediate transfusion of fresh whole blood or its equivalent in massively bleeding patients. Uncontrolled hemorrhage has been the leading cause of preventable death in 7–8% of combat casualties. This has put extra emphasis on the need for robust resources and an aggressive approach to resuscitation. Delays in transfusion of blood products by the over-reliance on volume expanders such as Ringer's lactate, hydroxyethyl starch, or dextran solutions run the risk of a significant increase in death rate. Their use not only runs the risk of prolonged hypoxemia, acidosis, and tissue necrosis, but also promotes the early depletion of platelets and key coagulation factors needed for hemostasis. Therefore, when faced with massive blood loss, the following guidelines should apply:

- Minimize the use of crystalloid or colloid expanders and begin aggressive transfusion as early as possible of type-specific red blood cells and fresh frozen plasma in a ratio of 1:1 or 2:1 at most.
- For every 10 U of red cells/plasma administer a 6-pack of stored platelets or a platelet pheresis unit (the latter is preferred because of the larger number of viable platelets).
- When component therapy is unavailable, transfuse fresh whole blood (unrefrigerated blood drawn within a few hours prior to administration from a type-specific donor).
- If bleeding is ongoing, consider the administration of rFVIIa before the patient becomes acidotic (pH <7.1).
- When faced with a life-threatening coagulopathy (disseminated intravascular coagulation [DIC]) and uncontrolled bleeding, administer both additional platelets and cryoprecipitate (fibrinogen).

When these guidelines were followed in combat support hospitals in Iraq and Afghanistan, the survivals of patients requiring massive transfusion increased to 75%–80%.

POINTS TO REMEMBER

There is a predictable physiological response to acute blood loss that reflects the loss of blood volume rather than the reduction in red cell mass. It is important, therefore, to estimate the volume lost from the patient's appearance and physical signs and immediately begin volume replacement.

Effective blood volume support can be attained using electrolyte solutions (Ringer's lactate and normal saline), colloid solutions (albumin, hydroxyethyl starch, and dextran), fresh whole blood, or red cells plus fresh frozen plasma.

When resuscitating with electrolyte solutions, a volume of 3–4 L must be infused to attain a blood volume expansion of 1,000 mL. This reflects the rapid equilibration of electrolyte with the extravascular space.

The need for red blood cell replacement must be determined according to the age and physiological status of the patient, the rate of blood loss, and the overall management plan, especially if the patient needs surgery with general anesthesia. Measurements of the hematocrit/hemoglobin are of limited value, especially in the first 24–48 hours when the plasma volume has yet to normalize.

The erythroid marrow's response to an acute bleed follows a predictable course. The release into circulation of a few immature marrow reticulocytes (polychromasia) driven by a rising tide of erythropoietin may be appreciated in the first 24–48 hours. A rise in the E/G ratio and the absolute number of reticulocytes (reticulocyte index) is seen by day 3–6 and peaks at day 7–10.

Iron deficiency, renal disease, marrow damage, or a concomitant inflammatory illness can dampen this response. While iron deficiency may not be immediately apparent, iron stores are limited and once exhausted will suppress erythroid precursor proliferation and, over time, will result in an iron-deficiency anemia. Therefore, treatment with oral or parenteral iron is required in all patients with significant acute or chronic bleeding.

Blood components available for transfusion include red blood cells, fresh frozen plasma, cryoprecipitate, pheresis or pooled random platelets, and, in some trauma centers, fresh whole blood.

Patients suffering from catastrophic blood loss and requiring massive transfusion need to be treated as soon as possible with either fresh whole blood or a balanced combination of red cells, fresh frozen plasma, and platelets. Large-volume electrolyte or colloid expander infusions should be avoided.

Allogeneic blood transfusion during surgery can be minimized using several techniques, including perisurgical erythropoietin administration, autologous blood storage, blood salvage, and in selected cases, normovolemic hemodilution.

BIBLIOGRAPHY

Adamson J: Perisurgical use of epoietin alfa in orthopedic surgery patients. Semin Hematol 1996;33:55(suppl 2).

Blumberg N: Allogeneic transfusion and infection: economic and clinical implications. Semin Hematol 1997;34:34.

Cazzola M, Mercuriali F, Brugnara C: Use of recombinant erythropoietin outside the setting of uremia. Blood 1997;89:4248.

Goldberg MA: Perioperative epoietin alfa increases red blood cell mass and reduces exposure to transfusions: results of randomized clinical trials. Semin Hematol 1997;34:41.

Goodnough LT et al: Transfusion medicine: blood conservation. N Engl J Med 1999;340:525.

Hoffman MR et al: Excessive bleeding in surgery and trauma: new concepts in coagulation theory and an updated treatment paradigm. Surg Rounds (suppl) 2002; October.

Lichtman MA et al: Williams Hematology, 7th ed. McGraw-Hill, 2006.

Nessen SC et al: War Surgery in Afghanistan and Iraq: A Series of Cases, 2003–2007. Office of the Surgeon General, Department of the Army, United States of America, 2008.

Thompson JF: Interoperative blood salvage. Haematol Rev 1992;7:55.

Tobias JD: Strategies for minimizing blood loss in orthopedic surgery. Semin Hematol 2004;41:145.

Weiskopf RB: Mathematical analysis of isovolemic hemodilution indicates that it can decrease the need for allogencic blood transfusion. Transfusion 1995;35:37.

HEMOLYTIC ANEMIAS · 11

CASE HISTORY · *Part I*

A 54-year-old woman presents with a 2–3 month history of increasing fatigue, dyspnea on exertion, and ankle edema. She denies any recent illness and her review of systems is basically negative, including any prior history of anemia. Examination reveals an anxious middle-aged woman with pale conjunctiva and slightly jaundiced sclera. Vital signs: BP - 150/60 mm Hg, P - 110 bpm, R - 20 bpm T - normal. Signs of congestive heart failure include inspiratory rales heard over both lung bases, cardiomegaly, a systolic murmur at the apex, and 2+ pitting edema in both ankles. There is no hepatosplenomegaly or lymphadenopathy.

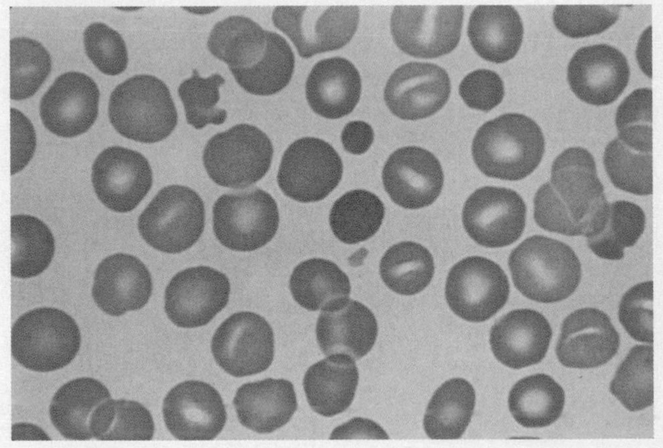

CBC: Hematocrit/hemoglobin - 18%/5 g/dL
MCV - 100 fL   MCHC - 36 pg   MCH - 33 g/dL
RDW-CV - 14%   RDW-SD - 53 fL
Reticulocyte count/index - 22%/>3
White blood cell count - 11,000/μL
Platelet count - 220,000/μL

Questions

- How should this anemia be described/classified?
- Are there additional tests that will confirm this classification and help identify a possible etiology?

The distinguishing feature of all hemolytic anemias is the **increased rate of adult red blood cell destruction.** Clinical presentation will vary according to the disease process. Some hemolytic anemias present as acute, self-limited episodes of red blood cell destruction, and others as chronic, well-compensated hemolytic states. Signs and symptoms of hemolysis will also differ according to the mechanism of red blood cell destruction. Sudden intravascular hemolysis results in hemoglobinemia and hemoglobinuria, whereas destruction limited to the extravascular monocyte-macrophage system may only be apparent from a fall in hemoglobin level and a rise in the serum bilirubin and lactic dehydrogenase (LDH) levels. Chronic, well-compensated hemolytic anemias are easily detected from the red blood cell production response (ie, increase in the reticulocyte index).

Red blood cell hemolysis can result because of environmental factors or an inherent defect in red blood cell structure or function. Even normal red blood cells can fall victim to environmental challenges such as mechanical trauma, infection, or autoimmune attack. Patients who inherit defects in membrane structure, hemoglobin stability, or metabolic function demonstrate both spontaneous shortening of red blood cell lifespan and a greater sensitivity to environmental factors.

NORMAL RED BLOOD CELL TURNOVER

Red blood cells are extremely pliable, resilient cells that survive for 100 or more days in circulation. Their capacity to survive is a tribute to the strength of the membrane and the metabolic pathways that supply the high-energy phosphate needed to maintain the membrane and keep hemoglobin in a soluble, reduced state (see Chapter 1). As red blood cells become older, however, metabolic pathways decay, oxidized hemoglobin accumulates, and oxidized phospholipids, especially phosphatidylserine, appear on the surface of the cell. A concomitant loss of flexibility interferes with the cell's ability to move through the microvasculature and initiates the process of removal by the monocyte-macrophage system via the CD36 receptor.

Role of the Spleen

The spleen plays a major role in red blood cell destruction (Figure 11–1). The structure of the spleen is a testing ground of cell flexibility and viability. Blood is delivered by terminal arterioles to the splenic red blood cell pulp, where the volume of plasma is reduced and the cell is subjected to a relatively hypoxic environment. This situation tests the metabolic pathways and, in older or diseased cells, results in a further loss of pliability. To escape and reenter circulation, the red blood cell must then squeeze through a 2–5 μm opening in the sinusoidal wall. In effect, this traps rigid cells and leads to phagocytosis and destruction by reticuloendothelial cells lining the sinusoids.

The uniform quality of red blood cell morphology on the blood film is a tribute to splenic function. The trapping-filtering mechanism of the spleen efficiently removes red blood cell inclusions including residual iron granules, nuclear remnants **(Howell-Jolly bodies)**, and any denatured hemoglobin **(Heinz bodies)**. Spleen reticuloendothelial cells also display receptors for the Fc fragment of immunoglobulin and the C3b component of complement. In patients with autoimmune hemolytic anemias, the spleen is the principal site of red blood cell destruction.

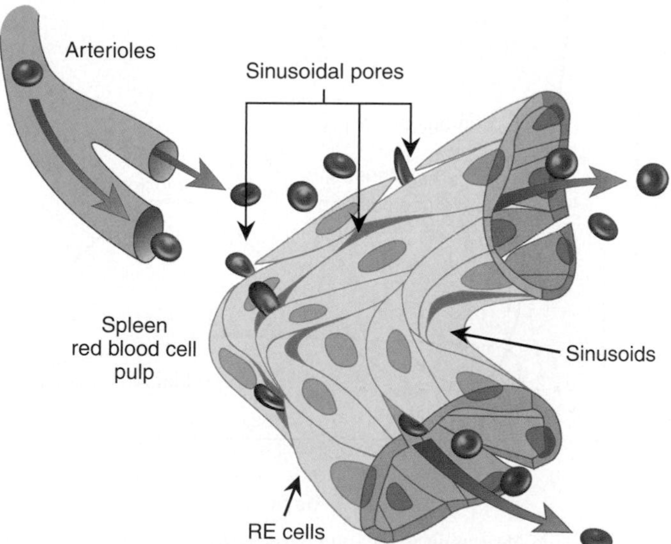

FIGURE 11–1. **Splenic function.** The anatomic structure of the spleen is ideal for testing the metabolic machinery and pliability of red blood cells. Within the splenic pulp, red blood cells are concentrated and their intracellular metabolic pathways stressed. The red cells must then pass through 2–5 μm pores to enter the sinusoidal system. Unusually rigid cells or a cell containing inclusion bodies will be unable to pass and will be destroyed by sinusoidal reticuloendothelial cells.

Pathways of Red Blood Cell Destruction

The pathways of red blood cell destruction effectively recover heme iron for new red blood cell production. This process is true whether the red blood cells break down in circulation **(intravascular destruction)** or by the normal reticuloendothelial cell pathway **(extravascular destruction)**. Destruction of senescent cells is largely limited to the extravascular pathway (Figure 11–2). Red blood cells are phagocytized by reticuloendothelial cells, the membrane is disrupted, and hemoglobin is broken down by lysozymal enzymes. Iron recovered from heme is then stored or transported back to the marrow for new red blood cell production. Amino acids are also recovered. At the same time, the protoporphyrin ring is metabolized to the tetrapyrrol **(bilirubin)** with the release of carbon monoxide. Bilirubin is subsequently transported to the liver, where it is conjugated and excreted into bile.

Intravascular red blood cell destruction follows a different pathway. Free hemoglobin either dissociates into α-β dimers that bind to haptoglobin or is oxidized to methemoglobin that

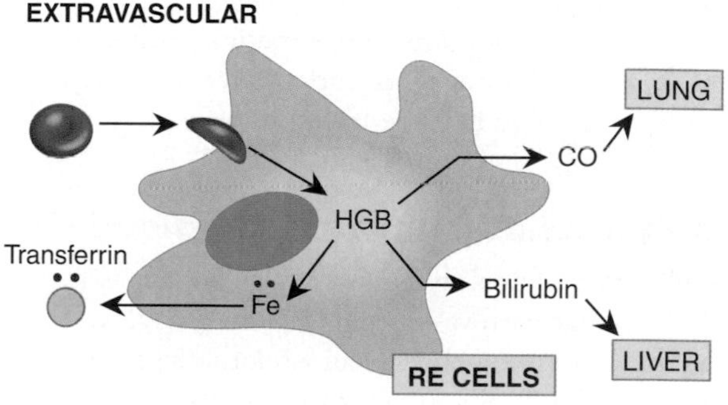

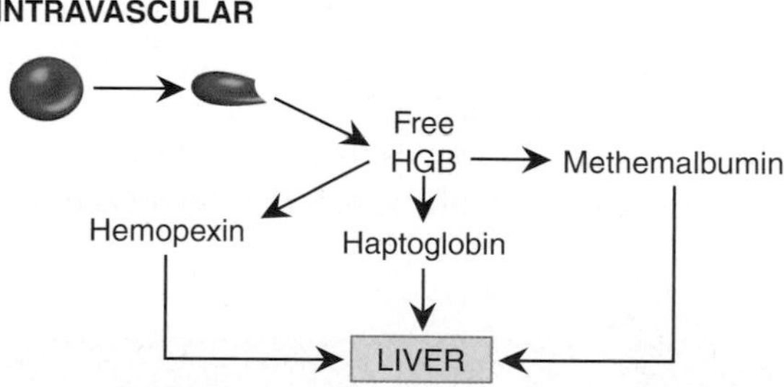

FIGURE 11–2. **Pathways of red blood cell destruction.** Red blood cell destruction can occur in the extravascular or intravascular space. With extravascular destruction, red blood cells are phagocytized by reticuloendothelial cells, the membrane structure is broken down, and the hemoglobin is reduced to its essential components. Iron is recovered for transport by transferrin back to the erythroid marrow. The porphyrin ring is broken, and a molecule of carbon monoxide is released. The remaining portion of the porphyrin ring is then transported as bilirubin to the liver for conjugation and excretion in bile. With intravascular red blood cell destruction, free hemoglobin binds either to haptoglobin or hemopexin or is converted to methemalbumin. These proteins are cleared by the liver, where the heme is broken down to recover iron and produce bilirubin.

then dissociates to release the heme group for binding with albumin and hemopexin. The binding step prevents immediate loss of the heme group by glomerular filtration and allows clearance by hepatocytes. The liver then breaks down the heme group to recover iron and produce bilirubin.

The **final common pathway** for both extravascular and intravascular red blood cell destruction is the conjugation of bilirubin by the hepatocyte, its excretion in bile, and the subsequent conversion by gut bacteria to urobilinogen and urobilin. These end products are excreted in both stool and urine.

Clinical Measurements of Red Blood Cell Destruction

The rate of red blood cell destruction can be assessed from measurements of several steps in the process. The most important clinical measurements are listed in Table 11–1. The **reticulocyte production index** provides an indirect measure of red blood cell destruction. When the reticulocyte index is greater than 3 times normal in a patient with a stable or falling hematocrit, the **destruction index** (the absolute number of red blood cells destroyed) can be assumed to be 3 times normal or higher. **Direct measurements of red blood cell lifespan** are possible using a ^{51}Cr red blood cell survival. **LDH and indirect bilirubin measurements** provide a qualitative measure of cell turnover. From a research standpoint, ferrokinetics, carbon monoxide excretion, and urobilinogen excretion have all been employed to quantitate red blood cell destruction.

Hemolysis and Abnormal Red Blood Cells

Very high levels of hemolysis can overwhelm the extravascular and intravascular pathways for heme iron recovery. There is a limit to the capacity of the reticuloendothelial system to clear abnormal red blood cells. When this capacity is exceeded, morphologically abnormal red blood cells appear in circulation. Depending on the cause of disease, these abnormal cells include microspherocytes, "bite" cells, fragmented red blood cells, and red blood cells with abnormal inclusion bodies. The presence of these cells in circulation suggests that either the capacity of the spleen is overwhelmed or splenic function is reduced as part of the disease process. Even normal subjects who have had a splenectomy will demonstrate abnormal forms. An overtaxed monocyte-macrophage system will also leak free hemoglobin back into circulation, resulting in a fall in serum haptoglobin level.

TABLE 11–1 • Measurements of red blood cell destruction

Indirect measurements
Changes in hematocrit
Reticulocyte production index
Serum lactic dehydrogenase (LDH)
Serum indirect bilirubin
Direct measurements
^{51}Cr red blood cell survival
Ferrokinetics
CO excretion
Urobilinogen excretion

Haptoglobin and Hemopexin Clearance Pathways

Intravascular hemolysis easily overwhelms haptoglobin and hemopexin clearance pathways. When hemoglobin binds to either haptoglobin or hemopexin, the complex is quickly cleared by the hepatocyte. The amount of hemoglobin that can be bound and removed depends on the rate of new haptoglobin and hemopexin production. Generally, intravascular lysis of more than 20–40 mL of red blood cells per day will effectively deplete both systems; haptoglobin levels will fall to undetectable levels (Figure 11–3). Once this occurs, free hemoglobin will be detected in both the patient's serum and urine, and methemalbumin levels will rise.

Recovery after an Intravascular Hemolytic Event

It is also important to recognize the pattern of recovery following an intravascular hemolytic event. As shown in Figure 11–3, following a self-limited intravascular hemolytic event, serum hemoglobin levels will drop rapidly as free hemoglobin is cleared

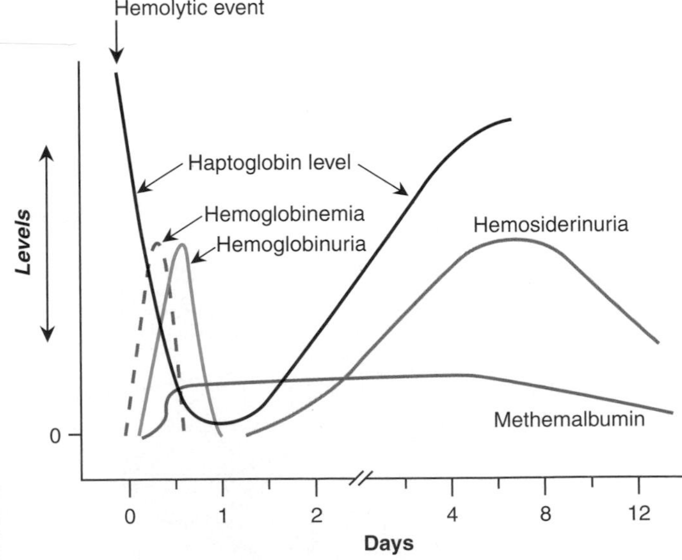

FIGURE 11–3. **Measurements of acute intravascular hemolysis.** Following an acute hemolytic event, measurements of plasma and urine hemoglobin, serum haptoglobin, serum methemalbumin, and urine hemosiderin follow a characteristic pattern. Hemoglobinemia, hemoglobinuria, methemalbuminemia, and a fall in the serum haptoglobin level are all present during the first 24 hours. If hemolysis does not continue, the patient will demonstrate a gradual return of the serum haptoglobin to normal and the appearance of hemosiderin in the urine for up to 7–10 days. Methemalbumin may be detectable for more than 1 week.

into urine. Hemoglobinuria will also be relatively short-lived. Haptoglobin levels then rise gradually over the next 24–72 hours. At the same time, methemalbumin levels in plasma will stay elevated for 5–10 days and patients will continue to shed tubular cells containing hemosiderin granules into urine for 1 week or more.

CLINICAL FEATURES

Most hemolytic anemias are associated with few specific symptoms or signs. **When anemia is severe,** patients will complain of increasing fatigue or exercise intolerance and may develop congestive heart failure. This is really no different from the clinical presentation seen with any severe anemia. In contrast, **acute intravascular hemolysis** may be associated with fever, chills, and severe lower back pain. This is most often seen in patients who receive incompatible or infected blood products. A severe intravascular hemolytic event with lysis of more than 20–40 mL of red blood cells will produce noticeable hemoglobinuria.

Since many hemolytic anemias are related to another disease state, a careful history and physical examination are always necessary. A search should be made for any evidence of autoimmune disease. Racial and family background are important. It is also important to try to document the chronicity of the anemia. Patients with congenital hemolytic anemias are frequently aware of other involved members in their family and may know the results of their own past blood counts.

Laboratory Studies

Diagnosis of a hemolytic anemia depends heavily on the laboratory. Any workup begins with several screening tests to classify the patient's disorder. This then provides a guide to the application of a larger number of specific tests of cell structure and function.

A. The Complete Blood Count

A complete blood count (CBC) with inspection of the film and measurement of the reticulocyte count is extremely valuable in both detecting a hemolytic anemia and pointing the way to diagnosis. An **acute hemolytic event** may only be heralded by a sudden fall in the patient's hemoglobin/hematocrit. **Chronic hemolytic states** are more easily detected. These patients have a moderate to severe anemia, a reticulocyte production index of greater than 3 times normal, and, in most cases, some abnormality of red blood cell morphology.

Most hemolytic anemias are normocytic, normochromic, although the presence of large numbers of microspherocytes on the blood film is accompanied by a rise in the mean corpuscular hemoglobin concentration (MCHC). Very high reticulocyte counts with marked polychromasia may be associated with a rise in the mean cell volume (MCV) to levels between 100 and 110 fL. An MCV greater than 110 fL is seen when the uncorrected reticulocyte count exceeds 25%–30%. This situation simply reflects the fact that when large numbers of marrow reticulocytes are added to the circulating normocytic red blood cell population, the MCV will rise. It will also be reflected in an increase in the red blood cell distribution width (RDW-SD).

TABLE 11–2 • Chronic hemolytic anemia erythropoietic profile

Red blood cell morphology	Normocytic, normochromic—abnormalities in red blood cell shape
Polychromasia	Present
Reticulocyte index	>3–5
Marrow E/G ratio	>1:1
Marrow morphology	Normoblastic
Serum iron/TIBC	Normal/normal
Serum bilirubin (mg/dL)	1–3
LDH (IU/mL)	>1,000

The full **erythropoietic profile of a chronic hemolytic anemia** is shown in Table 11–2. The marrow ratio of erythroid to granulocytic precursors (E/G ratio) is increased; red blood cell precursor morphology is usually normoblastic unless the patient becomes folic acid deficient. Iron studies demonstrate a normal serum iron and total iron-binding capacity, and a normal or slightly elevated ferritin level. Iron stores on the Prussian blue stain of the marrow are normal to somewhat increased. In patients with very high levels of red blood cell turnover, reticuloendothelial cells are filled with a finely granular, dustlike hemosiderin, which may reflect the rapid turnover of storage iron.

The **indirect bilirubin** and **serum LDH levels** are the most clinically useful measures of total red blood cell destruction. With significant hemolysis, the serum LDH level will quickly rise to levels in excess of 1,000 IU. Levels of 5,000 IU/mL or higher are not unusual. The indirect bilirubin level will increase to levels of 1–3 mg/dL in patients with significant hemolysis. Chronic elevations of the indirect bilirubin are also seen in patients with inherited defects in bilirubin conjugation (Crigler-Najjar and Gilbert disease).

B. Detection of Intravascular Hemolysis

The laboratory profile after an **acute intravascular hemolytic event** will vary according to the time elapsed. Acute hemolysis is associated with hemoglobinemia, hemoglobinuria, methemalbuminemia, and a rapid depletion of the serum haptoglobin level. Intravascular hemolysis several days prior to evaluation may only be detected by measurements of serum methemalbumin level and urine hemosiderin (see Figure 11–3).

1. Plasma hemoglobin level—Intravascular lysis of even small amounts of red blood cells (10–20 mL of packed red blood cells) will impart a pink tint to plasma for a few hours; more severe hemolysis will make plasma look like rosé or red wine (Figure 11–4). The amount of hemoglobin in plasma can be quantitated, but observation of the plasma for color changes will

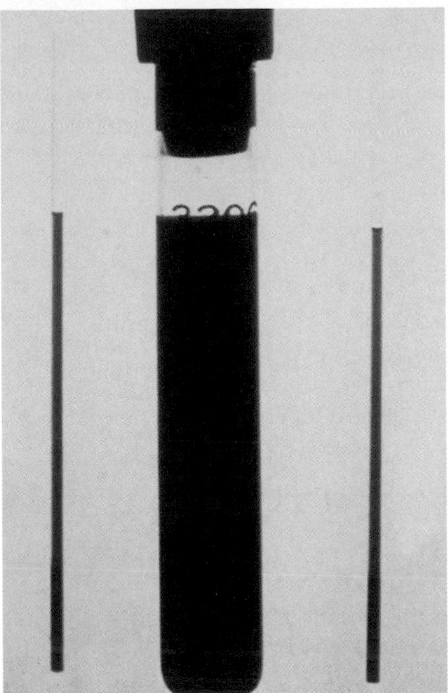

FIGURE 11–4. **Intravascular hemolysis.** Intravascular hemolysis of even a small amount of red blood cells will impart a pink to deep red tint to the plasma, as shown in this spun sample of heparinized blood.

usually suffice. A venous sample should be collected carefully using heparin or ethylenediaminetetraacetic acid (EDTA) as an anticoagulant, immediately centrifuged, and the color of the plasma observed. Quantitation of the plasma hemoglobin is performed using a dye such as benzidine or ortholidine, both of which turn blue in the presence of hemoglobin and hydrogen peroxide. A **plasma hemoglobin level of 50 mg/dL or higher** suggests intravascular hemolysis. It is at this point that the plasma first becomes pinkish. Once the level exceeds 150–200 mg/dL, plasma will be bright red (see Figure 11–4) and there will be accompanying hemoglobinuria.

Plasma hemoglobin levels below 50 mg/dL cannot be accurately measured and may be the result of phlebotomy-induced hemolysis. The Hemastix test used for detecting hematuria should never be used to screen for hemoglobinemia. It is much too sensitive and will invariably give a positive result, even in normal subjects.

2. Urine hemoglobin—Hemoglobinuria is suggested when the urine is red or brownish in color after centrifugation to remove intact red blood cells. A qualitative measurement is possible using the Hemastix but the Hemastix reaction does not distinguish hemoglobinuria from myoglobinuria. If the plasma hemoglobin level is elevated, it can be assumed that the pigment in urine is hemoglobin. If this is not the case, the 2 pigments must be separated using electrophoresis or differential solubility in ammonium sulfate.

3. Urine hemosiderin—Urine hemoglobin is reabsorbed by renal tubular cells and broken down to form hemosiderin.

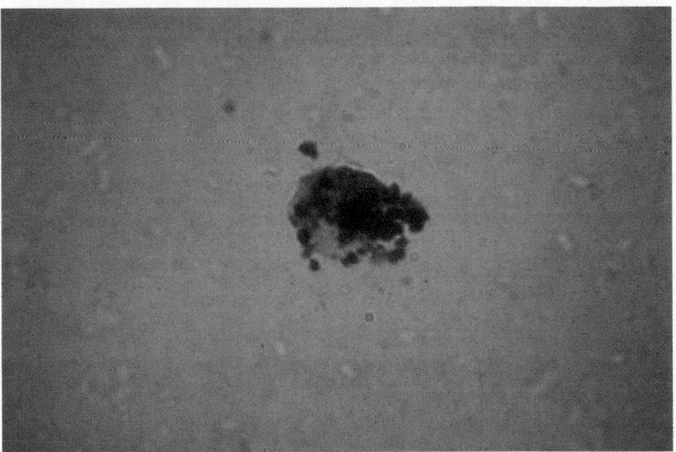

FIGURE 11–5. **Urine hemosiderin.** Detection of tubular cells containing visible iron granules on Prussian blue stain is a sensitive measure of recent intravascular hemolysis.

Following an intravascular hemolytic event, patients will shed tubular cells containing visible hemosiderin granules for several days to a week or more. This can be detected by performing a Prussian blue stain on the spun sediment of a random urine. A true positive should have distinct blue granules within intact tubular cells (Figure 11–5). Free iron outside of cells is generally a contaminant.

4. Serum haptoglobin—Haptoglobin is an α_2-globulin that binds in an equal molar ratio to free hemoglobin. The complex is then cleared from circulation by the liver. Both intravascular and severe extravascular hemolysis are associated with a depletion of the serum haptoglobin level. Normal serum haptoglobin is 50–200 mg/dL or higher in patients with inflammatory illness.

The serum haptoglobin level is easily quantitated by standard turbidometric methods and is often provided as a routine part of a serum protein profile. The pattern of behavior of the serum haptoglobin level after a hemolytic event is illustrated in Figure 11–3. It is possible to see a normal haptoglobin level immediately after the initiation of an intravascular hemolytic event, simply because the haptoglobin-hemoglobin complex has not yet been cleared from circulation. Conversely, abnormally low or absent haptoglobin levels are commonly seen in patients with liver failure or, rarely, due to genetic absence of the protein or a defect in binding sites on the molecule.

5. Methemalbumin—Following an intravascular hemolytic event of sufficient severity to deplete serum haptoglobin, increased amounts of methemalbumin may be detectable in plasma for several days (see Figure 11–3). Methemalbumin can be measured using a spectrophotometer from its absorption band at 625 nm. A more sensitive and quantitative measurement is possible using the Schumm test.

C. Detection of Extravascular Hemolysis

Several laboratory methods are used to detect and diagnose abnormalities of red blood cell membrane, hemoglobin, or intracellular metabolism that lead to an increased rate of extravascular

TABLE 11–3 • Laboratory methods in the diagnosis of extravascular hemolysis

Tests of hemoglobin stability
Hemoglobin electrophoresis Heinz body stains Isopropanol and heat denaturation tests
Tests of membrane structure
Osmotic fragility Autohemolysis test
Tests of metabolic machinery
Autohemolysis test G6PD screen/quantitative assay GSH assay Specific enzyme assays (eg, pyruvate kinase)
Tests of immune destruction
Direct and indirect antiglobulin tests (Coombs test or DAT) Cold agglutinin titer Complement levels Donath-Landsteiner test for PCH

hemolysis (Table 11–3). Some of these are provided as routine clinical tests, whereas others require the expertise of a special hematology laboratory.

1. Tests of hemoglobin stability—Many of the inherited hemoglobinopathies are associated with an increased rate of cell destruction. As discussed in Chapter 7, common hemoglobinopathies such as hemoglobin SS, CC, SC, and compound heterozygotes with thalassemia can be screened with high-performance liquid chromatography (HPLC) and then diagnosed using routine hemoglobin electrophoresis. In addition, **Heinz bodies** (intracellular inclusion bodies—Figure 11–6) may be detected using phase microscopy or a dried blood smear, with or without the supravital stains, brilliant cresyl blue and crystal violet, in patients with unstable hemoglobins or thalassemia. The isopropanol and heat denaturation tests are similarly used to detect patients with unstable hemoglobins.

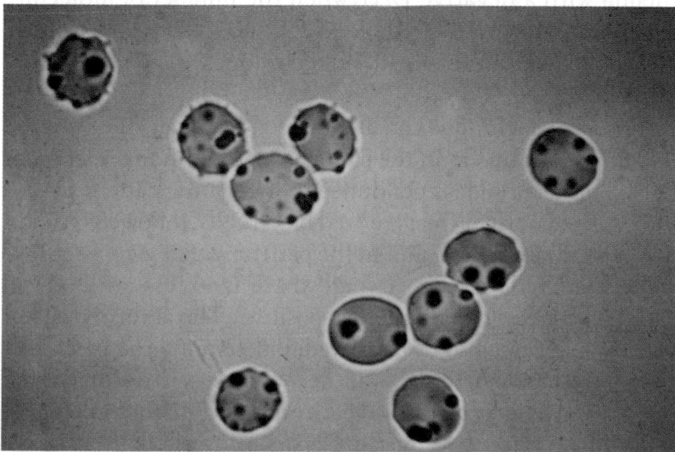

FIGURE 11–6. **Heinz bodies.** Heinz bodies—refractile intracellular hemoglobin precipitates—can be detected in patients with unstable hemoglobins, thalassemias, and G6PD deficiency.

2. Tests of membrane structure—The osmotic fragility and incubated autohemolysis tests are used to confirm the presence of the membrane structural defect seen in patients with hereditary spherocytosis. The **osmotic fragility test** involves subjecting the patient's red blood cells to an increasingly hypotonic environment (Figure 11–7). Normal red blood cells are resistant to hemolysis. This situation is also relatively true for fresh cells from patients with hereditary spherocytosis. Once the cells are incubated for 24 hours, however, the fragility of spherocytic red blood cells is far greater than that observed for normal red blood cells, and they consequentially lyse at higher salt concentrations than do incubated normal cells.

The **autohemolysis test** can help in diagnosing atypical cases of hereditary spherocytosis. This test is performed by incubating defibrinated whole blood with and without the addition of glucose for 48 hours, followed by the measurement of the plasma hemoglobin level (see Figure 11–7). Normal red blood cells show 2% lysis without glucose and even less when glucose is added to the incubated specimen. Hereditary spherocytosis patients show marked hemolysis without glucose, which is largely corrected when glucose is added. Intracellular enzyme defects also give abnormal test results for both the osmotic fragility and autohemolysis tests, but the hemolysis is less correctable by the addition of glucose.

3. Tests of metabolic machinery—Although the osmotic fragility and incubated autohemolysis tests provide a screening

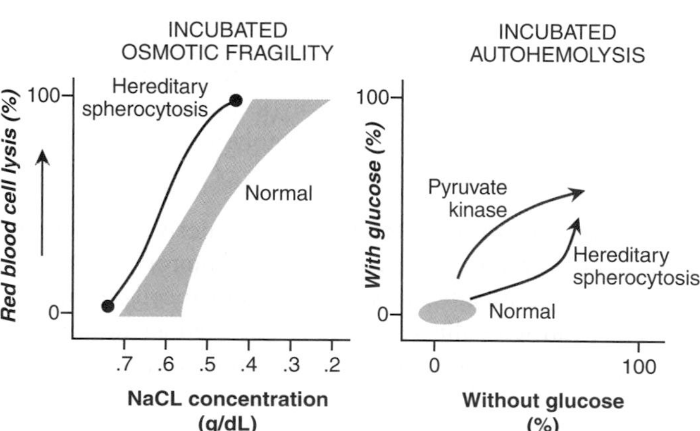

FIGURE 11–7. **Incubated osmotic fragility and autohemolysis tests.** Defects in red blood cell membrane structure (eg, hereditary spherocytosis) and intracellular metabolism (eg, enzymopathies) can be detected and classified using the incubated osmotic fragility and autohemolysis tests. Hereditary spherocytosis patients show a much greater tendency to cell lysis as the cells are suspended in solutions of decreasing salt concentration. This is enhanced by incubating the blood sample for 24 hours. The incubated autohemolysis test can distinguish between hereditary spherocytosis and pyruvate kinase deficiency based on sensitivity to lysis with and without glucose in the medium.

TABLE 11–4 • Causes of intravascular hemolysis

Blood transfusion
ABO mismatched transfusion
Infected blood
Thermal burns
Snake bites
Bacterial/parasitic infections
Clostridial sepsis
Malaria
Babesiosis
Bartonellosis
Mycoplasma pneumoniae
Mechanical heart valves
Paroxysmal hemoglobinuria
PNH
PCH

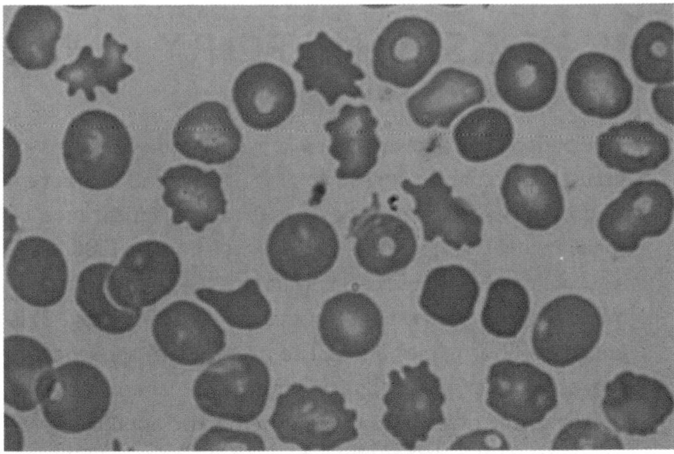

FIGURE 11–9. **Red cell fragmentation.** Schistocytes are commonly seen in patients with third-degree burns, mechanical heart valves, widespread malignancy, and DIC.

causes for acute intravascular hemolysis include severe thermal burns; snake bites; acute infections with ***Clostridium perfringens*, falciparum malaria, babesiosis, or bartonellosis;** and the appearance of a high-titer cold agglutinin. Low grade, chronic intravascular hemolysis is seen in patients with mechanical heart valves or paroxysmal nocturnal hemoglobinuria (PNH). Thrombotic complications can also occur with ongoing hemolysis; free hemoglobin in the plasma (hemoglobinemia) rapidly depletes nitric oxide (NO) and releases erythrocyte arginase, which further inhibits NO synthesis. This has major implications regarding smooth muscle function and clot formation.

Speed is essential in the diagnosis and management of these patients. Both plasma and urine should be examined immediately to document the intravascular nature of the hemolysis. Any obvious cause must also be identified without delay. For example, when a patient is receiving an ABO incompatible unit of blood, the transfusion must be stopped immediately and diuresis with fluids and mannitol initiated without delay. Similarly, patients with clostridial or severe parasitic infections will only survive if appropriate therapy is begun without delay.

When an intravascular hemolytic event is less severe, it will often escape detection for several days. In this situation, measurements of serum haptoglobin, methemalbumin, and urine hemosiderin will need to be used to confirm the intravascular nature of the hemolysis and provide information as to the rate and course of the process (see Figure 11–3). A self-limited hemolytic episode can be retrospectively diagnosed from the pattern of recovery of the serum haptoglobin level and the urine hemosiderin. The CBC and peripheral blood film can also provide important information. For example, in patients with mechanical heart valves, widespread malignancy, or chronic disseminated intravascular coagulation (DIC), the presence of fragmented red blood cells in circulation suggests ongoing hemolysis (Figure 11–9). As the patient improves, these cells tend to disappear. Red blood cell agglutination (Figure 11–10)—clumping of red cells in a disorganized mass—can be seen in patients with high-titer cold agglutinins, secondary to mycoplasma infection or, more rarely, an IgM paraprotein.

Acute Extravascular Hemolysis

A sudden fall in hemoglobin level without evidence of bleeding or intravascular hemolysis (hemoglobinemia or hemoglobinuria) suggests an **acute extravascular hemolytic event.** Once again, the clinical setting will provide valuable information as to the potential cause (Table 11–5). Acute extravascular hemolysis is frequently seen in association with drug therapy in normal individuals as well as patients with enzyme deficiencies, patients with autoimmune diseases, and after certain viral and bacterial infections. Patients who have a

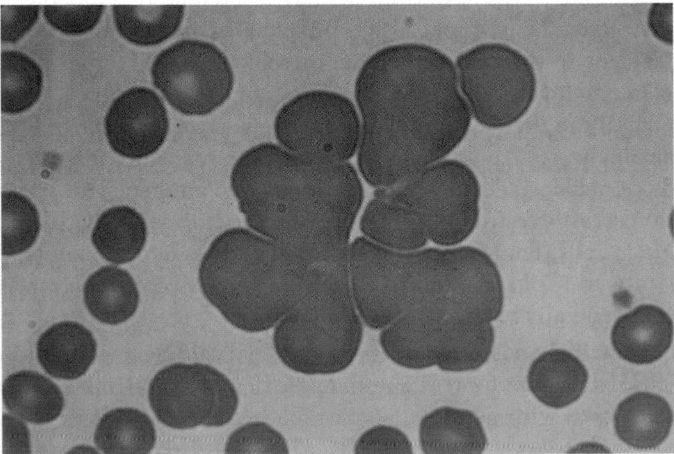

FIGURE 11–10. **Red cell agglutination.** Clumping of red blood cells in disorganized masses is typically seen with high-titer cold agglutinins.

TABLE 11–5 • Causes of extravascular hemolysis

Bacterial and viral infections
Malaria Babesiosis *Mycoplasma pneumoniae* Infectious mononucleosis
Drug-induced hemolysis
G6PD/GSH deficiency Autoimmune drug reactions Strong oxidant drugs/chemicals
Autoimmune hemolysis
Warm-reacting (IgG) AIHA Cold-reacting (IgM) AIHA
Hemoglobinopathies (see Chapter 7)
Membrane structural defect
Hereditary spherocytosis Hereditary elliptocytosis Acanthocytosis
Environmental disorders
Malignancy/DIC TTP/HUS (see Chapter 31) Eclampsia or preeclampsia

chronic, well-compensated hemolytic anemia can also demonstrate dramatic falls in their hemoglobin (hematocrit) secondary to an increased rate of red blood cell destruction or a sudden failure in red blood cell production (eg, parvovirus infection). The relationship of the sudden hemolysis to the chronic hemolytic state may not be apparent if the patient has not been previously diagnosed.

To diagnose an acute, extravascular hemolytic event, clinicians must have a high level of suspicion; otherwise, the event can go undetected for several days. This delay can make diagnosis much more difficult. It is also important to methodically consider and test for more common causes of extravascular hemolysis, especially infections, drugs, and autoimmune disease. Other conditions that must be considered in the differential diagnosis are microangiopathic (fragmentation) hemolysis secondary to malignancy, hemolytic uremic syndrome, and thrombotic thrombocytopenic purpura (see Chapters 31 and 35). In pregnant women, acute hemolysis may be observed late in the third trimester in association with eclampsia, preeclampsia, or HELLP syndrome.

A. Bacterial and Viral Infections

Extravascular hemolysis can occur with several bacterial, parasitic, and viral infections. Mild, self-limited destruction of older red blood cells in circulation is typical of almost all bacterial infections (see Chapter 4). This is not associated with ongoing hemolysis; septic patients typically present with a hypoproliferative anemia.

More severe hemolysis is seen in patients with malaria (Figure 11–11), babesiosis, bartonellosis, clostridial sepsis, and Epstein-Barr virus (EBV) and mycoplasma infections. The severity of the hemolysis in malaria patients depends on the organism involved. Most **patients with vivax and other non-falciparum malaria** have relatively mild extravascular hemolysis. However, up to 20% of patients with falciparum malaria can have severe intravascular hemolysis (black water fever). The patient's ABO blood type is a significant factor in determining both the incidence of infection and the severity of hemolysis. Type O patients are relatively resistant to both infestation and marked hemolysis, while type A individuals are at great risk of overwhelming infection, severe intravascular hemolysis, and cytokine-induced marrow suppression. In babesiosis, the severity of the anemia correlates with the percentage red blood cells seen to contain the organism; levels greater than 50% are associated with high morbidity and mortality. **Clostridial sepsis** can also be associated with severe, life-threatening intravascular hemolysis. A self-limited, usually mild hemolytic event is often seen during the convalescent phase of ***Mycoplasma pneumoniae*** in association with the appearance of high-titer polyclonal

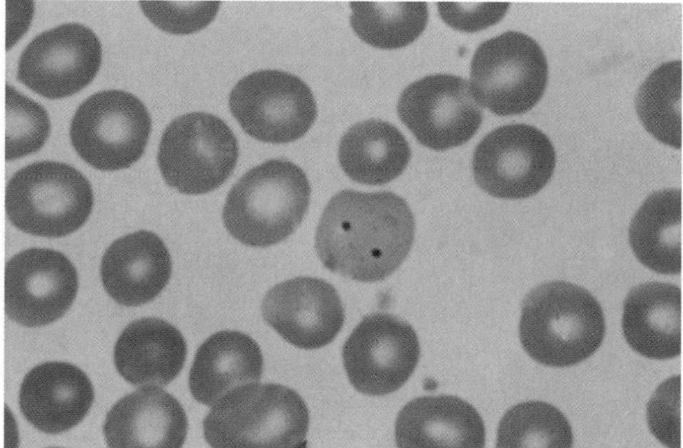

A

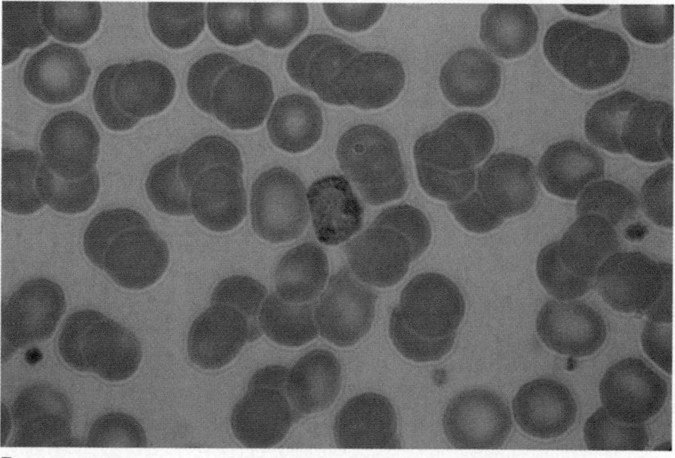
B

FIGURE 11–11. **Malaria.** Immature ring forms **(A)** and mature **(B)** trophozoites of Plasmodium vivax in adult red blood cells.

cold agglutinins. **Acute EBV infection (infectious mononucleosis)** can also produce an impressive hemolytic anemia secondary to marked cell-mediated immune response or proliferation/activation of the macrophage system.

B. Drug-Induced Hemolysis

Drugs induce hemolysis by an immune mechanism or by challenging metabolic machinery of the red blood cell. The latter is a very common scenario in patients with G6PD or GSH deficiency. Drugs associated with acute hemolysis in G6PD-deficient patients are listed in Table 11–6. They all share the characteristic of being oxidant compounds that overwhelm the phosphogluconate pathway, which results in denaturation of hemoglobin. Chemicals and drugs such as dapsone, phenylhydrazine, aniline dyes, and potassium or sodium chlorates can produce hemolysis in normal individuals by the same mechanism.

1. X-linked A-variant G6PD deficiency—The most common form of G6PD deficiency in the United States is the X-linked A-variant. Up to 10% of African American males are at risk. Typically, A-variant G6PD-deficient patients, who have normal basal hemoglobin levels, will demonstrate a decrease in the hemoglobin to 9–11 g/dL in association with an acute illness, often while taking 1 or more oxidant drugs (see Table 11–6).

The mechanism involved in G6PD deficiency is a failure to generate sufficient NADPH to maintain GSH levels and prevent hemoglobin oxidation. Intracellular aggregates of denatured hemoglobin, called **Heinz bodies** (see Figure 11–6), form and result in red cell trapping and destruction within the spleen. Hemolysis is self-limited once the population of older cells that have low G6PD levels are lost from circulation. In the A-variant form of the disease, younger red blood cells have normal or even high G6PD levels (reticulocytes). Therefore, as long as the patient is able to increase red blood cell production, the anemia will correct, even if the causative drug is continued.

The **ability of the patient to recover spontaneously** must be recognized both in diagnosis and management. If there is a delay in detecting the anemia, a hematologic evaluation can show a brisk reticulocytosis and return of the hemoglobin level toward normal. In addition, it is **not essential that all drugs with oxidant potential be withdrawn.** For example, in patients who require malarial prophylaxis, the drug(s) can be continued, recognizing that the patient will compensate with a sustained increase in red cell production. Patients (up to 5% of Ashkenazi Jews, Asians, and Mediterranean populations) with the Mediterranean form of G6PD deficiency or severe GSH deficiency are at risk for more severe hemolysis. Drug therapy or fava bean ingestion can precipitate a severe, even fatal hemolytic event with both extravascular and intravascular hemolysis. In such patients, the offending agent must be stopped.

2. Drug-induced immune hemolytic anemia—Drug-induced immune hemolytic anemia has been observed with several drugs (see Table 11–6). At least 4 different mechanisms can be involved, including the formation of antibodies specific to the drug, the induction of antibodies to natural antigens on the red blood cell membrane, the formation of an antigen-antibody complex, and the selective binding of the antibiotic to the cell membrane with formation of a complement-fixing antibody. **Penicillin** is the best example of the first phenomenon, because if given in high doses, it binds to the red blood cell membrane. If the patient then forms an antibody against the penicillin, red blood cells will be removed and destroyed by the monocyte-macrophage system. The hemolytic process is rapidly controlled by simply withdrawing the penicillin. Cephalosporins and semisynthetic penicillins show cross-reactivity with penicillin antibodies. Moreover, **second- and third-generation cephalosporins** have been associated with severe autoimmune hemolytic anemia and should be automatically discontinued in any patient who presents with a positive DAT. **Quinidine** can cause immune hemolysis as well as immune thrombocytopenia. The quinidine acts as the haptene for an incomplete anti–red blood cell antibody. Therefore, withdrawal of the drug stops the hemolysis.

α-Methyldopa is an example of a drug that somehow alters T-cell suppressor function to induce an autoantibody to the Rh antigens on the red blood cell membrane. Up to 40% of patients taking α-methyldopa will develop a positive DAT; however, very few patients (<1%) ever develop a hemolytic anemia. **Stibophen** appears to act by the formation of antigen-antibody complexes that bind to red blood cells and induce hemolysis. **Streptomycin** binds specifically to the M or D antigens on the red blood cell membrane. If patients develop a complement-fixing antibody to streptomycin, they can demonstrate hemolysis. A common theme in all patients with drug-induced immune hemolytic anemias is the presence of a positive DAT for IgG. Patients receiving streptomycin can show a positive DAT with both anti-IgG and anti-C3 sera.

The use of purine nucleoside analogues **(fludarabine and cladribine)** in the treatment of patients with malignant lymphoproliferative disorders has also been associated with the appearance of a warm antibody that causes some hemolysis. The mechanism behind this is unclear, though it has been proposed that a suppressed autoantibody to red cell membrane antigen(s) is released secondary to treatment-related T-cell lymphopenia.

TABLE 11–6 • Drugs associated with hemolysis

Oxidant drugs—G6PD deficiency
Antibiotics (nalidixic acid, nitrofurantoin, sulfa drugs, dapsone) Antimalarials (primaquine) Pyridium Doxorubicin
Immune mediated
Drug-specific antibodies—penicillin (cephalosporins, synthetic penicillins) Antibody-haptene (drug) combination (quinidine) Autoantibody to Rh antigens (α-methyldopa) T-cell immunomodulation (fludarabine, cladribine) Antigen-antibody complex (stibophen) Complement-fixing antibody (streptomycin)

It is important that therapy be immediately discontinued to avoid a fatal outcome.

C. Autoimmune Hemolytic Anemia

Autoimmune hemolytic anemias can be anticipated in such clinical situations as viral/bacterial infections and collagen vascular diseases and in association with lymphoproliferative disorders.

1. Patterns of hemolysis—Each clinical situation tends to have a predictable pattern of hemolysis. For example, patients who are recovering from ***M. pneumoniae*** can develop a high-titer cold agglutinin that results in an acute hemolytic episode over several days. **Patients with acute infectious mononucleosis** can develop an IgM cold agglutinin with anti-i specificity some weeks into the illness, associated with both hemolysis and thrombocytopenia.

If the clinician watches and documents the temporal nature of the hemolytic event, the diagnosis should be relatively easy. In both groups of patients, it should be possible to document a rise in the cold agglutinin titer, a negative anti-IgG DAT, and in some patients, a positive anti-C3 DAT. The demonstration of anti-i specificity in infectious mononucleosis patients is diagnostic. On occasion, **acute EBV infection** will stimulate proliferation and activation of the macrophage system with striking hemophagocytosis apparent in the marrow. These patients can exhibit pancytopenia and marrow hypoplasia, together with severe liver dysfunction and coagulopathies.

Acute and chronic extravascular hemolysis can accompany **collagen vascular disease** and lymphomas. **Patients with lupus erythematosus** will often present with a DAT-positive hemolytic anemia or immune thrombocytopenia or both. Autoimmune hemolytic anemia is an anticipated complication in the management of patients with **chronic lymphocytic leukemia,** a situation made worse by the possibility of inducing a warm antibody by treatment with fludarabine or cladribine (see section on drug-induced hemolytic anemias). Immune hemolysis has also been seen following stem cell and solid organ transplantation. However, the most common presentation of an immune hemolytic anemia is as an **autoimmune idiopathic hemolytic anemia (AIHA).**

2. Autoimmune idiopathic hemolytic anemia—AIHA patients usually have no clinical manifestations of other disease; their only finding is the extravascular hemolytic anemia. In most cases, the **erythropoietic profile** is typical of a relatively severe hemolytic anemia. The marrow E/G ratio is increased to greater than 1:1 and the reticulocyte index to greater than 3 times normal. Red blood cell morphology is generally normocytic, normochromic, although a varying number of cells may be spherocytic. Fragmentation is not observed and there is little evidence of poikilocytosis. Measurements of cell destruction (ie, the serum indirect bilirubin and LDH levels) are both increased. Patients with very severe AIHA can show reticulocytopenia in the face of marrow erythroid hyperplasia. In this situation, autoantibody is responsible for the rapid removal of newly released reticulocytes.

TABLE 11–7 • Antibody testing in AIHA

	DAT		
AIHA	**Anti-IgG**	**Anti-C3**	**Cold Agglutinins**
Warm-reacting antibody			
70%	Positive	Negative	<1:256
20%	Positive	Positive	
10%	Negative[a]	Weakly positive	
Cold-reacting antibody	Negative	Positive	1:512–1:10,000

[a]*The routine DAT (Coombs test) will not detect AIHA patients with small numbers of IgG molecules per red blood cell. However, much more sensitive testing can be done in specialty laboratories.*

AIHA is classified by laboratory testing as being secondary to either a warm-reacting (IgG) or cold-reacting (IgM) antibody. Rare patients present with a "mixed" AIHA in which both warm- and cold-reacting antibodies are detected. **Patients with a warm-reacting (IgG) AIHA** typically show IgG alone, although some express low levels of C3 (Table 11–7). **Patients with a cold-reacting (IgM) AIHA** will have a negative DAT for IgG and a positive test for C3, a surrogate marker for the presence of an IgM antibody.

3. Cold agglutinin hemolytic anemia—A small percentage of patients with IgM monoclonal proteins (see Chapter 26) will present with a high-titer cold agglutinin capable of causing extravascular red cell hemolysis and, rarely, acute episodes of intravascular hemolysis on exposure to cold. Unlike the transient anemia seen with polyclonal cold agglutinins (*M. pneumoniae*), monoclonal cold agglutinins are associated with more severe, chronic AIHA that is especially resistant to therapy. The typical polyclonal cold agglutinin IgM protein has I/i antigen specificity and variable temperature specificity. As a rule, low-titer cold agglutinins are inactive at temperatures above 20°C, while very high titer agglutinins show much wider thermal amplitudes (ie, they will bind to red cells and activate the complement cascade at temperatures even well above 25°C). Therefore, the titer and temperature of activation generally correlate with the severity of the patient's hemolytic anemia.

Chronic (Lifelong) Extravascular Hemolysis

Patients with inherited defects in cell membrane function, hemoglobin structure, or intracellular metabolism generally present with a lifelong history of anemia. Racial background and family history provide important clues to the nature of the anemia. The erythropoietic profile reflects a compensated hemolytic anemia with marked expansion of marrow erythroid progenitors (E/G ratio >1:1) and a reticulocyte production index that is 3 times normal or higher. Depending on the level of red cell production, the severity of the anemia can be quite variable. For example, patients with hereditary spherocytosis (HS), as long as they are healthy, can maintain an increased level of red cell production sufficient to nearly normalize their hemoglobin level.

The detection and diagnosis of a chronic hemolytic anemia is largely a laboratory exercise. It helps to have a well-organized approach to the workup, one that starts with simple tests available from the routine laboratory. From this viewpoint, the **examination of the peripheral blood film for abnormalities of red blood cell morphology** is the best starting point (Table 11–8). Unique red blood cell shape changes such as sickling, targeting, and spherocytosis are obvious clues to the cause of the hemolytic anemia. In fact, when taken in the context of the clinical picture, red blood cell morphology may be enough to make the diagnosis. If not, it at least guides the selection of additional confirmatory laboratory tests. It also helps to systematically **consider the most likely causes** of chronic hemolysis, grouped according to the broad categories of hemoglobinopathies, defects in membrane structure, abnormalities in intracellular metabolism, and disorders of the environment.

A. Hemoglobinopathies

Inherited abnormalities of hemoglobin structure and stability can result in a significant shortening of red blood cell lifespan. When severe, the erythropoietic profile will fit the picture of a chronic hemolytic anemia. Homozygous sickle cell disease is an excellent example of this presentation (see Chapter 7). Patients with thalassemia major or unstable hemoglobins can also have a hemolytic component to their disease. The laboratory detection and diagnosis of these conditions are discussed more extensively in Chapters 6 and 7. It involves the selective use of laboratory methods such as hemoglobin electrophoresis, brilliant cresyl blue and crystal violet stains for Heinz bodies, and the isopropanol and heat-stability screening tests.

TABLE 11–8 • Red blood cell morphology in the diagnosis of hemolytic anemias

Red Blood Cell Morphology	Possible Diagnoses	Confirmatory Tests
Sickle cells	Sickle cell anemia, SC disease, and S-β–thalassemia	Hemoglobin electrophoresis
Target cells	Hemoglobin C or SC disease, thalassemia, and severe liver disease	Hemoglobin electrophoresis
Spherocytes	Hereditary spherocytosis, autoimmune hemolytic anemia	Osmotic fragility, incubated autohemolysis, and DAT
Elliptocytes	Hereditary elliptocytosis	—
Stomatocytosis	Cirrhosis, malignancies, cardiovascular disease, and Rh antigen deficiency	—
Acanthocytosis	Cirrhosis/pancreatitis and abetalipoproteinemia	Lipoprotein assay
Fragmentation	Heart valves, DIC, malignancies, thermal burns, TTP, HUS	—

B. Membrane Structural Defects

Abnormalities in membrane protein composition can result in lifelong, well-compensated hemolytic anemia. Hereditary spherocytosis (HS) and hereditary elliptocytosis (HE) are the best clinical examples of this disorder.

1. Hereditary spherocytosis—HS is inherited in an autosomal dominant pattern in 60%–70% of patients and tends to have a similar clinical picture from generation to generation. Sporadic mutations of the dominant type make up another 20% of cases, whereas from 10%–15% of patients are classified as recessive. In the latter case, both parents have minor signs of disease and the patient presents with a much more severe anemia. HS is the most common inherited hemolytic anemia in Europe and the United States, with a frequency as high as 1 in 1,000–2,500 individuals. Multiple null and missense mutations and abnormalities in RNA processing result in unique mutations for each kindred.

The **principal molecular defect in HS** is a deficiency in spectrin or ankyrin or, less frequently, band 3 or protein 4.2, all of which are key membrane skeletal proteins. Most HS patients of northern European extraction demonstrate a silencing of the ankyrin gene, which then interferes with spectrin tethering and causes spectrin-rich vesiculation of the red cell membrane. This "vertical defect" results in a progressive loss of membrane lipid and surface area, as well as intracellular fluid leading to the formation of dense microspherocytes (see Chapter 1 and Figure 11–12). Clinically, HS is most often first detected because of the **presence of spherocytes on the peripheral blood film** and/or **an increase in the MCHC** to greater than 35% (a reflection of a disproportionate loss of membrane and intracellular fluid). The incubated osmotic fragility test can be used to confirm the HS membrane defect (see Figure 11–4).

Patients with HS can be clinically silent or have a compensated hemolytic anemia that ranges from very mild to quite severe. About a third of HS patients have a very mild form of the disease, with little or no anemia and a reticulocyte production index of 2–3 times normal but no higher. They have a fully compensated hemolytic "anemia" and may show few if any spherocytes on smear. The majority of HS patients, however, have a mild to moderately severe anemia, a reticulocyte index greater than 3, and prominent spherocytosis. They also have splenomegaly and may present with jaundice when their hemolysis is further increased in association with a viral or bacterial infection. These patients also complain of easy fatigability and a loss of vitality that is disproportionate to the severity of their anemia. Fewer than 5% of patients will present as neonates with a severe, life-threatening anemia. The latter are generally cases of autosomal recessive inheritance.

Regardless of the severity of the anemia, all HS patients are at risk for episodes of hemolytic or aplastic crisis and the development of pigment gallstones. Since the threat of gallstone cholecystitis is very high, laparoscopic cholecystectomy should

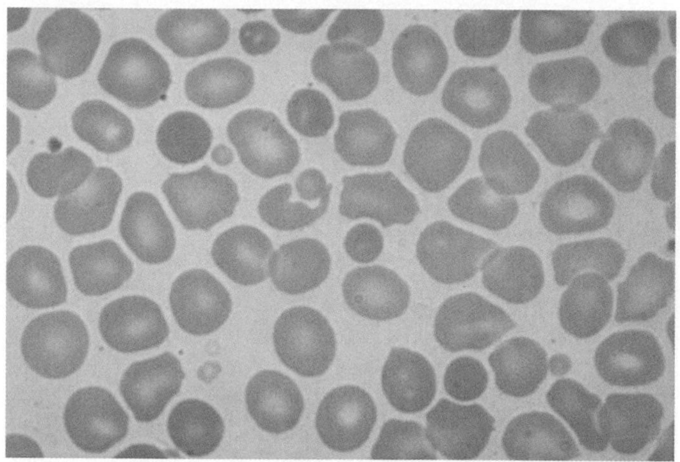
A

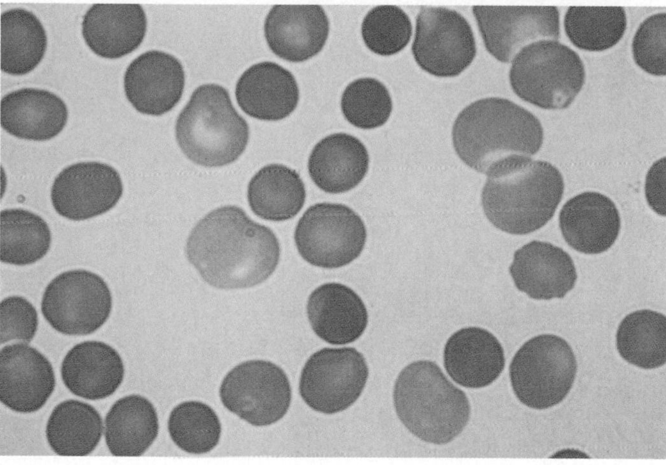
B

FIGURE 11–12. **Spherocytosis.** Patients with hereditary spherocytosis will exhibit varying numbers of microspherocytes in circulation, from relatively few **(A)** to overwhelming numbers **(B)**, depending on the severity of their disease.

be considered in most patients with moderately severe HS or those who develop biliary colic. An increase in hemolysis and transient worsening of the anemia (hemolytic crisis) is a recurrent problem with any viral or bacterial infection. Aplastic crisis is associated with parvovirus B19 infection. The virus attacks red cell precursors (Figure 11–13) and produces a profound but transient (10- to 14-day) failure in new red cell production with marked reticulocytopenia. Once antibody formation occurs, the parvovirus infiltration is cleared and the patient is immune to recurrences. Megaloblastic anemia can result from relative folic acid deficiency, since HS patients have an increased requirement for folate due to their high levels of red cell production.

2. Hereditary elliptocytosis—Patients with HE have an abnormality of the interaction of spectrin molecules, spectrin with the 4.1 protein, or with glycophorin C in the red cell membrane. This abnormality interferes with "horizontal stability" and pliability, making it difficult for the red blood cell to regain its biconcave shape after distortion in the microcirculation (see Chapter 1). HE is inherited as an autosomal dominant disorder

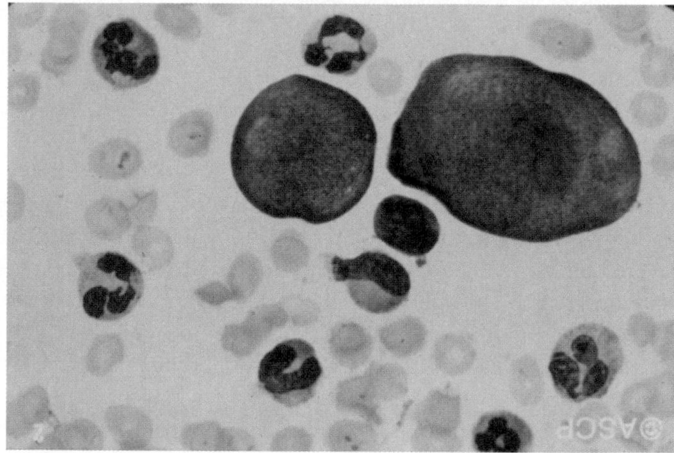

FIGURE 11–13. **Parvovirus infection.** Note the diagnostic finding of large nuclear inclusions in erythroid progenitors.

and is most prevalent in areas of endemic malaria. Depending on the origin of a patient's family, the frequency of HE can range from 3 in 100 to 1 in 4,000. Genetically, HE can result from a variety of mutations involving spectrin, protein 4.1, and the glycophorin C genes. Most patients with HE are heterozygous for one or another genetic mutation. Fewer than 10% of HE patients are homozygous or compound heterozygous and demonstrate severe hemolysis and marked anemia.

The **diagnosis of the most common heterozygous form of HE** is usually an incidental finding on a routine CBC. Most red blood cells on the peripheral blood film (50%–100%) have a uniform elliptical (oval) shape (Figure 11–14). Occasional rod-shaped cells may also be present. In contrast to other conditions where a few oval cells may be observed (eg, megaloblastic anemias), there is little or no poikilocytosis and the MCV is normal in HE. Rarely do patients with common HE variant develop significant hemolysis or anemia. In contrast, patients

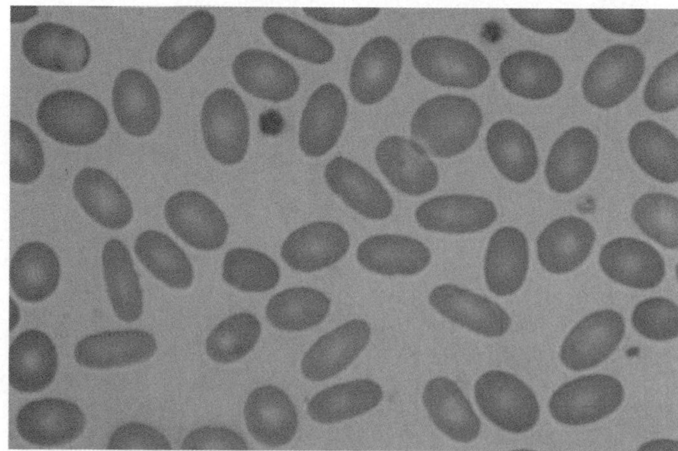

FIGURE 11–14. **Elliptocytosis.** Patients with hereditary elliptocytosis demonstrate a uniform population of oval-shaped cells that is virtually diagnostic of this condition.

with homozygous or compound heterozygous defects present with moderate to severe, even transfusion-dependent hemolytic anemias.

Other **less common forms of elliptocytosis** include spherocytic elliptocytosis (a phenotypic hybrid of HS and HE); Southeast Asian elliptocytosis (a band 3 mutation); and **hereditary pyropoikilocytosis (HPP).** Each has a somewhat different morphology. This is especially true of HPP, which presents as a severe hemolytic anemia with bizarre poikilocytes, budding red cells, and red cell fragments on smear. The name of the disorder is derived from the observation that the red cells have an unusual thermal instability pattern. The underlying defect, however, as in HE, involves a spectrin mutation. Southeast Asian elliptocytosis may have a protective effect against malaria.

3. Laboratory confirmation of HS/HE diagnosis— Characteristic morphology, coupled with a positive family history and an appropriate clinical presentation, can be enough to diagnose HS or HE. Laboratory confirmation is done using the **osmotic fragility and autohemolysis tests.** Direct assay of membrane proteins by **polyacrylamide gel electrophoresis** is only necessary when the clinical picture is atypical. If fragility of the patient's red blood cells is measured, it is important to order an **incubated** osmotic fragility test to bring out the underlying defect (see Figure 11–4).

4. Acanthocytosis—Acanthocytosis, another disorder of membrane structure, is seen in patients with abetalipoproteinemia (congenital absence of apolipoprotein-β) and as a complication of severe cirrhosis or pancreatitis. It results from accumulation of nonesterified cholesterol or sphingomyelin on the outer layer of the lipid membrane. This distorts the membrane configuration and produces a characteristic spiculated-spur shape of the acanthocyte (Figure 11–15).

5. Stomatocytosis—Stomatocytosis (Figure 11–16) is seen in patients with cirrhosis, neoplasms, cardiovascular diseases, and as an inherited defect characterized by marked reduction in the expression of Rh antigen on the cell membrane. Congenital stomatocytosis has been associated with vasoocclusive events, especially pulmonary hypertension. Osmotic fragility is increased, reflecting a loss of red cell membrane.

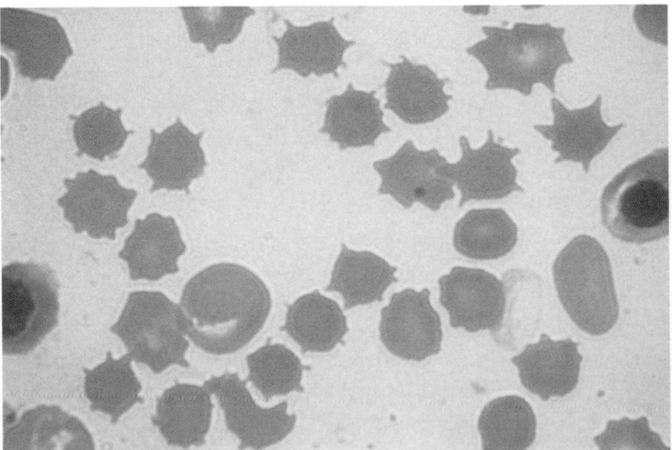

FIGURE 11–15. **Acanthocytosis.** The characteristic spiculated shape of the red blood cells is typical of acanthocytosis, typically seen with abetalipoproteinemia, and in patients with cirrhosis and/or pancreatitis.

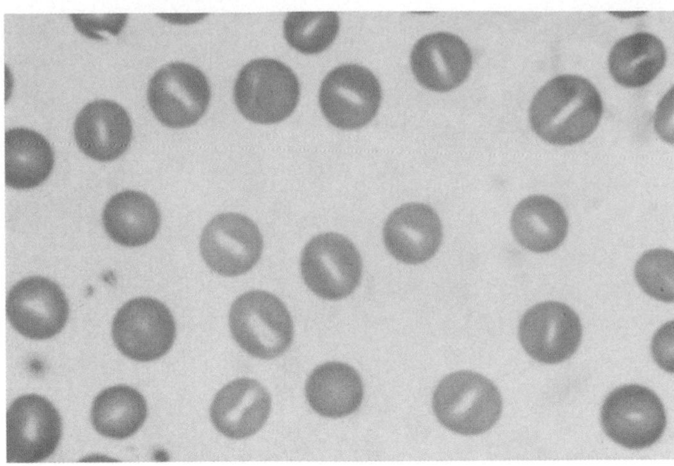

FIGURE 11–16. **Stomatocytosis.** Stomatocytes, cells with a mouth-shaped concavity, are seen as an inherited defect, as well as in patients with liver disease, neoplasms, and cardiovascular disease.

C. Intracellular Metabolic Defects

The principal metabolic pathways of the red cell are described in detail in Chapter 1. **Major functions of these pathways** include maintenance of protein integrity, membrane structure, and cell shape; the continuous reduction of heme-iron to its ferrous state; and production of appropriate amounts of 2,3-diphosphoglycerate (2,3-DPG). A deficiency in any one of the more than 20 enzymes involved in these pathways can result in a clinical abnormality. However, pyruvate kinase, hexokinase, glucose-6-phosphate isomerase, and phosphofructokinase are the enzymes most often linked to a clinically significant hemolytic anemia.

1. Pyruvate kinase deficiency—Pyruvate kinase deficiency **(PK)** is the most common of the Embden-Meyerhof pathway enzymopathies leading to defective glycolysis, adenosine triphosphate (ATP) depletion, and an increase in 2,3-DPG. PK is inherited as an autosomal recessive, missense or nonsense, mutation of a single gene (*PKLR*) on chromosome 1. While more than 160 different mutations have been reported, the clinical phenotypes are quite similar. Homozygous or compound heterozygous patients can present with an anemia that varies from extremely severe to a mild well-compensated hemolytic anemia (nonspherocytic hemolytic anemia). The more severe cases will present in childhood with a marked anemia and abnormal morphology: marked aniso- and poikilocytosis with red cell fragmentation and severely dehydrated cells—xerocytes. The reticulocyte count tends to be unusually high (often >30%–40%) due to an apparent delay in the breakdown of reticulocyte RNA. The incubated osmotic fragility test (see Figure 11–4) will generally distinguish PK from HS, since the PK xerocytes actually have a decreased osmotic fragility. A simple, highly sensitive screening test is also available to test for PK deficiency.

2. Glucose-6-phosphate isomerase—Glucose-6-phosphate isomerase **(GPI)** is the second most common enzymopathy responsible for a nonspherocytic hemolytic anemia. GPI deficiency is inherited as an autosomal recessive trait; homozygous or compound heterozygous patients present with an anemia of variable severity and, on occasion, a hemolytic crisis. GPI deficiency can also impact nonerythroid tissues, especially the central nervous system. The gene responsible for GPI (*GPI*) is located on chromosome 19.

3. Other enzymes in the Embden-Meyerhof pathway— Hexokinase, aldolase, phosphoglycerate kinase, and triosephosphate isomerase have been reported as rare causes of nonspherocytic anemia often in combination with a myopathy and neurologic dysfunction. **G6PD deficiency** is the most common of the phosphogluconate pathway enzyme defects (see discussion in the section Drug-Induced Hemolysis). **Glutathione reductase** and **phosphogluconate dehydrogenase deficiencies** are rare, but should be considered in circumstances of a well-documented oxidant-induced hemolysis when tests of G6PD are normal (see earlier discussion in this chapter under Drug-Induced Hemolysis).

D. Disorders of the Environment

Autoimmune hemolysis can also present as a chronic hemolytic anemia, the severity of which can be highly variable depending on the underlying disease process, the level of antibody production, and the activity of the antibody. Although this condition in most patients can be detected using routine polyspecific and monospecific DAT measurements, some patients will evade detection since they have relatively small amounts of antibody on the cell surface. Detection in these patients will require the expertise of a laboratory that uses sophisticated serological testing to detect very small amounts of cell-bound antibody.

As discussed in the section on intravascular hemolysis, mechanical heart valves can be associated with chronic fragmentation hemolysis. Hemolytic anemia is also an integral component of both hemolytic uremic syndrome and thrombotic thrombocytopenic purpura (see Chapter 31). One clue to an environmental disorder is the presence of fragmented cells **(schistocytes)** on the peripheral blood film; another is the appearance of both intravascular and extravascular hemolytic components to the disease.

THERAPY

The management of a patient with hemolytic anemia will vary according to the individual disease state. As a result, an accurate diagnosis is very important. There are also several therapeutic themes that apply to all hemolytic anemias, especially the chronic, well-compensated hemolytic states.

General Guidelines

Whatever the cause of increased destruction of circulating red blood cells, the **erythroid marrow has the capacity to compensate** by increasing production by more than 3- to 5-fold. This compensation is equal to a transfusion of a unit of red blood cells every 2–3 days. This fact, coupled with the innate ability of red blood cells to increase the oxygen delivery to tissues, allows patients to survive disease states where the red blood cell lifespan is as little as 10–20 days. The capacity to compensate depends, however, on the ability of the marrow to respond and the patient's cardiovascular status.

As with any anemia, an increase in red blood cell production depends on an adequate supply of essential substrates, a normal marrow structure, and an appropriate erythropoietin response. Patients who develop kidney or marrow damage as a part of their disease will be unable to respond and therefore will need transfusion to survive. **Adequate iron and folic acid supplies** are extremely important. The patient with intravascular hemolysis who loses iron into the urine will be unable to increase red blood cell production. All hemolytic anemia patients have an increased requirement for folic acid and need to be chronically supplemented (1 mg of folic acid twice a day by mouth). Otherwise, erythropoiesis will become ineffective and red blood cell production will decrease.

Intravascular Hemolysis

The success of treating intravascular hemolysis depends on the cause. In the case of transfusion of **ABO-incompatible blood,** the severity of the reaction will depend on the nature of the mismatch and the amount of blood transfused. The worst reactions are seen in type O patients who are mistakenly transfused with type A blood. If it is detected early and the transfusion is discontinued, little needs to be done other than providing sufficient fluid to induce a diuresis and prevent glomeruli and tubular

CASE HISTORY • *Part 3*

The finding of IgG on the patient's red cells (and potentially also in excess amounts in the plasma) is diagnostic for a (warm-antibody) autoimmune idiopathic hemolytic anemia (AIHA). The low cold agglutinin titer and absence of free hemoglobin in plasma rule out cold-antibody AIHA or intravascular hemolysis.

Questions

- How should this patient be managed?

damage. If there is a delay in detecting the reaction, the kidney is at risk for damage from both disrupted red blood cell membranes damaging the glomeruli and the excess of free hemoglobin that can result in acute tubular necrosis. In this situation, diuresis alone is not enough. The patient should also be treated with mannitol to encourage renal blood flow and decrease hemoglobin reabsorption. If renal shutdown does occur, patients can recover function with time. Transfusion of ABO-incompatible blood can result in severe hypotension, DIC, and the death of the patient.

The treatment of acute intravascular hemolysis associated with **bacterial or parasitic infections** must focus on the treatment of the primary infection. The hemolysis is usually not associated with renal failure. Transfusion may be necessary if the hemolysis is severe and, in the case of heavy infiltration of circulating red cells with malaria or babesia, exchange transfusion is indicated. **Chronic intravascular hemolysis in patients with PNH or mechanical heart valves** can result in iron deficiency and an iron-deficiency anemia (see Chapter 9). This condition may respond to routine iron therapy or may require transfusion. Therapy with eculizumab is indicated for PNH, while evaluation for a structural abnormality in a heart valve may reveal a correctable defect.

Extravascular Hemolysis

Management of acute or chronic extravascular hemolytic anemia involves both evaluating the patient's ability to physiologically compensate for the anemia and treating the specific condition. For example, acute self-limited hemolysis in patients with G6PD deficiency rarely needs treatment. The anemia that results is relatively mild, and the normal marrow production response will return the hemoglobin level to normal. The more important management issue is patient education regarding the drugs and chemicals that provoke hemolysis. On the other hand, patients with a more severe enzyme deficiency state or autoimmune disease can present with a life-threatening anemia. In this situation, transfusion, aggressive chemotherapy, or both will be required. As with the diagnostic workup, patient management needs to be organized according to the mechanism causing the hemolysis.

A. Hemoglobinopathies

The management of the patient with a hemoglobinopathy is discussed in Chapter 7. These patients require lifelong health care support and are at constant risk for both hemolytic and aplastic crises in association with various infections and systemic illness. If they have a severe anemia and require long-term transfusion therapy, they have to be simultaneously treated for iron overload.

B. Membrane Structural Defects

Patients with relatively mild hereditary spherocytosis or hereditary elliptocytosis maintain near normal hemoglobin levels and are generally in good health. Patients with more severe hereditary spherocytosis will be symptomatic. They are also at risk for recurrent hemolytic episodes in association with viral and bacterial infections and aplastic crisis with parvovirus (B19) infection. There is a role for splenectomy to improve red blood cell lifespan and decrease the severity of the anemia, since it almost always results in marked improvement. The patient feels better, the red blood cell lifespan returns to near normal, and the risk of gallstones and hemolytic crises is reduced. If possible, splenectomy should be avoided until after the first decade of life to decrease the risk of postsplenectomy sepsis. Partial splenectomy has been used in some centers to improve red cell lifespan without total loss of spleen phagocytic and immune functions.

After splenectomy, a sustained rise in the hemoglobin level and fall in transfusion requirement is observed, although the patients still demonstrate elevated reticulocyte counts. With partial splenectomy, the splenic remnant rapidly regrows, reaching normal splenic size by 1 year and twice normal size by 4–6 years. Because of this, a second total splenectomy is necessary in one-third of patients. Any patient who receives a splenectomy must receive *H. Influenzae*, meningoccal, and polyvalent pneumococcal vaccine prior to operation. If a total splenectomy is performed before age 10, the child should receive oral penicillin prophylaxis (125–250 mg penicillin per day by mouth).

Because **hereditary spherocytosis patients** are at risk for developing pigment gallstones, a prophylactic, laparoscopic cholecystectomy should be considered early in adult life. Elective cholecystectomy should definitely be performed if a patient has even one attack of cholecystitis or biliary colic because of the risk for recurrent disease.

C. Autoimmune Hemolysis

Management of patients with autoimmune hemolytic anemia will vary according to the nature of the disease process. For example, autoimmune red blood cell destruction associated with drug ingestion eventually stops after withdrawing the offending agent. When the autoimmune process complicates a lymphopoietic malignancy, control of the hemolysis will depend on effective treatment of the tumor. As for AIHA, the choice of therapy will depend on whether the hemolysis is owing to a warm- or cold-reacting antibody.

1. Warm-antibody AIHA—Several therapeutic options are available to treat warm-antibody AIHA. The first choice is always corticosteroids or, in the case of severe disease, steroids plus an immunosuppressive drug such as cyclophosphamide or rituximab.

a. Treatment with corticosteroids—Corticosteroids act by blocking the reticuloendothelial cell clearance of red blood cells coated with either IgG or C3 and the production of new IgG antibody. **Cyclophosphamide and rituximab** act as lympholytic agents to reduce antibody production.

Oral **prednisone** in a daily dose of 60–120 mg (1–1.5 mg/kg) is a typical starting regimen. It should be continued at this level for at least 2 weeks with daily measurements of the CBC and reticulocyte count. The patient's response will vary according to the severity and nature of the disease process. More than half of patients will show an increase in reticulocyte index and hemoglobin level within the first 1–2 weeks. Patients with severe AIHA can show little response or even a worsening of their anemia, however.

Subsequent management of the patient will depend on the observed response. If initial therapy is effective, the prednisone dose will need to be gradually tapered while closely monitoring the CBC. Warm-antibody AIHA will frequently relapse as the prednisone is tapered. Therefore, the taper should be gradual, reducing the daily dosage by increments of 10 mg or less at weekly intervals. As the dosage falls below 20 mg, there is a risk that severe hemolysis can recur suddenly, requiring an immediate return to a higher prednisone dose and the institution of other therapies. If the daily dosage can be brought below 15 mg/d, it may be possible to switch to an every-other-day schedule and thereby reduce the chance of significant side effects.

b. Treatment with combined chemotherapy or splenectomy— Patients who do not respond to steroid therapy or can't be tapered successfully are candidates for **combined chemotherapy** or splenectomy. Cyclophosphamide given in pulse doses of 1,000 mg intravenously on 1–3 occasions may be effective in some patients. It is very useful in patients who present with a severe hemolytic anemia that does not respond to prednisone therapy during the first 2–3 weeks. Rituximab, given in a dose of 375 mg/m^2 weekly for 3–4 weeks, has also been reported to reduce hemolysis in steroid resistant patients. **Splenectomy** can help in the long-term control of autoimmune hemolysis in the prednisone-refractory patient. It works both by removing the trapping function of the spleen and by reducing the level of antibody production. It should generally be performed after the patient is stabilized on chemotherapy. Splenectomy is not a cure by itself and will not eliminate the need for chemotherapy. It can, however, reduce the amount of prednisone, cyclophosphamide, or both needed to control the disease.

c. Other therapies—Warm-antibody AIHA can present as a severe, life-threatening anemia. In this situation, other therapies must be considered. **Transfusion with red blood cells** is clearly indicated, regardless of the difficulties encountered in adequately crossmatching the patient. An attempt should be made to find units of red blood cells that have the minimum activity on the indirect DAT, since it is unlikely that truly "compatible" blood will be identified. Patients can be transfused with type-specific blood when transfusion is required to save the patient's life. It can be anticipated that the survival of transfused red blood cells will be no better or no worse than the survival of the patient's own cells. In warm-antibody AIHA, there should be little or no risk of precipitating an intravascular hemolytic event.

Both intravenous immunoglobulin and plasmapheresis have been used with limited success in the treatment of AIHA. **Immunoglobulin** appears to work by acutely blocking the Fc receptors on reticuloendothelial cells, and perhaps by downregulating antibody production or increasing the fractional clearance of the antibody. If therapy is attempted, at least 5 days of 400 mg/kg/d of one of the commercially available immunoglobulin preparations should be given. If there is a response, it may not be observed for several days and can be short-lived. **Plasmapheresis** or extracorporeal absorption of IgG using an anti-staphylococcal protein-A-silica column may also be beneficial in the severely ill patient.

2. Cold-antibody AIHA—The treatment of a patient with cold-antibody AIHA is significantly different. Little needs to be done for those patients who develop a high-titer cold agglutinin following an infection with ***Mycoplasma*** or EBV virus other than to monitor the severity of the anemia and, if necessary, transfuse the patient. Patients with de novo cold agglutinin disease or lymphopoietic malignancy with a high-titer IgM antibody may respond to treatment with an **alkylating agent.** Usually, corticosteroids are of little benefit. When a patient's anemia is very severe, **plasmapheresis** can be lifesaving, because the major portion of the patient's IgM antibody is intravascular. The response to conventional agents (alkylating agents, interferon-α, purine analogs α is poor at best. Rituximab has been reported to be effective and well tolerated with an overall partial response rate of better than 50%.

As with warm-antibody AIHA, patients with cold-reacting IgM antibodies can receive **transfusions** without risk of precipitating a life-threatening hemolytic episode. However, any patients being treated or transfused at cold temperatures, such as those undergoing cardiac surgery, may be at risk for acute complement-mediated intravascular hemolysis. It is also very important to recognize the essential role of complement in IgM-driven AIHA. In fact, the severity of hemolysis in a patient with cold-antibody AIHA may be suppressed by the depletion of complement in the patient's plasma. In this situation, fresh complement provided as part of a red cell or plasma transfusion can result in a dramatic increase in hemolysis. Such a patient should receive transfusions of washed red blood cells that are free of complement.

CASE HISTORY • *Part 4*

This patient exhibits a severe, even life-threatening hemolytic anemia that requires immediate intervention. Immunosuppression using high-dose corticosteroids and, if needed, cyclophosphamide/rituximab should be started immediately and maintained until the hematocrit and reticulocyte index have normalized. Only then should therapy be slowly tapered while closely watching for signs of relapse. Transfusion of type-specific red blood cells may also be called for if the patient is highly unstable, even though the lifespan of the transfused red cells may be little better than that of the patient's own red cells. In patients who are refractory to immunosuppressive therapy, splenectomy may play a role.

Patients with cold agglutinin disease and a high thermal amplitude IgM antibody can demonstrate dramatic **cold sensitivity.** Even brief exposure of extremities to cold environments can result in an acute hemolytic episode. These patients need to learn how to avoid cold exposure. In addition, any blood product or intravenous fluid must be warmed prior to transfusion. Cold agglutinin disease is generally manageable but not curable. With time, patients become refractory to chemotherapy and transfusion dependent. In addition, the survival of transfused red blood cells becomes progressively shorter. This progression does not respond to splenectomy or other therapeutic options used in warm-antibody AIHA.

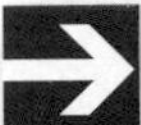

POINTS TO REMEMBER

Hemolytic anemias can present as an intravascular process with hemoglobinemia and hemoglobinuria, or a largely extravascular process where red cells are destroyed in the reticuloendothelial system (spleen, marrow, and liver).

Intravascular hemolysis is often transitory, such that when hemoglobinemia and hemoglobinuria are no longer present because of rapid free hemoglobin clearance, serial measurements of haptoglobin and methemalbumin levels, and the detection of hemosiderinuria may allow a retrospective diagnosis.

Extravascular hemolysis is associated with increases in LDH and indirect bilirubin levels and, when sustained, an impressive increase in red blood cell production as reflected in the reticulocyte count (reticulocyte index >3).

The differential diagnosis of a hemolytic episode/anemia is complex. Red cell morphology may provide a major clue (red cell fragmentation, spherocytosis, parasite infestation, etc). However, accurate diagnosis requires a number of laboratory tests to look for defects in hemoglobin stability, membrane structure, and metabolic pathways, as well as autoimmune disease and disorders of the environment.

The most common causes of acquired extravacular hemolysis are drug-induced hemolysis, especially the episodic hemolysis seen in patients with type A-G6PD deficiency who are exposed to oxidant drugs, and autoimmune idiopathic hemolytic anemia (AIHA).

Chronic (lifelong) extravascular hemolysis is the rule in patients with hemoglobinopathies (sickle cell anemia—see Chapter 7), membrane structural defects (hereditary spherocytosis, hereditary elliptocytosis, etc), and metabolic defects (pyruvate kinase deficiency, etc).

AIHA can be classified as secondary to an IgG antibody (warm-reacting antibody) or an IgM antibody (cold-reacting antibody) according to the pattern of the routine direct antiglobulin test (DAT or Coombs test) and a measurement of the cold agglutinin titer (IgM).

Treatment of warm-reacting antibody (IgG) AIHA patients depends in large part on the patient's primary diagnosis (ie, idiopathic AIHA or disorders such as lymphoma, chronic lymphocytic leukemia [CLL], lupus erythematosis, etc). Aggressive immunosuppression is usually effective, although chronic low-grade hemolysis may persist in some cases, requiring splenectomy.

Except for the transient IgM-related hemolysis seen with EBV or mycoplasma infections, patients with cold-reacting antibody AIHA tend to be much more resistant to therapy, even when associated with lymphoma.

BIBLIOGRAPHY

Tabbara IA: Hemolytic anemias: diagnosis and management. Med Clin North Am 1992;76:649.

Drug-Induced Hemolysis

Beutler E: Glucose-6-phosphate dehydrogenase (G6PD) deficiency. N Engl J Med 1991;324:169.

Membrane Structural Defects

Eber S, Lux SE: Hereditary spherocytosis: defects in proteins that connect the membrane skeleton to the lipid bilayer. Semin Hematol 2004;41:118.

Gaetani M et al: Structural and functional effects of hereditary hemolytic anemia-associated point mutations in the alpha spectrin tetramer site. Blood 2008;111:5712.

Gallagher PG: Hereditary elliptocytosis: spectrin and protein 4.1R. Semin Hematol 2004;41:142.

Liu SC et al: Alteration of the erythrocyte membrane skeletal ultra-structure in hereditary spherocytosis, hereditary elliptocytosis and pyropoikilocytosis. Blood 1990;76:198.

Palek J, Sahr KE: Mutations of the red blood cell membrane proteins: from clinical evaluation to detection of the underlying genetic defect. Blood 1992;80:308.

Enzyme Defects

van Wijk R, van Solinge WW: The energy-less red blood cell is lost: erythrocyte enzyme abnormalities of glycolysis. Blood 2005;106:4034.

Autoimmune Hemolysis

Berenstsen S et al: Rituxamib for primary chronic cold agglutinin disease: a prospective study of 37 courses of therapy in 27 patients. Blood 2004;103:2925.

Besa EC: Rapid transient reversal of anemia and long-term effects of maintenance intravenous immunoglobulin for AIHA in patients with lymphoproliferative disorders. Am J Med 1988;84:691.

Collins PW, Newland AC: Treatment modalities of autoimmune blood disorders. Semin Hematol 1992;29:64.

Engelfriet CP, Overbeeke MAM, vondem Borne AEGKR: Autoimmune hemolytic anemia. Semin Hematol 1992;29:3.

ANEMIA IN THE ELDERLY • 12

CASE HISTORY • *Part I*

A 77-year-old woman is brought to the Geriatric Center by her family for evaluation of increasing frailty, forgetfulness, and decreased ability to live independently and care for herself. She has a history of at least 2 falls and has lost approximately 15 lbs in the last 3 months. As part of her evaluation, she has a blood count with the following results:

CBC: Hematocrit/hemoglobin - 33%/11 g/dL
MCV - 96 fL　MCH - 34 pg　MCHC - 33 g/dL
RDW-CV - 14%
Reticulocyte count/index - 1.5%/~1
White blood cell count - 5,100/μL
Platelet count - 130,000/μL

• BLOOD SMEAR MORPHOLOGY

Generally normocytic, normochromic red blood cells with slight anisocytosis. No polychromasia and both white blood cell and platelet morphology are normal. Lymphocytes are decreased in number but with normal morphology.

Questions

- Is this patient anemic or does she fall into the appropriate range of normal for her age group?
- If a further workup is in order, what additional laboratory tests should be ordered?

Aging is associated with subtle physiologic changes in the hematopoietic system. Unlike the renal and reproductive systems, primary hematopoietic stem cell failure is very rare. Only the immune system demonstrates a predictable decrease in competence in the elderly (see Chapters 20 and 21). At the same time, the observed incidence of anemia, myelodysplastic disorders, and thrombotic events (see Chapter 36) is progressively greater with each passing decade. This is a result of the convergence of multiple factors, many of which are environmental in origin and are, therefore, reversible.

STEM CELLS AND THE AGING PROCESS

Hematopoietic stem cells (HSC) emerge early in embryonic development and, after residing in the fetal liver, spleen, and thymus, populate the bone marrow and lymph glands. Fetal HSC differ from adult HSC in their rate of proliferation, differentiation, cell surface markers, and regulatory control. While the majority of adult HSC are in the G_0 phase of cell division, they are capable of self-renewal and, despite a constant high level of differentiation needed to constantly repopulate the several lineages of mature blood cells, appear to gradually increase in number. In fact, based on mouse model experiments, there is a 2-fold increase in adult HSC in aging mice. Moreover, as demonstrated by serial transplant studies, these adult HSC are able to repopulate the marrow through 15–50 lifespans.

Adult HSC do age, although the mechanisms underlying the aging process are not well defined. Telomere length, DNA methylation, reactive oxygen species exposure, and accrued DNA damage have all been advanced as playing a role in this aging process. Because of this, individual HSC function decreases with age, while total capacity is made up for by the increased number of HSC. Changes in the marrow microenvironment are also important. The ratio of marrow precursor cells to fat cells decreases in the aging marrow, although rapid expansion of the erythroid marrow secondary to an increase in erythropoietin stimulation is still possible. However, the stromal cells and associated cytokines of the older marrow do appear to be less able to support repopulation following stem cell transplantation.

The pattern of HSC differentiation also changes with aging. The decline of the lymphopoietic cell lineages, particularly B-cell proliferation and differentiation, is the most dramatic, reflecting thymic involution and reduced cytokine levels. At the same time, granulopoiesis increases with age. This may reflect different demands on the immune system in the elderly. While young individuals are busy programming their adaptive immune systems, older adults face a greater threat from bacterial infections, and thus require a rapid granulocytic response.

ANEMIA IN THE ELDERLY

The **incidence of anemia** and associated comorbidities (functional disability, impaired cognition, increased episodes of hospitalization, and death) are reported to increase significantly after age 65. The prevalence by decade, based on the Third National Health and Nutrition Survey (NHANES III phases I and II data, 1988–1994), is illustrated in Figure12–1. The overall incidence of anemia for community-dwelling adults over age 65 was 11% for men and 10.2% for women, but progressively increased to levels exceeding 20% in individuals over age 80. Race/ethnicity also plays a role; the prevalence of anemia in non-Hispanic black men and women has been reported to be 2- to 3-fold higher, but is much less if patients with α-thalassemia, sickle cell trait, and iron deficiency are excluded.

The **prevalence of anemia depends, of course, on the definition of a lower limit of normal** for the hemoglobin in elderly men and women. Most survey studies have used the World Health Organization (WHO) definition of anemia—a hemoglobin less than 13 g/dL in men and less than 12 g/dL in women (Figure 12–2). The use of the lower cutoff point for elderly women, however, may not be as appropriate as it is for premenopausal women. It may, in fact, distort the incidence data, resulting in a falsely low estimate of anemic elderly women. If the less than 13 g/dL cutoff point is used for both sexes, the prevalence of anemia in women would be more than double and exceed levels in comparably aged men. There is a similar issue in regard to the criteria used for estimating anemia prevalence in African American and Hispanic populations.

The traditional definition of "anemia" for the purposes of anemia evaluation and treatment is not necessarily the same as that for predicting functional impairments in elderly populations. Recent epidemiological studies have suggested an independent association of lower hemoglobin levels with functional disabilities, including impaired mobility and cognitive function, as well as overall mortality. Moreover, the severity of the impairment appears to be a continuous function as the hemoglobin level declines below 13 g/dL.

Another argument for considering a higher hemoglobin level as the lower limit of normal is the observed increase in morbidity and mortality in elderly individuals with hemoglobin levels as high as 13–13.5 g/dL (NHANES III study). This was true regardless of the etiology of the anemia. The same is true for nursing home patients, where 50%–60% of long-term residents are "anemic" and demonstrate a 2- to 3-fold increase in morbidity and mortality as compared to non-anemic patients under similar circumstances. At the same time, there have been no organized studies of the impact of erythropoietin-induced higher hemoglobin levels on functional outcomes. Without such proof, the ability to convincingly separate the role of the hemoglobin level from the impact of other disease processes is lacking.

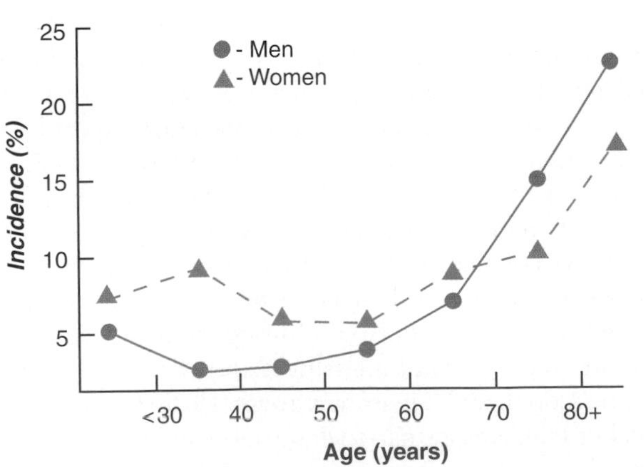

FIGURE 12–1. **Incidence of anemia by age.** The incidence of anemia in community-dwelling individuals increases progressively in the sixth, seventh, and eighth decades of life (based on the NHANES III survey data).

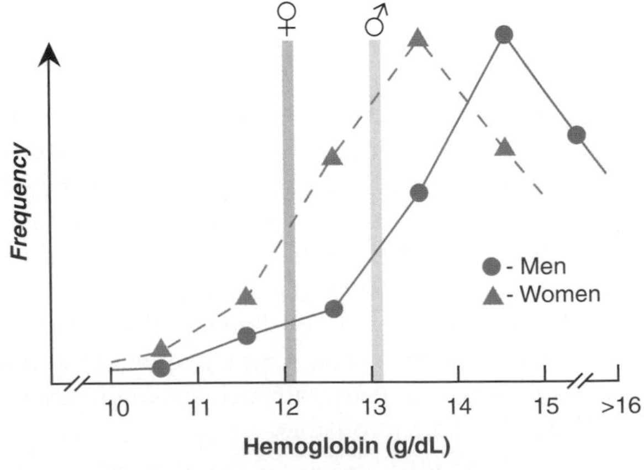

FIGURE 12–2. **Frequency distribution of hemoglobin levels in men and women, aged 65 and older.** Based on the NHANES III survey data, the recommended lower limits of normal (shown as vertical bars) are 13 g/dL in men and 12 g/dL in women. The use of a lower limit of normal (13 g/dL) in women would greatly increase the anemia frequency.

CASE HISTORY • *Part 2*

According to the NHANES III survey, this woman's hemoglobin level is below the lower limit of normal (<12 g/dL) for a community-dwelling woman in her 70s. At the same time, she has a very mild anemia with a hemogram that does not allow an accurate classification (see Chapter 2). In light of this, further evaluation should begin with a battery of tests, including, as a minimum, iron studies (serum iron, iron-binding capacity, and serum ferritin), both serum folate and cobalamin (B_{12}) assays, renal and thyroid function assays, and indirect measures of inflammation (sedimentation rate and C-reactive protein [CRP]).

These studies were drawn with the following results:

Serum iron - 40 μg/dL TIBC - 280 μg/dL Saturation - 14%
Serum ferritin - 55 μg/L
Serum folate - 5 ng/mL
Serum cobalamin - 220 pg/mL
Sedimentation rate - 60 mm/h (Westergren)
C-reactive protein - 3 mg/dL
Serum creatinine - 0.9 mg/dL
BUN - 23 mg/dL
Thyroid studies - within normal limits
Fasting blood glucose - 120 mg/dL

Questions

- Given the age of the patient and the above results, what are the possible etiological factors behind her anemia?
- What additional workup is in order?

TYPES OF ANEMIA

Anemia, as defined by the NHANES III study, is not a natural product of growing old, and therefore should not be ignored. As a practical matter, the "anemia of aging" is most often associated with 1 or more age-related illnesses, which helps guide the evaluation and treatment. The major types of anemia seen in the NHANES III survey of geriatric populations are listed with their relative frequencies in Table 12–1.

The apparently large proportion of elderly patients with anemia categorized as unexplained may be artifactual. The anemia of many individuals in this category may well represent an undiagnosed, slowly evolving dysplastic or sideroblastic anemia. These are often difficult diagnoses to make, requiring repeated blood studies over several years and several bone marrow aspiration/biopsies for morphology and cytogenetic studies (see Chapter 9). Therefore, a single time point survey could easily underestimate their prevalence.

TABLE 12–1 • Types of anemia seen in geriatric populations (NHANES III)

Etiology	Approximate Prevalence (%)
Anemia of chronic inflammation	20
Chronic renal disease	9
Renal disease with inflammation	5
Iron deficiency	17
Vitamin B_{12} and/or folate deficiency	15
"Unexplained" anemia	34

Anemia of Chronic Inflammation (Anemia of Chronic Disease)

Patients with chronic inflammatory conditions predictably demonstrate a mild to moderately severe anemia (see Chapter 4). The mechanisms involved include reduced red cell survival, impairment of the erythropoietin response, and a decrease in functional iron supply to the marrow secondary to **upregulation of the liver protein hepcidin**. Hepcidin and its response to inflammatory cytokines, especially interleukin 6 (IL-6), is the dominant mechanism. Increased blood levels of hepcidin are seen in association with many age-related illnesses—chronic infections, autoimmune disease, and some cancers. Still, even apparently healthy elderly patients can exhibit elevations of IL-6 and other proinflammatory cytokines and higher than normal hepcidin levels.

Since the anemia of inflammation, even when relatively mild, can be an especially strong predictor of morbidity and mortality in the elderly, a full workup is essential. This includes both proof of the nature of the anemia and a careful workup of associated disease processes, in as much as an inflammatory-based anemia will generally resolve once an underlying condition is treated successfully. The approach to anemia workup is discussed in detail in Chapter 4. In essence, the hematopoietic

characteristics of an inflammatory anemia are a hemoglobin level of 10–12 g/dL (mild to moderately severe anemia); normocytic to slightly microcytic red blood cell indices (mean cell volume [MCV] 80–90 fL); low reticulocyte index; and iron studies typical of inflammation, that is, decreased serum iron and iron-binding capacity (percent saturation of 10%–20%) and a normal to slightly elevated serum ferritin level. This pattern of iron studies distinguishes an inflammatory anemia (functional iron deficiency) from absolute iron deficiency where the iron-binding capacity is high, the percent saturation falls below 10%, and the serum ferritin is less than 15 μg/L (see Chapter 5).

As they become clinically available, direct measurements of blood IL-6 and hepcidin levels should increase the sensitivity and specificity for the differential laboratory diagnosis of an inflammatory-based anemia. It will also help distinguish components of inflammation from those of concurrent absolute iron deficiency and/or renal disease. At present, measurements of C-reactive protein (CRP) and sedimentation rate must serve as indirect indicators of an inflammatory state. Even when none of these studies are definitive, the importance of looking for an associated illness with an inflammatory component cannot be overemphasized. A patient with very mild inflammatory-based anemia may never show the distinctive changes in serum iron, iron-binding capacity, and serum ferritin, but nevertheless will respond to effective treatment of their primary disorder.

Chronic Renal Disease and Progressive Renal Failure

Chronic renal disease and progressive renal failure are associated with increasingly severe anemia. The potential mechanisms involved are several and include reduced red blood cell survival, impaired erythropoietin production, stem cell resistance to erythropoietin stimulation, and concurrent inflammation.

Progressive loss of renal mass is recognized as a predictable part of the aging process. The major loss involves the cortex and is associated with a falling glomerular filtration rate (GFR) and creatinine clearance as glomeruli are obliterated. By age 70–80, renal mass has decreased by 30% or more and the percent of hyalinized glomeruli can exceed 30%. The GFR declines progressively with aging, falling from approximately 140 mL/min/1.73m^2 at age 30 to 90–100 mL/min/1.73m^2 at age 80. At the same time, the serum creatinine level does not show a comparable increase, most likely related to the decrease in muscle mass in the elderly.

Renal vascular disease, hypertension, and diabetes are additive factors in the decline in renal function with age and also in predicting the frequency and severity of the patient's anemia. The NHANES III survey identified nearly 14% of anemic individuals over age 65 as suffering from chronic renal disease or the combination of renal disease and inflammation. At the same time, correlating the loss of renal function with the severity of anemia in the aged is difficult. While there is an apparent linear correlation between hemoglobin levels and creatinine clearance with aging, creatinine clearance by itself, once age is excluded, shows a relatively poor correlation with anemia incidence and severity. In fact, the creatinine clearance must fall to levels below 30% of normal before the incidence of anemia is significantly increased (Figure 12–3).

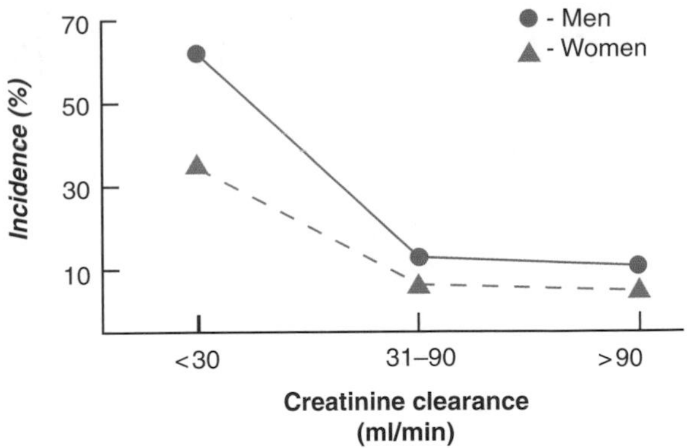

FIGURE 12–3. **Incidence of anemia in elderly individuals with renal failure.** The creatinine clearance must fall below 30 mL/min before the incidence of anemia in community-dwelling elderly is significantly increased.

Impairment of erythropoietin production has been advanced as the most likely mechanism responsible for renal disease–associated anemia in the elderly. Diabetic patients often develop anemia well before advanced renal failure, based on their vasculopathy and damage to the peritubular interstitial cells responsible for erythropoietin production. However, measurements of blood erythropoietin levels in nondiabetic, nonhypertensive populations have, in fact, shown an incremental rise in the erythropoietin level with advancing age, even in those who are thought to have the anemia of chronic renal disease. This would suggest the appearance of an age-related reduced sensitivity of the erythroid marrow to erythropoietin, cause unknown. This finding means that measurements of blood erythropoietin levels are of little value, but it does emphasize the need for greater diligence in identifying concurrent diabetes, hypertensive vascular disease, or chronic inflammatory conditions as important etiological cofactors.

While the exact sequence of events leading to the anemia of chronic renal disease remains to be defined, patients with moderate to severe anemia can be effectively treated with recombinant erythropoietin. Resistance to therapy is observed in some patients but relates more to the coexistence of an inflammatory disease and/or absolute iron deficiency and their impact on iron delivery rather than an outright failure in stem cell response.

Iron Deficiency

Iron deficiency was implicated as the sole etiological factor in up to 17% of community-based individuals over age 65 in the NHANES III survey. Iron-deficiency anemia in older individuals is most often the result of chronic blood loss, usually occult gastrointestinal bleeding. Therefore, a careful search for a bleeding site is mandatory (see Chapter 5). Inadequate nutrition may contribute as diets change and daily caloric intake falls, but diet is rarely the sole cause of an iron-deficiency anemia. Marked malabsorption of iron is seen in patients with severe disruption of duodenal function, as, for example, in celiac sprue (gluten-sensitive enteropathy) patients. In this situation, concomitant malabsorption of folic acid may cloud the laboratory presentation.

The diagnosis of an iron-deficient state is readily made from measurements of the serum iron, iron-binding capacity, percent saturation, and serum ferritin level. A visual assessment of marrow iron stores is possible using a Prussian blue stain of a marrow aspirate particle or biopsy specimen. Faced with negative iron balance, iron stores will be depleted first (absent stores on the marrow iron stain and a serum ferritin <15 μg/L), followed by a fall in the serum iron and an increase in the total iron-binding capacity, until the percent saturation is less than 10%. Changes in red cell morphology (microcytosis and hypochromia) only appear with worsening anemia, usually when hemoglobin levels are sustained below 10 g/dL. These several stages in the evolution of iron deficiency and iron-deficiency anemia are discussed in detail in Chapter 5. It is important to review this material, since iron-deficiency anemia can present either as a normocytic, normochromic (hypoproliferative) anemia or as a microcytic, hypochromic anemia depending on the severity and duration of the iron loss. Moreover, the classical changes in iron studies may be less definitive the milder the anemia.

Another major issue is the presence of a concomitant illness. Iron deficiency and the anemia of inflammation often coexist, making the diagnosis even more difficult. Measurement of the serum transferrin receptor has been used to help separate the 2 conditions, but is often not readily available nor has it been proven to be more reliable than the ferritin measurement. Once available, a measurement of the hepcidin level may help identify an underlying inflammatory component. At this time, the coexistence of iron-deficiency and chronic inflammatory anemia may only become clear when the patient fails to respond to iron therapy. Iron deficiency can also coexist with folate and/or vitamin B_{12} deficiency, especially in patients with malabsorption. This presentation can be very confusing, since one or another of the deficiencies will tend to dominate clinically. Even in the presence of marked iron deficiency, the patient may present with a macrocytic anemia secondary to folate or vitamin B_{12} deficiency. The underlying iron deficiency will only be detected as the patient is treated and fails vitamin therapy (see Chapters 5 and 8).

Vitamin B_{12} and/or Folic Acid Deficiency

Vitamin B_{12} and/or folic acid deficiency were implicated in up to 15% of the NHANES III survey group. In the case of folate deficiency, poor nutrition, malabsorption, and alcohol abuse can all play a role (see Chapter 8). **The primary manifestation of folate deficiency is a macrocytic anemia.** It can evolve quickly, especially in association with alcohol abuse, and can resolve just as quickly once a normal diet is reinstituted. The quickness of changes in serum **folate levels in alcoholic patients**, as a result of alcohol-induced metabolic blockade of the normal enterohepatic folate cycle, can make the diagnosis very difficult. Alcoholic patients with blood alcohol levels exceeding 100 mg/dL will invariably (unless on folate supplements) have a serum folate level less than 4 ng/mL. This will rapidly return to normal in patients with residual liver folate stores once alcohol is withdrawn and/or a normal diet is resumed.

Macrocytosis with little or no anemia can be a relatively common finding in elderly individuals who suffer from a poor diet, with or without alcohol intake. Dietary folic acid is primarily supplied by fresh vegetables and fruits in the diet; thus, subsistence on a daily diet of highly processed foods puts patients at risk. Furthermore, unlike vitamin B_{12}, folate stores in the liver are relatively small, making it possible for a pure dietary deficiency in folate to evolve within a few months of dietary restriction. The classic "tea and toast" diet of the elderly widow(er) is cited as a prime example of this scenario. Add to this diet several glasses of sherry each night, and low-grade macrocytosis, at times accompanied by a mild anemia, can be expected. Chronic liver disease has also been correlated with low-grade macrocytosis and target cells on the blood smear due to changes in red blood cell membrane cholesterol metabolism.

Elderly individuals are also at increased risk for **vitamin B_{12} deficiency** as a result of gastric/small bowel surgery, gastric atrophy with reduction in intrinsic factor levels, immune suppression of intrinsic factor activity, or malabsorption (parasite infestation, small bowel diverticulosis, celiac sprue, or regional ileitis). Faced with a reduced dietary vitamin B_{12} intake and age-related gastric atrophy, even the healthiest of elderly patients are at risk for negative vitamin B_{12} balance, resulting in gradual (over years) exhaustion of hepatic stores and a fall in blood cobalamin levels.

The clinical manifestations of vitamin B_{12} deficiency are diverse and involve both the hematologic and neurologic systems. Elderly individuals can present with a macrocytic anemia, a range of neurological abnormalities from early dementia to nonspecific neurological signs, or **"combined systems disease"** where a severe macrocytic anemia is accompanied by signs of dorsal column demyelination (positive Romberg, decreased position and vibratory sense, and dysesthesias).

Much has been made of measurement of **blood cobalamin level** as the gold standard for the detection and differential diagnosis of vitamin B_{12} deficiency. To make it reliable, the serum cobalamin level should be ordered together with a serum folate level. Both tests should be drawn without delay in patients presenting with a severe macrocytic anemia, prior to reinstituting a normal diet or, in the case of the alcoholic patient, before significant alcohol withdrawal (see Chapter 8). The normal range for serum cobalamin levels is said to be from 200–500 pg/mL. However, setting the lower limit of normal at less than 200 pg/mL has been challenged, based on the ability to detect "subclinical" cobalamin deficiency with the methylmalonic acid assay, a measure of functional metabolic deficiency (see Chapter 8). Because of this, the probability of a cobalamin level being abnormal may better be stated as follows:

- In the presence of a severe vitamin B_{12}–deficient macrocytic anemia, the serum cobalamin level will be less than 200 pg/mL 95%–97% of the time. From the opposite viewpoint, 60%–80% of individuals with serum cobalamin levels less than 200 pg/mL will have anemia or metabolic evidence (abnormal methylmalonic acid level) of vitamin B_{12} deficiency.

- When the serum cobalamin level is between 200 and 350 pg/mL, there is still a considerable chance of a metabolic abnormality suggestive of a subclinical deficiency state. From 30%–35% of apparently normal individuals with cobalamin levels in this range will have an abnormal methylmalonic acid level without hematologic abnormalities.
- The negative predictive value of tests for cobalamin deficiency is, however, a significant issue. In a single study of a group of ambulatory patients who appeared to improve hematologically or neurologically when given pharmacological doses of vitamin B_{12}, more than 50% had cobalamin levels greater than 300 pg/mL. Moreover, measurement of methylmalonic acid failed to identify apparently deficient patients 30%–45% of the time.

This raises major **concerns regarding the use of the cobalamin level and/or the test for methylmalonic acid for screening elderly patients** for vitamin B_{12} deficiency. The sensitivity and specificity of the tests are clearly not up to the task. Whether this is due to a failure of the commercially available tests for vitamin B_{12} deficiency or rapid changes in blood vitamin levels is unclear. One contributing factor may be the differential binding characteristics of circulating transcobalamin proteins (see Chapter 8). Whatever the cause, the end result is that many individuals will go undiagnosed and others will turn out to be false positives. This has resurrected the concept of performing a therapeutic trial using pharmacological doses of vitamin B_{12} (>100 μg daily by injection for several weeks) plus folic acid orally in elderly patients with a macrocytic anemia or a recent onset of dementia or unexplained neuropathy. It is not a welcome solution to a long-standing desire to have a highly sensitive and specific test for vitamin B_{12} deficiency in elderly patients. It also calls into question many past reports of the incidence and cause of neurological abnormalities in geriatric populations.

The treatment of vitamin B_{12} and folic acid deficiency is discussed in depth in Chapter 8. Proper management requires careful documentation of the patient's hematological and neurological responses to the vitamin. All too often, the hematological response can be dampened or defeated by the hidden presence of iron deficiency or inadequate iron stores. Any inflammatory illness will also inhibit the response. If 1 or both are not appreciated and dealt with judiciously, the whole basis of the diagnosis of vitamin B_{12} deficiency can be called into question. This can lead to disaster, since lifelong maintenance therapy with vitamin B_{12} is required to prevent irreversible neurological damage.

Elderly patients with a severe macrocytic anemia (hemoglobin <6 g/dL) are also at increased risk for cardiovascular failure and may need short-term transfusion support until vitamin therapy corrects their marrow defect.

Combined deficiencies of folic acid, vitamin B_{12}, iron, and rarely copper may be seen in patients with marked malabsorption as a result of extensive bowel surgery or celiac sprue. The hematological picture can be confusing at best, especially when iron deficiency is present. One or another of the deficiencies will usually dominate, so that, when the multiple deficiencies are involved, the true cause of the anemia will only be revealed when it fails to resolve with supplementation by iron alone or 1 or both vitamins. Copper deficiency has been reported in patients following bariatric surgery and extensive small bowel resections. The hematological picture of copper deficiency can be quite confusing. The anemia tends to be macrocytic but the marrow morphology most resembles a myelodysplastic anemia, and a neuropathy may be present suggesting vitamin B_{12} deficiency. Blood copper levels will make the diagnosis. The therapeutic response to copper supplements is quite slow; it can take several months before the anemia resolves and, like long-standing vitamin B_{12} deficiency, the neuropathy may not respond.

Unexplained Anemia

A third of anemic community-based individuals over age 65 are said to suffer from an unexplained anemia, that is, an anemia that does not fit into 1 of the above categories. Many such individuals may simply not be diagnosed due to the limitations of the survey screening approach. Others may be missed because their anemia is so mild that changes in red blood cell morphology, iron studies, and vitamin levels are not as helpful as with a more severe, long-standing anemia. Moreover, many of the physiological changes associated with aging—reduced renal or thyroid function, stem cell aging and erythropoietin resistance, reduced androgen levels, and undiagnosed low-grade inflammation—may play a more prominent, even multifactorial role in these individuals.

The incidence of evolving **myelodysplasia** almost certainly has been underestimated in past survey studies. The prevalence of dysplastic and sideroblastic anemias is known to greatly increase with age, predicting a significant etiological role. Why then did the NHANES III survey fail to identify this class of patients? One reason is the onset is typically very gradual with nonspecific symptoms and a minimal anemia and/or leukopenia or thrombocytopenia (see Chapter 9). Therefore, the diagnosis is usually only made after several years of monitoring the patient's routine blood counts, and then performing a bone marrow aspirate/biopsy for morphology and chromosomal analysis, once the anemia is relatively severe. Definitive diagnosis and classification of the dysplastic anemias depend on the marrow morphological abnormalities and characteristic genetic markers (see Chapter 9). These studies were not a routine component of the NHANES III survey.

FUNCTIONAL IMPLICATIONS

Anemia in the elderly has been associated with significant adverse functional outcomes. Increased frailty, decreased mobility, impaired cognitive function, and increased risk of hospitalization have all been correlated with worsening anemia regardless of etiology and presence of other disorders. The mechanism involved may well be an anemia-related limitation of aerobic exercise capacity, leading to exercise intolerance and

CASE HISTORY • *Part 3*

The most obvious clue from these test results is the abnormality in the serum iron profile (low serum iron, low total iron-binding capacity [TIBC], percent saturation of 14%, and normal serum ferritin), which suggests a significant inflammatory component to her anemia. The sedimentation rate and C-reactive protein provide further indirect evidence of an inflammatory component. This should stimulate a careful search for a coexistent inflammatory disorder.

A major difficulty in the evaluation of anemia in the elderly is the potential for more than 1 causative factor to be present at one time. This reflects the increased prevalence of renal functional decline/failure, diabetes, vitamin B_{12} malabsorption, reduced dietary folate intake, thyroid insufficiency, and chronic disorders with a significant inflammatory component. While inflammation may be the principle factor in this patient, the borderline serum cobalamin level raises the question as to vitamin B_{12} deficiency playing a role in her cognitive impairment and recent falls. Careful follow-up with repeated measurements of the complete blood count (CBC), iron studies, vitamin levels, and organ function are essential to solving this puzzle of multiple contributing factors. This is especially true when the patient is evolving to a myelodysplastic condition, where bone marrow aspirate/biopsy and chromosome studies are ultimately required to make the diagnosis and plan management.

physical deconditioning. Over time, a sense of fatigue and weakness, together with reductions in physical and social activities, would lead to an increased frailty and a lower resistance to concurrent illness. When the relationship of frailty to anemia is examined from the opposing direction, the prevalence of anemia in the "frail elderly" is increased 2- to 3-fold over comparably aged community-dwelling counterparts.

Anemia is said to be an independent variable in determining patient functional capacity and morbidity and mortality. Of course, separating the role of anemia from the impact of other illness in the individual patient can be difficult, if not impossible. Major declines in functional measures and an increase in morbidity and mortality are commonly associated with acute and chronic illness in elderly individuals. Can the components be separated, as a guide to management? It is now well documented that erythropoietin treatment of individuals with renal disease or cancer who have hemoglobins less than 10 g/dL will improve self-reported functional capacities and quality of life. Erythropoietin and growth factor therapies have also been shown to be of value in managing patients with myelodysplasia who require frequent red cell transfusion. However, this finding should not be automatically extrapolated to erythropoietin-based management of patients with "unexplained" anemias without greater clarity as to the etiology of the individual's anemia. In addition, given the expense of growth factor therapies, it is hard to defend such treatment of individuals with mild to minimal anemia where the relationship to functional impairments is less clear.

THERAPY

Treatment of the elderly individual with anemia should be targeted to the etiology. Iron- and vitamin-deficiency anemias should respond to the appropriate replacement therapy, as long as the underlying cause has been fully evaluated and resolved (see Chapters 5 and 8). This is most important in iron-deficient patients where chronic blood loss can be a sign of a gastrointestinal malignancy. Effective resolution of an inflammatory anemia also depends on identifying and treating the underlying cause, whether a bacterial infection, malignancy, or autoimmune disorder (see Chapter 4).

Patients with dysplastic and sideroblastic anemias will typically progress over time. While the anemia can be minimal early on, these patients predictably become more anemic and pancytopenic over many months or years. They will often require chronic transfusion support and, with malignant transformation, some form of chemotherapy, as well as treatment with growth factors, both erythropoietin and granulocyte colony-stimulating factor (G-CSF). Chronic renal disease patients are ideal candidates for recombinant erythropoietin therapy (see Chapter 4). This is especially true for dialysis-dependent individuals, where a hemoglobin level much below 11 g/dL is associated with functional impairment and decreased quality of life.

As for the elderly individual with an "unexplained" anemia, the question of appropriate treatment is still largely unanswered. Certainly, all due diligence must be exercised to detect a treatable cause. After that, much will depend on the severity of the anemia and the possibility for functional improvement. Transfusion therapy can be used to stabilize a severe anemia and permit short-term observation of the patient's ability to resume an active lifestyle. Recombinant erythropoietin therapy may be tried, though it will be expensive and the results are, to date, unpredictable. Very mild anemias, while reported to be associated with increased morbidity and mortality, are best left untreated until well-controlled studies define the role for erythropoietin therapy.

POINTS TO REMEMBER

Anemia in the elderly is not a reflection of adult hematopoietic stem cell failure or a major defect in the marrow environment. The majority of the anemias seen in geriatric populations are the same as those seen in younger adults—secondary to an inflammatory disorder; renal failure; deficiencies of iron, folic acid, or vitamin B_{12}; and the gradual onset of a myelodysplastic disorder.

The recommended standard for the diagnosis of anemia in older populations, based on the NHANES III survey data, is a hemoglobin level less than 13 g/dL in men and less than 12 g/dL in women. Based on this, the prevalence of anemia in community-dwelling individuals over age 65 is 11% for men and 10.2% for women, rising to over 20% by age 80 and even higher for nursing home patients.

The lower hemoglobin level in women may underestimate the prevalence of physiologically important anemia. If less than 13 g/dL is used as the lower limit of normal, more than 20% of elderly women will be diagnosed as anemic.

Successful diagnosis and management of anemia in the elderly depends on a careful evaluation of the hematopoietic profile, including iron and vitamin assays, and a search for contributing disease processes. Anemias associated with an inflammatory disorder; renal failure; iron or vitamin deficiencies; or evolving myelodysplasia are all amenable to treatment if accurately diagnosed.

The category of "unexplained" anemia (34% of anemic individuals in the NHANES III survey) needs to be better defined. Many in this category may be found to have evolving myelodysplasia, if a full evaluation with bone marrow aspirate/biopsy and cytogenetic studies are performed over time.

Anemia in the elderly is an independent variable affecting functional capacity (mobility, cognitive performance, frequency of hospitalizations) and overall morbidity and mortality.

Appropriate treatment of a deficiency state (iron, folic acid, vitamin B_{12}) and/or a related illness (blood loss, inflammatory disorder, renal failure, etc) will resolve the anemia and improve functional parameters. This has been best illustrated by the detailed studies of performance in renal disease patients receiving recombinant erythropoietin therapy.

Erythropoietin therapy in patients with "unexplained" anemia is not recommended. It is expensive and there is, as yet, no randomized study to support its effectiveness.

BIBLIOGRAPHY

Artz AS: Anemia and the frail elderly. Semin Hematol 2008;45:261.

Carmel R: Nutritional anemias and the elderly. Semin Hematol 2008;45:225.

Culleton BF et al: Impact of anemia on hospitalization and mortality in older adults. Blood 2006;107:3841.

Denny SD et al: Impact of anemia on mortality, cognition, and function in community-dwelling elderly. Am J Med 2006;119:327.

Ferrucci L et al: The origins of age-related proinflammatory state. Blood 2005;105:2294.

Grazit R et al: Hematopoietic stem cells and the aging hematopoietic system. Semin Hematol 2008;45:218.

Guralnick JM et al: Prevalence of anemia in persons 65 years and older in the United States: evidence for a high rate of unexplained anemia. Blood 2004;104:2263.

Lee EJ et al: Soluble transferrin receptor (sTfR), ferritin, and sTfR/log ferritin index in anemic patients with nonhematologic malignancy and chronic inflammation. Clin Chem 2002;48:1118.

Makipour S et al: Unexplained anemia in the elderly. Semin Hematol 2008;45:250.

Patel KV, Guralnick JM: Epidemiology of anemia in older adults. Semin Hematol 2008;45:210.

Prenninx BW et al: Anemia and decline of physical performance among older persons. Am J Med 2003;115:104.

ERYTHROCYTOSIS AND POLYCYTHEMIA VERA • 13

CASE HISTORY • *Part I*

A 50-year-old man presents with a history of worsening headaches, difficulty sleeping, and general malaise. Past history is positive for hypertension, chronic obstructive pulmonary disease, and a recent deep venous thrombosis. He has a more than 30-year history of smoking and poor weight control. Examination reveals an obese male (~280 lbs) with a ruddy complexion. Vital signs: BP - 160/95 mm Hg; P - 94 bpm; R - 18 bpm. Otherwise, his examination is unremarkable.

CBC: Hematocrit/hemoglobin - 59%/19.7 g/dL
MCV - 92 fL   MCH - 32 pg   MCHC - 33 g/dL
RDW-CV - 12%
WBC count - 14,500/μL
Platelet count - 280,000/μL

• SMEAR MORPHOLOGY

Normocytic and normochromic with normal white blood cell morphology. Platelets are abundant with some clumping.

Reticulocyte count/index - 1.0%/>1
Sedimentation rate - 10 mm/h (Westergren)

Questions

- What CBC abnormality is apparent?
- What tests are indicated to explore the cause?

Erythrocytosis and polycythemia are clinical terms used to describe an abnormally elevated hemoglobin (hematocrit) or red blood cell mass. As with anemia, the probability that a patient has an elevated hemoglobin level will depend on the distribution of "normal" hemoglobin levels for any population. This will differ according to age, gender, race, and for subjects living at different altitudes (see Chapter 1). Physiological changes can also result in an apparent increase in the hemoglobin/hematocrit without a concomitant change in red cell mass. Because the hemoglobin and hematocrit are simple ratios of the concentration of red blood cells to volume of plasma, an increase can result from a reduction in plasma volume without a true increase in red blood cell mass **(relative erythrocytosis)**.

Detection and accurate diagnosis of erythrocytosis is important regardless of its cause. Even modest increases in the hemoglobin/hematocrit level can have a major impact on whole blood viscosity. Depending on the patient's clinical condition, an increase in the hematocrit can significantly affect blood flow and oxygen delivery to tissues. Therefore, management involves both treating the primary condition and appropriately adjusting the patient's hematocrit to normal.

NORMAL ERYTHROPOIESIS AND BLOOD VOLUME CONTROL

The total number of red blood cells in circulation varies according to the patient's age, gender, race, and clinical condition. Just as the erythroid marrow increases red blood cell production in response to anemia, the number of red blood cells produced each day will increase in response to chronic hypoxia. The normal value for a patient must take these factors into account. The normal distribution of hemoglobin or hematocrit measurements will be different for men and women of different ages and for individuals living at higher altitudes (Figure 13–1). In addition, patients with mild to moderate hypoxia caused by lung disease will compensate by increasing the number of circulating red blood cells. Within limits, this physiologic response to decreased oxygen availability to tissues is an effective compensatory mechanism.

The **regulation of normal erythropoiesis and oxygen transport** are discussed in detail in Chapter 1. Specific derangements in hemoglobin-oxygen dissociation, erythropoietin production, and red cell progenitor growth regulation are associated with abnormal red cell production and, at times, an increase in red cell mass (volume) beyond physiologic limits.

The control of **plasma volume** follows its own rules. Oncotic protein production, salt and water metabolism, and vasomotor tone are key factors in regulating the amount of plasma in circulation. Clinical conditions such as severe dehydration or allergic reactions with loss of plasma proteins from the vascular compartment are associated with elevations in hemoglobin and hematocrit. Even though the red blood cell mass is not increased, a sustained reduction in plasma volume can significantly affect viscosity, blood flow, and oxygen delivery to tissues.

Major **increases in red blood cell mass**, as seen with polycythemia vera, may not be compensated for by a matched reduction in plasma volume. From a physiologic standpoint, this represents a choice between 2 bad situations. If an increase in red blood cell mass is accompanied by an equal reduction in plasma volume, the patient will experience an increase in blood viscosity. On the other hand, if plasma volume does not decrease, total blood volume will increase significantly, placing stress on the volume capacity of the vascular compartment.

The impact of changes in viscosity on blood flow and oxygen delivery to tissues is an important issue in polycythemia. Blood is a non-Newtonian suspension of cells and liquid plasma, such that whole blood viscosity is a complex function of the number of red blood cells suspended in the plasma, the deformability of those red cells, and, to a lesser extent, plasma viscosity. When the hematocrit increases to levels much above 50%–55%, whole blood viscosity rises exponentially, resulting in a decrease in blood flow, especially in vessels with low flow/shear rates, such as capillaries. Increased red cell rigidity or red cell agglutination has a similar effect. Because tissue oxygen delivery is theoretically the product of blood flow and the hemoglobin level, individuals with erythrocytosis are at risk for tissue hypoxia as viscosity increases (Figure 13–2). However, other factors come into play, including changes in vessel diameter, redirection of blood supply to selected tissues, and the response of the hemoglobin-oxygen dissociation curve to tissue hypoxia (see Chapter 1). Clinically, the most demonstrable impact of increased whole blood viscosity is on the brain, where a significant decrease in blood flow and oxygen supply is seen with a hematocrit much above 50%.

Individual organ blood flow is also affected by the blood gas concentration. For example, brain blood flow is very sensitive to CO_2 concentration. When the P_{CO_2} increases, cerebral vessels

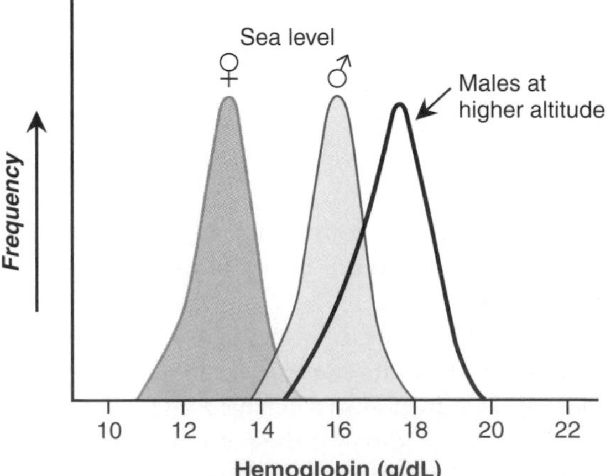

FIGURE 13–1. **Hemoglobin levels at sea level and higher altitudes.** Population distribution of hemoglobin levels for men and women at sea level will be significantly different from those seen for individuals living at higher altitudes or patients with chronic hypoxia.

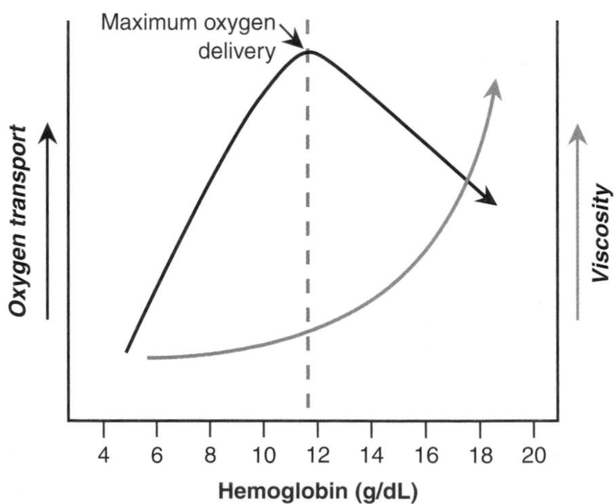

FIGURE 13–2. **The relationship of oxygen delivery to viscosity and the hemogobin level.** Tissue oxygen delivery is a product of blood flow and the hemoglobin/hematocrit level. As shown in this idealized curve, changes in hemoglobin/hematocrit are associated with changes in whole blood viscosity, which impacts on blood flow, so that there is a theoretical "optimal" point of maximal oxygen delivery corresponding to the normal range for hemoglobin of between 11 and 15 g/dL. Once the hematocrit rises much above 50%, viscosity increases exponentially, thereby reducing blood flow and oxygen transport/delivery. However, the actual supply of oxygen to any individual tissue will depend on the interaction of several other factors, including changes in vessel diameter, redistribution of blood flow, and the compensation provided by the hemoglobin-oxygen dissociation curve (see Chapter 1).

dilate. With sudden reductions in P_{CO_2}, vessels constrict and further limit the flow of more viscous blood to the brain. The interaction of blood viscosity with vessel reactivity is an important part of the compensation for chronic hypoxia, as seen in patients with chronic obstructive pulmonary disease. Although an increase in the hemoglobin/hematocrit in these patients is associated with increased blood viscosity, the impact on brain blood flow is in part compensated by their CO_2 retention and local vasodilation.

Clinical Features

The clinical signs and symptoms of an elevated hemoglobin/hematocrit vary depending on disease process and rate of onset. Expansion of the red blood cell mass requires weeks or even months of a sustained increase in red blood cell production. During this time, the patient's physiology has a chance to adapt. Therefore, patients with modest elevations in hemoglobin/hematocrit secondary to chronic lung disease, a hemoglobinopathy, or polycythemia vera will initially be asymptomatic. It is only **when the hemoglobin rises above 18–20 g/dL** that patients generally report symptoms such as chronic headaches, a general sense of malaise, and easy fatigability.

Hemoglobin levels greater than 20 g/dL can be life threatening. At this level, blood viscosity is so markedly increased that blood flow to vital organs is compromised. This also leads to an increased risk for both venous and arterial thrombosis with up to 40% of patients experiencing at least 1 thrombotic event during the course of their illness. The mechanism behind the hypercoagulable state may be nothing more than the increase in whole blood viscosity, although enhanced platelet–endothelial cell interaction may also play a role, especially when the platelet count is elevated. The most frequent sites of thrombosis are cerebral and intra-abdominal, including hepatic vein thrombosis. Conversely, patients with polycythemia vera can also present with life-threatening hemorrhage. This may relate to blood volume expansion and increased viscosity leading to spontaneous rupture of arterial vessels. There is also evidence that platelet function in polycythemia vera is defective. Untreated polycythemia vera patients are thus at risk for excessive bleeding with surgery or trauma.

Patients with a hemoglobin level in excess of 20 g/dL may be recognized from their general appearance. The increase in hemoglobin level and blood volume results in a noticeable facial plethora with prominent, bloodshot eyes and red to purplish mucous membranes. Vessels of the conjunctiva and ocular fundus appear dilated (Figure 13–3), and venous blood may appear desaturated. In addition, prominent cyanosis is observed in patients who are hypoxic.

The symptoms and signs associated with a primary disease process such as chronic obstructive pulmonary disease or congenital heart disease can point to the underlying cause of the erythrocytosis. Polycythemia vera patients can complain of **pruritus** (severe itching) occurring almost continuously or especially after a shower. This condition appears to relate to the mast cell proliferation seen with myeloproliferative disorders. Most polycythemia vera patients also have palpable splenomegaly.

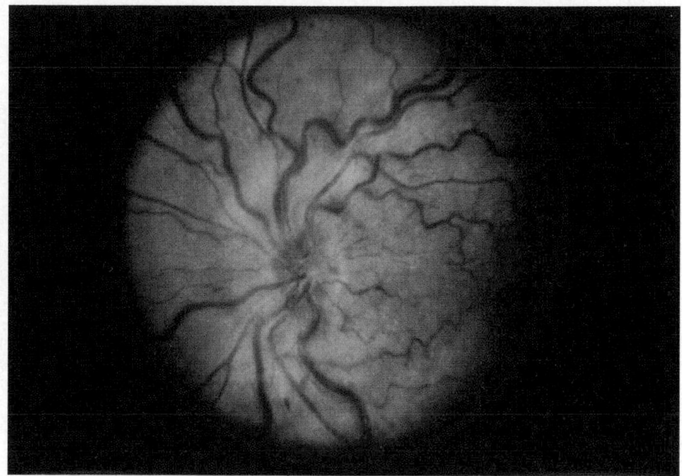

FIGURE 13–3. **Optic fundus in a patient with polycythemia vera.** Vessels in the conjunctiva and ocular fundus appear dilated and tortuous in the untreated polycythemia vera patient.

Laboratory Studies

A. Complete Blood Count

A routine complete blood count (CBC) will usually provide the entry point in the diagnosis of erythrocytosis and polycythemia vera. As a rule, the **upper limits for a normal hemoglobin for men and women living at sea level are 18.5 and 16.5 g/dL, respectively**. Patients who exceed these levels must have an increase in the red blood cell mass or a reduction in plasma volume. If the hemoglobin level is persistently above 20 g/dL in men and 18 g/dL in women, the patient almost certainly has a true increase in the red blood cell mass.

Other findings on the CBC can point directly to a diagnosis of polycythemia vera. The combination of a high hemoglobin level, leukocytosis, thrombocytosis, basophilia, sometimes accompanied by an increase in the leukocyte alkaline phosphatase, in a patient with symptoms and signs such as itching, headaches, malaise, and splenomegaly is virtually diagnostic for polycythemia vera. It reflects the fact that polycythemia vera is a clonal disorder affecting the stem cells responsible for all hematopoietic cell lines. This fact differentiates polycythemia vera from all other conditions where the increase in red blood cell mass results from a pure erythropoietin stimulus and other cell lines are not affected.

B. Red Blood Cell Mass and Plasma Volume Measurements

The circulating red blood cell mass can be directly measured using ^{51}Cr-labeled red blood cells. By injecting a known amount of labeled cells and measuring their subsequent dilution, it is possible to get an accurate measurement of the total red blood cell mass. In a similar fashion, ^{131}I-labeled albumin can be used to measure the plasma volume. Normal values for adult men and women are summarized in Table 13–1. It is important that both measurements be performed, because they vary independently according to the cause of the apparent erythrocytosis. Patients

TABLE 13–1 • Red blood cell, plasma, and total blood volumes ([mL ± 1 SD[a]]/kg)

	Red Blood Cell Volume	Plasma Volume	Total Blood Volume
Men	30 ± 5	35 ± 5	65 ± 8
Women	25 ± 5	35 ± 5	60 ± 7

[a]*The standard deviation for each volume measurement includes a ±5% coefficient of variation for the assay technique as well as individual subject variation. Falsely low values are observed in obese patients when results are expressed as milliliters per kilogram of measured body weight.*

with hypoxic erythrocytosis typically show a compensatory decrease in the plasma volume as the red cell mass expands, keeping the total blood volume close to normal. In contrast, untreated polycythemia vera patients most often present with increases in both red cell and plasma volumes, and therefore an increased total blood volume.

Unfortunately, these measurements are expensive, involve exposure to radioactivity, and are technically challenging. The wide coefficient of variation of the tests is another problem, making it difficult to establish a "normal" range of values. If the results are expressed according to weight, obese patients will appear to have smaller than normal red blood cell and plasma volumes (fat is relatively avascular). Even when calculated according to surface area, only those values that are more than 2 standard deviations from the normal mean value can be considered truly abnormal. It is inviting, therefore, to reserve these radiolabeling tests for those situations where the reason for an elevated hemoglobin/hematocrit level is unclear. Most often, this arises when the hemoglobin level is between 18 and 20 g/dL in men and 16 and 18 g/dL in women, and one is looking for an increased red cell mass masked by a simultaneous increase in plasma volume. When the hemoglobin is above these levels, the red blood cell mass is invariably increased.

C. Blood Gas Measurements

It is essential to measure an **arterial blood gas** in patients with suspected lung or heart disease. Sustained hypoxia sufficient to keep arterial oxygen saturation below 80% will, in a normally responsive patient, stimulate a hemoglobin increase to greater than 18 g/dL. Patients with congenital heart disease and pronounced right to left shunts show the most dramatic desaturation and highest hemoglobin levels (often exceeding 22 g/dL). A single blood gas determination in a chronic lung disease or sleep apnea patient may not accurately reflect the severity of the hypoxia. In this situation, repeated measurements over 24 hours or as part of a sleep apnea study may be necessary to evaluate the severity of the desaturation.

A direct measurement of **carbon monoxide concentration in blood (carboxyhemoglobin level)** is important in heavy smokers and individuals at risk of chronic environmental exposure to carbon monoxide. Carbon monoxide avidly binds to hemoglobin and displaces oxygen, effectively canceling the oxygen-carrying capacity of the molecule. Carboxyhemoglobin cannot be detected by pulse oximetry or standard blood gas measurement, and even high levels of carboxyhemoglobin will not be reflected by the calculated percent saturation.

Point mutations in globin structure can interfere with the respiratory motion of the hemoglobin molecule and binding of 2,3-diphosphoglycerate (2,3-DPG). Some of these hemoglobinopathies produce an increased hemoglobin-oxygen affinity, thereby stimulating a higher than normal hemoglobin level. This functional abnormality can be detected by **measurements of the hemoglobin P_{50} and intracellular 2,3-DPG levels.** A decrease in the P_{50} value to below 15 mm Hg is associated with increases in hemoglobin in excess of 18 g/dL (Figure 13–4). Up to half of these high-affinity hemoglobinopathies can be diagnosed by hemoglobin electrophoresis. Some of the unstable hemoglobinopathies also show decreased oxygen affinity as demonstrated by the P_{50} measurement (see Chapter 7).

D. Genetic Analysis

Between 10% and 20% of patients presenting with polycythemia vera will exhibit an abnormal marrow karyotype. The most common abnormalities are trisomies of 1q, 8, 9, or 9p, and deletions of 13q and 20q. However, none of these cytogenetic abnormalities are unique, and therefore they are not diagnostic of polycythemia vera. Over time with progression of disease, the frequency of chromosomal abnormalities increases, especially with evolution to myelodysplasia or acute leukemia. After 10 years, more than 80% of polycythemia vera patients will exhibit 1 or more chromosomal abnormalities.

The discovery of the **JAK2 gene mutation**, which is shared by several of the myeloproliferative disorders (polycythemia vera, essential thrombocytosis, and primary myelofibrosis), has provided an important diagnostic marker. JAK2 serves as the

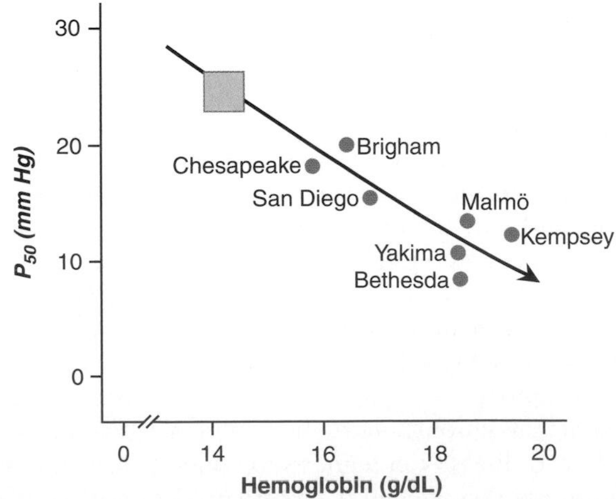

FIGURE 13–4. **Hemoglobinopathies associated with increased hemoglobin levels.** Inherited hemoglobin defects with an increased hemoglobin-oxygen affinity will demonstrate high hemoglobin levels. P_{50} values below 15 mm Hg are associated with hemoglobins greater than 18 g/dL

tyrosine kinase for both the erythropoietin and thrombopoietin surface receptors. This unique somatic mutation, a substitution of phenylalanine for valine (V617), results in enhanced tyrosine kinase activity and allows *JAK2* V617F-positive erythroid colonies to proliferate largely in the absence of erythropoietin. Upwards of 95% of patients with a clinical profile of polycythemia vera have been reported to carry the *JAK2* mutation, either in the heterozygous or homozygous form.

E. Erythropoietin and Stem Cell Assays

An accurate measurement of the **serum erythropoietin level** is possible by immunoassay. High-normal to elevated levels are typically seen with hypoxia, high oxygen-affinity hemoglobins, and erythropoietin-secreting tumors. As a note of caution, however, the normal range for the serum erythropoietin is from 4–26 mU/mL, so that a significant elevation in a patient may be present without exceeding the normal range. In untreated polycythemia vera patients, erythropoietin levels are usually depressed well below 4 mU/mL, even to the point of being undetectable.

Several physiological variables can interfere with the interpretation of any single erythropoietin level. For example, hypoxic patients will demonstrate a rapid return of the erythropoietin level to normal or even below normal when oxygen delivery to tissues is transiently improved. On the other hand, polycythemia vera patients who are treated with phlebotomy or who become iron deficient can show normal to elevated levels. The pattern of response of the erythropoietin level to phlebotomy can help identify the cause of the erythrocytosis (Figure 13–5). Patients with polycythemia vera or hypoxic erythrocytosis will show a normal or heightened increase in erythropoietin levels in response to phlebotomy, whereas patients with erythropoietin-secreting tumors fail to respond to a fall in the hemoglobin level.

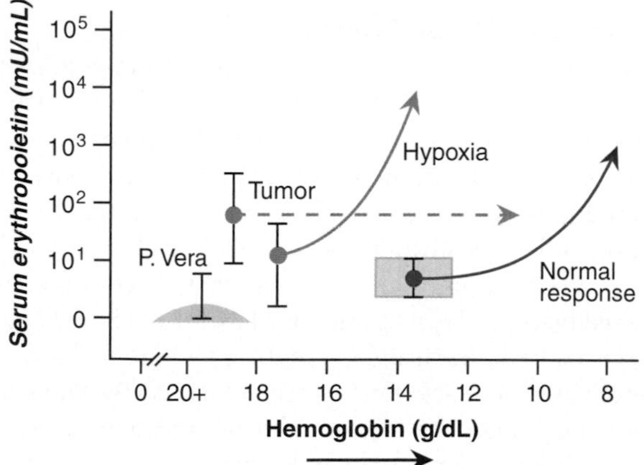

FIGURE 13–5. **Erythropoietin (EPO) measurements in patients with various forms of erythrocytosis.** When compared with the normal response, polycythemia vera patients present with below normal to absent serum EPO levels. Patients with polycythemia secondary to hypoxia or an erythropoietin-secreting tumor show high-normal to elevated levels. The response to phlebotomy is even more distinctive. Polycythemia vera patients essentially follow the normal curve, whereas patients with hypoxia show marked increases in serum erythropoietin levels even while the hemoglobin level is above normal. Patients with erythropoietin-secreting tumors generally show a suppressed response to phlebotomy since EPO production is autonomous.

Prior to the discovery of the *JAK2* marker, proof of polycythemia vera was possible using a **stem cell assay**. Expansion of burst-forming unit–erythroid (BFU-E) colonies in marrow culture normally requires exogenous erythropoietin. Polycythemia vera patients' BFU-E colonies grow in culture without added erythropoietin, demonstrating the loss of normal regulatory control of erythroid precursor proliferation. However, the BFU-E colony assay is difficult to standardize and lacks specificity. BFU-E growth patterns vary considerably among polycythemia vera patients, and the assay does not distinguish patients with erythropoietin receptor defects. For these reasons, detection of the *JAK2* mutation is now the gold standard for diagnosis.

F. Miscellaneous Studies

When the *JAK2* mutation is absent, several radiologic and laboratory studies can help in the differential diagnosis. **Examination of the marrow aspirate and biopsy** can provide evidence of myelocyte and megakaryocyte dysplasia in polycythemia vera patients. **Measurements of the serum vitamin B_{12} level and transcobalamin proteins** provide an indirect measure of granulocytic hyperplasia. Transcobalamins I and III, but predominantly transcobalamin III, tend to be increased.

In the case of secondary polycythemias, studies that help in diagnosing cardiopulmonary disease are integral to the definition of hypoxic erythrocytosis. These studies can include a range of **cardiac imaging studies, heart catheterization, and lung function studies. An intravenous pyelogram and computed tomography (CT) or magnetic resonance imaging (MRI) scans** of the head and abdomen will help rule out an erythropoietin-producing tumor or hydronephrosis of the kidney.

Iron studies, including **serum iron, total iron-binding capacity (TIBC), and serum ferritin levels**, are essential in the evaluation of any patient with erythrocytosis. Expansion of the red blood cell mass will deplete iron stores. In women, this may readily exhaust stores and result in iron-deficient erythropoiesis. Since a reduction in iron supply suppresses the proliferative capacity of the erythroid marrow, the interpretation of any elevation in hemoglobin/hematocrit must take into account iron balance. The appearance of microcytosis (low mean cell volume [MCV]) in a patient with a normal or only slightly reduced hemoglobin/hematocrit can be a clue to the diagnosis of polycythemia vera, especially in women. As discussed in Chapter 5, the microcytosis observed with iron-deficiency anemia is seen only when the hemoglobin falls below 10–11 g/dL. Microcytosis in the absence of anemia suggests polycythemia vera or a secondary erythrocytosis (hypoxia or tumor-driven BFU-E expansion).

DIAGNOSIS

The differential diagnosis of erythrocytosis is an excellent test of a clinician's diagnostic skill. Most often, the cause of an increased hemoglobin/hematocrit can be identified from the

CASE HISTORY • Part 2

The patient has a higher than normal hemoglobin, a modest leukocytosis, and a high normal platelet count. This meets the criteria for erythrocytosis, and because of the increase in leukocytes, raises the issue of polycythemia vera. At the same time, he is obese and suffers from chronic obstructive pulmonary disease, both of which are potential causes of hypoxic erythrocytosis. Because of the history of hypertension and smoking, it is also important to document his use of diuretics (decreased plasma volume) and level of carboxyhemoglobin as causes of relative and hypoxic erythrocytosis, respectively. A direct measurement of red cell mass and plasma volume may confirm a true increase in red cell mass, but his obesity will make the interpretation difficult.

Instead, the following tests were performed and their results are as follows:

Arterial blood gas, percent saturation - 91%
Carboxyhemoglobin - 4%
Serum EPO level - <1 mU/mL
JAK2 V617F mutation - present

Questions

- Do these results allow a definitive diagnosis of the etiology of his erythrocytosis/polycythemia?
- Are there other tests that need to be performed to help guide therapy?

clinical presentation, CBC, *JAK2* mutation, and evaluation of the patient's cardiopulmonary status. Measurements of red blood cell mass and plasma volume, hemoglobin-oxygen affinity, BFU-E hypersensitivity to erythropoietin, as well as other laboratory and radiologic studies, are only needed in rare cases where the clinical pattern of disease is confusing.

Polycythemia Vera

Polycythemia vera is a relatively uncommon disease with an incidence of approximately 2 per 100,000. It is a stem cell disorder (clonal myeloproliferative disorder) characterized by the production of an excessive number of mature hematopoietic cells, especially red blood cells. The mutational event appears to involve pluripotent stem cells of the marrow, although some patients demonstrate clonality for all cell lines except T cells and natural killer lymphocytes. Similar to the myelodysplastic anemias, polycythemia vera progresses with time to varying combinations of cell proliferation and cytopenia, myelofibrosis, distorted cell maturation, and even acute leukemia. Most patients, however, are diagnosed at a time when expansion of the red blood cell mass is the predominant feature.

The pathogenesis of polycythemia vera is still a bit of a mystery. The most prominent feature, the increase in red cell mass, is associated with the appearance of a clone of erythroid precursors that is able to grow in vitro in the absence or near absence of erythropoietin. It has now been shown that the somatic mutation **JAK2 V617F**, which results in an increase in tyrosine kinase activity, is in large part responsible for the uncontrolled proliferation of red cell precursors. *JAK2* V617F now serves as a key marker for the diagnosis of polycythemia vera: it has been shown to be present in 90%–95% of patients with a clinical picture consistent with polycythemia vera. At the same time, the *JAK2* mutation does not appear to be the sole event in the pathogenesis of the disease or its outcome.

The relationship of polycythemia vera to other myeloproliferative disorders is another area of uncertainty. The fact that a sizable number of patients with essential thrombocytosis and primary myelofibrosis also express the *JAK2* mutation strongly suggests a common role for the activated tyrosine kinase in the pathophysiology of each condition. What other mutations or factors are involved in determining the differences in these several disorders is a mystery. Moreover, the concept of polycythemia vera as a central disease process with possible evolution to myelofibrosis, marrow failure, and acute leukemia is hard to explain.

A. Major and Minor Criteria

Traditionally, the diagnosis of polycythemia vera was made based on a handful of clinical criteria (Table 13–2). Patients who live at sea level and present with very high hemoglobins (in excess of 20 g/dL in men and 18 g/dL in women) without evidence of lung or heart disease almost certainly have an increase in red cell mass. However, at lesser elevations of hemoglobin, changes in plasma volume can have a greater influence, so that direct measurements of the red blood cell mass using ^{51}Cr-labeled red blood cells and the plasma volume using ^{131}I-labeled albumin have been advanced as a more accurate way to detect an absolute increase in the red cell mass. Problems with this approach, as described in the methods section, include standard errors of the measurements, difficulty establishing a set of normal values based on weight or surface area, and the fact that not all hospitals/laboratories now offer the tests.

There is also the problem of relying on a major elevation of the hemoglobin and/or red cell mass as the lead-off major criterion for diagnosing polycythemia vera. Patients can present with only slightly elevated or even normal hemoglobin and red cell mass levels. One common scenario is the polycythemia vera patient who is also iron deficient, which sets a limit on erythroid expansion (see Chapter 5). These patients may be recognized by the

TABLE 13–2 • Polycythemia vera diagnostic criteria (2001)

Major criteria
Increased hemoglobin → >18.5 g/dL in men; >16.5 g/dL in women or red blood cell mass increase (^{51}Cr–red cell volume) → >36 mL/kg in men; >32 mL/kg in women
Normal arterial O_2 saturation
Palpable splenomegaly
No other explanation—renal disease, hypoxia, tumor, etc
Minor criteria
Thrombocytosis: >400,000 platelets/μL
Leukocytosis: >12,000 white blood cells/μL
Abnormal marrow karyotype
EPO level <4.0 mU/mL (or below normal reference range)
BFU-E hypersensitivity to EPO
Elevated leukocyte alkaline phosphatase[a]
Elevated serum B_{12} level: >900 pg/mL or elevated transcobalamin level (B_{12} binding capacity) >2200 pg/mL[b]

[a]*Difficult to standardize.*
[b]*Not specific to polycythemia vera.*

TABLE 13–3 • Proposed WHO revised criteria for polycythemia vera (2007)

Major criteria
Hemoglobin >18.5 g/dL in men, >16.5 g/dL in women, or an increase in red cell mass
Presence of the *JAK2* V617F or similar mutation (*JAK2* exon 12)
Minor criteria
Prominent leukocytosis, thrombocytosis, or bone marrow hypercellularity involving all cell lines
EPO levels: <4 mU/mL (or normal reference range)
BFU-E hypersensitivity to EPO

finding of significant microcytosis (MCV <70–80 fL) in the presence of a normal or near normal hematocrit. Coexistent chronic inflammation can play a similar role in suppressing iron supply and red cell production (see Chapter 4). Some patients may present with leukocytosis or thrombocytosis and only evolve to a full polycythemia vera picture over time. There is also the question of subclinical disease, where the *JAK2* gene mutation is detected months or years before clinical signs and symptoms develop.

With these exceptions in mind, the traditional set of diagnostic major and minor criteria (see Table 13–2) are clearly valid when full-blown polycythemia vera is present. A patient who demonstrates all of the **major criteria** (elevated hemoglobin/hematocrit or red blood cell mass, normal arterial oxygen saturation, and splenomegaly without another explanation) together with some or all of the **minor criteria** (thrombocytosis, leukocytosis, lower than normal to absent serum erythropoietin, elevated leukocyte alkaline phosphatase, and/or an elevated serum vitamin B_{12} or transcobalamin-binding capacity), almost certainly has polycythemia vera.

Given the ready availability of the test for the *JAK2* mutation, the approach to diagnosis of polycythemia vera, as well as primary myelofibrosis and essential thrombocytosis, can be greatly modified. Certainly, early measurement of the gene mutation can trump the relative importance of the other clinical criteria (Table 13–3).

B. Marrow Aspirate and Biopsy

Marrow examination is not necessary, and therefore not indicated in the workup of polycythemia vera, unless there are abnormalites of white cell morphology. If performed, marrow aspirate and biopsy will generally show a hypercellular marrow with expansion of all cell compartments. Megakaryocyte proliferation and dysplasia may be striking, with clusters ranging from micromegakaryocytes to very large, multinucleate cells. As the disease progresses, cellular elements tend to become more dysplastic and the marrow structure increasingly fibrotic, with an increase in reticulin and collagenous tissue and a corresponding decrease in overall cellularity.

C. Erythropoietin, Molecular Pathology, and Stem Cell Assays

Measurements of **serum erythropoietin and BFU-E growth patterns** can provide important information regarding the pathophysiology of erythrocytosis and polycythemia vera and are listed as minor diagnostic criteria. In general, erythropoietin levels are well below normal in untreated polycythemia vera patients, secondary to a suppression of normal erythropoietin production. With phlebotomy and return of the hematocrit/hemoglobin (red cell mass) to normal levels, erythropoietin levels and their response to anemia are within normal limits (see Figure 13–5). The assay of BFU-E growth potential in the absence of erythropoietin clearly demonstrates the physiological defect. However, this assay is problematic (as previously discussed) and not commonly available in most laboratories.

The detection of the **JAK2 V617F and other *JAK2* mutations** is a different matter. This abnormality is present in 90%–95% of patients with a clinical picture consistent with polycythemia vera. It is, therefore, of great value in confirming the diagnosis and serves as a major criterion in the recently **revised World Health Organization (WHO) criteria for the diagnosis of polycythemia vera** (see Table 13–3). There are, however, several unanswered questions regarding when to order the test. First of all, should it be ordered only when the hemoglobin and/or red cell mass are clearly elevated, or as a screening test in any patient with any unexplained cytosis? Next, if a patient who meets the traditional criteria for polycythemia vera but is not positive for the *JAK2* V617F or other *JAK2* mutation, does the patient have the disorder or should the patient be managed differently? Finally, since the mutation is detected in other myeloproliferative disorders, including essential thrombocytosis and primary myelofibrosis, it will always lack specificity as a stand-alone criterion.

D. Iron Studies

Iron studies are important in both diagnosing and managing polycythemia vera. The Prussian blue stain of the marrow aspirate shows a reduction in to complete absence of reticuloendothelial iron in virtually all cases, especially in women. Moreover, significant iron deficiency will restrict expansion of the red blood cell mass and lower the hemoglobin level. From a diagnostic viewpoint, this possibility must always be kept in mind, and measurements of serum iron, TIBC, and serum ferritin are important. When iron deficiency is severe, patients will present with normal to only slightly elevated hemoglobins but significant microcytosis.

Secondary Erythrocytosis

An increase in the red blood cell mass without evidence of changes in other hematopoietic cell lines is a normal physiologic response to hypoxia, regardless of cause. It can also result from increased autonomous production of erythropoietin by a diseased kidney or an extrarenal tumor.

A. Hypoxic Erythrocytosis

Individuals who live at high altitude exhibit an increase in their hemoglobin/hematocrit (see Figure 13–1). Up to altitudes of 7,000 ft, the increase in red blood cell mass is physiologically effective and not associated with any clinical abnormalities. At higher altitudes, humans are at risk for both acute and chronic mountain sickness. With rapid ascents, mountain climbers can acutely experience severe headaches, nausea, vomiting, and disorientation secondary to cerebral edema. This is secondary to hyperventilation, producing respiratory alkalosis, and can be largely prevented by the use of acetazolamide, dexamethasone, or both. Individuals who attempt to live at altitudes of 9,000–15,000 ft experience chronic mountain sickness. These individuals demonstrate much higher hemoglobin/hematocrit levels; chronic tissue hypoxia, especially during sleep; and significant problems maintaining nutrition and cardiopulmonary compensation.

Significant cardiopulmonary disease can also result in sufficient tissue hypoxia to induce erythrocytosis. The most dramatic example of this condition is in patients with congenital heart disease and cyanosis secondary to a major right to left shunt. These individuals can exhibit hemoglobin levels in excess of 22 g/dL (hematocrit >65%). Although such patients have very high whole blood viscosities, they appear to have surprisingly few problems with thrombosis or abnormal bleeding. Attempts to therapeutically reduce the hematocrit may be required if patients develop heart failure. Otherwise, patients may feel worse when their hemoglobin/hematocrit is lowered.

Pulmonary disease can also result in a hypoxic polycythemia. The most common clinical scenario is the very obese individual who develops **mechanical hypoventilation (Pickwickian syndrome)**. The intermittent nature of the hypoventilation must be recognized in the evaluation of these patients. A full sleep study may be necessary to document the extent of the patient's arterial desaturation. Most patients with **chronic obstructive pulmonary disease or interstitial lung disease** do not develop a significant erythrocytosis, which reflects the inhibiting effects of their illness.

A rare form of familial hypoxia-related polycythemia has been described in the Chuvash population of central Russia, as well as in a few families of Western European and Asian descent. It is inherited as an autosomal recessive disorder; affected individuals are typically homozygous for a mutation in the von Hippel-Lindau (*VHL*) gene on chromosome 3. The resulting defect involves the oxygen-sensing negative feedback loop responsible for moderating erythropoietin production. Because of this, erythropoietin levels are increased. Chuvash polycythemia presents early in life with a marked increase in the hemoglobin level (20–24 g/dL) and frequent thrombotic and hemorrhagic complications.

B. High-Affinity Hemoglobinopathies

Patients can develop erythrocytosis secondary to abnormalities in hemoglobin-oxygen binding. Most demonstrate an increase in hemoglobin-oxygen affinity owing to a mutational defect in globin structure or an abnormality in 2,3-DPG production or binding. More than 50 variants have now been described. They are recognized from their **lower than normal P_{50}** (normal P_{50} 26 mm Hg). Once the P_{50} falls much below 20 mm Hg, patients exhibit a significant increase in their red blood cell mass and hemoglobin levels (see Figure 13–3). **Patients with unstable hemoglobins** may also present with a normal hemoglobin level or mild hemolytic anemia, despite an oxygen-binding defect (see Chapter 7). A rare cause of secondary polycythemia is deficiency of 2,3-DPG secondary to an inherited defect in the DPG mutase gene localized to chromosome 7. An assay of DPG mutase will confirm the diagnosis. All patients with increased affinity hemoglobins appear well oxygenated, since their hemoglobin is fully saturated with oxygen. In contrast, patients **with methemoglobinemia, sulfhemoglobinemia, and hemoglobin M disease** (a group of mutant disorders where heme is stabilized in the ferric state) can present with a striking cyanosis owing to reduced hemoglobin-oxygen binding.

C. Methemoglobinemia

Hemoglobin is at constant risk for oxidation of its heme iron from the reduced ferrous to the ferric state to form methemoglobin. The normal methemoglobin reductase system helps maintain hemoglobin in its reduced state (see Chapter 1). The presence of ferric heme increases the oxygen affinity of ferrous heme, thereby shifting the oxygen dissociation curve to the left, resulting in a compensatory polycythemia.

There are 3 forms of hereditary methemoglobinemia—hemoglobin M disease, reduced (hydrogenated) nicotinamide adenine dinucleotide (NADH)-cytochrome b5 reductase deficiency, and cytochrome b5 deficiency. **Hemoglobin M** is a mutant hemoglobin (usually a His to Tyr substitution in the heme pocket) that is incapable of reversibly binding oxygen. These patients present with asymptomatic cyanosis and, in some cases, a mild hemolytic anemia. Two clinical phenotypes of **NADH-cytochrome b5 reductase deficiency** have been characterized: type I, where the defect is restricted to erythroid cells;

TABLE 13–4 • Drugs that cause methemoglobinemia

Analgesics (acetanilide, acetaminophen, phenacetin)
Cardiovascular drugs (nitrates, nitroprusside)
Local anesthetics (benzocaine, lidocaine, etc)
Antibiotics (sulfonamides)

and type II, where several tissues are involved. The type I defect is associated with mild cyanosis, whereas type II disease manifests severe cyanosis, mental retardation, and progressive encephalopathy.

Symptomatic methemoglobinemia can be seen in otherwise normal individuals who are exposed to strong oxidants in dyes, drugs (Table 13–4), solvents, and fertilizers, as well as in patients with congenital, heterozygous b5 reductase deficiency. Once the methemoglobin level exceeds 10%–20%, the patient appears visibly cyanotic and complains of symptoms such as headache, dyspnea, and dizziness. On measurement of the patient's blood gas, arterial blood will appear brownish in color and will not turn red when exposed to oxygen. Oxygen saturation will be reduced while the $\mathbf{PAO_2}$ (oxygen tension) is normal. Exposure to sulfa drugs, acetophenetidin, and acetanilide can result in irreversible production of sulfhemoglobin and similar symptoms once levels exceed 30%–40%.

Congenital methemoglobinemia can be treated by activating the NADPH-dependent reductase pathway with either ascorbic acid, 300–600 mg/d in 3–4 divided doses, or oral methylene blue, 60 mg 3–4 times a day. **Secondary symptomatic methemoglobinemia** is best treated with intravenous methylene blue, 1 mg/kg given over 5 minutes, and then repeated at 1 hour and every 4–6 hours, to a maximum dose of 7 mg/kg.

D. Increased Erythropoietin Production

Renal disease and several erythropoietin-secreting tumors have been associated with secondary polycythemia. Hydronephrosis, polycystic renal disease, renal cysts, and both benign and malignant renal tumors can result in increased production of erythropoietin. Uterine myomas, hepatomas, and cerebellar hemangiomas have also been shown to secrete erythropoietin. Mutations of the *VHL* gene are associated with hemangioblastoma, pheochromocytoma, renal carcinoma, and, in rare cases, polycythemia secondary to inappropriate production of erythropoietin by the tumor cells. Renal patients can develop erythrocytosis post-transplant that is unrelated to erythropoietin production. A role for angiotensin II as a red cell growth promoter has been postulated in this situation, based on the observation that angiotensin-converting enzyme inhibitors will reverse the erythrocytosis.

Surreptitious **use of recombinant erythropoietin by high-performance athletes** can also result in a hematocrit/hemoglobin in the polycythemia range. Measurements of serum erythropoietin levels in any of these patients may show a high normal to elevated value, certainly greater than would be expected if the patient had polycythemia vera. Blood doping is another strategy used by athletes to transiently increase their hemoglobin levels during a competition.

In patients with erythropoietin-secreting tumors, the normal erythropoietin response to anemia may be suppressed (see Figure 13–5). This situation is reminiscent of the adrenal suppression observed in patients with steroid-secreting adrenal adenomas. However, definitive diagnosis of a specific tumor or renal disease requires a careful search using appropriate radiologic and laboratory measurements. Any patient who is considered at risk for a nonhypoxic, secondary polycythemia should have an intravenous pyelogram, CT or MRI scans of head and abdomen, and both renal and liver function tests.

E. Erythropoietin Receptor Mutations

An acquired or congenital mutation of the erythropoietin receptor gene can lead to truncation of the cytoplasmic portion of the receptor and a failure to shut off signal transduction following erythropoietin binding. This has the same end result as abnormally high erythropoietin production.

Relative Erythrocytosis

Moderate elevations of hemoglobin level (16–18 g/dL in men or 14–16 g/dL in women) may be caused by a decrease in plasma volume without a true increase in red blood cell mass. **Acute elevations of hemoglobin/hematocrit** are observed in patients with severe dehydration secondary to salt and water deprivation, diarrhea, or excessive vomiting, or a combination of these. Overly aggressive use of diuretics can also be responsible. A sudden change in vascular permeability secondary to an allergic reaction can dramatically reduce the plasma volume, even to the point of increasing the hemoglobin to greater than 20 g/dL. Patients experiencing **allergic or anaphylactic reactions** also exhibit some combination of hives, bronchial spasm, angioneurotic edema, and orthostatic hypotension.

An elevated hemoglobin level may be seen in **patients with Cushing disease or pheochromocytoma**. With these conditions, the reduction in plasma volume appears to relate to a hormonally driven increase in vascular tone together with a reduction in the plasma volume. There is no true increase in the red blood cell mass. A similar mechanism has been postulated as the explanation for a condition referred to as **"stress" erythrocytosis**. This condition is recognized clinically as an elevation of the hemoglobin level in young to middle-aged males who smoke, are hypertensive, and live a high-pressure lifestyle. Smoking may be the most important factor in causing stress erythrocytosis. Patients who smoke a pack or more of cigarettes per day will have carboxyhemoglobin levels of 10% or higher. However, increased vascular tone and a reduction in plasma volume can also play a role. Stress erythrocytosis patients can show symptoms and signs related to increased blood viscosity and decreased brain blood flow. Even without a true increase in red blood cell volume, these patients have been shown to have reduced brain blood flows when their hemoglobins are above 17 g/dL.

CASE HISTORY • *Part 3*

Under the newest proposed guidelines for diagnosing polycythemia vera, the presence of a hemoglobin greater than 18.5 g/dL, together with a normal blood gas and presence of the *JAK2* V617F or similar *JAK2* exon 12 mutation, makes the diagnosis. The low to unmeasurable serum erythropoietin (EPO) level provides further support. At the same time, a single blood gas does not unequivocally rule out a component of hypoxia in this patient with chronic lung disease and obesity (Pickwickian syndrome) and may be reason enough for a sleep study with repeated blood gas measurements. A baseline set of iron studies is also in order.

Question

- What therapy should be initiated?

THERAPY

Effective management of the patient with polycythemia requires an accurate diagnosis. Although it makes sense to lower the hemoglobin level in patients with polycythemia vera or stress polycythemia, the increase in red blood cell mass in patients with hypoxic polycythemia is usually to the patient's physiologic advantage. In these settings, there has to be a very good reason to go against nature. Several side issues also require attention. Iron balance must be carefully assessed and appropriately managed. In patients with polycythemia vera, problems such as severe itching, erythromelalgia, thrombotic and bleeding complications, and symptomatic splenomegaly must be addressed.

Polycythemia Vera

The mainstay of effective treatment of the patient with polycythemia vera is the rapid and sustained reduction of the red blood cell mass. Aggressive phlebotomy is still the best way to achieve this reduction.

A. Phlebotomy Therapy

When a polycythemia vera patient is very symptomatic, phlebotomy should be performed daily or every other day, removing 200–500 mL each time, depending on the patient's hemodynamic status. When a patient is unable to tolerate a large-volume phlebotomy but needs a rapid reduction in hemoglobin level, a partial exchange transfusion can be performed by removing whole blood and reinfusing saline or a smaller volume of albumin or plasma. This procedure is most effective if the patient needs to be prepared for emergency surgery. The benefit of phlebotomy is 2-fold. It not only reduces the red cell mass and total blood volume acutely but, by stimulating an expansion of the plasma volume, also decreases viscosity. As whole blood viscosity returns to normal, the tendency to thrombosis is decreased. It is important to achieve a target hematocrit that is low enough to guarantee a return of the red blood cell mass to within normal limits. Otherwise, the patient will continue to be hypercoagulable. In general, this means phlebotomizing to a hematocrit below 45% in men and 40% in women. When the hematocrit is left at levels of 50% or higher, the patient is being undertreated.

Sustained reductions in red blood cell mass require that iron stores be exhausted. Otherwise, new red blood cell production will return the hemoglobin level to its original high level within a short period. Therefore, **phlebotomies must be continued until iron stores are exhausted** and the patient demonstrates a low serum iron and serum ferritin typical of iron-deficient erythropoiesis. A reduction in iron supply will suppress erythroid progenitor proliferation and limit new hemoglobin production. Of course, the drive to make new red blood cells can be so great that the patient's red blood cells will rapidly become microcytic and hypochromic, even while the hemoglobin is above 14–15 g/dL.

Success of long-term phlebotomy therapy will depend, therefore, on **management of the patient's iron balance**. The amount of iron ingested by the patient will determine the need for periodic phlebotomies. Patients must be educated regarding food and medicinal iron intake. Certainly, any iron supplement must be avoided because it will stimulate a rapid rise in the hemoglobin level. There are also downsides to being chronically iron deficient. Patients may complain of sore mouths, difficulty swallowing, spooning and splitting of the nails, a general loss of energy, and difficulty sleeping (see Chapter 5). This condition requires very careful treatment. Severely iron-deficient patients can be given 1–2 tablets of an oral iron preparation daily for 1 or 2 weeks at a time. This regimen can alleviate the symptoms of tissue iron deficiency without stimulating a major increase in the red blood cell mass. The patient must be monitored, however, and phlebotomized if the hemoglobin level rises.

B. Chemotherapy/Radiotherapy

Phlebotomy therapy alone may not be appropriate for all patients. Elderly individuals who cannot tolerate phlebotomy because of their cardiopulmonary status, symptoms associated with iron deficiency, or simply the logistics involved in monitoring therapy, are potential candidates for **radiotherapy**. Radioactive phosphorus (^{32}P) can be given as an intravenous bolus in a dose of 2–3 mCi/m^2 to a maximum dose of 5 mCi. Disease control is attained in up to 80% of patients with a single treatment, although some patients may need a retreatment after 3–6 months.

The downside of ^{32}P therapy is the **potential for marrow damage and the development of a hematologic malignancy**. A few patients will, unfortunately, trade their polycythemia for a transfusion-dependent anemia or pancytopenia.

Chemotherapy is an effective alternative to both phlebotomy and radiotherapy. It is preferred for patients who have very high platelet or granulocyte counts. Platelet counts in excess of 1 million/μL are associated with a higher incidence of both bleeding and thrombotic complications. This condition can be worsened by phlebotomy therapy, since iron deficiency will cause the platelet count to rise further and will increase red blood cell rigidity.

Of the possible **myelosuppressive drugs**, hydroxyurea has performed best in clinical trials. Other drugs including chlorambucil and busulfan, when given over a long period, are associated with an increased incidence of leukemia and pulmonary fibrosis.

1. Hydroxyurea—Most patients treated with hydroxyurea can be effectively controlled with a dose of 500–2,000 mg (1–4 tablets), given daily. Continuous, uninterrupted therapy is required. Hydroxyurea inhibits the synthesis of DNA and produces megaloblastic, ineffective hematopoiesis. It does not, however, decrease the number of stem cells capable of cell production. Therefore, even a short break in therapy can result in an immediate rebound production of all cell types.

Other **problems associated with hydroxyurea therapy** include gastrointestinal intolerance, stomatitis, hepatitis, rash, fever on occasion, and variable cytopenias. In some patients, anemia or leukopenia can set a limit to therapy despite a continued increase in the production of the other cell lines. The long-term management of hydroxyurea therapy, like phlebotomy therapy, is extremely demanding. Patients must be closely followed to guarantee compliance with the drug dosage and to monitor the CBC for side effects.

2. Interferon-α—Interferon-α has also been shown to be effective in the treatment of polycythemia vera. Compared with other therapies, it avoids hematologic complications associated with aggressive phlebotomy or hydroxyurea therapy, and it may delay the development of myelofibrosis if used early in the course of the disease. It also has proved to be of value in patients with pruritus. This may reflect a better control of megakaryocyte proliferation and platelet production by interferon. Beginning with a dose of 1 million units 3 times a week, the dose is gradually escalated to 3–5 million units 3 times a week. In some patients, periodic phlebotomy may still be needed if the dose tolerated by the patient does not give hematocrit control.

C. Management of Other Complications

Patients with polycythemia vera may report marked **pruritus** that is generalized but not associated with any specific skin lesion. This condition may correlate with a proliferation of mast cells and basophils or a release of prostaglandins and serotonin from platelets. Treatment of this condition can be a challenge. Antihistamines (diphenhydramine or hydroxyzine) may be effective when the condition is mild. When the condition is severe, however, the patient will need combined therapy aimed at both histamine and serotonin blockade with drugs such as doxepin, trifluoperazine, cyproheptadine, and cimetidine. If the pruritus appears to get worse with phlebotomy therapy, a short course of iron therapy may provide some relief. Interferon therapy may offer better control of pruritus in some intractable patients.

A few patients with polycythemia vera will complain of **erythromelalgia**, characterized by patchy, localized areas of burning pain and erythema of the skin. This condition is thought to be related to the platelet abnormality. Vascular injury with infarction, gangrene, or skin ulceration may be seen in severe cases. Treatment involves the use of hydroxyurea to lower the platelet count, platelet inhibitors such as aspirin, and vasodilator drugs.

Thrombocytosis and platelet dysfunction can result in either bleeding or thrombotic complications. The higher the platelet count, the more likely there will be a hemostatic defect. The most effective treatment is a sustained reduction in the platelet count using hydroxyurea. If the platelet count cannot be controlled, an antiplatelet agent such as aspirin or clopidogrel may be tried in patients with evidence of thrombotic disease. On the other hand, these agents should not be used in individuals who have a platelet function defect producing a prolonged bleeding time or bleeding tendency.

Gouty arthritis is seen in up to 10% of patients with polycythemia vera. Acute attacks should be managed similarly to primary gout with colchicine and phenylbutazone. Patients with very high uric acid levels who are at risk for recurrent episodes should be maintained on a dose of 300 mg of allopurinol per day.

D. Clinical Course

Although polycythemia vera can appear at any age, most patients present during their sixth or seventh decade. Often, the patient presents because of a transient ischemic attack or thrombotic stroke. The median survival for this group of patients is approximately 10 years. Related **causes of death** are thrombosis, acute leukemia, myelofibrosis with pancytopenia, or a complication of the illness such as hemorrhage, acute infection, or drug toxicity. When followed for over 10 years, 30% or more of patients will die of a thrombotic complication, most often a coronary or cerebral artery occlusion. Another 30% will die of cancer, with half of these developing myelofibrosis and acute myelogenous leukemia. The incidence of acute leukemia is 4-fold higher in patients who receive ^{32}P therapy or chemotherapy with the alkylating agent chlorambucil. It is most often an acute myeloid leukemia, which is resistant to antileukemic chemotherapy.

Patients who develop myelofibrosis go through a period where phlebotomy therapy is no longer necessary and then proceed to develop increasing splenomegaly and varying combinations of anemia, leukopenia, and thrombocytopenia. Blood film and marrow findings are similar to those of patients with primary myelofibrosis and include anisocytosis and poikilocytosis, teardrops, and nucleated red blood cells. The marrow shows progressive fibrosis with increased reticulin and collagen.

Secondary Erythrocytosis

Management of patients with secondary polycythemias will vary according to the specific cause. **Patients with mild hypoxic**

CASE HISTORY • Part 4

Given the fact that the patient's disorder (polycythemia vera) is largely restricted to the erythroid cell line, he is a candidate for phlebotomy therapy. Success will depend on the patient's iron balance, since phlebotomy-induced iron deficiency is required to limit red cell production in polycythemia vera. Therefore, periodic iron studies are important and the patient should not be given iron supplements of any kind. If phlebotomy is not effective, the patient would be a candidate for hydroxyurea therapy.

polycythemia should be left alone. The rise in the red blood cell mass helps compensate for their hypoxia despite the increase in viscosity. Patients who present with **an erythropoietin-producing tumor** should be treated for the tumor. In the case of the occasional **patient with a hemoglobinopathy associated with a very high hemoglobin level**, phlebotomy may be indicated, but only for symptomatic patients who have hemoglobins in excess of 22 g/dL.

Stress Erythrocytosis

Patients with stress polycythemia can show an impressive reduction in brain blood flow that is easily treated by phlebotomy. In most cases, removal of 300–500 mL of blood weekly for 3–6 weeks will be sufficient to lower the hemoglobin level to normal. This treatment will improve brain blood flow and will usually decrease complaints such as headache and generalized fatigue by the patient. Phlebotomy to the point of iron deficiency is unnecessary, whereas smoking cessation is recommended.

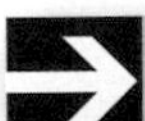

POINTS TO REMEMBER

The "normal" adult hemoglobin level varies according to age, gender, race, and whether an individual is living at an altitude well above sea level.

At higher than normal hemoglobin levels (>17 g/dL), whole blood viscosity increases dramatically, resulting in reduced blood flow to key organs, especially the brain.

Erythrocytosis is defined as an absolute increase in the red cell mass, which can usually be inferred when the hemoglobin is greater than 18.5 g/dL in men and greater than 16.5 g/dL in women. In situations where the plasma volume may be markedly reduced, a direct measurement of the red cell mass with ^{51}Cr-labelled red cells and the plasma volume with ^{131}I-labelled albumin may be required to make the diagnosis.

Polycythemia vera is a clonal disorder characterized by increases in 1 or more cell lines—erythrocytosis, leukocytosis, and/or thrombocytosis. At least 90% of clinically recognized polycythemia patients exhibit the *JAK2* V617F or other *JAK2* exon 12 gene mutation.

Polycythemia vera can be diagnosed based on several major and minor clinical criteria or in patients with clearly elevated hematocrits/hemoglobins (increased red cell mass) from the presence of the *JAK2* gene mutation. Since other myeloproliferative disorders (primary myelofibrosis and essential thrombocytosis) share the *JAK2* mutation, it is not specific for polycythemia vera.

Secondary erythrocytosis is seen in patients with hypoxia from chronic lung disease, congenital heart disease, high-affinity hemoglobinopathies, methemoglobinemia, erythropoietin-producing tumors, renal cystic disease, and erythropoietin receptor mutations.

Relative erythrocytosis, due to a reduction in the plasma volume, is seen in patients with severe salt and water dehydration, overdose/use of diuretics, Cushing disease, pheochromocytoma, and allergic or anaphylactic reactions with loss of plasma proteins from the vascular space.

"Stress" erythrocytosis is a modest increase in the hemoglobin/hematocrit level, most often seen in middle-aged males who smoke (elevated carboxyhemoglobin levels), are hypertensive, and live a high-pressure lifestyle.

The treatment of erythrocytosis has as its primary goal the reduction of the hematocrit/hemoglobin to levels below 45%/15 g/dL, to improve whole blood viscosity and reduce complications such as thrombosis and increased bleeding tendency.

Polycythemia vera is readily controlled in most patients with periodic phlebotomy sufficient to induce iron deficiency and limit red cell production or, in patients with marked leukocytosis or thrombocytosis, chemotherapy—either hydroxyurea or γ-interferon may be required. Patients with generalized pruritus or erythromelalgia will usually require chemotherapy.

The median survival of uncomplicated polycythemia vera patients exceeds 10 years. Causes of death include thrombotic events, myelofibrosis with pancytopenia, and acute myelogenous leukemia, especially in patients treated with chlorambucil or ^{32}P therapy.

BIBLIOGRAPHY

Polycythemia Vera

Baskurt OK, Meiselman HJ: Blood rheology and hemodynamics. Semin Thromb Hemost 2003;29:435.

Finazzi G, Barbui T: How I treat patients with polycythemia vera. Blood 2007;109:5104.

Fruchtman SM et al: From efficacy to safety: a Polycythemia Study Group report on hydroxyurea in patients with polycythemia vera. Semin Hematol 1997;34:17.

Gordeuk VR et al: Congenital disorder of oxygen-sensing: association of the homozygous Chuvash polycythemia VHL mutation with thrombosis and vascular abnormalities but not tumors. Blood 2004;103:3924.

Kippel S et al: Quantification of PRV-1 mRNA distinguishes polycythemia vera from secondary erythrocytosis. Blood 2003;102:3569.

Landaw SA: Acute leukemia in polycythemia vera. Semin Hematol 1986;23:156.

Marchioli R, for Gruppo Italiano Studio Policitemia: Polycythemia vera: the natural history of 1213 patients followed 20 years. Ann Intern Med 1995;123:656.

Muller EW et al: Long-term treatment with interferon-α 2b for severe pruritus in patients with polycythemia vera. Br J Haematol 1995;89:313.

Najean Y, Rain JD: The very long-term evolution of polycythemia vera: an analysis of 318 patients initially treated by phlebotomy or 32P between 1969 and 1981. Semin Hematol 1997;34:6.

Najean Y, Rain JD: Treatment of polycythemia vera: use of 32P alone or in combination with maintenance therapy using hydroxyurea in 461 patients greater than 65 years of age. The French Polycythemia Study Group. Blood 1997;89:2319.

Silver RT: Interferon α: effects of long-term treatment for polycythemia vera. Semin Hematol 1997;34:40.

Spivak JL: Polycythemia vera: myths, mechanisms, and management. Blood 2002;100:4272.

Spivak JL, Silver RT: The revised World Health Organization criteria for polycythemia, essential thrombocytosis, and primary myelofibrosis: an alternative proposal. Blood 2008;112:231.

Tartarsky I, Sharon R: Management of polycythemia with hydroxyurea. Semin Hematol 1997;34:24.

Tefferi A et al: Proposals and rationale for revision of the World Health Organization diagnostic criteria for polycythemia, essential thrombocythemia, and primary myelofibrosis: recommendations from an ad hoc international expert panel. Blood 2007;110:1092.

Secondary Erythrocytosis

Brown MM, Wade JPH, Marshall J: Fundamental importance of arterial oxygen content in the regulation of cerebral blood flow in man. Brain 1985;108:81.

Gregg XT, Prchal JT: Erythropoietin receptor mutations and human disease. Semin Hematol 1997;34:70.

Perloff JK et al: Adults with cyanotic congenital heart disease: hematologic management. Ann Intern Med 1989;109:406.

DISORDERS OF PORPHYRIN METABOLISM • 14

CASE HISTORY • *Part I*

A 45-year-old housepainter presents with several weeks of worsening abdominal pain, headache, insomnia, and difficulty gripping his paint brush. His past history and review of systems (ROS) is positive for smoking, alcoholism, and reactive depression. Vital signs: BP - 165/95 mm Hg, P - 84 bpm, R - 16 bpm. Examination is positive for grayish staining of the gum line, hepatomegaly, diffuse abdominal tenderness without rebound, and 2+ weakness of wrist extensors bilaterally.

CBC: Hematocrit/hemoglobin - 36%/12 g/dL
MCV - 87 fL MCH - 30 pg MCHC - 31 g/dL
RDW-CV - 12%
WBC count - 6,500/μL
Platelet count - 160,000/μL

• SMEAR MORPHOLOGY

Normocytic and normochromic red cells, a few hypochromic cells, and occasional "shift cells" with questionable stippling. Normal white blood cell and platelet morphology.

Reticulocyte count/index - 4%/1.5–2.0

Questions

- What condition(s) is suggested from this presentation and complete blood count (CBC) findings?
- What additional history and laboratory tests are needed to confirm the diagnosis?

The **porphyrias** are caused by inherited defects in the heme biosynthetic pathway that result in excess production of porphyrin precursors. Depending on the type of excess porphyrin produced, patients can experience severe photosensitivity, nerve damage, liver disease, and anemia. Detection requires a high level of suspicion and skill in using the laboratory. Accurate diagnosis is important because there are now effective therapies for several of these defects.

NORMAL PORPHYRIN SYNTHESIS

The normal heme biosynthetic pathway is shown in Figure 14–1. The initial step is condensation of glycine and succinyl-CoA to form **δ-aminolevulinic acid (δ-ALA)**, which is catalyzed by a mitochondrial enzyme, ALA synthase. This is the only enzyme step that requires a cofactor, in this case, pyridoxal-5-phosphate (vitamin B_6).

The next several steps include formation of porphobilinogen, uroporphyrinogen III, and coproporphyrinogen III, which are catalyzed by cytosolic enzymes. The final three steps in the sequence depend on mitochondrial enzymes (coproporphyrinogen oxidase, protoporphyrinogen oxidase, and ferrochelatase). Chelation of iron to protoporphyrin IX depends on an adequate supply of iron; deficient patients accumulate excess protoporphyrin in their red blood cells.

Porphyrin synthesis is regulated by the activity of ALA synthase and the end product, heme. Levels of transcription and

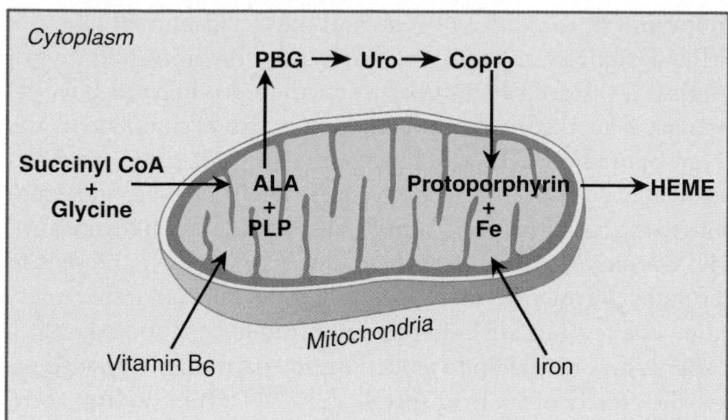

FIGURE 14–1. **The normal heme biosynthetic pathway.** The first step in the synthesis of heme is the condensation of glycine and succinyl-CoA with pyridoxal 5-phosphate as the coenzyme to form δ-aminolevulinic acid (δ-ALA). This process is carried out in mitochondria catalyzed by the enzyme ALA synthase. The subsequent formation of porphobilinogen, uroporphyrinogen III, and coproporphyrinogen III occurs in the cell cytoplasm. The final steps of protoporphyrin production and the assembly of protoporphyrin IX and iron to form heme depend on mitochondrial enzymes.

translation of ALA synthase in mitochondria are a function of the heme concentration. This is especially true for liver porphyrin synthesis where any reduction in free heme owing to inhibition of heme synthesis or accelerated heme breakdown induces a major increase in hepatic ALA synthase. Defects in any one of the intermediate enzymes in the heme biosynthetic pathway also result in an excess production of porphyrin precursors proximal to the enzyme defect, even while heme synthesis is maintained.

CLINICAL FEATURES

The most prominent clinical findings associated with excess production of porphyrin precursors are cutaneous photosensitivity and nervous system dysfunction. Patients with **porphyria cutanea tarda (PCT)** generally present with photosensitivity problems, including appearance of vesiculo/bullous eruptions on the face and hands; white, plaquelike scar formation; hyperpigmentation; and excess hair formation over the face. Symptoms and signs of liver disease and excessive iron loading are also common. **Erythropoietic protoporphyria (EPP)** patients experience variable photosensitivity beginning in childhood, characterized by marked itching, burning, erythema, and angioneurotic edemalike swelling of exposed skin areas. Unlike PCT, vesicle formation is uncommon and scarring and hirsutism are not seen. Neuropathic presentations are more typical of patients with **acute intermittent porphyria (AIP), variegate porphyria (VP), hereditary coproporphyria (HCP),** and **lead poisoning**. Acute intermittent porphyria patients present with recurrent bouts of severe, poorly localized abdominal pain, peripheral and cranial motor neuropathies, seizures, and psychotic episodes. Photosensitivity is not seen with AIP, but does occur in VP and HCP patients.

TABLE 14–1 • Patterns of porphyrin excretion

	δ-ALA/PBG	URO	COPRO	PROTO
Acute intermittent porphyria	↑↑/↑↑	↑	NL	NL
Porphyria cutanea tarda	NL	↑↑	↑	NL
Hereditary coproporphyria	↑/↑	±	↑	NL
Variegate porphyria	↑/↑	↑[a]	↑[a]	↑[a]
Erythropoietic protoporphyria	NL	NL	NL	↑↑[b]
Lead poisoning	↑/NL	NL	↑↑	↑[b]

[a]*Excretion predominantly in stool.*
[b]*Levels increased in red blood cells.*

Laboratory Studies

Measurements of **porphyrin precursors** in urine and stool provide the key to diagnosis. **Other laboratory studies** of importance in the evaluation of a porphyria patient include the routine complete blood count (CBC); serum iron, total iron-binding capacity (TIBC), and ferritin levels; and liver function studies. In patients with neurologic damage, **electroencephalography and electromyography studies** can be important.

Accumulation and excretion of porphyrin precursors in red blood cells, urine, and feces for the various disease states are summarized in Table 14–1. **Screening for excess porphyrin excretion** is best carried out when the patient is symptomatic. This situation is especially true for measurements of δ-ALA and porphobilinogen in patients with AIP, HCP, and VP. Porphyrin excretion is highest when the patient is experiencing a neurologic crisis, especially during an attack of abdominal pain. Protoporphyrin measurements in patients with EPP and lead poisoning are easily carried out using a **standard red blood cell zinc protoporphyrin assay**. Detection of elevated porphyrin levels in patients with VP requires a **stool assay**.

The CBC can be abnormal in patients with EPP and lead poisoning. Mild hemolysis and a tendency to hypochromia have been observed. Lead poisoning is associated with prominent stippling of red blood cells on the peripheral blood film and the appearance of ringed sideroblasts in the marrow. It is easily diagnosed by direct measurement of lead levels in blood. **Measurements of serum iron, TIBC, and serum ferritin levels** are essential in patients being evaluated for PCT. Excessive liver iron loading leading to cirrhosis is a prominent manifestation of this disease. When iron studies are equivocal, **liver biopsy** may be needed to fully evaluate the severity of the cirrhosis and the accumulation of iron in hepatocytes.

DIAGNOSIS

Differential diagnosis of porphyria is not difficult once the possibility of its existence is considered. Only 5 major, inherited

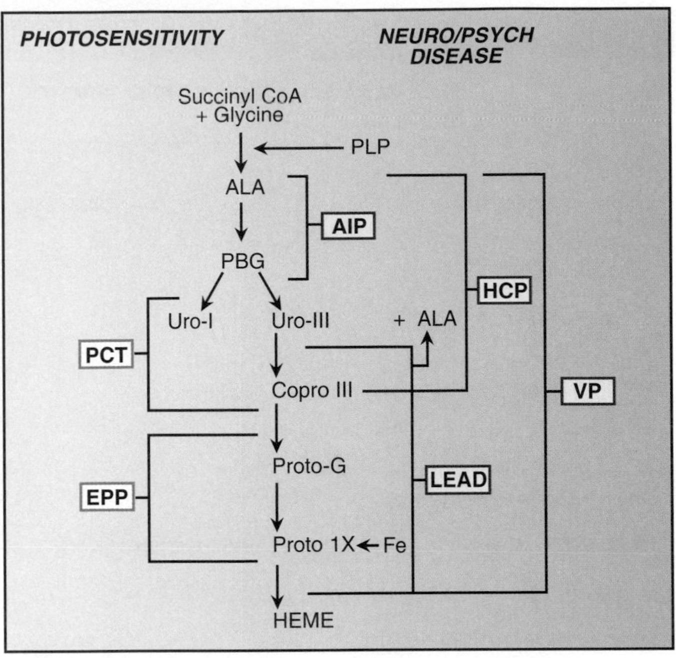

FIGURE 14–2. **Differential diagnosis of the porphyrias and lead poisoning.** PCT and EPP present with symptoms and signs of increased photosensitivity. In both situations, excess porphyrins produced include the uroporphyrins, coproporphyrins, and protoporphyrins. These are highly fluorescent molecules that are found both in red blood cells and in urine and stool. In contrast, AIP, HCP, VP, and lead poisoning present with symptoms and signs of neurologic dysfunction, especially recurrent episodes of abdominal pain and both cranial and motor nerve dysfunction. The common factor in these conditions is the excretion of excess amounts of δ-ALA and porphobilinogen. Those conditions (HCP and VP) where there is also excretion of uroporphyrins, coproporphyrins, and protoporphyrins show a mixed picture of neurologic dysfunction and photosensitivity.

forms of porphyria plus lead poisoning need to be considered (Figure 14–2). Two of these (PCT and EPP) typically present with **photosensitivity problems**, whereas the others (AIP, HCP, VP, and lead poisoning) present with **neurologic abnormalities**. The specific diagnosis of the individual type of porphyria is usually obvious from the clinical presentation and routine studies of porphyrin excretion. Actual assay for the enzyme defect is unnecessary.

Porphyria Cutanea Tarda

Porphyria cutanea tarda (PCT) results from a deficiency of hepatic uroporphyrinogen decarboxylase enzyme (URO-D). It is the most common of the porphyrias and can either be inherited as an autosomal dominant trait or occur sporadically, often in association with hepatitis C virus (HCV) infection or chemical exposure.

The *URO-D* gene has been located at p34 on chromosome 1. Two forms of PCT are observed clinically. **Familial PCT patients** (approximately 25% of patients with PCT) are heterozygous for mutations of the *URO-D* gene and have half-normal levels of URO-D activity and protein. While most heterozygotes do not express a disease phenotype, when they do, hepatic URO-D activity is markedly reduced and porphyrins accumulate in the liver. **Sporadic PCT**, which accounts for most cases, has been associated with HCV infection, excess alcohol intake, and exposure to estrogens. From 60%–90% of sporadic PCT cases are anti-HCV positive, and most of these have HCV mRNA present in serum by polymerase chain reaction, indicating an active infection. The level of URO-D protein in the liver of sporadic PCT patients is normal despite reductions in enzyme activity, suggesting the presence of a liver-specific URO-D inhibitor. Iron accumulation in hepatocytes appears to play a key role in this inhibition of URO-D activity and may reflect concurrent abnormalities in the *HFE*, *HAMP*, *or HJV* genes or gene expression. Homozygosity for the *HFE C282Y* hereditary hemochromatosis mutation (see Chapter 15) is seen in up to 20% of PCT patients. Dysregulation of *HAMP* with reduced levels of hepatic hepcidin, somehow related to HCV infection, alcohol intake, or estrogen use, may be responsible for the remainder.

The characteristic clinical feature of PCT is marked **photosensitivity** with the appearance of vesiculo/bullous eruptions of the face and hands, hyperpigmentation, and excessive hair growth on the face. Some patients develop marked thickening and scarring of the skin reminiscent of scleroderma. Most PCT patients also show **manifestations of liver disease**. In some cases, the appearance of jaundice and mild to moderately advanced cirrhosis can be the event that brings the patient to medical attention. **Excess tissue iron loading** with elevation of the serum iron and serum ferritin levels can also be the first clue to the diagnosis. All patients with PCT should have a full evaluation of liver function including iron studies, and should be considered for a liver biopsy to document both the severity of hepatocellular damage and the level of iron loading of hepatocytes.

A study of **porphyrin precursor excretion in urine** confirms the diagnosis. PCT patients show an excessive excretion of uroporphyrinogens I and III, and to a lesser extent coproporphyrinogen; δ-ALA and porphobilinogen levels are never increased.

Erythropoietic Protoporphyria

Erythropoietic protoporphyria (EPP) patients present during childhood with complaints of **itching, burning, and angioneurotic edemalike swelling of skin that occurs almost immediately with sunlight exposure**. Unlike PCT patients, EPP patients tend not to have vesiculo/bullous eruptions or skin scarring. In addition, EPP patients are not at risk for liver disease, iron loading, or neurologic dysfunction.

EPP results from the autosomal dominant inheritance of a deficiency (10%–30% of normal) in the ferrochelatase (heme synthetase) enzyme. This inhibits the final step in heme production and results in an accumulation of protoporphyrin IX in marrow erythroid precursors and adult red blood cells. It does not result, however, in a significant anemia, although red blood cells may be slightly microcytic and hypochromic. A measurement of **red blood cell zinc protoporphyrin levels or**

demonstration of marked fluorescence of marrow precursors can be used to confirm the diagnosis of EPP.

Congenital Erythropoietic Porphyria

Congenital erythropoietic porphyria (CEP) is inherited as an autosomal recessive deficiency of uroporphyrinogen synthase. Type I isomers of both uro- and coproporphyrins accumulate in marrow precursors, mature red cells, and plasma, and are excreted in both urine and stool. Cutaneous photosensitivity is severe, leading to progressive disfigurement of hands and face. Hypertrichosis and reddish-brown staining of the teeth with the fluorescent porphyrins is a prominent feature and has been advanced as the basis for the "werewolf" myth. A hemolytic anemia with splenomegaly, most likely as a result of the high levels of red cell porphyrins, is also a component of the disorder. The diagnosis may be confirmed by the pattern of porphyrin excretion and measurement of uroporphyrinogen synthase activity.

Acute Intermittent Porphyria

Acute intermittent porphyria (AIP) is caused by the autosomal dominant inheritance of a deficiency in porphobilinogen deaminase. It is a relatively common form of porphyria and classically presents with recurrent episodes of poorly defined, **diffuse abdominal pain**. The severity of the presentation can, unfortunately, lead to an unrevealing exploratory laparotomy before the diagnosis is made. Other **neurologic abnormalities** include proximal motor neuropathies with axonal degeneration and loss of reflexes, cranial nerve damage (most often cranial nerves VII and X), bulbar paralysis, and seizures. Acute psychosis during exacerbations of the illness is also seen. **Rarer manifestations of AIP** include cardiac arrhythmias, inappropriate antidiuretic hormone (ADH) secretion with hyponatremia, and chronic hypertension.

AIP is rarely seen before puberty and tends to be more common in women. This situation may relate to the **tendency for hormones and drugs to induce acute exacerbations of the disease.** Birth control pills that contain high levels of progesterone and pregnancy are known to induce AIP attacks. Several drugs, including barbiturates, sulfonamide antibiotics, anticonvulsants, and alcohol, also increase the production of δ-ALA and porphobilinogen. Finally, a sudden decrease in caloric intake with dieting or illness can precipitate an attack.

Laboratory diagnosis of AIP is straightforward. A urine sample should be obtained while the patient is symptomatic, especially during an attack of acute abdominal pain, to screen for δ-ALA and porphobilinogen. The excretion of both products should be markedly increased. Screening between attacks is not as reliable, even though most AIP patients do have at least some elevation of both products at all times. Attempts to increase excretion by starvation or drug administration are not advised.

Variegate Porphyria

Variegate porphyria (VP) is caused by an inherited deficiency in protoporphyrinogen oxidase, which is a much less common form of porphyria, being most prevalent in Finnish and South African populations. It can present with **neurologic abnormalities** similar to those of AIP, or **skin manifestations** more typical of PCT. In both cases, the disease tends to be milder. An occasional patient can present with **abdominal pain attacks** as severe as those seen in AIP patients, however.

Laboratory diagnosis of VP requires assay of porphyrin precursors in stool. Protoporphyrin and coproporphyrinogen levels are increased at all times; δ-ALA, porphobilinogen, and uroporphyrinogen levels are increased during attacks of abdominal pain. Assays of porphyrin precursors in urine are inadequate to make the diagnosis.

Hereditary Coproporphyria

Hereditary coproporphyria (HCP) is caused by an inherited defect in coproporphyrinogen oxidase. It is a very uncommon form of porphyria but presents with **symptoms and signs similar to a mild AIP**. Some patients also complain of mild photosensitivity. Diagnosis is confirmed by demonstrating very **high levels of coproporphyrinogen III in urine**, as well as δ-ALA and porphobilinogen during attacks of abdominal pain.

Lead Poisoning

Lead-poisoned patients can present with symptoms and signs that mimic the neurologic abnormalities seen with AIP. Attacks of **severe, diffuse abdominal pain with episodes of paralytic ileus** are the most common manifestation of acute lead intoxication. **Motor neuropathies and central nervous system damage** are also observed. Chronic low-level lead exposure can lead to hypertension, hyperuricemia, interstitial nephritis, and renal failure. In contrast to AIP, patients with severe lead toxicity usually are anemic. This reflects the greater effect of lead on the erythroid precursor heme biosynthetic pathway. Even low-level lead poisoning should be screened for **in all children and adults whose occupation puts them at risk**.

Several of the heme synthesis enzymes are inhibited by lead, including ALA synthase and dehydrase; heme synthase (ferrochelatase); uroporphyrinogen decarboxylase; and coprophyrinogen oxidase. Tests of urinary porphyrins will demonstrate excess excretion of δ-ALA without a comparable increase in porphobilinogen. Coproporphyrin III levels are also increased, not because of the toxic effect of lead on the coproporphyrinogen oxidase enzyme per se, but perhaps due to induction of an alternate metabolic pathway of coproporphyrin production.

With **chronic lead toxicity**, the routine CBC will show a modest normocytic, hypochromic anemia with mild hemolysis and an increase in the reticulocyte index and lactic dehydrogenase (LDH). The red blood cell zinc protoporphyrin level is elevated (usually more than 250 μg/dL), and red blood cell stippling should be obvious on blood films prepared from fresh, finger-stick blood. An ethylenediaminetetraacetic acid (EDTA) anticoagulated blood film is not as reliable, since EDTA can make the stippling disappear. Stippling is related to the inhibition of pyrimidine 5′-nucleotidase by lead. Accumulation of pyrimidine nucleotides inhibits the depolymerization of ribosomal RNA in reticulocytes, resulting in visible dust-like

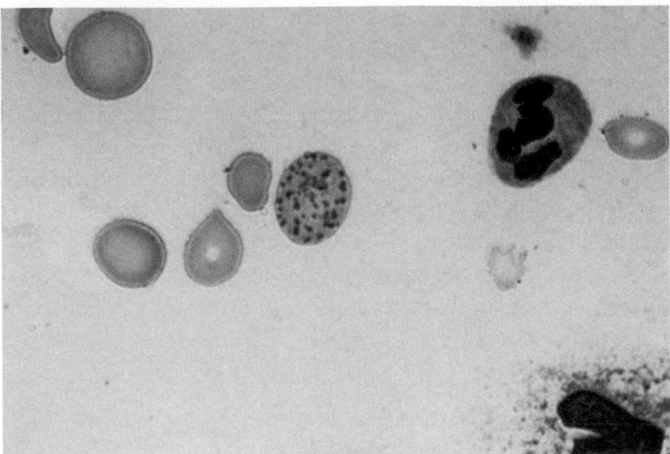

FIGURE 14–3. **Stippling.** Fine, dust-like basophilic stippling of newly produced red cells is commonly seen in symptomatic lead-poisoned patients. A fresh finger stick blood sample should be used to make the smear, since EDTA anticoagulant can make the stippling disappear. Of course, a direct measurement of the blood lead level is diagnostic.

particles in new red cells (Figure 14–3). Severe, chronic lead poisoning can also lead to the appearance of ringed sideroblasts in the marrow (see Chapter 9).

The diagnosis is confirmed by a measurement of a blood lead level. Symptomatic disease with anemia in adults is usually accompanied by an increase in blood lead to levels well in excess of 50 μg/dL (2.4 μmol/L). Hypertension, renal disease, and learning disabilities in children have been associated with lead levels of 7–35 μg/dL, well below the Occupational Safety and Health Administration (OSHA) requirement of maintaining a blood lead level less than 40 μg/dL in workers exposed to high levels of environmental lead.

THERAPY

There are effective treatments for the major forms of porphyria, including AIP, PCT, and EPP, as well as for lead poisoning. Effective management of infected patients also involves educating the patient regarding risk factors that can increase the severity of the disease process.

Porphyria Cutanea Tarda

PCT patients with cirrhosis and iron loading should be **aggressively phlebotomized** to deplete their excess tissue iron. Generally, the magnitude of the iron overload is less than that seen in idiopathic hemachromatosis and removal of 500 mL of blood every 1–2 weeks for 6 months is usually sufficient. Patients should also be advised to **avoid alcohol**. These 2 precautions can prevent further hepatocellular damage and result in a decrease in light sensitivity. In some patients, even the cutaneous thickening and scarring will appear to improve.

Treatment with low-dose **chloroquine** (125 mg twice weekly) has also been recommended for treatment of PCT. The mechanism of action is unclear, however. Chloroquine that is concentrated in the liver may complex with the porphyrin or stimulate an increased release from hepatocytes or both. **Interferon therapy** may play a role in patients with active HCV infections. Reports have suggested that the level of porphyrin excretion and the progression of liver disease can be reduced.

Acute Intermittent Porphyria

Effective management of patients with AIP requires **close attention to factors that can precipitate attacks or worsen an ongoing attack**. Drugs and hormones that lead to increased production of δ-ALA and porphobilinogen must be avoided. Most narcotics are safe for pain control, and both chlorpromazine and diazepam (Valium) are appropriate to control nausea and vomiting. Since fasting worsens an AIP attack, patients

CASE HISTORY • *Part 2*

House painters are at increased risk of acute and chronic lead poisoning, especially when involved with scraping or burning old paint or applying a lead-containing product. This patient's presentation—abdominal pain, headache, sleep disturbance, and a motor neuropathy, together with a gum "lead line," hypertension, and abdominal tenderness—strongly supports the diagnosis of acute lead poisoning. The anemia also fits the picture. Usually, the anemia is normocytic and normochromic (slight hypochromia may be seen) with evidence of low-grade extravascular hemolysis. Fine basophilic stippling of newly produced red cells is a characteristic finding (best seen on a fresh finger stick sample).

The firm diagnosis of lead poisoning is best made on the basis of the blood lead level. This patient was found to have a blood lead of 85 μg/dL (4 μmol/L), a level associated with both symptomatic disease and anemia. Other confirmatory tests include the erythrocyte zinc protoporphyrin level (acute lead poisoning is associated with levels >250 μg/dL), and increased urine levels of δ-ALA and coproporphyrin III, without a concomitant increase in porphobilinogen.

should receive a **high-carbohydrate diet**: at least 300 g of carbohydrate per day, either enterally or parenterally.

Since heme will downregulate δ-ALA and porphobilinogen synthesis, patients can be effectively treated with **intravenous infusions of hematin** given in a dose of 1–4 mg/kg once or twice daily. Hematin will significantly decrease ALA and porphobilinogen production. The onset of action is somewhat slower than glucose loading, and a full clinical response may not be seen for 48–72 hours. Hematin is primarily indicated for treatment of severe neurologic diseases or a major abdominal pain attack. Excessive doses of hematin can cause renal tubular damage.

Erythropoietic Protoporphyria

Children with relatively mild EPP can be managed by protecting them from direct sunlight. **β-Carotene** given in doses of 120–180 mg/d in adults can help. **Cholestyramine** may be used to interrupt the enterohepatic circulation of protoporphyrin. For patients who have relatively severe hemolysis, **splenectomy** will help decrease the level of red blood cell turnover and lessen protoporphyrin production.

Lead Poisoning

The first and most important step in treating lead poisoning is to **identify and eradicate exposure**. The next step is to use **chelating agents** to mobilize lead and encourage excretion into urine. The principal agents available include calcium disodium versenate, penicillamine, and dimercaprol. Acutely ill patients should receive a 5-day course of 12–24 mg/kg of dimercaprol per day and 0.5–1.5 g/m^2 of edetate calcium disodium per day. After a pause of 2–3 days, this regimen can be repeated until the patient is asymptomatic and demonstrates a blood lead level less than 40 μg/dL. Penicillamine given in a dose of 20–40 mg/kg but not more than 1 g/d can be given over several months to further deplete the bone lead pool.

POINTS TO REMEMBER

Defects in the heme synthetic pathway result in an excess production of porphyrin precursors, even while heme synthesis is maintained.

Excessive levels of porphyrins are most often associated with cutaneous photosensitivity and neuropathies.

Porphyria cutanea tarda patients present with variable photosensitivity, vesiculo/bullous eruptions, scarring, hirsutism, liver disease, and iron loading. The first indication of the disease may be a presentation resembling hemachromatosis with advancing cirrhosis.

Erythropoietic porphyria patients present in childhood with complaints of itching, burning, and edema immediately upon sunlight exposure, but no permanent scarring. Congenital erythropoietic porphyria patients have severe photosensitivity, scarring to the point of disfigurement, and staining of teeth and bones with fluorescent porphyrins. They also have a hemolytic anemia and splenomegaly.

Acute intermittent porphyria, variegate porphyria, hereditary coproporphyria, and lead poisoning present with various neuropathies, seizures, and psychotic episodes.

Lead poisoning is a major environmental hazard and is associated with inhibition of a number of heme biosynthetic pathway enzymes. Patients present with neuropathies, especially abdominal pain and wrist drop, hypertension, renal failure, and a mild hemolytic anemia.

The various porphyrias can be easily distinguished using their patterns of urinary porphyrin excretion.

BIBLIOGRAPHY

Ajioka RS et al: Down-regulation of hepcidin in porphyria cutanea tarda. Blood 2008;112:4723.

Bulaj ZJ et al: Hemochromatosis genes and other factors contributing to the pathogenesis of porphyria cutanea tarda. Blood 2000;95:1565.

Cribier B et al: Porphyria cutanea tarda and hepatitis C viral infection: a clinical and virologic study. Arch Dermatol 1995;131:801.

Kushner JP: Laboratory diagnosis of the porphyrias. N Engl J Med 1991;324:1432.

McManus JF et al: Five new mutations in the uroporphyrinogen decarboxylase gene identified in families with cutaneous porphyria. Blood 1996;88:3589.

Najahi-Missaoui W, Dailey HA: Production and characterization of erythropoietic protoporphyric heterodimeric ferrochelatases. Blood 2005;106:1098.

HEMOCHROMATOSIS • 15

CASE HISTORY • *Part I*

A 47-year-old man presents with palpitations, shortness of breath, and marked asthenia. Past history and review of systems (ROS) are positive for more than 10 years of arthralgia/arthritis of both small and large joints, progressive loss of libido, and recent weight loss. Vital signs: BP - 135/80 mm Hg, P - 96 bpm, R - 16 bpm. Examination reveals a tanned, anxious white male; irregular pulse without cardiomegaly or murmurs; slight hepatomegaly; no obvious joint deformity; and testicular atrophy. Initial studies:

CBC: Hematocrit/hemoglobin - 42%/14 g/dL
MCV - 90 fL MCH - 32 pg MCHC - 33 g/dL
White blood cell count - 7,200 /µL with a normal differential
Platelet count - 190,000/µL

• SMEAR MORPHOLOGY

Normocytic and normochromic with normal white cell morphology.

Reticulocyte count/index - 1%/1.0
Blood chemistries: Fasting glucose - 150 mg/dL
Slightly elevated AST and ALT
Serum iron - 270 µg/dL TIBC - 300 µg/dL
Serum ferritin - 2,360 µg/L
ECG - Atrial fibrillation, left bundle hemiblock and strain pattern

Questions

- Given the patient's history and laboratory findings, what diagnosis comes to mind?
- What additional laboratory tests are indicated?

Excessive iron loading of tissues **(hemochromatosis)** can result from a primary genetic defect or as a complication of liver disease and certain anemias. Genetic predisposition to excess iron absorption **(hereditary hemochromatosis)** is especially prevalent in European populations; approximately 1 of every 8 individuals of Celtic or Northern European stock is heterozygous for the most common ***HFE* gene defect**, while 1 of 200 is homozygous. In addition, a number of other less common genetic defects involving steps in the regulation of iron absorption and storage have now been identified by genetic analysis in non-European populations. Patients with liver disease, pancreatic dysfunction, and certain erythropoietic disorders can also demonstrate significant iron loading, leading to tissue damage.

NORMAL IRON BALANCE

The major pathways of iron metabolism are described extensively in Chapter 5. Most of the body's iron is incorporated in hemoglobin, myoglobin, and iron-containing enzymes (see Table 5–1). The amount of iron bound to the transport protein, transferrin, is only 3 mg. Reticuloendothelial iron stores vary according to the patient's sex and diet. Adult males have up to 1,000 mg of reticuloendothelial iron stores, whereas children and menstruating females rarely have more than 200 mg.

Iron Storage, Transport, and Absorption

Iron is stored intracellularly as ferritin and hemosiderin. **Ferritin synthesis** is regulated according to iron availability by a system of cytoplasmic iron binding proteins (IRP-1 and -2) and a noncoding, mRNA iron regulatory element (IRE). With iron deficiency, binding of IRP to the mRNA IRE inhibits the translation of isoferritins. When abundant, iron blocks binding and promotes an increased synthesis of ferritin. In the absence of organ damage, primarily liver damage, serum ferritin is in equilibrium with tissue stores, and therefore can be used as an indirect indicator of total body iron stores.

Mucosal cells of the small intestine play a key role in maintaining iron balance. Iron transport involves several pathways (Figure 15–1). Heme iron appears to enter mucosal cells directly, where it is metabolized to release ferric iron, while mucin-bound iron binds to β_3 integrin in the membrane, which is then internalized and complexed with mobilferrin to form a ferrous iron compound referred to as paraferritin. A nonspecific duodenal iron transporter, **DMT1** (also called DCT1 or Nramp2), is responsible for uptake of ferrous iron from the intestinal lumen. Iron is then bound to cytosolic metal-binding proteins and can accumulate in the mucosal cell as ferritin or be transported into the plasma. Transport systems involved in the export of enterocyte iron to plasma include **hephaestin**, a copper-dependent ferroxidase, and **ferroportin**.

The **efficiency of iron transport varies** according to the type of iron ingested and body needs. **Mucosal cells regulate iron absorption** according to the level of iron stores as mediated by the liver-produced proteins **hepcidin, HFE, and transferrin receptor 2 (TFR2)**. Clinically, the control of iron absorption is exquisite. As body iron stores expand, hepcidin levels increase and, by binding to ferroportin, block iron transport. As stores shrink, hepcidin levels fall and absorption increases. HFE and TFR2 also appear to play a role in downregulating iron absorption, although the exact nature of their interactions with hepcidin is still a mystery. It is clear, however, that *HFE* and *TFR2* genetic defects result in excess iron absorption and tissue damage.

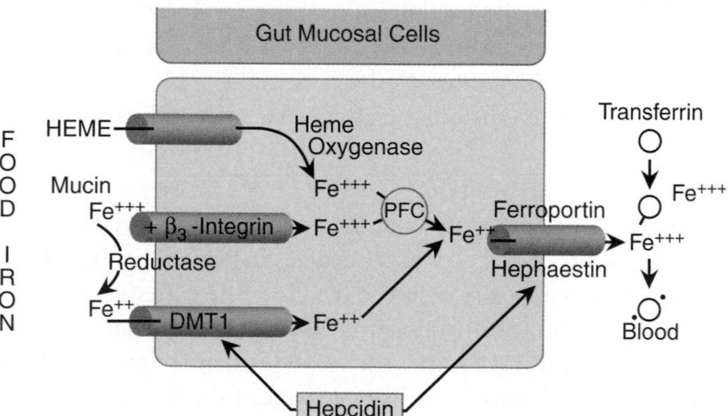

FIGURE 15–1. **Iron absorption.** Food iron is absorbed by any 1 of 3 pathways. Heme iron is transported directly into intestinal mucosal cells, where it is metabolized, releasing ferric iron. Free ferric iron is brought into solution at an acid pH, bound to mucin, and then picked up and transported complexed to β_3-integrin. Membrane ferric reductase also generates ferrous iron, which is then transported by the DMT1 pathway. Intracellular ferric iron is held in a paraferritin complex (PFC) until released for transport as ferrous iron across the basolateral membrane. This is facilitated by hephaestin (a ceruloplasmin homolog) and plasma ceruloplasmin and appears to be somehow regulated by HFE protein.

In a normal adult male, where iron losses per day are usually less than 1 mg and stores approach 1,000 mg, only a small portion of available dietary iron is absorbed. In contrast, a menstruating female needs to absorb up to 4 mg per day to compensate for menstrual losses. Absorption can increase to levels of 40–60 mg per day in the patient with severe iron-deficiency anemia who is receiving maximum oral iron therapy. The level of erythropoiesis also affects absorption. For example, patients with thalassemia who have high levels of ineffective erythropoiesis consistently show increased iron absorption.

Dietary Content of Iron

Dietary content of iron is also an important variable in determining the level of iron absorption and stores in humans. In Western cultures, most available iron comes from meats and meat by-products; much less comes from vegetable sources. Moreover, unlike developing countries, very little iron is incorporated in the diet from cooking in iron utensils or contamination by dirt. Thus, the content of iron in the Western diet is relatively low, only 6 mg per 1,000 kcal, providing the adult male with between 15 and 20 mg of iron per day, but only 8–15 mg per day to the adult female. This situation puts the adult female at a considerable disadvantage and helps explain the absence of significant reticuloendothelial iron stores in menstruating women. Childbearing presents an additional challenge and almost certainly produces iron deficiency unless iron supplements are provided.

Genetic Control of Iron Absorption and Transport

Some 5 genes have now been identified that play some role in iron transport and iron overload (Table 15–1). The *HFE* gene, localized to chromosome 6, was the first to be identified. Together with hepcidin, its protein HFE plays a key role in downregulating iron absorption. Inherited mutations of the *HFE*

TABLE 15–1 • Genes involved in iron absorption and transport

Gene	Location	Function
HFE	6q21	Essential for hepcidin production by liver
HJV (hemojuvelin)	1q21	May help regulate hepcidin production
HAMP (hepcidin)	19q13	Regulatory hormone for iron absorption and RE cell release
TFR2 (transferrin receptor 2)	7q22	Involved in regulation of hepcidin production
SLC40A1 (ferroportin)	2q32	Cell membrane iron transporter

gene are the principal cause of the adult form of **hereditary hemochromatosis** and typically are associated with both an increased level of iron absorption and excessive accumulation of iron in vital organs.

Three other genes—*HJV* (hemojuvelin), *TFR2* (transferrin receptor 2), and the gene responsible for ferroportin production—also appear to play important roles in iron absorption and cellular uptake. Mutations in both the *HJV* and *TFR2* genes have been shown to cause juvenile hemochromatosis.

CLINICAL FEATURES

Symptoms and signs of iron overload reflect the sensitivity of the liver, pancreas, anterior pituitary, joints, and heart to iron toxicity. The original description of **hereditary hemochromatosis** (most commonly the ***HFE* gene mutation**) used the term "bronze diabetes" to highlight the **darkening of the skin** and the appearance of **insulin-dependent diabetes** as 2 prominent characteristics of iron overload. As listed in Table 15–2, **cirrhosis, gonadal failure, arthritis, and cardiac failure** were also described as prominent findings. The clinical expression of the disease is similar for men and women, despite a proposed protective effect of menstrual iron losses. The mean age of presentation (48–50 years) is the same, and the iron load is only slightly less (a mean of 5.5 g for women versus 8.6 g for men). Postmenopausal women have the same level of iron loading as men.

The pattern of clinical disease tends to correlate with the level of iron accumulation. Patients with hereditary hemochromatosis are usually asymptomatic until 7 g or more of excess iron has accumulated. The **first symptoms and signs are asthenia (unexplained chronic fatigue)**, arthralgia, loss of libido, impotence (or amenorrhea), and a subtle change in skin color secondary to an increase in melanin pigment. However, these complaints are relatively nonspecific when it comes to identifying patients at risk. In large prospective screening studies, none of these symptoms or signs was significantly more common in homozygote hemochromatosis patients when compared with normal controls. **Clinical findings associated with advanced liver, pancreas, and heart damage** tend to occur beginning with iron accumulations of 10–15 g or more.

TABLE 15–2 • Clinical findings in hemochromatosis

Arthralgia/small and large joint arthritis
Gonadal failure
Testicular atrophy/impotence
Amenorrhea
Skin pigmentation
Cardiac failure/arrhythmias
Diabetes
Cirrhosis
Abdominal pain

Arthropathy of Iron Overload

The arthropathy of iron overload is generally not severe when it first appears and is often confused with rheumatoid or osteoarthritis since it involves multiple joints, including small joints of the hands and feet, and several large joints, including the knees, hips, and shoulders. Although joint x-rays are initially normal, with progression, films of the hands show osteopenia, cartilage loss (usually most pronounced in the second and third metacarpal phalangeal joints), cyst formation in metacarpal heads and, on occasion, the development of osteophytes. When large joint arthritis is pronounced, x-rays show chondrocalcinosis with linear and punctate calcification of the lateral meniscus. Large joints can also show cartilage loss, a narrowing of the joint space, and cystic erosions leading to a severe destructive arthritis.

It is important to **consider iron overload in the differential diagnosis of early arthritis.** Studies of patients presenting with hereditary hemochromatosis have shown a delay of 4–10 years between the patient's first arthritic complaints and the correct diagnosis. Even longer delays to diagnosis have been reported in patients who do not go on to develop other organ damage. However, it is also important to recognize the nonspecific nature of a complaint of arthralgias reaching back over many years.

Gonadal Failure and Amenorrhea

Another early manifestation of iron overload is gonadal failure owing primarily to iron loading of the anterior pituitary. Male patients may experience a loss of libido progressing to impotence with testicular atrophy, whereas women will complain of amenorrhea. Neither of these complaints is responsive to phlebotomy therapy.

Heart Disease

Heart disease, presenting as either congestive heart failure or a cardiac arrhythmia, can be a manifestation of iron overload. **Congestive failure** is usually biventricular in nature but may resemble constrictive pericarditis with jugular venous distention, hepatomegaly, and ascites. Patients may also present with **atrial fibrillation, supraventricular tachycardia, or a conduction defect**.

Diabetes and Hepatic Cirrhosis

When there is a delay in diagnosis, patients can develop symptoms and signs of diabetes and hepatic cirrhosis. The **diabetes** is caused by iron deposition in the β cells of the pancreas and islet cell dysfunction. Insulin resistance is observed and patients usually require insulin therapy. The earliest manifestation of **liver toxicity** is an elevation in liver enzymes (alanine aminotransferase and aspartate aminotransferase) and later serum bilirubin. Iron tends to concentrate in the parenchymal cells in the periportal areas of the liver. With time, these cells are destroyed and replaced by fibrous tissue, leading to cirrhosis (Figure 15–2). One-third or more of patients with iron overload–induced cirrhosis will go on to develop **hepatocellular carcinoma (hepatoma)**. This condition occurs late in the disease and is not prevented by iron removal. The clinical appearance of hepatoma is signaled by weight loss, fever, worsening liver function, and right upper quadrant pain.

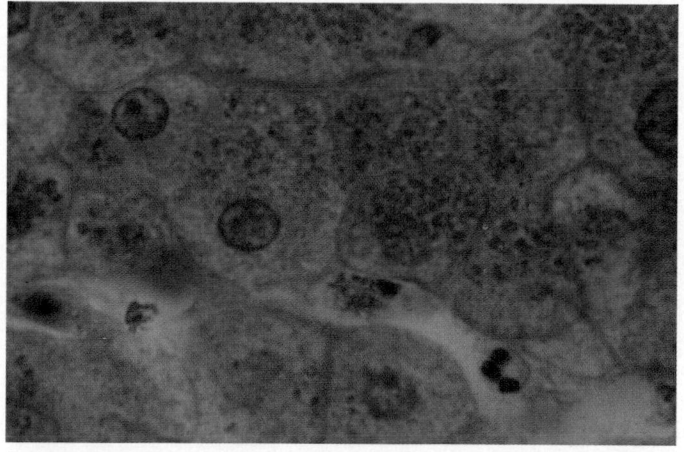

A

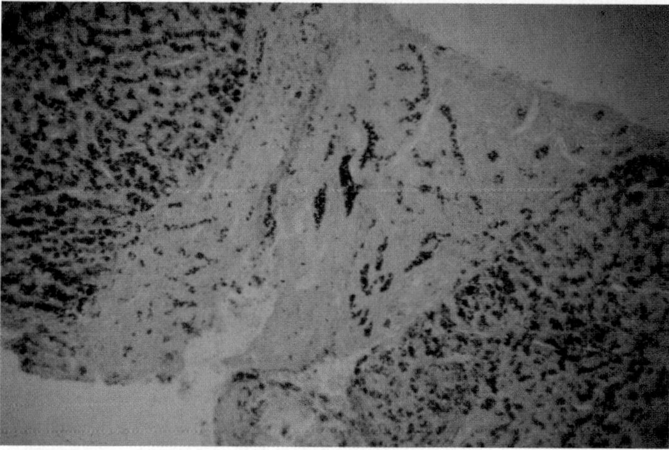

B

FIGURE 15–2. **Liver biopsy and iron overload.** Even without Prussian blue stain, heavy deposits of iron are visible in hepatocytes as golden-red granules **(A)**. With Prussian blue, both the extent and location of the iron deposits is clearly visible **(B)**. This liver needle biopsy section also shows significant fibrosis and architectural damage consistent with progressive cirrhosis.

Unusual Presentations of Hemochromatosis

Hemochromatosis appears in the differential diagnosis of systemic illness not only because the constellation of symptoms and signs involves several organs, but also because of several unusual presentations. Excessive iron loading has been associated with **coronary artery disease** and **acute myocardial infarction** in patients at a relatively young age. This does not seem to relate to a concomitant lipidopathy; iron overload may be an independent risk factor. **Right upper quadrant abdominal pain** prior to development of cirrhosis has been reported as a presenting complaint. Although it may mimic acute cholecystitis, it is not associated with an unusual tendency to gallstone formation. **Skin pigmentation secondary to increased melanin formation and iron deposition in the skin** is another interesting component of the disease. In those patients who develop severe pituitary failure, skin pigmentation may be accompanied by a thinning and wrinkling of the skin that suggests Addison disease.

Susceptibility to Infections

Hemochromatosis patients appear to have a greater susceptibility to infections with organisms such as ***Listeria, Yersinia enterocolitica,*** and ***Vibrio vulnificus***. This may reflect an increased growth potential of these organisms in patients with higher than normal serum iron (SI) levels or represent a side effect of iron overload on leukocyte and reticuloendothelial cell phagocytic and lytic activities. Hemochromatosis patients receiving iron-chelating therapy have also been reported to be more susceptible to ***Escherichia coli*** and ***Staphylococcus aureus*** septicemia. Again, the explanation for this susceptibility is unclear.

Laboratory Studies

The SI, total iron-binding capacity (TIBC), and serum ferritin levels are the mainstays in the laboratory diagnosis of iron overload (Table 15–3). Other important studies in the differential diagnosis and in the evaluation of organ toxicity include bone marrow aspirate, liver biopsy, and the detection of a mutant *HFE* gene.

TABLE 15–3 • Body iron balance

		Iron Overload States	
	Normal Males	**Hematopoietic Disease**	**Hemochromatosis**
Erythron iron (mg)	2,400	<2,000	2,400
Serum iron (SI)	Normal	Increased	Increased
Transferrin saturation (%)	<50	>50	>50
Reticuloendothelial stores	3+	>4+	3+
Serum ferritin (μg/L)	100	>500	>1,000
Liver iron	Normal	Increased iron in Kupffer cells and hepatocytes	Increased iron in hepatocytes only

A. Serum Iron/Ferritin Studies

The **normal SI** ranges from 50–150 μg/dL with a percent saturation of the TIBC of less than 45%. Patients with clinical signs and symptoms of hereditary hemochromatosis typically show an increase in the percent saturation to greater than 45% very early in their disease process, which reflects the failure in the regulation of iron transport from the reticuloendothelial cell to transferrin. Children and women may not demonstrate a higher than normal saturation, however, because of the relative depletion of their iron stores. In addition, any concomitant inflammatory disease can still increase hepcidin levels and block the delivery of iron from the reticuloendothelial cell, thereby reducing the percent saturation to below 45%.

Although the SI provides information as to the flow of iron to tissues, the **serum ferritin level** is the best indirect measure of total body iron stores. (The log serum TfR/ferritin ratio is more accurate in the diagnosis of iron deficiency and the anemia of inflammation; see Chapters 4 and 5). With certain exceptions, the serum ferritin correlates well enough that it can be used to estimate total body iron load (Figure 15–3). Each microgram per liter of serum ferritin equates to approximately 10 mg of iron stores. Thus, a normal adult male with a serum ferritin of 100 μg/L generally has 1,000 mg of iron stores. **Hereditary homozygous hemochromatosis patients with organ damage** will usually have serum ferritin levels in excess of 1,000–2,000 μg/L, representing an iron load of greater than 10–20 g. The correlation of the ferritin level can fail at higher levels of iron loading (>20 g) because of a limit to isoferritin production, as well as in patients with complicating illness, especially inflammatory conditions. Very high levels of serum ferritin are seen in patients with **acute hepatic necrosis** where large amounts of intracellular ferritin are released into circulation.

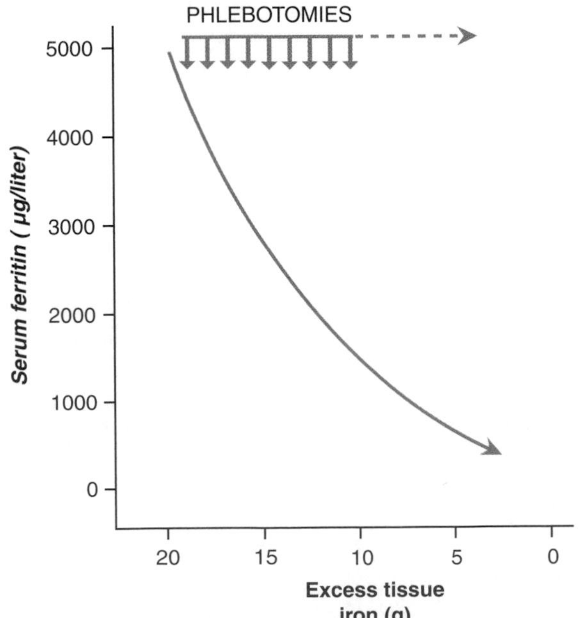

FIGURE 15–3. **Serum ferritin levels and body iron content.** The serum ferritin level provides an indirect measure of the total amount of iron in tissues. As a patient with hemochromatosis is phlebotomized, the fall in serum ferritin can be used to estimate the progress in iron unloading.

Modest elevations of serum ferritin to 150–300 μg/L are typically seen in non-hemochromatosis patients with **acute and chronic inflammatory states, liver disease, and certain tumors**. Patients with **aplastic anemia or ineffective erythropoiesis** (thalassemia major, megaloblastic and dysplastic anemias) also exhibit both high SI levels with elevated percent saturations and high ferritins. In the case of ineffective erythropoiesis, this reflects an increase in iron absorption with tissue iron loading, as well as increased red cell turnover. Repeated transfusion will also elevate the serum ferritin level because each unit of red blood cells contributes 200 mg of iron to stores. In light of these several causes of ferritin elevations, the serum ferritin has a high sensitivity but relatively low specificity for identifying homozygous hemochromatosis patients. Therefore, it has fallen out of favor as a screening or diagnostic test. At the same time, it can be extremely useful in tracking the successful removal of iron during phlebotomy therapy in hemochromatosis.

B. Marrow Iron Studies

A marrow aspirate or biopsy stained with Prussian blue provides information regarding both the level of reticuloendothelial iron stores and the incorporation of iron into hemoglobin (see Figure 2–17). **Patients with iron overload secondary to a hematopoietic disorder or repeated blood transfusion** typically show a marked increase in marrow iron stores. In fact, the amount of iron in each cell increases to where it obscures normal cellular landmarks. In contrast, patients with **hereditary hemochromatosis** show relatively normal amounts of reticuloendothelial cell iron.

A careful **inspection of marrow erythroid precursors** is also important. Patients with defects in globin production (the thalassemias) or mitochondrial function (the sideroblastic anemias) show excessive accumulation of iron in the cytoplasm of basophilic, polychromatophilic, and orthochromatic normoblasts. In thalassemia, excess iron tends to be distributed throughout the cell cytoplasm. Sideroblastic anemias are characterized by precursors with a ring or collar of large iron granules just around the nucleus. These "ringed sideroblasts" are the result of iron deposition in the perinuclear mitochondria (see Figure 9–3).

C. Liver Biopsy

Tissue iron loading and cirrhotic changes are best assessed by liver biopsy (see Figure 15–2). Using the Prussian blue stain, it is possible to characterize the distribution of iron in hepatocytes and Kupffer cells. Patients with **hereditary hemochromatosis** show iron deposits in hepatocytes and bile duct epithelium with lesser amounts in Kupffer cells. Hepatocytes in the periportal area are the most heavily involved. **Fibrosis progressing to cirrhosis** will generally reflect the amount of excess total body iron and the duration of the illness.

Organ damage can be correlated with a quantitative analysis of iron concentration per gram of dry weight liver tissue.

Normal individuals have hepatic iron concentrations of 1–2 mg/g dry weight tissue, whereas hemochromatosis heterozygotes have concentrations of 3–7 mg/g. Liver damage begins once the iron load exceeds 7 mg/g and may advance rapidly once the concentration exceeds 15 mg/g. This correlates with total body iron loads of 10–20 g. In the presence of hepatitis C infection, iron overload can be particularly damaging to the liver, even at lower liver iron concentrations.

Patients with **iron overload secondary to hematopoietic disorders, excessive transfusion, or alcohol-induced increased absorption** tend to show a greater deposition of iron in Kupffer cells with less involvement of the hepatocytes. Moreover, excessively transfused patients will not develop cirrhosis until iron loads are far greater than 20–30 g. This situation would appear to reflect the fact that the normal monocyte-macrophage system is able to trap most of the excess iron and prevent hepatocyte loading.

Patients with **certain hematopoietic disorders** such as thalassemia can show hepatocyte damage at a relatively early age. Because of their high levels of ineffective erythropoiesis, these patients usually demonstrate high SI levels and transferrin saturations of greater than 60% beginning early in childhood. This opens the pathway for parenchymal cell loading despite a normally functioning monocyte-macrophage cell system. They are also at increased risk of hepatitis C infection, which, in conjunction with transfusion-related iron loading, will accelerate liver damage.

D. Other Diagnostic Tests

Patients with marked iron deposition in the liver can be detected by computed tomography (CT) scan or magnetic resonance imaging (MRI). In the latter case, there is a marked attenuation of the T2 signal producing a black image. As a supplement to the SI and serum ferritin levels in screening for iron overload, urinary excretion of iron after parenteral injection of an iron chelator (deferoxamine) is sensitive to both reticuloendothelial cell and tissue iron loading. A dose of 10 mg/kg of deferoxamine is given by subcutaneous injection, and urine is collected for 24 hours to measure total iron content.

E. Genetic Testing

Missense mutations of the *HFE* gene on chromosome 6 are responsible for 60%–100% of the cases of adult hemochromatosis worldwide (85% of cases in the United States). The *HFE* gene is closely linked to the HLA-A and -B loci. On average, 73% of patients with the disease will be HLA-A3. HLA-A11, -B7, and -B14 have also been associated with the disease. However, the gold standard test for the diagnosis of hereditary hemochromatosis is the **direct detection of the defective *HFE* gene**. More than 80% of symptomatic patients are now thought to be homozygous for the single point mutation, **Cys^{282}Tyr (*C282Y*)**, whereas another 3%–5% are compound heterozygotes, **Cys^{282}Tyr/His^{63}Asp (*C282Y/H63D*)**. Homozygous H63D patients exhibit significant iron overload but do not appear to develop the full clinical picture of hemochromatosis. A third mutation, designated *S65C*, has now been identified. In combination with *C282Y* (*C282Y/S65C* compound heterozygotes), *S65C* has been associated with mild hemochromatosis.

Additional mutations involving any 1 of the 5 *HFE* genes are anticipated, since 10%–30% of adult patients do not have an identifiable *HFE* gene mutation. Other genetic mutations associated with excessive iron loading and tissue damage include the ***HJV*, *TFR2*, *SLC40A1*, and *HAMP* gene loci**.

DIFFERENTIAL DIAGNOSIS

The typical patterns of body iron balance measurements for normal males, patients with iron-loading hematopoietic diseases, and hereditary hemochromatosis are summarized in Table 15–3. The classification of iron overload states is shown in Table 15–4. The diagnosis of a hematopoietic disorder with iron loading is relatively easy. Hematopoietic disorders are usually apparent from the patient's past medical history and routine blood count. Severe tissue iron overload is **associated with the more severe anemias**, such as heavily transfused marrow damage, aplastic or dysplastic anemias, and congenital defects in globin production (the thalassemias). The diagnosis of inherited defects in iron absorption leading to iron overload is a bigger challenge, not only in regard to the early detection of a defect, but also in the differential diagnosis of the underlying mechanism.

CASE HISTORY • *Part 2*

The patient has symptoms, signs, and laboratory results that would suggest a diagnosis of hereditary hemochromatosis. The normal hemogram rules against a hematological disorder associated with iron overload. The serum iron is elevated for a percent saturation of 90% and the serum ferritin is greater than 1,000 μg/L, indicating the potential for significant tissue iron overload. The skin pigmentation, cardiac arrhythmia, abnormal fasting blood glucose and liver chemistries, testicular atrophy, and history of arthralgias/arthritis, all suggest iron-related organ damage and are typically seen in patients with HFE-hemochromatosis.

Questions

- Are other studies needed to document the diagnosis?
- Given the pattern of inheritance, should family members be evaluated?

TABLE 15–4 • Classification of iron overload states

Hematopoietic disorders
Thalassemia Sideroblastic anemias Dysplastic/megaloblastic anemias Pyruvate kinase deficiency G6PD deficiency
Secondary iron overload
Transfusion hemosiderosis Porphyria cutanea tarda Alcoholic cirrhosis South African (Bantu) hemochromatosis
Inherited defects
Classic (HFE) hemochromatosis (Type 1) Juvenile hemochromatosis (Type 2) Transferrin receptor 2 deficiency (Type 3) Ferroportin deficiency (Type 4) African iron overload

Anemia Diagnosis

The accurate diagnosis of the particular hematopoietic disorder is the key to the detection and management of complicating iron overload. Patients with β-thalassemia major are at highest risk for tissue iron loading. These individuals are always identified soon after birth, so that the iron-loading manifestation of their disease is anticipated as a part of the treatment of their hematologic disease. Patients with **acquired, dysplastic anemias** present later in life; more than 80% are diagnosed after age 60. Their tendency to iron loading varies and depends on both their transfusion requirement and the nature and duration of their disease. Patients with **refractory anemia with ringed sideroblasts (RARS)** have the highest propensity to tissue iron loading. This correlates primarily with their level of ineffective erythropoiesis and the need for repeated transfusions, although some patients may also be *HFE* heterozygotes. Whether this increases their tendency to iron loading is unclear. RARS patients are usually recognized from the inspection of the Prussian blue stain of a marrow aspirate. The presence of ringed sideroblasts, ineffective erythropoiesis, and high SI and serum ferritin levels are clear indicators of a propensity for tissue iron loading.

Regardless of the nature of the anemia, a history of **transfusion dependence**, that is, a transfusion requirement of 2–3 U of red blood cells each month for a year or more, will predictably result in iron overload. Since each unit contains 200–250 mg of iron, the patient will receive 6–10 g of iron each year.

Iron Studies

In light of the frequency of ***HFE*** mutations in Caucasian populations, it has been recommended by some that all adult Caucasians should be routinely screened for laboratory evidence of iron loading. A **rise in the percent saturation of transferrin** is the most reliable indicator of iron overload; 70%–80% of homozygous men and 40%–45% of homozygous women will have levels greater than 50%. The **serum ferritin level** may be slightly more sensitive but is also less specific. Several disease states, including a number of hematopoietic disorders, liver disease, and inflammatory conditions, can result in serum ferritin elevations. However, a ferritin level greater than 1,000 μg/L should always stimulate a full evaluation for tissue iron loading. **Quantitative analysis of hepatic iron content** together with histologic examination for parenchymal cell versus Kupffer cell loading is perhaps the gold standard, but liver biopsy hardly lends itself well to screening and should be reserved for patients with abnormal liver chemistries.

HFE Genotype Analysis

The majority of adult patients presenting with a clinical picture of hereditary hemochromatosis are homozygous for the C282Y mutation (C282Y/C282Y). The most common compound mutation is the *C282Y/H63D* heterozygote. However, the clinical penetrance of the *C282Y/H63D* heterozygote, as well as other infrequent mutations (*IVS3 + 1G-T*, *I105T*, and *S65C*) is less than 1%–2% of that of the homozygous genotype. Therefore, **genetic testing can be used to rapidly confirm the diagnosis** of hereditary hemochromatosis secondary to an *HFE* mutation—better than 80% of patients who present with clinical manifestations of classic hemochromatosis will be positive. It obviates liver biopsy unless, because of elevated liver chemistries, there is a need to evaluate the patient for cirrhosis.

Genotyping has replaced HLA testing in pedigree studies. It is the most sensitive and specific approach to detecting family members with a potential for developing clinical disease. However, the clinical penetrance of the several *HFE* gene mutations is quite low; phenotypic disease is observed in less than 10%–30% of male and less than 1% of female probands. Therefore, the accurate determination of risk of clinical disease in screened family members will still require periodic monitoring of iron studies and liver function. It should be emphasized that genetic testing should never be undertaken without the consent of the patient and individual family members, and then only after counseling. Considering the cost of the testing and the potential implications of a positive finding on insurability, it is also reasonable to restrict genetic testing to patients and family members with phenotypic disease.

Genotypic analysis is **not recommended for population screening.** While it is highly specific for the diagnosis of symptomatic HFE hemochromatosis, carriers of the defect are not at risk. Even more importantly, the majority of *C282Y* homozygotes will have normal iron studies and will never develop clinically significant iron overload. In part, this reflects the fact that hepcidin levels in patients with HFE hemochromatosis are actually normal or only slightly decreased. The symptom-producing metabolic error, therefore, has more to do with a failure to upregulate hepcidin production in the face of iron excess and increasing body iron stores. Because of this, children, women, and young males, in whom iron requirements tend to meet or exceed dietary supply, are physiologically protected from iron loading.

Even in adult males, the penetrance is extremely low. At least 5 studies of disease-related morbidity in homozygous (*C282Y*) hemochromatosis patients have now shown phenotypic penetrance of less than 1%. The incidence of symptoms and signs associated with iron overload (eg, fatigue, arthralgias, impotence, arrhythmias) in fact appears to be no higher for homozygous *C282Y* patients than that reported by normal controls. Markers of liver function (aspartate aminotransferase [AST] and alanine aminotransferase [ALT] levels) and fibrosis (biopsy or serum collagen IV levels) may be somewhat more sensitive but not necessarily more specific. Whereas from 5%–25% of homozygous *C282Y* patients detected in screening programs have abnormal liver chemistries and/or histology, the contribution by other disease states (eg, alcoholic liver disease, hepatitis, porphyria cutanea tarda) is unclear in reported studies. Therefore, as a side issue, even those patients who appear to fit the clinical picture of hereditary hemochromatosis must be evaluated to rule out other diseases that can lead to excessive iron loading or contribute to iron-induced organ damage.

Other Genotypes/Phenotypes

Several genotypes/phenotypes not linked to the *HFE* gene have now been described (see Tables 15–1 and 15–4). One of these, **juvenile hemochromatosis**, is caused by a mutation(s) on chromosome 1 of the ***HJV* (hemojuvelin)** or, less commonly, the ***HAMP* (hepcidin)** gene. Both mutations result in low to unmeasurable levels of hepcidin and the tendency to iron loading is far greater than that seen with *HFE* mutations. Patients present in the second or third decade with hypogonadism, arrhythmias, and cardiac failure. Liver biopsy to measure the iron burden and determine the extent of liver damage is important. Juvenile hemochromatosis will respond to phlebotomy therapy and should be initiated at an early age.

So-called type 3 hemochromatosis is a rare condition resulting from a mutation of the **TFR2 gene that regulates transferrin receptor 2.** TFR2 is expressed only in hepatocytes and appears to respond to the level of diferric transferrin to somehow help regulate iron uptake, but the exact mechanism involved is still unclear. The resulting phenotype is indistinguishable from *HFE*-related hemochromatosis, although, like *HJV* and *HAMP* mutations, it tends to present earlier and be somewhat more severe.

Type 4 hemochromatosis, **ferroportin deficiency**, results from an autosomal dominant mutation of the *SLC40A1* gene. Unlike other types of hemochromatosis, affected patients show predominant iron loading of macrophages, rather than hepatocytes. Moreover, although serum ferritin levels are elevated, transferrin saturations are normal or only slightly increased. Type 4 patients tolerate phlebotomy therapy poorly, becoming anemic while the serum ferritin level remains high. This suggests a defect largely limited to the role of ferroportin in managing macrophage iron transport.

Hereditary hyperferritinemia-cataract syndrome is another autosomal dominant genetic disorder that should not be confused with hemochromatosis. Involved family members present with ferritin levels of 500–1,000 μg/L or higher and congenital nuclear cataracts. The underlying mechanism is an increased synthesis of serum L-ferritin secondary to a mutation of the L-ferritin IRE on chromosome 19. These patients do not demonstrate tissue iron loading. Phlebotomy therapy soon produces an iron-deficiency anemia, and is therefore contraindicated.

Other rare abnormalities of iron metabolism include hereditary aceruloplasminemia secondary to a mutation of the ceruloplasmin gene on chromosome 3, and "dysmetabolic hepatosiderosis," a syndrome characterized by mild to moderate iron excess in patients with insulin-resistant diabetes. In both cases, serum ferritin levels are elevated but the percent saturations of transferrin are normal. Like patients with ferroportin deficiency, aceruloplasminemia is associated with an apparent defect in iron export from macrophages. Aceruloplasminemia patients present with dementia, ataxia, and extrapyramidal signs secondary to iron accumulation in brain tissue and neurodegeneration. This condition is readily diagnosed by demonstration of an undetectable serum ceruloplasmin level.

Iron Overload in African Descendents

Iron overload in African Americans and sub-Saharan Africans is **not the same as hereditary hemochromatosis in Caucasian populations**. It is not associated with the *C282Y* gene mutation. Rather, several factors may play a role, including a high incidence of hepatitis, ingestion of alcoholic beverages containing large amounts of iron, ferroportin deficiency, and a second, as yet unidentified, iron-loading gene that is not the same as the hemochromatosis *HFE* gene defect. Furthermore, the pattern of iron deposition in the liver is different. Both hepatocytes and Kupffer cells show excess iron accumulations in black patients, in contrast to the restriction of iron loading to the hepatocytes in HFE hereditary hemochromatosis in whites.

The **onset of clinical disease can be subtle** in black patients, so the level of clinical suspicion must be especially high. Evaluation of suspected iron overload in black patients should include not only serum ferritin and transferrin saturation measurements, but also a liver biopsy. The range of percent saturations can be lower than that seen in whites, falling below 50%, even with significant iron overload. While testing for the *C282Y* mutation is appropriate to exclude the *HFE* mutation, a normal test should not deter a full evaluation, including liver biopsy.

Other High-Risk Conditions

Patients with **alcoholic liver disease, cirrhosis with portacaval shunt, porphyria cutanea tarda, and aplastic anemia** are also at risk for iron loading and tissue toxicity even without a genetic abnormality. Usually, the etiologic relationship of the disease state to the iron loading is clear. However, some patients with end-stage liver disease and a strong alcoholic history may represent a diagnostic dilemma as to whether the iron loading or the alcohol damage came first. Genetic testing can be very valuable in this situation in Caucasians.

CASE HISTORY • Part 3

The patient should be tested for the *HFE C282Y* gene mutation, the most common mutation associated with hereditary hemochromatosis. If, as suspected, he is homozygous for the *HFE* gene mutation (*C282Y/C282Y*), this will confirm the diagnosis. A liver biopsy should also be considered to evaluate the iron distribution in hepatocytes and Kupffer cells and document the presence of cirrhotic changes. Family screening, either by genetic testing or iron studies, should be discussed with the patient. Since the penetrance of the *HFE* gene mutation is quite low, serial iron studies in potentially at-risk adult male relatives makes the most sense and saves on expense.

Question

- What treatment is indicated?

THERAPY

Effective treatment of iron overload requires **early detection and aggressive iron unloading**. A high SI with greater than 50% saturation of the TIBC or a serum ferritin level greater than 1,000 μg/L must not be ignored, even when it is discovered in an otherwise healthy patient. Moreover, the fact that the patient is young or female should not be used as an excuse to delay the diagnostic workup. With the discovery of the *HFE* gene, it is now easy to confirm the diagnosis and, if desired, screen family members of the patient with HFE hemochromatosis. Even though the penetrance of the *HFE* gene is quite low, homozygous *C282Y* family members should be followed with serial SI, TIBC, and ferritin levels, and phlebotomy therapy initiated at the earliest sign of iron overload. Heterozygotes are not at risk for clinically significant iron overload, unless they also have a condition such as alcoholic cirrhosis, porphyria cutanea tarda, or an iron-loading anemia.

The first rule of good management is to **aggressively treat any patient with iron overload**. The hereditary hemochromatosis patient with a ferritin level in excess of 1,000 μg/L (10 g or more of excess body iron) deserves maximum therapy. When the iron loading is even greater and organ damage, especially cardiac and liver disease, is present, as much iron as possible should be removed in the shortest possible time. Otherwise, the organ damage will put the patient at risk of death from heart failure, a cardiac arrhythmia, or irreversible liver damage.

Effects of Iron Removal

Rapid removal of iron can **reverse organ damage**. Cardiac arrhythmias and heart failure tend to respond early in the course of treatment. Improvement in liver function can also be seen, even though liver fibrosis will not significantly reverse and patients will still exhibit complications of their cirrhosis. Moreover, hemochromatosis patients are at increased risk for the development of a primary hepatic malignancy. One-third of patients will go on to die of a hepatoma. This is true even for patients who have been aggressively treated and had their excess iron removed by either phlebotomy or chelation therapy.

Iron removal has **less of an effect on the other manifestations of the disease**. Islet cell function is not restored, even though the patient's insulin-dependent diabetes may be somewhat easier to control. The gonadal failure caused by iron loading of the anterior pituitary is generally irreversible, and patients may require hormonal replacement. The patient's arthropathy may actually worsen during therapy and any joint destruction will be irreversible. Finally, the darkening of skin color will gradually lessen over several years.

Choice of Therapy

The therapeutic approach to hemochromatosis is influenced by the cause of iron loading, the age of the patient, and the amount of the iron overload. The 2 mainstay treatments are **phlebotomy** and the administration of **deferasirox and deferoxamine**. Whenever possible, phlebotomy therapy is preferred, especially in patients with hereditary hemochromatosis who have no difficulty increasing red blood cell production to compensate for the phlebotomy-induced anemia. In patients with iron overload due to thalassemia or RARS, the primary defect in red blood cell production rules against this approach. In this situation, **chelation therapy** is the only alternative.

Monitoring of Iron Intake

Attention must also be paid to the patient's iron intake. Medicinal iron, including the ingestion of iron as part of an over-the-counter vitamin preparation or dietary supplement, must be avoided. Patients should be counseled and given a list of approved vitamin preparations. Dietary restriction is less of an issue. Although many vegetables are high in iron content, the bioavailability of this iron is low. Most absorbable iron in Western diets comes from meats and meat by-products. Commercial beer and wines do not contain excess iron. Even patients with the most severe HFE hemochromatosis will only absorb 2–5 mg of iron per day or 500–1,500 mg per year on a normal diet. Therefore, once their iron load has been reduced, these patients will require only 2–6 phlebotomies per year to prevent excess iron reaccumulation.

Phlebotomy Therapy

The quickest and least complicated way of removing iron is phlebotomy. In a patient with a hematocrit of between 35% and 45%, the removal of 500 mL of whole blood will remove approximately 200 mg of iron. If the patient is estimated to have 10 g of excess body iron, 50 or more phlebotomies will need to be performed to return their total body iron load to normal. To achieve this goal in a reasonable period of time, phlebotomies must be scheduled at least once or twice each week. This rate of blood loss may not be tolerated at the beginning of therapy, especially when the patient is older or of small body size. In this situation, 200–300 mL of blood should be initially removed until the patient's red cell production increases. Less-frequent phlebotomies can be scheduled in patients with smaller iron loads (a serum ferritin level <1,000 μg/L). However, reducing the rate of phlebotomy in hemochromatosis patients with organ damage, especially cardiac disease, is poor management—the maximum frequency must be maintained.

A. Measurement of the Amount of Iron Removed

The amount of iron removed can be estimated from the number of phlebotomies. For every 5 phlebotomies, approximately 1 g of excess iron will be removed. The serum ferritin level can also be used to monitor the effectiveness of therapy (see Figure 15–3). Early in the course of phlebotomy therapy, the serum ferritin level may fluctuate and even appear to increase. However, as stores fall to 10 g or less, the serum ferritin generally provides a good measure of total body iron. The SI and percent saturation of TIBC can then be used as end points to indicate successful iron unloading. HFE hemochromatosis patients generally show little change in these latter measurements until their iron load is nearly depleted.

The challenge comes when patients are nearly depleted of their excess iron. At this point, they should be more closely monitored with measurements of complete blood count (CBC), SI, and serum ferritin levels. The **ideal end point** is a serum ferritin less than 50–100 μg/L and a normal SI with less than 50% saturation of the TIBC in a patient who is not anemic or microcytic. Overly aggressive phlebotomy can easily induce a microcytic, hypochromic anemia secondary to iron deficiency, whereas too little will allow the SI to remain high, with a greater than 50% saturation of the TIBC and the risk of continued tissue iron loading.

Hemochromatosis patients may show **fluctuating measurements of the serum ferritin level and SI** near the end of unloading therapy. This situation reflects a problem with mobilization of some of the excess iron, so that the phlebotomies get ahead of the rate of release. In this circumstance, the frequency of phlebotomy should be reduced to allow time for iron to mobilize from tissues. The other challenging problem is the propensity of some patients with hemochromatosis to **increase their SI levels to greater than 50% saturation of their TIBC** even with small accumulations of excess iron. In these patients, serum ferritin levels will need to be reduced to below 40–50 μg/L to keep the SI level within the normal range, even at the risk of a slight anemia. In an occasional patient who does not follow the predicted response, a repeated liver biopsy can help document the effectiveness of therapy.

B. Patient Compliance

Although there are few complications with phlebotomy therapy, patient compliance can be an issue. Patients will need to be encouraged to **keep up with the phlebotomy schedule**. They should also **maintain a diet with adequate protein** to support albumin production, and they should receive a **folic acid supplement**. Once the excess iron load has been removed, it is possible to prevent reaccumulation with a low-iron diet. It is usually more convenient, however, to simply have the patient donate a unit of blood 4 times a year.

C. Treatment of Porphyria Cutanea Tarda

Phlebotomy therapy also works very well in treating porphyria cutanea tarda. Usually, the iron load is considerably less and a series of weekly or every-other-weekly phlebotomies over 4–6 months will result in a significant clinical improvement both in terms of the skin disease and liver chemistries. It is important, however, to be sure that the patient does not have hereditary hemochromatosis, where the iron load is much greater. Therefore, these patients should also be closely monitored with repeated SI, serum ferritin levels, and repeated liver biopsies to document improvement.

Iron Chelation Therapy

Excess body iron can also be removed with chelation therapy. Deferoxamine is an effective iron chelator for parenteral use. The disadvantages of deferoxamine are its high cost and the need for continuous subcutaneous or intravenous administration. Deferoxamine is the drug of choice, however, when rapid iron unloading is indicated. An oral chelating agent, deferasirox, can be used to prevent iron loading in patients with thalassemia when given long term.

A. Deferoxamine

Although deferoxamine has a lower binding affinity for iron than transferrin, it can successfully compete for excess iron stored in tissue cells. When injected subcutaneously or intravenously, it is rapidly taken up by the hepatocytes, excreted into bile, and reabsorbed by the intestine. At low doses, most of the iron-laden deferoxamine is excreted in urine. At higher doses, it also appears in stool.

Since deferoxamine is not absorbed orally and has a very short half-life, effective therapy requires that it be **administered either subcutaneously or intravenously by continuous infusion**. To achieve a level of therapy equivalent to 2 phlebotomies each week, the patient should receive an infusion of 40–50 mg/kg of deferoxamine administered over 10–12 hours each night by continuous infusion pump, 5–7 nights each week. Vitamin C, given orally prior to infusion, will enhance iron excretion. Deferoxamine can be made up in a small enough volume that any of the portable pump technologies can be employed. When subcutaneous therapy is used, the drug can be administered with a small-gauge butterfly needle placed just under the skin.

Patients who receive more than 4 g or more than 50 mg/kg/d of deferoxamine are at risk for an optic neuropathy characterized by increased retinal pigmentation, central scotoma, and night blindness. Less frequently, patients may develop high-tone deafness. These nerve toxicities appear to be dose dependent and can improve if the dosage is reduced. Serial auditory and visual

CASE HISTORY • *Part 4*

Treatment should be immediate and aggressive. If tolerated, twice weekly phlebotomy is in order and will successfully reduce body iron to normal levels over 6–12 months. If the patient is unstable (life-threatening arrhythmias or congestive heart failure) or does not tolerate phlebotomy, subcutaneous or high-dose intravenous deferoxamine therapy should be considered.

measurements should be performed whenever high-dose deferoxamine therapy is employed. The only other complication of deferoxamine therapy is an increased risk of sepsis from organisms such as ***Yersinia*** and ***S. aureus***.

B. Oral Chelators

Patients with hematological disorders who are unable to tolerate phlebotomy can be treated chronically with the new oral chelator, deferasirox (see Chapter 6). Deferasirox, given in a dose of 20–30 mg/kg/d, can prevent and even reduce iron overload in transfusion-dependent children with thalassemia. It is also recommended in any patient receiving frequent transfusions over more than a year. Another useful oral chelator is **deferiprone**, a bidentate α-ketohydroxypyridine. It has a higher binding affinity for iron than deferoxamine and is capable of removing iron from tissue cells and transferrin. Deferiprone is rapidly absorbed, appearing in blood within minutes, where it is metabolized to the inactive glucuronide. The ability of deferiprone to mobilize iron from transferrin and iron pools within parenchymal and reticuloendothelial cells is a potential advantage over deferoxamine, especially in the treatment of patients with cardiac dysfunction secondary to iron overload. Combination therapy with deferoxamine may have an added or even a synergistic effect because of the somewhat different binding characteristics of the drugs.

CLINICAL COURSE

Survival of patients with iron overload is clearly improved by early diagnosis and effective phlebotomy or chelation therapy. Five-year survivals in patients with **untreated hereditary hemochromatosis** have been reported to be as low as 15%–20%. Aggressively treated patients clearly do better, although the extent of organ damage at diagnosis is a major factor. The cumulative survival rate of **patients without cardiac, pancreas, or liver damage** is the same as that for the general population, whereas **patients with cirrhosis or diabetes** follow the survival rates of patients with these same disorders secondary to other causes.

Patients who are not aggressively treated are at risk of an early death from **cardiac complications**. Cardiac disease is also the major manifestation of iron overload in thalassemic patients. Hereditary hemochromatosis patients are at risk for the development of a **liver neoplasm**, either a primary hepatoma or bile duct carcinoma, and up to one-third will die of hepatic malignancy. This condition is usually seen in patients who have evidence of cirrhosis, but all hereditary hemochromatosis patients are at increased risk, and the chance of developing malignancy is not diminished by phlebotomy or chelation therapy.

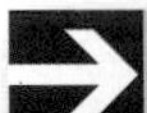

POINTS TO REMEMBER

Increased iron absorption, saturation of the iron-binding capacity of transferrin, and loading of key organs (liver, heart, pituitary, and skin) is the hallmark of hemochromatosis.

Hereditary hemochromatosis is primarily the result of a mutation of the *HFE* gene, although other mutations (*HJV*, hemojuvelin; *HAMP*, hepcidin; *TFR2*, transferrin receptor 2; and *SLC40A1*, ferroportin) are involved in rare cases.

Hematologic disorders (thalassemia, dysplastic/sideroblastic anemias, aplastic anemia, multiple transfusions), alcoholic liver disease, and porphyria cutanea tarda are also associated with iron overload.

Patients with organ iron overload, especially HFE hemochromatosis, who are left untreated will develop diabetes, cirrhosis, testicular atrophy/amenorrhea secondary to anterior pituitary failure, cardiac arrhythmias and cardiac failure, progressive darkening of the skin, and hepatomas.

Early clues to an iron overload condition include an increase in the serum iron to the point of full saturation of the iron-binding capacity and a serum ferritin in excess of 500 μg/L. Symptomatic HFE hemochromatosis patients will almost always have a serum ferritin well above 1,000 μg/L (reflecting a total body iron load of >10 g).

HFE hemochromatosis patients often report several years of a nondeforming arthralgia/arthritis involving small and large joints; a loss of libido or amenorrhea can be another early sign of organ damage.

The definitive diagnosis of clinically significant HFE hemochromatosis requires the detection of the *C282Y/C282Y* genotype (infrequently the *C282Y/H63D* and *C282Y/S65C* compound mutations). Liver biopsy is also indicated in patients with very high ferritin levels and abnormal liver chemistries to look for cirrhosis.

Treatment of HFE hemochromatosis patients presenting with evidence of organ damage, especially arrhythmias or cardiac failure, should be immediate and aggressive.

Phlebotomy, deferoxamine given intravenously or subcutaneously, and the new oral chelator deferasirox are all effective in reducing iron loading. If tolerated, aggressive phlebotomy and/or intravenous deferoxamine should be used in patients with life-threatening cardiac complications. Deferasirox is especially useful in preventing iron loading in thalassemia patients who require frequent transfusions.

Twice weekly phlebotomy should remove 10 g or more of total body iron within 6–12 months and return the ferritin and serum iron levels to within normal limits.

Adult male family members of HFE hemochromatosis probands should be screened for the *C282Y/C282Y* genotype (heterozygotes are not at risk for iron overload) or with serial iron studies to detect iron loading. Since the clinical penetrance of the *HFE* homozygous mutation is very low, monitoring the percent saturation of transferrin (>50% is abnormal) and/or the serum ferritin (>500 μg/L is abnormal) is preferred by many clinicians.

BIBLIOGRAPHY

Clinical Features

Ajioka RS, Kushner JP: Hereditary hemochromatosis. Semin Hematol 2002;39:235.

Andersen RV et al: Hemochromatosis mutations in the general population: iron overload progression rate. Blood 2004;103:2914.

Beutler E et al: Penetrance of the 845G6A (C282Y) HFE hereditary hemochromatosis mutation in the USA. Lancet 2002;359:211.

Bulaj ZJ et al: Clinical and biochemical abnormalities in people heterozygous for hemochromatosis. N Engl J Med 1996; 335:1799.

Camaschella C et al: Juvenile hemochromatosis. Semin Hematol 2002;39:242.

Cazzola M et al: Hereditary hyperferritinemia-cataract syndrome: relationship between phenotypes and specific mutations in the iron-responsive element of ferritin light-chain mRNA. Blood 1997;90:814.

Ganz T: Hepcidin, a key regulator of iron metabolism and mediator of anemia of inflammation. Blood 2003;102:783.

Gordeuk V et al: Iron overload in Africa. N Engl J Med 1992;326:95.

Mendler MH et al: Insulin resistance–associated hepatic iron overload. Gastroenterology 1999;117:1155.

Moirand R et al: Clinical features of genetic hemochromatosis in women compared to men. Ann Intern Med 1997;127:105.

Mura C, Raguenes O, Ferec C: HFE mutations analysis in 711 hemochromatosis probands: evidence for S65C implication in mild forms of hemochromatosis. Blood 1999;93:2502.

Olynk JK et al: A population-based study of the clinical expression of the hemochromatosis gene. N Engl J Med 1999; 341:719.

Phatak PD et al: Hereditary hemochromatosis: time for targeted screening. Ann Int Med 2008;149:270.

Pietrangelo A: Hereditary hemochromatosis: a new look at an old disease. N Engl J Med 2004;350:2383.

Ponka P: Rare causes of hereditary iron overload. Semin Hematol 2002;39:249.

Therapy

Barton JC et al: Management of hemochromatosis. Ann Intern Med 1998;129:932.

Liu DY et al: Oral iron chelators: development and application. Clin Haematol 2002;15:369.

Mourad FH et al: Comparison between desferrioxamine and combined therapy with desferrioxamine and deferiprone in iron overload thalassemia patients. Br J Haematol 2003; 121:187.

Porter JB: Practical management of iron overload. Br J Haematol 2001;115:252.

SECTION II
White Blood Cell Disorders

NORMAL MYELOPOIESIS · 16

Normal myelopoiesis is essential to normal host defense. It involves the regulated production of new myeloid cells, including neutrophilic, eosinophilic, and basophilic granulocytes, as well as monocytes and macrophages. The process is driven by several growth factors that control both the rate of cell production and their subsequent function. Thus, an understanding of normal myelopoiesis requires knowledge of individual cell characteristics and the expected responses of these cells to disease states.

MYELOID STEM CELLS

The myeloid cells share a common progenitor known as the **colony-forming unit–granulocyte, monocyte (CFU-GM)**. This cell arises from earlier progenitors, which are capable of giving rise to myeloid, megakaryocytic, and lymphoid lineages, and ultimately from the multipotent stem cell, which is capable of differentiation into all hematopoietic cell lines (Figure 16–1). The progeny of the CFU-GM are capable of differentiating toward granulocytes or monocytes and macrophages. There is a well-recognized pattern of morphology that can be used to evaluate the later stages of differentiation of the myeloid cell lines (Figure 16–2).

MYELOID GROWTH FACTORS

The several myeloid growth factors that are known to influence the differentiation of the CFU-GM are shown in Figure 16–1. These growth factors interact with membrane receptors of the cytokine receptor superfamily, including interleukin (IL)-3, IL-5, and granulocyte macrophage colony-stimulating factor (GM-CSF). These receptors share a common β chain, which explains the overlap of responses resulting from stimulation by these cytokines. They lack specific tyrosine kinase activity. Upon ligand binding, the common β chain and specific α chain dimerize and are able to trigger **progenitor cell transcription factor proteins Jak-STAT, RAS, NF-κB, and PI3-kinase**, which control the expression of the genes involved in cell differentiation. Thus, in order for a progenitor cell to proceed down a unique pathway of differentiation, it must express 1 or more transcription factors that, when activated by a growth factor receptor, in turn activate the family of genes required for that pathway.

The **marrow microenvironment (stromal cells)** also plays an important role in cell differentiation and growth factor response. Current methods of studying the marrow structure are still too crude, however, to clearly identify these interrelationships. Still, similar to the response of erythropoiesis to anemia, there are definable limits to the production of myeloid cells in response to infection. Unlike the situation in the erythroid line in which there is a single predominant growth-regulating hormone, erythropoietin, the myeloid growth factors exhibit more complex interactions that do not lend themselves to the simple concept of a feedback regulatory loop.

Most studies of myeloid growth factors have involved use of single or multiple factors given in soluble form so that progenitor cells are exposed to a uniform concentration of growth factor throughout their environment. It is likely that this is not the physiologic mode of action of these substances. Their **principal functions may be more restricted to the local microenvironment**, interacting primarily on surfaces of cells and seldom being present in soluble form. With development of new **immunoassays to detect low levels of humoral growth factors in plasma**, it is possible to show increased levels of granulocyte colony-stimulating factor (G-CSF), GM-CSF, and monocyte colony-stimulating factor (M-CSF, or CSF-1) in response to infections and inflammation.

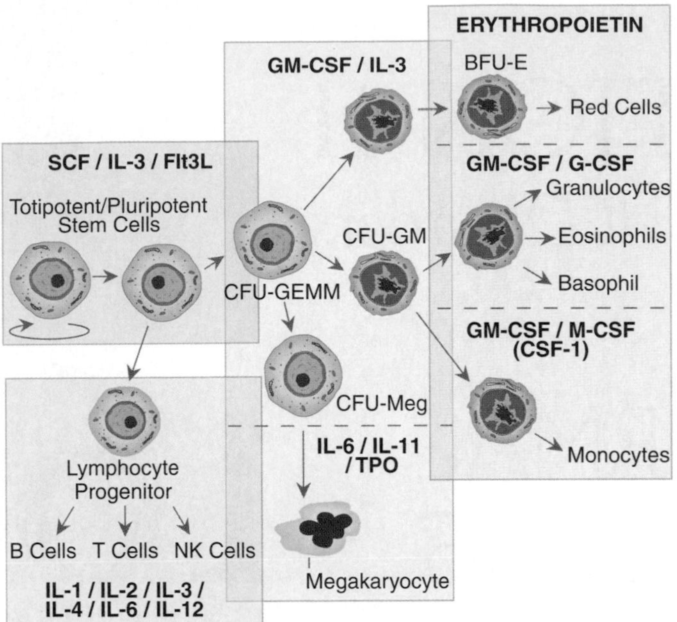

FIGURE 16–1. **Stem cell differentiation and growth factors.** The central differentiation pathway from totipotent stem cell to committed progenitors is regulated by numerous interleukins and growth factors. With the exception of erythropoietin, none of these factors is entirely specific for a single lineage. They interact with each other and have broad effects at several stages of the differentiation pathways.

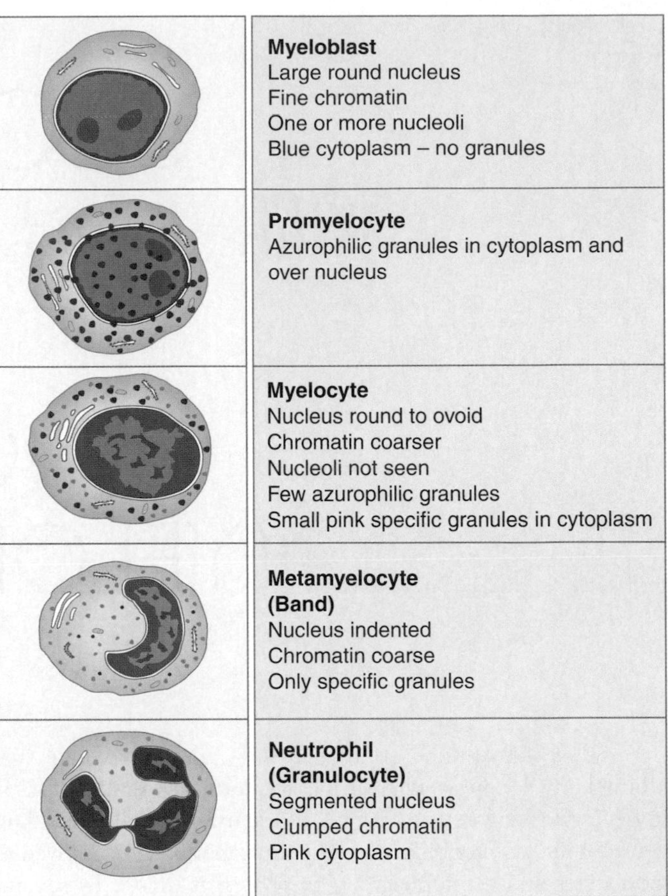

FIGURE 16–2. **The sequence of neutrophil differentiation—morphology.** Neutrophils have several stages of differentiation that are easily distinguished by morphology. Changes in staining properties of the granules, the shape of the nucleus, and the chromatin pattern can be used to distinguish each stage, although intermediate stages are commonly seen in normal and abnormal marrow.

Thus, myeloid progenitors are probably responding to fluctuating mixtures of growth factors presented in their microenvironment.

Abnormalities in production and regulation of these growth factors may lead to the development of **myeloproliferative diseases**. In particular, there is a cluster of genes on the long arm of chromosome 5 that includes the genes for GM-CSF, IL-3, M-CSF, the receptor for M-CSF (fms), IL-4, IL-5, and others. Deletions in this region are associated with a myelodysplastic syndrome with unique characteristics (the 5q minus syndrome) (see Chapter 9). Additionally, conditions mimicking leukemia can result from inappropriate secretion of these growth factors by several types of malignant conditions, including thyroid, gastric, lung, and gallbladder cancers (GM-CSF); Hodgkin disease; and T-cell lymphomas (IL-5). Myeloid growth factors also affect the functional activity of mature cells. The **clinical role of growth factors** can be thought of as 2-fold. In most cases, they stimulate proliferation and increase the numbers of 1 or more myeloid cell subtypes. In addition, many of them can affect the function of the myeloid cells, increasing or decreasing phagocytosis, locomotion, and the ability to kill pathogens.

Granulocyte Macrophage Colony-Stimulating Factor

GM-CSF is a 22-kDa molecule that stimulates the production of colonies containing neutrophils, eosinophils, and monocytes. It has a similar effect clinically by causing an increased number of the same cells. It also significantly augments the function of mature neutrophils, eosinophils, and monocytes, and appears to be responsible for such systemic effects of inflammation as fever and malaise. It has been shown to be active in mobilizing progenitor cells into the periphery for peripheral blood stem cell harvesting. GM-CSF is produced by several cell types including lymphocytes, myeloid cells themselves, endothelial cells, and fibroblasts. Its production is stimulated by inflammatory cytokines such as IL-1, tumor necrosis factor, and bacterial endotoxin. GM-CSF also may play a role in stimulating megakaryocyte colony formation and, together with erythropoietin, promotes burst-forming unit–erythroid growth.

The cell surface receptors for GM-CSF belong to a superfamily of related molecules that includes the receptors for GM-CSF, G-CSF, IL-3, IL-6, and erythropoietin as well as others. In the case of GM-CSF, it is clear that most myeloid cells (including many myeloid leukemias) express the receptor and are capable of binding the molecule. A possible autocrine activity of GM-CSF in promoting autonomous growth of leukemic cells has been suggested. Hypersensitivity of myeloid progenitors to GM-CSF in vitro is a diagnostic hallmark of **chronic juvenile myelomonocytic leukemia.**

Granulocyte Colony-Stimulating Factor

G-CSF is a 19- to 20-kDa molecule that, in cell culture systems, stimulates production of granulocyte colonies. It is secreted by a variety of cell types, including endothelial cells and fibroblasts.

Clinically, it promotes the production of granulocytes with fewer systemic effects than GM-CSF. G-CSF also tends to inhibit migration, while strongly activating mature granulocytes. It is widely used in the mobilization of CD34$^+$ stem cells into the circulation for the purposes of transplantation, in promoting more rapid recovery of granulocytes following intensive chemotherapy, and in the treatment of chronic severe neutropenia associated with recurrent infections. When given to normal individuals, G-CSF demonstrates a dose-dependent leukocytosis. A 3- to 4-day course of filgrastim, 6 μg/kg subcutaneously, results in an 8-fold increase in the number of circulating granulocytes and monocytes. Long-acting formulations of pegylated G-CSF are currently available; these simplify dosing and possibly improve efficacy. In the clinic, **Sweet syndrome (acute neutrophilic dermatitis)** is likely to result from G-CSF overproduction or, rarely, therapeutic infusion.

Monocyte Colony-Stimulating Factor

M-CSF (also designated as CSF-1) has its primary effect on macrophage colonies. Its clinical activity has not been extensively explored to date. In animal studies, it promotes monocytosis and activation of monocytes and macrophages, and causes moderate to severe thrombocytopenia. The mechanism of the latter is uncertain. Its receptor is the product of the *CFEMS* oncogene that is expressed on mononuclear phagocytes and shows increased expression in some tumors, particularly ovarian carcinoma. It also stimulates osteoclastogenesis and has a local role in bone development and remodeling. It is heavily glycosylated and, unlike the other colony-stimulating factors (CSFs), is found circulating in blood and in urine from which it may be purified. Despite its effects in activating phagocytes, it is has not found utility in combating infectious diseases or tumors.

Interleukin-3

This molecule was originally called multi-CSF. It stimulates the production of neutrophils, monocytes, eosinophils, basophils, and platelets, and augments the function of mature eosinophils and monocytes. It has systemic side effects similar to those of GM-CSF. IL-3 works together with erythropoietin in the differentiation and proliferation of precursors for erythropoiesis. In the laboratory, it is most effective when used in combination with other CSFs, where it shows marked synergy. It is unique among the CSFs because it appears to be produced only by T lymphocytes, hence its reclassification as an interleukin. It has not yet found clinical utility.

Stem Cell Factor (c-kit Ligand, Steel Factor)

In cell culture systems, this molecule has activities similar to those of IL-3 because it enhances the growth of multiple lineages and appears to have its major activity on very early progenitors. It has been studied for a possible clinical role to improve the mobilization of stem cells for transplantation, perhaps in combination with other cytokines.

Interleukin-5

IL-5 is the most specific cytokine involved in eosinophil differentiation, marrow release, and survival. Increased levels of IL-5 are associated with helper T-cell and natural killer (NK) cell activity, and both mast cells and eosinophils themselves may secrete IL-5 as part of the allergic response.

Interleukin-6

IL-6 is another factor that has multilineage effects and appears to act primarily on early progenitors. One of its most profound effects in animals is to increase platelet production. However, it is unlikely to find clinical utility in this role because recently developed analogs of thrombopoietin (both peptide and non-peptide mimetics, see Chapter 31) have greater activity in the stimulation of platelet production.

Interleukin-11

This factor also has multilineage effects in vitro. When given to patients it has 2 major clinical effects: one is to increase the rate of platelet production; the other is to promote fluid retention by the kidney. IL-11 is approved for use in decreasing the degree of thrombocytopenia induced by chemotherapy. When used in this way, it must be accompanied by diuresis to prevent excessive fluid retention. Its usefulness for treatment of thrombocytopenia could be reconsidered owing to the availability of new analogs of thrombopoietin (see Chapter 31).

Flt3 Ligand

Flt3 ligand is active on the Flt3 membrane receptor (*fms-like tyrosine kinase*), and structurally closely related to M-CSF and c-kit, with which it shares structural homology and biological effects. It synergizes with other hematopoietic growth factors and interleukins to stimulate the proliferation of stem cells, myeloid progenitors, dendritic cells, and natural killer cells. It is capable of expanding CD34$^+$ cells both in vivo and in vitro.

Chemokines and Their Receptors

A large family of more than 50 small molecules with highly conserved structure, most of which are coded together on chromosome 4, have been called chemokines (originally chemotactic cytokines). They are classified into groups according to their structure. The 2 major groups are CXC and CC in which the Cs stand for conserved cysteine residues and the X indicates the presence of another amino acid between the cysteines (CXC) or its absence (CC). Corresponding receptors for these chemokines are designated CXCR and CCR. There are several of each kind of receptor with complex and overlapping ligand-binding properties. The general function of chemokines is to direct migration of cells. They have an important role in immune surveillance, tissue development, and angiogenesis. Recent work has underscored the importance of many of these chemokines and their receptors (in particular CXCR4) in the regulation of hematopoiesis and the control of leukocyte migration out of the marrow. Others enhance stem cell survival and suppress apoptosis; still others control homing and migration of myeloid cells. Many drugs directed at these receptors are currently under development. Examples are antagonists to the HIV co-receptors CCR5 and CXCR4 aimed at blocking the entry of the virus into CD4 cells, and one, plerixafor, which antagonizes interactions with CXCR4, has recently received orphan drug status for enhancing mobilization of $CD34^+$ stem cells for transplantation.

Myeloid Cell Function

Myeloid cells may be thought of as having 3 basic functions. The first is the **ability to migrate out of the circulation into tissues** at sites of infection, damage, or inflammation. The mechanisms by which they do this have recently been shown to involve 3 classes of adhesion molecules (Figure 16–3). The first, **leukocyte adhesion molecule (L-Selectin)**, belongs to the selectin class of adhesion molecules and mediates the low-affinity interaction of myeloid cells with endothelium, promoting both margination and a rolling motion along the walls of blood vessels. The second, the **integrin class of adhesion molecules**, mediates a strong interaction of myeloid cells with subendothelial matrix proteins. Third is a mucin-like surface molecule called **P-Selectin glycoprotein ligand (PSGL-1)**. This is expressed on myeloid cells and binds to P-Selectin, which is exposed on activated or damaged endothelial cells. This interaction is essential for the migration of the cells out of the blood vessel and into the tissues. The direction of migration is determined by chemotactic factors, many of which, such as the C5b complement component, are well characterized. Drugs designed to interfere with these interactions hold promise of being a new class of powerful anti-inflammatory agents.

The second major function of myeloid cells is **phagocytosis**. Cells' ability to ingest a particle depends on the nature of the adhesive interactions with the cell surface. Some particles, such as bacteria, seem to have natural surface substances that trigger the phagocytic reaction; others must first be **coated with antibody or complement components (opsonized)** before they can be recognized by phagocytes. Once ingested, particles are isolated in phagocytic vacuoles that fuse with some of the granules within the cell's cytoplasm forming phagosomes. Within these organelles, the particles are subjected to degradation by enzymes and oxidants that kill infectious particles. The ability of myeloid cells to perform phagocytosis and killing of intracellular particles is subject to considerable regulatory control. Thus "activated" cells have markedly enhanced capabilities. Activated status can be achieved by exposure to cytokines, CSFs, and the products of granule release by other myeloid cells.

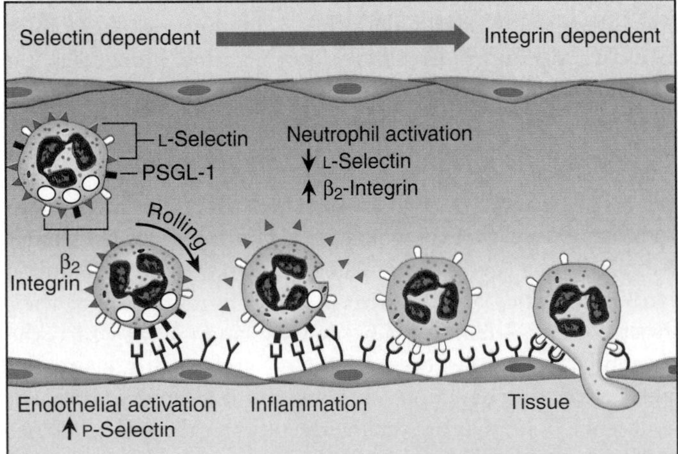

FIGURE 16–3. **The role of adhesion molecules in margination and migration of neutrophils.** Two major classes of adhesion molecules on neutrophils are the selectins and the integrins. L-Selectin on the neutrophil and P-Selectin on activated endothelial cells are primarily responsible for the loose adhesion of the cell to the endothelium, which leads to rolling and margination. When cells are activated by inflammation, L-Selectin is shed, P-Selectin increases, and β_2-integrin is upregulated, leading to strong adherence of the cell and finally to migration through the endothelium into the tissues.

The third function of myeloid cells is the **release of granule contents**, so-called **exocytosis**. The granules found within myeloid cells are their most clearly defining morphologic feature. Depending on the individual cell type, the granules contain digestive and hydrolytic enzymes and substances capable of mediating the entire range of the inflammatory response. These include chemotactic factors, activators of the complement system, activators of the coagulation system and the fibrinolytic systems, substances that affect vascular permeability and blood flow, and enzymes that are capable of breaking down extracellular matrix proteins. By releasing the content of their granules, myeloid cells trigger and sustain the inflammatory response, recruiting more myeloid cells to the site, and modulating the other components of the organism's reaction to infection, malignancy, and injury.

The **normal myeloid response to a host challenge** hinges on the function of individual myeloid cells. Disease states can be defined according to the capacity and effectiveness of each of these key functions for each of the myeloid cell types. It is important, therefore, to understand the individual characteristics of the myeloid cells.

Neutrophils (Granulocytes)

The mature neutrophil, or granulocyte, is easily recognized by its unique morphology (see Figure 16–2). On the stained film, the cell takes on a nearly round shape with a diameter of 12–16 μm, which is nearly twice that of the red blood cell. The most distinguishing feature is the **segmented nucleus**, where 2–3 lobes of dense nuclear material are separated by thin, hairlike connections. The other most distinguishing feature is the **large number of granules in the cytoplasm**. Normally this includes a small number of azurophilic, or primary, granules and a greater number of specific, or secondary, granules. **Granule formation is a useful marker** of cell differentiation. Primary granules appear during the promyelocyte stage, whereas specific granules appear during the myelocyte and metamyelocyte stages. By the time the cell reaches maturity, the number and staining properties of the primary granules become less prominent, and the nucleus gradually assumes the lobed configuration.

The granule contents of the neutrophil are a visual demonstration of its functional capabilities (Table 16–1). Primary granules contain abundant myeloperoxidase. This serves as an excellent

TABLE 16–1 • Functions and granule contents of myeloid cells

Cell Type	Function	Related Granule Contents
Neutrophils	Degradation of pathogens	Lysozyme
		Esterases
		Cathepsin G
		Proteinases
	Generation of oxidants	Peroxidase
	Tissue degradation	Elastase
		Collagenase
Monocytes	Same as neutrophils	
	Clot dissolution	Plasminogen activator
Eosinophils	Same as neutrophils	
	Killing of parasites	Major basic protein
Basophils	Immediate hypersensitivity	Histamine
	? Clot inhibition	Heparin
		Glycosaminoglycans

histochemical marker for this series; neutrophilic precursors can be differentiated from other myeloid cells by their **strong peroxidase staining** (Table 16–2 and Figure 16–4). Monocytes are also positive but to a far lesser degree. **Leukocyte alkaline phosphatase** is present in mature neutrophils and is markedly increased in most inflammatory states. A reduction of leukocyte alkaline phosphatase is seen in some malignancies, notably **chronic myelogenous leukemia (CML)**, but is now rarely used as a confirmatory test in making this diagnosis because of the utility of *BCRABL1* testing. **Lysozyme (muramidase)** is present in neutrophils (and monocytes) but not eosinophils and basophils. Finally, the pattern of staining for carbohydrate-containing granules using periodic acid–Schiff stain and 2 esterase stains (naphthol AS-D chloracetate and α-naphthyl acetate or butyrate) can help **distinguish neutrophils from monocytes** (see Table 16–2 and Figure 16–4). Neutrophils stain positively with **naphthol AS-chloracetate** (specific esterase) but weakly with **α-naphthyl acetate or butyrate** (nonspecific esterase) as a substrate. **Monocytes give the opposite reaction**, that is, a weak or negative reaction with the specific esterase stain but a strong positive reaction to the nonspecific esterase stain.

Myeloid cells can also be categorized according to their **immunologic markers** (Figure 16–5). The marker system is not as extensive as that for the lymphocyte cell line; it is only possible to divide neutrophils into rough stages of immature and mature. The characteristic marker of very immature myeloid cells is **CD34**, and the characteristic markers of more mature myeloid cells are **CD13 and CD33**. CD34 is lost very early, and the later markers appear simultaneously at a fairly early stage. Thus, these markers are not terribly useful in categorizing the maturation sequence of neutrophils. The later acquisition of mature markers such as **CD11b and CD16** (the latter an Fc receptor for immunoglobulin) occurs at the metamyelocyte and granulocyte stages.

Monocytes

Mature monocytes also have a distinctive morphology (Figure 16–6). They tend to be somewhat larger than neutrophils with a more irregular cell border on a stained film. The nucleus appears as a horseshoe-shaped structure with chromatin that is less dense than that seen in mature neutrophils. The cytoplasm is a grayish-blue color and contains sparse numbers of pink to purplish granules. When blood is collected in ethylenediaminetetraacetic acid (EDTA) (purple-topped tube) for laboratory testing, monocytes develop **multiple vacuoles** in the cytoplasm, providing a useful marker of this cell type. Histochemically, monocytes are **best identified by their strong staining with nonspecific esterase**. They stain far less intensely than neutrophils for peroxidase, specific esterase, and acid phosphatase (see Table 16–2). They are rich in lysozyme (muramidase), and very high levels of muramidase can be detected in the urine of patients with monocytosis or monocytic leukemia.

The differentiation of monocytes is less well defined morphologically. It is difficult to distinguish monocyte precursors in the marrow.

A. Immunologic Markers

Immunologic markers of monocytes are similar to those of the neutrophils with the exception of the acquisition of CD14 and the strong expression of class II histocompatibility antigens (HLA-DR) (see Figure 16–5). CD14 is a relatively late marker, and many leukemic cells that appear morphologically and

TABLE 16–2 • Histochemical stains for myeloid cells

Cell Type	Myeloperoxidase	Specific Esterase	Nonspecific Esterase	Periodic Acid–Schiff
Neutrophil	4+	3+	1+	4+
Monocyte	2+	1+	3+	2+
Lymphocyte	—	—	±	±

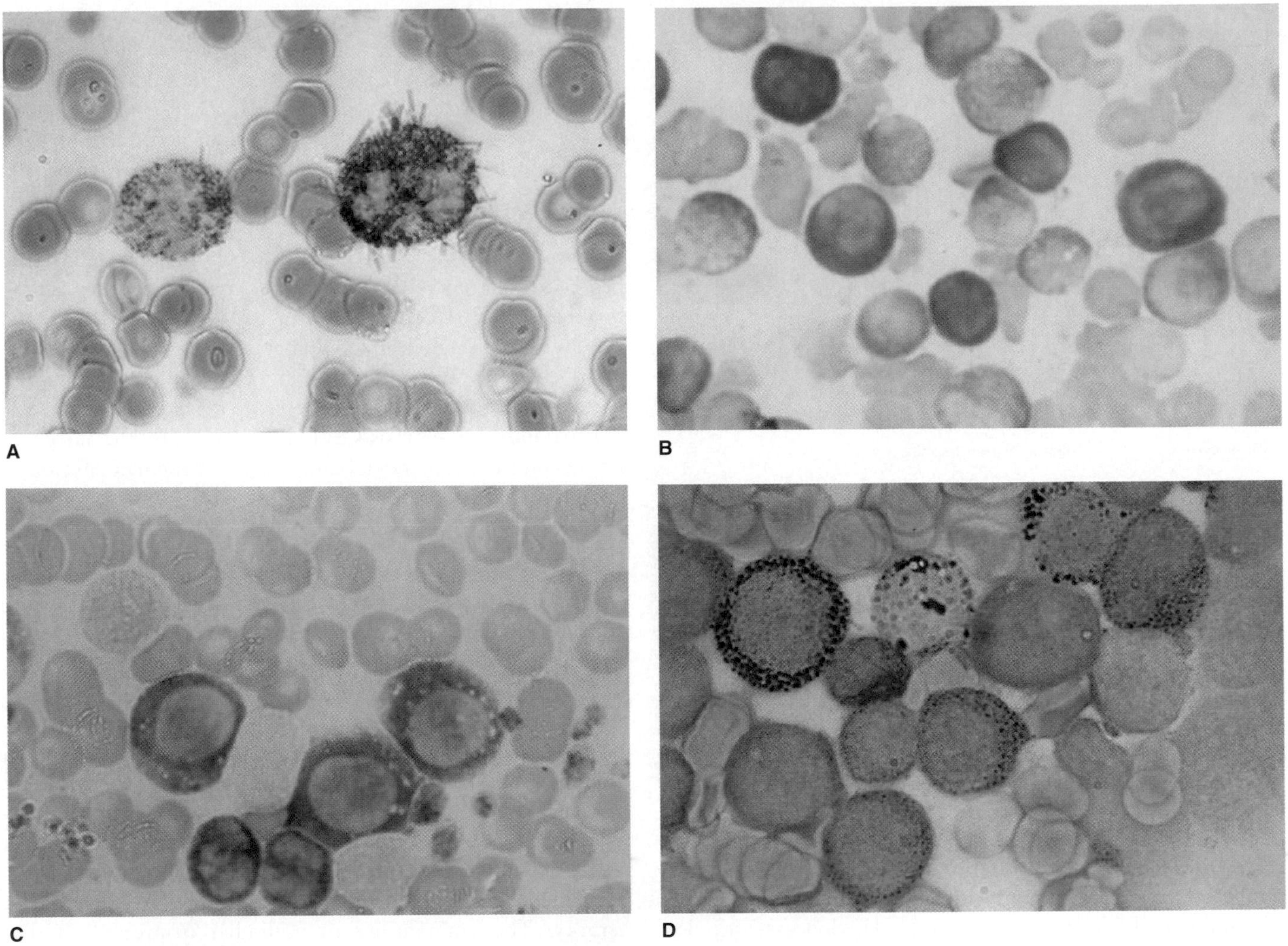

A B C D

FIGURE 16–4. **Histochemical stains for myeloid cells. A:** Peroxidase stain—myeloblasts staining positively (dark blue) for peroxidase. **B:** Combined esterase stain—differential staining of monoblasts (red) and myeloblasts (blue) in myelo-monocytic leukemia. **C:** Nonspecific esterase stain—monoblasts staining positively (red cytoplasmic granules) in acute monoblastic leukemia. **D:** Periodic acid–Schiff (PAS) stain—blasts stain positively for PAS (bright red granules) in erythroleukemia and acute lymphoblastic leukemia.

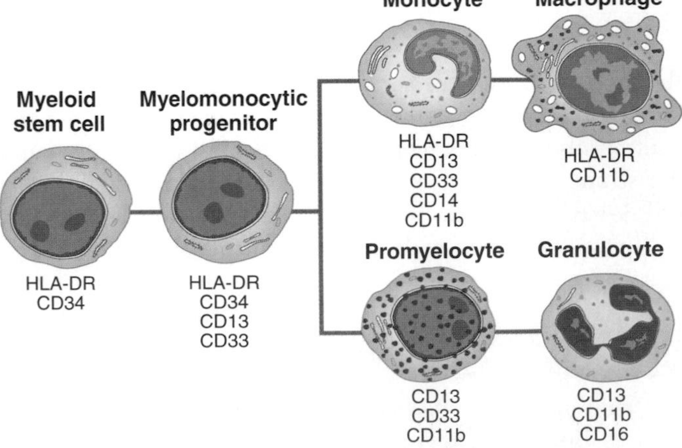

FIGURE 16–5. **The sequence of neutrophil differentiation—immunologic markers.** Immunologic markers, identified by monoclonal antibodies, can be used to define a maturation sequence for the myeloid cells. Although such markers are most useful in distinguishing very early progenitor cells from mature cells, they do not define the intermediate stages as clearly as morphology.

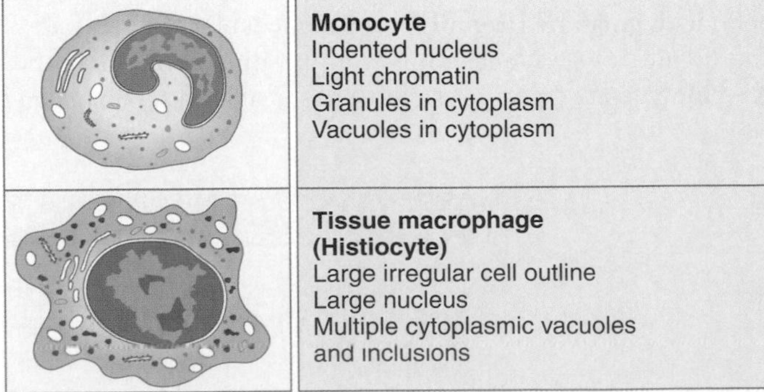

FIGURE 16–6. **Monocyte and macrophage morphology.** The major functions of monocytes are phagocytosis, killing, granule release, and the processing and presentation of antigen to lymphocytes.

histochemically to be monocytes lack CD14. Of importance is the presence of small amounts of the CD4 molecule on the surface, which serves as a target for HIV. In addition, monocytes have abundant receptors for immunoglobulin Fc receptors, CD16 (FcRIII), CD32 (FcRII), and CD64 (FcRI), and are normally coated with considerable plasma immunoglobulin. They also express complement receptors (CD11b, CD18), and toll-like receptors, which are innate immune recognition structures of foreign pathogens.

B. Functions of Circulating Monocytes

Functions of circulating monocytes parallel those of the granulocytes. Mature monocytes are capable of migration, chemotaxis, phagocytosis, killing, and granule release. They have an important additional role in the immune system. Circulating monocytes and their progeny, tissue-bound macrophages, are both capable of processing and presenting antigens to lymphocytes.

An additional, closely related cell type, **the dendritic cell**, is found in the skin and in germinal centers of lymph nodes. Dendritic cells are specialized in the antigen presentation function. They are derived from hematopoietic stem cells and appear to differentiate from monocytes. They reside in the skin (Langerhans cells) and in the respiratory and gastrointestinal mucosa where they are maximally exposed to potential pathogens. They internalize antigenic particles, such as bacteria and viruses, partially degrading the molecular components of the antigen and then exposing the degraded and denatured products on their surface noncovalently attached to HLA class II molecules. Dendritic cells then migrate to the lymphoid tissues where this molecular complex is recognized by the T cells as antigenic (Figure 16–7). This antigen presentation function is shared by dendritic cells, macrophages, and B cells (see Chapter 20); however, dendritic cells appear to be highly specialized and very potent in antigen presentation. Cultured dendritic cells, and agents that stimulate their function, are being evaluated in the immunotherapy of malignant diseases with improved vaccines. All antigen-presenting cells (APCs) express a variety of co-stimulatory molecules such as CD40, CD70, and CD86 (see Figure 16–7), which augment and modulate the response of the immune cells. Drugs and antibodies that inhibit these interactions are being developed.

In addition, so-called **"co-stimulatory" molecules** have been shown to greatly augment the interaction between APCs and T lymphocytes. These include CD28 (T cells) and B7 (APCs), CD154 (T cells) and CD40 (APCs), and CD2 (T cells) and CD58 (APCs). Disruption of these interactions using antibodies and recombinant molecules shows considerable promise as a strategy for immunosuppression.

Monocytes also appear to be more capable than neutrophils in **killing intracellular pathogens** such as ***Listeria monocytogenes***, as well as mycobacteria and yeasts. When activated, they are also able to **kill** many types of **tumor cells**. Finally, monocytes **express surface structures that encourage their interaction with platelets** and result in the incorporation of monocytes into thrombi. The purpose of this interaction is unclear; however, monocytes are a source of plasminogen activator and may play a role in limiting clot formation or promoting clot dissolution.

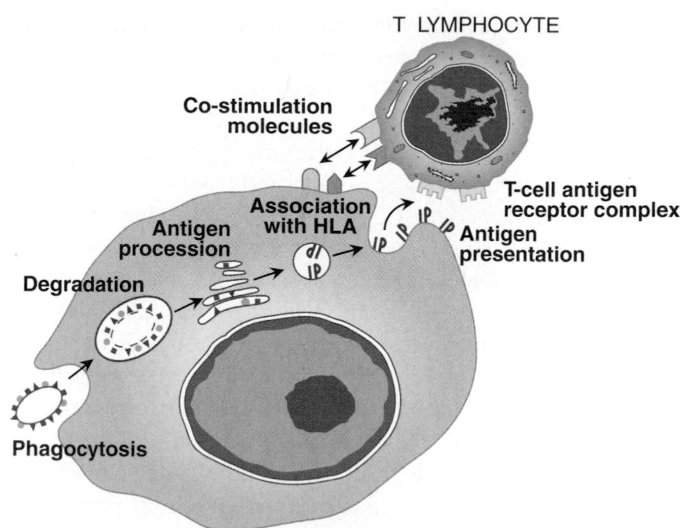

FIGURE 16–7. **Antigen presentation by macrophages and dendritic cells.** In addition to their role in phagocytosis and killing of pathogens, macrophages play a central role in the immune system by processing antigen and presenting it to the lymphocytes in a manner that facilitates the recognition of foreign material and triggers the immune response. Dendritic cells use the same mechanism portrayed here to present antigen very efficiently. This process involves partial degradation of the antigen, transport to the cell surface, and attachment to the major histocompatibility (HLA) molecules. Lymphocytes recognize foreign antigen as a molecular modification of the normal HLA antigens. Although both macrophages and B cells can perform this antigen-presenting role, the dendritic cells are more highly specialized as "professional" antigen presenters, and are becoming the targets of immunotherapy. The important role of the co-stimulatory molecules in the induction of immunity and tolerance is also being exploited therapeutically.

Eosinophils

The eosinophil is easily recognized either in the marrow aspirate or on the stained blood film (Figure 16–8). Their size is similar to a neutrophil and the nucleus is typically bilobed, even though cells with 3 segmented lobes may be observed. The most distinguishing characteristic, however, is the large number of **bright orange to red specific granules that fill the cell's cytoplasm** to the point of obscuring the margins of the nucleus. When viewed through an electron microscope, the granules contain a crystal composed of an extremely alkaline protein called **major basic protein**.

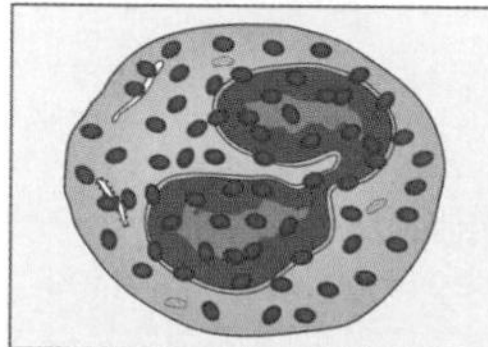

Eosinophil
Bilobed nucleus
Abundant red granules

FIGURE 16–8. **Eosinophil morphology.** The major function of eosinophils appears to be the defense against multicellular parasites mediated by the release of the highly toxic major basic protein in their granules. In addition, they are capable of scavenging immune complexes and may play a role in the suppression of humoral immune reactions.

Although the **principal function of the eosinophil is to kill parasites**, the cell also contains peroxidase and other enzymes similar to those of neutrophils. The production of eosinophils is stimulated by several cytokines, including IL-1, IL-3, and IL-5, as well as by GM-CSF, but IL-5 is the most specific growth factor. Their production and function seems to be more closely tied to the immune system, helper T-cell and NK-cell activity, than the typical antibacterial response of neutrophils.

Eosinophils are **phagocytic** and can kill organisms by phagosome formation. At the same time, when the eosinophil must deal with an organism such as a helminth that is too large to engulf, it will release its granules directly onto the surface of the organism. Eosinophils also appear to be **involved in immediate-type hypersensitivity reactions**. They are capable of neutralizing histamine and may play a role in downregulating allergic reactions. When stimulated to excessive levels, eosinophils, perhaps by release of their granules, **can give rise to tissue damage and endomyocardial fibrosis**.

Basophils

Basophils and marrow mast cells are equally distinctive morphologically because of their basophilic granules (Figure 16–9). However, the granules of basophils and mast cells are not identical and it is still unclear just how they are related. Circulating basophils are easily recognized on stained films as cells whose internal structure is largely occluded by a **dense mass of large, deep-purple granules**. The cells often appear somewhat smaller than neutrophils. In patients with basophilia, however, the granules may be relatively sparse, revealing a nucleus that resembles that of a monocyte more than a neutrophil. The size of the individual granules is the tip-off; they are much larger than the primary granules of the neutrophils.

Circulating basophils appear to play a **major role in immediate-type hypersensitivity reactions both as triggering and effector cells**. Their granules contain abundant proteoglycans and histamine. They express high-affinity Fc receptors for IgE and are triggered to release their granule contents by crosslinking of their surface-bound IgE by antigens. Basophils also produce other mediators of acute hypersensitivity such as leukotrienes. Clinically, basophil granule release is **manifested as urticaria, rhinitis, asthma, and anaphylaxis**. Tissue mast cells also play a role in the hypersensitivity response. In addition, **mast cells** contain large amounts of heparin that may serve to maintain blood and extracellular fluid flow, especially in the marrow. Mast cells in the marrow are closely located to vessels and sinusoids.

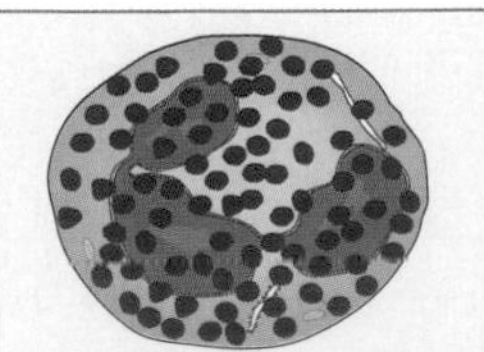

Basophil
Segmented nucleus
Cytoplasm filled by large, dark granules

FIGURE 16–9. **Basophil morphology.** The major role of basophils and mast cells is the release of vasoactive compounds in response to immunologic stimuli mediated by the crosslinking of IgE.

Cytokines responsible for basophil production may be similar to those that stimulate eosinophil production. Basophils provide a **useful marker for certain myeloproliferative disorders**, particularly CML. Leukemias restricted to basophils or mast cells are very rare. Marrow and tissue mast cells are increased in the benign disorder urticaria pigmentosa and the clonal malignancy progressive systemic mastocytosis. Symptoms of these disorders are related to the release of histamine and leukotrienes from the cells, resulting in angioedema, pruritus, and hypotension.

MYELOID CELL KINETICS

The kinetics of cell production, egress from the marrow, and survival in circulation is best illustrated by neutrophils. As with red blood cell production, **marrow biopsy** can be used to evaluate overall cellularity of the pool of leukocyte/monocyte progenitors, whereas a **marrow aspirate** provides information regarding cell differentiation. Overall, there should be approximately 3 myeloid precursors or mature granulocytes for every recognizable erythroid precursor. The normal ratio of erythroid to granulocytic precursors (E/G ratio) is 1:3. Moreover, in the normal basal state, about one-third of all cells observed in a marrow aspirate are mature granulocytes that are being stored and awaiting release in response to an infection-related cytokine.

Figure 16–10 illustrates the relative sizes of the neutrophil precursor compartments, the transit times, and the storage pool

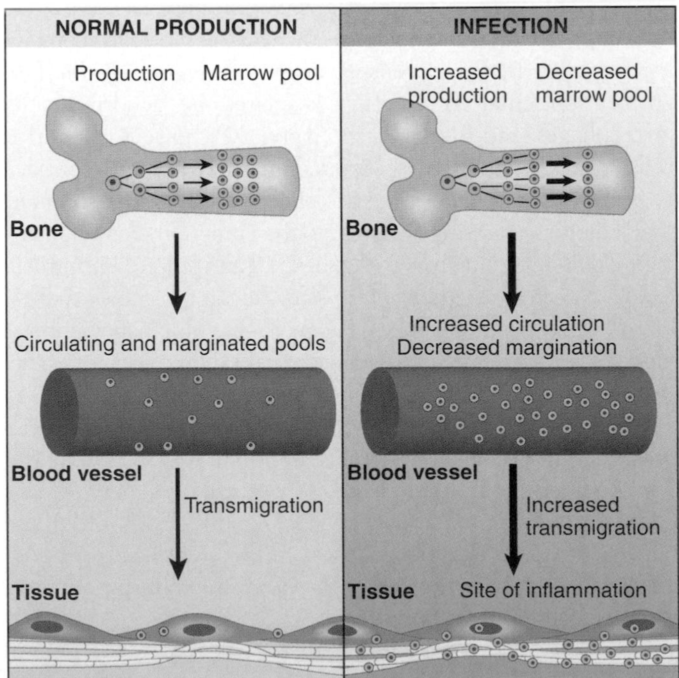

FIGURE 16–10. **Neutrophil kinetics in the basal state and in infection.** There are several distinct compartments of neutrophils within the body. These are the proliferating and storage pools in the marrow, the marginated and circulating pools in the blood vessels, and finally those neutrophils in the tissues at the site of inflammation. Infection triggers increased production, depletion of the marrow storage and marginated pools, increase in the circulating pool, and increased transmigration into the tissues.

for both the normal and infected states. Approximately 1×10^9 neutrophils/kg/d are produced by the **normal adult marrow**, and the total time spent in proliferation, maturation, and marrow storage is estimated to be between 5 and 14 days. **With a severe infection**, however, the maturation time may be shortened to as little as 48–72 hours. This process reflects a shift of the marrow storage pool into circulation, a phenomenon that can be recognized on inspection of the marrow aspirate as a disappearance of mature neutrophils from the specimen even while the E/G ratio shows an increase in the immature granulocyte compartment.

Factors Affecting the Number of Circulating and Stored Neutrophils

Once neutrophils enter circulation, they rapidly equilibrate with the marginated neutrophil pool of approximately equal size. The partition between the marrow storage pool, the circulating neutrophils, and the marginal pool is in constant flux. The number of neutrophils in circulation can increase dramatically in **response to infection** as a result of a shift of neutrophils out of the marrow storage pool that exceeds any increased egress of neutrophils from circulation into the tissues. **Administration of glucocorticoids** will also change the partition by releasing marrow granulocytes into circulation, changing the size of the marginal pool, and slowing the rate of egress into tissues. **Sudden exertion** with release of catecholamines will also change the pool partition and can double or even triple the blood neutrophil count. Finally, **African American subjects** may have significantly lower neutrophil counts because of variations in the pool sizes, with otherwise normal neutrophil production and delivery into tissues.

Circulating granulocytes leave circulation in a random fashion with an average **disappearance time of 6–7 hours**. Once they enter tissue they do not return to circulation, and their survival depends on their reason for homing to that site. At best, it is less than 2–3 days. In response to an infection, they release cytokines, which encourage additional granulocyte migration.

Estimates of Myeloid Cell Production

Even though the kinetics of neutrophil production and survival in circulation are complex, it is possible clinically to estimate myeloid cell production from the count of mature and immature cells in circulation. **Modern automated counters** provide an accurate measurement of the total leukocyte count and a relatively accurate differential count of neutrophils, metamyelocytes (bands), monocytes, eosinophils, basophils, and lymphocytes (see Chapter 2 and Figure 2–2). A **white blood cell differential** can also be performed by direct counting of a stained blood film. Since a smaller number of cells are counted, the error of this measurement is far larger than that of the automated differential. However, automated counters are often unable to accurately classify abnormal cell types, and such methodologic errors result in flags that must be taken into account before releasing differential results.

Normal values for the leukocyte count and differential are summarized in Table 16–3. Clinical laboratories generally report the absolute number of leukocytes and a percent differential of the individual cell types. The **clinician is advised to calculate and use the absolute number** in determining whether the patient has too few or too many cells of a certain type in circulation. This measurement is most important for the accurate identification of a neutropenia or lymphopenia (see Chapter 20). It is also true in the case of monocytosis, eosinophilia, and basophilia. A **significant monocytosis** is defined as an absolute monocyte count of greater than 1,000/μL (1.0×10^9/L); significant **eosinophilia** is greater than 450/μL (0.45×10^9/L), whereas **basophilia** is defined as greater than 50 basophils/μL (0.05×10^9/L).

TABLE 16–3 • The normal leukocyte count

Cell Type	Percent	Absolute Count
Leukocytes		5–11,000/μL ($5–11 \times 10^9$/L)
Neutrophils	45–75	4–6,000/μL ($4–6 \times 10^9$/L)
Metamyelocytes (bands)	0–5	
Monocytes	5–10	500–1,000/μL ($0.5–1 \times 10^9$/L)
Eosinophils	0–5	<450/μL ($<45 \times 10^9$/L)
Basophils	0–1	<50/μL ($<0.05 \times 10^9$/L)
Lymphocytes	10–45	1,500–4,000/L ($1.5–4 \times 10^9$/L)

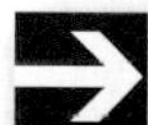

POINTS TO REMEMBER

Myeloid cells—granulocytes (neutrophils), monocytes, eosinophils, and basophils—differentiate from a common progenitor, CFU-GM, under the influence of the growth factors: GM-CSF, G-CSF, and M-CSF. The marrow environment also plays a key role in supporting cell proliferation and differentiation.

A number of interleukins (IL-3, IL-5, IL-6, IL-11), as well as stem cell factor and Flt3 ligand play a role in stem cell growth and development.

These factors in most cases influence not only the growth and development of the myeloid cells but also their function.

Myeloid cells have 3 functions—the ability to migrate into tissues, phagocytosis, and the release of granule contents (exocytosis). Each of these functions plays a key role in the management of a bacterial infection and the resulting inflammatory response.

Individual myeloid cell types also have unique functions. Neutrophils and monocytes are primarily dedicated to fighting bacterial infections; monocytes also have the ability to process and present antigens to lymphocytes; eosinophils are capable of killing parasites; while basophils play a major role in immediate-type hypersensitivity reactions.

The several types of myeloid cells can be readily distinguished by their morphology, different staining characteristics using the special stains for myeloperoxidase, specific and nonspecific esterase, and periodic acid–Schiff reaction, and immunologic markers.

Many automated counters can perform a 3- or 5-part differential (neutrophils, lymphocytes, monocytes, eosinophils, and basophils) using their light scatter characteristics (see Chapter 2 and Figure 2–2). Abnormal white blood cell elements (blasts, promyelocytes, and metamyelocytes) can also be identified, but generally require a microscopic examination to confirm their cell type and quantity.

An examination of the blood smear is essential for any patient with an abnormal automated counter result, whether it involves the absolute number of each cell line (see Table 16–3) or the presence of abnormal cells.

A bone marrow examination is also essential whenever the number of 1 or more cell lines in circulation is below or above the normal range and/or abnormal cells are present, without a clear clinical explanation. The marrow provides a powerful tool for distinguishing abnormalities in progenitor proliferation and differentiation.

Neutrophil proliferation, maturation, and storage in the marrow takes 5–14 days. They then spend less than 12 hours in circulation before entering tissue sites, never to return. With a severe infection, the storage pool is rapidly emptied into circulation, raising the neutrophil count to levels as high as $15–30 \times 10^3/\mu L$. This predictable response, as well as the appearance of immature neutrophils (metamyelocytes or bands), can be used clinically as an indicator of a bacterial infection, but clinicians must recognize that this finding is nonspecific and, furthermore, cannot be used to determine resolution of infection.

BIBLIOGRAPHY

Anderlini P et al: Biologic and clinical effects of granulocyte colony-stimulating factor in normal individuals. Blood 1996;88:2819.

Bainton DF: Morphology of neutrophils, eosinophils and basophils. In: MA Lichtmann et al. (eds.): Williams Hematology, 7th ed. McGraw-Hill, 2006, 831–845.

Berliner N: Understanding myelopoiesis. Lessons from congenital neutropenia. Blood 2008;111:5427.

Broxmeyer HE: Regulation of hematopoiesis by chemokine family members. Int J Hematology 2001;74:9.

Charo IF, Ransonhof RM: The many roles of chemokines and chemokine receptors in inflammation. New Engl J Med 2006;354:610.

Delves PJ, Roitt IM: The immune system, Part II. N Engl J Med 2000;343:108.

Hogan SP, Rosenberg HF, Moqbel R, et al: Eosinophils: biological properties and role in health and disease. Clin Exp Allergy 2008;38:709.

Kaushansky K: Lineage-specific hematopoietic growth factors. N Engl J Med 2006;354:2034.

Malech HL: The role of neutrophils in the immune system: an overview. Methods Mol Biol 2007;412:3.

Metcalf D: Hematopoietic cytokines. Blood 2008;111:485.

Middleton J et al: Leukocyte extravasation: chemokine transport and presentation by the endothelium. Blood 2002; 100:3853.

Min B, Paul WE: Basophils and type 2 immunity. Curr Opin Hematol 2008;15:59.

Möhle R, Kaénz Lothar: Hematopoïetic growth factors for hemetopoïetic stem cell mobilisation and expansion. Semin Hematol 2007;44:193.

Obata K, Mukai K, Tsujimura Y, et al: Basophils are essential initiators of a novel type of chronic allergic inflammation. Blood 2007;110:913.

Ravetch JV, Bolland S: IgG Fc receptors. Annu Rev Immunol 2001;19:275.

Serbina NV, Jia T, Hohl TM, Pamer EG: Monocyte-mediated defense against microbial pathogens. Annu Rev Immunol 2008;26:421.

Shivdasani RA, Orkin SH: The transcriptional control of hematopoiesis. Blood 1996;87:4025.

Smith CW: Production, distribution, and fate of neutrophils. In: Lichtmann MA et al. (eds.). Williams Hematology, 7th ed. McGraw-Hill, 2006, 855–861.

Tacke F, Randolph GJ: Migratory fate and differentiation of blood monocyte subsets. Immunobiology 2006;211:609.

Uematsu S, Akira S: Toll-like receptors and innate immunity. J Mol Med 2006;84:712.

Wagner DD, Frenette PS: The vessel wall and its interactions. Blood 2008;111:5271.

Wedemeyer J, Galli SJ: Mast cells and basophils in acquired immunity. Br Med Bull 2000;56:936.

QUANTITATIVE AND QUALITATIVE DISORDERS OF NEUTROPHILS • 17

CASE HISTORY • *Part I*

A 54-year-old woman with poorly controlled hypertension while on a beta-blocker is started on hydrochlorothiazide. A month later she returns for a blood pressure check and describes several days of a sore throat, fever, and chills. On examination she has a temperature of 39.5°C, a pharyngeal exudate, and submaxillary lymphadenopathy. A complete blood count (CBC) with differential is ordered STAT.

CBC: Hematocrit/hemoglobin - 40%/13 g/dL
WBC - 4.1 × 10^3/uL
Differential - Neutrophils 10% Monocytes 15%
Lymphocytes 75%
Platelet count - 150 × 10^3/uL

• SMEAR MORPHOLOGY

Normocytic, normochromic red cells without aniso- or poikilocytosis. White cells are sparse, comprised mostly of normal-appearing lymphocytes, with a few normal-appearing neutrophils; no early neutrophil precursors (bands, myelocytes, or blasts) are seen. Platelets are normal.

Questions

- Given the CBC findings, what are the absolute numbers for each of the white cell lines and what abnormality is present?
- What further workup is needed—both history and laboratory testing?

Quantitative disorders of neutrophils are frequently encountered in clinical practice but seldom present a diagnostic problem. For example, granulocytosis, which is an acute increase in the number of mature and immature granulocytes in circulation, is an anticipated part of the normal response to any infection. Eosinophilia and monocytosis are seen in association with allergic and inflammatory conditions. On the other hand, granulocytopenia can occur as a side effect of drug administration or as a component of the pancytopenia seen with severe marrow damage. It is an anticipated complication of cancer chemotherapy.

Qualitative disorders of neutrophil function are much less common. Again, they can occur as a complication of drug therapy. Those that result from genetic defects in granulocyte adhesion, migration, or lysozyme function are a greater diagnostic challenge.

NORMAL RESPONSE OF NEUTROPHILS TO INFECTION

The kinetics of normal neutrophil production and destruction are described in Chapter 16. In response to infection or presentation of a foreign antigen, several cytokines (tumor necrosis factor [TNF]-α, interleukin [IL]-1, granulocyte colony-stimulating factor [G-CSF], granulocyte macrophage colony-stimulating factor [GM-CSF], monocyte colony-stimulating factor [M-CSF], and IL-3) are released that affect the kinetics of neutrophil production and the distribution of cells within the circulation and tissues. A single mediator of inflammation cannot be identified; however, the broad effects of TNF-α illustrate how the reaction is coordinated. Administration of TNF-α essentially duplicates all of the signs and symptoms of sepsis, including fever, hypotension, and acute respiratory distress syndrome/pulmonary edema. It is associated with concomitant changes in other cytokines that mediate the reaction to infection, such as IL-1, which stimulates the immune system, and the colony-stimulating factors (CSFs), which stimulate granulocyte production and function. Interestingly, experimental blockade of TNF-α can ablate most of the inflammatory effects of sepsis and, in some models, can prevent death from septic shock.

The earliest response to an infection is the emigration of granulocytes out of circulation and into the site of bacterial invasion. Granulocytes close to the infected area respond to local chemotactic factors by increasing their rate of margination and migration. They also trigger the full inflammatory response with further release of cytokines capable of stimulating marrow-progenitor proliferation.

The rapidity and magnitude of the rise in the number of circulating granulocytes in response to infection is impressive. Within hours of the onset of a severe infection, the granulocyte count can increase by 2- to 4-fold. Initially, this increase represents a change in the partition between the marginated and circulating pools of granulocytes and the delivery of new granulocytes from the marrow pool (Figure 17–1). In the basal state, mature granulocytes spend 5–6 days in the marrow before entering circulation. With severe infection, this transit time can be shortened to a day or less with release of immature granulocytes (bands or metamyelocytes). With the stimulus of G-CSF, there is a proliferation of committed progenitors and a further shortening of the time delay in precursor maturation. Finally, the response is made more effective by shortening the transit time of granulocytes through the circulation to increase the rate of delivery to a tissue site.

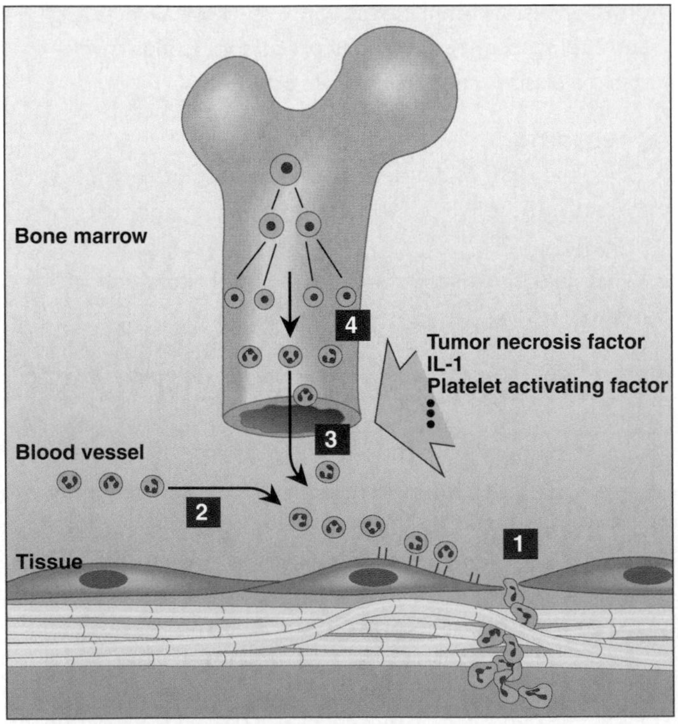

G-CSF, GM-CSF, and M-CSF (CSF-1) can all play a role in the sustained increase in granulocyte and monocyte production. The primary effect of G-CSF is to stimulate the committed granulocyte precursor pathway. GM-CSF and M-CSF promote both granulocyte and monocyte production. As illustrated by measurements of plasma cytokine levels in neutropenic patients, these growth factors appear in sequence, according to the severity of the infection and the rate of use of mature cells. The level of G-CSF rises first. Increases in the levels of GM-CSF and M-CSF occur somewhat later and are most pronounced in patients who become granulocytopenic. They have a wider impact on cell production and are responsible for the increase in the number of circulating monocytes in patients with severe granulocytopenia. In addition to their role as growth factors, they also enhance the phagocytic and cytotoxic functions of granulocytes and monocytes.

FIGURE 17–1. **Granulocyte response to infection.** The response to infection includes (1) an increase in cell adherence and migration out of circulation; (2) demargination of cells more remote to the site of infection; (3) a shift of the marrow granulocyte pool into circulation; and (4) a severalfold increase in proliferation of committed progenitors. The response is mediated by cytokines including tumor necrosis factor, IL-1, and platelet-activating factor, among others.

NEUTROPHILIA

Clinically, neutrophilia is defined in adults as an absolute granulocyte count in excess of 7×10^9/L (7,000 segmented granulocytes plus bands/μL), while newborns have normal values up to 25,000/μL and infants and children up to 8,500/μL. The major causes of neutrophilia are listed in Table 17–1. Tissue damage, inflammation, and bacterial infection stimulate the normal response pattern of neutrophils to a foreign antigen. This pattern includes changes in cell production, marrow release, and rate of entry into tissues. Other causes of neutrophilia involve changes in only 1 or 2 of the steps in the kinetic response. For example, the granulocytosis observed with stress is caused by a shift in the pool of marginated granulocytes. The increase in granulocyte count

TABLE 17–1 • Etiology of neutrophilia

Cause	Mechanism
Infections/inflammation/ tissue damage	Increased production, marrow granulocyte pool release, demargination
Myeloproliferative disease	Increased production
Stress/metabolic disorders (ketoacidosis, eclampsia, etc)	Demargination
Steroid therapy/endotoxin, cigarettes, lithium salts	Marrow granulocyte pool release, demargination, decreased egress
Growth factor therapy (G-CSF, GM-CSF)	Increased production, change in egress
Splenectomy	Decrease in splenic pool

observed in patients with myeloproliferative diseases such as polycythemia vera or chronic myelogenous leukemia (CML) is the product of uncontrolled cell production typical of a clonal malignancy.

Clinical Features

An increase in the granulocyte count by itself does not produce specific symptoms or signs, except when the count exceeds 100,000/μL in patients with CML. In this situation, marked leukostasis in the spleen can result in splenic infarction. Sudden activation of granulocytes in the circulation can lead to stasis in the lungs with a drop in oxygen diffusion capacity. When present in very large numbers, granulocytes can also accumulate in the skin to produce nontender, purplish nodules (chloromas). Unlike immature blasts, mature granulocytes do not invade brain tissue.

The clinical features associated with moderate granulocytosis are those of the primary disease. With an acute bacterial infection, the patient is usually febrile and has evidence of a tissue infection (ie, lung infiltrate, abscess, cellulitis). Similarly, noninfectious inflammatory diseases are accompanied by clinical features particular to the individual condition.

Laboratory Studies

A routine complete blood count (CBC) and white blood cell (WBC) differential may be all that is needed to diagnose the common causes of granulocytosis. The CBC provides an accurate measurement of the total WBC count, whereas the differential provides a measure of the number of mature granulocytes, metamyelocytes (band forms), monocytes, and eosinophils. In the basal state, the absolute number of bands should be less than 500 cells/μL. Severe infection or inflammation is associated with an increased release (shift) of marrow metamyelocytes into circulation. Reactive monocytosis (monocyte counts >1,000/μL) is seen in patients with active tuberculosis, subacute bacterial endocarditis, and generally as the first sign of recovery in severe transient granulocytopenia. Parasitic infestations are typically associated with an elevated eosinophil count, whereas basophilia (a basophil count >50/μL) is seen in patients with myeloproliferative diseases, especially CML.

A marrow aspirate can provide additional supporting information. The shift of marrow granulocytes into circulation and the proliferation of myelocytic precursors are easily detected on inspection of the marrow aspirate film (Figure 17–2). In the basal state, mature granulocytes make up one-quarter or more of the cells in the marrow. This number is dramatically reduced in patients with acute infection. In addition, the number of early myelocytic precursors increases to shift the ratio of erythroid to granulocytic precursors (E/G ratio) to below 1:3 (expansion of the myelocytic portion of the marrow).

Changes in individual cell morphology can also help in the diagnosis. The appearance of metamyelocytes (bands) in circulation is one sign of a reactive granulocytosis secondary to cytokine stimulation. Another is the appearance of granulocytes with prominent azurophilic granules, so-called toxic granulation. The leukocyte alkaline phosphatase stain coupled with bone marrow chromosomal analysis and specific molecular markers are also of value in distinguishing reactive granulocytosis from a malignant state. Although patients with CML present with varying combinations of granulocytosis, toxic granulation, Döhle bodies, and basophilia, the condition is also accompanied by a decrease in leukocyte alkaline phosphatase activity. In contrast, leukemoid reactions in patients with infection or inflammation demonstrate an elevated leukocyte alkaline phosphatase. Bone marrow karyotypes from CML patients demonstrate the distinctive translocation of the *C-ABL* oncogene from chromosome 9 to chromosome 22 with the reciprocal transposition of the terminal portion of chromosome 22 to chromosome 9 (the Philadelphia chromosome defect). Even more sensitive for diagnosing CML is the BCR-ABL fusion product, which can be detected and quantitated from peripheral blood leukocytes via reverse transcriptase polymerase chain reaction (RT-PCR).

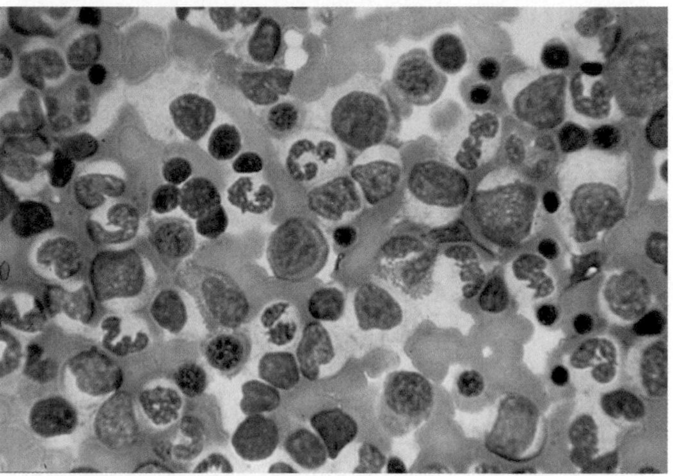

FIGURE 17–2. **Granulocytic hyperplasia.** Marrow aspirate specimen showing an erythroid/granulocytic ratio less than 1:3, suggesting a proliferation of myeloid elements associated with granulocytosis.

Diagnosis

The diagnosis of granulocytosis associated with an acute infection, inflammation, or major tissue damage is generally straightforward. Major bacterial infections are associated with granulocyte counts of 10,000–30,000/μL, together with an increase in the number of band forms. Although a count in excess of 30,000/μL is unusual, very high counts may be observed in patients with deep-seated infections, abscess, or peritonitis. As a rule, granulocyte counts of 50,000/μL or higher indicate a noninfectious, primary myeloproliferative malignant disease process. The appearance of very immature myelocytic cells in circulation and accompanying change in other cell lines (eg, increased or decreased platelets or red blood cells) are also signs of myeloproliferative or myelodysplastic diseases.

Changes in pool kinetics can result in modest increases in the granulocyte count (see Table 17–1). After splenectomy, patients will chronically demonstrate neutrophil counts of 10,000–15,000/μL. Acute stress in association with trauma, hemorrhage, marked hypoxia, or ketoacidosis will produce a self-limited granulocytosis. This condition involves a catecholamine-induced shift of the marginated granulocyte pool into circulation.

Granulocytosis is an expected side effect of glucocorticoid therapy that interferes with the egress of granulocytes from circulation into tissues. There is a clear dose-response relationship since patients who are receiving 60–100 mg of prednisone per day will run WBC counts of 15,000–20,000/μL. Higher doses of prednisone can make the WBC count reach levels of 30,000/μL or higher, which is characterized by a marked increase in the percentage of granulocytes, together with a reduction in lymphocytes and eosinophils. Treatment with lithium salts and cigarette smoking are other causes of mild sustained granulocytosis. G-CSF and GM-CSF are also capable of producing a marked granulocytosis. In this case, the primary cause of the increased count is increased marrow production. However, G-CSF also influences the rate of egress of granulocytes from circulation. Daily administration of large doses of either cytokine can raise the granulocyte count to levels in excess of 100,000/μL.

EOSINOPHILIA

Clinically significant eosinophilia is defined as a sustained absolute eosinophil count of greater than 1,000–1,500/μL. Table 17–2 lists the various disease states associated with eosinophilia.

TABLE 17–2 • Etiologies of eosinophilia

Allergic disorders
Asthma
Allergic vasculitis—polyarteritis nodosa
Angioneurotic edema
Dermatologic disorders
Eczema
Psoriasis
Dermatitis herpetiformis
Pemphigus
Parasitic diseases
Protozoan infections—toxoplasmosis, amebiasis
Metazoan infections—nematode, trematode, and cestode infestations; scabies
Gastrointestinal disease
Ulcerative colitis/regional enteritis
Eosinophilic gastroenteritis
Malignancies
Hodgkin disease/B- and T-cell lymphomas
Myeloproliferative disorders
Carcinomatosis
Eosinophilic granuloma
Hypereosinophilia
Familial eosinophilia
Hypereosinophilic syndrome (HES)
Eosinophilic leukemia
Loeffler syndrome

Moderate eosinophilia is commonly seen with a wide spectrum of disorders, including parasitic infestations, systemic allergic disorders, collagen vascular diseases, various forms of dermatitis, drug reactions, and tumors. Hodgkin disease and both B-cell and T-cell non-Hodgkin lymphomas can present with eosinophilia. Even when there is no obvious sign of an underlying lymphoma, up to 25% of patients with apparent idiopathic eosinophilia will have an expanded clone of aberrant T-cells, which produce high levels of IL-5.

Hypereosinophilia (an eosinophil count of 2,000–5,000/μL or higher) is chronically associated with tissue damage secondary to the release of the eosinophil's major basic protein. Irreversible **endomyocardial fibrosis** producing a restrictive cardiomyopathy can be anticipated in patients who maintain eosinophil counts greater than 5,000/μL. One exception is familial eosinophilia, an autosomal dominant disorder, where organ damage is seen in a minority of affected family members. In patients with **eosinophilic leukemia, idiopathic hypereosinophilic syndrome (HES), or Loeffler syndrome**, eosinophil counts can reach 20,000–100,000/μL. Widespread **organ dysfunction and rapidly progressive heart disease** can be anticipated with these conditions, and aggressive treatment with both corticosteroids and hydroxyurea is recommended. Leukapheresis can be used acutely to lower the eosinophil count. Recently there have been reports that tyrosine kinase inhibitors may be effective in patients with idiopathic hypereosinophilic syndrome that is associated with the t(1;4)(q44;q12) *FIP1L1-PDGFα* recombination.

NEUTROPENIA

Clinically, neutropenia is defined as an absolute granulocyte count below 2,000/μL in Caucasians or 1,500/μL in those of African descent. It is not until the granulocyte count falls below 500/μL, however, that the patient is at significant risk for bacterial or fungal infections. The major causes of neutropenia in the adult involve abnormalities in cell production and autoimmune destruction. Changes in pool kinetics play less of a role.

Clinical Features

The symptoms and signs of neutropenia depend on the actual level of granulocytes. When the absolute number of granulocytes is between 500 and 2,000/μL, it is unlikely that the patient will develop a serious bacterial infection. The moderately neutropenic patient may be unable, however, to mount an adequate defense. When challenged by infection, the associated increase in WBC utilization can result in a rapid fall in the granulocyte count. This situation puts the patient at risk for spread of the infection and life-threatening bacteremia.

Once the count falls below 500/μL, the patient is at significant risk for infections of the skin, mouth (teeth and periodontal tissue), pharynx, and lung. As the count falls below 100/μL, the risk of bacterial sepsis and fungal infections increases dramatically.

Laboratory Studies

The CBC and WBC differential are the key measurements in diagnosing and managing the neutropenic patient. It is important to focus on the absolute granulocyte count and not the total WBC count. Most patients with granulocytopenia will still have normal or near normal numbers of lymphocytes, which may keep the total WBC count above 2,000/μL. Attention should also be given to the number of monocytes. A reactive monocytosis is often observed in patients with drug-induced or cyclic neutropenia. A small increase in the number of monocytes to levels of 500–1,000/μL can significantly reduce the risk of fatal bacteremia.

The marrow aspirate is the other key test in determining the cause and future course of a neutropenia. Usually, a simple marrow aspirate to look at the marrow E/G ratio and the maturation of myelocyte precursors is adequate. Production defects are associated with a uniform loss of myelocytes at all stages of maturation. The aspirate appears hypocellular with the remaining cell elements limited to red blood cell precursors, lymphocytes, plasma cells, and mast cells. Patients with drug-induced neutropenia often demonstrate "a maturation arrest" where relatively normal-appearing early myelocytic precursors do not progress to more mature myelocyte, metamyelocyte, and granulocyte stages. Folic acid and vitamin B_{12} deficiency can also produce a maturation abnormality, characterized by megaloblastic morphology and the appearance of mature granulocytes with an increased number of nuclear lobes (hypersegmented nuclei with more than 5 lobes).

If an adequate marrow aspirate cannot be obtained, a marrow biopsy is required. In patients with severe marrow damage secondary to malignancy, drug damage, or idiopathic aplasia, the marrow biopsy is preferred for the evaluation of total cellularity and structural damage. Patients with myelofibrosis, hairy-cell leukemia, and paroxysmal nocturnal hemoglobinuria will frequently have a dry tap on aspiration, and therefore can only be diagnosed by biopsy.

Other tests that can help pinpoint the diagnosis include cytogenetics (for clonal malignancies of the hematopoietic system), tests for paroxysmal nocturnal hemoglobinuria (see Chapter 9), including flow cytometric evaluation of glycosylphosphatidylinositol (GPI)-linked glycoproteins (CD59/55), serum folic acid and vitamin B_{12} levels (megaloblastic pancytopenia), and assays for antineutrophil antibodies (collagen vascular disease). The Rebuck skin window test to assess the egress of granulocytes into tissues, and turnover measurements are possible using radiolabeled granulocytes. However, these latter measurements are usually limited to the research laboratory. Measurements of circulating cytokine levels (G-CSF, GM-CSF, and M-CSF) by immunoassay are becoming available, but their role in diagnosing clinical conditions is yet to be determined.

TABLE 17–3 • Etiologies of neutropenia in children

Cause	Mechanism
Newborns	
Alloimmune neonatal neutropenia	Immune destruction (NA alloantibodies)
Infections	Production defect and increased utilization
Maternal drug ingestion	Production defect
Congenital neutropenias Benign (chronic idiopathic neutropenia) Kostmann syndrome Immunodeficiency states Chédiak-Higashi syndrome Shwachman-Diamond syndrome Autoimmune disease	Production defect
Infants and young children	
Infections	Increased utilization
Drug ingestion	Production defect
Vitamin deficiency (vitamin B_{12} folate/copper)	Production/maturation defect
Hematopoietic malignancy	Production defect
Cyclic neutropenia	Intermittent failure of marrow proliferation

Diagnosis

A. Neutropenia in Newborns and Children

Several neutropenic syndromes are observed in newborns and young children (Table 17–3). Neonatal sepsis is perhaps the most common cause of severe neutropenia within the first few days of life. A reversible immune neutropenia can be observed in children born to mothers with autoimmune disease, or as a consequence of alloimmunization against specific neutrophil antigens (mainly the NA1/2 system). Other causes of transient neonatal neutropenia occur as a result of maternal hypertension, drug ingestion, or both. Persistent neutropenia can occur as a result of defects in neutrophil production, maturation, or survival.

Cyclic neutropenia, an autosomal dominant condition, is a particularly well-studied cause of childhood neutropenia. This disorder is characterized by recurrent episodes of neutropenia, which are not always associated with infection and occur in regular cycles of 3–4 weeks. Each episode is characterized by 1 week of reduced granulocyte production, followed by a reactive monocytosis and then a spontaneous recovery of normal granulocyte production. The granulocytopenia can be severe enough to result in recurrent, severe bacterial infections that require aggressive antibiotic therapy. As the child grows older, the cyclical nature of the WBC production can diminish, thereby resulting in a chronic severe granulocytopenia. The postulated mechanism behind cyclic neutropenia is a defective feedback mechanism with a decreased capacity of precursors to respond to growth factors such as G-CSF. Constitutional mutations, most of them inside exons 4 and 5 of the neutrophil elastase gene

(*ELA2*) at 19q3 have been recognized as the hallmark of cyclic neutropenia, and are now available by genetic testing.

Kostmann syndrome, an autosomal recessive disorder of neutrophil maturation, is another cause of severe congenital neutropenia. These patients appear to have a normal population of early progenitors, but impaired maturation is related to excessive early apoptosis. They are at risk for severe, life-threatening infections. Most patients with Kostmann syndrome have been shown to have mutations of the G-CSF receptor or the *ELA2* gene. Although most of the former do respond to therapy with G-CSF, the latter are associated with poor responsiveness to growth factor and an increased risk of developing myelodysplastic syndrome (MDS) or acute myeloid leukemia (AML). Recently, the *HAX1* mutation, the normal product of which is a mitochondrial protein with BCL2 homology, has been identified in some pedigrees of Kostmann disease.

Shwachman-Diamond syndrome is a rare autosomal recessive disorder characterized in infancy by the association of exocrine pancreatic insufficiency, maturation defects, insulin-dependant diabetes mellitus, neutropenia, impaired chemotaxis, and an increased risk of transformation to AML.

Neutropenia can be associated with lymphocytopenia and hypogammaglobulinemia in myelocathexis. WHIM combines warts, hypogammaglobulinemia, infections, and myelocathexis, and results from mutations of the *CXCR4* gene (see Chapter 16). Both syndromes are characterized by hypersegmented neutrophils with a pyknotic nucleus and cytoplasmic vacuoles.

Chédiak-Higashi syndrome is an autosomal recessive disorder with moderate neutropenia, a distinctive appearance of circulating granulocytes containing very large azurophilic granules in all myelocytic lineages, and a high susceptibility to bacterial infections.

TABLE 17–4 • Etiologies of neutropenia in adults

Cause	Mechanism
Drug induced	Production, maturation, and survival defects
Autoimmune disease	Increased destruction (antineutrophil antibodies)
Hypersplenism	Increased splenic pooling, destruction
Hematopoietic malignancy Leukemias Hodgkin disease T-cell malignancies (LGL, etc)	Production defects
HIV-1 infection (AIDS)	Production, maturation, and survival defects
Congenital Neutropenia in blacks Chronic idiopathic neutropenia	 Maturation defect, increased margination Production defect

B. Neutropenia in Adults

The principal causes of neutropenia in adults are listed in Table 17–4. Acquired defects in marrow production are very common and often can be anticipated as, for example, with cancer chemotherapy and in the treatment of AIDS patients with zidovudine (AZT). This result reflects the impact of specific

CASE HISTORY • *Part 2*

The calculation of the absolute values for each of the cell types shows the following:

Neutrophils - 410/μL
Monocytes - 710/μL
Lymphocytes - 3,000/μL

In light of the normal red cell and platelet counts, the patient has an isolated absolute neutropenia of considerable severity. The slight elevation of the monocytes is generally a compensatory response to severe neutropenia. The absence of early white cell precursors, especially primitive blasts, on the stained smear rules against leukemia and suggests acute drug or toxin damage limited to the neutrophil cell line. In this regard, a careful follow-up history may identify a putative drug or chemical agent that has a known association with neutropenia.

The workup also requires an immediate bone marrow aspirate and biopsy to evaluate both cell number and morphology. In this patient's case, the marrow revealed a marked reduction in myelocyte, metamyelocyte, and mature leukocyte forms; a few early normal-appearing blasts were still present. E/G ratio was greater than 1:1. Erythroid precursors and megakaryocytes appeared normal. No tumor, granulomas, or fibrosis were apparent on biopsy.

Given her history of recently starting a chlorothiazide, a class of drugs associated with acute but reversible neutropenia, the most likely diagnosis is a drug-related neutropenia.

Questions

- How should this patient be managed?
- Should her apparent infection be treated, and if so, with what regimen?
- Would she benefit from the administration of a growth factor?

drugs on stem cell and early myelocytic progenitor proliferation. In most cases, the marrow will recover once the drug(s) are withdrawn.

Many drugs have been associated with occasional idiosyncratic neutropenia, with 2 distinct mechanisms. In the first, toxicity is dose related, and not always restricted to the neutrophil lineage. The most prominent drugs associated with this are the injectable gold salts, chloramphenicol, antithyroid medications (carbimazole and propylthiouracil), analgesics (indomethacin, acetaminophen, and phenacetin), tricyclic antidepressants, and the phenothiazines. The second mechanism is immuno-allergic (ie, dose independent) and specific for the neutrophilic lineage, inducing a profound neutropenia (agranulocytosis) that is self-limited, for example, recovery occurs within 10 days provided the offending drug is stopped. The most frequently recognized drugs in this setting are sulfonamides, ß-lactam antibiotics, antihistamine/H2 blockers, ticlopidine, and levamisole. Virtually any drug can, on occasion, produce severe, life-threatening neutropenia. Therefore, whenever neutropenia occurs in the course of medical treatment, the possibility that it is drug induced must be considered.

"Autoimmune" neutropenia is observed with collagen vascular or autoimmune disease. The 2 most common associations are systemic lupus erythematosus (SLE), where the neutropenia occurs alone or is accompanied by thrombocytopenia, and rheumatoid arthritis (Felty syndrome), where neutropenia in association with splenomegaly is common. Because the arthritic component of the disease process may be subtle, the appearance of either of these combinations should trigger a careful evaluation for collagen vascular disease as a first step in the differential diagnosis. Other causes of splenomegaly and neutropenia include lymphoma, hairy cell leukemia, myeloproliferative disease, and severe liver disease with portal hypertension. In all of these situations, it is often difficult to decide whether the granulocytopenia is owing to sequestration alone versus an additional autoimmune component. Splenomegaly may also have an impact on marrow production. Although this connection is not well understood, splenectomy in cases of Felty syndrome and in selected patients with myelofibrosis has been reported to significantly improve neutrophil production.

Acute, life-threatening granulocytopenia can occur in patients with overwhelming sepsis. A falling count in a patient with pneumococcal sepsis or peritonitis is, of course, a bad prognostic sign. It reflects a rate of granulocyte use that exceeds the ability of the marrow to produce new cells. Alcoholic patients are especially susceptible to infection-induced granulocytopenia. In this setting, both folic acid deficiency and the direct toxic effect of alcohol on marrow precursors cripples the patient's ability to produce new cells in response to infection.

Some patients will present with "idiopathic" neutropenia, without any obvious cause. Usually, the reduction in the number of circulating granulocytes is relatively mild and not associated with life-threatening infections. When the granulocytopenia is accompanied by abnormalities of other blood elements (anemia and thrombocytopenia), it is likely the patient is developing a myeloproliferative bone marrow disorder (see Chapter 9).

Lymphoproliferative disease, especially T-suppressor cell malignancies (large granular lymphocyte [LGL] disease) (see Chapter 22) can also present with granulocytopenia and an increased incidence of skin and mucous membrane infections. Human immunodeficiency virus (HIV) infection is a common cause of T-cell dysfunction. In these patients, the loss of the T-helper subset and overexpression of the T-suppressor subset is associated with abnormalities of neutrophil production and function.

NEUTROPHIL DYSFUNCTION

Patients can present with normal numbers of circulating granulocytes but demonstrate a defect in cell function (Table 17–5). This results from distinct mechanisms involving humoral defects (antibody or complement) leading to impaired chemotactic signals, and abnormalities of cell adhesion, mobility, and granule activation that diminish bacterial killing. The most common causes of poor granulocyte function fit in the acquired category. Patients with metabolic diseases, especially diabetes mellitus, or those who are alcoholics or have uremia or collagen vascular diseases under treatment with corticosteroids can be shown to have mild to moderate defects in granulocyte function. Most often, this defect reflects a decreased responsiveness of

TABLE 17–5 • Etiologies of neutrophil dysfunction

Cause	Mechanism
Congenital defects	
Leukocyte adhesion defect	Decreased adherence (CD11/CD18 deficiency)
Lazy leukocyte syndrome	Decreased motility
Chédiak-Higashi syndrome	Decreased motility, phagocytosis
Immunoglobulin/complement deficiency states	Decreased phagocytosis
Kartagener syndrome (immotile cilia syndrome)	Decreased chemotaxis, motility
Specific granule deficiency	Decreased chemotaxis, killing
Chronic granulomatous disease	Decreased killing
Acquired defects	
Drug induced (prednisone, etc)	Decreased migration
Alcoholism	Decreased motility, phagocytosis
Metabolic disorders (diabetes, uremia, malnutrition, autoimmune disease, glomerulonephritis)	Decreased adhesion, motility, and phagocytosis
HIV infection	Decreased motility, phagocytosis, and killing; poor monocyte function
Myeloproliferative disorders	Decreased phagocytosis and killing

the cell to chemotactic signals and a demonstrable reduction in the rate of egress into a site of tissue infection. In diabetic patients, the level of diabetic control may correlate with the functional defect. Patients with myeloproliferative disorders can also demonstrate a functional defect of their granulocytes with or without granulocytopenia. Patients presenting with recurrent pyogenic infections are frequently suspected of having neutrophil dysfunction, but most cases do not demonstrate any specific defect.

The most defined disorders of neutrophil dysfunction are genetic in nature. Some are characterized by structural changes in the cell that can be easily observed on blood films (Chédiak-Higashi syndrome), whereas others involve biochemical abnormalities detectable by immunophenotyping. The latter includes leukocyte adhesion deficiency (LAD), in which neutrophils lack an important adhesive molecule (the CD11/CD18 integrin) that mediates the binding of the cell to the subendothelium and its subsequent migration out of the vasculature. At least 2 types of LAD have been described. In LAD type 1, leukocytes roll normally but do not adhere or migrate out of the circulation, while LAD type 2 patients demonstrate defects both in rolling and adhesion. Recently, a child with a defective cell surface adhesion factor, E-Selectin, has also been described. Clinically these defects result in an accumulation of granulocytes in circulation and an inability of cells to migrate to the site of infection. Patients have recurrent infections, but do not form pus.

Chronic granulomatous disease (CGD) is another genetic disorder in which the granulocytes lack the ability to generate reactive oxygen species because of a defect in a single enzyme system, nicotinamide adenine dinucleotide phosphate (NADPH) oxidase. CGD patients present in infancy or later in childhood with severe, often recurrent abscesses, infectious dermatitis, and pneumonia. Tissue biopsies show multiple microscopic granulomas, giving the syndrome its name. The patient's granulocytes are capable of migrating to a site of infection and ingesting organisms, but they are unable to kill them. Therefore, *Staphylococcus aureus* and certain gram-negative bacteria (*Burkholderia cepacia, Serratia marcescens*) that are normally killed by granulocyte phagocytosis and lysosome digestion are responsible for most of the infections in these patients. Invasive *Aspergillus* infections (especially *Aspergillus* pneumonia) are common and life threatening, whereas infections by other fungal strains (eg, *Candida, Nocardia*) are less common. Inflammatory bowel disease is another infrequent manifestation of CGD.

A defect in any one of the 6 genes encoding the components of NADPH oxidase can result in CGD, but 70%–80% of cases have an X-linked recessive form of the disease, so that the majority of CGD patients are males. It is a relatively rare condition, affecting 1 out of every 200,000 births. Management strategies have included long-term administration of Bactrim and interferon-γ with some success. Bone marrow transplantation has been curative in a small number of children.

Diagnosis

Patients suspected of neutrophil dysfunction should always have an evaluation of their immune system, specifically serum immunoglobulin (IgA, IgG, IgM, and IgE) levels and complement because a lack of antibody production can result in poor opsonization and phagocytosis, yielding the same symptoms as primary neutrophil dysfunction. In addition, phenotypic analysis of the neutrophils, with special attention to the expression of CD11 and CD18, and the selectins, should be performed. Structural abnormalities of neutrophils are best determined by careful examination of the blood film. Subtler neutrophil defects such as abnormal phagocytosis or chemotaxis can be evaluated by research testing, such as the Rebuck skin window and measurement of phagocytosis of beads or bacteria.

Chronic granulomatous disease has traditionally been diagnosed by observing the ability of neutrophils to reduce nitroblue tetrazolium to form purple intracellular crystals following a phagocytic stimulus. Recently, fluorescence-based tests for the generation of superoxide and other reactive oxygen species have become available.

Therapy

Patient management needs to reflect the specific cause of the abnormality in neutrophil number or function. The granulocytosis of patients with infections or inflammatory states will respond to the treatment of the primary condition. Marked increases in the granulocyte count as a result of a clonal malignancy need to be treated aggressively with appropriate chemotherapy and leukapheresis (see Chapters 18 and 19). The management of patients with neutropenia or a qualitative disorder of granulocyte function can benefit significantly from antibiotic therapy and the appropriate use of recombinant G-CSF, whereas more specific treatments such as interferon-γ and stem cell transplantation may have specific indications.

A. Antibiotic Therapy

Most patients with neutropenia or a functional defect of granulocytes present with recurrent infections of skin, mucous membranes, and upper and lower respiratory systems. The organisms responsible for the infections are the common organisms found on the skin and mucous membranes. Patients will develop recurrent staphylococcal skin infections, gingivitis, periodontitis, sinusitis, and pharyngitis with common enteric organisms. Because of this, prophylaxis is not very effective. Rather, patients should be aggressively treated with cidal antibiotics that are specific for the site and type of infection. Careful culture and sensitivity testing of bacterial isolates are extremely important to successful therapy.

B. Growth Factor Therapy

Whenever possible, the cause of the neutropenia should be addressed with appropriate therapy. Any drugs that may be responsible for a production defect should be withdrawn and drugs that can further suppress neutrophil production (eg, Bactrim, H2 blockers, tricyclic antidepressants) must not be given. Patients with hematopoietic malignancies or autoimmune disease need to be treated with chemotherapy with or without marrow transplantation. These therapies provide the most effective long-term management strategy.

CASE HISTORY • *Part 3*

The first step in this patient, as always, is to stop *all* drugs, immediately! As for her infection, it appears limited (not septic), so she should be cultured and treated with an appropriate oral antibiotic. Given that she almost certainly has a reversible suppression of her myelopoiesis (very early blasts and myelocyte forms still present in the marrow), she should be monitored over the next 2–3 weeks with frequent CBCs. It takes roughly 5–7 days for a new generation of neutrophils to proliferate and mature enough to migrate into the blood stream. Although the use of a growth factor, such as G-CSF, may add little to the recovery rate (only a day or two earlier), it should be considered if she is slow to recover or her infection worsens.

Recombinant G-CSF (filgrastim) and GM-CSF can help in managing the neutropenic patient. The strategy for the use of these growth factors varies for each condition. It is now routine to use G-CSF as a part of marrow transplantation and multidrug chemotherapy protocols to encourage the more rapid return of granulocyte production (5–10 μg/kg/d subcutaneously [SC] until the granulocyte count exceeds 10,000/μL). A long-acting form of G-CSF (pegfilgrastim) is now available and offers a more convenient dosing schedule consisting of a single 6-mg dose given SC with each chemotherapy cycle. It should not be given in the period between 14 days before to 24 hours after cytotoxic therapy. The duration of absolute neutropenia in patients receiving ablative chemotherapy and autologous marrow transplantation for lymphoma can be significantly reduced, thereby shortening the length of time patients spend on antibiotics, the risk of life-threatening bacteremia, and the incidence of fungal infections.

Children with cyclic neutropenia clearly benefit from G-CSF therapy (5 μg/kg/d SC or less to keep the granulocyte count above 1,500/μL). Although treatment with growth factor does not stop the cycling of the granulocyte count, it does decrease the severity of the granulocytopenia. By not allowing the granulocyte count to fall to below 1,000/μL, children stop having recurrent infections. G-CSF therapy has also been approved for the reversal of the neutropenia associated with HIV infection (1–4 μg/kg/d SC) and the prevention of worsening neutropenia with therapy (300 μg/d). The use of growth factors in managing patients with qualitative disorders of granulocyte function still needs to be determined.

POINTS TO REMEMBER

The earliest response to a bacterial infection and tissue inflammation is the outward migration of neutrophils from circulation to the tissue site. This is rapidly followed by a release of neutrophils from the marrow storage pool, with the response level (increase in blood neutrophil count) being dependent on the stimulus.

The levels of specific growth factors—G-CSF, GM-CSF, and M-CSF—determine the subsequent proliferation of the various granulocyte cell types (neutrophils, monocytes, and eosinophils).

Neutrophilia is defined as an absolute neutrophil count of greater than 7×10^3/μL (7,000/μL). Modest increases are typical for minor infections, while increases to levels of up to 50,000/μL are seen with peritoneal sepsis and deep abscess formation.

Monocytosis is defined as an absolute monocyte count of greater than 1,000/μL. Modest increases are seen in patients with severe neutropenia or major sepsis; higher levels are seen in patients with subacute bacterial endocarditis and miliary tuberculosis.

Eosinophilia is defined as an absolute count of greater than 1,000/μL. However, more modest levels of eosinophilia are seen with drug reactions, allergies, and skin disease. Higher levels are seen with certain parasitic infestations and tumors, especially lymphomas. Hypereosinophilia (>2,000–5,000/μL) is generally a sign of eosinophilic leukemia and is associated with tissue damage (hypereosinophilic syndrome).

Basophilia is defined as an absolute count of greater than 50/μL. Basophilia is most often seen in patients with polycythemia vera and chronic myelogenous leukemia. Mast cell disease is a form of leukemia and is associated with major complications related to the release of mast cell granules.

Neutropenia is broadly defined as an absolute count of less than 1,000/μL. However, the clinical implications of neutropenia worsen as the count falls much below 500/μL. An absolute count below 100/μL conveys significant risk of bacterial sepsis.

Modest neutropenia is often seen with drug toxicity, vitamin deficiency (folate, vitamin B_{12}, alcoholism), HIV, and autoimmune disease. Severe neutropenia is more often associated with leukemia, myelofibrosis, and cyclic neutropenia.

Neutrophil dysfunction is defined as a defect in 1 or more of the critical steps in neutrophil function—chemotaxis, adherence, migration, motility, phagocytosis, and bacterial killing. There are a number of congenital defects in neutrophil function, all of which are relatively rare. Important acquired defects include drug-induced disorders (especially from high-dose steroid therapy), alcoholism, metabolic disorders (diabetes, uremia, autoimmune disease), HIV, and myeloproliferative disorders.

In evaluating a patient with a quantitative disorder of any hematopoietic cell, such as neutrophils, it is important for the clinician to carefully consider whether any of the other cell lines (such as red cells or platelets) are affected. If it is clear that only 1 cell line is affected, the most likely etiologies are drug-induced or autoimmune disorders, whereas when all 3 cell lines are affected, etiologies such as myeloproliferative disorders or malignancies are more likely.

BIBLIOGRAPHY

Andersohn F, Konzen C, Garbe E: Systematic review: agranulocytosis induced by nonchemotherapy drugs. Ann Intern Med 2007;146:657.

Berliner N: Understanding myelopoiesis. Lessons from congenital neutropenia. Blood 2008;111:5427.

Borregard N, Boxer L: Disorders of neutrophil function. In: Lichtmann AM et al (eds): William's Hematology. McGraw-Hill, 2006; 921–955.

Boxer LA: Role of neutrophils in genetic disorders of phagocyte function leading to IBD. J Pediatr Gastroenterol Nutr 2008;46(Suppl 1):E17.

Boxer L, Dale DC: Neutropenia: causes and consequences. Semin Hematol 2002;39:75.

Burks EJ, Loughran TP Jr: Pathogenesis of neutropenia in large granular lymphocyte leukemia and Felty syndrome. Blood Rev 2006;20:245.

Capsoni F, Sarzi-Puttini P, Zanella A: Primary and secondary autoimmune neutropenia. Arthritis Res Ther 2005;7:208.

Dagher MC, Pick E: Opening the black box: lessons from cell-free systems on the phagocyte NADPH-oxidase. Biochimie 2007;89:1123.

Dale DC: Neutropenia and neutrophilia. In: Lichtmann AM et al (eds): William's Hematology. McGraw-Hill, 2006; 907–919.

Dale DC, Bolyard AA, Schwinzer BG, et al: The Severe Chronic Neutropenia International Registry: 10-year follow-up report. Support Cancer Ther 2006;3:220.

Dinauer MC: Chronic Granulomatous Disease and Other Disorders of Phagocyte Function. Hematology (ASH educational book). 2005; 89–95.

Elloumi HZ, Holland SM: Diagnostic assays for chronic granulomatous disease and other neutrophil disorders. Methods Mol Biol 2007;412:505.

Falagas ME, Vardakas KZ, Samonis G: Decreasing the incidence and impact of infections in neutropenic patients: evidence from meta-analyses of randomized controlled trials. Curr Med Res Opin 2008;24:215.

Galli SJ, Metcalfe DD, Arber D, Dvorak A: Basophils and mast cells and their disorders. In: Lichtmann AM et al (eds): William's Hematology. McGraw-Hill, 2006; 879–897.

Gotlib J: Chronic eosinophilic leukemia/hypereosinophilic syndrome. Cancer Treat Res 2008;142:69.

Gotlib J, Cross NC, Gilliland DG: Eosinophilic disorders: molecular pathogenesis, new classification, and modern therapy. Best Pract Res Clin Haematol 2006;19:535.

Heuser M, Ganser A, Bokemeyer C: Use of colony-stimulating factors for chemotherapy-associated neutropenia. Review of current guidelines. Semin Hematol 2007;44:148.

Heyworth PG, Cross AR, Curnutte JT: Chronic granulomatous disease. Curr Opin Immunol 2003;15:578.

Horwitz MS, Duan Z, Korkmaz B, Lee HH, Mealiffe ME, Salipante SJ: Neutrophil elastase in cyclic and severe congenital neutropenia. Blood 2007;109:1817.

Kuderer NM, Dale DC, Crawford J, Lyman GH: Impact of primary prophylaxis with granulocyte colony-stimulating factor on febrile neutropenia and mortality in adult cancer patients receiving chemotherapy: a systematic review. J Clin Oncol 2007;25:3158.

Lichtman MA: Classification and clinical manifestations of neutrophil disorders. In: Lichtmann AM et al (eds): William's Hematology. McGraw-Hill, 2006; 899–905.

Rosenzweig SD, Holland SM: Phagocyte immunodeficiencies and their infections. J Allergy Clin Immunol 2004; 113:620.

Ryser MF, Roesler J, Gentsch M, Brenner S: Gene therapy for chronic granulomatous disease. Expert Opin Biol Ther 2007;7:1799.

Segel GB, Halterman JS: Neutropenia in pediatric practice. Pediatr Rev 2008;29:12.

Seger RA: Modern management of chronic granulomatous disease. Br J Haematol 2008;140:255.

Sessler CN, Perry JC, Varney KL: Management of severe sepsis and septic shock. Curr Opin Crit Care 2004;10:354.

Simon H et al: Abnormal clone of T-cells producing interleukin-5 in idiopathic eosinophilia. N Engl J Med 1999; 341:1112.

Smith OP: Shwachman-Diamond syndrome. Semin Hematol 2002;39:95.

Urban C, Zychlinsky A: Netting bacteria in sepsis. Nat Med 2007;13:403.

Waedlaw A: Eosinophils and their disorders. In: Lichtmann AM et al (eds): William's Hematology. McGraw-Hill, 2006; 863–878.

THE ACUTE MYELOID LEUKEMIAS · 18

CASE HISTORY • *Part I*

A 28-year-old man, previously in excellent health, presents with a 2-week history of fatigue and worsening fever. He has been convinced by his family to seek medical attention because of noticeable pallor and the recent onset of a petechial rash on his extremities. His physical examination is remarkable for pallor, the petechial rash, pharyngitis, and gingivitis. He does not have lymphadenopathy or hepatosplenomegaly, and the remainder of the examination is unremarkable.

CBC: Hematocrit 19% WBC 32,000/μL
Differential: Neutrophils - 0% Monocytes - 2%
Lymphocytes - 13% Cells identified by an automated counter as immature - 85%
Platelets: 14,000/μL

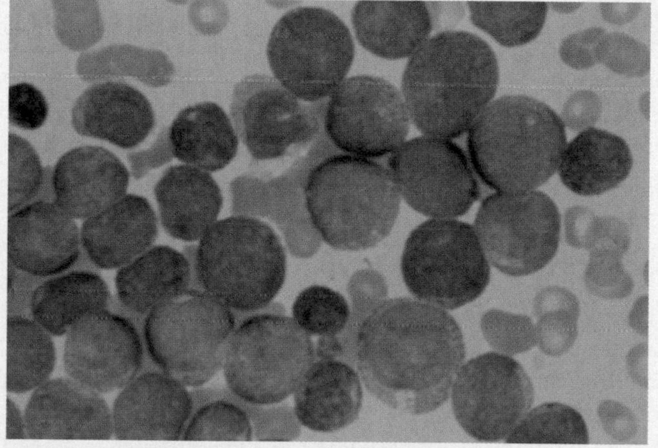

• SMEAR MORPHOLOGY

Mature neutrophils are not seen. Platelets are markedly decreased, but red cell morphology is normal. The immature cells are large, with an open nuclear chromatin pattern, prominent nucleoli, and few granules. In rare cells, one or more red staining, rod-shaped objects can be found (Auer rods).

Questions

- What further history, examination, and laboratory evaluation is indicated?
- What should be the pace of this workup?

The acute myeloid leukemias (AMLs) are clonal malignancies that are characterized by the appearance of increased numbers of immature myeloid cells in the marrow and blood. The fundamental oncogenic event takes place at the level of a very early progenitor cell, which results in a leukemic stem cell with self-renewal and multipotential properties. Still, the malignant progeny are often capable of considerable differentiation. This has led to classification schemes that emphasize the morphologic characteristics of the cell, patterned after the classification of normal myeloid cells.

AML can present as an acute, catastrophic illness in a patient who is otherwise healthy. Alternatively, it can be the final outcome of a myeloproliferative disease such as chronic myeloid leukemia, polycythemia vera, or primary myelofibrosis or a myelodysplastic syndrome (see Chapters 9, 13, and 19). Despite the differences in onset and morphologic appearance, the AMLs generally have a similar clinical presentation, prognosis, and treatment.

The yearly estimated incidence of AML in the United States is 12,000 new cases, two-thirds of which will die from the disease.

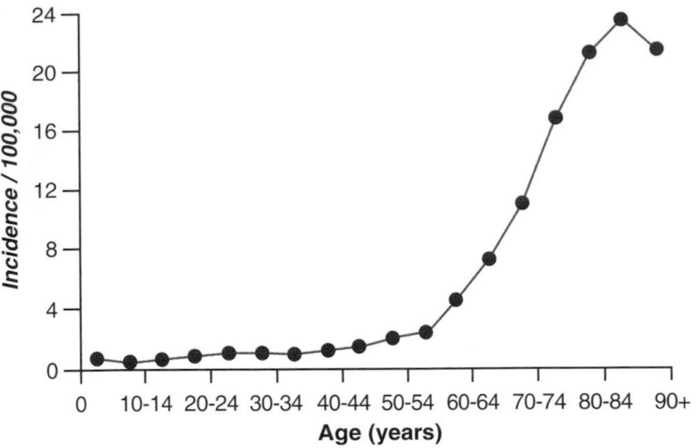

FIGURE 18–1. AML age-specific incidence rates: 1998–2002 (NCI-SEER program). The incidence of AML increases steadily with age. Most cases are seen in the sixth, seventh, and eighth decades.

As shown in Figure 18–1, the **incidence is clearly age related:** most patients are adults, and the median age of onset is 70 years. In elderly patients, the disease frequently presents as evolution from a myelodysplastic syndrome, whereas in younger patients, de novo AML is more common.

LEUKEMIA CLASSIFICATION

The original classification scheme for AML was the French-American-British (FAB) system, which began as a purely morphologic classification. However, over the years it has been bolstered by immunohistochemical and immunologic data, using markers for different stages of myeloid differentiation. Even with this information, the overriding principle of leukemia classification continued to be the placement of the malignant cell in the normal scheme of hematopoietic cell differentiation. The most recent modification of the **classification of AML, proposed by a World Health Organization (WHO) conference**, goes a step further. It takes into account both **genetic information and whether AML arises de novo or evolves from a myelodysplastic syndrome** (Table 18–1). This approach is likely to continue to evolve in the future as new information regarding cell biology, therapeutic response, and outcome becomes available. Gene-expression profiling using microarray technology and molecular genetics are expected to have a major impact on future leukemia classification. However, some of these techniques are still far from routine in nonacademic hospitals and may be time-consuming. Considering the need for urgent results to make treatment decisions, blood and bone marrow morphology and immunophenotyping remain critical components for AML diagnosis.

TABLE 18–1 • The WHO/FAB classification of acute myeloid leukemias

AML with genetic abnormalities			
AML with t(8;21) or inv(16)			
AML with eosinophilia and inv(16) or t(16;16)			
AML with 11q23 abnormalities			
APL with t(15;17) and variants			
AML with multilineage dysplasia/infidelity			
Evolution from myelodysplasia (MDS)			
Without antecedent MDS but dysplasia in at least 50% of cells in 2 or more lineages			
AML secondary to therapy-related MDS			
Radiation/alkylating agent related			
Topoisomerase II inhibitor related			
All others			
AML not otherwise categorized—FAB classification			
Cell Type	**FAB**	**Description**	**Incidence (%)[a]**
Undifferentiated	M0/1[b]	Blasts with no differentiation	20
Myeloblastic	M2	Blasts with early granulocytic differentiation	30
Promyelocytic	M3	Clear promyelocytic characteristics	10
Myelomonocytic	M4	A mixture of granulocytic and monocytic characteristics	25
Monocytic	M5	Clear monocytic characteristics	10
Erythroleukemic	M6	Blasts with erythroid characteristics	4
Megakaryocytic	M7	Blasts with megakaryocytic properties	1

[a]*Percentage of FAB-classified AML cases.*
[b]*M0 is only recognized by lack of positivity for peroxidase activity, usually in association with C34, CD13, and CD33 expression, whereas M1 has a similar immunophenotype but reacts at least minimally (>3% of blasts) for myeloperoxidase content.*

Morphologic Classification

The maturation of normal myeloid cells in the marrow is based on morphologic criteria (see Figure 16–2). Several characteristics of this maturation sequence are used in classifying the leukemic cell line. The first of these is the appearance of cytoplasmic granules in the maturing granulocytes. The most primitive (undifferentiated) myeloblasts have no granules and are difficult to distinguish from lymphoblasts. The earliest cells that can be identified as myelocyte progenitors contain primary (nonspecific) granules that appear as relatively large, purple (azurophilic) granules on the Wright-Giemsa stain. As the cell line matures to the promyelocyte stage, primary granules become abundant and partially obscure the nucleus (Figure 18–2A), but some patients with promyelocytic leukemia have a microgranular morphology. Malignant myeloblasts and promyelocytes can also contain abnormal rod-shaped granules known as **Auer rods** (see Figure 18–2B). When present, Auer rods are by far the best

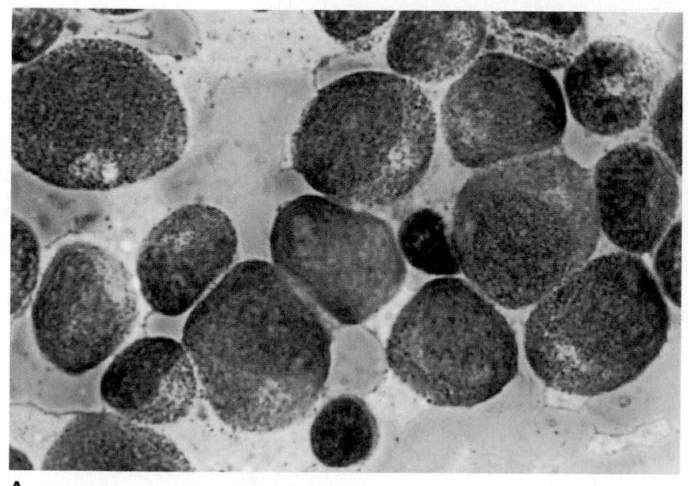

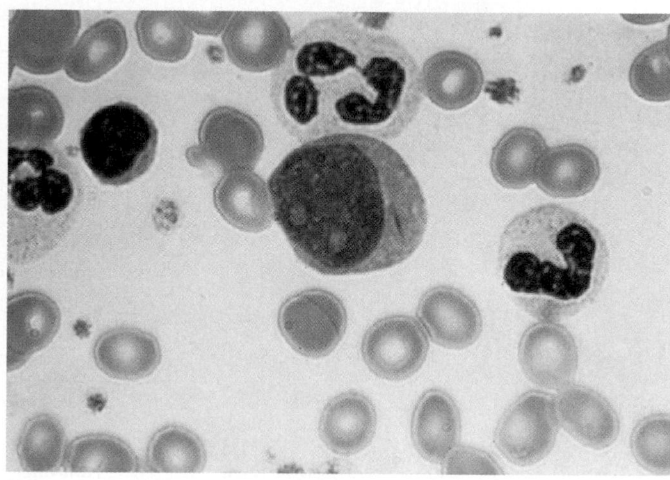

FIGURE 18–2. **A: Promyelocytic leukemia.** Promyleocytic (M3) leukemia is characterized by a uniform population of malignant cells with a heavy concentration of primary granules in the cytoplasm. **B: Auer rods.** A sensitive marker for myeloblasts is the presence of 1 or more rod-shaped granules (Auer rods) in the cytoplasm.

criterion for identifying leukemic myeloid cells in the granulocytic lineage. As myelocytes mature further, they acquire secondary granules that are smaller and more heterogeneous in their staining properties. When cells follow the monocytic differentiation pathway, cytoplasmic granules are never as prominent as those in granulocytes. They are smaller, scantier, and remain pink to purple. The categorization of some leukemias as myelomonocytic reflects the immature cells as having characteristics of both granulocyte and monocyte lineages. Finally, the rare acute eosinophilic and basophilic (mast cell) leukemias are readily identified based on their distinctive granules within the cytoplasm.

Histochemical stains help to confirm the specific granule content of a malignant cell line. The peroxidase and specific esterase stains detect the primary granules of myeloid cells. In contrast, the nonspecific esterase stain detects the esterase activity of monocytes and is only weakly positive in immature myeloid cells. Both the alkaline phosphatase and periodic acid–Schiff (PAS) stains give a strong reaction with mature granulocytes. These stains are used in conjunction with conventional morphology in the FAB classification system (see Table 18–2 and Figure 16–4).

The second most important morphologic criterion in the detection of a myeloid leukemia is the morphology of the nucleus. The chromatin of immature cells such as myeloblasts is characterized by a very fine, lacy pattern. As the cell matures, the chromatin becomes progressively more coarse or clumped. Moreover, the nature of the clumping is different in granulocytes, lymphocytes, and monocytes. The nucleus in the granulocyte lineage first folds at the metamyelocyte stage and then becomes segmented, whereas the nucleus of the developing monocyte remains indented or horseshoe shaped. **Nucleoli** are another sign of immaturity. They are invariably present in immature blasts and are lost during normal maturation. Leukemic cells frequently have a nuclear chromatin pattern that is finer and more immature appearing than that of a corresponding normal cell. They can also demonstrate multiple, abnormally large nucleoli that persist even as the cell cytoplasm matures.

Immunologic Classification

Several normal immunologic markers on myeloid cells can be detected by monoclonal antibodies. There are no markers that

TABLE 18–2 • Histochemical stains in the FAB classification of AML

			Combined Esterase		
Cell Type	**FAB**	**Peroxidase**	**Specific**	**Nonspecific**	**+NaF**
Undifferentiated	M0	0	0	0	—
Minimal differentiation	M1	<3+	0–1+	0	—
Myeloblastic	M2	4+	4+	0	—
Promyelocytic	M3	4+	4+	1–2+	1–2+
Myelomonocytic	M4	3–4+	3+	3+	1–2+
Monocytic	M5	0–1+	0–1+	4+	0
Erythroleukemia	M6	0	0	0	—

TABLE 18–3 • Immunologic markers on myeloid cells and leukemias

CD	Other Names	Normal Cells	Utility in AML
13	My7	Mono and myeloid	Distinguish AML from ALL
14	My4	Mature monocytes	Monocytic leukemias
15	My1	Mono and myeloid	Distinguish AML from ALL
33	My9	Mono and myeloid	Most consistent marker in AML
34	My10	Progenitor cells only	Most primitive marker
41	GPIIb/IIIa	Megakaryocytes	Megakaryocytic leukemia
42	GPIb	Megakaryocytes	Megakaryocytic leukemia
45	HLE	All leukocytes	Decreased intensity on leukemic cells
90	Thy-1, theta	Nonlymphoid cells	
117	c-Kit	Progenitor cells	Expressed on leukemic stem cells, not on normal hemopoietic stem cells
123	IL-3R α chain	Pluripotent and progenitor cells	
—	HLA-DR	Mono and myeloid	Nearly always present on AML and ALL but not in APL
—	Glycophorin	Erythrocytes	Erythroleukemia

by themselves are completely specific for malignant myeloid cells. Therefore, the immunologic classification of a leukemia, like the morphologic classification, is an exercise in matching the malignant cell line to the normal pattern of hematopoietic cell differentiation.

The most commonly used immunologic markers for myeloid cells are summarized in Table 18–3. They are most useful in distinguishing myeloid from lymphoid leukemias and in helping determine the lineage of the myeloid leukemias. The immunologic classification of an acute leukemia does not always correlate with the morphologic appearance. For example, cells expressing monocyte markers may or may not have a morphology that suggests monocytic leukemia, and the degree of maturation suggested by the surface markers may not match morphologic features such as cytoplasmic granules and nuclear chromatin. **Myeloid leukemias can also show lineage infidelity** in that they express aberrant markers that are normally not present on the same cell or because they lack markers that should be present on the cells of a given lineage. It is common to find heterogeneous expression of markers within the leukemic population. A patient who has nearly 100% blasts by morphology may show only 50% $CD34^+$ blasts by marker studies. This condition usually reflects variations in the intensity of expression of these markers but can also indicate true clonal diversity within the leukemic population. Recently, leukemic stem cells have been identified as $CD34^+$, $CD38^-$, $CD71^-$, $HLADR^-$, $CD90^-$, and $CD117^-$, with absence of the latter 3 allowing clear-cut differentiation from normal hematopoietic stem cells. Finally, phenotyping acute myelogenous leukemia can occasionally identify **a unique signature of the malignant clone, which can help with residual disease assessment** once a remission is obtained.

Cytogenetic Abnormalities

More than a third of AMLs show some cytogenetic abnormality (Table 18–4) by karyotype. There is a great deal of diversity, however, in the types of abnormalities observed, and as yet, there are only a few robust correlations between cytogenetic markers and either prognosis or response to therapy.

A common abnormality in AML, present in about 10% of cases, and associated with a relatively poor prognosis, is trisomy of chromosome 8. The **t(8;21) translocation or inv(16), seen in 40% of M2 AMLs, is associated with a somewhat better prognosis**. Abnormalities of chromosome 11 are often found in secondary M4 and M5 AMLs after **exposure to topoisomerase II inhibitors**, whereas abnormalities of chromosome 16 are associated with a variant of M4 that shows pronounced eosinophilia and is associated with a relatively good prognosis. Prognostically adverse cytogenetic findings include −5/del(5q), −7, abnormal 3q, t(9;22), and complex karyotypes.

An important example of the importance of detecting cytogenetic abnormalities is the translocation between chromosomes 15 and 17 [t(15;17)] that can be detected in most cases of promyelocytic leukemia. It involves 2 genes, 1 on chromosome 15 known as *PML* and the other on chromosome 17 that is a receptor for retinoic acid, a cofactor known to induce differentiation in many cell types. The translocation, known as *PML-RARα* functions as

TABLE 18–4 • Acute myeloid leukemias with recurrent cytogenetic abnormalities

Abnormality	Approximate Frequency	Genes Involved	Prognostic Significance
t(8;21)(q22;22)	40% of M2 AML	*AML1/ETO*	Favorable
t(15;17)(q22;q11–22) (Promyelocytic)	10% of AML	*PML/RARα*	Favorable
inv(16)(p13q22) or t(16;16) (p13;q11)	Most M4 with abnormal marrow eosinophils	*AML1/MYH11X*	Favorable
11q23 abnormalities	6%–8% of primary AML and 85% of secondary AML	*MLL* (mixed lineage leukemia)	Intermediate or unfavorable
del(5q) or monosomy 5	More common in older patients and secondary AML	Growth factor cluster	Unfavorable
Trisomy of chromosome 8	10% of AML	*? AML1*	Unfavorable

an oncogene by inhibiting cell differentiation and causing an arrest in development at the promyelocytic stage. From a therapeutic standpoint, the function of the *PML-RARα* oncogene can be inhibited by **all-trans retinoic acid (ATRA)**. This has been applied with great effectiveness in the treatment of promyelocytic leukemia and has led to a higher rate of remission and disease-free survival.

Molecular Genetics

Recently, new methods have provided insights at a molecular level and revealed a significant amount of heterogeneity in both the cytogenetically normal and abnormal acute myeloid leukemias.

Genetic abnormalities associated with the leukemic clone affect intracellular signaling molecules, which regulate cell proliferation and survival or transcription factors involved in hematopoietic differentiation. Besides their pathogenic significance, these mutations impact the prognosis (Table 18–5). For instance, even in the presence of a normal karyotype, internal mutations of the tyrosine kinase receptor FLT3, seen in 30%–40% of patients with AML, are associated with higher initial white blood cell (WBC)/blast counts and shorter remissions and survivals. However, there is still some heterogeneity within this group of patients, depending on the number of mutant alleles, the impact of the mutations on tyrosine kinase activity, and the interference with coexisting mutations such as *NPM1* or others.

By contrast, *CEBPA* mutations are found in patients with more favorable outcomes. Similarly, among the so-called core-binding factor AMLs (*AML1/ETO*, *AML1/MYH11X*: see Table 18–4), associated mutations of *c-KIT* appear to influence

TABLE 18–5 • Relevant gene mutations in cytogenetically normal AML

Gene	Function	Pronostic Impact	Expected Therapeutic Impact
FLT3	Tyrosine kinase	ITD: worse; TKD: better	Yes, trials with inhibitors ongoing
NPM1 (nucleophosmin)	Pleiotropic	Favorable with FLT3^{-}	Interference with RA
CEBPA	Transcription factor	Favorable	Elusive
MLL	Histone methyltransferase	Unfavorable	Histone deacetylase and methyltransferase inhibitors
N-RAS	Intracellular signalling	Neutral	Efficacy of high dose Ara-C
WT1 (Wilms tumor gene 1)	Differentiation factor	Unfavorable	Elusive

ITD, internal tandem duplication; RA, retinoic acid; TKD, tyrosine kinase domain.

outcome and also constitute potential targets for specific molecular inhibitors. Gene expression profiling (see Chapter 23) can isolate well-defined gene clusters, the majority of which correlate with the main cytogenetic abnormalities. Some clusters characterize patients without abnormal karyotypes and help to refine diagnosis and prognostic classifications. Deregulated expression can result from gene mutations such as *EVI1*, *ERG*, and *MN1*, which confers some heterogeneity among these groups. Another approach using miRNA expression appears to characterize a molecular signature of high-risk, cytogenetically normal AML.

In addition to offering new insights into the molecular mechanisms of malignant transformation, these approaches pinpoint targets for specifically tailored treatments based on the molecular disease characteristics in each patient.

CLINICAL FEATURES

The AMLs usually present with some **combination of granulocytopenia, anemia, thrombocytopenia, and the appearance of immature cells** (blasts) in blood and marrow. The disease can present at any age but is uncommon in children. The classic presentation of AML in an otherwise healthy patient is most often seen in young adults. Older patients can present with atypical aspects such as a preexisting myelodysplastic syndrome or a slow onset of the disease (smoldering leukemia). The incidence of AML increases dramatically after age 50; the median age of onset overall is now 64 years owing to the late evolution of myelodysplastic syndrome (MDS) patients.

AML in younger patients usually presents as a catastrophic illness. The entire clinical history is seldom more than a few weeks long and is characterized by the sudden appearance of fatigue, fever, bacterial infections of the upper respiratory tract, bone pain, and various bleeding manifestations. These are signs and **symptoms associated with marked anemia, granulocytopenia, and thrombocytopenia**.

Less common presentations are seen in patients with various subtypes of AML or monocytic leukemia. Rarely, an AML patient will present with an apparently isolated tumor mass of myeloblasts, known as a **chloroma**, involving the spinal column or orbit, or other unexpected locations such as the urinary tract, digestive system, or biliary tract. Monocytic leukemia is more frequently associated with **malignant cell infiltrates** in skin, gingiva, and the central nervous system. Patients with high levels of primitive blasts (>100,000/μL) can present with a **leukostasis** syndrome characterized by ischemia of multiple organs and both pulmonary and central nervous system dysfunction (Ball disease). This situation is a true hematologic emergency and needs to be treated immediately with combination chemotherapy and leukapheresis to prevent severe morbidity or death.

Most patients with AML develop bleeding because of thrombocytopenia. Therefore, the most common bleeding manifestations are petechiae, gum bleeding, nose-bleeds, and in women, menorrhagia. Patients with acute promyelocytic leukemia have more complex abnormalities, combining thrombocytopenia with consumptive coagulopathy. They can present with significant prolongations of their prothrombin time (PT) and partial thromboplastin time (PTT) secondary to ongoing disseminated intravascular coagulation (DIC). These patients can have more prominent bruising and much more severe mucous membrane bleeding.

Physical findings in the AML patient include pallor from the anemia, skin and mucous membrane bleeding from thrombocytopenia, and aphthous ulcers, gingivitis, and pharyngitis from neutropenia. Massive marrow infiltration results in generalized bone pain and, on occasion, sternal tenderness. Lymphadenopathy and hepatosplenomegaly are seen in less than 20% of adult patients, and mediastinal lymphadenopathy is extremely rare.

Laboratory Studies

The key to the diagnosis of any leukemia is the study of blood and marrow morphology. When AML presents as a precipitous illness in a young or middle-aged adult, the blood film morphology may be enough to make the diagnosis. A complete workup should always include a marrow aspirate and biopsy for routine morphology, histochemical staining, and both immunophenotyping and chromosomal/cytogenetic analysis. In patients who present with extensive bruising or severe mucous membrane bleeding, a full coagulation profile should be obtained to look for DIC.

A. Complete Blood Count

The complete blood count (CBC) will demonstrate varying combinations of anemia, granulocytopenia, and thrombocytopenia, together with the appearance of abnormal immature cells (blasts) in circulation. The total number of blasts will vary from a small percentage of the circulating cells to an overwhelming, uniform population of primitive blasts, often exceeding 50,000/μL. The loss of other normal cell elements helps make the diagnosis. The malignant event responsible for proliferation of the leukemic cell line also blocks normal granulocyte, red blood cell, and platelet production. At the same time, small numbers of normal lymphocytes may still be present; coupled with the absence of granulocytes, this suggests myeloid involvement in the leukemic process.

Up to 10% of **leukemias can present without recognizable blasts** on blood smears, that is, as pancytopenia. In this situation, marrow aspirate and biopsy invariably supply the diagnosis. In patients who gradually evolve to AML as an endpoint of a myeloproliferative or myelodysplastic disorder, the pattern of cytopenia may be quite variable. In addition, some of these patients will demonstrate a macrocytic anemia, marked poikilocytosis with nucleated red blood cells on the peripheral film, or both.

B. Marrow Aspirate and Biopsy

A marrow aspirate should be obtained in all patients. Sufficient material should be collected for routine morphology and histochemical staining, immunophenotyping, and chromosomal analysis. This process will require several aspirations and may involve several placements of the marrow aspirate needle.

A marrow biopsy core is useful to determine overall cellularity, the distribution of the malignant process, and any tendency to fibrosis. Rarely, an AML patient will present with a packed or even necrotic marrow that defies aspiration. In this case, the biopsy is critical.

C. Histochemical Stains

Histochemical staining of blood and marrow aspirate films is an integral part of the FAB classification of leukemia (see Table 18–2). The most commonly used stains are:

1. Peroxidase stain—This stain detects the myeloperoxidase enzyme contained in the primary granules of **myeloid cells**. In the presence of hydrogen peroxide, myeloperoxidase releases free oxygen that can then be detected with benzidine or 3-amino-9-ethyl carbazole. The latter reagent gives a reddish-brown reaction product, whereas the benzidine reagent produces a bluish-black product. Myeloperoxidase is abundant in nearly all mature and immature myeloid cells and is also present in monocytes to a small extent. Recently, it has become possible to detect myeloperoxidase using a monoclonal antibody and flow cytometry. The increased sensitivity of this method has proved very useful in identifying even very immature myeloid leukemias that appear to be peroxidase negative by histochemistry.

2. Combined esterase stain—This stain uses 2 substrates, α-naphthyl acetate and naphthol ASD chloracetate, to **distinguish myelocytes from monocytes**. The chloracetate esterase stain (specific esterase) identifies the primary and secondary granules in myeloid cells. It gives a negative or very weak reaction in monocytes. Furthermore, it is resistant to treatment with sodium fluoride. The α-naphthyl acetate stain (nonspecific esterase) produces a strong reaction in monocytes, which is positive to a lesser and varying degree in mature and immature myeloid cells. The monocyte reaction is inhibited by sodium fluoride.

3. Periodic acid–Schiff (PAS) stain—This stain involves the oxidation of carbohydrates by periodic acid to aldehyde products. Mature myeloid cells stain intensely red; myeloblasts are usually negative. The PAS stain is therefore useful in **separating AML from acute lymphocytic leukemia**; lymphoblasts can show heavy block-like staining.

D. Immunophenotyping and Cytogenetics

Both blood and marrow specimens should be collected for immunophenotyping and cytogenetic studies. The most important immunologic markers on myeloid cells and their usefulness in the diagnosis and management of AML are listed in Table 18–3. Chromosomal analysis should be performed using high resolution banding techniques in order to identify common translocations. The most important cytogenetic abnormalities are listed in Table 18–4. This type of information is particularly useful in the case of very immature leukemias in which it can be difficult to distinguish between myeloid and lymphoid lineage. The distinctive phenotype and genotype of the malignant cell line can also be used once the patient enters remission to detect relapse and new mutations at the earliest possible time. The new WHO/FAB classification of the myeloid leukemias (see Table 18–1) recognizes cytogenetic abnormalities as a key factor in the classification of AML. In fact, even in patients with nondiagnostic morphologies and few blasts, the presence of one of these distinctive mutations will make the diagnosis.

E. Other Laboratory Studies

The growth of the myeloid cell tumor mass is associated with several metabolic abnormalities. When blast counts are high in blood, factitious hypoglycemia, as a result of in vitro glucose consumption, is prevented by blood sampling with fluoride in the tube. Similarly, blood gases should be sampled using a cooled syringe maintained at low temperature until analysis. The serum **lactic dehydrogenase (LDH) level is elevated** in most patients without significant changes in other liver chemistries. An elevation mirrors the rate of growth and turnover of the leukemic cells. Another indirect measure of myeloid cell proliferation is the level of vitamin B_{12} binding proteins, specifically transcobalamin III. In patients with myelomonocytic or monocytic leukemia, a high tumor burden is associated with an increased excretion of muramidase (lysozyme) in urine. This process can result in potassium wasting and hypokalemia. Finally, up to 20% of patients may have an elevated serum uric acid level.

CASE HISTORY • *Part 2*

The patient is admitted and his further workup is completed within the next few hours. Further history reveals no personal or family history of hematologic diseases. He has 3 siblings, all in good health. A dental examination reveals an apical abscess in 1 molar.

A bone marrow aspirate is obtained and examined for morphology, histochemical staining, and flow cytometry. Samples are sent for cytogenetics and molecular genetics. The marrow contains a nearly uniform population of cells resembling those seen in the blood. Some of the blasts contain neutrophilic granules, and some contain Auer rods (see Figure 18–2B). Histochemistry shows the blasts to be strongly peroxidase positive, and positive for specific esterase, but all other stains are negative. Flow cytometry shows the blasts to express low levels of CD45, and to be strongly positive for CD34, CD13, and HLA-DR. They are weakly $CD33^+$ and negative for CD14 and CD64 and all lymphoid-specific markers.

Upon review of these data the leukemia is classified as acute myeloid leukemia FAB M2.

Questions

- What initial therapeutic steps should be taken?
- What longer-term interventions should be planned?

DIAGNOSIS

An important element in diagnosing AML is the speed of the workup. This is especially true when AML presents as a precipitous illness in an otherwise healthy young adult, because successful management depends on the early initiation of appropriate chemotherapy. The time element is less important in patients who gradually evolve from a myeloproliferative or myelodysplastic disease into AML. In this situation, it can be to the patient's advantage to delay therapy until it is absolutely necessary.

It is very important to determine whether the AML is secondary to some other factor such as previous chemotherapy or radiation exposure. **AML is the most common form of secondary malignancy** following previous tumor therapy. For example, the risk of AML in patients treated for Hodgkin disease with combination radiation/chemotherapy is 3%–10% at 10–15 years. In addition, the incidence of AML as the final outcome in patients with myeloproliferative/dysplastic diseases, such as RAEB (refractory anemia with excess blasts), polycythemia vera, and myelofibrosis may be increased by treatment with specific chemotherapeutic agents. Both aplastic anemia and AML have also been associated with benzene exposure. These relationships are important since secondary AML generally carries a worse prognosis. The patient may be slow to achieve remission, relapse rapidly, or fail to recover normal hematopoiesis following chemotherapy.

Because of the need for a rapid workup and treatment decision, the initial classification of a myeloid leukemia is most often based on cellular morphology and histochemical staining, using the FAB system (see Table 18–1). The key decision points are the following:

- Does the patient have acute myelocytic versus acute lymphocytic leukemia?
- To which FAB category does the patient belong?

Therapy can and should be initiated based on this information. It is unnecessary and unwise to delay treatment if the results from immunophenotyping and molecular analysis are not available within 24–48 hours. Although these results may affect long-term management and prognosis, they are not important in guiding the initial treatment decision once an AML M3 has been definitively ruled in or out.

The patient should also be routinely evaluated for a **coagulopathy**. This process is very important in patients with **acute promyelocytic leukemia (M3)**. Many of these patients present with ongoing DIC and a severe bleeding tendency, which can worsen in the early phases of treatment. A full coagulation profile including a platelet count, PT, PTT, thrombin time, fibrinogen level, fibrin split product or d-dimer level, and both antithrombin and α_2-antiplasmin levels should be measured prior to initiating chemotherapy.

The final classification of the patient's leukemia will reflect the studies of morphology, immunophenotype, and cytogenetics, and the relationship to preexisting preleukemic states (see Table 18–1). The most important and predictive categories are:

Acute Myeloid Leukemia with Genetic Abnormalities

Approximately 30% of patients presenting with de novo AML will fall into this category. Patients with t(15;17), t(8;21), and inv(16) abnormalities generally have distinctive clinical/morphologic findings and the most favorable prognosis (see Table 18–4). Acute promyelocytic leukemia [t(15;17)] has the best prognosis when treated with combination ATRA and chemotherapy. Other abnormalities are associated with less favorable outcomes, including –5/del(5q), –7, abnormal 3q, t(9;22), and complex karyotypes. Patients with myelodysplasia-related AML may have cytogenetic abnormalities, most often balanced translocations of 11q23 and 21q22, but the antecedent history helps with the diagnosis.

Acute Myeloid Leukemia with Multilineage Dysplasia

This diagnosis is easily made when there is a well-established history of myelodysplasia, extending back more than 6 months. When the patient presents without a history of myeloproliferative illness or myelodysplasia, it can be made when the blast count in marrow and blood is over 20%, and more than 50% of 2 myeloid lineages are dysplastic. The presence of cytogenetic abnormalities, especially complex karyotypes, helps confirm the diagnosis.

Acute Myeloid Leukemia Secondary to Therapy-Related Myelodysplasia

Two types of therapy-related myelodysplasia evolving to AML are recognized in the WHO classification—radiation/alkylating agent induced and topoisomerase II inhibitor related. The former is usually seen 4–7 years after exposure and correlates with the severity and duration of exposure, especially with combination radiation/chemotherapy regimens. These patients often present with a myelodysplasia evolving to AML. They have a high incidence of chromosome 5 and 7 abnormalities and can be extremely resistant to AML induction chemotherapy.

Topoisomerase II inhibitor–related leukemia generally presents 3–5 years after exposure without a myelodysplastic phase, but often with a prominent monocytic component to the morphology. The most common chromosomal abnormalities include translocations of 11q23 and 21q22. These patients respond well to chemotherapy and have survivals comparable to de novo AML patients.

Acute Myeloid Leukemia Not Otherwise Categorized

In the absence of a distinctive clinical presentation or cytogenetic abnormality, AML patients are classified according to their morphologic/histochemistry and immunophenotypic characteristics. This is the original FAB classification approach (see Table 18–1). More than 50% of de novo AML patients still fall within this category, although it is anticipated that future gene-expression profiling studies (*NPM1*, *ITD/FLT3*, and *CEBPA*) will lead to a further subclassification based on genetic and/or molecular biology abnormalities.

CASE HISTORY • *Part 3*

After thorough cultures, the patient is hydrated and begun on allopurinol, the infected tooth is extracted, and empiric antibiotic therapy is begun. He is begun on prophylactic antifungal and antiviral therapy and, within the first 24 hours of admission, he is begun on chemotherapy.

Several days later, the results of the cytogenetics are available showing a t(8;21) translocation. His parents and siblings are asked for blood samples to begin histocompatibility testing.

THERAPY

Therapy for AML should begin promptly after the diagnosis is made. Because the disease is rapidly progressive, any delay can decrease the chance of therapeutic success. In elderly patients, the possibility of a sustained remission is far less, and in the case of extreme age or debilitation, only symptomatic therapy may be indicated. Age by itself is not a contraindication to therapy, and a sustained remission can be achieved even in patients older than 70 years of age. However, while complete remission rates in patients under age 50 years average 70%, older patients show overall rates of less than 40%–50% and survivals of less than 12 months. This can be attributed to a higher incidence of unfavorable cytogenetics, multidrug resistance protein (MDR1) expression, and functional drug efflux.

Other **adverse prognostic factors**, besides age, include AML resulting from prior chemotherapy or myelodysplasia, an initial blast count in excess of 20,000/μL, an elevated LDH, and a poor initial performance status. Patients who fall in a favorable prognostic group, with a better than 85% chance of a remission and low relapse rate, are younger and have either a t(15;17), t(8;21), or inv(16) mutation. Unfavorable cases have mutations involving more than 2 chromosomes, a deletion or abnormality of the long arm of chromosome 3 or 5, 11q23 translocation, or monosomies of chromosomes 5 or 7. Regardless of age, these patients have a survival rate of less than 20% at 5 years.

Predictable complications such as anemia, thrombocytopenia, coagulopathy, or infection should never delay therapy since they are unlikely to improve until a remission is obtained. They should be treated with appropriate transfusions and antibiotics at the same time that chemotherapy is begun. The goal of therapy is to ablate the leukemic cell line and allow normal progenitor cells to repopulate the marrow. This process will require a period of marrow aplasia and marked granulocytopenia that can extend for 1–4 weeks or even longer. Because of this, leukemia therapy must be carried out in a hospital setting, preferably in a dedicated cancer nursing unit.

General Guidelines

Reliable vascular access is essential and usually requires placement of an indwelling catheter (eg, Hickman-Broviac catheter). The patient should be hydrated and receive allopurinol 300–600 mg/d by mouth or intravenous rasburicase to prevent hyperuricemia as tumor cells are lysed. Serum electrolytes and CBCs need to be monitored on a daily or every-other-day basis. In those patients who are at risk for DIC, a full coagulation profile should be measured daily for the first several days of chemotherapy to assess platelet, fibrinogen, and coagulation factor levels. If bleeding is life threatening, the patient should be treated with platelet transfusions and infusions of cryoprecipitate to correct hypofibrinogenemia (fibrinogen levels <100 mg/dL). In patients with promyelocytic leukemia, prophylactic anticoagulation with heparin is no longer indicated, owing to the quick reversal of DIC with ATRA treatment.

In the absence of severe cardiovascular disease, the hematocrit should be kept in the vicinity of 25%–30% to decrease the frequency of red blood cell transfusions. Prophylactic platelet transfusions should only be given when the platelet count falls below 10,000/μL in the patient with little or no bleeding, or 20,000/μL if the patient has significant mucous membrane bleeding or tends to bleed from venipuncture sites.

The treatment of ongoing infection must be very aggressive, and potential sources of infection should be eliminated. For example, infected teeth should be pulled, abscesses drained, and foreign bodies such as infected intravenous catheters removed and replaced. Good nursing care of the mouth, skin, and rectum is very important. Oral prophylaxis to prevent infection using an oral fluoroquinolone such as ciprofloxacin can be used. It is well tolerated and preserves the anaerobic gastrointestinal flora, thereby avoiding the problem of fungal overgrowth in the intestinal tract. It also appears to be effective in reducing the frequency of systemic infections with gram-negative bacteria.

Aside from local, nonresorbable antifungal therapy to limit yeast colonization of the gastrointestinal tract as a source for systemic candidiasis, prophylaxis against yeast infections is based on oral fluconazole or second-generation azoles (itraconazole, voriconazole, posaconazole), which are started from the completion of the chemotherapy regimen and maintained until myeloid reconstitution. However, this precaution is counterbalanced by the possible induction of resistant strains of Candida species. Empiric antiviral therapy has also been recommended. Acyclovir, 250 mg/m^2 (5 mg/kg) intravenously every 8 hours, or famciclovir, 500 mg given orally every 8 hours during marked granulocytopenia, has been suggested for patients who are known to be at risk for recurrent herpes simplex oral lesions. Patients should also be tested for their cytomegalovirus (CMV) status.

CMV-negative patients should receive only CMV-negative or adequately leukodepleted blood products to avoid transmission of an acute CMV infection. Ganciclovir, given in a dose of 5 mg/kg twice daily, may be effective prophylaxis for CMV infection in those who are CMV seropositive.

Empiric Antibiotic Therapy

If patients are not already febrile at the time of diagnosis, they soon become febrile with treatment. They should have thorough cultures to identify specific organisms. But even before a specific site of infection is identified, they need to receive prompt empiric antibiotic therapy (Table 18–6). The choice of antibiotics will depend to some extent on what organisms are seen in each institution. The usual approach is to provide broad-spectrum coverage for both gram-negative and gram-positive organisms. A popular combination of antibiotics for this purpose is an aminoglycoside (gentamicin, tobramycin, or amikacin) together with an antipseudomonal penicillin (carbenicillin, ticarcillin, mezlocillin, or piperacillin) or a wide-spectrum cephalosporin.

If pseudomonas infection is considered unlikely, a double β-lactam combination or Bactrim plus an antipseudomonal β-lactam can be used. This offers the one advantage for decreasing the risk of ototoxicity or nephrotoxicity. At the same time, it is not as effective in coverage of Pseudomonas aeruginosa. Single-drug therapy with ceftazidime, imipenem, or newer cephalosporins is a third alternative. It has the disadvantage of poor coverage for anaerobes and gram-positive bacteria and runs the risk of inducing β-lactam resistance.

Once initiated, antibiotic coverage must be continued throughout the period of granulocytopenia, until the absolute granulocyte count is greater than 500/μL. This is true even if the patient becomes afebrile during therapy. For most patients, the opposite will be true. Their fever will be poorly controlled, and in fact many patients will, after a brief period of improvement, experience recurrent chills and fever spikes. A careful examination of the patient, repeated chest x-ray, and blood cultures should be obtained with each episode of chills and fever, and the clinician should look for a drug-resistant bacterium or fungus. However, even when an organism cannot be isolated, other antibiotics should be added to the regimen. Vancomycin should be started as empiric therapy for Staphylococcus. If this has little or no effect after 4–6 days, antifungal therapy should be initiated for a presumptive fungal infection.

TABLE 18–6 • Empiric antibiotic therapy

Prophylaxis
Gastrointestinal tract
Nystatin suspension 20 mL swish and swallow or clotrimazole troche PO qid
Norfloxacin 400 mg PO q12h
Herpes simplex prevention
Acyclovir 250 mg/m^2 IV q8h
Initial fever
Culture negative
IV aminoglycoside (gentamicin or amikacin) + third-generation cephalosporin (cefepime, ceftazidine, ceftriaxone) or ureidopenicillin (piperacillin)[a]
Culture positive for Staphylococcus (possible catheter infection) or no response after 2 days
IV vancomycin
Uncontrolled or relapsing fever after 4–6 days
Culture negative
Empirical amphotericin B or voriconazole or echinocandin (caspofungin)
Culture positive for fungus
Amphotericin B or extended-spectrum azole or echinocandin (caspofungin)

[a]*Alternatives in patients who can't tolerate aminoglycosides: double β-lactam or Bactrim plus a β-lactam, or imipenem/meropenem monotherapy.*

Remission Induction

Chemotherapy protocols are in a constant state of evolution, and the specific regimen to be used may depend on the protocol in a given institution. Chemotherapy for AML can be divided into several phases: **remission induction, consolidation, and maintenance**. Marrow transplantation must also be considered as an important option for the younger AML patient.

The gold-standard remission induction protocol is treatment with cytosine arabinoside and an anthracycline. A typical protocol would include cytosine arabinoside 100–200 mg/m^2 daily for 7 days and either daunorubicin 40–60 mg/m^2 or idarubicin 12–13 mg/m^2 for the first 3 days. This will ablate the leukemic marrow in most patients. If after 7–10 days a repeated bone marrow biopsy shows residual leukemic blasts, the regimen should be repeated. Ideally, the patient should undergo a 1- to 3-week period of severe pancytopenia followed by a return of normal hematopoiesis (Figure 18–3). Once a complete remission is achieved, the patient's blood and marrow morphology should appear normal. The frequency of complete remission in AML is currently reported as 60%–80% overall; patients under the age of 50 years have a better chance of reaching a complete remission.

GM-CSF and G-CSF have been used after induction chemotherapy to shorten the duration of severe neutropenia with only modest success—length of stay reductions of 3–4 days. At the same time, they significantly increase the cost of therapy. Growth factors can be given, however, without fear of decreasing the complete remission rate or promoting early relapse. To date, attempts to use growth factors to enhance the effect of chemotherapy by increasing the number of cells in S phase have not been successful. Whether growth factors can be used to increase drug dose intensity with consolidation, resulting in a better outcome, is still not clear.

Specific treatments are indicated in promyelocytic leukemia (M3). All-trans retinoic acid (ATRA) restores differentiation in myeloid cells and is capable of inducing remission in 70%–90% of cases. This correlates with the presence of the

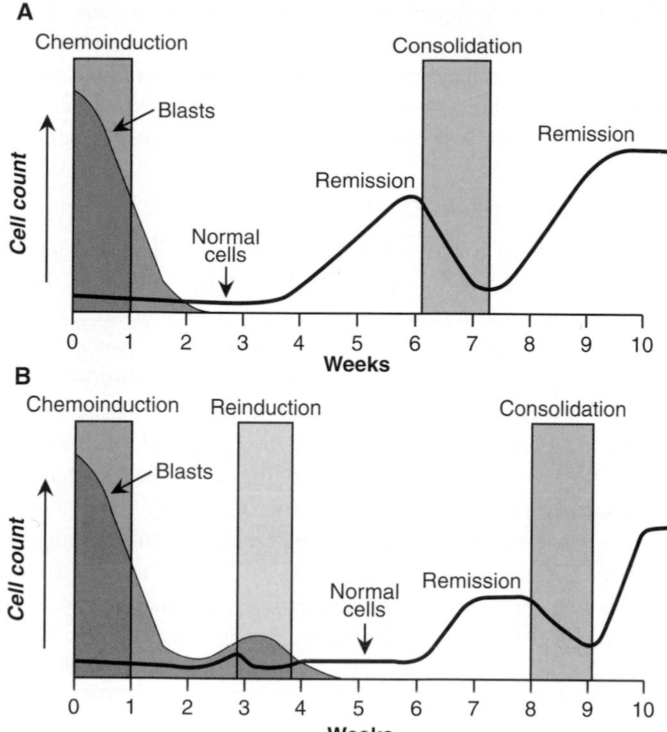

FIGURE 18–3. **Remission induction and consolidation.** The patient is initially treated with 2 or more drugs to eradicate the leukemic cell line. The sequence of drug therapy will depend on the patient's response as follows: **A:** Sixty percent or more of patients will achieve a complete remission with the first chemoinduction course of therapy. They can then be consolidated with a second course of therapy after 6–7 weeks. **B:** Patients who do not achieve remission with the initial chemoinduction will need a second course of (reinduction) therapy to achieve a complete remission.

15:17 chromosomal translocation (*PML-RARα*) involving the receptor for retinoic acid. ATRA given in a dose of 45 mg/m^2/d orally can be used to induce the patient, unless the WBC is high (>10,000/μL). In this situation, an initial treatment with hydroxyurea to first reduce the count or combined ATRA and chemotherapy is indicated. Once remission is attained on ATRA, the patient should be consolidated with 2 cycles of chemotherapy (daunorubicin and cytarabine) followed by maintenance therapy. Maintenance with ATRA (45 mg/m^2/d given orally in divided doses every 12 hours) has been reported to give the best prognosis, up to an 80% disease-free survival at 5 years. Treatment failures and relapsed patients may respond well to **arsenic trioxide** and stem cell transplantation therapies (see below). Complications of ATRA therapy include hyperleukocytosis and an acute syndrome of fever, weight gain, respiratory distress with pulmonary infiltrates, and acute renal failure (retinoic acid [RA] syndrome). The syndrome will usually resolve rapidly with dexamethasone 10 mg twice a day for several days.

Intrathecal therapy with cytarabine-methotrexate and steroids is restricted to patients with abnormal spinal fluid or high-risk features of leptomeningeal involvment at presentation, such as M5 variety and hyperleukocytosis at presentation.

Postinduction and Maintenance Therapy

Once the patient achieves remission residual leukemic cells are nevertheless present as shown by the frequency of relapse. The goal becomes to purge the residual disease and maintain the remission. There are 3 options at this time: chemo-immunotherapy–based consolidation, intensification with autologous stem cell support, and allogeneic stem cell transplantation. The choice of these treatment options has to take into account the patient's age and general status, the prognostic characteristics of the specific malignant clone, and the availability of a suitable donor. The karyotype at the time of diagnosis is the strongest prognostic indicator. Patients with more favorable genotypes [t(15;17), t(8;21), or inv(16)] may not benefit from early transplantation in the face of transplant-related complications and death. Conversely, patients with adverse genotypes should be transplanted as soon as possible because their response to chemotherapy is unacceptably poor.

Intensive consolidation and maintenance chemotherapy includes consolidation with 3–4 courses of high-dose cytosine arabinoside, which has proven efficacy with a low relapse rate for patients with favorable cytogenetics, such as t(8;21) or inv(16). For patients with unfavorable prognostic factors and who are ineligible for transplant programs, post-remission protocols have been evaluated. They involve the repeated use of cytosine arabinoside plus an anthracycline with the addition of 6-thioguanine, vincristine, prednisone, cyclophosphamide, and other drugs in combination designed to minimize the development of drug resistance in the leukemic cell line. Unfortunately, no one combination has emerged as a front-runner. Most centers report a median duration of complete remission of 12–18 months and a 2- to 3-year survival rate of 20%–40%. Long-term survivals depend on patient age and individual prognostic factors; 5-year survival ranges from up to 65% in younger adults with favorable genotypes to 10–15% in older adults with unfavorable ones.

Allogeneic Stem Cell Transplantation

Experimental and clinical data clearly demonstrate that allogeneic stem cell transplants trigger an antileukemic allogeneic effect (**graft versus leukemia**), which is an important part of the cure strategy. If the patient is under 55–60 years of age, does not have favorable cytogenetics, and has a histocompatible sibling who is willing to donate marrow, full myeloablative allogeneic marrow transplantation is the best option. For patients older than 55–60 years of age, reduced intensity conditioning regimens (nonmyeloablative) offer a suitable alternative. The overall probability of disease-free survival after 5 years following allogeneic transplantation is approximately 45%. Patients between 15 and 35 years of age have disease-free survivals of greater than 70% (Figure 18–4). This rate is a significantly better result than that achieved with conventional chemotherapy.

Patients who have relapsed and receive transplants in second or subsequent remission have survivals of 20%–40%. However, only 10%–15% of patients meet the requirements for allogeneic transplantation, and even with the advent of the nonrelated marrow donor program, fewer than 30% of patients can be matched to a suitable donor. Moreover, the use of an unrelated donor

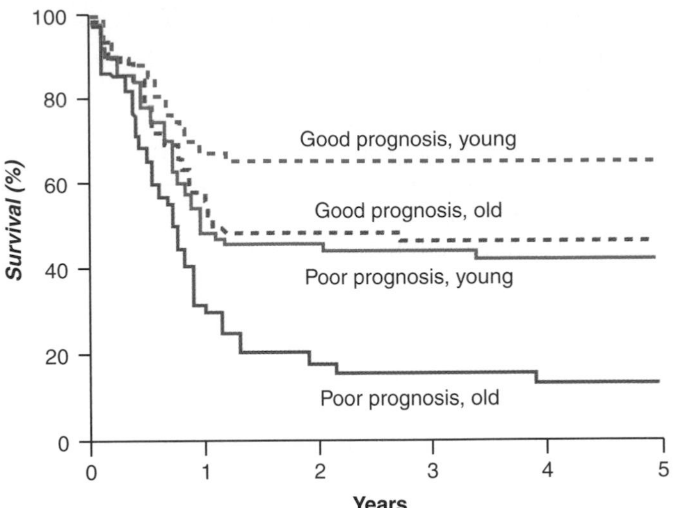

FIGURE 18–4. **Allogeneic bone marrow transplantation in AML.** Younger patients who respond well to chemotherapy and receive transplants in first remission have an excellent chance of long-term disease-free survival. Older patients, patients with less-responsive tumors, and those who receive transplants later in the disease process have less successful results. Patients with severe GVHD also have a poor prognosis.

increases the risk of severe, life-threatening **graft-versus-host disease** (GVHD). Recent data suggest that high-dose chemotherapy with autologous stem cell transplantation offers results nearly as good as allogeneic transplantation and better than conventional chemotherapy. This alternative may be considered for patients who do not have a matched donor.

Autologous Marrow Transplantation

For patients with intermediate or high-risk AML, in the absence of an HLA-matched donor, a chemotherapy protocol consisting of intensive consolidation followed by prolonged maintenance therapy can be offered. The 3-year relapse-free survival is around 40% with this procedure. Patients treated in first remission with autologous transplantation have a higher relapse rate than those undergoing allogeneic transplantation, but have a similar overall survival because of the decrease in procedure-related mortality associated with autologous transplantation. Both forms of transplant appear to be superior to conventional chemotherapy. In second remission, autologous stem cell transplantation is a welcome option whatever the nature of the AML for patients where a suitable donor is lacking.

Treatment of Relapse

Once the patient relapses, the prognosis is poor. It is frequently difficult to achieve a second or third remission. As a rule, if the first remission was a relatively long one (6–12 months), then standard induction therapy is used a second time. Newer drugs such as etoposide and mitoxantrone, as well as high-dose cytosine arabinoside, are alternatives. When the patient is younger and in good health, an autologous marrow transplantation as a part of the treatment of a first relapse may increase the chances of a second remission. Early results with the use of allogeneic or autologous transplantation to salvage relapsed patients suggest long-term survival rates of 20%–25%, which appear to be slightly better than those for conventional chemotherapy.

In patients who are unresponsive to these approaches, there are 2 salvage options. One is the drug gemtuzumab ozogamicin (Mylotarg) combining a monoclonal antibody (to CD33) with a cytotoxic antibiotic (calicheamicin) that has been shown to have efficacy in killing leukemic cells. Recent trials including this drug in the induction regimen have shown improved remission rates in young adults. For patients with promyelocytic leukemia who are refractory to ATRA and chemotherapy or who relapse, treatment with arsenic trioxide 0.15 mg/kg/d may be effective (85% complete response rate in small series). Its major complications are an increase in the QTc interval, and a syndrome resembling the RA syndrome. If the patient with acute promyelocytic leukemia (APL) relapses more than once, subsequent remissions are usually short and nearly always eventually fatal.

Emerging Therapies

Several innovative therapies are under active investigation, including agents active in many of the systems involved in leukemic cell biology: farnesyltransferase (inhibition of RAS^+ leukemias), histone deacetylase (restoration of maturation),

CASE HISTORY • *Part 4*

The patient becomes pancytopenic, fevers continue despite negative cultures, and about 14 days after induction chemotherapy his white count begins to recover with the appearance of normal monocytes and neutrophils. A repeat marrow examination shows markedly reduced numbers of myeloid cells, but evidence of normal myeloid maturation and no increase in blasts. Over the next few weeks, the patient recovers completely, with a normal CBC and normal marrow examination.

Histocompatibility studies show that he is a good match to one of his siblings. Due to his young age, and the availability of a well-matched donor, he is referred to a transplant center for allogeneic transplantation consideration. With his relatively favorable cytogenetics, he might also have been managed without immediate transplantation. This latter option would have been especially feasible if there had been comorbidities or lack of a suitable donor.

FLT3 and other tyrosine kinase inhibitors, demethylating agents (5-azacytidine, decitabine) antibody-toxin conjugates, anti-CD45 radiolabeled antibodies in combination with bone marrow transplantation, anti-*Bcl2* antisense nucleotides, desoxynucleoside analogs (clofarabine), MDR-1 reversing agents, and tumor vaccines.

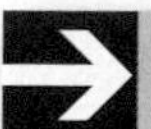

POINTS TO REMEMBER

Acute myeloid leukemia in younger patients has an abrupt onset and progresses very rapidly. Diagnosis and initiation of therapy must be carried out quickly.

In older patients or those with a history compatible with a myelodysplastic syndrome, the disease often progresses much more slowly but is also much less responsive to therapy.

When presented with an acute leukemia the 2 most important determinations to be made are to distinguish acute myeloid from acute lymphoid leukemia, and to determine the subtype of myeloid leukemia, particularly to identify promyelocytic leukemia.

Promyelocytic leukemia is often accompanied by severe thrombocytopenia and diffuse intravascular coagulation, which responds rapidly, however, to treatment with ATRA.

Patients with AML have markedly impaired host defenses at presentation and will be rendered pancytopenic for many days by their induction chemotherapy. They are, therefore, at high risk for infections. The use of prophylactic and empiric antibiotic therapy as well as aggressive treatment of any potential site of infection is critical.

Cytogenetic and molecular genetic analysis, while very important for planning the long-term management of an AML patient, are not needed for initial therapy, which should not be delayed for these results.

Following induction chemotherapy, decisions regarding the use and timing of additional chemotherapy, allogeneic bone marrow transplantation, or autologous transplantation will depend on a number of factors, including age, physical status, availability of matched marrow donor(s), level of remission following initial chemotherapy, morphological classification, cytogenetics, and time to relapse.

BIBLIOGRAPHY

Diagnosis

Falini B, Nicoletti I, Bolli N, et al: Translocations and mutations involving the nucleophosmin (NPM1) gene in lymphomas and leukemias. Haematologica 2007;92:519.

Fröhling S et al: Prognostic significance of activation FLT3 mutations in younger adults (16 to 60 years) with acute myeloid leukemia and normal cytogenetics: a study of the AML Study Group Ulm. Blood 2002;100:4372.

Garzon R, Volinia S, Liu CG, et al: MicroRNA signatures associated with cytogenetics and prognosis in acute myeloid leukemia. Blood 2008;111:3183.

Grimwade D, Haferlach T: Gene-expression profiling in acute myeloid leukemia. N Engl J Med 2004;350:1676.

Haferlach T, Bacher U, Kern W, Schnittger S, Haferlach C: Diagnostic pathways in acute leukemias: a proposal for a multimodal approach. Ann Hematol 2007;86:311.

Harris NL et al: The World Health Organization classification of hematological malignancies. Report of the Clinical Advisory Committee meeting, Arlie House, Virginia, November 1997. Mod Pathol 2000;13:193.

Kaleem Z, Crawford E, Pathan MH, et al: Flow cytometric analysis of acute leukemias. Diagnostic utility and critical analysis of data. Arch Pathol Lab Med 2003;12:42.

Nimer SD: Is it important to decipher the heterogeneity of "normal karyotype AML"? Best Pract Res Clin Haematol 2008;21:43.

Olsen RJ, Chang CC, Herrick JL, Zu Y, Ehsan A: Acute leukemia immunohistochemistry: a systematic diagnostic approach. Arch Pathol Lab Med 2008;132:462.

Paschka P, Marcucci G, Ruppert AS, et al: Wilms tumor 1 gene mutations independently predict poor outcome in adults with cytogenetically normal acute myeloid leukemia: a cancer and leukemia group B study. J Clin Oncol 2008;26:4595.

Porcu P, Cripe LD, Ng EW, Bhatia S, Danielson CM, Orazi A, McCarthy LJ: Hyperleukocytic leukemias and leukostasis: a review of pathophysiology, clinical presentation and management. Leuk Lymphoma 2000;39:1.

Radich JP: Molecular classification of acute myeloid leukemia: are we there yet? J Clin Oncol 2008;26:4539.

Renneville A, Roumier C, Biggio V, et al: Cooperating gene mutations in acute myeloid leukemia: a review of the literature. Leukemia 2008;22:915.

Schlenk RS, Döhner K, Krauter J, et al: Mutations and treatment outcome in cytogenetically normal acute myeloid leukemia. N Engl J Med 2008;358:1909.

Slovak ML et al: Karyotypic analysis predicts outcome of preremission and postremission therapy in adult acute myeloid leukemia: a Southwest Oncology Group/Eastern Cooperative Oncology Group study. Blood 2000;96:4075.

Stone RM, Mayer RJ: The unique aspects of acute promyelocytic leukemia. J Clin Oncol 1990;8:198.

Valk PJM, Verhaak RGW, Beijen MA, et al: Prognostically useful gene-expression profiles in acute myeloid leukemia. N Engl J Med 2004;350:1617.

Vardiman JW, Harris NL, Brunning RD: The World Health Organization (WHO) classification of the myeloid neoplasms. Blood 2002;100:2292.

Therapy

Amadori S, Stasi R: Integration of monoclonal antibodies and immunoconjugates into the treatment of acute myeloid leukemia. Curr Opin Hematol 2008;15:95.

Appelbaum FR: Incorporating hematopoietic cell transplantation (HCT) into the management of adults aged under 60 years with acute myeloid leukemia (AML). Best Pract Res Clin Haematol 2008;2:85.

Blum W, Marcucci G: New approaches in acute myeloid leukemia. Best Pract Res Clin Haematol 2008;21:29.

Bow EJ: Of yeasts and hyphæ: a hematologist's approach to antifungal therapy. Hematology (ASH educational program book). 2006; 361–367.

Breems DA, Löwenberg B: Acute myeloid leukemia and the position of autologous stem cell transplantation. Semin Hematol 2007;44:259.

Craddock CF: Full-intensity and reduced-intensity allogeneic stem cell transplantation in AML. Bone Marrow Transplant 2008;41:415.

Dombret H et al: Established practice in the treatment of patients with acute promyleocytic leukemia and the introduction of arsenic trioxide as a novel therapy. Semin Hematol 2002;39:8.

Estey EH: Older adults: should the paradigm shift from standard therapy? Best Pract Res Clin Haematol 2008;21:61.

Freifeld A et al: A double-blind comparison of empirical oral and intravenous antibiotic therapy for low-risk febrile patients with neutropenia during cancer chemotherapy. N Engl J Med 1999;341:305.

Fröhling S, Schlenk RF, Stolze I, et al: CEBPA mutations in younger adults with acute myeloid leukemia and normal cytogenetics: prognostic relevance and analysis of cooperating mutations. J Clin Oncol 2004;22:624.

Jurcic JG, Soignet SL, Maslak AP: Diagnosis and treatment of acute promyelocytic leukemia. Curr Oncol Rep 2007;9:337.

Kern WV et al: Oral versus intravenous empirical antimicrobial therapy for fever in patients with granulocytopenia who are receiving cancer chemotherapy. N Engl J Med 1999;341:312.

Kolb H et al: Graft-versus-leukemia reactions in allogeneic chimeras. Blood 2004;103:767.

Laughlin MJ, Eapen M, Rubinstein P, et al: Outcomes after transplantation of cord blood or bone marrow from unrelated donors in adults with leukemia. N Engl J Med 2004;351:2265.

Leith CP et al: Acute myeloid leukemia in the elderly: assessment of multidrug resistance (MDR1) and cytogenetics distinguishes biologic subgroups with remarkably distinct responses to standard chemotherapy. A Southwest Oncology Group study. Blood 1997;89:3323.

Marcucci G, Radmacher MD, Maharry K, et al: MicroRNA expression in cytogenetically normal acute myeloid leukemia. N Engl J Med 2008;358:1919.

Neubauer A, Maharry K, Mro´ zek K, et al: Patients with acute myeloid leukemia and RAS mutations benefit most from postremission treatment with high-dose cytarabine: a Cancer and Leukemia Group B study. J Clin Oncol doi:10.1200/JCO.2007.14.0418

Oliansky DM, Appelbaum F, Cassileth PA, et al: The role of cytotoxic therapy with hematopoietic stem cell transplantation in the therapy of acute myelogenous leukemia in adults: an evidence-based review. Biol Blood Marrow Transplant 2008;14:137.

Rocha V, Labopin M, Sanz G, et al: Umbilical cord-blood vs bone marrow transplant from unrelated donors in adults with acute leukemia. N Engl J Med 2004;351:2276.

Rowe JM: Consolidation therapy: what should be the standard of care? Best Pract Res Clin Haematol 2008;21:53.

Sanz MA: Treatment of acute promyelocytic leukemia. Hematology (ASH educational book). 2006; 147–155.

Schiffer CA: Hematopoietic growth factors as adjuncts to the treatment of acute myeloid leukemia. Blood 1996;88:3675.

Soignet S et al: United States multicenter study of arsenic trioxide in relapsed acute promyelocytic leukemia. J Clin Oncol 2001;19:3852.

Stasi R: Gemtuzumab ozogamicin: an anti-CD33 immunoconjugate for the treatment of acute myeloid leukaemia. Expert Opin Biol Ther 2008;8:527.

Tallman MS et al: All-trans-retinoic acid in acute promyelocytic leukemia: long-term outcome and prognostic factor analysis from the North American Intergroup protocol. Blood 2002;100:4298.

Tse WW, Zang SL, Bunting KD, Laughlin MJ: Umbilical cord blood transplantation in adult myeloid leukemia. Bone Marrow Transplant 2008;41:465.

Wang ZY, Chen Z: Acute promyelocytic leukemia: from highly fatal to highly curable. Blood 2008;111:2505.

Zittoun RA et al: Autologous or allogeneic bone marrow transplantation compared with intensive chemotherapy in acute myelogenous leukemia. N Engl J Med 1995;332:217.

CHRONIC MYELOGENOUS LEUKEMIA AND THE MYELOPROLIFERATIVE DISORDERS • 19

CASE HISTORY • *Part I*

A 67-year-old woman is referred for evaluation of anemia. She complains of gradually increasing fatigue and has recently noticed some abdominal distention and weight loss. She also describes difficulty eating a full meal due to early satiety.

Her past history is remarkable for the fact that several years ago she had been told by her gynecologist that she had very good blood counts with an elevated hematocrit and a tendency to a high white count. These findings were never evaluated. She had 2 uneventful pregnancies with no history of thrombosis or bleeding.

On examination she appears somewhat cachectic and pale. Her abdominal examination is remarkable for hepatomegaly and striking splenomegaly; the spleen tip is palpated nearly at the pelvic rim.

CBC: Hemoglobin/hematocrit - 7 g/dL/23%

WBC count - 3,500/μL with a decreased neutrophil percentage, but otherwise relatively normal leukocyte differential

Platelet count - 60,000/μL

• SMEAR MORPHOLOGY

Numerous "teardrop" red cells are noted, as well as occasional nucleated red cells. White cells appear decreased in number with no morphological abnormalities. Platelets are also decreased in number, and giant platelets are seen.

Questions

- What aspects of this case would lead the clinician away from a routine anemia workup?
- How many hematopoietic cell lines appear to be involved in this disorder?
- What additional laboratory studies are indicated?

Chronic myelogenous leukemia (CML) and the various myeloproliferative disorders are all clonal malignancies of the hematopoietic stem cell. In contrast to acute leukemia, they tend to have a more protracted clinical course as the malignant cells maintain the ability to mature during the chronic phase of the disease. Even if they present primarily as a proliferation of 1 cell line, cells of the granulocytic, erythrocytic, and megakaryocytic lineages can be shown to arise from the same abnormal clone. Moreover, overlapping between these disorders is frequent, either at presentation or during the disease course, providing a challenge to the clinician in the classification and management of the disease state.

The diseases that are commonly classified as myeloproliferative disorders are displayed in Table 19–1. The list traditionally

TABLE 19–1 • Classification of myeloproliferative diseases

Chronic myelogenous leukemia (*BCR-ABL* positive)
Chronic myelogenous leukemia (*BCR-ABL* negative)
Chronic neutrophilic leukemia
Primary myelofibrosis
Primary (essential) thrombocythemia
Polycythemia vera (see Chapter 13)
Chronic eosinophilic leukemia
Chronic myelomonocytic leukemia (CMML)
Juvenile chronic myelomonocytic leukemia

includes chronic myelogenous leukemia, primary myelofibrosis, polycythemia vera, and essential thrombocythemia. A number of other conditions can, however, share characteristics with the myeloproliferative disorders. Chronic myelomonocytic leukemia, previously categorized as a primary myelodysplastic syndrome, is now considered more in the spectrum of myeloproliferative diseases. In addition, several of the dysplastic anemias share features with the myeloproliferative disorders, including the refractory anemias with excess blasts, and some instances of aplastic anemia (see Chapters 3 and 9). Chronic eosinophilic leukemia is also now recognized as a well-defined clonal entity.

CLASSIFICATION

The clinical diagnosis of a myeloproliferative disorder is usually made based on the morphologic pattern of cell involvement (Table 19–2). The names of the several disorders mirror their morphologic abnormalities. Thus, CML is characterized by uncontrolled expansion of the myeloid cell lines, whereas essential thrombocythemia shows prominent megakaryocyte expansion with excessive platelet production. Polycythemia vera (see Chapter 13) is an example of a clonal malignancy resulting in uncontrolled red blood cell production as the predominant feature. All 3 conditions can share morphologic features, however, which makes the diagnosis more difficult. For example, it is not unusual for polycythemia vera patients to have increased granulocyte and platelet counts. In fact, the platelet count can increase to levels in excess of 1 million/μL, similar to levels in the patient with essential thrombocythemia.

Primary myelofibrosis generally presents with decreased levels of cell production, and varying combinations of anemia, leukopenia, and thrombocytopenia. Marrow histology is very important in discerning myelofibrosis. A dramatic increase in reticulin fibers and collagen, together with a loss of normal hematopoietic cells, provides the basis for diagnosis. Myelofibrosis can appear de novo or develop as part of another myeloproliferative disorder. Therefore, the interpretation of the morphologic findings must be made in light of the patient's clinical course.

TABLE 19–2 • Morphologic patterns of the myeloproliferative disorders

Disease	Morphologic Characteristics
Chronic myelogenous leukemia	Marked increase of myelocytes in marrow and blood Absolute basophilia Normal or increased platelet count Increase in megakaryocytes
Primary myelofibrosis	Moderate to marked normocytic anemia with nucleated red blood cells and "teardrop" forms Marrow fibrosis (increase in reticulin and collagen) Increase in megakaryocytes
CMML	Modest increase in monocytes Increase in "blast" forms in marrow and blood Marrow hyperplasia with increase in myelomonocyte precursors
Primary thrombocythemia	Normal red blood cell, granulocyte counts Marked increase in platelet count, marrow megakaryocytes
Chronic eosinophilic leukemia	Marked increase of mature and immature eosinophils in blood and marrow

CYTOGENETIC ANALYSIS

Cytogenetic analysis is of particular value in CML and chronic eosinophilic leukemia. The identification of a morphologically abnormal chromosome, the Philadelphia (Ph^1) chromosome, more than 30 years ago was a landmark in the use of chromosomal analysis in CML diagnosis. The implications of this neo-chromosome have become clear with time. The Ph^1 chromosome is actually a translocation of the Abelson proto-oncogene from chromosome 22 to the long arm of chromosome 9, t(9;22), resulting in a *BCR-ABL* fusion gene (Figure 19–1).

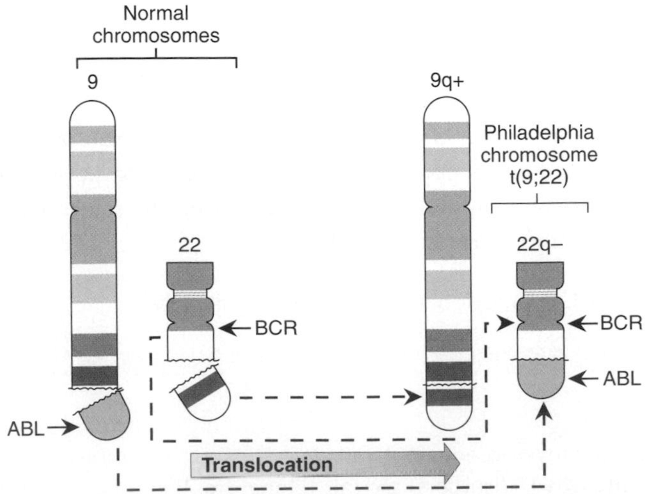

FIGURE 19–1. **The *BCR-ABL* translocation in CML.** The fundamental genetic lesion in CML results in the translocation of the *ABL* oncogene, normally on chromosome 9, to the *BCR* gene on chromosome 22 and is recognized karyotypically as the Philadelphia chromosome. The resulting *BCR-ABL* gene product plays a role in the malignant transformation of the hematopoietic stem cell.

TABLE 19–3 • Common cytogenetic/karyotypic abnormalities in myeloproliferative disorders

Syndrome	Abnormality
CML—chronic phase	t(9;22) (Ph[1] chromosome)
CML—blastic phase	Extra Ph[1] chromosome Isochromosome 17 Monosomy 7 Trisomy 8, 19
Primary myelofibrosis	Trisomy 1q, 8 Deletions 13q, 20q
Chronic eosinophilic leukemia	t(1;4); t(5;12)

According to the precise breakpoint in the *BCR* gene (m-BCR, M-BCR, or μ-BCR), 3 types of recombinant fusion genes can be recognized, each with a different protein expression (p190, p210, and p230, respectively). The expression of p190 is seen in Ph[1]-positive acute lymphocytic leukemia (ALL) (see Chapter 25), whereas p210 is the most commonly observed translocation in CML, while p230 is infrequently associated with an atypical form of CML, chronic neutrophilic leukemia. These proteins all display tyrosine kinase activity. This appears to activate multiple intracellular signaling pathways, including the RAS, PI3-K, and c-MYC pathways, to both increase progenitor cell proliferation and decrease myeloid cell apoptosis and cell adhesion. In the early phases of the disease the malignant cells retain the ability to differentiate, giving rise to increased numbers of apparently normal granulocytes. However, over time, there is a progressive failure to differentiate, resulting in increasing numbers of immature cells and even blasts appearing in blood; blasts can be of either myeloid or lymphoid lineage. Other types of cytogenetic translocations can be observed in otherwise typical CML. Some recombine *BCR* with *ABL* through complex translocations and hence test as *BCR-ABL* positive. Others recombine *BCR* with non-*ABL* gene partners as, for example, the fusion of *BCR* with *FGFR1* (t(8;22) CML). Such rare cases are classified as *BCR-ABL*–negative CML.

Chronic eosinophilic leukemia is another well-characterized example of myeloproliferative disease resulting from a definitive chromosomal translocation, t(1;4)(q44;q12), which fuses the *FIP1L1-PDGFRA* genes and in turn promotes a fusion protein with tyrosine kinase activity. Translocations involving the platelet growth factor receptor family such as t(5;12)(q33;p13) (*EVT6-PDGFRB*) give rise to a similar phenotype. Karyotypic abnormalities have also been described in several of the other chronic myeloproliferative disorders. Some of the most common of these are shown in Table 19–3.

MOLECULAR DIAGNOSIS

The recent discovery of mutations inside the Janus kinase gene (*JAK2 V617F*) has shed new insight on the pathophysiology of *BCR-ABL*–negative myeloproliferative diseases and modified our diagnostic accuracy for these diseases. The *JAK2 V617F* mutation is shared by the granulocytic, erythroid, megakaryocytic, and monocytic lineages, but is usually absent from lymphocytes. It is detectable in DNA from blood in nearly all cases of polycythemia vera, and approximately 50%–65% of patients with myelofibrosis or primary thrombocythemia. In this setting, the *JAK2* mutation confirms a strong link between these disorders. However, some features remain poorly explained, such as the various clinical syndromes associated with this single mutation. Experimental data with *JAK2* transgenic mice indicate that the mutant *V617F*/wild-type *JAK2* ratio determines the clinical phenotype. In any case, the *JAK2* mutation helps considerably in the diagnosis and classification of patients presenting with a myeloproliferative picture.

CLINICAL FEATURES

The clinical presentation of a patient with a myeloproliferative disorder will reflect the pattern of abnormalities in cell production and function. Early in the disease process, CML patients demonstrate dramatic increases in the number of mature and immature myelocytes in circulation and tissues. The CML patient may complain of abdominal discomfort secondary to massive splenomegaly. White blood cells accumulate in the spleen to the point where they jeopardize the normal blood supply. This condition can result in splenic infarction, presenting clinically as moderate to severe left upper quadrant pain made worse with deep inspiration. Patients generally have abdominal tenderness with or without peritoneal signs, and in some cases, a friction rub is heard over the spleen with respiration. CML patients may also seek medical attention because of a worsening anemia or, rarely, because of easy bruising and abnormal bleeding.

Patients with severe myelofibrosis usually present with symptoms and signs of severe anemia or pancytopenia. Myelofibrotic patients can demonstrate impressive splenomegaly, especially when there is significant extramedullary hematopoiesis. Unlike CML patients, myelofibrosis patients do not often present with splenic infarction, even when the spleen is so enlarged that it extends to the iliac crest. Myelofibrosis patients can exhibit thrombocytopenia or thrombocytosis with platelet dysfunction sufficient to result in purpura and both mucous membrane and gastrointestinal bleeding. Petechial eruptions are less common.

Patients with primary thrombocythemia are usually asymptomatic. Slight splenomegaly is frequent when clinical examination is carefully done. Microcirculation symptoms such as livedo reticularis, burning palms, and erythromelalgia (painful red digits) are often present and are very suggestive of the diagnosis when alleviated by aspirin. Bleeding of mucous membranes or thrombosis are serious complications that can disclose hitherto latent disease.

Laboratory Studies

The complete blood count (CBC) and marrow aspirate and biopsy are key studies in the diagnosis of these disorders.

A. Complete Blood Count

The CBC provides an accurate measure of the absolute numbers of the red blood cell, white blood cell, and platelet components.

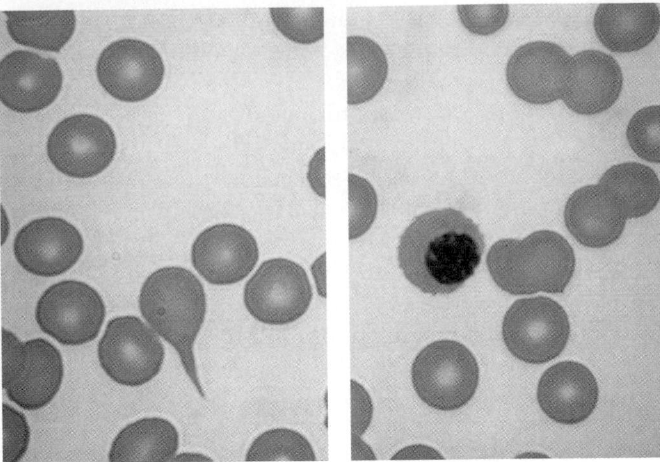

FIGURE 19–2. **Teardrop and nucleated red cells.** A teardrop-shaped red blood cell (left panel) and a nucleated red blood cell (right panel) are typically seen with myelofibrosis and extramedullary hematopoiesis.

It also will reveal increased numbers of immature myeloid progenitors in circulation. Inspection of the blood film can be very helpful, since automated counters (although flagging samples as abnormal) are insensitive to the specific appearance of the blasts and subtle differences between immature myelocytes and monocytes. Furthermore, film inspection will permit a more careful evaluation of red blood cell morphology. This helps in the diagnosis of myelofibrosis, where the appearance of teardrop red blood cells, schistocytes, and nucleated red blood cells is characteristic of progressive fibrosis of the marrow and extramedullary hematopoiesis in the liver and spleen (Figure 19–2).

B. Special Stains

Special stains are not as useful in the diagnosis of myeloproliferative disorders as they are in acute leukemia. An absolute basophil count using a toluidine blue stain is occasionally of value in diagnosing CML. The normal basophil count should be less than 50/μL; CML patients almost always have basophil counts in excess of 50–100/μL. At presentation, most CML patients have low to absent levels of leukocyte alkaline phosphatase. This finding is not unique to CML, and is now considered an obsolete diagnostic criterion.

C. Marrow Aspirate and Biopsy

Except for obtaining a karyotype, the marrow aspirate is of little interest in the chronic phase of the myeloproliferative diseases, as morphological changes show no more than hypercellularity, which cannot be used to distinguish between disorders. However, the aspirate provides essential information during the course to assess blastic transformation. On the other hand, the marrow biopsy is essential to the diagnosis of the myeloproliferative disorders. The marrow biopsy provides information regarding the overall cellularity and changes in marrow structure. Diagnosis of myelofibrosis depends on the demonstration of increased amounts of reticulin fibers and collagenous tissue. Both a silver stain for reticulin fibers and a trichrome stain for collagen can help in detecting early changes in marrow structure (Figure 19–3).

D. Chromosomal Studies

Karyotyping of metaphase cells in the marrow is important, primarily to distinguish CML from the other myeloproliferative disorders (see Table 19–3). Karyotyping of peripheral blood in the chronic phase is usually nondiagnostic as it contains few if any myeloid cells capable of entering metaphase, which are lost in maturation beyond the promyelocyte stage. The most common karyotypic abnormalities seen are listed in Table 19–3. More sensitive molecular genetics techniques are now available that can detect small numbers of abnormal cells. They have been used to detect residual disease in treated CML patients. For example, the *BCR-ABL* fusion gene transcript can be identified in small numbers of cells using **reverse transcriptase**

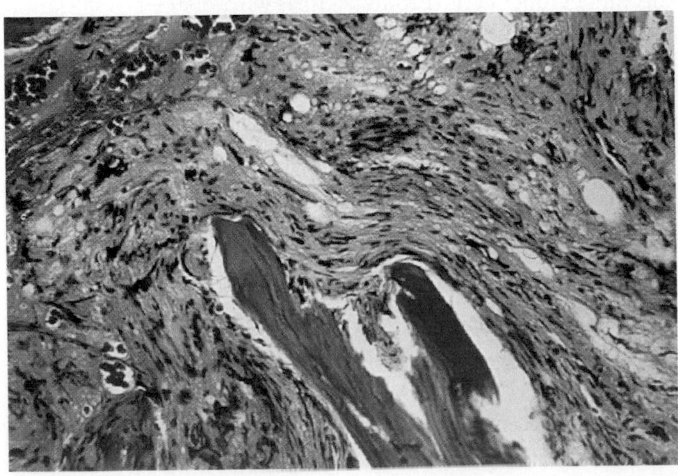

A

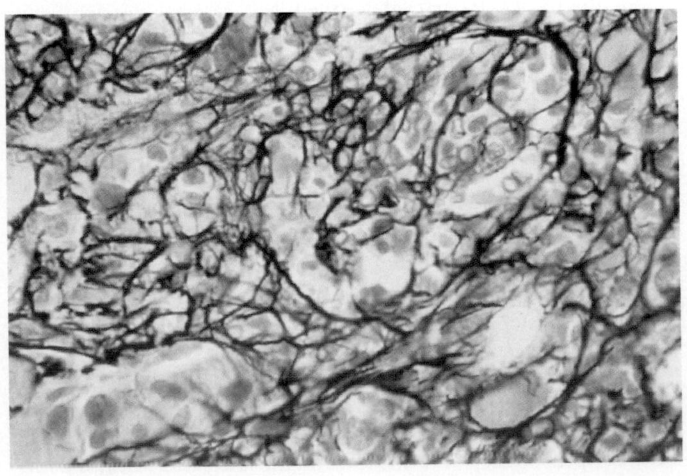

B

FIGURE 19-3. **Myelofibrosis.** Marrow precursors and fat cells are completely replaced by a dense infiltration of collagen (**A:** hematoxylin-eosin stain) and reticulin fibers (**B:** silver stain).

polymerase chain reaction (RT-PCR), with DNA and RNA blotting techniques, and also via specific DNA probes. RT-PCR is capable of detecting CML cells in about 1 in 10,000 cells, making this assay a robust diagnostic and follow-up tool for quantitating the response to therapy.

E. Other Laboratory Tests

Other ancillary laboratory signs of increased proliferation of cells typical of myeloproliferative disorders include an increase in the **vitamin B_{12} binding proteins** (transcobalamins I and III) and, as a consequence, very high vitamin B_{12} levels. **Uric acid and lactic dehydrogenase (LDH) levels** may also be increased in patients with large tumor burden.

DIFFERENTIAL DIAGNOSIS

The diagnosis of the individual myeloproliferative disorders is guided by their clinical presentation and the routine CBC, which helps to select the most appropriate follow-up laboratory tests.

TABLE 19–4 • Chronic myelogenous leukemia hematopoietic profile in chronic phase

Complete blood count (CBC)
Hemoglobin: normal or slightly decreased
White blood cell count: markedly increased (50,000–200,000/μL)
Increased numbers of metamyelocytes, myelocytes, promyelocytes, and blasts in circulation
Platelet count: normal or increased
Basophil count: greater than 50/μL
Marrow
Hypercellular (decreased fat)
E/G ratio: 1:4–1:10 (myelocytic hyperplasia)
Increased numbers of megakaryocytes
Variable fibrosis, increase in reticulin is moderate in chronic phase
Special studies
Ph^1 chromosome; present in more than 90% of patients
BCR-ABL recombinant transcript (RT-PCR) is the gold standard

CHRONIC MYELOGENOUS LEUKEMIA

Chronic myelogenous leukemia (CML) is a disease of middle age; the peak incidence is in the fifth decade of life. It is observed, however, in younger and older individuals. CML is a leukemia that may be induced by environmental factors such as radiation exposure, either accidental or for diagnostic or therapeutic purposes.

CML patients may first be detected from a **routine CBC** or because of **nonspecific complaints** such as weight loss, fatigue, night sweats, abdominal fullness, or episodes of abdominal pain. They usually do not have abnormal bleeding or an increased tendency to infections. On physical examination, most CML patients have **splenomegaly**, whereas less than a third have hepatomegaly. Patients with very large spleens and acute left upper quadrant abdominal pain may have experienced splenic infarction and may demonstrate a splenic friction rub.

Laboratory Studies

A. Complete Blood Count

The complete blood count (CBC) usually points to the diagnosis (Table 19–4). The number of circulating mature and immature granulocytes can be markedly increased. Counts of 50,000–200,000/μL or higher are common. While most of these cells are mature granulocytes, lesser percentages of metamyelocytes, myelocytes, promyelocytes, and even a few blasts are typically present. The spectrum of cells in circulation closely resembles the maturation sequence of the myelocyte lineage in the marrow. An **increase in the basophil count** to levels greater than 50/μL is frequent, and higher levels have worse prognostic significance. Some CML patients may also show an impressive eosinophilia, although this is not diagnostically specific.

At presentation, CML patients are usually not very anemic. In fact, their hemoglobin level can be normal or even slightly elevated. Similarly, the **platelet count** may be low, normal, or elevated. With higher platelet counts, platelet function can be abnormal and associated with a tendency to bruising. Although the malignant event responsible for CML involves the most primitive hematopoietic stem cell, there is usually no early evidence of lymphocyte dysfunction. Late in the course of the disease, some patients (between 20% and 30%) may present with a picture clinically similar to those with de novo acute lymphocytic leukemia (ALL).

B. Other Tests

Even when the clinical diagnosis is obvious, the patient's **marrow should be studied** for the presence of the t(9;22)-(q34;q11) translocation to form the *BCR-ABL* hybrid gene (Ph^1 chromosome) and other **chromosomal abnormalities**. The fusion mRNA that results is translated in the majority of cases into a chimeric **p210** protein. This protein functions as a tyrosine kinase that interacts with RAS, a guanosine triphosphate-binding protein responsible for cell proliferation and differentiation. By standard banded karyotype technique, approximately 5%–10% of CML patients will appear to be apparently Ph^1 negative. Although true *BCR-ABL*–negative CML rarely exists, mostly when translocations involve unusual gene partners, most of the apparently Ph^1-negative patients actually can be shown by fluorescence in-situ hybridization (FISH) or molecular techniques to still demonstrate *BCR-ABL* fusion products.

Even though the **t(9;22) translocation** is the hallmark of CML, it is also detected in 10%–20% of adults and 2%–5% of children with ALL. Most of these patients have a unique breakpoint **BCR-ABL translocation** resulting in a smaller **p190** fusion protein. Expression of p190 can also be associated with a pronounced monocytosis in some patients. Another more rare CML variant, Ph^1-positive chronic neutrophilic leukemia with thrombocytosis, demonstrates a novel breakpoint *BCR-ABL* translocation with a **p230** protein product.

Phases of CML and Genetic Factors

Initially, CML is a slowly progressive disease. The excessive proliferation of marrow progenitors, the expansion of the mature granulocyte and platelet pools, and the tendency to hepatosplenomegaly are the major manifestations of the clonal defect. Early release of marrow granulocytes and their precursors, and reduced apoptosis also play a role in producing the very high peripheral white blood cell counts. **Prognostic features at the time of diagnosis** include age, splenomegaly, platelet count, number of blasts or metaphases in the marrow, extent of basophilia and eosinophilia, and chromosomal abnormalities other than the Ph^1 chromosome. The International Collaborative CML Prognostic Factors Project Group proposed and validated a CML prognostic scoring system using these variables in patients treated with interferon. Young age, moderate splenomegaly, normal platelet count, and lower levels of eosinophils, basophils, and marrow blasts predict a median survival time of better than 90 months. Older patients (>60 years) and those with more massive splenomegaly, platelet counts less than 15,000/μL or greater than 700,000/μL, higher blast counts in the marrow, eosinophilia, and basophilia fall into intermediate- or high-risk groups with median survivals of 67 and 43 months, respectively. However, the value of this scoring system has to be reconsidered in the tyrosine kinase inhibitor (TKI) era. Patients who have received imatinib as initial therapy show survivals of 89% at 60 months, with a projected overall median survival of 15 years. The main prognostic factor appears now to best relate to the absolute level of residual disease as assessed by RT-PCR, and the stability of this result over time. Besides the level of molecular response, the so-called **"phase of the disease"** process is also important to both overall survival and planning therapy.

A. Chronic Phase

As long as the granulocyte and platelet counts are close to normal levels, such patients are generally asymptomatic. This is referred to as the **chronic phase** of CML. Depending on the mix of prognostic features and response to TKI treatment, this phase can last anywhere from less than 1 year (poor prognostic factors and/or little response to TKI) to more than a decade (complete molecular remission after TKI).

B. Accelerated Phase

In the past, the average chronic phase of CML lasted for 3–5 years (now longer with the advent of TKI therapy) before symptoms and signs of more aggressive disease (the **accelerated phase**) appear. At this latter point, the patient will note fatigue, weight loss, night sweats, and at times, bone pain. Hepatosplenomegaly worsens, with progressive abdominal discomfort, and control of the proliferation of both granulocytes/myeloid precursors and platelets becomes much more difficult. Counts rise to high levels, which places the patient at risk for widespread tissue infiltration by white blood cells. Patients can develop lymphadenopathy and nodular tumors of the skin **(chloromas)** that on biopsy have the appearance of marrow tissue. Some patients may also exhibit progressive fibrosis of the marrow that further stimulates the development of extramedullary hematopoiesis and tissue infiltrates.

C. Blast Crisis

As the disease progresses, the number of blasts in the marrow and peripheral blood continues to increase. After less than 1 year in the accelerated phase, most patients will evolve to an acute leukemia-like picture, referred to as a **blast crisis**. The number of blasts needed to declare a blast crisis is unclear. However, once the patient demonstrates other manifestations of leukemia, including worsening anemia, thrombocytopenia, and a sufficient loss of mature granulocytes to put the patient at risk for infections, there is no question that the patient is in the final phase of CML. Secondary genetic changes, including mutations in the p53 and/or Rb genes, are common at this point and may help explain the loss of myeloid differentiation.

D. Genetic Tests

Most terminal leukemias in CML involve the myeloid lineage, although 20%–30% are lymphoblastic in nature. Since the latter are more responsive to ALL-specific chemotherapy regimens, it is important to **phenotype the blasts to characterize their lineage**, whether myeloid or lymphoid. **Genotyping** is also important. Cytogenetic changes including isochromosome 17; monosomies or trisomies of chromosomes 7, 8, and 19; additional translocations; and the appearance of an extra Ph^1 chromosome occur in 50%–80% of patients (see Table 19–3). Trisomy 8 is the most common finding in patients undergoing transformation to blastic stage. The appearance of multiple chromosomal defects is another poor prognostic sign.

Detection of the *BCR-ABL* translocation product by RT-PCR is now recommended to assess the patient's response to therapy. The RT-PCR assay for minimal residual disease is the most sensitive measure of the effectiveness of treatment. Up to 80% of bone marrow transplant patients will demonstrate a negative assay for the *BCR-ABL* RNA. Similarly, patients treated with imatinib frequently achieve complete molecular remission, that is, RT-PCR negativity (Figure 19–4). In contrast,

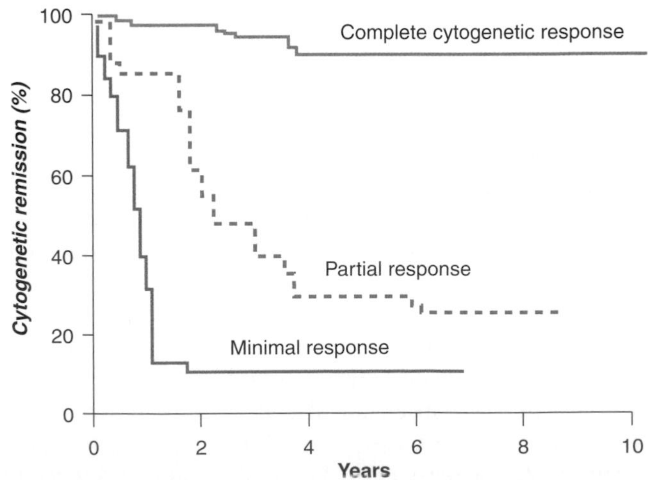

FIGURE 19–4. **Survival curves in CML.** The quality of remission in CML depends on the degree to which cells carrying the cytogenetic abnormality can be eliminated. Tests for residual cells carrying the *BCR-ABL* translocation make it possible to distinguish patients with markedly different outcomes. It is likely that these survival curves are being improved by the widespread use of imatinib.

most patients treated with interferon show residual disease even after a year of therapy. Furthermore, a cytogenetic relapse (increase in product by RT-PCR) will usually precede a recognizable clinical relapse, so the molecular follow-up is important for early detection and changes in therapy. Resistance to imatinib as well as other TKIs, another important indicator of relapse, has been shown to be related to various mutations in the tyrosine kinase domain of *ABL*, the most resistant being the *T315I* mutation.

PRIMARY MYELOFIBROSIS

Myelofibrosis can present as a de novo, primary illness or as a secondary manifestation of CML, polycythemia vera, or tumor infiltration of the marrow (see Chapter 3). Primary myelofibrosis, similar to CML and polycythemia vera, is a disease of the middle-aged and older patient populations. Studies of glucose-6-phosphate dehydrogenase (G6PD) isoenzymes, cytogenetic abnormalities, and more recently, the detection of the *JAK2* mutation in half of the patients tested have shown that it is a clonal malignancy involving all hematopoietic cell lineages. However, although marrow fibrosis is its most distinguishing feature, the malignant change does not involve the fibroblasts and marrow reticuloendothelial cells. Instead, the **fibrosis** appears to be a late reaction to the initial proliferation of the malignant stem cell line, especially the proliferation of megakaryocytes, and is **associated with the release of several growth factors** (transforming growth factor-β, platelet-derived growth factor, interleukin [IL]-1, and fibroblast growth factor). Recently, high levels of thrombopoietin have been demonstrated in patients with myelofibrosis, suggesting perhaps a cause for the megakaryocyte expansion. As further evidence of the key role of megakaryocytes, even advanced marrow fibrosis has been shown to reverse with bone marrow transplantation or 2-chlorodeoxyadenosine (2-CDA) therapy.

Patients with **primary myelofibrosis**, like CML patients, present with **nonspecific symptoms** and signs of easy fatigability, malaise, abdominal distention, and at times, abdominal pain. **Marked splenomegaly**, sometimes filling the abdomen and extending to the pubic rim, results from extramedullary hematopoiesis and is a hallmark of the disorder. Spleen enlargement can even induce hemodynamic changes mimicking high-output cardiac failure. Patients frequently complain of a dragging sensation in the abdomen, left upper quadrant tenderness or pain, and early satiety. At the same time, they appear to be less prone to splenic infarction than CML patients. Patients with rapidly progressive, acute myelofibrosis can complain of **bone pain** and bone tenderness, especially over the sternum.

Laboratory Studies

A. Complete Blood Count

The routine **CBC** helps distinguish the myelofibrotic from the CML patient (Table 19–5). Patients with myelofibrosis present with a moderate to severe normochromic, normocytic anemia with prominent anisocytosis and poikilocytosis. Nucleated red blood cells and teardrop red blood cells on the peripheral film are characteristic of myelofibrosis and suggest extramedullary hematopoiesis in the spleen (see Figure 19–2). Giant platelets and dysplastic leukocytes **(Pelger-Huët anomaly)** may also be present (Figure 19–5).

TABLE 19–5 • Myelofibrosis hematopoietic profile

Complete blood count (CBC)
Hemoglobin: moderate to severe normocytic anemia
Red blood cell morphology: prominent aniso-/poikilocytosis, with nucleated red blood cells and "teardrop" cells
White blood cell count: near normal
Platelet count: normal to increased or decreased
Marrow (biopsy)
Patchy cellularity: islands of hypercellular marrow
Increased reticulin and collagen
Marked increase in megakaryocytes
Special studies
JAK2 mutation present in approximately 50% of patients; 5% have the *MPL W515* mutation
Ph^1 chromosome: absent unless fibrosis is a late complication of CML

Unlike CML, the myelofibrotic patient will present, especially early in the disease, with a normal or only moderately increased **leukocyte count**. With disease progression, the white blood cell count can fall to subnormal levels as a result of both poor production and increased destruction by the spleen. The **platelet count** may be low, normal, or high when the patient first presents. With treatment and disease progression, platelets can fall to very low levels or increase dramatically to levels in excess of 1 million/μL. Marked thrombocytosis (platelet counts of several million) is commonly observed in patients who have had a therapeutic splenectomy.

B. Marrow Biopsy

Definitive diagnosis of myelofibrosis rests with the marrow biopsy. The marrow is often difficult or impossible to aspirate and a core biopsy is required. Depending on the stage of the disease process, a biopsy can show variable distortions of the marrow structure ranging from complete fibrous replacement (see Figure 19–3A) to patchy losses of hematopoietic and fat cells with islands of residual hyperplastic marrow. Proliferation of immature and abnormal-appearing megakaryocytes can be impressive. Both **trichrome and silver stains** should always be performed to better define the amount of collagen and reticulin fibers in the marrow structure. Increases in reticulin and collagen will depend on the severity and progression of the disease process (see Figure 19–3B).

Myelofibrosis can develop as a **secondary manifestation** in other myeloproliferative disorders. This course is infrequent **in CML** but more common in other *JAK2*-positive diseases such as polycythemia vera and essential thrombocythemia. In this setting, the appearance of the peripheral blood and marrow is similar to that of idiopathic myelofibrosis. Proliferation of megakaryocytes is a prominent component, suggesting a key role for megakaryocyte

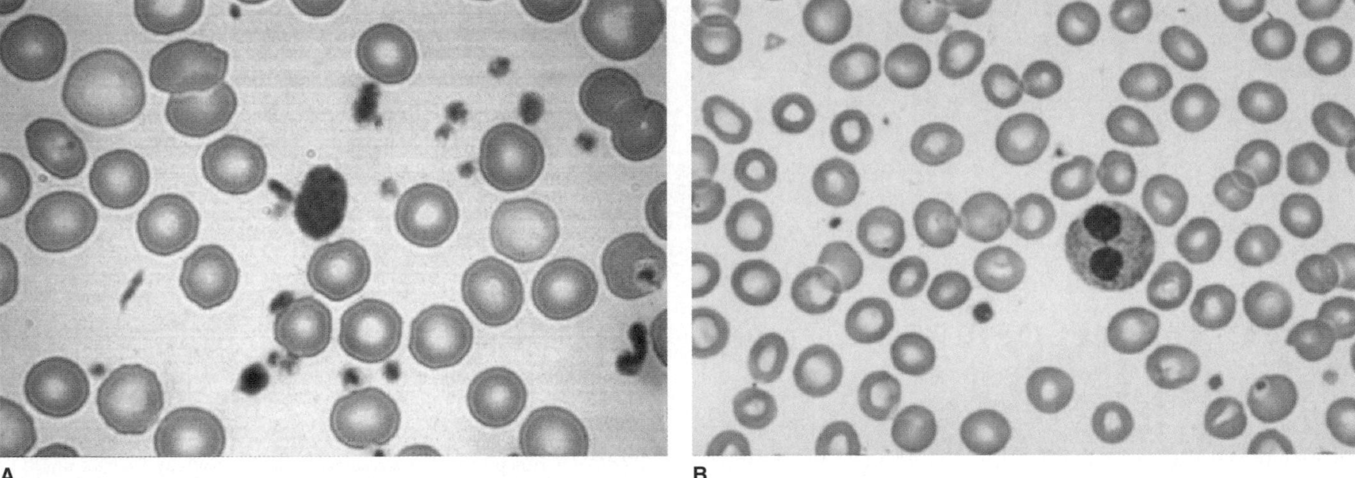

FIGURE 19–5. **Giant platelets and pseudo–Pelger-Huët anomaly.** Giant platelets **(A)**, together with a marked increase in the platelet count are seen in myeloproliferative disorders, especially thrombocythemia. The Pelger-Huët anomaly **(B)**, characterized by dumbbell-shaped nuclei, is seen both with myelodysplastic and myeloproliferative disorders.

and platelet growth factors in stimulating the fibrosis. Patients with widespread malignancies or disseminated tuberculosis can also develop significant marrow fibrosis. It is essential, therefore, to both culture for mycobacterium and carefully inspect the marrow biopsy for nests of malignant cells (Figure 19–6).

Systemic mastocytosis (mast cell leukemia) can present with a hematologic picture similar to that of idiopathic myelofibrosis. Some clinical details, however, help to distinguish these 2 disorders: reddish-brown cutaneous infiltrates, a Darier sign (development of an itchy, red hive upon stroking the skin), diarrhea, and the characteristic radiological appearance of osteoporosis will suggest mastocytosis. Diagnosis is established on finding mast cell infiltrates in the skin or bone marrow biopsy, and most of the patients display a *C-KIT* mutation at codon 816 in cell-sorted samples. T- and B-cell lymphomas, especially hairy-cell leukemia, can also present with some features of myelofibrosis, especially splenomegaly.

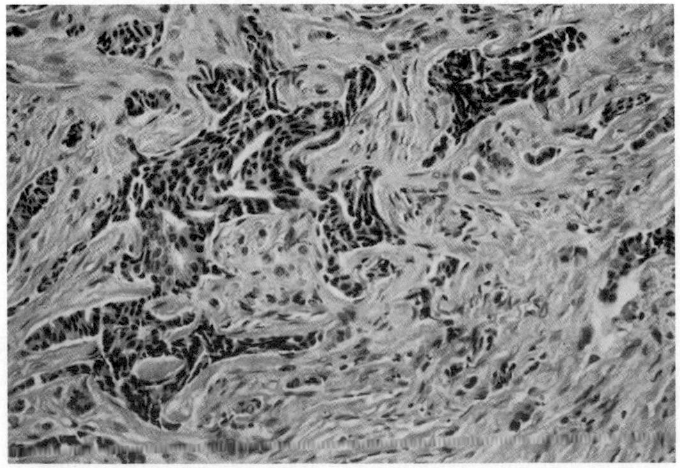

FIGURE 19–6. **Metastatic cancer.** Marrow biopsy specimen infiltrated with metastatic breast cancer and reactive fibrosis (H&E stain).

C. Other Tests

The *JAK2* mutation is present in nearly 50% of patients with primary myelofibrosis. This test, when positive, greatly facilitates the diagnosis. **Chromosomal analysis** is a less rewarding exercise in the diagnosis of idiopathic myelofibrosis. Although chromosomal abnormalities occur in about 30% of patients (see Table 19–3), they do not show a predominant karyotype. Other laboratory measurements follow the pattern of other myeloproliferative disorders. For example, these patients can show an increase in **LDH and blood uric acid levels**. In patients with very high platelet counts, it may be possible to demonstrate **defects in platelet aggregation**. A few patients may manifest a hypercoagulable state. On bone films, osteocondensation or mixed sclerotic and lytic lesions are frequent, which can sometimes mimic bone metastases.

Disease Course

Most patients with idiopathic myelofibrosis follow a protracted course with a median survival between 5 and 8 years. Adverse factors for survival are the *JAK2 V617F* mutation and myelofibrosis arising in the course of polycythemia vera or essential thrombocythemia. Because it is a disorder of older patients, death may result from unrelated causes; only one-third or less of patients will actually die of complications resulting from their hematopoietic disorder. Unlike CML, a small subset (10% or less) of patients will progress to acute leukemia.

PRIMARY THROMBOCYTHEMIA

Primary thrombocythemia (essential thrombocythemia or thrombocytosis) is defined by the presence of a markedly elevated platelet count (600,000/μL–>1 million/μL) in the absence of any other cause of a reactive process. The *JAK2* mutation, which is present in 40%–50% of patients, greatly facilitates the diagnosis. For patients who are *JAK2* negative,

CASE HISTORY • Part 2

A bone marrow aspirate is attempted but is not successful. A biopsy specimen shows marked increase in reticulin and fibrosis as well as increased numbers of dysplastic megakaryocytes.

Cytogenetic and molecular genetic analyses show no evidence for a Philadelphia chromosome or the *BCR-ABL* translocation; however, molecular analysis shows the presence of the *JAK2 V617F* mutation.

Based on these findings a diagnosis of primary myelofibrosis can be made. At the same time, the history of elevated red cells and white cells in the past suggests the possibility that this could represent evolution of a process that may have been active for many years, such as polycythemia vera. The finding of the *JAK2* mutation is compatible with either diagnosis.

Questions

- What are the therapeutic priorities for this patient?
- What is the prognosis at this juncture?

thrombocythemia is a diagnosis of exclusion, which means that any known cause of reactive or clonal thrombocytosis must be considered. This includes iron deficiency, chronic inflammatory disorders, chronic infectious diseases, hyposplenia, and solid malignancies, as well as the other stem cell myeloproliferative disorders such as polycythemia vera, CML, and idiopathic myelofibrosis. In the case of thrombocytosis secondary to inflammation or neoplasia, IL-6 appears to be a primary mediator responsible for overexpression of thrombopoietin mRNA. From the perspective of relative incidence, more than 80% of patients presenting with a platelet count greater than 500,000/μL will have reactive thrombocytosis.

Primary thrombocythemia has been shown by G6PD isoenzyme studies, and more recently by the presence of the *JAK2* mutation, to be a clonal disorder involving all of the hematopoietic cell lines in most patients. The underlying disease mechanism involves a defect in the *c-Mpl* thrombopoietin receptor. This includes both a decreased expression and abnormal binding of thrombopoietin, resulting in higher than normal thrombopoietin levels and, because of this, increased megakaryocyte proliferation.

Most patients with primary thrombocythemia are first detected on routine CBC while they are still asymptomatic. When the **platelet count reaches very high levels**, the most common symptoms are those associated with bleeding owing to platelet dysfunction or the appearance of a hypercoagulable state with thrombosis and microvascular ischemia. During the course of the disease, some 50% of patients will experience at least 1 venous or arterial thrombotic event, ranging from distal vessel thromboses to strokes and coronary artery occlusions to unusual presentations such as Budd-Chiari syndrome or skin necrosis. Patients with higher platelet counts will complain of vasomotor symptoms such as headaches, dizziness, syncope, visual disturbances, paresthesias, acrocyanosis, livedo reticularis, palmar burning, and digital erythromelalgia. These events are related to platelet activation and usually are responsive to treatment with aspirin and a reduction in the platelet count. Patients will have some splenic enlargement, but it is never as prominent as that seen in CML or idiopathic myelofibrosis. The very high platelet counts can result in **splenic infarction and a loss of splenic function**. This will result in the appearance of Howell-Jolly bodies, nucleated red blood cells, and target cells on the peripheral film (see Chapter 2).

Laboratory Studies

A routine **CBC** and **marrow examination** may distinguish primary thrombocythemia from CML, polycythemia vera, and idiopathic myelofibrosis. The very high peripheral platelet count is not accompanied by major changes in the white blood cell or red blood cell lines, although an absolute basophilia is observed in some patients. The marrow may be normocellular or hypercellular, with a normal ratio of erythroid to granulocytic precursors and a normal display of myelocytic precursors. At the same time, the number of megakaryocytes should be dramatically increased. Their morphology is usually normal, but it is common to see large aggregates of megakaryocytes dispersed throughout the marrow aspirate and biopsy. An artifactual hyperkalemia is frequent, due to loss of potassium from the excess platelets in vitro following blood drawing.

For *JAK2*-negative patients, a primary thrombocythemia diagnosis is reached after exclusion of other disease states. The laboratory evaluation should include **iron studies** to rule out iron deficiency or an inflammatory state; **chromosomal analysis** to rule out CML and myelodysplasia, especially the 5q minus syndrome where elevated platelet counts are frequent; and a **bone marrow biopsy** to exclude a diagnosis of myelofibrosis. Polycythemia vera patients with marked thrombocythemia can present with a normal hemoglobin level and red blood cell mass, or even anemia secondary to acute and chronic blood loss. These patients may be recognized because of the marked disparity between the severity of their microcytosis and their mild degree of anemia (see Chapters 5 and 10). Rarely, polycythemia vera will not be detected until after iron replacement is initiated and the hemoglobin level rapidly increases.

Spontaneous in vitro formation of megakaryocyte colonies **(CFU-MK)** in the absence of added growth factors has been reported in patients with primary thrombocytosis. While this has been previously suggested as a diagnostic test for the disease, the phenomenon has also been observed in patients with other myeloproliferative disorders and has been largely replaced by the *JAK2* mutation evaluation.

Disease Course

The overall life expectancy of patients with essential thrombocytosis is near normal (median survival 10–15 years). However, older adults (over age 60) and patients with a history of thrombosis and a platelet count greater than 1.5 million/µL are at a significant increased risk of thrombohemorrhagic complications and need to be treated. Transformation into polycythemia vera, myelofibrosis, or acute leukemia, even with prolonged chemotherapy, is seen in fewer than 5% of patients. There would appear, therefore, to be little downside to extended chemotherapy with hydroxyurea.

CHRONIC EOSINOPHILIC LEUKEMIA

For a long time, cases presenting with very high eosinophil blood counts have been classified as hypereosinophilic syndromes, as their specific cause remained elusive. Recently, chromosomal data obtained in some patients with this presentation have revealed the presence of a recurrent translocation t(1;4)(q44;q12) involving the gene for the receptor of the platelet derived growth factor α (*PDGFR-α*) with a hitherto unknown partner gene (*FIP1L1*). The fusion protein that results from this rearrangement has tyrosine kinase activity.

Patients are generally young adults, more frequently men. The presentation is often asymptomatic for a long period of time. The diagnostic criteria are persistent elevated eosinophil counts above 1,500/µL, absence of known cause of hypereosinophilia, and possible signs of organ damage related to toxicity of eosinophil granule constituents on tissues, the most severe being endomyocardial fibrosis, which can result in a restrictive cardiomyopathy and tricuspid insufficiency. Neurologic manifestations, both central and peripheral; lung infiltrates; skin lesions; and mucous membrane ulcerations are less prominent symptoms.

Laboratory Studies

Blood hypereosinophilia is a constant, isolated, and prominent feature. Eosinophil values are generally above 5,000/µL. Other cell lines are normal. Marrow aspiration shows isolated eosinophil hyperplasia, but a mild fibrosis is frequent on marrow biopsy. Serum tryptase is elevated. Cytogenetic studies have shown the most frequent abnormality being the t(1;4)(q44;q12) translocation and, less commonly, translocations involving chromosome 5 at the site of *PDGFR-β*. In these latter forms, the disease often shares features with chronic myelomonocytic leukemia (see below).

Disease Course

The course is highly dependent on stage and treatment efficacy. Patients responding to treatment with tyrosine kinase inhibitors have a protracted benefit with stabilization, regression, and sometimes disappearance of symptoms. In other cases, however, when tissue symptoms are present prior to instituting therapy, the disease quickly progresses to fatal heart failure or acute leukemia.

CHRONIC MYELOMONOCYTIC LEUKEMIA

Overlapping the myeloproliferative and the myelodysplastic syndromes, chronic myelomonocytic leukemia (CMML) presents in adult (especially elderly) patients as an insidious disease, with manifestations including fatigue, easy bruising, and splenomegaly. The CBC and blood film show an admixture of immature myelocytes and monocytes (>10,000/µL), together with quantitative and qualitative modifications of red cells, neutrophils, and platelets, as generally observed in myelodysplastic syndromes. The combined esterase stain (see Chapter 16) clearly confirms the mixed population of myelocytes and monocytes, even when the cells are immature with few granules. Hyposegmented neutrophils (pseudo–Pelger-Huët abnormality) and mild eosinophilia are frequent. The marrow aspirate shows granulocytic and monocytic hyperplasia, and sometimes a mild increase in myeloblasts. Marrow karyotyping is abnormal in one-third of patients, mainly with translocations recombining 5q33 (*PDGFR-β*) with several gene partners. The fusion products behave as tyrosine kinases and can display sensitivity to TKIs.

Disease Course and Prognosis

CMML has a highly variable course. As discussed in Chapter 9, CMML may have a relatively benign course. Some elderly patients can remain alive and asymptomatic for relatively long periods of time. On the other hand, some patients, especially those with chromosomal abnormalities, more rapidly develop pancytopenia, and 20% of cases evolve over time into an acute myeloid leukemia (AML)-like picture.

JUVENILE MYELOMONOCYTIC LEUKEMIA

Juvenile myelomonocytic leukemia (JMML), observed in young children less than 4–5 years of age, has a presentation similar to adult CMML. However, its mechanism appears quite different as cells in vitro display a high sensitivity to granulocyte macrophage colony-stimulating factor (GM-CSF), which is a hallmark of the disease. Several mutations involving RAS signaling pathways have been described. Infants present with failure to thrive, fever, recurrent infections, and mucous membrane bleeding. Spleen enlargement is almost constant, as well as maculopapular or xanthomatous skin lesions. Blood films show a picture similar to adult CMML. Cytogenetics is either normal or infrequently shows recurrent abnormalities, the most frequent being monosomy 7. The disease displays poor sensitivity to chemotherapeutic regimens and the overall survival is generally less than 3–4 years, unless a stem cell transplant can be performed.

THERAPY

The most important elements of good management of a patient with a myeloproliferative disorder are the accurate diagnosis of the condition and a sense of when to treat the disease. Since many patients are elderly at the time of presentation, aggressive chemotherapy and marrow transplantation are often not feasible. Therefore, watchful waiting with blood product support and single-drug chemotherapy are often more appropriate. The selection of drugs also varies according to the individual disease process. This is especially true for CML, for which TKI therapy has become increasingly effective.

Chronic Myelogenous Leukemia

Until the late 1970s–1980s, CML outcome was invariably lethal as treatment was limited to drugs such as hydroxyurea or busulfan that were unable to eradicate the Ph^1-positive malignant clone. During the last 20 years, 3 treatment modalities, that is, allogeneic bone marrow transplantation, interferon-α, and more recently the TKIs have demonstrated their ability not only to reduce but even to eradicate the malignant clone. In fact, true remissions (Ph^1 negative) and durable disease-free survivals can be achieved when patients are treated with imatinib, interferon-α, or allogeneic marrow transplantation. Success depends on several factors including the patient's age, the timing of the treatment according to the phase of the disease, and the innate responsiveness of the CML. In essence, younger patients who are diagnosed and treated early in the chronic phase of their illness and who have a very responsive leukemic stem cell do the best. Control of *BCR-ABL* residual disease is most likely dependent on an effective immune response against the *BCR-ABL* clone. This is best illustrated by the presence of cytotoxic T cells directed against CML-specific epitopes in patients maintained in stable, complete molecular responses after interferon or allogeneic transplantation, as well as the graft versus leukemia effect that can be induced by donor lymphocyte infusions in allogeneic stem cell recipients.

A. BCR-ABL Tyrosine Kinase Inhibitors

A specific inhibitor of the Ph^1 chromosome *BCR-ABL* tyrosine kinase, **imatinib mesylate** (Gleevec), has shown significant activity in both the chronic and blast phases of CML and in the treatment of Ph^1-positive ALL. A large multicenter trial has compared imatinib 400 mg/d to interferon plus cytarabine in previously untreated patients in chronic phase. Long-term results from this trial show that 87% of patients receiving imatinib are in complete cytogenetic response at 60 months, and the estimated overall survival is 89%, reaching 95% when only CML-related deaths are considered. Imatinib has also been shown to be effective in patients who have failed interferon-α therapy. In addition, responses have been reported in more than 50% of patients with myeloblastic crises and 70% of patients with lymphoblastic crises or Ph^1-positive ALL. However, unlike chronic-phase patients, most blastic crisis patients relapsed while receiving therapy. Adverse side effects are described as minimal and include nausea, myalgias, edema, diarrhea, and in some patients, abnormal bleeding.

Because of its low toxicity and effectiveness in the early phases of CML, imatinib has now become the treatment of choice. Current trials support the use of high-dose imatinib, 400 mg orally twice a day, both because of its greater efficacy in inducing a complete molecular remission (absence of *BCR-ABL* RNA) and as a way to reduce the development of resistance. When the response is incomplete or because of resistance to imatinib (Ph^1-positive cells persist in the marrow or less than a 3-log reduction in RNA product in blood), higher-dose imatinib therapy may be more effective but yields poorer hematologic tolerance, which, in some patients, can be mitigated by the use of growth factors. A better approach to higher dose imatinib is the use of one of the newer tyrosine kinase inhibitors.

Second-generation TKIs have now reached the clinic. They offer improved efficacy and can overcome some of the resistance mechanisms resulting from mutation within the tyrosine kinase domain. **Dasatinib**, a "dual inhibitor" as it inhibits TKs together with src kinase, is roughly 300 times more active in vitro when compared with imatinib and displays activity against most of the resistant mutated clones, with the exception of *T315I*. In a pivotal study, patients insensitive or intolerant to imatinib experienced 52% major cytogenetic responses. The recommended optimal dosage is 100 mg once a day. Tolerance is good, although some patients have developed pleural effusions that resolved with stopping the drug or reducing its dose. **Nilotinib** is equally active on non-*T315I* resistant cells, and the results observed in imatinib-resistant patients compare with those of dasatinib. The recommended dosage is 400 mg twice a day. Both drugs are currently under study for first-line treatment of CML. **Bosutinib** is another "dual inhibitor" currently being tested in phase II/III trials. Finally, MK-0457, an Aurora kinase inhibitor, appears to be promising as it retains activity against *T315I* mutations.

Patients can develop resistance to the effects of imatinib, especially when it is given at lower doses. Several mechanisms of resistance have been identified, with mutations within the tyrosine kinase activity site being the most frequent. Some of these mutations can be overcome with a dosage increase or switch to another TKI such as dasatinib, nilotinib, or bosutinib. However, a mutation in codon 315 induces an invariable resistance to TKIs, and therefore is associated with a poor response and prognosis.

Long-term control of the malignant clone with imatinib is a major issue in as much as patients stopping imatinib while in complete remission (Ph^1-negative for 2 years) have experienced molecular relapse. This observation supports the concept of continuous TKI treatment, or combining it with other treatment modalities that are capable of suppressing residual disease, such as allogeneic bone marrow transplantation. Of note, previous treatment with imatinib does not alter the morbidity and outcome of stem cell transplantation when patients switch to this procedure.

B. Interferon-α

Prior to the success of imatinib, interferon-α was the preferred drug in the initial treatment of the chronic phase of CML. It now must be considered a poor second choice. Interferon therapy can improve overall survival by about 20 months when compared with hydroxyurea or busulfan therapy. Normalization of the CBC can be achieved in 70%–80% of patients and a Ph^1-negative remission in up to 30% of patients. However, residual malignant cells can still be detected by polymerase chain reaction (PCR) measurement of the *BCR-ABL* translocation. Still, a complete cytogenetic response does predict a more durable remission.

The effectiveness of interferon therapy correlates with the maximum dose tolerated by the patient. Lower-dose regimens (2×10^6 U/m^2 given subcutaneously or intramuscularly 3 times per week) will improve the blood counts in most patients but will not produce a complete cytogenetic response. A dose of 5×10^6 U/m^2 given 3 times a week or, if tolerated, daily is needed to achieve a complete cytogenetic response. The rate of response is slow. If the initial granulocyte count exceeds 100,000/μL, the patient should be first treated with hydroxyurea (see below) to lower the count to below 20,000/μL. The hydroxyurea should then be continued during the first 2–3 months to prevent a count rebound. Interferon therapy is best started at a reduced dose, 3×10^6 U/d for 1–2 weeks followed by 5×10^6 U/d for another 1–2 weeks, before escalating to full dose. Otherwise, the patient will show poor tolerance for the interferon.

Patients are slow to respond to interferon. Therapy must be given continually for 1 year or more because the maximum response may not occur for 12–18 months. A major downside is when interferon is given for more than 6 months, the success rate of a subsequent marrow transplant may be significantly reduced. Therefore, a **decision regarding transplantation needs to made in the first 6 months** and the transplant completed during the first year. Transplantation should be seriously considered when a significant hematologic remission is not reached by 6 months. If a major cytogenetic remission is achieved, the interferon should be continued for 2–3 years. The patient should then be followed off therapy using a sensitive assay (PCR or FISH assay) for the re-emergence of Ph^1-positive cells. The projected 6- to 8-year survival rate for patients with major cytogenetic responses is better than 85%, and the 10%–20% mortality with transplantation is avoided.

Interferon-α therapy is associated with several side effects. With each injection, patients experience a flu-like syndrome with fever, chills, and anorexia. **Severe, persistent fatigue, depression, weight loss**, and the **appearance of autoimmune-mediated organ damage** (cardiomyopathy, collagen vascular disorders, hypothyroidism, hemolysis, and thrombocytopenia) will require **dose reductions**. As a rule, the dose administered will need to be cut by 25%–50% when there is evidence of organ damage or severe leukopenia or thrombocytopenia (absolute leukocyte count below 2,000/μL or platelet count below 60,000/μL). Up to 20% of patients will not be able to tolerate the drug. Rarely, severe organ damage, especially cardiac disease with arrhythmias or congestive failure, will require discontinuation of the drug.

C. Hydroxyurea

Hydroxyurea has been used in the past to treat CML. However, it is now obsolete, and with few exceptions has little or no place in the treatment strategies of CML. However, hydroxyurea continues to be used in the treatment of other myeloproliferative disorders, primarily for palliation and relief of symptoms due to splenomegaly and reduction of extremely elevated platelet and leukocyte counts, and therefore is briefly discussed here.

Hydroxyurea is an inhibitor of DNA synthesis and acts by blocking cell division and marrow precursor maturation. It does not affect the malignant stem cells, and therefore does not produce a cytogenetic remission. Because hydroxyurea blocks maturation of all hematopoietic cell lines, patients become markedly megaloblastic and develop a peripheral macrocytosis. It can be very effective in the treatment of patients with very high granulocyte counts (>100,000/μL) in myeloproliferative disorders. Given as an oral dose of 2–8 g/d, hydroxyurea will rapidly reduce the granulocyte count, generally within 48–72 hours. In a similar fashion, hydroxyurea will reduce the platelet count in primary thrombocythemia patients whose platelet counts rise to levels above 1 million/μL. Hydroxyurea in doses less than 2 g per day has few if any side effects, but its long-term use can be limited by its impact on red cell and leukocyte production.

D. Bone Marrow Transplantation

1. Allogeneic marrow transplantation—Allogeneic marrow transplantation was recommended as first-line therapy for younger CML patients with a matched sibling donor before the era of TKIs. It is not without risk; the procedure itself carries a risk of 5%–20% acute mortality. In addition, survivors have to deal with some degree of GVHD in order to achieve the 50%–75% chance of a prolonged disease-free survival when transplanted during the chronic phase.

The best results are achieved when transplantation is carried out early in the chronic phase of CML. Once the disease progresses, the chance of an effective transplant decreases dramatically. When the patient has had the disease for more than 2 years, a positive result can be expected less than 50% of the time. If the disease enters the accelerated phase, the results fall to nearer 20%–40%, and patients in blastic crisis have only a 15%–20% chance of achieving any significant remission. The preparative regimen also makes a difference; patients who achieved a Ph^1-negative remission with TKI therapy do the best.

2. Unrelated HLA-matched donor transplants—Unrelated HLA-matched donors have been used extensively in the marrow transplantation of CML patients. In the ideal situation, unrelated donor transplants appear to be as or more effective than an HLA-matched sibling transplant: disease-free survival is 75% if the transplant is done in the first year. It is self-evident, however, that patients who use the unrelated donor pool for their transplant will often have progressed further in their disease, been exposed to more chemotherapy, and be somewhat older. Because of a higher rate of transplant-associated deaths, overall disease-free survival for patients receiving transplants from unrelated donors is approximately 30%–40% at 5 years, and there is a significantly higher incidence of severe GVHD.

Late relapses are seen in CML patients with transplants, suggesting that transplantation will never result in a guaranteed cure. This situation may reflect a persistence of the rare leukemic stem cell or an environmental factor that leads to reemergence of the clone. The antileukemic effect of acute and chronic GVHD also plays a role. Patients who receive T-cell–depleted marrow transplants have a 5-fold increased risk of relapse. This is also true for twin transplants and for patients who receive immunosuppressive therapy for their GVHD. It is perhaps the best example of the **graft-versus-leukemia (GVL)** effect of donor lymphocytes.

In patients who relapse following transplant, **donor lymphocyte transfusions** have been used successfully to reinduce remission. From 70%–90% of patients with a hematologic or cytogenetic relapse will respond, usually after a 2- to 3-month course of multiple transfusions of donor T cells. Patients who develop grade 2 or higher GVHD as a result of the therapy do best, demonstrating a better than 90% remission rate. The mechanism behind this effect is still unclear. Experimental data would suggest, however, that the T-cell GVL effect is distinct from the GVHD effect, and that infusions of CD8 (suppressor) T-cell–depleted donor lymphocytes will give the GVL effect with far less GVHD.

3. Autologous marrow transplantation—Attempts to use autologous marrow transplantation have not been effective in CML. In this case, the inability to completely eradicate the malignant cell line with chemotherapy and the absence of a GVL effect may guarantee failure. However, it has been observed that during culture in vitro, the Ph^1-containing stem cells may not survive as well as normal stem cells.

4. Non-myeloablative allogeneic transplantation—An alternative approach to full allogeneic transplantation is being investigated. It consists of reduced doses of myelosuppressive drugs followed by relatively large infusions of donor stem cells. This results in partial engraftment of donor cells (mixed chimerism) with reduced severity of GVHD but preservation of the GVL effect of the donor immune cells. Another investigative approach is to follow allogeneic transplantation with infusions of donor lymphocytes, the intent being to augment the GVL phenomenon without significantly worsening GVHD. Results with these approaches can compare with full myeloablative stem cell transplants. They offer the opportunity to extend the indications for stem cell transplantation in CML for patients who are up to 65–70 years old.

E. Choice of the Appropriate Therapy

The TKIs are now the recommended first-line treatment for management of CML. Patients treated with imatinib during the chronic phase of their illness achieve maximum control of their hematologic abnormalities with minimal side effects. Second-generation TKIs are suitable for patients with imatinib intolerance or resistance with the exception of the *T315I* mutation. These TKIs have completely replaced interferon and stem cell transplant as initial treatments in the chronic phase of CML. However, for patients in accelerated or blastic phase, allogeneic stem cell transplantation is recommended as soon as possible, after a short course of imatinib at a higher dose (600–800 mg/d), with the aim of improving hematological status before the transplant procedure.

Myelofibrosis

Patients with myelofibrosis are classically managed conservatively. Most often, the disease process follows a chronic, slowly progressive course, and patients can simply be observed. **Symptomatic anemia** will respond adequately to periodic red blood cell transfusion, unless the patient develops hypersplenism with an increased rate of red blood cell destruction. Patients who develop **hypersplenism** may be candidates for **splenectomy**. Splenectomy may also play a role in decreasing the rate of progression of the marrow fibrosis. It is difficult, however, to predict the outcome of a splenectomy. Often, the patient's condition is worsened both by a spread of the extramedullary hematopoiesis to the liver and other tissues and a post-splenectomy rise in the platelet count to levels in excess of 1 million/μL. Splenectomy is most successful in those patients with symptomatic splenomegaly, with overt portal hypertension, and progressive, transfusion-dependent anemia. Severe thrombocytopenia and a hypocellular marrow are adverse indicators for response to splenectomy. Splenic irradiation has been used effectively to control the splenomegaly and hypersplenism. Ninety percent of patients will respond to repeated irradiation. However, splenic irradiation is associated, at times, with severe myelosuppression, even aplastic anemia.

Marrow transplantation has been used successfully in young patients with myelofibrosis. Of interest, the marked fibrosis of the marrow can be reversed if the patient's malignant cell lines are eliminated and a successful transplant is achieved. The number of patients who are reasonable candidates for transplantation is relatively small, however. Since myelofibrosis is an illness of middle-aged and older patients, the risk of procedural death and severe GVHD is also very high. It has been reported that **2-CDA therapy** will also result in a decrease in marrow fibrosis. Non-myeloablative allogeneic transplantation may have something to offer to this older patient population. Very promising results have recently been observed with a novel *JAK2* inhibitor (referred to as INCB018424) and tipifarnib, a farnesyltransferase inhibitor, in both primary and secondary myelofibrosis, the latter including post–polycythemia vera or essential thrombocythemia patients.

Primary Thrombocythemia

Age greater than 60 years, a history of at least 1 thrombotic event, or platelet counts greater than 1–1.5 × 10^6/μL are adverse prognostic signs that dictate a need for treatment. Patients with primary thrombocythemia can usually be controlled with **chemotherapy**. Several single-agent drug regimens have been used, including hydroxyurea, anagrelide, interferon-α, and in selected cases, alkylating agents. Since the course of the disease can be prolonged, **hydroxyurea** may be considered the drug of choice. Although its use is associated with the development of both anemia and granulocytopenia, the fears of hydroxyurea-induced acute leukemia or myelodysplasia in patients receiving long-term therapy have not been confirmed. The use of regimens containing alkylating agents is discouraged because of the higher risk of secondary malignancies.

Anagrelide can be effective in resistant patients. If one begins with a daily oral dose of 0.5 mg 2–4 times per day and

CASE HISTORY • Part 3

The presence of cachexia and weight loss, as well as significant anemia and marked splenomegaly, suggest that this patient has severe myelofibrosis and a poor prognosis. Treatment priorities include red cell transfusions to alleviate the anemia. However, the effectiveness of transfusion therapy may be in jeopardy since her low WBC and platelet counts suggest hypersplenism may be playing a role in her disease. As a result she should be evaluated for splenectomy with a careful consideration of her suitability as a surgical candidate. Splenic irradiation is a possible alternative. She is at the upper limit of the age range for allogeneic stem cell transplantation, but this could be considered once she has improved symptomatically. Of course, transplantation will depend on her overall medical evaluation and the availability of a matched donor or the possibility of a non-myeloablative transplant protocol.

then escalating the dose by 0.5 mg/d at 1- to 2-week intervals, the platelet count should fall below 600,000/μL within 1 month. Continuous maintenance is required, since like hydroxyurea, anagrelide interferes with platelet maturation, not megakaryocyte proliferation. Side effects are frequent and include headache, fluid retention, diarrhea, nausea, abdominal pain, and, in elderly patients, congestive heart failure. Patients with known heart disease should be given the drug with caution. In a recent trial comparing anagrelide plus aspirin to hydroxyurea plus aspirin, anagrelide was associated with a significant excess of arterial thrombosis, bleeding, and myelofibrotic transformation, and thus should be considered as second-line therapy.

Interferon can be used in hydroxyurea or anagrelide failures, but at considerable cost and toxicity. Treatment is initiated with 3 million units subcutaneously 3 times a week.

Use of **antiplatelet agents** other than aspirin in the treatment and prevention of thrombotic events is somewhat controversial. **Aspirin** is effective in patients with recurrent thromboses, especially arterial thrombi or microvascular ischemia. It is contraindicated in patients with a history of abnormal or gastrointestinal bleeding.

Chronic Eosinophilic Leukemia

Steroids (prednisone) have remained for a long time the effective treatment of hypereosinophilic syndrome. Responding patients are expected to have a 70% survival rate. However, steroid side effects or resistance lead to a need for alternative drugs including hydroxyurea, vincristine, methotrexate, or other cytotoxic agents. More recently, recombinant interferon-α, cyclosporine, and anti–IL-5 monoclonal antibodies have demonstrated efficacy. However, the recent discovery of imatinib-sensitive cases, especially but not only in patients demonstrating *PDGFR-α* translocations, has led to trials of imatinib. Complete response, including molecular ones, can be achieved with moderate doses of imatinib (100–400 mg/d), which now appears to be the treatment of choice in these cases.

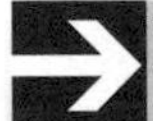

POINTS TO REMEMBER

The myeloproliferative disorders are all clonal disorders of the hematopoietic stem cell. Although they usually present with disease expression in a single cell line, all hematopoietic cell lines are affected to some extent. Over time, this can result in a variable disease course and considerable overlap of clinical findings.

CML is unique in that its pathogenesis depends upon the presence of the *BCR-ABL* fusion protein, which has tyrosine kinase activity. Based on this, treatment with the tyrosine kinase inhibitor imatinib has shown great clinical success. In fact, it has revolutionized the treatment of CML.

A small proportion of CML patients will become resistant to imatinib. They may respond to an increased dose of imatinib or, even better, one of the newer tyrosine kinase inhibitors—dasatinib, nilotinib, or bosutinib—if the *T315I* mutation is not present.

Polycythemia vera (see Chapter 13), primary myelofibrosis, and primary thrombocythemia share the *JAK2* mutation. This is of considerable value in diagnosis and is a potential future therapeutic target.

When the *JAK2* mutation is not detected, the diagnosis becomes largely one of exclusion. The differential diagnosis of polycythemia vera is discussed in detail in Chapter 13. Myelofibrosis is frequently seen with the progression of disease in polycythemia vera, CML, and refractory anemia with excess blasts (RAEB) patients and in association with systemic tuberculosis and solid tumors (breast, lung, and prostate) metastatic to the bone marrow.

There is a considerable overlap between the myeloproliferative disorders and the myelodysplastic disorders (see Chapter 9). Evolution from a dysplastic state (RAEB) to a myeloproliferative state, either CMML or AML, is a relatively common occurrence.

Treatment goals for all of the myeloproliferative disorders begin with preventing vascular events (thrombosis or bleeding) followed by relief of symptoms due to anemia, thrombocytosis, and organomegaly, and then to improving survival and possible cure. Only successful allogeneic stem cell transplantation is currently known to be curative.

BIBLIOGRAPHY

Cytogenetics and Molecular Characterization of Chronic Myeloproliferative Diseases

Haferlach T, Bacher U, Kern W, Schnittger S, Haferlach C: The diagnosis of BCR/ABL-negative chronic myeloproliferative diseases (CMPD): a comprehensive approach based on morphology, cytogenetics, and molecular markers. Ann Hematol 2008;87:1.

Pardanani A: JAK2 inhibitor therapy in myeloproliferative disorders: rationale, preclinical studies and ongoing clinical trials. Leukemia 2008;22:23.

Smith CA, Fan G: The saga of JAK2 mutations and translocations in hematologic disorders: pathogenesis, diagnostic and therapeutic prospects, and revised World Health Organization diagnostic criteria for myeloproliferative neoplasms. Hum Pathol 2008;39:795.

Tefferi A: The history of myeloproliferative disorders: before and after Dameshek. Leukemia 2008;22:3.

Tiedt R, Hao-Shen H, Sobas MA, et al: Ratio of mutant JAK2-V617F to wild-type Jak2 determines the MPD phenotypes in transgenic mice. Blood 2008;111:3931.

Chronic Myelogenous Leukemia

Azam M, Latek RR, Daley GQ: Mechanisms of autoinhibition and STI-571/imatinib resistance revealed by mutagenesis of BCR-ABL. Cell 2003;112:831.

Burchert A, Wölfl S, Schmidt M, et al: Interferon-alpha, but not the ABL-kinase inhibitor imatinib (STI571), induces expression of myeloblastin and a specific T-cell response in chronic myeloid leukemia. Blood 2003;101:259.

Calabretta B, Perrotti D: The biology of CML blast crisis. Blood 2004;103:4010.

Druker BJ et al: Activity of a specific inhibitor of the BCR-ABL tyrosine kinase in the blast crisis of chronic myeloid leukemia and acute lymphoblastic leukemia with the Philadelphia chromosome. N Engl J Med 2001;344:1038.

Druker BJ et al: Efficacy and safety of a specific inhibitor of the BCR-ABL tyrosine kinase in chronic myeloid leukemia. N Engl J Med 2001;344:1031.

Druker BJ, Guilhot F, O'Brien SG, et al: Five-year follow-up of patients receiving imatinib for chronic myeloid leukemia. N Engl J Med 2006;355:2408.

El-Zimaity MHT, Kantarjian H, Talpaz M, et al: Results of imatinib mesylate therapy in chronic myelogenous leukaemia with variant Philadelphia chromosome. Brit J Haematol 2004; 125:187.

Giralt S et al: CD8-depleted donor lymphocyte infusion as treatment for relapsed chronic myelogenous leukemia after allogeneic bone marrow transplantation. Blood 1995;86:4337.

Goldman JM: How I treat chronic myeloid leukemia in the imatinib era. Blood 2007;110:2828.

Goldman JM, Melo JVl: Chronic myeloid leukemia: advances in biology and new approaches to treatment. N Engl J Med 2003;349:1451.

Hasford J et al: Prognosis and prognostic factors for patients with chronic myeloid leukemia: nontransplant therapy. Semin Hematol 2003;40:4.

Hehlmann R, Hochhaus A, Baccarani M, European LeukemiaNet: Chronic myeloid leukaemia. Lancet 2007;370:342.

Hochhaus A, Druker B, Sawyers C, et al: Favorable long-term follow-up results over 6 years for response, survival, and safety with imatinib mesylate therapy in chronic-phase chronic myeloid leukemia after failure of interferon-treatment. Blood 2008;111:1039.

Kantarjian HM et al: High-dose imatinib mesylate therapy in newly diagnosed Philadelphia chromosome-positive chronic phase chronic myeloid leukemia. Blood 2004;103:2873.

Kantarjian HM, Cortes JE, O'Brien S, et al: Long-term survival benefit and improved complete cytogenetic and molecular response rates with imatinib mesylate in Philadelphia chromosome–positive chronic-phase chronic myeloid leukemia after failure of interferon. Blood 2004;104:1979.

Kantarjian H, Schiffer C, Jones D, Cortes J: Monitoring the response and course of chronic myeloid leukemia in the modern era of BCR-ABL tyrosine kinase inhibitors: practical advice on the use and interpretation of monitoring methods. Blood 2008;111:1774.

Kavalerchik E, Goff D, Jamieson CH: Chronic myeloid leukemia stem cells. J Clin Oncol 2008;26:2911.

Kolb H et al: Graft-versus-leukemia effect of donor lymphocyte transfusions in marrow grafted patients. Blood 1995; 86:2041.

Martinelli G: Atypical chronic myeloproliferative disorders: genes and imatinib-sensitive targets. Semin Hematol 2007;44:S1.

Molldrem JJ, Lee PP, Wang C, et al: Evidence that specific T lymphocytes may participate in the elimination of chronic myelogenous leukemia. Nat Med 2000;6:1018.

Oehler VG, Gooley T, Snyder DS, et al: The effects of imatinib mesylate treatment before allogeneic transplantation for chronic myeloid leukemia. Blood 2007;109:1782.

Press RD, Love Z, Tronnes AA, et al: BCR-ABL mRNA levels at and after the time of a complete cytogenetic response (CCR) predict the duration of CCR in imatinib mesylate–treated patients with CML. Blood 2006;107:4250.

Rousselot P, Huguet F, Rea D, et al: Imatinib mesylate discontinuation in patients with chronic myelogenous leukemia in complete molecular remission for more than 2 years. Blood 2007;109:58.

Savage DG, Szydio RM, Goldman JM: Clinical features at diagnosis in 430 patients with chronic myeloid leukemia seen at a referral centre over a 16 year period. Br J Hematol 1997;96:111.

Schiffer CA: BCR-ABL tyrosine kinase inhibitors for chronic myelogenous leukemia. N Engl J Med 2007;357:258.

Talpaz M, Shah NP, Hagop Kantarjian. et al: Dasatinib in imatinib-resistant philadelphia chromosome–positive leukemias. N Engl J Med 2006;354:2531.

Myelofibrosis

Abgrall JF, Guibaud I, Bastie JN, et al: Thalidomide versus placebo in myeloid metaplasia with myelofibrosis: a prospective, randomized, double-blind, multicenter study. Haematologica 2006;91:1027.

Barosi G, Hoffman R: Idiopathic myelofibrosis. Semin Hematol 2005;42:248.

Campbell PJ, Griesshammer M, Dôhner K, et al: V617F mutation in JAK2 is associated with poorer survival in idiopathic myelofibrosis. Blood 2006;107:2098.

Kröger N, Thiele J, Zander A, et al: Rapid regression of bone marrow fibrosis after dose-reduced allogeneic stem cell transplantation in patients with primary myelofibrosis. Exp Hematol 2007;35:1719.

Mesa RA, Camoriano JK, Geyer SM, et al: A phase II trial of tipifarnib in myelofibrosis: primary, post-polycythemia vera and post-essential thrombocythemia. Leukemia 2007;21:1964.

Tefferi A: Pathogenesis of myelofibrosis with myeloid metaplasia. J Clin Oncol 2005;23:8520.

Essential Thrombocythemia

Finazzi G, Harrison C: Essential thrombocythemia. Semin Hematol 2005;42:230.

Gisslinger H: Update on diagnosis and management of essential thrombocythemia. Semin Thromb Hemost 2006;32:430.

Harrison CN, Campbell PJ, Buck G, et al: Hydroxyurea compared with anagrelide in high-risk essential thrombocythemia. N Engl J Med 2005;353:33.

Schafer AI: Thrombocytosis. N Engl J Med 2004;350:1211.

Chronic Eosinophilic Leukemia

Bain B: Cytogenetic and molecular genetic aspects of eosinophilic leukaemias. Brit J Haematol 2003;122:173.

Martinelli G, Rondoni M, Ottaviani E, Paolini S, Baccarani M: Hypereosinophilic syndrome and molecularly targeted therapy. Semin Hematol 2007;44:S4.

NORMAL LYMPHOPOIESIS AND THE LYMPHATIC SYSTEM · 20

Normal lymphopoiesis is an essential component in host defense. It involves the proliferation and function of several types of lymphoid cells including **B cells**, which are the antibody-producing cells; **T cells**, which carry out cell-mediated immune functions and are largely responsible for regulatory control of the immune system; and the **natural killer (NK) cells**, which function more in a macrophage-like role in host defense against infection and malignancy. An understanding of normal lymphopoiesis requires knowledge of individual cell characteristics and expected responses of these cells to disease states.

LYMPHOID STEM CELLS

The earliest lymphoid stem cell is derived from the totipotent stem cell pool of the marrow. However, both B cells and T cells then mature in other lymphoid tissues. The thymus plays a major role in developing T cells. Precursors leave the marrow and migrate to the thymus, where they develop into immunocompetent cells. It is in the environment of the thymus that the T cell develops its critical ability to distinguish self from non-self and where errors in development form the basis for most, if not all, autoimmune disease. The stages of T-cell development in the thymus are well defined and form the basis for the clinical approach to the classification of T-cell malignancies.

B-cell development takes place in the marrow and peripheral lymphoid tissues, the lymph nodes, and spleen. The stages of B-cell development are not as clearly defined as those of T cells, forming more of a continuum leading to the end stage plasma cell. In addition to their classical role in the production of antibodies, B cells also serve as **antigen-presenting cells**. They have the ability to localize and process antigens from the environment and to present these antigens to other cells of the immune system just like macrophages. Regulatory T cells largely control their development and function. Therefore, it is sometimes difficult when presented with a disease secondary to immune dysfunction to assign root cause to the B- or T-cell system simply because the 2 systems are so intimately intertwined.

The Immune Network

One important concept for disorders of the immune system is the **"immune network."** Cells of the immune system make no basic distinction between internal antigen (ie, a component of self) and external antigen (ie, a pathogen or molecule arising from mutation or transplantation). All chemical structures in the body, including proteins, carbohydrates, and to a lesser extent lipids, are recognized by immune cells. This includes the components and products of the immune cells themselves. The "immune network" is balanced in such a way, however, that those cells that recognize self-antigens are suppressed but not eliminated, and those cells recognizing foreign antigens are stimulated but not allowed to become predominant. Thus, the immune system can be looked on as a balanced network of positive and negative interactions that is controlled by intertwined feedback systems (Figure 20–1).

Although we understand the principles that control the immune network, and have some clear examples of how it functions, it is too complex to describe completely. Autoimmunity is a necessary, even critical part of the immune system. Disease results from a disruption of the normal balance, that is, emergence of uncontrolled autoimmunity, inappropriate suppression of the ability of cells to recognize a foreign antigen, or uncontrolled proliferation of 1 or more clones of lymphocytes. However, simple disease explanations, such as "too many suppressor cells" or "too few helper cells," are viewed with great skepticism because they do not present the complete clinical picture of immune dysfunction.

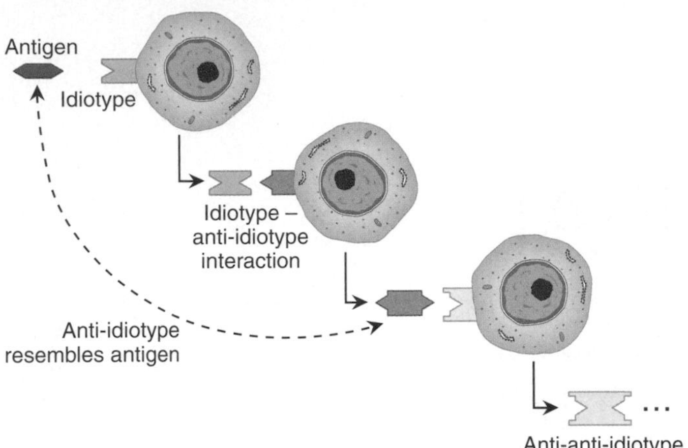

FIGURE 20–1. **The "immune network."** The immune network consists of a cascade of interacting cells with specificity for antigen and for each other. The first cell that responds to antigen creates an antibody that is itself antigenic for other cells. The idiotype of this antibody stimulates production of "anti-idiotype" antibodies that resemble, antigenically, the original antigen. This series of interactions continues and results in a balanced network of stimulatory and suppressive interactions that control the immune system.

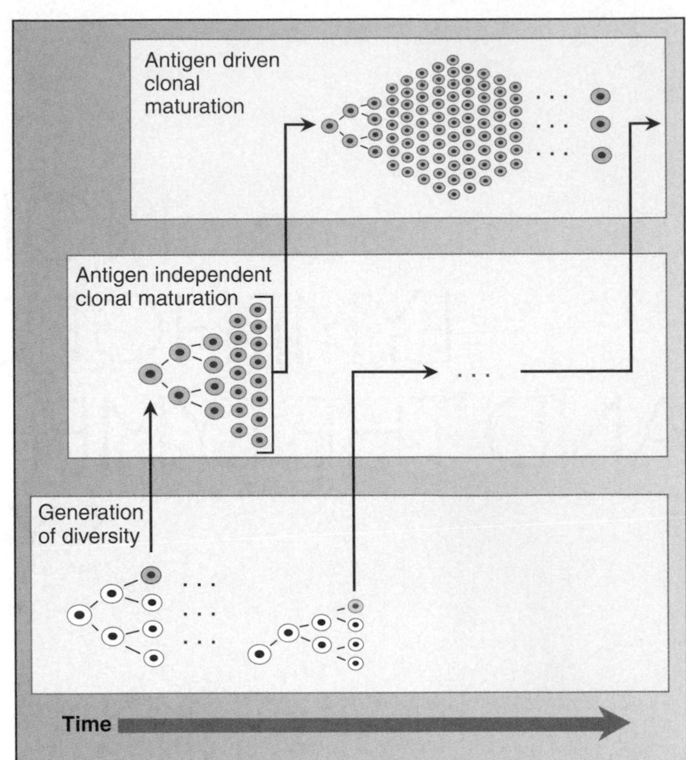

FIGURE 20–2. **Lymphocyte development.** Both B and T cells develop along a multidimensional pathway. On the first level is the continuous process of gene rearrangement, taking place in lymphoid progenitors, which results in the generation of the diverse repertoire of the immune response. This process begins in the fetus and continues throughout life. As cells with new specificities arise, their development moves to the level of antigen-independent clonal maturation, which results in the production of a clone of cells with the same specificity capable of recognizing a specific antigen. Although all of the cells of a given specificity will have the same antigen-receptor molecules, they may differ in other respects depending on their stage of maturation at this level. Finally, when the cells of a given clone encounter specific antigen, they begin to mature on a new level with the result that they give rise to both the fully differentiated cells of the immune system (plasma cells in the case of B cells, and effector T cells) and also to memory cells. As the antigen-driven clonal expansion fades, the memory cells survive and are capable of mounting a secondary response should antigen reappear.

Lymphoid Cell Development

Another important concept in development of the immune system is that it is not a linear process. Development of erythrocytes or neutrophils is normally characterized by a series of recognizable steps in maturation with no possibility of return to a more immature cell form or independent clonal expansion. This characteristic has served as the foundation for classifying myeloproliferative disorders. This is not true, however, for lymphoid cells. Both B cells and T cells develop in a 3-dimensional manner (Figure 20–2). This complex maturation can be simplified to a linear, recognizable morphologic pathway (Figure 20–3). However, unlike myelocytes, developing lymphoid cells, by the process of gene rearrangement, are able to program themselves to respond to a wide variety of antigens. This results in the appearance of clones of lymphocytes with the ability to recognize and react to a specific antigen. Whenever these cells encounter that antigen, they are stimulated to begin a new round of proliferation and differentiation typical of the mature immune response, both cellular and humoral.

This complex pattern of proliferation and differentiation makes it difficult to determine the history and future of a lymphoid cell simply from its morphology. For example, an activated, proliferating T-cell can be a cell that has never encountered antigen but is proliferating in the normal course of expanding the number of antigen-reactive cells. On the other hand, it may be a T-cell that has recently encountered antigen and is proliferating to give rise to programmed cytotoxic effector and memory cells. Or it may be a cell that has undergone an oncogenic mutation and is on the way to produce a lymphoma. In each case, we would call such a cell a blast, and the morphologic, immunologic, and cytogenetic tools that we now have could not distinguish between the several possibilities. In order to clinically define the condition, whether benign or malignant, the entire pattern of the disease process must be examined.

LYMPHOID GROWTH FACTORS

Several growth factors **(interleukins)** that regulate the development and function of lymphocytes have now been identified. The precise regulatory roles of each of the interleukins still need to be defined. It is apparent that they function in a complex and overlapping way to control lymphocyte development. In some cases, interleukins affect other cell lineages as, for example, the role of interleukin-3 in myelocyte and erythrocyte production. Thus, the descriptions that follow are not meant to be exhaustive but simply to provide examples of the roles of some of these growth factors in cell development and function.

Interleukin-1

Interleukin-1 (IL-1) is produced by several different cell types and has a wide range of effects as part of acute and chronic inflammation. For example, IL-1 induces proliferation of thymocytes and

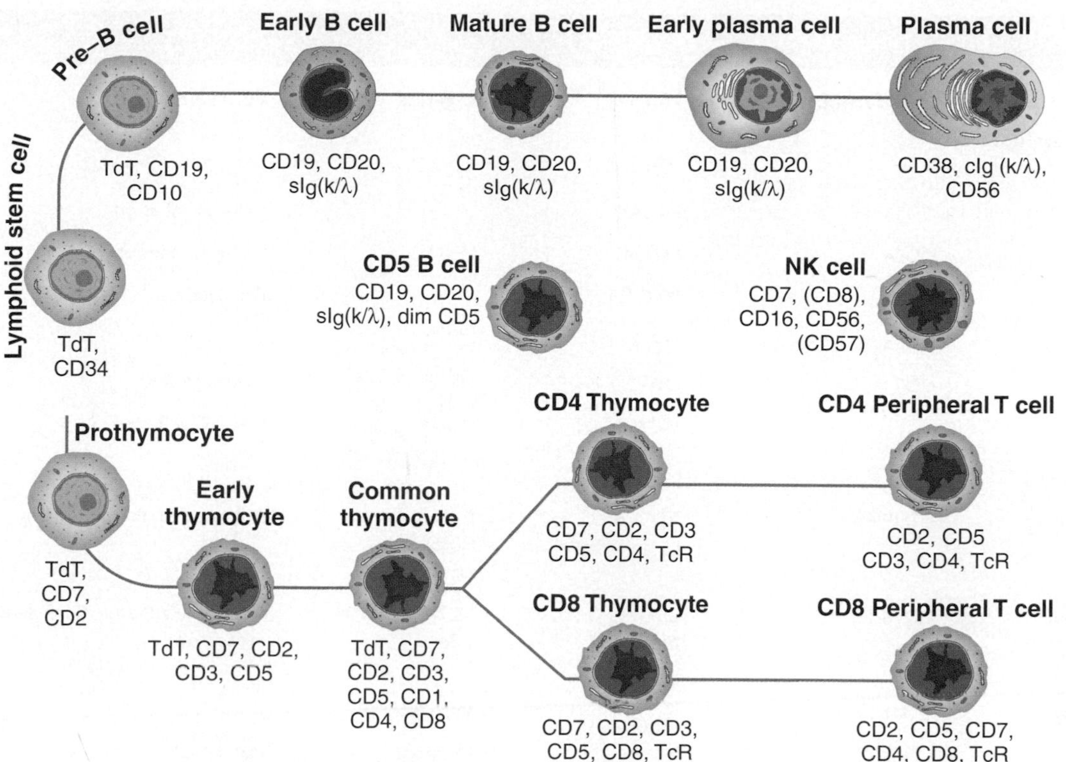

FIGURE 20–3. **Morphologic and phenotypic differentiation of B and T cells.** The lymphocytic stem cell can differentiate along a B- or T-cell pathway, characterized by changes in morphology and cell phenotype. Surface markers can be helpful in diagnosing lymphoproliferative disorders, malignancies of the B- and T-cell lines, and immune deficiency states (sIg, surface immunoglobulin; cIg, cytoplasmic immunoglobulin).

fibroblasts, activates osteoclasts to enhance bone reabsorption, increases levels of acute phase reactants, and activates neutrophils. It also stimulates the production of IL-2 by T cells and synergizes with myeloid growth factors to stimulate marrow stem cells.

Interleukin-2

Interleukin-2 (IL-2) is the interleukin most clearly associated with lymphoid functions. It is produced by activated T cells and in turn stimulates the proliferation and differentiation of both T and B cells. It serves to amplify the immune response and is required for T-cell responses and the stimulation of NK cells. The measurement of IL-2 and its receptors has been used to monitor the activity of the immune system. Drugs and antibodies that inhibit IL-2 or block its receptors may play a role as immunosuppressive agents. On the other hand, IL-2 itself has been used therapeutically as an antitumor agent.

Interleukin-3

Interleukin-3 (IL-3) is a growth factor for B cells. It induces proliferation of antigen-activated B cells, increases antibody synthesis, and synergizes with IL-2. It also stimulates the proliferation of T cells, predominantly of the CD8 subtype. IL-3 plays a synergistic role in early myeloid and erythroid progenitor proliferation and differentiation (see Chapters 1 and 16).

Other Interleukins

Several other interleukins are now being investigated. **Interleukin-5** appears to induce B-cell maturation with its major effect on IgA production. Its major clinical effect in humans is on eosinophil differentiation. **Interleukin-6** affects B-cell growth and differentiation but also stimulates the growth of hepatocytes and neurons. IL-6 plays a major role in regulating hepcidin expression as a part of the anemia of inflammation (see Chapter 4). **Interleukin-7** has stimulatory effects on early B cells and may affect lymphoid progenitors of both B- and T-cell pathways. **Interleukin-11** functions as a generalized hematopoietic growth factor and may have a role in thrombopoiesis. **Interleukin-12** has potent stimulatory effects on lymphoid cells, especially cytotoxic T cells. It is being investigated in the treatment of infectious disease, immunodeficiency, and autoimmunity.

Both lymphocytes and myeloid cells are also capable of producing interferons as a part of host defense. The **interferons** function as stimulators of T- and NK-cell function. At the same time, they have a suppressive effect on hematopoiesis, reducing red blood cell and white blood cell proliferation at the same time they stimulate cell functions such as cytotoxicity and phagocytosis.

LYMPHOCYTE ADHESION MOLECULES

In addition to the growth factors, several adhesion molecules govern the migration, localization, and function of lymphocytes and other blood cells. These appear to fall into several families of related molecules (Table 20–1).

TABLE 20–1 • Major families of adhesion molecules

Family	CD Numbers	Names	Ligands	Functions
Immunoglobulin-like				
	CD56	N-CAM		Cell-cell adhesion
	CD54	I-CAM1	LFA-1	Cell-cell adhesion
	CD31	PE-CAM		On platelets
	CD58	LFA-3	LFA-2	T-cell signaling
	CD2	LFA-2	LFA-3	T-cell signaling
		V-CAM	VLA-4	Cell-cell adhesion
Integrins				
β1 family	CD29/49	VLA1-6	Collagen Fibronectin Laminin	Adhesion to matrix proteins
β2 family	CD18/11	LFA-1 MAC-1 p150,95	I-CAM1 C3bi	Leukocyte adhesion Complement receptor
β3 family	CD61/51		Vitronectin	
	CD61/41		Fibrinogen	Platelet–platelet adhesion
Selectins				
	CD62P	P-Selectin	Carbohydrate	Platelet–leukocyte adhesion
	CD62E	E-Selectin	Carbohydrate	Leukocyte–endothelial cell adhesion
	CD62L	L-Selectin	Carbohydrate	Lymphocyte–endothelial cell adhesion

Immunoglobulin Super Family

The **immunoglobulin (Ig) super family** contains molecules that are structurally related to immunoglobulins. In general, these molecules appear to be involved with cell-cell adhesive interactions, although in some cases they also serve as receptors for soluble complement components.

Integrins

The **integrins** are a large family of heterodimers with closely related structures. They derive much of their diversity from different combinations of the 2 component molecules, the α- and β-chains. They mediate interactions between cells and molecules of the vascular subendothelium and serve as receptors for coagulation proteins such as fibrinogen and factor VIII.

Selectins

The **selectins** are molecules that are structurally related to lectins that bind to carbohydrates. They are involved in interactions between leukocytes, platelets, and endothelial cells, playing a key role in granulocyte adhesion and egress from circulation (see Chapter 16).

Cadherins

The **cadherins** are a family of molecules that bind to themselves. They appear to be involved largely in the interaction of cells within tissues. They play an essential role in the immune network, controlling lymphocyte circulation and their function in immune surveillance. They act as homing receptors to govern migration of lymphocytes into lymph nodes and Peyer patches.

The **L-Selectin** molecule plays a role in the binding of lymphocytes to the high endothelial venules of lymph nodes. Another molecule, **CD44**, has been implicated in the preferential binding of gut-associated lymphocytes to the endothelium of Peyer patches. These molecules are expressed on mature migratory lymphocytes but not immature thymocytes or marrow lymphocytes.

B CELLS

Lymphocytes can be characterized according to their functional differentiation, surface phenotype, and gene rearrangement pattern. Each of these needs to be considered when diagnosing an immune deficiency state or clonal malignancy.

Functional Differentiation

A. Antibody Production

The principal role of the B cells in the immune system is to produce antibodies. Early in its development, the B cell acquires, by rearrangement of its immunoglobulin genes, the ability to make a specific antibody. It subsequently displays a small sample of this antibody on its surface (about 100,000 molecules per cell). This antibody serves as an **antigen receptor** for the B cell. Whenever the cell encounters that antigen that binds to the receptor, it is stimulated to begin a process of differentiation leading to the conversion of the B cell into a plasma cell. The **plasma cell** is then a stable factory for manufacturing a constant amount of the same antibody for excretion. This capability of B cells to recognize antigen and respond with production of antibody is to some extent autonomous, although it is markedly influenced by interactions with T cells, which also recognize the same or closely related antigens. B-cell responses are augmented by the "helper" T cells and are suppressed by interactions with "suppressor" T cells.

B. Augmentation of the Immune Response

Augmentation of the immune response involves several mechanisms. The antibody receptor of B cells can interact directly with antigen to trigger B-cell differentiation. B cells are also capable of internalizing some of the antigen and processing it in the same way that macrophages process antigen by digestion with proteases. The cell then re-expresses partially degraded and denatured antigen on the surface for recognition by T cells. Thus, **B cells have an antigen-presenting function** that stimulates T-cell activity.

C. Maturation Sequence

Once B cells are triggered by antigen, they undergo a **maturation sequence** leading to changes in class, but not specificity, of antibody they produce. Early in the immune response, B cells give rise largely to IgM antibodies. With maturation, there is an increase in the proportion of B cells producing IgG, IgA, and IgE. This occurs by a process called **class switching** that involves further alteration at the DNA level and by RNA splicing. The end result is production of **memory B cells**. These cells are capable of recognizing antigen upon re-exposure so as to give rise to an accelerated (secondary) immune response consisting of a magnified production of IgG.

D. Tolerance to Antigens

There are also defined mechanisms by which B cells fail to respond to a given antigen, that is, demonstrate **"tolerance."** A first mechanism is an active **suppression of the response mediated by T cells** that recognize the same or similar antigen and actively suppress the response. A second mechanism is **clonal deletion**, in which all of the B-cell clones capable of interacting with antigen are destroyed.

Suppression is the normal mechanism by which an organism prevents its immune system from responding to self-antigens. It is an active, continuous process that requires the proper functioning of the immune network. A failure in network control gives rise to autoimmune disease. Immune deficiency or tolerance can also develop because of **clonal deletion**. It can result because of a lymphoid malignancy or following chemotherapy. This is not necessarily irreversible. The continuous process of regeneration of diversity by gene rearrangement at the level of the lymphoid progenitor cells will eventually give rise to new clones capable of responding to specific antigens. Thus, no form of tolerance is likely to persist for the life of the patient.

Phenotypic Classification

The normal sequence of maturation and phenotypic expression of B cells is illustrated in Figure 20–3. The listed antigenic markers are those that are most often used clinically in categorizing disease processes. There are many other markers that are not indicated because they are not unique or are of unknown significance.

A. Pre–B Cell

The earliest recognizable B cell, the **pre–B cell**, is recognized by the presence of cytoplasmic μ heavy chain but no light chain, together with an absence of intact immunoglobulin on its surface. Its surface markers consist of CD19 (but not CD20), HLA-DR, CD34, and CD10 (CALLA). The cell also expresses the nuclear enzyme **terminal deoxynucleotide transferase (TdT)**, which may be one of the enzymes involved in the gene rearrangement process. This stage of B-cell maturation matches the level of cell development seen in the most common form of acute lymphoblastic leukemia.

B. Mature B Cell without Antigen

As the B cell matures, it loses CD34 and TdT and acquires surface immunoglobulin, first IgM alone and then IgM plus IgD. It also acquires CD19 and then CD20. This process takes place in the marrow and in lymph nodes and spleen. It results in a mature B cell that has not yet been exposed to antigen with phenotypic markers of CD19, CD20, HLA-DR, sIgM, and sIgD. This is the most common B cell found in the lymphoid tissues of adults.

C. Mature B Cell with Antigen

Once a B cell encounters antigen, it continues to express CD19 and CD20, but expression of surface immunoglobulin now includes IgM, IgG, IgA, or IgE. In addition, these cells can express any number of activation antigens. One antigen that has become of some importance in the classification of lymphomas (see Chapter 22) is **CD23**, which serves as a receptor for the Fc portion of IgE and appears on some activated B cells. This variability in the normal response is reflected in the diversity of phenotypes seen with B-cell lymphomas. For the purposes of clinical diagnosis, the most consistent and reliable markers for mature B cells at any stage of development are CD19, CD20, and the expression of κ- and λ-immunoglobulin light chains on the cell surface.

D. Plasma Cell

Once B cells differentiate to become plasma cells, they devote nearly all of their synthetic energy to immunoglobulin production and cease expression of other B-cell markers. Therefore, the best marker for plasma cells is the abundance of **cytoplasmic immunoglobulin** and the intense surface expression of **CD38**, an activation marker involved in signaling leading to activation and proliferation of lymphoid cells.

E. CD5-Positive B Cell

A major B-cell subset that does not fit easily into the sequence of B-cell development is characterized by the expression of **CD5**. This antigen is also expressed by T cells. CD5-positive B cells are abundant in the fetus and represent 10%–20% of B cells in the adult. They express CD19, CD20, sIgM, and sIgD much like conventional B cells. An expansion of this subset of B cells is associated with a production of autoantibodies in diseases such as rheumatoid arthritis and systemic lupus erythematosus. This is also the phenotype associated with chronic lymphocytic leukemia and mantle cell lymphoma.

Gene Rearrangement Pattern

The lymphoid stem cell gives rise to the earliest recognizable B cell in the marrow, fetal liver, and spleen. This pre–B cell has already undergone the process of gene rearrangement of both its immunoglobulin heavy- and light-chain–variable regions. The rearrangement normally proceeds in an orderly fashion in which the cell rearranges each of its genes in sequence until it either produces a pair of functional heavy- and light-chain genes or has failed. Because of the uncertainties of splicing the rearranged DNA segments, there is a significant probability that some rearrangements will not give rise to functioning molecules. Even when it is successful, there is a good chance that the gene product will be slightly different from that encoded by the original germ-line gene sequences. This process of **"generation of diversity"** gives rise to an enormous variety of different antibodies produced by the mature immune system.

From a clinical point of view, studies of the gene rearrangement pattern are important in diagnosing lymphoproliferative diseases. They can be used to answer 2 important questions:

- Are the malignant cells B, T, or NK cells?
- Do the cells belong to a single clone, which would strongly suggest malignancy?

Although these questions can in part be answered using immunologic markers, they are more directly answered by **analyzing the gene structure of the cells**. Gene rearrangement is independent of the stage of maturation of the lymphocytes since it is the first defining event in a cell's life. In addition, gene rearrangement is unaffected by any of the later events in the life of the lymphocytes such as antigen exposure. Thus, it defines clonality in an irrefutable way.

Recently, information about the genetic structure of malignant B cells has begun to provide prognostic, as well as diagnostic, information. It has been observed that some cases of **chronic lymphocytic leukemia (CLL)** have relatively unrearranged (germ-line) immunoglobulin heavy-chain genes (98%–100% germ-line homology) and thus most likely represent naive B cells that have not previously encountered antigen. This subset of CLL patients has a significantly worse prognosis than those patients in whom the heavy-chain genes have undergone significant somatic mutation (<97% homology) as described above.

T CELLS

As with B cells, T cells can be characterized according to their function, surface phenotype, and gene rearrangement pattern. Clinically, classification of the cell type and function is essential for understanding an immune deficiency state or diagnosing a malignancy.

Functional Differentiation

There are 2 fundamental roles for T cells in the immune system. The first is their **regulatory role**. They modulate the function of all of the cellular components of the immune system, including macrophages, other T cells, and B cells. The second is their role as **effectors of cellular immunity**. They are responsible for carrying out delayed-type hypersensitivity reactions, cytotoxicity, and both graft and tumor rejection, that is, all of the immune functions that are not mediated by antibodies.

A. Antigen Recognition and "Altered Self"

T cells directly recognize antigen using receptors that are similar to the immunoglobulin antigen receptors of B cells. However, rather than recognizing native, soluble antigen, they respond to antigen processed by macrophages, dendritic cells, or B cells and presented on the surface of the cell in association with the **major histocompatibility complex (MHC) molecules** (HLA-A, HLA-B, and HLA-DR). By way of this close association, the T cell actually senses an alteration of the normal cellular histocompatibility molecules (ie, an **"altered self"**). This concept is integral to the proper functioning of the immune system.

B. Cytokine Secretion and Suppression of Immune Response

Once a T cell recognizes a specific antigen, it secretes cytokines that increase the activity of macrophages, recruit more T cells, and augment the function of B cells. Thus, T cells are responsible for initiating the immune and inflammatory response to an antigen. In addition, once the immune response is exhausted, usually by elimination of the antigen, T cells have an important role in signaling the termination of the response. The suppression of the immune response is an active process mediated by T cells.

In the absence of normal balanced T-cell function, an immune response once initiated will not terminate even after the antigen is eliminated. This **failure of suppression** is central to many, if not all, autoimmune diseases. It is important to recognize that the "helper" and "suppressor" functions are not restricted to specific subsets of T cells, as was once thought, but are distributed throughout the T-cell system. A given clone of antigen-reactive T cells will contain both helper and suppressor functions. The dominance of one over the other will depend on the antigenic stimulus, its concentration, and complex interactions within the immune network.

C. Role in Inflammation and Cytotoxicity

The effector functions of T cells are important in initiating inflammation and for killing other cells **(cytotoxicity)**. The secretion of cytokines such as IL-1, which recruit and activate other cells of the inflammatory response, in part mediates **inflammation**. T cells also mediate the local delayed hypersensitivity reaction, for example, as seen when antigen is injected into the skin (the **tuberculin reaction**). The induration and erythema result when T cells recognize the tuberculin protein on the surface of local macrophages and then initiate the recruitment of other T cells, macrophages, neutrophils, and monocytes to the site.

The **cytotoxic function** of T cells is initiated when a programmed T cell recognizes foreign histocompatibility antigens, viral antigens, or tumor-associated antigens on the surface of a target cell. The lymphocyte is then stimulated to secrete cytoplasmic granules that contain enzymes to lyse the target cell. This reaction is at the basis of T-cell elimination of transplanted tissue, tumors, and virus-infected cells. Cytotoxicity is not restricted to a specific subset of T cells. Instead, many if not all T cells are capable of cytotoxicity when appropriately activated by cytokines such as IL-2.

Phenotypic Classification

The differentiation sequence of T cells is illustrated in Figure 20–3. The list of phenotypic markers shows those most often used in the clinical classification of T cells. By the time T-cell markers are first expressed, the cell has already undergone rearrangement of the receptor genes. The presence of TdT as a nuclear marker, and the presence of the common progenitor cell marker CD34, are not unique to the T cell but are shared with the pre–B cell. **CD7** is the earliest marker that characterizes a T-cell lineage.

The CD7 marker is conserved throughout T-cell development; however, it is most strongly expressed on immature T cells and is the best marker for T-cell acute lymphocytic leukemia. **CD2** is the marker originally described as the sheep erythrocyte rosette receptor. It also appears early and is highly conserved. It has a role in signaling activation of the T cell. Early T cells express cytoplasmic but not surface CD3. The **CD3** marker is the best marker for mature T cells and is an integral part of the complex of molecules that constitute the T-cell antigen receptor.

The most abundant cell in the thymus, the **common thymocyte**, expresses a wide array of markers that are common to all T cells, including CD1, CD2, CD3, CD5, and CD7. This panel of markers is useful in differentiating normal from abnormal mature T cells. Malignant T cells are often revealed by the absence (or low expression) of 1 or more of these markers. The only unique distinguishing characteristic of the common thymocyte is the simultaneous presence of CD4 and CD8.

Later in thymic differentiation, the **maturing T-cell loses either CD4 or CD8**, thereby declaring itself as a member of one of the 2 major subsets referred to as **helper (CD4 positive)** and **suppressor (CD8 positive)** T cells. The actual role of these 2 antigenic molecules has to do with the recognition of HLA class II or class I (respectively) histocompatibility molecules and is not directly related to helper or suppressor function.

Mature T cells leave the thymus and circulate in the periphery as **either CD4 or CD8 subsets**. This distinction is very useful clinically. Attempts to further subdivide T cells with finer functional distinctions or markers have not proved to be clinically useful. For example, although most peripheral T cells (80%–90%) use a pair of receptor molecules referred to as the α/β-receptor, 10%–20% of cells use a different pair known as the γ/δ-receptor. γ/δ T cells are more often found in skin, but the functional significance of this is not yet clear. The exclusive presence of γ/δ T cells in a tumor mass may suggest clonality, but this is only occasionally useful because of the predominance of the α/β subset in many T-cell lymphomas.

Mature T cells also express an array of new antigens when activated. The most frequently noted antigens are the reappearance of **HLA-DR** and the new expression of the **IL-2 receptor (CD25)**. In general, these activation markers are found on cells activated by exposure to antigen. They have also been described on malignant T cells, however. The effector stage of T-cell maturation is not distinguished by any unique markers. Although CD57 is found on cytotoxic T cells, it is not unique and can be present in both reactive and clonal T cells.

Classification by Cytokine Production

In addition to classification by phenotype, recently T cell subsets have been classified by their ability to secrete different combinations of cytokines. The two best defined subsets are the Th1 and Th2 subsets of helper T cells. Th1 cells are characterized by the secretion of interferon and tumor necrosis factor beta. These cells function primarily to augment cellular immunity and cytotoxicity. Th2 cells are characterized by the production of IL-4, 5, 6, 10, and 13 and function primarily to augment the humoral (antibody) immune system. Further expansion of this classification system may occur, for example, recently a Th17 subset has been described which primarily secretes IL-17 and appears to function in both autoimmunity and inflammation.

Gene Rearrangement Pattern

Although the receptors of T cells are different from those of B cells, the principles that govern their genetics are very similar. Thus, T cells undergo a process of sequential rearrangement of their T-cell receptor genes that is analogous to the rearrangement of the B-cell immunoglobulin genes. Identification of rearranged gene sequences by polymerase chain reaction and Southern blot analysis is important clinically in the diagnosis of malignancy. Since studies of T-cell surface markers are poor indicators of malignancy, proof of clonality rests in showing a common gene rearrangement pattern.

NK CELLS

Approximately 10% of circulating lymphocytes do not fall into the T- or B-cell categories, by either surface markers or genetic analysis. These NK cells **share some properties of T cells and macrophages**. They are very active in cytotoxicity and have been shown to be important in host defense, especially against tumors and virus-infected cells. They appear early in ontogeny and reappear as a larger percentage of circulating lymphocytes following ablation of the immune system (eg, following marrow transplantation). They may, therefore, be thought of as the more primitive relatives of the true immune system.

NK cells do not have antigen-specific receptors, and they do not show evidence of immune memory. Their ability to kill target cells is not affected by prior exposure to antigen, thus the name **natural killer** cells. NK cells have receptors for MHC class I molecules that are inhibitory, that is, they recognize and kill cells that are deficient in MHC class I expression. Target cells expressing low levels of HLA-A and -B are, therefore, better targets for NK-cell killing. Many tumor cells and virus-infected cells share this property of low-level class I expression. The actual act of killing by NK cells is similar or identical to that of activated macrophages and cytotoxic T cells, involving the release of toxic substances (perforin, granzyme) from cytoplasmic granules.

NK cells bind to soluble antibody and are thus capable of attaching to and killing any cell expressing antigen recognized by that antibody. This property of being "armed" by antibody (antibody-dependent cytotoxicity) is shared with monocytes and macrophages. NK cells also **respond to and are activated by IL-2**. IL-2–activated NK cells, referred to as **lymphokine-activated killer** cells, have been used effectively in the treatment of certain malignancies.

CHANGES IN THE IMMUNE SYSTEM WITH AGING

A large number of changes in the immune system have been described with advancing age. Taken together these changes have been termed "immunosenescence." Experimental evidence suggests that many of these changes are not necessarily inevitable or degenerative, and many may be under genetic control. Thus the rate and severity of these changes is highly variable and their clinical significance in any given patient is often difficult to determine. In addition, the evaluation of immune function in the elderly is complicated by the frequent presence of other conditions that may add to the severity of the immune defect or mask the symptoms of infections and autoimmune processes associated with immunosenescence.

Every component of the immune system can be involved in this process. There may be a loss of the self-renewal capacity of hematopoietic stem cells committed to the renewal of immune progenitors. There is also a decrease in the number and functional capacity of phagocytic cells and NK cells as well as a decrease in the ability of antigen-presenting cells to function. B cells decrease in number and there is a decrease in the diversity and affinity of antibodies produced. T-cell production, which primarily takes place in the thymus in young persons, is affected by thymic involution with a decrease in the output of naive T cells. This is associated with a decrease in the T-cell repertoire, decreased lymphokine production, decreased proliferation in response to antigen challenge, and decreased cytotoxic activity.

It is reasonable to assume that in total these changes would render some older individuals more susceptible to infections, less able to destroy virus-infected and transformed (malignant) cells, and more likely to develop autoimmune disorders. However, in general, there are no easily available tests that can evaluate the degree of immunosenescence, and thus its role in individual patients is largely a matter of speculation.

LYMPHATIC "ORGAN" SYSTEM

The lymphatic system is comprised of **an intricate network of bone marrow stem cells, circulating B and T cells, lymphatic vessels, lymph nodes, and spleen** (Figure 20–4). Lymphoid cells are released from the marrow as B cells or travel to the thymus where they are programmed as T cells. These cells then travel as part of the blood circulation to tissues, lymph nodes, spleen, or back to the marrow. Lymphocytes are highly mobile and easily transit in and out of tissues, returning via dedicated lymphatic channels to lymph nodes and eventually the blood stream via the thoracic duct. Each lymph node serves as a miniature factory for processing antigen and supporting B-cell proliferation, differentiation, and programming to produce a singular antibody. The spleen serves both as a sophisticated filter to remove cellular material and organisms from blood and to program B cells to produce antibodies against antigens. In every respect, therefore, the circulating B and T cells, lymphatic vessels, lymph nodes, and spleen together function as an **immunologic organ**.

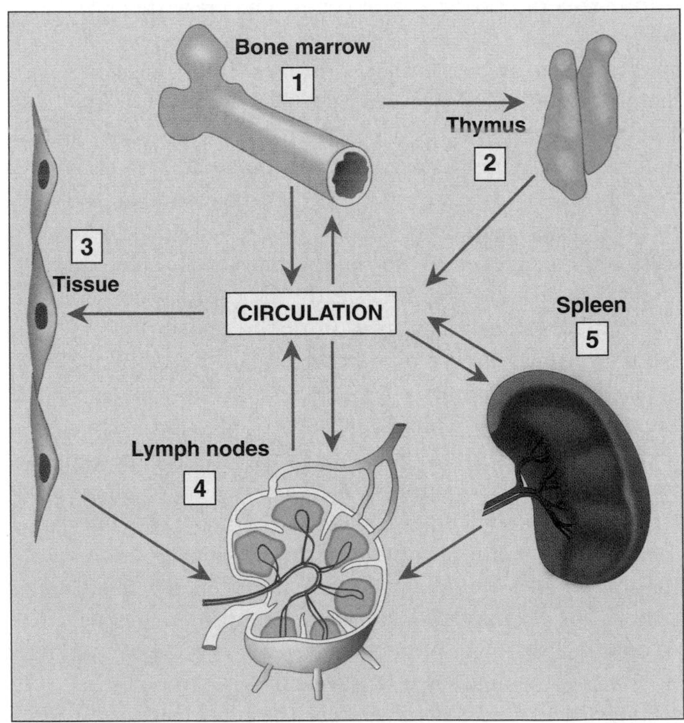

FIGURE 20–4. **The lymphatic "organ" system.** Marrow lymphoid precursors provide a renewable source of unprogrammed B cells (1), some of which then travel to the thymus to be programmed as T cells (2). Circulating B cells and T cells enter tissues via the blood stream and leave via lymphatic vessels connected to regional nodes (3). Lymph nodes act as miniature factories responding to foreign antigen by guiding B-cell proliferation and differentiation to develop a clone of mature lymphocytes programmed to produce a singular antibody (4). The spleen acts as both a filter and an active participant in the immune response to certain bacteria and parasites (5).

Lymph Nodes

The basic structure of the individual lymph node is **an array of B-cell lymphoid follicles**, surrounded by regulatory T cells and supplied by lymphatic and blood vessels. Lymph nodes are connected to the lymphatic circulation by afferent and efferent lymphatic vessels, and to the blood circulation by a dedicated arteriole-venule with capillary loops perfusing the follicular structure (Figure 20–5). Antigenic material entering the node via lymphatic channels is processed and, under the control of regulatory T cells, stimulates the proliferation and differentiation of B cells within the follicular centers and the eventual release of a clone of programmed B cells. Dendritic cells and macrophages, which arise from myeloid precursors, play a crucial role in processing and presenting antigens to the cells of the immune system (see Chapter 16).

Virtually **every body tissue and organ has a lymphatic pathway of vessels connected to a set of regional lymph nodes**, many of which can actually be palpated during a routine physical examination (Figure 20–6). Others are located well out of reach and can only be assessed using sophisticated imaging studies. These regional lymph node collections respond acutely to infections involving their respective tissue or organ, often to an extent that the nodes become easier to palpate, so-called lymphadenopathy. Other causes of lymphadenopathy include tumors of a lymphatic cell line (B- and T-cell lymphomas), metastatic tumors (breast, prostate, lung), and chronic infection (eg, tuberculous granulomas) seeded from the blood stream or, more commonly, via the regional lymphatic channel drainage.

Lymphadenopathy

Lymphadenopathy may be the first sign of a malignancy, especially the presence of a solid tumor or lymphoma. For this reason, the examination of any patient should always include a careful assessment of all palpable node sites (submandibular, submaxillary, occipital, cervical, supraclavicular, axillary, epitrochlear, and inguinal; see Figure 20–6). The examination should look for the **degree of enlargement, any tenderness, and whether the nodes are soft or hard, separate or matted together, uniform or irregular in size and shape, freely movable or fixed to surrounding tissues**. In some areas (supraclavicular, axillary) any palpable node is highly suspect, while in others (submandibular, inguinal) the presence of multiple pea-sized ("shotty") lymphadenopathy is routinely seen in patients with poor dental hygiene or foot care, respectively. Suspicious lymphadenopathy requires that individual nodes exceed 1 cm in diameter and/or be associated with changes in physical qualities.

The most likely causes of lymphadenopathy vary for each of the superficial node groups (Table 20–2 and see Figure 20–6).

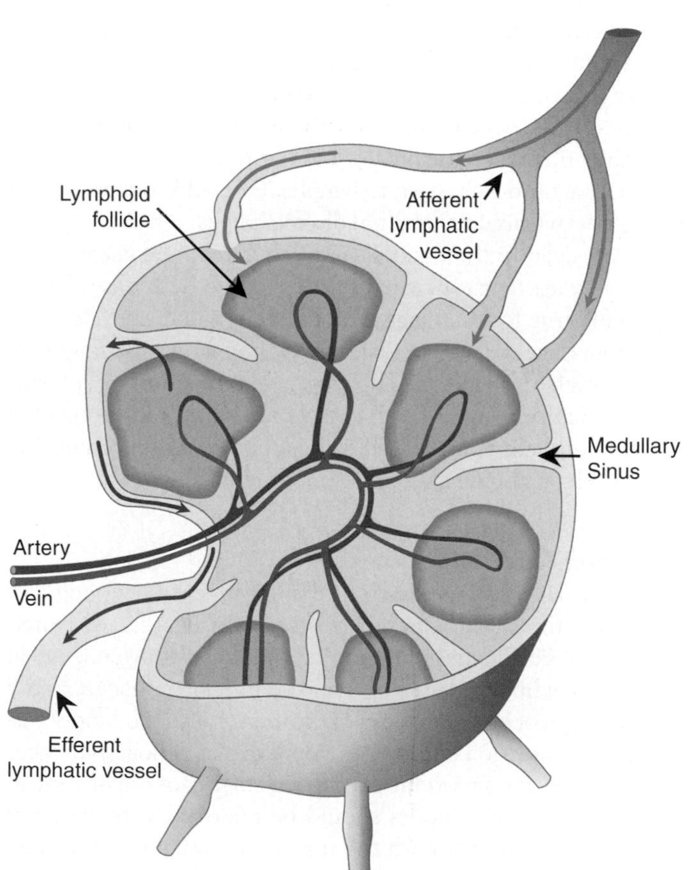

FIGURE 20–5. **Lymph node architecture.** The normal lymph node is basically a collection of lymphoid follicles where B-cell proliferation and differentiation in response to antigenic stimuli is carried out under T-cell control. Each node has a set of afferent lymphatic vessels that carry B cells/antigen to the node and efferent vessels, which return programmed B cells to the blood stream via the thoracic duct. Blood supply is provided by arteriole-capillary-venous loops, which perfuse each follicle to deliver oxygen and nutrients.

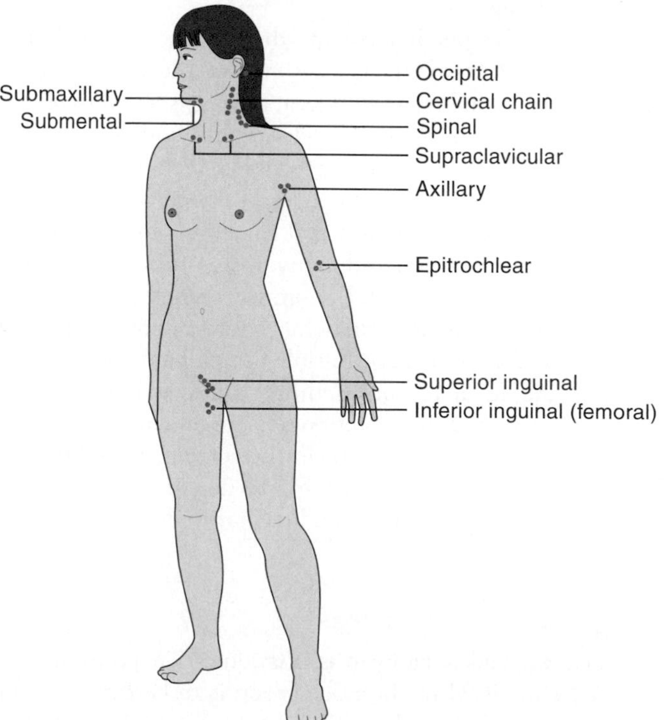

FIGURE 20–6. **Regional lymph node distribution.** A number of regional lymph node groups (as shown) can be palpated on the routine physical examination.

TABLE 20–2 • Causes of lymphadenopathy by major nodal group

Location	Drainage Area	Causes of Adenopathy
Submaxillary/submandibular	Lower face/mouth/submaxillary gland	Viral and bacterial infections; tongue, tonsil, mucous membranes
Occipital	Scalp/head	Rubella/scalp infections
Cervical	Pharynx, larynx, thyroid	Viral and bacterial infections/ lymphomas/carcinomas
Right supraclavicular	Mediastinum/lungs/esophagus	Mediastinal/lung tumors; sarcoidosis/ tuberculosis
Left supraclavicular	Mediastinum/abdomen (thoracic duct)	Mediastinal/gastric/testicular tumors
Axillary	Breast/arm	Viral and bacterial infections; breast cancer/lymphoma
Inguinal	Feet/legs/perineum	Viral and bacterial infections/ venereal disease; lymphoma

The most obvious differences relate to their area of drainage. Submandibular and submaxillary nodes respond to diseases of the mouth (lips, tongue, teeth), while inguinal nodes respond to disorders involving the feet, legs, and perineum. There is also the incidence and nature of the disease process. Bilateral, recurrent lymphadenopathy involving the submaxillary and cervical node groups is commonly seen with viral and bacterial pharyngitis. The predictability of this finding in patients with pharyngitis makes further workup unnecessary. The same is true for lymphadenopathy associated with a bacterial cellulitis, although the presence of lymphadenopathy suggests a spread beyond the local area of infection.

Malignant lymphadenopathy, whether due to lymphoma, leukemia, or solid tumor metastasis, often is the first sign of disease. Hodgkin lymphoma presents at an early stage with unilateral involvement of a single node group, most often in the cervical region. More advanced Hodgkin lymphoma is heralded by involvement of 2 or more contiguous node groups. In contrast, non-Hodgkin lymphoma and leukemia generally present with widespread disease, and many, if not most, node groups show a uniform enlargement. By contrast, a single palpable node in the supraclavicular area can herald a tumor of the lung, mediastinum, stomach, or testis. Multiple firm to hard nodes matted together and fixed to surrounding tissues usually indicates metastatic cancer. Documentation of metastatic involvement of regional nodes is a key element in the staging of solid tumors. This requires both careful imaging to detect enlargement of nodes in the pelvis, abdomen, and mediastinum, and confirmatory biopsy of suspicious nodes.

Diagnostic Procedures

Localized lymphadenopathy in association with a specific inflammatory lesion distal to the node group is to be expected and requires no further workup. Persistent non-tender, pea-sized ("shotty") lymph nodes in the submaxillary, cervical, axillary, or inguinal areas are almost always associated with a past infection, poor dental hygiene, or repeated trauma to the hands or feet. Age can also be a major clue. Rubella in unimmunized children is associated with occipital adenopathy, while the college student is likely to present with adenopathy secondary to streptococcal pharyngitis or infectious mononucleosis. These situations rarely require further evaluation, unless the lymphadenopathy persists after the primary disease process has resolved.

The diagnostic approach to lymphadenopathy, not associated with an active viral or bacterial disease, needs to be very aggressive. Any delay in the workup can result in a missed diagnosis or, at the very least, an unwanted progression of the disease. This is especially true for the diagnosis of Hodgkin and non-Hodgkin lymphomas, where diagnosis and treatment at an early stage correlate with better survival. Therefore, "watchful waiting" of lymphadenopathy is not in order; the patient should be quickly biopsied and clinically staged using a combination of imaging studies, blood chemistries, and tumor markers.

A. Lymph Node Biopsy

The most definitive approach to the diagnosis of lymphoma or metastatic tumor is the biopsy of an obviously enlarged lymph node. Superficial node groups can be sampled readily under local anesthesia, while mediastinal and abdominal lymphadenopathy may be approached laparascopically. Sentinel node biopsy following the injection of a breast nodule with a radioactive tracer or dye is now an important part of the staging of breast cancer. One or more intact nodes should be removed with minimal trauma so as to not disturb the nodal architecture. Immediate processing is important with samples taken for frozen section, flow cytometry, and formalin fixation for hematoxylin and eosin (H&E) and histochemical staining. A cut section of the node can also be used to prepare a touch prep smear for Wright stain examination of individual cell morphology. As discussed in Chapters 23 and 24, the diagnosis and classification of a lymphoma depends on the assessment of both overall architecture and individual cell morphology.

B. Fine Needle Aspiration

In patients with an inflammatory lymphadenopathy, a fine needle aspirate may be used in the office setting to sample cell type and identify bacterial suppuration by culture. It is less satisfactory for the diagnosis of metastatic tumor or lymphoma, since it can easily miss foci of tumor or may not allow for an adequate assessment of cell phenotype by flow cytometry or nodal architecture by histology.

C. Imaging Studies

The diagnosis and staging of a lymphoma or a solid tumor requires a full assessment of all node groups and a search for evidence of tissue/organ invasion. Computed tomography (CT) scan, magnetic resonance imaging (MRI), positron emission tomography (PET) scan, bone scan, and ultrasonography can all play a role. The sequence of testing will depend on the likely diagnosis. Lymphangiography, where contrast material is injected into an afferent lymphatic vessel in the foot and then tracked as it diffuses into pelvic and abdominal nodes, was used in the past to diagnose and stage Hodgkin disease. Theoretically, an irregular pattern of contrast staining of individual nodes caused by fibrosis (nodular sclerosis subtype of Hodgkin disease) can identify nodal involvement, even in the absence of adenopathy. In addition, imaging studies are now routinely used to guide biopsies.

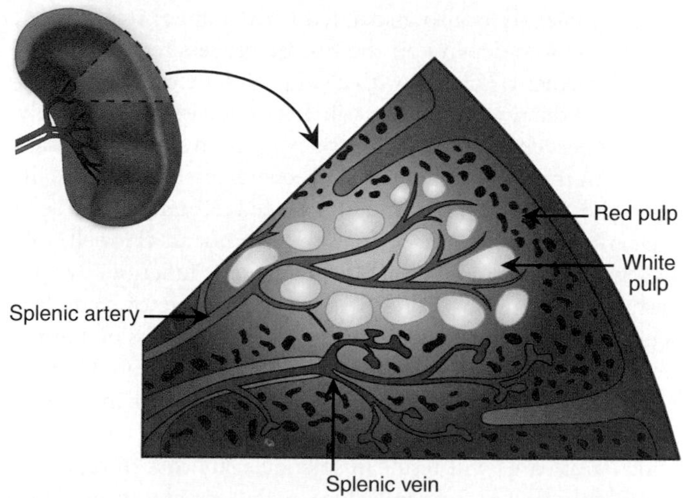

FIGURE 20–7. **Splenic architecture.** The spleen is a highly efficient filter. Blood cells delivered by the splenic artery are metabolically stressed and tested for pliability by having to pass through 2–3 μm pores to reach the splenic sinusoids of the red pulp and subsequently return to the general circulation. Senescent red cells and cells containing inclusions are phagocytosed by macrophages lining the sinusoids. Antigen derived by this process is processed and used to stimulate B-cell production and programming in the white pulp. Unlike lymph nodes, the spleen has only efferent lymphatic vessels to return programmed lymphocytes to the circulation.

D. Blood Chemistries, Marrow Aspirate and Biopsy, and Tumor Markers

Depending on the putative diagnosis, clinical staging requires a search for disease involving other tissues or organs. Favored sites of widespread (stage IV) disease are the liver, bone marrow, and brain. In the case of lymphoma patients, bilateral bone marrow aspirates/biopsies for both morphology and flow cytometry are essential since the marrow is an active player in the lymphatic circulation/system. Certain lymphomas, especially B-cell lymphomas in AIDS patients, can first appear in the brain. Metastatic carcinomas tend to favor the liver, lung, bone, and brain, with each tumor type having a typical pattern of spread. Tumor markers specific for some solid tumors can also help in diagnosis and management as an indirect measure of tumor mass.

Spleen

The spleen is also part of the lymphatic system. Its principle function is the filtration and destruction of senescent or abnormal cells and the trapping of blood borne pathogens. At the same time, the spleen participates in the proliferation, differentiation, and programming of B cells in response to antigen delivered from the filtration process. The structure of the spleen is illustrated in Figure 20–7. It is located in the left upper quadrant just under the diaphragm. The spleen in a normal adult weighs approximately 200 g and is perfused by a dominant splenic artery at a rate of 150–200 mL of blood per minute. Unlike lymph nodes, there are no afferent lymphatic channels entering the spleen. However, efferent vessels that track the venous drainage connect to the celiac lymph nodes and subsequently back to the blood stream via the thoracic duct.

The anatomical structure of the spleen is designed to test the pliability and survivability of circulating red blood cells and to remove intracellular inclusions. As illustrated in Figure 11–1, red cells entering the spleen are concentrated and their intracellular metabolic pathways stressed, followed by a mandatory pass through 2–5 μm pores to reach the sinusoids of the splenic red pulp. Rigid cells or cells containing inclusions (nuclear fragments, hemoglobin crystals, encapsulated bacteria, and parasites) will be unable to pass the test and either be phagocytosed or have their inclusion bodies removed. The adjacent "white pulp" of the spleen serves the same function as the follicles of lymph nodes. Antigen presented by macrophages stimulates B-cell growth and programming to produce singular, targeted antibodies.

A. Splenomegaly

Normally the spleen is not palpable, although 2%–3% of otherwise healthy individuals will have a just barely palpable spleen that does not change over time. As a rule of thumb, the spleen must double in size to be palpable. Very large spleens (4–5 kg or more) can reach well below the costal margin, seemingly filling the abdomen and even approaching the iliac crest. Marked splenomegaly is usually symptomatic due to compression of the adjacent stomach (early satiety, postprandial discomfort) or because of splenic infarction as the splenic mass outstrips its blood supply. The latter is associated with left upper quadrant pain, tenderness to palpation, and, in some cases, rebound tenderness with an audible friction rub. Infarcts adjacent to the diaphragm can present as pleurisy or referred pain to the neck and shoulder.

Splenomegaly is also associated with changes in function, which may also depend on the disease process responsible for the enlargement. Patients with a congenital hemolytic anemia, such as hereditary spherocytosis, will develop modest splenomegaly, which is best characterized as work hypertrophy of the filtration system. In this situation, filtration becomes less efficient, resulting in the appearance of abnormal-shaped red cells and red cell fragments and even intracellular nuclear remnants (Howell-Jolly bodies) in circulation that signify poor splenic function. By contrast, hematopoietic disorders associated with extramedullary hematopoiesis and the appearance of large numbers of marrow precursors in the spleen generally do not demonstrate Howell-Jolly bodies, but the marrow precursors will appear in circulation. Space-occupying infiltrates of the spleen (lymphoma, Gaucher disease) will result in splenomegaly that disrupts the normal filtration process and additionally decreases intrasplenic pools of platelets and granulocytes, increasing CBC counts. Finally, splenomegaly is a common complication of portal hypertension in patients with advanced cirrhosis and is often associated with moderate cytopenia.

B. Hypersplenism

From a clinical standpoint, it can be useful to characterize splenic functional defects as either hyper- or hyposplenism. Hypersplenism is defined as an increase in cell clearance involving some combination of red cells, white cells, and platelets. Increased red cell destruction can result in a worsening anemia and an increased transfusion requirement. Patients with portal hypertension and splenomegaly commonly have a pancytopenia secondary to increased trapping and destruction of all cell types. As a rough approximation, the severity of the pancytopenia correlates with the size of the spleen.

C. Hyposplenism

Hyposplenism is seen with space-occupying diseases such as lymphoma and Gaucher disease, repeated infarction (sickle cell anemia), or as a result of splenectomy. It is characterized by a buildup in circulation of distorted red cells, red cell fragments, Howell-Jolly bodies, and nucleated red cells, all elements that should have been removed by splenic filtration. In addition, both the white cell and platelet counts can increase as a result of the loss of intrasplenic pooling. This is most pronounced for the platelet count, which can increase to levels in excess of 1 million/μL in patients with myeloproliferative disorders (see Chapter 19). Complete loss of splenic function (asplenia) is associated with an increased incidence of life-threatening sepsis, most often due to infections with encapsulated bacteria (pneumococcus, hemophilus). This is a significant management issue in patients who have sickle cell anemia or have been splenectomized at an early age (see Chapters 7, 11, and 24).

POINTS TO REMEMBER

The immune system consists of a complex network of intertwined feedback interactions resulting in a balance between augmentation and suppression of the immune response to both self and nonself antigens. Alterations of this network can lead to autoimmunity or tolerance.

The immune system is constantly generating and regenerating the ability to respond to antigen through a process of gene rearrangement taking place in lymphocyte precursors.

Due to the complex pattern of differentiation in the lymphoid system the morphology of individual cells is frequently not helpful in diagnosis. The overall pattern of a lymphoproliferative process as well as phenotypic and genetic indications of clonality must be considered.

Lymphocytes secrete a large number of cytokines and growth factors that influence the function of all of the cells of the hematopoietic system.

B cells are responsible for recognition of antigen and production of antibodies (humoral immunity). Clonality among B cells is best indicated by expression of immunoglobulin light chains and by genetic analysis.

T cells are responsible for regulation of the immune network, cytotoxicity, and regulation of the inflammatory response (cellular immunity). Clonality among T cells is best indicated by genetic analysis.

NK cells are capable of killing certain malignant and virus-infected target cells by a mechanism similar to that of T cells but they do not show immunological memory.

In general, the function of the immune system decreases with age, but the extent and rate of this process is highly variable and difficult to measure.

Careful and systematic evaluation of the lymphoid system—the lymph nodes and spleen—is critical to many hematologic diagnoses.

BIBLIOGRAPHY

Cambier J: Immunosenescence: a problem of lymphopoiesis, homeostasis, microenvironment and signalling. Immunol Rev 2005;205:5.

Chin YH, Sackstein R, Cai JP: Lymphocyte homing receptors and preferential migration pathways. Proc Soc Exp Biol Med 1991;196:374.

Fackler MJ, Strauss LC: Lymphohematopoiesis: role of growth factors in leukemogenesis and therapy. Hematol Oncol Clin North Am 1990;4:849.

Ferrer R: Lymphadenopathy: differential diagnosis and evaluation. Amer Fam Physician 1998;58:1313.

Friedman AM: Evaluation and management of lymphadenopathy in children. Pediatr Rev 2008;29:53.

Gordon J, Cairns JA: Autocrine regulation of normal and malignant B lymphocytes. Adv Cancer Res 1991;56:313.

Haberman TM, Steensma DP: Lymphadenopathy. Mayo Clin Proc 2000;75:723.

Hamblin TJ et al: Unmutated Ig VH genes are associated with a more aggressive form of chronic lymphocytic leukemia. Blood 1999;94:1848.

Hehn ST et al: Utility of fine-needle aspiration as a diagnostic technique for lymphoma. J Clin Oncol 2004;22:3046.

Henney CS: The interleukins as lymphocyte growth factors. Transplant Proc 1989;21:22.

Mebius RE, Kraal G: Structure and function of the spleen. Nat Rev Immunol 2005;5:606.

Weng NP: Aging of the immune system: how much can the adaptive immune system adapt? Immunity 2006;24:495.

William BM, Corazza GR: Hyposplenism: a comprehensive review. Part I: basic concepts and causes. Hematology 2007;12:1.

William BM et al: Hyposplenism: a comprehensive review. Part II: clinical manifestations, diagnosis, and management. Hematology 2007;12:89.

LYMPHOPENIA AND IMMUNE DEFICIENCY • 21

CASE HISTORY • *Part I*

A 23-year-old woman presents with recurrent episodes of sinusitis, a well-documented pneumococcal pneumonia at age 17, and a chronic productive cough for over a year; the latter has not responded to several courses of antibiotics. She has lost 10 lbs over the last 6 months and feels chronically ill. Her sexual history includes unprotected sex with at least 5 different males over the last 4 years.

On examination, she is afebrile with normal vital signs but appears poorly nourished and chronically ill. She has palpable, slightly enlarged, non-tender cervical lymph nodes and a palpable spleen without hepatomegaly. Chest examination is remarkable for prominent rhonchi and crackles throughout the lower lung fields, without signs of pleural fluid or consolidation. Fingers appear to be slightly clubbed. A routine complete blood count (CBC) is drawn and chest film obtained:

CBC: Hematocrit/hemoglobin - 33%/11 g/dL
MCV - 93 fL MCH - 31 pg MCHC - 33 g/dL
WBC count - 10,900/μL
Differential: Neutrophils - 7,500/μL
Lymphocytes - 2,450/μL
Monocytes - 850/μL
Eosinophils - 100/μL
Platelets - 35,000/μL
Chest film: Nonspecific scarring in both lower lobes. No evidence of consolidation or pleural fluid.

Questions

- Do the history and physical examination suggest a diagnosis?
- What abnormalities are apparent from the CBC?
- What additional workup is in order?

The immune system, consisting of both the adaptive (T and B cells) and the innate (natural killer [NK] cells, macrophages, and myeloid effector cells) components as described in Chapter 20, is carefully balanced and interactive; thus, immune dysfunction of any kind is frequently associated with the combination of impaired defense against pathogens, autoimmunity, and increased risk of malignancy.

Constitutional or primary immune deficencies are relatively rare disorders, affecting mainly young infants. **Acquired immune deficiency** has become a more dominant issue with the advent of the human immunodeficiency virus (HIV) epidemic. The diagnosis and treatment of HIV and its associated life-threatening complications (AIDS) has become a major occupation for many medical subspecialties, including hematology. One of the early clues to an acquired immunodeficiency state is the development of absolute lymphopenia. At the same time, patients may manifest profound immune defects with normal or even elevated lymphocyte counts.

NORMAL LYMPHOCYTE KINETICS

The pathways of lymphocyte development are described in detail in Chapter 20. **Lymphocytes** arise from progenitors in the

TABLE 21–1 • The normal distribution of lymphocyte subsets in blood

Subset	Percentage	Absolute Count (cells/μL)
Lymphocytes		1,500–4,000
T cells	65–75	1,300–1,500
B cells	10–15	200–300
NK cells	10–20	200–400
CD4 T cells	35–45	700–900
CD8 T cells	30–40	600–800

marrow and develop in the lymphoid organs including, for **T cells**, the thymus and lymph nodes, and for **B cells**, the marrow and lymph nodes. Circulating lymphocytes in blood are not representative of all lymphocytes, but rather are particular subsets that circulate for specific reasons (Table 21–1).

Blood lymphocytes consist predominantly of T cells (70%–80%) that are in a constant state of circulation from blood through the lymph nodes, tissues, and lymphatics, and back to blood. They exit the blood in specialized post-capillary venules within the lymph nodes, percolate through the nodes, and then return via the lymphatics. T cells are also found in perivascular locations in tissues throughout the body; T cells can live for months to years under normal conditions. Their role in the immune system may be thought of as spreading the immune response against a particular antigen throughout the body.

B cells are much less common in blood (10%–15%) and do not appear to circulate through the tissues as do T cells. There is some evidence that many of the B cells found in blood are a distinct class of B cells, although this is not well established. Since they account for about 50% of the lymphocytes in the nodes, the relatively small numbers that circulate probably serve a special purpose. Blood B cells appear to be enriched for $CD5^+$ cells that have been implicated in autoimmunity. B cells, like T cells, are relatively long-lived and when fully differentiated to plasma cells, they no longer circulate but are confined to lymphoid tissues and marrow.

Natural killer (NK) cells (10%–15% of circulating lymphs) share some properties of macrophages and also express antigens and functions that are similar to those of T cells. They appear to mediate a type of immunity that is less antigen-specific than that of T and B cells, and they lack the property of immunologic memory. They may be thought of as more primitive than T or B cells. Nevertheless, they appear to be a major host defense mechanism against viral infections and some tumors. The fact that very few patients have been described with severe defects of NK-cell function may be testimony to their importance in host defense. Their lifespan and circulation patterns are not well defined.

CLINICAL FEATURES

Significant **lymphopenia or lymphocyte dysfunction** is usually suspected because of repeated episodes of infection. Pyogenic, gram-positive bacterial infections suggest a defect in antibody production, which may or may not be accompanied by hypogammaglobulinemia. Since an antibody specific for even a complex bacterial antigen usually represents far less than 10% of the total circulating immunoglobulin, it is difficult to detect a failure of specific antibody production by measuring total immunoglobulins. In fact, there would appear to be a feedback mechanism that increases the levels of other immunoglobulins in the face of many forms of immunodeficiency such that an affected patient may well have elevated immunoglobulins.

Repeated episodes of viral, fungal, or other opportunistic infections suggest a defect in T-cell function or number. Again, the number of T cells reacting specifically against any one antigen represents a very small proportion of the total T-cell pool, so profound T-cell defects may not be reflected by lymphopenia or decrease in any T-cell subset. Thus, clinical evaluation of any patient suspected of immune deficiency must rely on a detailed medical history to define the nature and frequency of infections, a family history to identify a possible genetic disorder, and a careful examination for signs or symptoms suggestive of a lymphoproliferative disorder.

Laboratory Studies

The laboratory evaluation of these patients should include a routine complete blood count (CBC) and white blood cell differential, a measurement of the major lymphocyte subsets in the blood, and a quantitative measurement of each of the major immunoglobulin classes. The distribution of lymphocyte subsets in the blood and the absolute number of cells for each subset are listed in Table 21–1. **Absolute lymphopenia** is defined as a count less than 1,500/μL. Even when the total lymphocyte count is normal, however, a deficiency of one of the lymphocyte subsets can result in significant immune deficiency.

Measurement of total levels of the major immunoglobulin classes (IgG, IgM, IgA) is relatively insensitive to the detection of immune deficiency. A more sensitive measure of the ability of the immune system to make specific antibodies can be obtained by quantitating levels of antibody against antigens that the patient is known to have encountered. This can be done by measuring antibody titers against known infectious agents (*Candida*, mumps, rubella, Epstein-Barr, herpes, or cytomegalovirus) or by measuring antibody levels before and after intentional immunization (Pneumovax, tetanus toxoid, hepatitis B).

Laboratory testing of **T-cell function** will depend on the level of laboratory services available. Skin testing with antigens such as *Candida* and purified protein derivative of tuberculin (PPD) can be used, but their interpretation is highly subjective and a lack of responsiveness may indicate generalized suppression of the inflammatory response rather than a specific immune defect. The ability of T cells to proliferate in vitro in response to mitogens such as phytohemagglutinin, soluble antigens such as tetanus toxoid, or allogeneic T cells (the mixed lymphocyte response) provides a more quantitative and reproducible measure of T-cell function. The ability of T cells to kill allogeneic cells after exposure in vitro (so-called cell-mediated lympholysis) is a measure of the ability of T cells to both respond to an

CASE HISTORY • *Part 2*

The patient's history is notable for repeated sinus and bronchopulmonary infections, resulting in chronic bronchitis with permanent scarring and bronchiectasis. Her CBC shows normocytic, normochromic anemia, an elevated neutrophil count, a lower than normal lymphocyte count, and increases in both monocytes and eosinophils. She also has moderately severe thrombocytopenia.

Together, these findings would suggest an inherent inability to handle common bacterial infections, especially encapsulated organisms including *Haemophilus influenzae*, *Moraxella catarrhalis*, and *Streptococcus pneumoniae*, despite antibiotic therapy. This must raise questions regarding the state of her immune system, whether she is suffering from an inherited or, given her age and sexual history, perhaps an acquired immunodeficiency. Based on this history, measurements of B- and T-cell subsets and function are in order. Results are as follows:

Quantitative immunoglobulins: Normal albumin; markedly reduced IgG and IgA levels; normal IgM; no monoclonal immunoglobulin detected
Flow cytometry: Blood T-cell CD4/CD8 ratio is inverted at 0.25; the number of CD27$^+$ (memory) B cells is reduced, but there is no evidence for monoclonal B-cell lymphoproliferative disease.
HIV antibody: Negative
Anti-platelet antibody: Positive

Questions

- What inherited or acquired immune defect is suggested by these test results?
- Would additional tests help with the diagnosis? What therapy is indicated?

antigen and to generate fully differentiated effector cells. It is also possible to measure the ability of T cells to produce cytokines such as interleukin-2 (IL-2) in response to soluble antigen or allogeneic cells. NK-cell function is usually measured by the ability of lymphocytes to kill certain tumor cell targets or virus-infected cell lines.

CONGENITAL IMMUNODEFICIENCY DISORDERS

Several inherited immunodeficiency disorders may be diagnosed during the first few years of life. They present with recurrent bacterial and fungal infections and are often associated with 1 or more congenital abnormalities (Table 21–2). These disorders have allowed some insight into the normal processes involved in lymphoid maturation and helped to identify specific causal gene mutations and dysfunctions.

Immunodeficiency Syndromes

Children with immunodeficiency syndromes present with recurrent infections involving a variety of organisms including viruses, fungi, and protozoans, or inflammatory diseases. According to the type, primitive immune deficiencies can impair both B- and T-cell function, antibody production, phagocytosis, complement activation, and innate immunity.

Severe combined immunodeficiency disease (SCID), involving both the T- and B-cell systems, is now known to arise from several distinct mutations or dysfunction of genes critical for the normal maturation of the the immune system, including mutations in the γ chain shared by IL-2, -4, -7, -9, -15, and -21 receptors; *Jak3*, *IL7R*, *CD45*, *CD3D*, *RAG-1* and *RAG-2*, Artemis and *ADA* genes. The most common of these is **adenosine deaminase deficiency (ADA)**. The lack of this enzyme results in the accumulation of adenosine metabolites that inhibit the growth and function of T cells, and to a lesser extent B cells. Some of these patients will respond to exogenous adenosine deaminase provided by red blood cell transfusion or the administration of stabilized preparations of the enzyme. The treatment of choice, however, is gene transplantation, which involves transfecting autologous hematopoietic progenitor cells with the adenine deaminase gene followed by reimplantation. Recently, it has been recognized that some children and adults with mild to moderate lymphopenia and immune deficiency may be partially ADA deficient. Since this is potentially treatable, measurement of erythrocyte ADA should be done in suspected cases.

Other causes of combined immunodeficiency include the **X-linked hyper-IgM syndrome**, the **Omenn syndrome** (absence of class II HLA antigens necessary for antigen presentation), and other defects in T-cell development or function. Because of the central role of the T cells in the immune system, any defect in T-cell development will result in profound immunodeficiency involving both T- and B-cell function. The **Wiskott-Aldrich syndrome** includes a defect in the CD43 (sialophorin) antigen found on both platelets and lymphocytes. CD43 is apparently involved with T-cell activation, and the defect does shorten the survival of both T cells and platelets. These patients have recurrent pyogenic infections. They are also at risk for developing lymphomas. Marrow transplantation, which is designed to

TABLE 21-2 • Congenital immunodeficiency disorders

Disease	Major Manifestation	Abnormality	Therapy
T- and B-cellular immunodeficiencies			
Severe combined immunodeficiency	Recurrent viral, bacterial, fungal, and protozoan infections	Absent or very low T and B cells. Low serum Ig. Several mechanisms and genetic transmission modes	Marrow transplantation
Omenn syndrome	Erythrodermia, eosinophilia, splenomegaly	T and B cells present or slightly decreased. Low serum Ig. Missense mutations in *RAG-1/2* genes	Marrow transplantation
ADA (adenosine deaminase) deficiency	Recurrent viral, bacterial, fungal, and protozoan infections	Progressive decrease of T and B cells. Low serum Ig. Mutation in *ADA* gene	Gene transfer (autologous stem cell transplantation)
X-linked hyper-IgM syndrome	Opportunistic infections, neutropenia, thrombocytopenia, hemolysis, liver abnormalities	T and IgM, IgD bearing B cells normal. High serum IgM, low serum IgG. Mutations in the *CD40* ligand gene	*CD40L* gene transfer
Predominant antibody deficiencies			
X-linked hypogammaglobulinemia	Pyogenic infections in infancy; absent IgM, IgA, IgD, and IgE; very low IgG	B cells absent	IV gamma globulin Antibiotics
IgA deficiency	Usually asymptomatic, very low IgA. Reactions to transfusion of blood and plasma products	Normal or decreased B cells. Serum IgA absent	None
Common variable immunodeficiency	Recurrent upper-aiways and skin pyogenic infections	B cells normal or decreased. Serum IgG decreased	Immunoglobulins and antibiotics
Other immunodeficiency syndromes			
Thymic aplasia (DiGeorge syndrome)	Hypoparathyroidism, abnormal facies, opportunistic infections	Decreased T cells	Fetal thymus transplant
Chronic mucocutaneous candidiasis	Chronic *Candida* infection, multiple endocrinopathies	Normal T cells but failure to respond to *Candida* antigens	Antibiotics
Ataxia-telangiectasia	Telangiectasia, neurologic abnormalities, recurrent sinopulmonary infections	Decreased T cells, often low IgA levels, mutation in *ATM* gene	Antibiotics
Wiskott-Aldrich syndrome	Eczema, thrombocytopenia, recurrent pyogenic infections	Abnormal or decreased CD43 on lymphocytes and platelets	Marrow transplantation

replace both lymphoid and hematopoietic progenitors, will correct both the thrombocytopenia and the immune deficiency state.

Ataxia-Telangiectasia

Ataxia-telangiectasia is an autosomal recessive disorder that has been shown to result from mutations of a gene known as *ATM*. Current information suggests that the product of this gene plays a role in monitoring the genome for the presence of DNA damage and protecting the cell from abnormal genetic rearrangements resulting during repair. Patients with this disease have an overall incidence of malignancy of 38% despite a reduced lifespan, and 85% of these are lymphoid leukemias or lymphomas. Most lymphomas demonstrate genetic rearrangements involving the immunoglobulin and T-cell-receptor loci that normally undergo rearrangement (see Chapter 23). Thus, abnormal regulation of the gene rearrangement process resulting from mutation of *ATM* may be the root cause of both the immunodeficiency and the high incidence of lymphoproliferative disease in these patients. There is some evidence that, even in the heterozygous (carrier) state, *ATM* mutations may result in a generally increased incidence of malignancy, including breast cancer.

Defects in Immunoglobulin Production

Children with defects in immunoglobulin production generally present with recurrent, severe pyogenic infections once their maternally acquired antibody is lost at approximately 5–6 months of age. Infants with **congenital hypogammaglobulinemia**, the most common form of which is X-linked, demonstrate a profound decrease in all classes of immunoglobulin and a near total absence of B lymphocytes. They are especially susceptible to encapsulated organism infections. Children with **solitary IgA deficiency** are usually asymptomatic. They do not have pyogenic infections but are at lifelong risk for anaphylaxis if they receive repeated transfusion of blood products containing IgA.

Other Defects in the Immune System

Other defects in immunity are associated with a failure in one of the steps in the immune reaction. Disruption of one or more steps in the complement system is one example. **Hereditary angioedema** is the consequence of C1 inhibitor deficiency. A closely related disease, **acquired angioneurotic syndrome**, is observed in patients with monoclonal gammopathies who develop antibodies to the C1 esterase molecule. Defects in the first steps of the classical pathway (C1-C4-C2-C3) are associated with lupus-like syndromes. Later defects in the lytic complex (C5-9) can increase sensitivity to *Neisseria* infections. Specific mutations can also lead to inflammatory disorders including **familial Mediterranean fever, hyper-IgD syndrome, and tumor necrosis factor (TNF) receptor–associated periodic syndrome**, characterized by recurrent fever, serositis, and joint inflammation.

ACQUIRED IMMUNODEFICIENCY DISORDERS

Acquired immunodeficiency must be considered whenever a patient has recurrent bacterial, viral, or fungal infections. It can occur at any age and may or may not be obviously associated with other disease. In addition to the well-defined immunodeficiency disorders listed in Table 21–3, several other common clinical conditions are accompanied by a relative immunodeficiency, including advanced age, malnutrition, and chronic inflammatory states associated with autoimmunity or infection.

Hypogammaglobulinemia

Acquired hypogammaglobulinemia or **common variable immunodeficiency (CVID)** is frequently diagnosed in young adults and is characterized by progressive loss of immunoglobulins, despite the presence of near-normal lymphocyte subsets, after a prolonged period of normal immune function. Some cases have been attributed to increased levels of suppressor T-cell function, but many cases go unexplained. CVID is usually sporadic but may occur in several members of the same family, raising the issue of an inherited mutation that is somehow uncovered by environmental factors.

CVID patients usually present in their second or third decade with recurrent encapsulated organism infections, especially *H. influenzae* and *S. pneumoniae*, involving the upper and lower airway—recurrent sinusitis, pneumonia, and chronic bronchitis progressing to bronchiectasis. They can also develop gastrointestinal abnormalities, including gastric mucosal atrophy with vitamin B_{12} malabsorption, inflammatory bowel disease, and bacterial overgrowth with chronic diarrhea. Small and large joint polyarthritis is sometimes seen, suggesting an autoimmune component. Alopecia areata and sarcoid-like granulomas of the skin are also reported. Weight loss is common, and CVID patients typically have widespread lymphadenopathy and splenomegaly. As with other immunodeficiency states, CVID patients are at increased risk of developing autoimmune disease and malignancy.

The most prominent laboratory finding in CVID patients is the markedly reduced levels of serum IgG, IgA, and, in up to 50% of patients, IgM. They may also exhibit an inflammatory anemia (see Chapter 4), and both leukocytosis and monocytosis in response to chronic infection. Autoimmune thrombocytopenia may also be seen. Flow cytometry most often shows a decrease in memory B cells ($CD27^+$) and diminished expression of CD45RO on T cells in circulation, suggesting poor development of memory T cells.

TABLE 21–3 • Acquired immune deficiency disorders

Disease	Major Manifestation	Cellular Abnormality	Therapy
Common variable hypogammaglobulinemia (CVID)	Recurrent pyogenic infections at any age, autoimmune disorders	Hypogammaglobulinemia with normal numbers of B and T cells	IV immunoglobulins
Chronic graft-versus-host disease	Desquamation, hepatosplenomegaly, lymphadenopathy, diarrhea, recurrent infections	Activated T cells	Immunosuppression with steroids, methotrexate, cyclosporine
Secondary to lymphoproliferative disease	Opportunistic or recurrent pyogenic infections	Most common in chronic lymphocytic leukemia and multiple myeloma; may be seen in any lymphoma	Chemotherapy for underlying disorder
Imunosuppressive drugs (cyclosporine, purine analogs, anti-T monoclonal antibodies)	Opportunistic infections, transfusion-related GVHD, EBV-associated lymphoma	Decreased CD4 T cells	Irradiation of blood products. Prevention of viral and protozoan infections
AIDS	Opportunistic infections	Decreased CD4 T cells	Antiretroviral drugs

Acquired hypogammaglobulinemia is also a frequent component of underlying autoimmune disease, protein-losing enteropathies, nephrotic syndrome, and the progression of a clonal malignancy of B cells such as chronic lymphocytic leukemia (CLL) or multiple myeloma.

Chronic Graft-Versus-Host Disease

Graft-versus-host disease (GVHD) is a common complication of allogeneic marrow transplantation. The syndrome is characterized by skin disease, diarrhea, hepatic dysfunction, and immunosuppression. It results from the reaction of the engrafted immune system against host histocompatibility antigens. Young patients who receive fully HLA-compatible marrow transplants usually have mild or no GVHD, but older patients can develop life-threatening disease. It can occur even following transplants that are fully HLA compatible owing to differences at minor histocompatibility loci.

Conversely, patients who are immune deficient for any reason are also at risk for acute GVHD acquired from viable lymphocytes in **unirradiated transfusion products** such as whole blood, red cells, and platelets. This form of GVHD is usually fulminant and carries a high mortality. Any patient thought to have significant immune dysfunction (eg, receiving myeloablative chemotherapy) should be transfused with irradiated blood products to prevent this dreaded complication.

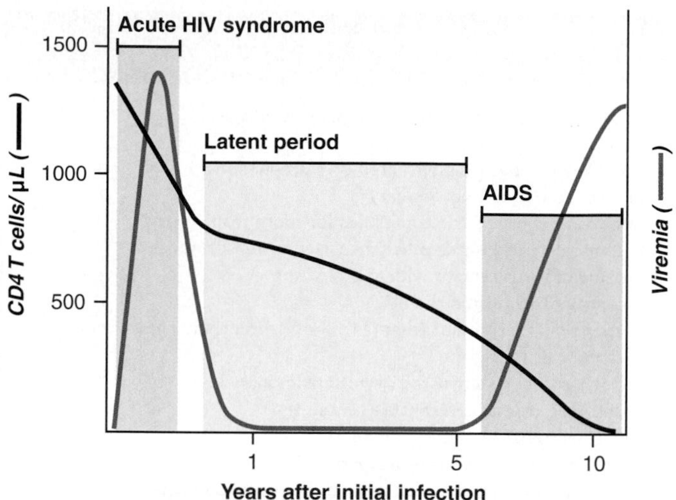

FIGURE 21–1. **The course of HIV infection.** Initial infection by HIV can be accompanied by an acute viral syndrome, after which the disease enters a prolonged latency phase with no symptoms and no immunologic abnormality. During this time, viral antigen and antiviral antibody can be detected, but there is little viremia. Progression of the disease is characterized by a progressive fall in the CD4 T-cell level and the onset of overt immunodeficiency with AIDS-specific diseases (see Table 21–4).

Acquired Immune Deficiency Syndrome

By far the most common immune deficiency syndrome is acquired immune deficiency syndrome (AIDS), secondary to infection by HIV. In the United States, the estimated incidence rate was 22.8 per 100,000 population, with 56,300 new infections in 2006. This retrovirus is transmitted by sexual contact, intravenous drug abuse, blood and blood product transfusion, and potentially by other body fluids. The virus binds to and infects $CD4^+$ cells, that is, T lymphocytes, macrophages, and dendritic cells.

A. Course of Infection

The course of infection is illustrated in Figure 21–1. Three to six weeks following infection, most patients experience a clinical syndrome with fever, malaise, rash, myalgias, and lymphadenopathy, referred to as **acute mononucleosis-like syndrome**. However, contrasting with Epstein-Barr virus (EBV) mononucleosis syndrome, an increase in the number of reactive blood lymphocytes is not present. In fact, the absolute blood lymphocyte count may be decreased. This syndrome is caused by acute viremia and the development of an immune response, with formation of circulating antibody-virus complexes. Diagnosis of the HIV infection is typically made on the basis of the detection of viral antigens, antibodies, or both. However, it is important to remember that serodiagnosis has 2 limitations: it remains negative during the first weeks following primary contact, and it can be falsely positive in infants born from infected mothers due to passive transfer of maternal antibodies. In these 2 circumstances, detection of viral RNA or p24 antigen are the only means to make the diagnosis.

With the appearance of the immune response, the acute viremia ceases and a period of latency begins that may last for several years. During the latency period, the patient remains asymptomatic or may display little more than generalized mild lymphadenopathy. During this period the infection persists and progresses and the patient is capable of infecting others. Virus can be demonstrated in the patient's lymph nodes, as well as in T lymphocytes and macrophages. The exact mechanism by which the virus is able to continue to exist and proliferate within the lymph nodes during the latency period is under intense investigation. As the HIV infection evolves, the progression of the viral replication and subsequent destruction of T cells is reflected by an increase in the viral load in plasma, as assessed by the number of RNA copies. In addition, the ratio of CD4 to CD8 T cells decreases due to progressive loss of CD4 T cells. Once the CD4 T-cell level falls below 200/µL, the patient is at high risk for opportunistic infections.

After a latency period of 5–10 years, the patient gradually becomes symptomatic because of deterioration of the immune system. The diagnosis of AIDS depends on 2 elements. The first is the demonstration of the antibody to HIV indicating previous infection, and the second is the appearance of 1 or more AIDS-defining illnesses (Table 21–4). A staging classification for the progression of AIDS has been proposed (Table 21–5). It combines the quantitation of the CD4 T-cell level and the presence or absence of complicating illness.

B. Hematologic Manifestations

In addition to the expected lymphopenia, AIDS patients usually show varying combinations of anemia, granulocytopenia, and

TABLE 21–4 • AIDS-defining illnesses (AIDS indicator conditions)

Candidiasis of bronchi, trachea, lungs, or esophagus
Cervical cancer, invasive
Coccidioidomycosis, disseminated or extrapulmonary
Cryptococcosis, extrapulmonary
Cryptosporidiosis, chronic intestinal for more than 1 month
Cytomegalovirus disease other than liver, spleen, or nodes
Cytomegalovirus retinitis with loss of vision
Encephalopathy related to HIV
Herpes simplex, chronic ulcers (>1 month), bronchitis, pneumonitis, or esophagitis
Histoplasmosis, disseminated or extrapulmonary
Isosporiasis, chronic intestinal (>1 month)
Kaposi sarcoma
Lymphoma, high-grade or primary in brain
Mycobacterium, any strain, disseminated or extrapulmonary
Mycobacterium tuberculosis, any site
Pneumocystis carinii pneumonia
Pneumonia, recurrent
Progressive multifocal leukoencephalopathy
Salmonella septicemia, recurrent
Toxoplasmosis of brain
Wasting syndrome owing to HIV

thrombocytopenia. Anemia can be anticipated as the disease progresses. It is usually a hypoproliferative anemia with normocytic, normochromic morphology; low reticulocyte count; and iron studies typical of inflammatory disease. However, Coombs-positive autoimmune hemolytic anemia, megaloblastic anemia secondary to vitamin B_{12} or folic acid malabsorption, and pure red cell aplasia with parvovirus infection must be considered. In addition, anemia concomitant with AZT (zidovudine) treatment will progress during AIDS therapy and become macrocytic. The use of erythropoietin in treating the anemia of AIDS is discussed in Chapter 4.

Both neutropenia and thrombocytopenia can occur early in the disease process. They may also occur as a result of treatment with antiviral drugs, infection, or as a manifestation of neoplasia.

TABLE 21–5 • Staging classification for AIDS

CD4 T-Cell Levels	Asymptomatic	Symptomatic, No AIDS Indicator Conditions	AIDS Indicator Conditions Present
	A	B	C
>500/μL	A1	B1	C1
200–499/μL	A2	B2	C2
<200/μL	A3	B3	C3

Note: Categories A3, B3, C1, C2, and C3 meet the criteria for AIDS case surveillance. The other categories are pre-AIDS syndromes.

Early in the progression of the disease, an examination of the marrow frequently shows normal or increased cellularity, compatible with peripheral destruction rather than failure of production. However, as complicating illnesses appear and patients demonstrate infectious processes such as mycobacterial or fungal infections, marrow hematopoiesis becomes disordered and may sometimes show a life-threatening hemophagocytic syndrome. In addition, the marrow may be directly affected by invasive lymphoma or Kaposi sarcoma.

Another complication of AIDS is the development of a high-grade B-cell lymphoma. Indeed, AIDS-related lymphoma is rapidly becoming a major cause of non-Hodgkin lymphoma. Patients with symptomatic HIV infection have an incidence of lymphoma of 2%–6% per year, and a greater than 100-fold increased risk compared with HIV-negative individuals. Despite the advent of highly active antiretroviral therapy, the incidence of HIV-associated non-Hodgkin lymphoma has not declined.

A large proportion (30%–60%) of AIDS-related lymphomas is associated with the EBV genome and may be related to activation of EBV in the immunodeficient patient. Interestingly, the HIV genome is seldom found in the lymphoma. This apparent role of EBV is similar to that observed in post-transplant lymphoproliferative disease and in some patients with congenital immunodeficiency disorders. However, AIDS-related lymphoma is usually of higher grade than post-transplant lymphomas, and more often involves a *c-myc* rearrangement. About 20% of AIDS-related lymphomas also show the *c-myc*–associated small noncleaved Burkitt histology. In general, the prognosis for AIDS patients who develop a lymphoma is poor, although some do respond to conventional multiagent therapy and experience remissions lasting several years. The central nervous system component of their disease must be recognized and treated early. In addition, the patient's course of therapy is very often complicated by opportunistic infections.

Immunodeficiency Secondary to Lymphoproliferative Disease

Most of the lymphomas are associated with relative immunodeficiency due to disruption of the normal lymph node architecture and aberrant secretion of cytokines, such as IL-1, IL-2, and IL-6, that regulate the normal immune response. Chronic lymphocytic leukemia (see Chapter 22) and Hodgkin disease (see Chapter 24) are often accompanied by a profound immunodeficiency. In CLL, the defect impairs the production of normal antibody responses, leading to recurrent pyogenic infections. In Hodgkin disease, the defect is primarily in T-cell responses, leading to anergy and increased susceptibility to viral infections such as herpes zoster, to transfusion-associated GVHD, and to secondary malignancies. Patients with Hodgkin disease can have a profound immune defect even when only small amounts of tumor are present, and even after successful therapy. The defect can also continue for years in patients who have been cured of their Hodgkin disease. In addition, most of the therapies used in the treatment of the lymphoproliferative diseases induce additional immune defects of varying severity and duration.

Post-Transplant Immunodeficiency

Patients who receive immunosuppressive therapy for prevention or treatment of organ rejection following transplantation are at increased risk for lymphoproliferative disease. The intensity of the immunosuppressive therapy is an important factor; patients who receive cyclosporine and the monoclonal anti-thymocyte antibody OKT3 are at special risk. In virtually all cases, the lymphoproliferative disease is associated with EBV infection.

Three types of post-transplant lymphoproliferative disorders have been described. The first is a polyclonal proliferation of plasmacytoid lymphocytes in the oropharynx or lymph nodes. EBV infection can be demonstrated in multiple genomic sites without immunoglobulin-gene rearrangements or oncogene activation. This type of disease is more responsive to chemotherapy and may spontaneously regress if immunosuppressive therapy is discontinued. Another form is a polymorphic lymphoproliferative disorder, presenting in nodal or extranodal sites, secondary to a monoclonal EBV infection. The third type presents as a widely disseminated B-cell lymphoma, immunoblastic lymphoma, or multiple myeloma with alterations in tumor-suppressor and oncogenes.

THERAPY

Treatment of congenital immunodeficiencies is directed at replacing the missing or dysfunctional component of the immune system, if possible. Although it is possible to supply adequate amounts of antibody to replace B-cell function, it is not possible to replace defective T-cell function except by transplanting a new T-cell system. For acquired immunodeficiencies, treatment is directed at the underlying disorder. With the rapid development of cytokine and growth factor therapy, it may be possible in the future to direct therapy toward improving or augmenting the function of the immune cells themselves.

Gamma Globulin

Defective B-cell function and hypogammaglobulinemia can be effectively treated by replacing the antibody with intravenous immunoglobulin (IVIG). These preparations are obtained from very large numbers of donors and thus contain antibodies representative of the normal immune response. They have few serious side effects and can be given in large amounts. There is some evidence that intravenous immunoglobulin, because it arises from a large pool of donors, may contain enough anti-idiotypic antibody or antibody to histocompatibility antigens that it may actually have some immunosuppressive characteristics. However, its advantages at replacing missing antibodies for patients with B-cell dysfunction far outweigh this drawback.

The recommended dose of IVIG is 100–200 mg/kg every 3–4 weeks. The dose and frequency of administration should be adjusted to achieve near normal levels of serum IgG. It should not be given to patients with isolated IgA deficiency due to the risk of anaphylaxis. In addition to IVIG, some patients may require chronic or intermittent prophylactic antibiotics to prevent recurrent infections. Bactrim is most commonly used in this setting.

Marrow Transplantation

Children with congenital defective T-cell function can only be treated with marrow transplantation. In severe combined immunodeficiency disease (SCID), the lack of a normal immune system means that there is no need to condition the patient with immunosuppressive therapy prior to the transplant. If a matched donor is available the donor's immune system will replace the defective system, resulting in a stable chimeric state in which the lymphoid cells arise from the donor and the remainder of the hematopoietic cells are of recipient origin.

Drugs for Patients with AIDS

The treatment of AIDS is directed at suppressing the growth of the retrovirus. In recent years, many new drugs have become available, which can be classified according to their mechanisms of action (Table 21–6). With the availability of these new classes of antiviral drugs, it is now possible to give patients therapy with 2 or 3 drugs with different mechanisms of action directed at specific viral genotypes (highly active antiretroviral treatment [HAART]). HAART is highly successful at suppressing HIV growth and is now being used at a much earlier stage of the disease. Many combinations of drugs have been tested so

TABLE 21–6 • Approved HIV antiretroviral single drugs

Mode of Action	Drug Name
Inhibitors of entry	Enfurvirtide Maraviroc
Anti-integrase	Raltégravir Elvitégravir
Reverse trancriptase inhibitors, nucleosidic	Abacavir Didanosine Emtricitabine Lamivudine Stavudine Zalcitabine Zidovudine
Reverse trancriptase inhibitor, nucleotidic	Tenofovir
Reverse trancriptase inhibitors, non-nucleosidic	Delaviridine Efavirenz Nevirapine Integrase
Protease inhibitors[a]	Amprenavir/ritonavir Atazanavir/ritonavir Darunavir/ritonavir Fosamprenavir/ritonavir Indivavir/ritonavir Nelfinavir Ritonavir Saquinavir/ritonavir Tripanavir/ritonavir Lopinavir/ritonavir

[a]*Ritonavir, as an inhibitor of cytochrome P450 CYP3A4 enzyme, reduces the metabolism of concomitantly administered protease inhibitors.*

CASE HISTORY • Part 3

The patient has a marked defect in immunoglobulin (IgG and IgA) production, which would explain the susceptibility to recurrent upper and lower airway infections with encapsulated organisms. The absence of a monoclonal immunoglobulin (M component) would rule out multiple myeloma, and the negative HIV antibody assay rules against AIDS as a primary diagnosis. The findings of a reduced number of circulating CD27$^+$ memory B cells and an autoimmune thrombocytopenia strongly suggest the diagnosis of common variable immunodeficiency (CVID), the most prevalent form of inherited immunodeficiency. Flow cytometry can also demonstrate a decrease in CD45RO$^+$ memory T cells, but this is a nonspecific finding.

CVID patients should receive maintenance intravenous immunoglobulin (IVIG) as replacement therapy. She will also require aggressive evaluation and treatment for her bronchiectasis. Her prognosis will depend more on the course of her chronic lung disease than the CVID itself, and her autoimmune disease (immune thrombocytopenia) should be readily controlled with IVIG but could require more aggressive therapy (see Chapter 31).

far. Combinations of 2 nucleoside reverse transcriptase inhibitors plus either efavirenz (non-nucleosidic reverse transcriptase inhibitor) or a ritonavir-boosted protease inhibitor are usually recommended for initial therapy.

The decision to begin therapy depends on the presence of clinical manifestations of AIDS-related illness and the level of CD4 T cells. The standing recommendation has been to treat patients with symptomatic disease and/or CD4 levels less than 350/μL. Some patients with CD4 greater than 350/μL may also be candidates, depending on the clinical setting and the level of viral genome in their blood. Patients with high viral loads (>100,000 copies per milliliter) now receive therapy long before their CD4 count has fallen into the immunosuppressed range. Such early combination therapy can lead not only to a dramatic fall in viral load, but also to a recovery of CD4 T cells with improvement in immunologic function.

The current goal of treatment is to obtain a plasma HIV-1 RNA titer below 50 copies/mL within 6 months and to maintain this result thereafter. This may require substitution of drugs due to intolerance or decreased efficacy. While results are encouraging, it is not yet clear to what extent the immune system can reconstitute itself with control of the HIV viral load. It can be anticipated that longer survival and delayed onset of viral drug resistance will increase the number of patients surviving with partial immunologic defects.

POINTS TO REMEMBER

Immunodeficiency should be suspected in patients with a history of recurrent or persistent infections. A high level of suspicion is frequently necessary to make the correct diagnosis.

Important elements of the diagnosis include the types of infections and the duration of the symptoms. These help distinguish between antibody production defects (recurrent pyogenic infections) and T-cell defects (fungal and viral infections), and also between acquired and congenital disorders.

Beyond measurement of immunogobulin levels and lymphocyte subsets in the blood, testing for immune defects is not well standardized and often falls in the realm of the research laboratory.

Although HIV infection frequently presents with hematologic signs and symptoms, its treatment has become highly complex and specialized, with a major focus on the eradication/control of the viral load as a route to decreasing the complications and progression of AIDS.

Patients being treated for other hematologic disorders, particulary the lymphoproliferative diseases, often have severe acquired immune defects secondary to their treatment. In addition, patients receiving significant post-transplant immunosuppression must be vigilantly screened for post-transplant lymphoproliferative disorder as a result of EBV infection.

BIBLIOGRAPHY

Binder V, Albert MH, Kabus M, Bertone M, Meindl A, Belohradsky BH: The genotype of the original Wiskott phenotype. N Engl J Med 2006;355:1790.

Buckley RH: Molecular defects in human severe combined immunodeficiency and approaches to immune reconstitution. Annu Rev Immunol 2004;22:625.

Buckley RH: Primary immunodeficiency or not? Making the correct diagnosis. J Allergy Clin Immunol 2006;117:756.

Cavazzana-Calvo M, Hacein-Bey S, de Saint Basile G, et al: Gene therapy of human severe combined immunodeficiency (SCID)-X1 disease. Science 2000;288:627.

Deeg HJ, Antin JH: The clinical spectrum of acute graft-versus-host disease. Semin Hematol 2006;43:24.

Fleisher TA, Oliveira JB: Functional and molecular evaluation of lymphocytes. J Allergy Clin Immunol 2004;114:227.

Hall HI, Song R, Rhodes P, et al: Estimation of HIV incidence in the United States. JAMA 2008;300:520.

Hammer SM, Eron JJ Jr, Reiss P, et al: Antiretroviral treatment of adult HIV infection: 2008 recommendations of the International AIDS Society—USA panel. JAMA 2008;300:555.

Levine AM: Acquired immunodeficiency syndrome related lymphoma: clinical aspects. Semin Oncol 2000;27:442.

Mounier N, Spina M, Gabarre J, et al: AIDS-related non-Hodgkin lymphoma: final analysis of 485 patients treated with risk-adapted intensive chemotherapy. Blood 2006;107:3832.

Navarro WH, Kaplan LD: AIDS-related lymphoproliferative disease. Blood 2006;107:13.

Notarangelo L, Casanova JL, Fisher A, et al: Primary immunodefiency diseases: an update. J Allergy Clin Immunol 2004; 114:677.

Notarangelo LD, Lanzi G, Peron S, Durandy A: Defects of class-switch recombination. J Allergy Clin Immunol 2006; 117:855.

Notarangelo LD, Miao CH, Ochs HD: Wiskott-Aldrich syndrome. Curr Opin Hematol 2008;15:30.

Ozsahin H et al: Adenosine deaminase deficiency in adults. Blood 1997;89:2849.

Rudd CE: Disabled receptor signaling and new primary immunodeficiency disorders. N Engl J Med 2006;354:1874.

Simon V, Ho DD, Quarraisha AK: HIV/AIDS epidemiology, pathogenesis, prevention, and treatment. Lancet 2006;368:489.

Stebbing J, Gazzard B, Douek DC: Where does HIV live? N Engl J Med 2004;350:1872.

Thrasher AJ: Gene therapy for primary immunodeficiencies. Immunol Allergy Clin North Am 2008;28:457.

Tosi MF: Innate immune responses to infection. J Allergy Clin Immunol 2005;116:241.

Wen L, Atkinson JP, Giclas PC: Clinical and laboratory evaluation of complement deficiency. J Allergy Clin Immunol 2004;113:585.

World Health Organization (WHO): Interim proposal for a WHO Staging System for HIV Infection and Disease. Wkly Epidemiol Rec 1990;65:221.

CHRONIC LYMPHOCYTIC LEUKEMIA AND OTHER LEUKEMIC LYMPHOPROLIFERATIVE DISEASES • 22

CASE HISTORY • *Part I*

A 68-year-old man who has been in good health presents with the recent onset of marked fatigue and shortness of breath. He gives no history of an increased frequency of infections, nor any bleeding tendency, and has no family history of hematologic disorders. Examination is remarkable for pallor and the presence of multiple firm, freely movable, nontender nodes in the neck, axilla, and groin. The spleen and liver are not palpable.

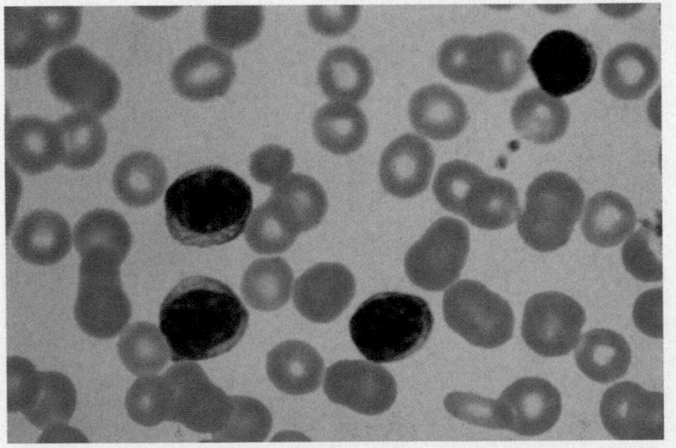

CBC: Hematocrit/hemoglobin - 18%/6 g/dL
MCV - 88 fL MCH - 33 pg MCHC - 36 g/dL
WBC count - 20,500/μL
Differential: Neutrophils - 18%
Lymphocytes - 80%
Monocytes - 1%
Eosinophils - 1%
Platelet count - 30,000/μL
Reticulocyte count/index - 14%/3
Coombs test positive

Questions

- What abnormalities are apparent from the CBC?
- What further laboratory tests should be obtained?

The most common lymphoproliferative disorder in Western countries is B-cell chronic lymphocytic leukemia (CLL). At the same time, there are a number of other lymphoproliferative disorders that present with a leukemic component and need to be differentiated from CLL. Understanding and diagnosing the various lymphoproliferative disorders requires familiarity with the normal lymphocyte subsets, which are described in Chapters 20 and 21.

B-CELL CHRONIC LYMPHOCYTIC LEUKEMIA

B-cell CLL typically has a long course, and therefore is considered the least "malignant" of the lymphoproliferative disorders. B-cell CLL is almost entirely a disease of older adults (median age 65-68 years, with 90% over 40 years of age). CLL demonstrates major **genetic and environmental influences** in different populations. In the United States, the incidence among white populations is 5 and 2.5/100,000 for males and females, respectively. By contrast, B-cell CLL is a very infrequent disease in Asians, including longstanding US immigrants. Recent studies have explored the interaction between genetic factors and hitherto undefined environmental factors in the initiation of the CLL B-cell clonal expansion. In European populations, the nature of genes from the variable heavy chain (IgV_H) selected during the process of recombination of the variable (V), diversity (D), and joining (J) regions of the immunoglobulin genes in CLL clones have clearly shown differences from polyclonal cells in specific IgV_H frequencies.

The major clinical manifestation of CLL is an increase in the number of circulating lymphocytes. The patient with CLL may also have varying degrees of lymphadenopathy, ranging from little at all to massive involvement. With the increasing availability of lymphocyte marker studies, CLL is being diagnosed earlier and in younger patients. In fact, small collections of clonal B cells with the characteristic surface markers of B-cell CLL (CD19, CD20, and CD5 positive) can be found in otherwise normal individuals with normal blood counts (<5000 lymphocytes/μL) in 3% to 4% of individuals over age 40 and in 5.1% older than 60. The frequency of small populations of circulating monoclonal CLL B cells is even higher in family members of CLL patients (~13%), suggesting an inherited susceptibility. This does not translate, however, into a comparable increase in the incidence of actual clinical disease in family members. Some other stimulus, such as repetitive antigenic stimulation, may be required.

The **distinction between CLL and small-cell lymphocytic lymphoma** is largely semantic. Patients presenting with a marked increase in circulating lymphocytes and less adenopathy are diagnosed as having CLL, whereas patients presenting with prominent adenopathy and/or a tumor mass of monoclonal $CD19^+$ $CD5^+$ B cells with near normal white blood counts are diagnosed as having small cell lymphoma. Lymph node biopsy demonstrates a "small cell" or "diffuse well-differentiated" lymphocytic lymphoma (see Chapter 23). However, even when the lymphocyte count is normal, such patients will have detectable circulating $CD19^+$ $CD5^+$ lymphoma cells and thus can be said to have small cell lymphoma/CLL. From a clinical standpoint, there is little difference between patients presenting with tissue lymphoma and those presenting only with chronic leukemia, and these should be considered varying manifestations of the same disease.

CLL may also present with major immunologic or hematologic abnormalities. The most common are a **B- or T-cell immunodeficiency state** resulting in recurrent infections, autoimmune hemolytic anemia or thrombocytopenia, and, less often, pure red cell aplasia. Thus, CLL must be considered in the differential diagnosis of patients with any of these disorders and must be ruled in or out by analysis of blood counts and lymphocyte markers. It is not uncommon to find patients with a normal level of circulating lymphocytes that are, nevertheless, largely CLL cells.

Clinical Features

B-cell CLL is often discovered on a routine blood count in an otherwise asymptomatic patient. B-cell CLL patients may also present with **nonspecific symptoms** of malaise, easy fatigability, weight loss, and night sweats. Symptoms appear to correlate with overall tumor load. In symptomatic patients, widespread lymphadenopathy, splenomegaly, or, in some cases, tonsillar enlargement are almost always apparent on examination. The nontender lymph nodes are typically multiple, slightly to moderately enlarged, involve all palpable nodal sites, and are not matted or fixed to surrounding tissue. Even bulky lymph node enlargement does not usually result in compressive symptoms unless the CLL is transforming to a more aggressive form of large cell lymphoma (Richter transformation).

The increase in the number of circulating B cells does not correlate with the clinical presentation. Most patients with CLL are asymptomatic despite the presence of impressive numbers of circulating lymphocytes. Even at levels up to 100,000–300,000/μL, the lymphocytosis never results in microcirculatory leukostasis, nor does it impinge on the production of other hematopoietic cell lines. Anemia, thrombocytopenia, and neutropenia are more likely due to disease progression within the marrow, autoimmune complications, hypersplenism, or treatment side effects.

B-cell CLL patients can also present with symptoms of immune deficiency. Hypogammaglobulinemia is observed in more than half of patients during the course of the disease, exposing patients mainly to pulmonary bacterial infections. T-cell deficiency is more often the result of treatment, and increases the risk of viral and opportunistic infections (see Chapter 21). Autoimmune manifestations such as autoimmune thrombocytopenia, Coombs positive hemolytic anemia, or pure red cell aplasia are also frequent in CLL.

Laboratory Studies

Accurate diagnosis of B-CLL is based on the **CBC, bone marrow examination, and flow cytometric immunophenotyping of the B cells**. The typical CBC pattern is an increase in the number of mature-appearing lymphocytes in circulation to more

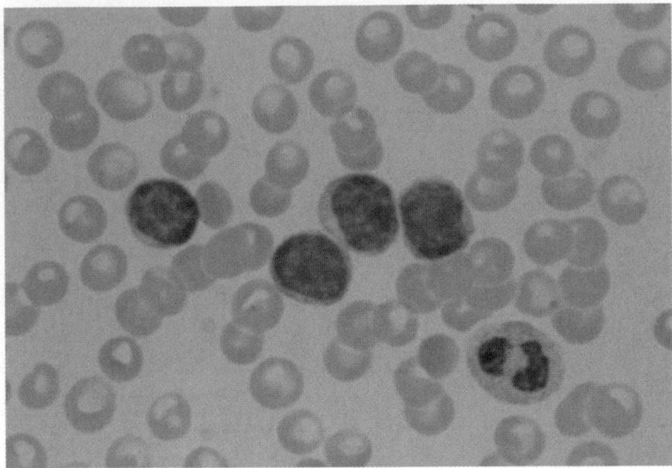

FIGURE 22–1. **CLL Lymphocytes.** A group of mature-looking B lymphocytes in chronic lymphocytic leukemia.

than 5000/μL (Figure 22–1) with little or no impact on the red blood cell, granulocyte, or platelet counts. Smudge cells—nuclear fragments resulting from shearing—are frequently observed on smears; adding albumin to blood before making a peripheral smear will preserve intact lymphocytes for morphologic evaluation. The bone marrow generally shows a diffuse infiltration of small, mature-appearing lymphocytes, largely obscuring all other hematopoietic cell lines. Still, the **definitive diagnosis** requires immunophenotyping.

In typical CLL, CD19 B-cells express CD5, dim CD20, and CD23, together with abnormally low surface amounts of monotypic sIg; κ/λ analysis is consistent with a monoclonal population. The sIg involved is usually IgM or IgD or both, rarely IgG; and always only a single immunoglobulin light chain, either κ or λ, is present (see Chapter 26). Thus, the finding of an increased number of B cells expressing CD5 and CD23, with low levels of sIg and a single immunoglobulin light chain, has been considered diagnostic of B-cell CLL (Figure 22–2). The Matutes scoring system expands on this use of markers to make the distinction between typical CLL and other leukemias of lymphoid origin (Table 22–1). The system takes into account low sIg density and low CD79b levels, and expression of CD5 and CD23 (for each of the characteristics, score 1 when present and 0 when absent). Most typical B-cell CLL patients have scores of 4; scores less than 4 should prompt consideration of a different lymphoproliferative disorder in combination with other phenotypic markers.

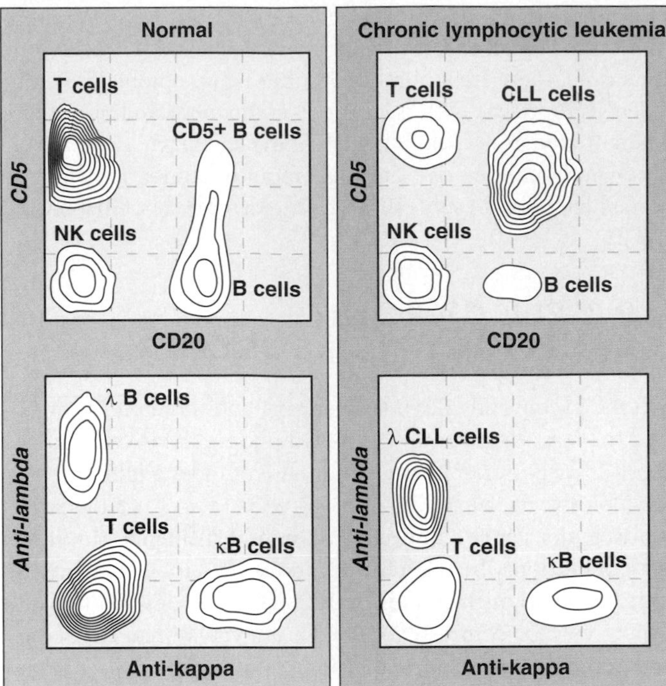

FIGURE 22–2. **Marker studies in CLL.** CD20, a B-cell marker, and CD5, a T-cell marker, distinguish between normal T cells ($CD5^+$ $CD20^-$) and normal B cells ($CD5^-$ $CD20^+$). A subset of normal (polyclonal) B cells also expresses lower levels of CD5 ($CD5^+$ B cells). B-cell CLL is characterized by a predominance of $CD5^+$ B cells which express monoclonal immunoglobulin light chains on their surface, in this case λ light chain, at levels lower than normal.

A. Immunoglobulin Gene Rearrangement

All B-cell CLLs show rearrangements of one or both immunoglobulin heavy chain genes and expression of either the κ or λ immunoglobulin light chain gene. Although testing for these rearrangements is both extremely sensitive and specific, it is

TABLE 22–1 • Immunophenotype in B-cell CLL and other lymphoproliferative disorders

	sIg	CD5	CD23	CD79b	FMC7	CD22	CD10
B-cell CLL	↓	+	+	↓	-	↓	-
B-cell prolymphocytic leukemia	+	±	±	+	+	+	±
Mantle cell lymphoma	+	+	-	+	+	±	–
Follicular center cell lymphoma	+	-	±	+	+	+	+
Splenic marginal zone lymphoma	+	–	–	+	+	+	–

usually unnecessary in the patient who presents with lymphocytosis or lymphadenopathy with sufficient cells for immunophenotyping. Gene rearrangement may rarely be of value in situations where the immunophenotype is nondiagnostic and can recognize clonal cells with a sensitivity ranging from 10^{-2}–10^{-5} depending on whether the technique uses consensus sequences or clone-specific probes, respectively. However, with immunophenotyping, multichannel flow cytometers provide comparable detection sensitivity.

In approximately 50% of CLL patients the IgV_H genes show low levels of somatic mutation (more than 98% homology with germline genes), whereas the remainder display significant somatic hypermutations (less than 98% homology). A greater degree of somatic mutation has been associated with a better prognosis. CLL with unmutated genes (98% or more homology) has a median survival of 8–10 years, with therapy being required at a median of 3 years, whereas the hypermutated genotype (<98%) is associated with a 25-year median survival and much longer interval to therapy. Surrogate markers for the unmutated genotype include high percentages (>30%) of CLL cells expressing surface CD38 and/or high levels of cytoplasmic expression of ZAP-70, a protein involved in intracellular signaling from the antigen receptor (see Chapter 20). While these features are of significance for prognosis, they tend to impact only on the care of relatively younger CLL patients who may die from complications of CLL rather than comorbidities of advanced age.

B. Cytogenetic Analysis

In the past, obtaining cytogenetic analysis of CLL cells was difficult owing to their very low proliferation in response to mitogens. However, recent studies using improved mitogenic strategies have provided informative karyotypes in 80%–85% of patients. Fluorescence in-situ hybridization (FISH) technology, using a selected set of four probes for the more frequent chromosomal abnormalities, reveals a similar frequency of abnormalities. In practice, the two techniques complement one another. For instance, FISH better recognizes the 13q deletion, but not translocations or complex karyotypes, which are powerful prognostic indicators. A variety of chromosomal abnormalities have been described, the most common being deletions on chromosomes 11q, 13p, and 17q; trisomy 12; and both balanced and unbalanced translocations. CLL patients with $17p^-$, $11q^-$, or multiple cytogenetic abnormalities have a shorter survival. The $17p^-$ abnormality may involve loss of the **p53 gene**, which is important in the tumor response to purine nucleoside analogues.

C. Other Laboratory Studies

Other important laboratory studies for CLL include **serum protein electrophoresis** to detect a possible M component (about 5% of cases) and to provide an overall screen of immunoglobulin production (see Chapter 26). CLL patients can present with diffuse hypogammaglobulinemia or may develop hypogammaglobulinemia during the course of their disease; quantitative levels will confirm this. A Coombs test should be obtained in any CLL patient who presents with anemia. In patients with very large tumor burdens, elevated **serum lactic dehydrogenase (LDH), β_2-microglobulin, and uric acid levels** are expected.

Differential Diagnosis

Many of the B-cell lymphomas have an accompanying leukemic component, that is, circulating lymphoma cells. Therefore, if adenopathy is a prominent aspect of the clinical presentation, a node biopsy is indicated to rule out a more aggressive form of lymphoma. The presence of high-density sIg similarly indicates that the physician is not dealing with typical B-cell CLL. Disorders such as **hairy cell leukemia, prolymphocytic leukemia,**

CASE HISTORY • *Part 2*

The blood smear shows microspherocytes, polychromasia (shift reticulocytes), and numerous small lymphocytes. Platelets are markedly decreased. Severe anemia with spherocytosis and polychromasia on smear and a very high reticulocyte count/index is typical of a hemolytic anemia, almost certainly in this case, an autoimmune hemolytic anemia, since the Coombs test is positive. The very low platelet count may also be a sign of autoimmune thrombocytopenia. Not to be ignored is the marked increase in mature-appearing lymphocytes (absolute count >16,000/μL). This strongly suggests a lymphoproliferative disorder, especially B-cell CLL. To evaluate this, immunophenotyping and chromosomal analysis were performed with the following results:

• IMMUNOPHENOTYPE

Most of the lymphocytes are identified as $CD19^+$ B cells, which are $CD20dim^+$, $CD5^+$, and $CD23^+$, with low levels of surface IgM and IgD and exclusively expressing low levels of κ light chain. Small numbers of phenotypically normal B cells ($CD5^-$) and T cells are present.

• CYTOGENETICS

FISH reports a deletion on chromosome 13p.

Questions

- What is the diagnosis and stage of disease?
- What additional workup is indicated?
- How should this patient be managed?

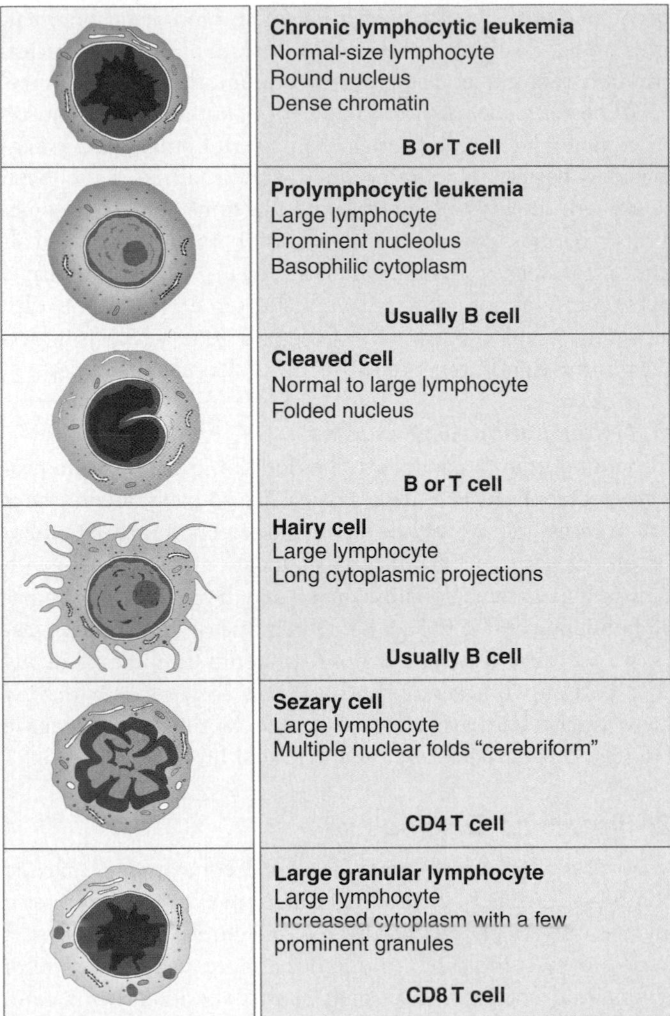

FIGURE 22–3. Morphology in CLL versus other circulating lymphoma cells. The morphologic appearance of typical CLL cells is indistinguishable from that of normal B and T lymphocytes. Several morphologically distinctive forms of lymphocytic lymphomas with leukemic involvement, however, correlate to some extent with their immunophenotype.

and **leukemias involving large cell, less well-differentiated lymphomas** are usually distinguished on the basis of immunophenotyping and morphology (Figure 22–3 and Table 22–1). **Mantle cell lymphoma** is another B-cell malignancy that expresses CD5 but is distinguished from CLL by the absence of CD23, the presence of larger cells, and by a much more aggressive course. Seventy percent of mantle cell lymphomas show a t(11;14) translocation involving the bcl-1 locus, which results in the **overexpression of cyclin D1**—a critical regulator of the cell division cycle.

Therapy

The treatment of B-cell CLL with chemotherapy with or without transplantation is never curative. Therefore, the choice and timing of therapy depend heavily on the stage of the disease. A majority of patients present with little more than an elevated lymphocyte count and follow a protracted clinical course. Others, however, progress rapidly and develop anemia, leukopenia, thrombocytopenia, and hypogammaglobulinemia with a propensity to life-threatening infections. CLL can also undergo transformation to a much more aggressive form of lymphoma such as **diffuse large cell lymphoma with massive splenomegaly (Richter syndrome)** or prolymphocytic leukemia. Transformation of CLL should be suspected if the patient's course appears to change abruptly, or when the proportion of larger, nucleated cells (especially prolymphocytes) increases in blood.

TABLE 22–2 • Rai and Binet staging systems for B-cell CLL

Level of Risk	Rai Staging System	Binet Staging System	Percentage of Patients	Overall Survival
Low	Stage 0-1	Stage A	50%-55%	>120 mo
Intermediate	Stage 2	Stage B	25%-30%	60-80 mo
High	Stages 3-4	Stage C	15%	20-60 mo

Two slightly different staging systems, Rai and Binet, have been recommended for staging the patient with CLL (Table 22–2), and both rely on physical examination and CBC findings. In the Rai system, patients are classified as stage 0 (lymphocytosis without clinical symptoms), 1 (lymphocytosis with lymphadenopathy), 2 (lymphocytosis with splenomegaly), 3 (anemia with Hb <11 g/dL whatever the other signs), and 4 (thrombocytopenia <100,000/μL whatever the other signs). In the Binet system, patients with Hgb greater than 10 g/dL and platelets greater than 100,000/μL and limited lymphadenopathy and/or splenomegaly are classified as stage A, while those with normal counts but more extensive lymphadenopathy and splenomegaly are classified as stage B. Stage C is defined by either Hgb less than 10 g/dL or platelets less than 100,000/μL. The distribution of patients according to stage and level of risk for progression and associated illness and the overall survivals for each group are shown in Table 22–2.

Other **prognostic factors** for determining prognosis and planning therapy include lymphocyte doubling time, IgV_H mutational status, cytogenetic abnormalities, expression of CD38 and ZAP-70, and tumor burden as indicated by an elevated LDH, β_2-microglobulin, or both.

Although there is **no curative therapy**, recent advances in chemotherapy have led to a substantial number of complete responses and prolonged disease-free survival. In general, treatment is directed toward palliation of symptoms with minimal morbidity. As a general rule, treatment should be deferred in patients without symptoms (eg, fever, weight loss, night sweats, fatigue, bulky adenopathy) and without complications such as thrombocytopenia, anemia, or infections. Chemotherapy directed entirely at lowering the lymphocyte count will be effective, but there is no evidence that it prolongs life or slows progression. Chemotherapy certainly increases morbidity owing to infection and the possible risk of treatment-related second malignancies.

A. Drug Therapy

Several first-line treatment options are available. **Chlorambucil,** an oral alkylating agent, can be given to outpatients with excellent tolerance and little impact on blood counts, other than the absolute lymphocyte count. Various continuous or intermittent schedules have been used, aimed at an average dose of 40–70 mg each month. It generally takes 6–12 months to obtain a response in 60%–70% of patients, lasting less than 20 months in all but a few patients. The possible long-term risk of developing myelodysplastic syndromes remains unclear in CLL patients treated with this drug.

Fludarabine is a purine analog available only for intravenous use in the United States (orally in the European Union). It is administered monthly for 5 consecutive days at a dosage of 25 mg/m^2/d, usually for 6 courses. Overall response rates are 75%, with a mean duration of 25 months. Cladribine, another purine analog, displays similar efficacy.

Alemtuzumab is a recombinant monoclonal antibody active against the CD52 epitope, shared by CLL B cells and normal T cells. It is administered through IV or subcutaneous routes. Efficacy is impressive on blood lymphocytosis and splenomegaly, but less marked on bulky lymphadenopathy. Interestingly, anti-CD52 retains efficacy even in patients with p53 mutations. Treatment with alemtuzumab is associated with a common "first dose effect" consisting of rigors, fever, hypotension, and respiratory distress. This syndrome can be severe in as many as 14% of patients receiving this drug.

Combining **fludarabine with cyclophosphamide, mitoxantrone,** and/or **rituximab** appears to result in higher response rates, including complete and sometimes molecular remissions, and longer event-free survival when compared with chlorambucil or fludarabine alone. However, side effects and toxicity are more frequent with these combinations; combinations including purine analogs and alemtuzumab deplete the blood CD4 cells for months. Complete response rates following first-line therapy vary by drug and drug combination—less than 5% with chlorambucil, 20% with fludarabine, 40% with fludarabine plus cyclophosphamide, and nearly 60% when rituximab is combined with these 2 drugs. Duration of responses parallel these results. However, the relationship between response and outcome remains unclear. All trials to date conclude that the overall survival is similar whatever first-line regimen is administered.

In clinical practice, the current recommendation is to select a treatment that is well tolerated and preserves comfort and quality of life, especially in elderly patients. For younger patients, the optimal approach to therapy is still being studied, with the goal of improving response rate and duration, and, if possible, long-term outcomes. Once the patient's disease process transforms into a more aggressive lymphoproliferative disorder, combination chemotherapy is indicated but can only delay progression. Targeted radiotherapy can also help to reduce bulky lymphadenopathy.

B. Intensive Therapy

In the younger patient with adverse prognostic factors, intensification with **autologous stem cell rescue** is currently being assessed in large prospective trials. Poor stem cell harvest is a limitation in 30% of patients, because of the infiltration and damage to the marrow by malignant lymphocytes. Whatever benefit can be expected, this procedure is not going to be curative. On the other hand, **allogeneic stem cell transplantation** is potentially curative in CLL. However, its application is limited by the patient's age and tolerance, and the availability of a compatible donor. The use of reduced conditioning regimens appears promising, making it possible for patients aged up to 65 years to undergo this procedure. Allogeneic stem cell transplantation is currently considered the therapy of choice for younger patients with refractory disease, especially with p53 (17p) mutations.

C. Complications

CLL patients will, with progression of their disease, develop manifestations of autoimmune disease, especially hemolytic anemia and thrombocytopenia. When severe, both can be treated with corticosteroids, starting with a high dose of prednisone, 60–90 mg orally daily, and then tapering to a minimal daily or every-other-day maintenance dose. Pure red cell aplasia, an uncommon complication, usually responds to cyclosporin.

With progression, some CLL patients will develop hypogammaglobulinemia and experience repeated infections with encapsulated organisms, especially involving the respiratory tract. These can be life-threatening and should be aggressively treated with broad-spectrum antibiotics; even a simple bronchitis can progress to pneumonia if treatment is delayed. The propensity to recurrent infections can, in part, be decreased by administering intravenous gamma globulin (IVIG, 400 mg/kg every 3 weeks). However, owing to its expense, prophylactic IVIG should be reserved for patients with severe hypogammaglobulinemia. Immunization with hemophilus and pneumococcal vaccines early in the disease process may also help to reduce the incidence of infection.

PROLYMPHOCYTIC LEUKEMIAS

Prolymphocytic leukemias differ from B-cell CLL in morphology, phenotype, and clinical course.

B-Cell Prolymphocytic Leukemia

B-cell prolymphocytic leukemia (B-PLL) is a more malignant, more aggressive variant of B-cell CLL. Clinically, B-PLL presents with bulky lymphadenopathy, prominent splenomegaly, and very high lymphocyte counts. Lymphocyte morphology is distinctive; most lymphocytes (>55%) in circulation are medium sized but are clearly larger than the typical small B lymphocyte, and each displays a prominent nucleolus. Such cells can be observed in advanced cases of CLL, but predominant prolymphocytes in CLL signify transformation. The immunophenotype of de novo B-PLL cells differs from B-cell CLL by absence of CD23, expression of FMC7, and strong expression of sIg (Table 22–1). Deletions of 11q23 and 13q14 with loss of the retinoblastoma gene are common. Treatment with combination chemotherapy, including alemtuzumab and purine analogs, generally result in incomplete and transient responses.

CASE HISTORY • Part 3

The patient has the typical clinical and phenotypic presentation of B-cell CLL, complicated by an associated autoimmune hemolytic anemia and, most likely, autoimmune thrombocytopenia. In the absence of the associated autoimmune abnormalities, the patient would be categorized as Rai stage I or Binet stage B since the lymphocyte count is not greatly elevated, nor is the lymphadenopathy striking. If the hemolytic anemia had not developed and brought this patient to medical attention, he might have had undiagnosed CLL for many years. However, in light of the anemia and thrombocytopenia, the patient is a Rai 3 or Binet C stage CLL with a poor prognosis.

With typical findings in the blood, and evidence of a strong marrow response to the anemia, a bone marrow aspiration/biopsy is not necessary, but if carried out it would show extensive infiltration with small lymphocytes and likely erythroid hyperplasia. A lymph node biopsy is also not needed to confirm the diagnosis of CLL, unless transformation to a more aggressive lymphoma is suspected because of rapid node enlargement or compression. If a node were biopsied in this case, the pathological diagnosis would be diffuse small cell lymphoma.

This patient's immune hemolytic anemia and thrombocytopenia should be treated with prednisone (1 mg/kg/d), transfusions if bleeding or cardiac failure is a problem, and folic acid supplementation. Simultaneous treatment of the CLL with chemotherapy is clearly indicated and should help decrease the levels of anti–red cell/anti-platelet antibodies. Initial therapy with chlorambucil alone or fludarabine in combination with cyclophosphamide to provide immunosuppression would be a good choice. Fludarabine as a single agent is contraindicated due to reports of fatal exacerbation of hemolytic anemia. Combined therapy with rituxan can be effective, and in refractory patients splenectomy can reduce both red cell and platelet destruction.

T-Cell Prolymphocytic Leukemia

T-cell prolymphocytic leukemia (T-PLL) presents in adults with very high counts of medium-sized lymphocytes, notable for their scanty cytoplasm, a convoluted nucleus with open chromatin, and a prominent central nucleolus. On examination, T-PLL patients typically have diffuse, bulky lymphadenopathy, hepatosplenomegaly, and skin infiltrates. Their immunophenotype is typical for a mature T cell (expressing CD3, CD4, CD5, and CD7). Most cases are $CD4^+/CD8^-$, but some can express a $CD4^+/CD8^+$ or $CD4^-/CD8^+$ phenotype. Mutation in the *ATM* gene (11q23) is frequently observed, as well as *TCL1* gene overexpression. Clonality of the disease can be ascertained by study of the T-cell receptor genes or abnormal T-cell immunophenotyping.

T-PLL is a very aggressive disease with median patient survivals of less than 10 months. Few treatments are effective. Among them, pentostatin, and more recently the monoclonal antibody, alemtuzumab, have provided high response rates, but unfortunately of short duration. Consolidation with high dose therapy and autologous stem cell support or allogeneic stem cell transplantation can improve the outcome in some patients.

ADULT T-CELL LEUKEMIA/ LYMPHOMA

The adult T-cell leukemias share several clinical characteristics. Most striking is a propensity to involve the skin such that they are often included in a heterogeneous group of peripheral T-cell lymphomas (see Chapter 23). However, some of these cases will present with a leukemic picture and distinctive features.

Clinical Features

Adult T-cell leukemia/lymphoma (ATLL) was first described in Japan, where it represents the most common form of lymphocytic leukemia. Similar cases have now been recognized in the Caribbean, Great Britain, and worldwide. ATLL is associated with human T-cell leukemia virus-1 (HTLV-1) infection. Infection of T cells by this retrovirus results in a long period of latency, followed by either their destruction or uncontrolled lymphocyte proliferation in 1%–3% of infected patients. The clinical expression is highly variable. Some patients present with little more than lymphocytosis and/or chronic lymphadenopathy, while others follow a more aggressive course with subacute leukemia, hypercalcemia, myeloma-like lytic bone lesions, and skin infiltrates. The morphology of the malignant cells in which the nuclear shape is typically "flowerlike" can make the diagnosis.

Mycosis fungoides is due to an epidermal infiltration of monoclonal $CD4^+$ T cells, often with an associated leukemic T cell population. When the leukemia is prominent and the cells have a characteristic nuclear morphology (ie, a folded or "cerebriform" nucleus), the disease is referred to as **Sézary syndrome** (Figure 22–4). Unlike ATLL, this cutaneous T-cell lymphoma is not associated with HTLV-1. Many patients with mycosis fungoides/Sézary syndrome can present with exfoliative dermatitis or patchy plaque-like or nodular infiltration. Pruritis is a prominent complaint and is usually constant and severe. Infection of

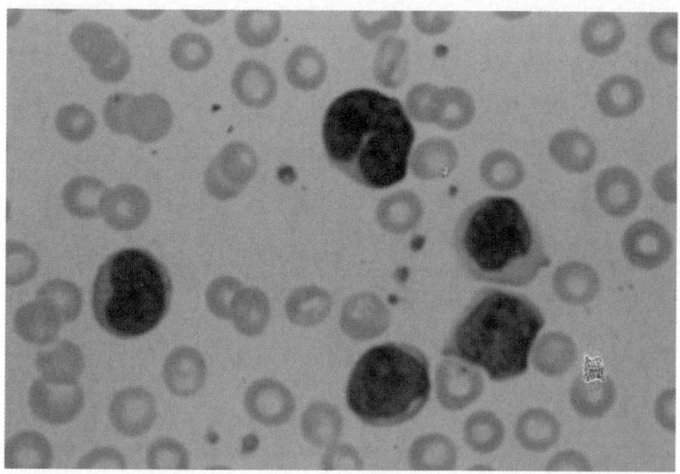

FIGURE 22–4. **Sézary cells.** Lymphocytes with convoluted or cerebriform nuclei (Sézary cells) in a patient with advanced mycosis fungoides/cutaneous T-cell lymphoma.

the skin lesions is also common and can be life-threatening (see Chapter 23).

Laboratory Studies

Unlike B-cell CLL, there is **no constant immunologic marker for ATLL T cells that indicates clonality**. The cells express an activated mature T-cell phenotype, CD3/CD4/CD25 and are HLA-DR positive. One useful clue can come from examining several different T-cell–associated markers. Normal mature $CD4^+$ T cells also express CD2, CD5, and CD7, while a malignant T-cell population may lack one or more of these markers or express them in abnormal amounts. In addition, normal resting $CD4^+$ T cells do not express HLA-DR or CD38; intense expression of these activation markers may indicate that the cells are clonal. The definitive test for clonality among the T-cell disorders is to examine for **rearrangement of the T-cell receptor genes**. Most malignant T cells will have a clonal rearrangement of the *TCR-β* and/or -γ genes that can be detected either by restriction mapping and Southern blotting or by polymerase chain reaction (PCR).

Therapy

The course of aggressive ATLL is almost always fatal, generally in the year after diagnosis. Some responses have been recorded with treatments combining recombinant interferon and zidovudine. By contrast, cutaneous T-cell lymphoma with Sézary syndrome may respond to aggressive chemotherapy, photopheresis, or the combination.

LARGE GRANULAR LYMPHOCYTIC LEUKEMIA

Occasionally, patients with what appears to be typical ATLL will prove to have a proliferation of $CD3^+$ $CD8^+$ T cells. These cases can be distinguished only by immunophenotyping, although leukopenia, especially neutropenia, may be clinically evident. This $CD8^+$ T-cell disorder has been given various names, the most common of which are **large granular lymphocytic (LGL) leukemia or T γ-lymphocytosis**. However, LGL lymphoproliferations constitute a heterogeneous group of disorders, including transient or chronic benign LGL expansions and true T-cell LGL leukemias.

Clinical Features

LGL leukemia patients generally present with, at most, a modest lymphocytosis together with granulocytopenia, aplastic anemia, or pancytopenia. There is evidence that $CD8^+$ T cells are capable of directly inhibiting one or more aspects of hematopoiesis and that this gives rise to this unique clinical presentation. In contrast to B-cell CLL, where hematopoietic failure is not seen until there is extensive marrow infiltration with malignant cells, the offending $CD8^+$ T cells may never be present in large numbers within the marrow during the course of LGL. Approximately 25% of LGL patients will also have preexisting systemic autoimmune disorders such as rheumatoid arthritis, lupus erythematosus, Sjögren syndrome, or autoimmune cytopenias. In this setting, the presentation can be very similar to Felty syndrome.

Laboratory Studies

The malignant cells ("large granular lymphocytes") resemble "atypical lymphocytes" of the type sometimes seen in infectious mononucleosis. They are larger than normal lymphocytes, with a more open chromatin pattern and a few prominent azurophilic granules in their cytoplasm. **Marker studies** show expression of the normal T-cell lineage markers CD3 and CD8. In addition, they typically express CD57 and activation markers such as HLA-DR and CD38; some cases will aberrantly express the adhesion molecule CD56. In some cases, cells have low or absent expression of the CD5 that should be present on normal T cells.

This morphology and phenotype are associated with activated cytotoxic T cells, which resemble and are sometimes confused with $CD3^-$ NK cells because they share morphologic characteristics and markers such as CD57. Gene rearrangement studies have shown definitively, however, that the cells are $CD3^+$ T cells. The entity of true natural killer NK-cell ($CD3^-$ $CD16^+$ $CD56^+$) leukemia is rare. Although morphologically very similar, NK leukemic cells do not show rearrangement of T-cell receptor genes and do not express CD3. The presentation is much more acute, often with neurologic signs, and the course is much more aggressive.

Therapy

The course of LGL leukemia is highly variable. Some patients appear to have little or no progression of the lymphoproliferative process and may only need to be treated for their anemia or granulocytopenia, whereas others have a more aggressive course resulting in progression to florid lymphoma and/or lymphocytic leukemia. Up to one-third of patients may require only supportive therapy, including hematopoietic growth factors, for anemia or recurrent infections owing to granulocytopenia. Others respond to single-agent treatment with methotrexate, cyclosporin, chlorambucil, or cyclophosphamide, with or without prednisone, or purine analogs. With transition to more aggressive disease, combination chemotherapy can be effective; however, the response rate is poor and brief in duration.

HAIRY CELL LEUKEMIA

Hairy cell leukemia (HCL) was named for its unusual cell morphology. The malignant B lymphocytes have very long filamentous cytoplasmic projections that are sometimes difficult to see in dried stained films but are prominent in wet mounts observed by phase microscopy. HCL has also been called "leukemic reticuloendotheliosis," perhaps because of the tendency for the malignant cells to infiltrate the marrow, liver, and spleen.

Clinical Features

Like many of the chronic lymphoid neoplasms, this disorder occurs most commonly in adults and frequently has a unique clinical presentation characterized by extensive marrow involvement with pancytopenia and prominent splenomegaly. Lymphadenopathy is uncommon and should make the diagnosis of HCL questionable. It is more often seen in males than females (4 to 5:1).

Laboratory Studies

The so-called "hairy" cell has been the subject of considerable investigation. Some HCL cases have cells with properties of both lymphocytes and macrophages in that they can be mildly phagocytic and have markers associated with macrophages. Careful marker studies, gene rearrangement, and microarray studies have shown, however, that they are mature clonal B cells. A normal counterpart of hairy cells has not been identified, and the oncogenic process that results in the development of the disease is unknown. The **most useful markers** for hairy cells, in addition to the usual lineage-specific B-cell markers (CD19, CD20, and a single light chain), are the absence of CD5, CD10, and CD23, and the strong presence of CD11c, CD22, and CD103.

Patients with HCL often present with mild to moderate pancytopenia. The number of abnormal lymphocytes in circulation is often low, and automated cell counters class the cells as normal lymphocytes. A careful inspection of the blood film is, therefore, mandatory to detect the classic **hairy cell** (an intermediate-sized lymphocyte with a large nucleus and filamentous projections of cytoplasm; Figure 22–5). Cytochemistry, specifically the **tartrate-resistant acid phosphatase stain** (see Figure 22–5), can be used to confirm the presence of hairy cells in circulation, with characteristic polar brownish-red deposits surrounded by unstained cytoplasm. Cytochemistry, however, has largely been supplanted by immunophenotyping for clonal CD11c$^+$ CD103$^+$ B cells. Variant HCL is defined by its presentation with elevated white counts and large numbers of leukemic cells; variant disease is more aggressive.

The diagnosis of HCL can also be made on the **histology of the marrow or spleen**. When the marrow is infiltrated by hairy cells, it usually cannot be aspirated because the cells tend to adhere to marrow structural cells. A marrow biopsy specimen will reveal a typical morphologic pattern, characterized by a diffuse infiltration with each cell nucleus separated by a large, clear cytoplasmic area, the so-called "fried egg" appearance. This is very different from the diffuse infiltration of small lymphocytes seen in B-cell CLL.

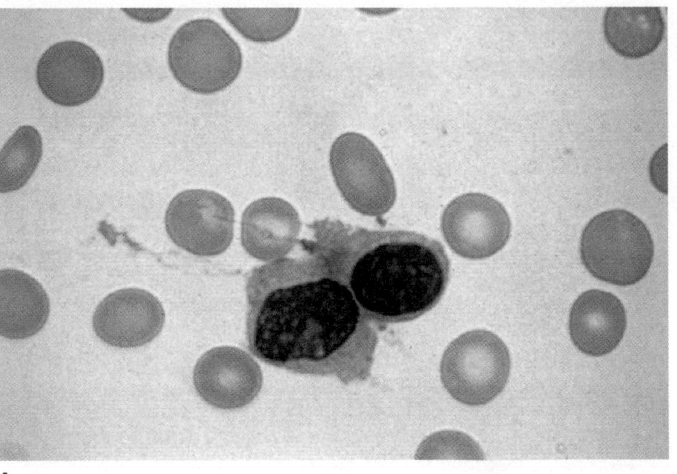
A

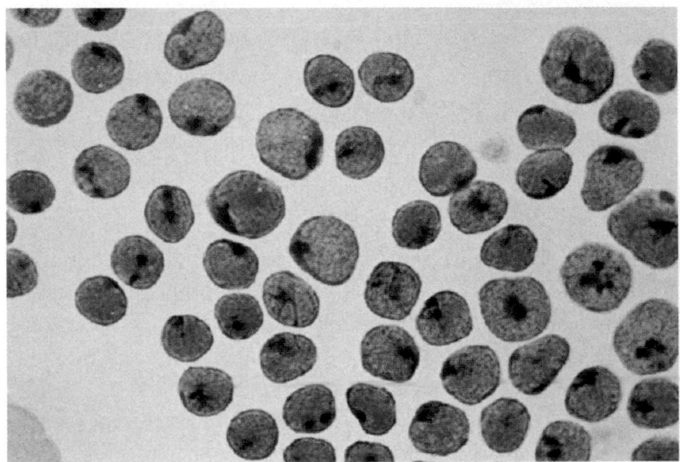
B

FIGURE 22–5. **Hairy cell leukemia. A:** Hairy cells in peripheral blood (clonal CD103$^+$ B cells) demonstrate their characteristic filamentous cytoplasm. **B:** Polar staining (red-brown) for acid phosphastase is seen in the cytoplasm of T-cell lymphoma cells; this staining is tartrate-resistant in hairy cell leukemia B cells.

Therapy

The outlook for patients with HCL has changed dramatically over the last 2 decades. Until the mid 1980s, HCL was a lethal disease. Most of the patients experienced infectious complications from which they died within 5 years after diagnosis. Currently, when recognized early and treated effectively, HCL is an indolent disorder with survival exceeding 80% at 5 years.

HCL responds very well to therapy with **interferon**, with complete or partial response rates of about 80% but without evidence for cure. Even higher complete remission rates and prolonged relapse-free survival are obtained with **pentostatin** (deoxycoformycin) and with **2-CdA**. **Fludarabine** has shown similar results and has been effective in patients who have failed treatment with other agents. Anti-CD20 monoclonal antibody (rituximab) has also demonstrated some efficacy in HCL.

Purine analogues are now preferred to interferon as initial therapy, despite the depletion of CD4 cells, which can take as long as 1 year to replenish. Overall survival is 80%–90% at 5 years for each of these drugs, even with the variant form of HCL. Given the low incidence of the disease, and the reduced death rates with these treatments, it will be virtually impossible to determine if one of the agents can provide substantially longer survival. Moreover, patients who relapse or are refractory can successfully move from one drug to another or may respond to rituximab, obscuring the impact of each drug on survival.

Prior to the use of these drugs, splenectomy was considered the initial therapeutic step owing to a high frequency of apparent remissions. **Splenectomy** is now considered only as a palliative option in patients with massive splenomegaly or severe hypersplenism. If the patient is not a candidate for surgical splenectomy, **splenic irradiation** is an alternative.

POINTS TO REMEMBER

B-cell chronic lymphocytic leukemia (B-CLL) is the most common lymphoproliferative disease in Western countries.

B-CLL occurs predominantly in the elderly and frequently presents with little more than an elevated lymphocyte count and modest lymphadenopathy. Diagnosis is relatively easy based on the clinical picture and immunophenotype.

With disease progression, B-CLL patients are at risk for autoimmune complications (hemolytic anemia, thrombocytopenia) and recurrent infections secondary to hypogammaglobulinemia.

B-CLL can transform to a more aggressive large cell lymphoma with splenomegaly (Richter syndrome) or even to an aggressive prolymphocytic leukemia, with both entities preserving their $CD19^+$ $CD5^+$ $CD23^+$ dim surface Ig immunophenotype. De novo B-cell prolymphocytic leukemia lacks CD23 and strongly expresses surface Ig.

Younger patients with CLL should be studied for IgV_H, CD38, and ZAP-70 expression to determine if their disease fits a more aggressive genotype. B-CLL responds well to chemotherapy, although even a complete response/remission does not translate into a prolonged survival. Only allogeneic bone marrow transplantation can achieve cure and is reserved for young patients with a matched sibling donor.

T-cell leukemias are much less common than B-CLL in the United States and Europe. ATLL is a $CD4^+$ T-cell neoplasm with an aggressive course and associated with HTLV-1 infection. Other $CD4^+$ T-cell malignancies most often present as a more indolent infiltrative skin disease (cutaneous T-cell lymphoma/mycosis fungoides) without significant lymphadenopathy, but patients can have leukemic presentations (Sézary syndrome).

$CD3^+$ $CD8^+$ $CD57^+$ T-cell (large granular lymphocytic) leukemia classically presents with pancytopenia, secondary to marrow depression of other hematopoietic lines. LGL leukemia is often associated with preexisting autoimmune disease. Like all T-cell neoplasms, large granular lymphocytic leukemia is confirmed to be clonal if T-cell receptor studies show gene rearrangement.

Hairy cell leukemia is a B-cell lymphoma that presents in the elderly with pancytopenia and splenomegaly and relatively few hairy cells in the blood. Thus, a high degree of suspicion may be needed to make the diagnosis by classic CD11c/CD103 immunophenotyping. Hairy cell leukemia responds very well to chemotherapy with purine analogues, making early diagnosis critical.

BIBLIOGRAPHY

Bartlett NL, Longo DL: T-small lymphocyte disorders. Semin Hematol 1999;36:164.

Binet JL, Caligaris-Cappio F, Catovsky D, et al: Perspectives on the use of new diagnostic tools in the treatment of chronic lymphocytic leukemia. Blood 2006;107:859.

Catovsky D, Richards S, Matutes E, et al: Assessment of fludarabine plus cyclophosphamide for patients with chronic lymphocytic leukaemia (the LRF CLL4 Trial): a randomised controlled trial. Lancet 2007;370:230.

Diamandidou E, Cohe PR, Kurzock R: Mycosis fungoides and Sézary syndrome. Blood 1996;88:2385.

Dighiero G, Hamblin TJ: Chronic lymphocytic leukaemia. Lancet 2008;371:1017.

Doehner H, Stilgenbauer S, Benner A, et al: Genomic aberrations and survival in chronic lymphocytic leukemia. N Engl J Med 2000;343:1910.

Dungarwalla M, Matutes E, Dearden CE: Prolymphocytic leukaemia of B- and T-cell subtype: a state-of-the-art paper. Eur J Haematol 2008;80:469.

Eichhorst BF, Busch R, Hopfinger G, et al: Fludarabine plus cyclophosphamide versus fludarabine alone in first-line therapy of younger patients with chronic lymphocytic leukemia. Blood 2006;107:885.

Gale RP, Cozen W, Goodman MT, Wang FF, Bernstein L. Decreased chronic lymphocytic leukemia incidence in Asians in Los Angeles County. Leuk Res 2000;24:665.

Ghia P, Stamatopoulos K, Belessi C, et al: Geographic patterns and pathogenetic implications of *IGHV* gene usage in chronic lymphocytic leukemia: the lesson of the *IGHV3-21* gene. Blood 2005;105:1678.

Golomb HM: Hairy cell leukemia: treatment successes in the past 25 years. J Clin Oncol 2008;28:2607.

Hallek M, Cheson BD, Catovsky D, et al: Guidelines for the diagnosis and treatment of chronic lymphocytic leukemia: a report from the International Workshop on Chronic Lymphocytic Leukemia (IWCLL) updating the National Cancer Guidelines Institute-Working Group (NCI-WG) 1996. Blood 2008; 111:5446.

Hamblin TJ et al: Unmutated IgV_H genes are associated with a more aggressive form of chronic lymphocytic leukemia. Blood 1999;94:1848.

Hillmen P, Skotnicki AB, Robak T, et al: Alemtuzumab compared with chlorambucil as first-line therapy for chronic lymphocytic leukemia. J Clin Oncol 2007;25:5616.

Hoffman MA: Clinical presentation and complications of hairy cell leukemia. Hematol Oncol Clin N Am 2006;20:1065.

Lamy T, Loughran TP: Clinical features of large granular lymphocyte leukemia. Semin Hematol 2003;40:185.

Matutes E: Adult T-cell leukemia/lymphoma. J Clin Path 2007;60:1373.

Matutes E: Immunophenotyping and differential diagnosis of hairy cell leukemia. Hematol Oncol Clin N Am 2006;20:1051.

Mayr C, Speicher MR, Kofler DM, et al: Chromosomal translocations are associated with poor prognosis in chronic lymphocytic leukemia. Blood 2006;107:742.

Rawstron AC, Bennett FL, O'Connor SJM, et al: Monoclonal B-cell lymphocytosis and chronic lymphocytic leukemia. N Engl J Med 2008;359:575.

Shanafelt TD, Geyer SM, Kay NE: Prognosis at diagnosis: integrating molecular biologic insights into clinical practice for patients with CLL. Blood 2004;103:1202.

Taylor G: Molecular aspects of HTLV-1 infection. J Clin Path 2007;60:1392.

Thomas DA et al: Rituximab in relapsed or refractory hairy cell leukemia. Blood 2003;102:3906.

NON-HODGKIN LYMPHOMAS • 23

CASE HISTORY • *Part I*

A 46-year-old man seeks evaluation of a non-tender mass that he recently discovered in his left axilla. He notes that it seems to have been enlarging rapidly over the past 3 weeks. He is otherwise feeling well, with no weight loss, fever, or chills, and has no significant past medical history, nor any family history of hematologic disease.

On examination, in addition to the 5–6 cm mass that the patient noted, multiple 1- to 2-cm lymph nodes are found in both axillae and in the cervical region. All of these are non-tender, mobile, and rubbery in texture. There is no hepatosplenomegaly or palpable abdominal masses; the only other finding of significance is the presence of mild bilateral pitting edema in the lower extremities.

The patient's complete blood count (CBC) is entirely normal; no abnormal cells are noted on examination of the blood smear.

Question

- What diagnostic procedures are indicated?

The **non-Hodgkin lymphomas (NHLs)** are disorders characterized by malignant proliferation of B or T lymphocytes. From a clinical standpoint, lymphomas generally present as tumors of the lymphoid system—the lymph nodes, Waldeyer ring, spleen, blood, and marrow. However, since lymphocytes by their nature are heterogeneous and have access to nearly every anatomic site, the NHLs may present with involvement of any organ, including the central nervous system. With advances in clinical and pathological staging techniques, the ability to accurately diagnosis a specific NHL disorder and **predict the course of the disease** in an individual patient has greatly improved. It has also made it possible to plan an optimal course of treatment.

The etiological mechanisms involved in lymphomagenesis are yet to be fully understood. Environmental factors, including radiation, chemical exposures, and both viruses and bacteria (human T-cell lymphotrophic virus type 1 [HTLV-1], hepatitis C virus [HCV], Epstein-Barr virus, *Helicobacter pylori*, and *Campylobacter jejunii*) clearly play a role in many of the NHL subtypes. Genetic predisposition is also a major factor. This is best illustrated by the recurrent genetic abnormalities observed in NHL disorders, including translocations or mutations involving proto-oncogenes, signal transduction factors, cell cycle regulation, and apoptotic pathways. Epigenetic factors are almost certainly another important etiological mechanism in NHL.

The importance of accurate diagnosis and effective management of lymphomas has been heightened by their increasing incidence, the association of lymphomas with immune deficiency states, and concomitant improvements in therapy. The incidence in Western countries has more than doubled in the last 20 years not only because of the association of B-cell lymphomas with AIDS, but also likely due to greater exposure to chemical agents in the environment.

NHL in general is very **responsive to therapy**, and in most cases the physician can offer the patient with NHL both improved survival and quality of life. It is a paradox that the NHL patient with the most aggressive form of the disease can actually be offered the possibility of a cure, whereas the patient with indolent lymphoma may never be cured despite a relatively long survival.

Because lymphoma cells tend to be very mobile, silently involving not only lymphoid organs but nearly every part of the body, the concepts of staging, remission, and relapse are far more fluid than with solid tumor malignancies. With increasingly sensitive **means of detecting lymphoma cells**, it is frequently possible to demonstrate their presence throughout the body in patients previously thought to have localized disease. Similarly, it is frequently possible to detect lymphoma cells in patients who appear by usual criteria to be in complete remission. Patients with NHL will sometimes undergo prolonged periods of quiescent disease punctuated by periods of increased disease activity. In general these patients must be followed up carefully, with a constant suspicion that minor symptoms may indicate progression or relapse.

DIAGNOSIS

Ultimately, a diagnosis of NHL depends on finding clonal lymphoid cells that are destroying the normal architecture of the lymphoid tissues or invading non-lymphoid tissues, or both. Detection of lymphoma in its early stages can be more of a challenge. It is difficult, probably impossible, to recognize a single lymphocyte as malignant based on morphology alone, because normal lymphocytes are capable, through dedifferentiation, proliferation, and differentiation in the course of a normal immune response, to display morphological changes mimicking malignancy. A reactive lymph node contains activated lymphocytes that look as malignant as any lymphoma cell.

Thus, in order for one to accurately diagnose lymphoma, an adequate **tissue biopsy** is absolutely required to display a large area of cells for collective morphology. Lymphoma can be suspected on the basis of cytologic examination of blood, marrow, effusions, and aspirates, but the physician should always make every attempt to obtain a good surgical biopsy of involved lymphoid or non-lymphoid tissue in order to be certain of the diagnosis. When multiple sites are available for biopsy, one should avoid those sites where normal reactive nodes are frequently found, such as the groin and the axilla. The surgical biopsy should always be considered as the first step of the pathology workup, in order to provide to the pathologist optimal samples for an accurate diagnosis.

With the availability of **immunologic and genetic tests for clonality**, one can make a strong presumptive diagnosis of lymphoma on the basis of the finding of clonal and immunophenotypically abnormal lymphocytes involving multiple sites, such as marrow and blood, but the finding of clonality does not absolutely prove malignancy, and clonality alone yields no information regarding prognosis. Therefore, a diagnosis based solely on these criteria should be viewed with caution, and tissue confirmation should always be sought, if possible.

CLASSIFICATION

Over the years, several different classifications of lymphomas—the Rappaport, Lukes-Collins, and Lennert classifications, and subsequently the International Working Formulation—have been proposed as guides to the classification and treatment of the non-Hodgkin lymphomas. These systems were based almost entirely on morphologic criteria. The Working Formulation was an advance because it emphasized the clinical behavior of the various lymphomas, grouping them into low, intermediate, and high grades based on their clinical aggressiveness. Inclusion of immunological and genetic characteristics have allowed better definition and revealed new entities, as described in the **Revised European American Classification (REAL)**, and most recently in the consensus classification sponsored by the **World Health Organization (WHO)**, which closely follows the REAL system. The WHO classification is summarized in Table 23–1.

TABLE 23–1 • Lymphoma classification

B-Cell Neoplasms	T-Cell and NK-Cell Neoplasms
Precursor B-cell neoplasms	**Precursor T-cell neoplasms**
B lymphoblastic leukemia/ lymphoma	T lymphoblastic leukemia/ lymphoma Blastic NK/T lymphoma
Mature B-cell neoplasms	**Mature T-cell neoplasms**
CLL/small lymphocytic lymphoma B-cell prolymphocytic leukemia Lymphoplasmacytic lymphoma Splenic marginal zone lymphoma Hairy cell leukemia Plasma cell myeloma Solitary plasmacytoma of bone Extra-osseous plasmacytoma Extranodal marginal zone B-cell lymphoma of mucosa-associated tissue (MALT) Nodal marginal zone B-cell lymphoma Follicular lymphoma Mantle cell lymphoma Diffuse large B-cell lymphoma Mediastinal (thymic) large B-cell lymphoma Intravascular large B-cell lymphoma Primary effusion lymphoma Burkitt lymphoma/leukemia	T-cell prolymphocytic leukemia T-cell large granular lymphocytic leukemia Aggressive NK-cell leukemia Adult T-cell lymphoma/leukemia Extranodal NK/T-cell lymphoma, nasal type Enteropathy-type T-cell lymphoma Hepatosplenic T-cell lymphoma Subcutaneous panniculitis-like T-cell lymphoma Mycosis fungoides Sézary syndrome Primary cutaneous anaplastic T-cell lymphoma Peripheral T-cell lymphoma, unspecified Angioimmunoblastic T-cell lymphoma
B-cell proliferations of uncertain malignant potential	**T-cell proliferations of uncertain malignant potential**
Lymphomatoid granulomatosis Post-transplant lymphoproliferative disorder, polymorphic	Lymphomatoid papulosis

TABLE 23–2 • Frequencies of non-Hodgkin lymphoma subtypes in the United States

Diagnosis	Frequency (%)
Diffuse large B-cell lymphoma	31
Follicular lymphoma	22
Marginal zone B-cell lymphoma, MALT type	8
Peripheral T-cell lymphoma	7
Small lymphocytic lymphoma	6
Mediastinal large B-cell lymphoma	6
Mantle cell lymphoma	6
Anaplastic T-cell lymphoma	2
Lymphoblastic lymphoma	2
Burkitt-like lymphoma	2
Marginal zone B-cell lymphoma	1
Lymphoplasmacytic lymphoma	1
Burkitt lymphoma	<1

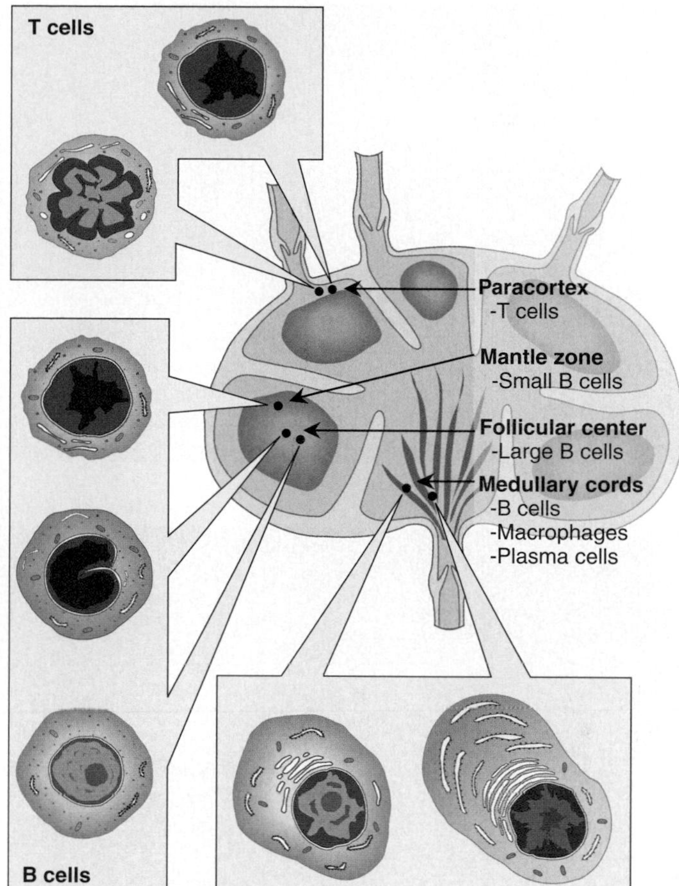

FIGURE 23–1. **The normal architecture, histology, and phenotype of a lymph node.** The major lymphocyte subsets are distributed through the lymph node in characteristic regions. Follicular centers contain predominantly large proliferating B cells, whereas the mantle zones of the follicles contain smaller B cells in the resting state. Interfollicular regions and the paracortex contain predominantly T cells. Macrophages are located in the follicular centers and in the medulla of the node. Antigen and circulating T cells enter via the cortical afferent lymphatics. Antigen-stimulated T cells reenter the circulation via the efferent lymphatics. Disruption of the normal lymph node architecture is one of the major causes of immunodeficiency in lymphoma.

The **WHO system** defines the lymphomas according to their pathological, immunological, and genetic features. At the same time, as regards the clinical picture, this classification does not always translate into specific prognostic indications or treatment recommendations. It is likely that the situation will improve as data from gene expression studies emerge and are incorporated into classifications, as they will provide insights into clinical and genetic correlations and clues to the development of targeted treatments.

The frequencies of the more common NHLs are listed in Table 23–2. When a patient presents with lymphoma it is important to obtain as much prognostic information as possible on the basis of multiple features including histology, cytology, immunophenotyping, cytogenetics, molecular genetics, and anatomic stage or extent of disease.

Histologic Features

The normal architecture of a lymph node and the phenotypic and cytologic features of the lymphocytes found in various regions are illustrated in Figure 23–1. The histologic description of lymphoma focuses on the overall architecture of a lymphoid or non-lymphoid tissue. Perhaps the most useful histologic finding is whether there is **nodular (or follicular) versus diffuse morphology** (Figure 23–2). Those lymphomas showing the formation of nodules, reminiscent of normal lymphoid follicles, tend to be more indolent and have a better prognosis than those showing diffuse infiltration. This distinction is true regardless of the details of the individual cells and regardless of the immunophenotype of the lymphoma. Therefore, the first question the clinician should ask in diagnosing an NHL is whether the lymph node biopsy shows a nodular (follicular) or diffuse histology. This distinction can only be made on the basis of an adequate lymph node biopsy since nodular versus diffuse patterns are difficult to determine when examining extranodal sites.

Cytologic Features

The cytologic classification of a lymphoma depends on the appearance of the individual cells. Cells may be described as well differentiated versus poorly differentiated (Rappaport classification) or as large versus small, with folded or "cleaved" nuclei (Luke-Collins classification and International Formulation). In general, small, well-differentiated cells are seen with more indolent lymphomas, whereas large, poorly differentiated cells are typical of high-grade, aggressive lymphomas. However, this classification is weakened by the frequent presence of cells of many descriptions scattered throughout the lesion. Overall, the

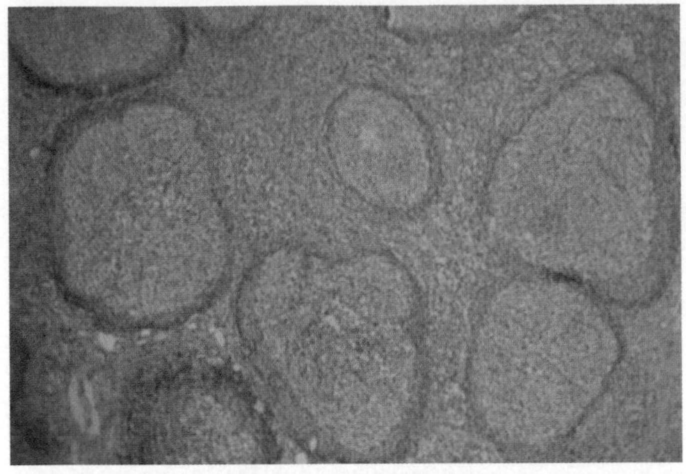

A

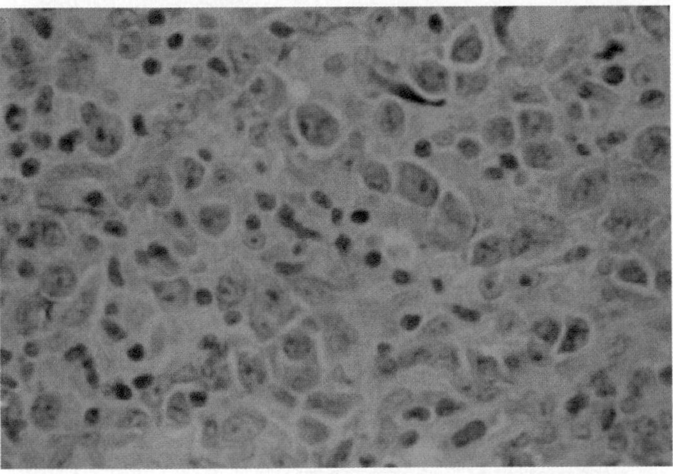

B

FIGURE 23–2. **Follicular/nodular versus diffuse histologic patterns in lymphoma.** Lymph node section, under low-power magnification, showing the distorted follicular architecture typical of a follicular/nodular (small cell) lymphoma **(A)**. High-power view of a diffuse, large B-cell lymphoma **(B)**. Note the diffuse infiltrate of enlarged lymphocytes with prominent nuclei (malignant B cells) overwhelming a smaller population of small reactive lymphocytes.

cytologic description of the cells is not as strongly associated with prognosis as is the histologic description (nodular versus diffuse).

Immunologic Features

The immunologic classification of NHL requires the use of immunologic markers, genetic analysis, or both (see Chapters 20 and 22) to determine whether the cells are of B- or T-cell origin and to indicate clonality. Most (approximately 80%) NHLs are of B-cell origin. **Clonality in a B-cell lymphoma** is most easily indicated by uniform expression of a single light-chain class of surface immunoglobulin (κ or λ); more complex molecular studies will detect the presence of immunoglobulin gene rearrangement. **Clonality of the T-cell lymphomas** is suggested by a characteristic abnormal pattern of CD expression, often with deletion of the normal T-cell markers, but T-cell clonality is most reliably demonstrated by genetic analysis for T cell–receptor gene rearrangement.

Immunophenotypic analysis of lymphomas is particularly useful in distinguishing between a reactive process and a lymphoma. It is not uncommon for a lymph node biopsy to show a lymphocyte proliferation that could be a normal reactive process rather than a lymphoma. Since the reactive process is characterized by a heterogeneous collection of T and B cells arising from multiple clones of different progenitor cells, it is easy to distinguish immunologically from a lymphoma, where most cells are of one phenotype and belong to a single clone. This approach is possible using either immunohistochemical studies on fixed material, or by flow cytometry on gently disrupted cells from a biopsy or a fine needle aspirate.

Cytogenetic Features

Specific NHL subtypes can also be classified based on **nonrandom chromosomal translocations** (Tables 23–3 and 23–4). Many gene partners can contribute to lymphoma transformation. One common feature is that they frequently involve the genes responsible for the coding of the immunologic receptors for antigen on the lymphocytes. For the B cells these are located on chromosome 14q32 (the immunoglobulin heavy chains) and on chromosomes 2 (κ immunoglobulin light chain) and 22 (λ immunoglobulin light chain). For the T cells, the α, β, and γ subunit genes of the T cell–receptor, located respectively in 14q12, 7q35, and 7q14, are often involved. Most of these mutations result in the juxtaposition of an immunologic receptor gene and its controlling elements next to a proto-oncogene, resulting in overexpression of the oncogene product. The best examples are the t(14;18) (q32;q21) translocation, which brings the immunoglobulin heavy chain locus next to the *BCL-2* proto-oncogene, and the translocations that bring the c-*myc* oncogene next to immunoglobulin genes on chromosomes 14, 2, or 22. The *BCL-2* abnormality occurs in at least 80% of nodular lymphomas, and the c-*myc* translocation is characteristic of Burkitt lymphoma. *BCL-2* is a gene associated with the inhibition of programmed cell death (apoptosis). Thus, its overexpression in lymphomas leads to prolongation of the lifespan of the cells and their accumulation to the detriment of the patient. The expression of bcl-2 has also been associated with poor overall survival. Other examples are illustrated by the t(11;14) in mantle cell lymphoma, involving the cyclin *D1* gene, and deregulation of *BCL-6* in large B-cell lymphomas and *c-myc* in Burkitt lymphoma, which are associated with uncontrolled cell proliferation.

Since immunoglobulin or T cell–receptor genes are always rearranged as a part of the normal differentiation process of B and T lymphocytes (see Chapter 20), it is reasonable to conclude that the defect in lymphoma is often owing to an abnormal rearrangement. This is confirmed by the observation that most of the translocations in B-cell lymphomas involve the J and S sequences of the immunoglobulin genes that are the sites of normal rearrangements. Most of the common genetic alterations seen in lymphomas can be detected by polymerase chain reaction (PCR) techniques or by fluorescence in-situ hybridization.

TABLE 23–3 • Morphologic, immunophenotypic, and genetic features in the WHO classification of the most frequent B-cell neoplasms

Disease	Morphology	Immunophenotype	Karyotype	Involved Genes
CLL/small lymphocytic lymphoma	Small, round lymphocytes	Dim sIg (μ,δ) CD5/19/23$^+$, FMC7$^-$	No specific karyotype (see Chapter 22)	
Lymphoplasmocytoid variant	Small lymphocytes with plasmacytoid features	cIgM$^+$ IgD$^-$, CD19/20/22$^+$ CD 5/10/23$^-$, CD38^{++} clonal	t(9;14) (50%)	*Pax 5* (9q13) Controls B-cell proliferation and differentiation
Mantle cell	Small to medium irregular lymphocytes	sIgM, sIgD$^+$ CD5/19$^+$ CD10$^\pm$, CD23$^-$	t(11;14) (70%)	*BCL-1* (11q13) Controls the cell cycle
Follicular center cell	Small, medium, or large irregular, cleaved cells	sIgM, sIgD$^+$ CD10/19$^+$ CD5$^-$	t(14;18) (70%–95%)	*BCL-2* (18q21) Inhibits apoptosis
Diffuse large B cell	Large, irregular cells	sIgM, sIgD$^\pm$ CD19/20$^+$, often CD10$^+$	3q27 (30%)	*BCL-6* (3q27) Germinal center maturation
Burkitt lymphoma	Medium round cells with abundant cytoplasm	sIgM^{++} CD19/20$^+$/10^{++} CD5/23$^-$	t(8;14), t(2;8), or t(8;22) (100%)	*c-myc* (8q24) Transcription factor, controls proliferation, differentiation, and apoptosis
MALT lymphoma	Small or large "monocytoid" lymphocytes	sIgM, sIgD$^+$ CD19, 20$^+$ CD5/10/23$^-$	Trisomy 3 (60%), t(11;18) (25%) of extranodal cases	*API2, MLT* Inhibition of apoptosis

Note: By definition, all have rearranged Ig genes.

Gene-Expression Profiling

Gene-expression profiling using microarray technology (Figure 23–3) is now being explored as a way of both understanding lymphomagenesis and better classifying the non-Hodgkin lymphomas. For example, it has been reported that small-cell lymphocytic lymphoma, marginal zone B-cell lymphoma, and mantle cell lymphoma can be reliably distinguished using a 44-gene microarray more than 95% of the time, a considerable improvement over traditional histopathology. Using a cDNA microarray analysis, large B-cell lymphomas can also be divided into 3 distinct groups with regard to patterns of gene expression that appear to correspond to survival after chemotherapy. In one series, the measurement of 6 gene patterns (*LMO2, BCL6, FN1, CCND2, SCYA3*, and *BCL-2*) was reported to reliably identify patients with very poor 5-year survivals (<27%). The future clinical utility of microarray patterns will be dependent on prospective studies showing an impact on outcome.

CLINICAL FEATURES

The clinical manifestations of lymphoma can be considered under several general categories, which are discussed further under the Laboratory Studies section. The first category includes those effects caused by enlargement of lymphoid tissues; the second includes the immunologic sequelae of the lymphoma; the third includes those effects caused by invasion of non-lymphoid tissues, particularly marrow; and the last includes the metabolic and humoral effects of the lymphoma.

Enlargement of Lymphoid Tissues

Most patients with lymphoma present with **painless enlargement of lymph nodes or spleen** or both. The effects of node enlargement vary from the cosmetic to such critical complications as obstruction of airway or major vessels, compression of the stomach, or obstruction of the intestines. In general the node enlargement is gradual and painless. Lymphomatous infiltration seldom results in an inflammatory response, and thus symptoms such as fever, weight loss, and night sweats are less common than in Hodgkin lymphoma.

A common clinical situation is the patient who presents with 1 or more **enlarged nodes** and a history compatible with a recent **viral infection**. Although the only way to confidently rule out lymphoma is to take a biopsy of the node, one is usually reluctant to do this immediately. This is especially true when the node enlargement has been sudden or painful (tender), suggesting a reactive process more than a lymphoma. If the node feels very hard to palpation or is fixed to underlying tissues, metastatic carcinoma is more likely than lymphoma. In general a reactive process will subside over a few weeks. A node that persists longer than this, and is painless, firm, or grows in size, must undergo biopsy. Lymphomatous nodes can also undergo fluctuating enlargement. A history of recurrent enlargement of a node is as compatible with lymphoma as is persistent enlargement. It is also possible to obtain a history of previous node biopsies that were correctly read as reactive only to be followed by an ultimate biopsy correctly read as lymphoma. Therefore, a previous benign biopsy should not weigh against repeating the biopsy of a suspicious node.

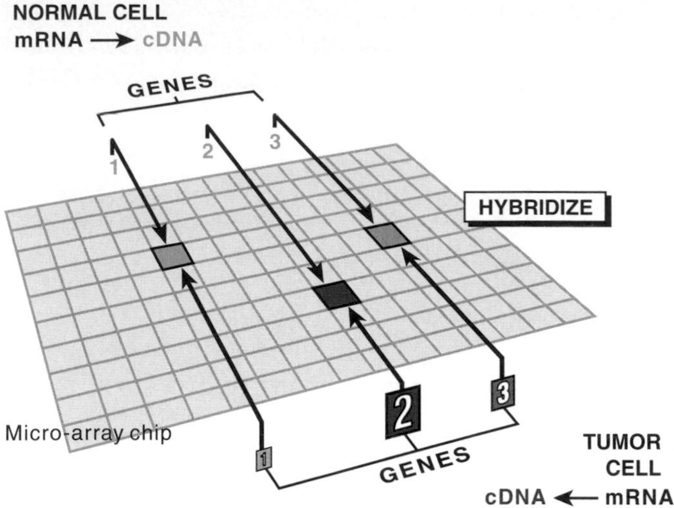

FIGURE 23–3. **Measuring gene expression by cDNA hybridization on microarray chips.** Microarray chip technology makes it possible to determine the presence and level of activity of genes from a target malignant cell line. In one commonly used format, the normal cDNA and the abnormal cDNA (tumor cell derived) are prepared such that they fluoresce at different wavelengths, eg, the normal cDNA as green and the abnormal cDNA as red. The 2 cDNA preparations are competitively hybridized on the chip. If the particular gene is comparatively underexpressed by the abnormal cells (1), the corresponding spot will be green. If the abnormal cells have upregulated the gene (2), the corresponding spot will be red; if the normal and abnormal cells equally express the gene product (3), the corresponding spot will be yellow. Computer analysis of the arrays can identify families of genes that are coordinately upregulated or downregulated in abnormal cells. These patterns of gene expression have been used to confirm and enhance the classification of leukemias and lymphomas. It is hoped that this technology will become the basis for treatment decisions, especially as drugs are developed to target specific genetic abnormalities.

Multifocal Versus Localized Disease

Nodal involvement in NHL is usually **multifocal**, with involved nodes separated by groups of normal nodes, and with early dissemination throughout the body. Thus, the concept of orderly progression of disease from one node group to another, although useful in Hodgkin lymphoma, has little use in NHL.

However, a few patients do present with **localized disease**, often in unusual locations. **Large cell B-cell lymphomas** can present in one node area or present as extranodal disease such as primary brain, testicular, breast, kidney, salivary, intestinal, or osteolytic bone tumors. **Gastrointestinal lymphomas** can be localized and, if disseminated, tend to preferentially involve gut-associated lymphoid tissue (see mucosa associated lymphoid tissue lymphomas later in the chapter).

Interestingly, low- and intermediate-grade lymphomas are almost always disseminated at the time of presentation. Although the tumor masses associated with **B-cell lymphomas** tend to follow the anatomic distribution of the lymph nodes and lymphatics, **T-cell malignancies** are more likely to show a wider tissue distribution. T-cell malignancies resulting from clonal expansion of CD4-positive T cells generally involve the skin, sometimes with their major manifestation being skin infiltrations (mycosis fungoides). This situation reflects the natural propensity of CD4 T cells to migrate through the subepidermal layers of the skin. Both T- and B-cell lymphomas can have a blood (leukemic) component. The **T-cell lymphomas and B-cell chronic lymphocytic leukemia (CLL)** (see Chapter 22) are the most likely to result in high circulating lymphocyte (lymphoma cell) counts, whereas other lymphomas usually have a minor, if any, circulating component that may not be reflected in the absolute lymphocyte count.

Other Clinical Features

A detailed history and physical examination are very important in evaluating the patient with NHL. **Exposure to toxic chemicals, chemotherapeutic or immunosuppressive agents, or ionizing radiation** can have epidemiologic importance, especially in the younger patient. **HIV infection** is a clear risk factor. A careful physical examination to look for **other enlarged lymph nodes** is essential for any patient presenting with a suspicious node. In addition to the common sites, involvement of retroclavicular nodes, Waldeyer ring, and thoracic and retroperitoneal nodes should be sought by physical examination and imaging studies. Renal and hepatic function tests should be done; however, in the absence of obstruction, involvement of these organs with lymphoma is frequently not reflected by chemistries. Both B- and T-cell lymphomas can present with symptomatic hypercalcemia.

Laboratory Studies

As mentioned in the preceding section, a detailed history and physical examination are important in identifying many manifestations of NHL. The evaluation of patients suspected of having lymphoma should include **examination of blood and marrow** for the presence of lymphoma cells as judged by morphology, **cell surface markers**, and **genetic analysis**. Sixty to eighty percent of lymphoma patients have involvement of blood, marrow, or both when sensitive techniques are used. This is true even when the complete blood count is perfectly normal. **Renal and hepatic function tests** should also be done.

A. Blood and Marrow Testing

Most patients with NHL do not develop profound marrow dysfunction even when the marrow is partially infiltrated with malignant cells. **Immunophenotypic testing** of blood and marrow is best performed after the disease has been diagnosed by biopsy so that the extent of the lymphoma's involvement is known. For example, if the lymphoma is of B-cell origin and is expressing λ immunoglobulin light chains on biopsy, this information can be confirmed by immunophenotypic testing of B cells in blood and marrow.

Many patients with B-NHL have at presentation or soon develop an **immune deficiency** that is characterized by diffuse hypogammaglobulinemia or by a poor response to new antigens or infections (or both). However, a significant number of NHL patients, particularly those with T-NHL, may have diffuse or even specific hypergammaglobulinemia, while a minority of B-NHL (about 5%) show a monoclonal serum immunoglobulin

(M component). Increased susceptibility to viral infection and reactivation of viruses such as herpes zoster may occur even prior to the onset of overt symptoms of lymphoma or chemotherapy, likely as a result of depression of cell-mediated immunity. Some lymphomas, particularly low-grade B-NHL and CLL, may demonstrate autoantibodies directed against red blood cells or platelets, resulting in Coombs-positive hemolytic anemia or immune thrombocytopenia.

B. Tests for Lymphomatous Infiltration of Non-lymphoid Organs

The possibility of lymphomatous infiltration of non-lymphoid organs should always be suspected. Because lymphoma seldom elicits an inflammatory response as it invades, the involvement can be extensive before the patient becomes symptomatic. The most common involvement is seen in skin (especially T-cell lymphomas), lung, the gastrointestinal (GI) tract, the liver, bone and marrow, the kidney, and the central nervous system (CNS). Attention should be paid to all of these sites in evaluating a patient with lymphoma, and any otherwise unexplained findings should be fully evaluated by laboratory and radiologic techniques. Liver involvement, for example, may be revealed by **computed tomography (CT) scan** despite normal **liver chemistries**. Because the patient with lymphoma is subject to unusual and opportunistic infections, one is often faced with a difficult clinical distinction between infection and lymphomatous infiltration, for example, in the lung. These distinctions may require **biopsy** to resolve.

Positron emission tomography (PET scanning) is now recognized to be critically useful in the initial staging, and even more so in follow-up, of lymphoma patients. Because PET detects regions of increased metabolic activity, it is sometimes more sensitive than CT or magnetic resonance imaging (MRI) in locating sites of lymphoma and in distinguishing between active tumor and residual scarring following treatment. However, the avidity for 18FDG is variable in different histologic subtypes: F-FDG-PET identified more than 97% of disease sites of large cell non-Hodgkin lymphoma, 91% of follicular lymphomas, 82% of mucosa associated lymphoid tissue (MALT) lymphomas, and 50% of small cell lymphocytic (SCLL) and splenic marginal zone lymphomas (SMZL). Follow-up PET-scans during treatment have been recognized as powerful predictors of treatment efficacy and long-term outcome. Attempts to modify treatment according to early response are currently being explored.

C. Serum Assay Tests for Metabolic and Humoral Effects

Some patients with lymphoma develop profound marrow dysfunction even when the marrow cannot be shown to be heavily involved with lymphoma. However, more common is the presence of significant numbers of lymphoma cells in the marrow with relatively normal blood counts. Anemia and thrombocytopenia are more often seen as side effects of myeloablative therapy than as presenting features. Because lymphocytes produce a variety of cytokines with diverse effects on other cells, patients with lymphoma can display generalized **metabolic and systemic symptoms**. Most common are unexplained fever, weight loss, night sweats, and chills; less common are hypercalcemia and hypoglycemia. Lactic dehydrogenase (LDH) and β_2-microglobulin levels in serum reflect tumor burden and activity and have strong prognostic significance at diagnosis.

CHARACTERISTICS OF INDIVIDUAL B-CELL LYMPHOMAS

Some types of B-cell lymphoma have relatively specific profiles of clinical presentation, histology, cell phenotype, and cytogenetic abnormalities. The following descriptions highlight the more important disease states. Table 23–3 summarizes the features of many of these lymphoma types while CLL, B-cell prolymphocytic leukemia, and hairy cell leukemia are described in Chapter 22, and plasma cell myeloma and lymphoplasmocytic lymphomas are described in Chapter 26.

Follicular (Nodular) Lymphomas

The nodular, or follicular, lymphomas make up about 20% of all cases of NHL. **Follicular lymphomas** typically occur in middle-aged or elderly adults. They usually present as a slow-growing, non-tender enlargement of lymph nodes, taking months to years to become clinically apparent. More than 75% of patients have disseminated disease at presentation, and 50% or more have marrow involvement. They tend to be resistant to curative chemotherapy, but even so, often have an indolent course, especially when small cells predominate. With time, the follicular lymphomas can exhibit a change in histology and evolve to a more high-grade tumor class with a concomitant worsening in prognosis.

Once a diagnosis is made from a node or tumor mass biopsy, a **search for evidence of disseminated disease** should be undertaken, using studies of blood and marrow for cell morphology, immunophenotypic markers, and gene rearrangement. These hematologic studies will often be positive. Staging is based on clinical examination and thoraco-abdominal CT imaging. A greater precision for staging is unnecessary unless it appears that the disease may truly be localized.

These are B-cell tumors, and their nodular pattern of growth is reminiscent of their origin in the germinal center. The presence of larger cells or a mixture of diffuse and nodular architecture suggests a more aggressive variant of the disease. The characteristic **cell phenotypes** are summarized in Figure 23–4. These cells correspond to the phenotype of maturing lymphocytes of B-cell type (see Chapter 20).

The B-cells display characteristic **immunoglobulin gene rearrangements**. Most will display a t(14:18) **chromosomal translocation**, which places the *BCL-2* proto-oncogene under the influence of the immunoglobulin heavy chain gene locus. The use of PCR technology to detect immunoglobulin gene rearrangements and the *BCL-2* translocation permits the detection of very small numbers of malignant cells in clinical specimens.

Follicular lymphomas are considered to be low-grade NHLs. However, there is a great heterogeneity in the course of individual patients. For a better prognostic assessment, a Follicular

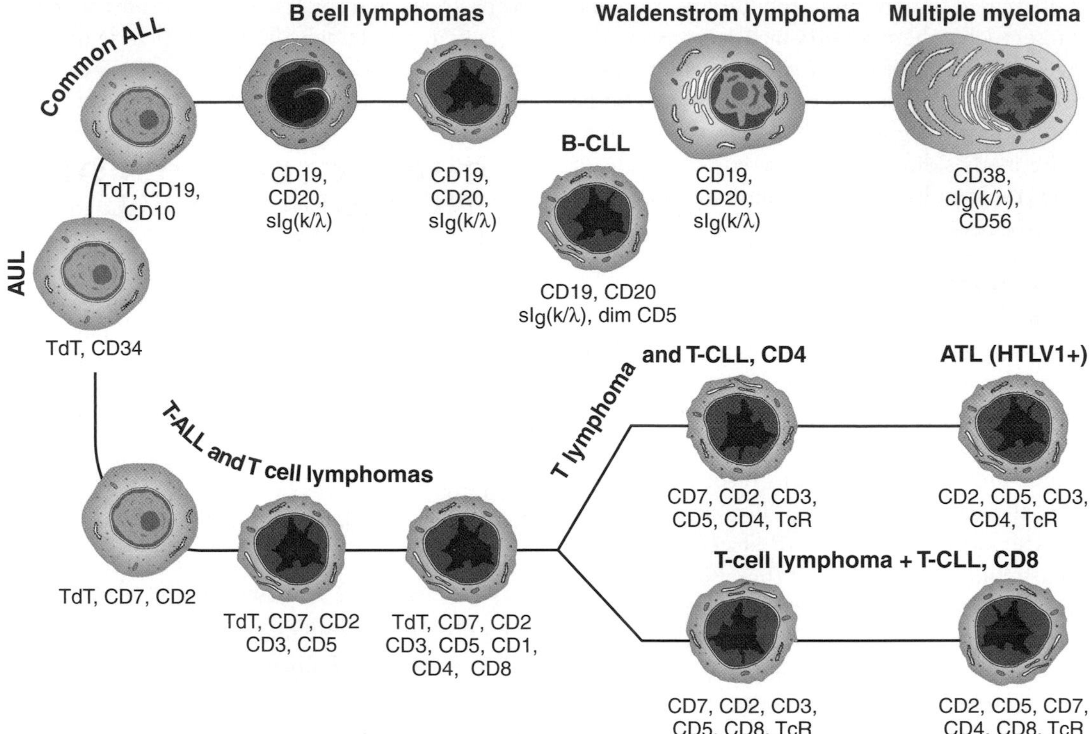

FIGURE 23–4. **Characteristic phenotypes of B- and T-cell lymphomas.** Patterns of normal lymphocyte differentiation (see Figure 20–3) can be used as a basis to visualize the relationships between the various NHL entities. Although the phenotypes of the lymphomas bear some resemblance to their normal developmental counterparts, there are numerous differences that make the comparisons only approximate.

Lymphoma International Prognostic Index (FLIPI) has been designed, based on the following 5 features with significant prognostic impact: age above 60 years, Ann Arbor stage III/IV (see Table 24–2 for description of this staging system), elevated LDH, hemoglobin less than 12 g/dL, and more than 5 nodal sites, with each feature scored as 1 when present (Table 23–4).

In addition, recent studies of gene expression profiling in follicular lymphomas have identified specific signatures with prognostic significance, delineating groups of patients with overall survivals ranging from 3.9–13.6 years.

Small Cell Lymphocytic Lymphoma

This B-NHL is characterized by a diffuse infiltration of small, noncleaved lymphocytes. SCLL is the tissue-based variant of B-cell CLL, almost always associated with a leukemic phase when blood lymphocytes are subjected to sensitive methods of analysis like flow cytometry or clonality assays. The presence of the CD5 marker and low levels of surface immunoglobulin are characteristic. Its presentation and response to therapy are identical to that of CLL. In some cases, it evolves over time to a more aggressive variant of lymphoma similar to the Richter transformation in CLL (see Chapter 22).

TABLE 23–4 • The Follicular Lymphoma International Prognostic Index

Score	Risk	% Patients	% 5-Year Survival	% 10-Year Survival
0–1	Good	36	91	71
2	Intermediate	37	78	51
3	Poor	27	53	36

Lymphoplasmocytoid Variant

The lymphoplasmocytoid variant is frequently associated with a serum monoclonal IgM protein (M component) that leads to its being considered as a tissue variant of Waldenström macroglobulinemia (see Chapter 26).

Marginal Zone Lymphomas

The marginal zone lymphomas encompass 3 clinical presentations, including nodal marginal zone, splenic marginal zone, and extranodal with masses in the respiratory or GI system, involving subepithelial, mucosa-associated lymphoid tissue (MALT tumors). **Nodal marginal zone lymphomas** do not differ from follicular lymphomas with regard to clinical presentation, outcome, and management. Patients with **MALT tumors** generally have a history of autoimmune disease or chronic antigenic stimulation. Sites of presentation include the GI tract, especially the stomach, and also salivary glands, skin, lung, thyroid, and orbit. Gastric MALT lymphoma (Figure 23–5A) commonly presents with symptoms of dyspepsia, anorexia, epigastric pain, and GI bleeding. Its pathogenesis is related to ***Helicobacter pylori*** infection, and some 70% of cases will show regression of the tumor with eradication of *H. pylori* using combined antibiotic and antacid or proton pump inhibitor (PPI) therapy. This has led to the use of antibiotic and acid blockade as first-line therapy. Sustained responses are seen reliably in patients with stage I disease (endoscopic appearance of gastritis), whereas chemotherapy and gastrectomy may be needed in gastric MALT patients who present with more advanced disease.

Splenic marginal zone lymphoma appears to be another distinct entity, although much less commonly. Interestingly, some splenic marginal lymphomas (SMZL) have been recognized to arise from chronic antigen stimulation such as with HCV infection, and treatment directed at the virus may lead to regression of the lymphoma. SMZL is distinguished by variable lymphocytosis (10,000–40,000/μL) with the appearance of villous lymphocytes in both blood and marrow, moderate to marked splenomegaly, and often the presence of a small M component (either IgG or IgM) of less than 30 g/L. Constitutional symptoms are rare, and the LDH level tends to be normal at presentation. Spleen histology shows giant follicles with some red pulp infiltration, but not to the degree seen in hairy cell leukemia. By immunophenotype, the tumor cells are surface light chain restricted, positive for CD20 and CD79a, negative for CD25 and CD103 (unlike hairy cells), and negative for CD5 and CD23 (unlike CLL cells). No consistent or unique chromosomal abnormalities have been reported. Recent data from gene expression studies have identified unique profiles in marginal zone lymphomas, which may eventually be clinically diagnostic.

Mantle Cell Lymphoma

Mantle cell lymphoma (MCL) is recognized by definitive histologic and immunogenetic features. Malignant cells arise from the mantle zone or perifollicular area, and present as small- to

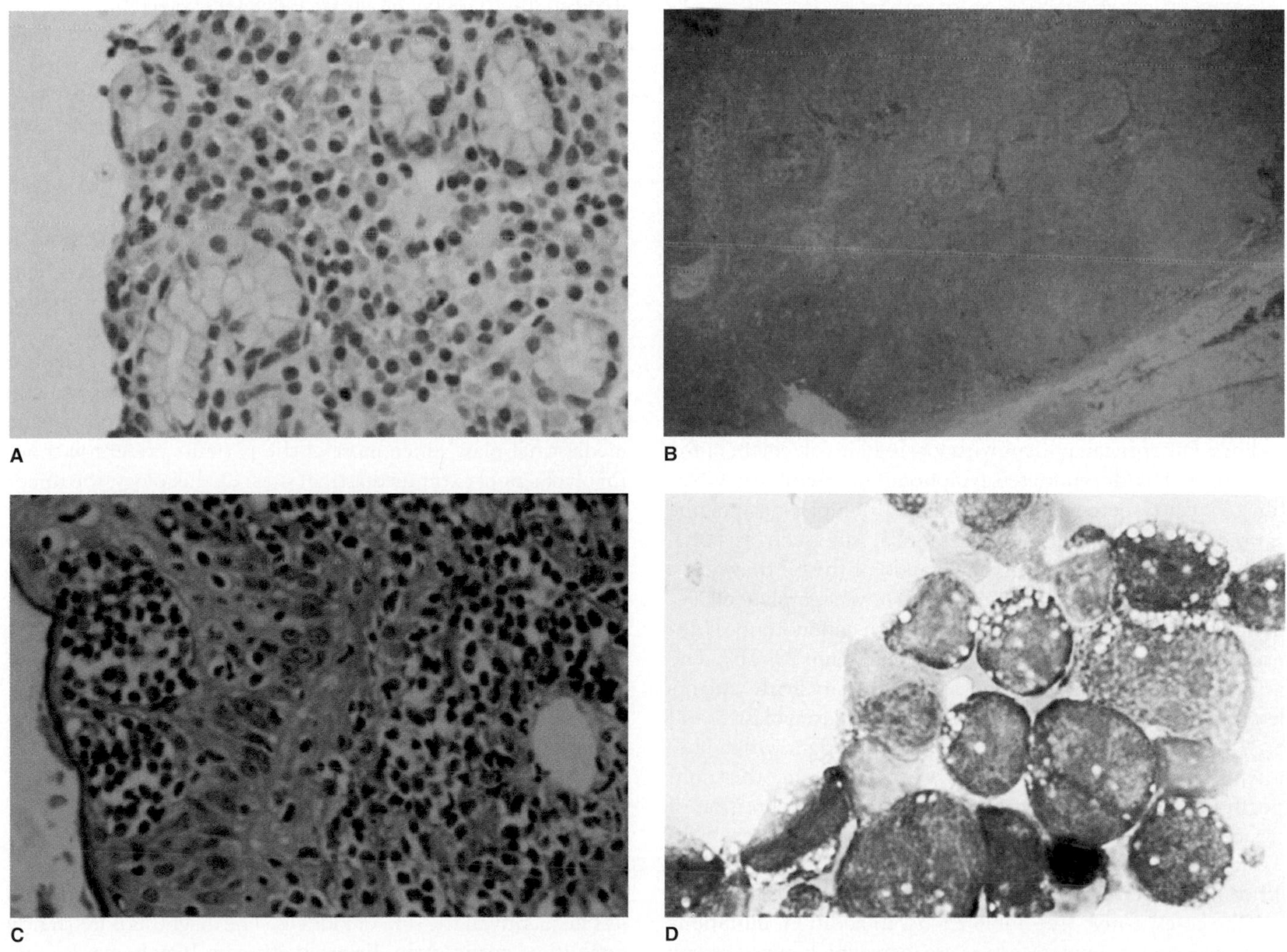

FIGURE 23–5. **Various lymphoma histologies. Gastric lymphoma MALT type (A)**—high-power view of malignant B cells and plasma cells in the gastric mucosa. **Mantle cell lymphoma (B)**—low-power view showing vaguely nodular architecture and an enlarged mantle zone. **Mycosis fungoides (C)**—skin biopsy showing an intraepidermal Pautrier microabscess. **Burkitt lymphoma (D)**—heavily vacuolated immature lymphocytes shown under high power.

medium-sized lymphocytes with a round, irregular nucleus, which is sometimes cleaved. They display a follicular or diffuse pattern (Figure 23–5B). This lymphoma is characterized immunophenotypically by the presence of CD5 (like CLL), but unlike CLL, it does not express CD23. Most mantle cell lymphomas have a t(11;14) translocation that involves the *BCL-1* proto-oncogene (see Table 23–3) and strongly express cyclin *D1* mRNA by reverse transcriptase polymerase chain reaction (RT-PCR), even in t(11;14)-negative cases. Many patients present with a disseminated illness with a leukemic spread at diagnosis, resulting in possible confusion with CLL. Lymphomatoid polyposis coli is also associated, and colonoscopy is part of the clinical evaluation of MCL. Although considered a relatively indolent lymphoma, MCL responds poorly to treatment and has a median survival of only 3–4 years, much less than most CLL patients. A blastic variant has an even poorer prognosis and is frequently associated with CNS infiltration and neurologic symptoms. When immunophenotypic analysis is unable to distinguish CLL from MCL, cyclin *D1* and t(11;14) analyses are required.

TABLE 23–5 • The International Prognostic Index system for "aggressive" lymphomas[a]

Score	Risk	% Patients	% Complete Responders	% 5-Year Overall Survival
0–1	Low	35	87	73
2	Intermediate low	27	67	51
3	Intermediate high	22	55	43
4–5	High	16	44	26

[a]*These results have not yet been updated with recent improvements in staging (PET scans) or treatment (monoclonal antibodies).*

Diffuse Large B-Cell Lymphoma

The large B-cell lymphoma patient frequently presents with 1 or more rapidly developing tumor masses involving nodal or extranodal sites. As is typical of most NHL, the mass is non-tender and does not cause inflammation or interfere with organ function except by compression. Retroperitoneal disease can obstruct venous drainage of the legs, resulting in edema and thrombophlebitis.

Staging studies should involve a large-volume biopsy of the tumor for histology and phenotyping. Marrow and blood studies for morphology, immunophenotype, chromosomal analysis, and B-cell gene rearrangements should be obtained to confirm disseminated disease. Cerebrospinal fluid examination and imaging of the CNS are indicated in patients with neurologic findings. Patients can present with localized involvement of the brain or widely disseminated lymphoma involving the CNS. Ten to twenty percent of the large cell lymphomas may be limited to a single node or extranodal site such as bone, Waldeyer ring, thyroid, lachrymal glands, or the GI tract.

The **typical large-cell tumor mass** shows complete effacement of normal lymphoid architecture with a monotonous (diffuse) infiltrate of large lymphocytes (see Figure 23–2B). The large cells display some morphological diversity, with variants described as centroblastic, immunoblastic, plasmablastic, and large anaplastic. These cells are all of B-cell origin with a phenotype (often $CD10^{+}$) not distinctly different from other nonspecific or follicular NHL except for increased expression of surface immunoglobulin in many cases. Many of these lymphomas have chromosomal rearrangements that involve ***BCL-6***, either alone or in combination with involvement of ***BCL-2*** and, in some cases, ***c-myc*** (see Table 23–3). In addition, **mutations of the p53** tumor-suppressor gene are seen, which have a strong impact on prognosis. This complex genetic background may explain the clinical heterogeneity that characterizes this disease. This heterogeneity has been confirmed recently by several studies of gene expression patterns.

The prognosis of large B-cell lymphomas is now assessed by using an international prognosis index (IPI) based on 5 statistically significant and independent factors: age above 60 years, Ann Arbor stage III/IV (see Table 24–2 for a description of this staging system), poor performance status (Eastern Cooperative Oncology Group [ECOG] ≥2), 2 or more extranodal sites, and above normal LDH, with each positive feature scoring as 1. Table 23–5 shows the overall survival according to the number of unfavorable factors at presentation.

Diffuse large B-cell lymphomas have some rare, though unique, presentations. **Mediastinal (thymic) large B-cell lymphoma** is a tumor arising from thymic medullary B cells and accounts for more than 2% of NHL cases. It usually presents in a young adult woman as a bulky mediastinal mass with superior vena cava syndrome, and infiltration of the pleura, pericardium, lungs, and chest wall. Diagnosis is based on direct biopsy of the mediastinal mass, since most of the patients present without involvement of extra-mediastinal sites. On histology, the tumor is characterized by a diffuse infiltrate of large cells with clear cytoplasm and some sclerosis. The cells express CD20, but often lack sIg. The most frequent karyotypic abnormalities are 9p+ (75%), 2p+, and XXY. The 9p24 gain affects the *JAK-2* locus. Gene expression arrays have shown profiles more reminiscent of the nodular sclerosing forms of Hodgkin disease than diffuse large B-cell NHL. Despite an aggressive presentation and course, the outcome seems to be better when compared with other presentations of diffuse large B-cell NHL.

Intravascular lymphoma is a rare presentation of large B-cell NHL, in which the tumor cells are found within the vascular lumen, with little if any appreciable tissue involvement. This affects elderly patients, with an aggressive course and short survival. Occlusive symptoms are seen in the CNS and lung, and less frequently in the skin or kidneys. The diagnosis is frequently established postmortem. **Primary effusion lymphoma** is a rare B-cell variant observed in HIV patients (see below). **Primary cutaneous B-cell lymphomas** include follicular center cell, marginal zone, and large cell subtypes. While they share most of the histologic and immunophenotypic features characteristic of their nodal counterparts, the large cell type has unique characteristics when it is localized on the legs. It presents in elderly patients as palpable, sometimes ulcerated lesions with a diffuse infiltration of the dermis by large cells, which lack the characteristic CD10 expression and the t(14;18) translocation. The course is usually aggressive.

Burkitt Lymphoma

Burkitt lymphoma is a very aggressive NHL of B-cell origin. The characteristic histology is that of a diffuse infiltrate of small, non-cleaved lymphocytes interspersed with large cells imparting a "starry sky" appearance under low-power magnification (Figure 23–5D). The vacuoles in these cells responsible for the starry sky appearance stain positively for fat using the oil red O stain. Burkitt cells express a B-cell immunophenotype with CD19/20/22/10 positivity, but monotypic sIg expression, and are negative for terminal deoxynucleotide transferase (TdT), which distinguishes Burkitt NHL from precursor B-cell acute lymphocytic leukemia (ALL). Burkitt NHL is associated with a unique chromosomal rearrangement involving translocation of the *c-myc* proto-oncogene on chromosome 8 to one of the immunoglobulin gene loci, the most common being t(8;14) (see Table 23–3).

Burkitt lymphoma presents as 3 distinct variants. The first was described in 1958 by the British surgeon Dennis Burkitt in Uganda. It occurs endemically in African children as a tumor mass localized to the jaw or retroperitoneum with involvement of bone, kidney, ovaries, and CNS. This endemic form led to the discovery of the Epstein-Barr virus (EBV) in Burkitt lymphoma tumor specimens. In Western countries, Burkitt lymphoma is a non-endemic disease of children and young adults with no clear connection to EBV. It most often presents as a rapidly growing tumor of abdominal lymph nodes, although marrow and CNS involvement are found in 30% of children and 15% of adults at diagnosis. Progression to a leukemic phenotype is frequent (see Chapter 25). Burkitt lymphoma is also a complication of immunodeficiency, mainly in the setting of HIV infection (see below).

B-Cell Lymphoma in AIDS Patients

An increasing incidence of B-cell lymphomas is being seen in AIDS patients. These NHL are strongly associated with EBV and may also show rearrangements involving *c-myc* and mutation of p53. Many of these NHL involve the brain. Clinical staging is important in planning treatment and should be carried out without delay. Patients with a single tumor mass and low LDH have the best prognosis. Bulky tumor in the abdomen imparts a worse prognosis, and involvement of either marrow or the CNS, together with a high LDH, predict a high failure rate even with aggressive chemotherapy. The incidence of AIDS-related NHL has not changed with the introduction of highly active antiretroviral therapy (HAART). This is in contrast to the marked reduction in the incidence of Kaposi sarcoma.

Primary effusion lymphoma is a complication of human herpesvirus 8 (HHV-8) infection in AIDS patients, characterized by a unique clinical presentation involving the serous cavities of pleura, peritoneum, and pericardium. The malignant cells display the pan-lymphocyte CD45 cell marker, but most B-cell markers (CD19/20/79a) and T-cell markers (CD3/CD4/CD8) are absent. However, the cells are of B-cell origin since Ig gene rearrangement is consistently found. The prognosis is poor.

Post-Transplant Lymphoproliferative Disorders

Post-transplant B-cell lymphomas are seen in patients receiving chronic immunosuppressive therapy for solid organ or hematopoietic stem cell transplantation. The incidence is variable according to the duration of the immunosuppression and ranges from less than 1% in hematopoietic stem cell recipients

CASE HISTORY • *Part 2*

Even though the majority of the lymphadenopathy found on examination is not impressive, the presence of a large, non-tender nodal mass in the axilla, without a history of a recent infection or injury to that hand/arm, requires immediate surgical biopsy with removal of adequate tissue for histologic, flow cytometric, and genetic analysis.

The nodal biopsy is performed, and pathological review reveals a diffuse, large B-cell NHL in the nodal mass, while 2 small adjacent nodes show only reactive changes. A bone marrow aspirate and biopsy are also performed. Flow cytometric immunophenotyping demonstrates $CD19^+$ $CD20^+$ $CD10^+$ KAPPA-restricted monoclonal B cells in both marrow and blood. The marrow biopsy confirms paratrabecular lymphocytic proliferation with diffuse large cell morphology.

Renal and hepatic function tests show only a moderately elevated LDH (624 U/L). However, CT imaging of the abdomen shows the presence of an intrahepatic mass and several enlarged nodes in the retroperitoneum. A subsequent PET scan confirms the presence of sites of increased uptake in the axillae, the liver, and the retroperitoneum.

Question

- What is this patient's International Prognostic Index score and associated prognosis?

to 2%–5% in heart, liver, and lung transplant recipients. They generally arise from host cells after solid organ transplantation, whereas donor origin is the rule after allogeneic hematopoietic stem cell transplantation. **Post-transplant lymphoproliferative disorders (PTLD)** present mainly as tumors of extranodal sites. Early-onset **PTLD** are usually related to EBV infection, are polyclonal or oligoclonal, and may frequently resolve with discontinuation of immunosuppression, whereas late-onset **PTLD** are true monoclonal malignancies of the diffuse, large B cell (Burkitt-like type). Most of the monoclonal B cells in the latter are derived from germinal center B cells.

Lymphoblastic Lymphoma

Precursor lymphoblastic lymphoma represents another high-grade malignancy with diffuse histology. This condition is a disease of younger adults and children. It often presents with a bulky, rapidly growing mediastinal mass. The marrow and CNS are frequently involved. On biopsy, the mass consists of a diffuse infiltrate of cells with convoluted nuclei and little cytoplasm. The phenotype of the cells is most often that of a pre–B or T cell. This tumor shares characteristics with ALL and is treated with a similar regimen (see Chapter 25). Patients presenting with lymphoblastic lymphoma frequently have a leukemic component to their disease and have a clinical course more like overt ALL than NHL.

Lymphomatoid Granulomatosis

This variety of lymphoma has been described under several designations in the past, including polymorphic reticulosis and Liebow-Carrington disease, and finally has been determined to be an EBV-driven NHL of B-cell origin. It presents mainly in adults as an extranodal disease involving lungs, skin, kidneys, and nerves, and clinically is reminiscent of Wegener granulomatosis.

T-CELL LYMPHOMA CLASSIFICATION

As techniques for diagnosing clonal lymphoid malignancies have improved, especially the ability to detect rearrangements of the B- and T-cell antigen receptor genes, an increasing number of tumors of T-cell origin have been identified. **Clinical clues** to the presence of a T-cell malignancy include the presence of constitutional (B-type) symptoms, leukopenia or aplastic anemia (or both), disseminated disease with marrow involvement, hepatosplenomegaly, lung and skin involvement, and hypercalcemia.

Several subtypes of T-cell NHL have been identified. These are defined largely by their clinical profiles. Four main primary presentations are distinctive within this category, that is, leukemic, nodal, cutaneous, and non-cutaneous extranodal T-cell lymphoproliferations. However, the ultimate diagnosis of a T-cell lymphoma requires studies of **cell surface markers and T cell–receptor gene rearrangement**. The latter is the only certain way of proving a clonal origin for T cells since a normal T-cell immunophenotype occurs in many T-NHLs. However, the array of surface markers can be helpful in that T-cell NHL will frequently lack normal antigen expression (eg, CD7), express cytoplasmic (but not surface) CD3, and sometimes demonstrate aberrant T-cell markers (eg, CD25) or dual positivity for (or absence of) both CD4 and CD8.

Many T-cell lymphomas are characterized by a pleomorphic cell population, often including large numbers of macrophages. This diverse cell population is probably recruited to the site of the tumor by production of cytokines by the malignant T cells. In addition, production of these cytokines explains the common occurrence of inflammatory signs and symptoms.

Leukemic T-Cell Lymphomas

Disorders in this category present as leukemic proliferations. Prolymphocytic T-cell leukemia, T-cell large granular lymphocyte leukemia, and adult T-cell leukemia/lymphoma are described in Chapter 22, and T-cell ALL is discussed in Chapter 25.

Nodal T-Cell Lymphomas

Most patients presenting with **peripheral nodal T-cell lymphomas**, which are diffuse small- or large-cell NHLs with the phenotype of mature T cells, have constitutional symptoms (fever, chills, weight loss) suggesting active cytokine production by the malignant cells. Widespread lymphadenopathy is the rule, and many patients have involvement of extranodal sites, marrow, blood, liver, spleen, lung, or skin.

A. Angio-immunoblastic T-Cell Lymphoma

Also referred as **angio-immunoblastic lymphadenopathy**, angio-immunoblastic T-cell lymphoma is a disease of the elderly accounting for 4%–6% of all lymphomas. Patients present with generalized lymphadenopathy, hepatosplenomegaly, skin rashes, arthritis, pleural effusions, and constitutional symptoms. There is a polyclonal B-cell expansion with hypergammaglobulinemia, and in some cases autoantibodies, resulting in Coombs-positive hemolytic anemia or thrombocytopenia. The EBV genome is integrated in nearly 100% of lymph node T cells. The course of the disease is aggressive. A very similar presentation has been described in rare patients treated with the hydantoin drugs.

B. Anaplastic Large Cell Lymphoma

This variety of lymphoma accounts for 2%–3% of all NHLs. It has been previously referred as Ki-1 lymphoma, as these T cells express Ki-1 antigen (CD30). Malignant cells are large, undifferentiated "anaplastic" cells, which have sometimes been confused in the past with Reed-Sternberg cells of Hodgkin lymphoma. Anaplastic large cell lymphoma has 2 different presentations, differing in their expression of the ALK kinase (Table 23–6). ALK-positive cases present in young men with lymphadenopathy and extranodal sites, and constitutional symptoms, and have a better prognosis, whereas ALK-negative cases present in the sixth decade and have less extranodal involvement, but a poorer outcome.

C. Peripheral T-Cell Lymphoma, Unspecified

This variety is the most frequent type of T-cell NHL in Western countries, accounting for 5%–7% of all NHLs. It presents in

TABLE 23–6 • Immunophenotypic and genetic features of T-cell neoplasms

Disease	Morphology	Immunophenotype	Karyotype	Involved Genes
Leukemic presentation				
T-cell prolymphocytic leukemia	Prolymphocytes or small lymphocytes (variant)	CD2, 3, 5, 7^{+} CD25^{-} CD4^{+}8^{-} > CD8^{+}4^{-} > CD4^{-} 8^{-}	Inv 14 (q11;q32) (75%) T(14;14)	*ATM* mutations (11q23) *TCL1* overexpressed (14q32)
Large granular lymphocyte	Lymphocytes with abundant cytoplasm and azurophilic granules	CD2, 3^{+}, 5$^{\pm}$ CD8, 16, 57^{+} CD4, 56, 25^{-}	No recurrent abnormality	Unknown
Adult T-cell leukemia/ lymphoma	Highly variable "flower-like" nuclear shape	CD2, 3, 5, 25^{+} CD7^{-}, CD4^{+}8^{-}	Complex	Integrated *HTLV-I*
Precursor T lymphoblastic	Medium-sized blastic cells	CD7^{+} CD2, 3, 5$^{\pm}$ CD4, 8^{+} or CD4, 8^{-}	14q11.2, 7q35, 7p14-15	*Myc* (8q24) *TAL1* (1p32) *RBTN1* (11p15) *RBTN2* (11p13) *HOX11* (10q24)
Nodal presentation				
Anaplastic large-cell lymphoma	Large blastic pleomorphic cells	CD2, 3, 5, 7$^{\pm}$ CD25$^{\pm}$, CD30^{+}	t(2;5)(p23;q35) t(1;2)(q25;p23) t(2;3)(p23;q21) t(2;22)(p23;q11)	*ALK* (2p23) *NPM* (5q35) *TPM3* (1q21) *TFG* (3q21) *CLTCL* (22q11)
Angio-immunoblastic T-cell lymphoma	Small- to medium-sized plasma cells, immunoblasts	CD4^{+} CD8$^{\pm}$, CD10^{+}	Trisomy 3, 5, +X	Integrated *EBV*
Peripheral T-cell lymphoma	Small- to medium-sized irregular lymphocytes	CD2, 3, 5, 7$^{\pm}$ CD4 and/or 8^{+}	Complex No recurrent abnormality	Unknown
Extranodal presentation				
Cutaneous T-cell lymphoma	Small and large cells with cerebriform nuclei	CD2, 3, 5^{+}, 7$^{\pm}$ CD4^{+}8^{-}, CD25$^{\pm}$	No recurrent abnormality	Unknown
Hepatosplenic γ/δ T-cell lymphoma	Small- to medium-sized atypical lymphocytes (red pulp infiltration in spleen)	CD2^{+}, CD3^{+}, CD4^{-}, CD5^{-}, CD7$^{\pm}$, CD8^{-}, CD16$^{\pm}$, CD38^{+}, CD56^{+}	Isochromosome 7q	Unknown
Nasal T/NK lymphoma	Small-, medium-, or large-sized atypical lymphocytes	CD2^{+} 16^{+} 56^{+} 57^{+} Surface CD3^{-} Cytoplasmic CD3^{+}	No recurrent abnormality	Integrated *EBV*
Enteropathic T-cell lymphoma	Small, medium, and large cells	CD3/7^{+}CD5^{-} CD103^{+}	LOH[a] 9p21	Integrated *EBV* in some regions

Note: By definition, all have rearranged TCR genes.
[a]*Loss of heterozygosity.*

elderly patients with bulky lymphadenopathy, constitutional symptoms, and usually disseminated disease. The proliferating cells are pleomorphic, varying from small, cleaved cells to large, immunoblastic ones. Some cases include epithelioid cells, which characterize a lympho-epithelioid variant, the so-called "Lennert lymphoma." Patients demonstrating the p53 mutation have a poorer prognosis.

Cutaneous T-Cell Lymphomas

Lymphomas of the skin are not always T-cell malignancies; B-cell lymphomas and Hodgkin disease can also initially present with cutaneous involvement. As a reflection of this, classification schemes for the cutaneous lymphomas have been proposed by the WHO and the EORTC (European Organization for Research and Treatment of Cancer). The classification is summarized in Table 23–7.

A. Sézary Syndrome and Mycosis Fungoides

T-cell malignancies can also present as skin disease **(cutaneous T-cell lymphoma/mycosis fungoides/Sézary syndrome; see Figures 22–4 and 23–5C)**. The presenting skin lesions of mycosis fungoides vary from eczematous or psoriatic-appearing

TABLE 23–7 • Classification of cutaneous lymphomas

Cutaneous T-cell and NK lymphomas
Sézary syndrome and mycosis fungoides Primary cutaneous CD30$^+$ lymphoproliferative disorders Subcutaneous panniculitis-like T-cell lymphoma Primary cutaneous peripheral T-cell lymphoma, unspecified (CD4$^+$, CD8$^+$, γ/δ),
Cutaneous B-cell lymphomas
Cutaneous marginal zone lymphoma of MALT type Primary cutaneous follicle center lymphoma Primary cutaneous diffuse large B-cell lymphoma Intravascular large B-cell lymphoma

lesions to plaques with sharply demarcated margins. Cutaneous lesions are severely pruritic and eventually develop into painless nodules that ulcerate and become infected. Many patients will develop generalized erythroderma progressing to exfoliation. Survival can range from a few months to several decades, depending on the extent of blood, nodal, and visceral disease. When the disease is limited to the skin, median survival is more than 10 years. However, most patients will progress to stage IV with involvement of lymph nodes and visceral organs. Blood and marrow involvement is characterized by the appearance in the circulation of small or large CD4$^+$ T lymphocytes with highly convoluted (cerebriform) nuclei. Their presence signifies progression to Sézary syndrome.

On skin biopsy, the CD4$^+$ T-NHL typically show a lymphocytic or mixed cell infiltrate immediately under the epidermis, and the epidermis is actually invaded by clusters of lymphocytes producing unique lesions called **Pautrier microabscesses** (see Figure 23–5C). This pattern (so-called epidermotropism) is quite different from that seen with cutaneous B-NHL, where the cells tend to congregate in the lower dermis, leaving a clear subepidermal zone. T cell–receptor gene rearrangement analysis can be used to identify the clonal T-cell nature of the infiltrate in unclear cases.

B. Cutaneous CD30$^+$ Lymphomas

Cutaneous CD30$^+$ lymphomas account for 30% of the cutaneous T-cell lymphomas, encompassing the primary cutaneous anaplastic large cell lymphomas and lymphomatoid papulosis. Patients with **primary cutaneous anaplastic large cell lymphomas** present with cutaneous nodules evolving quickly to ulceration, characterized by non-epidermotropic infiltrates of large anaplastic cells expressing CD4 and CD30; unlike cells from the nodal or systemic forms (see above), the malignant T cells lack the EMA and ALK proteins, and the t(2;5) translocation. The nodules can disappear, even without treatment, but recurrences are usually observed. Nevertheless, the overall prognosis is quite favorable.

In **lymphomatoid papulosis**, the clinical presentation is very similar, but infiltrates in skin lesions display scarce CD30$^+$ large T cells among a reactive, polymorphic non-tumor infiltrate. Prognosis is usually good. However, in a minority of patients lymphomatoid papulosis evolves to mycosis fungoides, large cell lymphoma, or Hodgkin lymphoma.

C. Subcutaneous Panniculitis-Like T-Cell Lymphoma

Subcutaneous panniculitis-like T-cell lymphoma (SCPTCL) presents as violaceous plaques or skin infiltrates, characterized by an infiltration of subcutaneous fat by a mixture of small to large cells, and frequent hemophagocytosis by adjacent macrophages. Most of the patients have associated systemic symptoms such as fever, lung infiltrates, hepatosplenomegaly, jaundice, and pancytopenia. This presentation is closely related to a systemic hemophagocytic syndrome, which worsens the prognosis.

Other Extranodal T-Cell Lymphomas

γ/δ T-cell lymphoma results from a proliferation of morphologically small- to medium-sized atypical lymphocytes, which are non–major histocompatibility complex (MHC)-dependent cytotoxic T cells; this entity is associated with a 7q– abnormality and preferential involvement of the liver, spleen (red pulp), and marrow. Following the first descriptions as a hepatosplenic lymphoma (the so-called γ/δ hepatosplenic T-cell lymphoma), similar proliferations have been observed in the skin, and similar hepatosplenic presentations have been reassigned as α/β T-cell proliferations. Most patients with γ/δ T-NHL are middle-aged males, and many are subject to immunosuppression for solid-organ transplantation. There is no associated viral infection. Clinically, patients present with hepatosplenomegaly, autoimmune cytopenia, and no lymphadenopathy. Constitutional

CASE HISTORY • *Part 3*

This patient has stage IV disease—tumor masses in multiple nodal sites plus the liver and detectable clonal B cells in both the marrow and blood. His LDH is also elevated. Based on these findings, his FLIPI score is 3 (see Table 23–4), placing him in the intermediate- to high-risk category with a probability of 5-year survival somewhat less than 50%. However, despite the aggressive presentation, this patient's lymphoma subtype is potentially curable.

Question

- How should this patient be treated?

symptoms and elevated LDH are common. The course is progressive and the prognosis quite poor, as most of the patients die within 1 year despite treatment.

Enteropathy-like T-cell lymphoma arises most frequently in adults with celiac disease, who have a 1% risk of developing this complication. The malignant T cells are transformed monoclonal, intraepithelial T lymphocytes. The risk of this complication is reduced when patients are compliant with a gluten-free diet. Prognosis is quite poor as only 10% of patients survive 5 years.

Nasal T/NK lymphoma, formerly referred to as **polymorphic reticulosis** or **lethal midline granuloma**, presents clinically as angio-invasive and angio-destructive infiltrates with necrosis localized to the nasal, palatal, and/or facial structures, or associated with skin, lung, or kidney infiltrations clinically reminiscent of Wegener granulomatosis. This last presentation has also been referred to as lymphomatoid granulomatosis or Liebow-Carrington disease. Malignant T cells usually express EBV transcripts and display an admixture of NK and T antigens (see Table 23–6). The lesions respond transiently to chemotherapy and/or local irradiation, but recurrence is frequent and the prognosis is quite poor.

THERAPY AND CLINICAL COURSE

The success rate in treating lymphoma is, of course, related to grade of disease and prognostic factors. For practical purposes, treatment decisions are based on a stratification of lymphomas according to their grade of malignancy as proposed initially by the Working Formulation for Clinical Usage (Table 23–8).

TABLE 23–8 • Working formulation for clinical use and its B and T cell counterparts

Working Formulation	B-Cell Neoplasms	T-Cell Neoplasms
Low grade		
Small lymphocytic	B-cell CLL/SLL Marginal zone, mucosa associated (MALT) Mantle cell	Large granular lymphocytic Adult T-cell lymphoma/leukemia
Plasmacytoid	Lymphoplasmacytic Marginal zone (MALT)	
Follicular, small cell, and mixed cell	Follicular, grades I and II Mantle cell Marginal zone (MALT)	
Intermediate grade		
Follicular, large cell Diffuse, small cell	Follicular, grade III Mantle cell Follicular center, diffuse small cell Marginal zone (MALT)	Large granular lymphocytic Adult T-cell lymphoma/leukemia Angio-immunoblastic Angiocentric
Diffuse, mixed cell	Large B-cell lymphoma Follicular center, diffuse small cell Lymphoplasmacytoid Marginal zone (MALT) Mantle cell	Peripheral T-cell lymphoma Adult T-cell lymphoma/leukemia Angio-immunoblastic Angiocentric Intestinal T-cell lymphoma
Diffuse, large cell	Diffuse large B-cell lymphoma	Peripheral T-cell lymphoma Adult T-cell lymphoma/leukemia Angio-immunoblastic Angiocentric Intestinal T-cell lymphoma
High grade		
Large-cell immunoblastic	Diffuse large B-cell lymphoma	Peripheral T-cell lymphoma Adult T-cell lymphoma/leukemia Angio-immunoblastic Angiocentric Intestinal T-cell lymphoma Anaplastic large cell
Lymphoblastic	Precursor B-cell lymphoblastic	Precursor T-cell lymphoblastic
Burkitt lymphoma	Burkitt lymphoma	Peripheral T-cell lymphoma

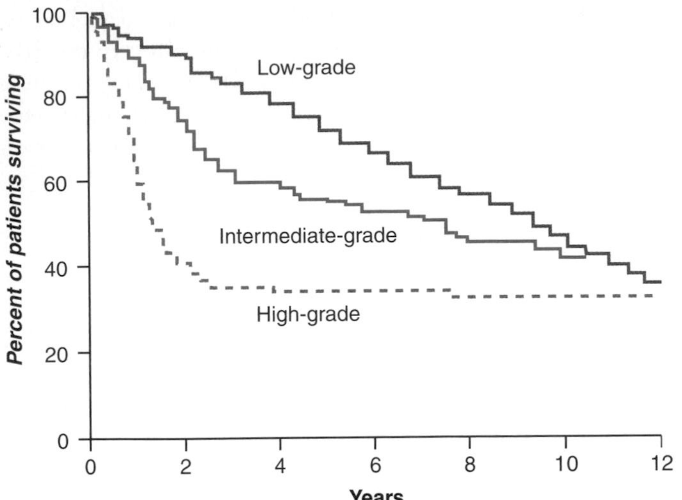

FIGURE 23–6. **Survival curves in lymphomas.** The success rate in treating high-grade lymphomas depends on the age of the patient, the tumor burden, the histologic characteristics of the lymphoma, and both the presence of complicating illness and performance status.

Despite the fact that this formulation is not really a classification of lymphomas, it introduces 2 important concepts. First, the **low-grade lymphomas**, which present in older patients as widely disseminated disease, generally have an indolent course and long-term outcome is poorly influenced by treatment. Second, **high-grade lymphomas** present more often with limited extension and are curable with aggressive treatment.

The most common low-grade lymphoma is **follicular (small cell) lymphoma**, whereas **diffuse, large cell lymphoma** is the most common high-grade lymphoma. The prognostic factors and predicted survivals for follicular and large cell lymphomas are summarized in Tables 23–4 and 23–5. Patients with follicular lymphomas often have a good prognosis in terms of their long-term survival but are very rarely cured, ultimately dying of their disease. Conversely, patients with diffuse, large cell lymphomas, who have a very poor prognosis and a much shorter average survival when untreated, can often be cured by aggressive therapy (Figure 23–6).

NHL therapy must also be tailored according to the disease subtype, the presence of complicating illness, and the age and performance status of the individual patient. In many institutions these patients will be treated according to strict research protocols. This permits continuous improvement in therapy design as new regimens for radiotherapy, chemotherapy, monoclonal antibodies, and hematopoietic stem cell transplantation are introduced. Successful treatment of the lymphoma also requires a high-quality blood transfusion service to provide red blood cell and platelet support, and expert management of immunocompromised patients.

Radiation Therapy

Radiation therapy is very effective in destroying sites of bulky disease. Relatively low doses (2,000 cGy) will result in spectacular regression of a localized tumor mass. However, since NHL is most often a disseminated disease, chemo-immunotherapy combinations have shown greater efficacy, such that the role of radiotherapy is now restricted to palliation or directed at restricted sites of symptomatic disease in elderly patients.

Treatment of Low-Grade Lymphomas

Low-grade lymphomas are usually **extremely indolent**, with long periods of regression or stable disease interrupted by periods of increased disease activity. No evidence exists that aggressive chemotherapy can cure these patients. Thus, a conservative therapeutic approach is indicated, ranging from no therapy at all during quiescent periods to the use of minimal chemotherapy or radiotherapy designed to control flare-ups and eliminate symptoms. Most of these patients will survive for more than 10 years, requiring only brief periods of treatment or none at all. If treatment is indicated, it has traditionally been restricted to local radiotherapy of bulky symptomatic disease or a mild chemotherapy regimen such as oral chlorambucil or cyclophosphamide alone, or a cyclophosphamide-vincristine-prednisone regimen (Table 23–9).

The availability of 2 new and more effective chemotherapy drugs—**fludarabine** and **2′ chlordeoxyadenosine (2-CdA)** has modified this treatment approach. Both have proved effective in

TABLE 23–9 • Some typical chemotherapeutic regimens for lymphoma

Regimen	Drug Dosage and Schedule
Single agent	
Cyclophosphamide	100 mg PO qd
Chlorambucil	4–12 mg PO qd
Fludarabine	25 mg/m^2 IV days 1–5
CVP repeated q3 weeks	
Cyclophosphamide	400 mg/m^2 PO days 1–5
Vincristine	1.4 mg/m^2 IV day 1
Prednisone	100 mg/m^2 PO days 1–5
CHOP repeated q3 weeks	
Cyclophosphamide	750 mg/m^2 IV day 1
Adriamycin	50 mg/m^2 IV day 1
Vincristine	1.4 mg/m^2 IV day 1
Prednisone	100 mg PO days 1–5
R-CHOP repeated q3 weeks	
Rituximab	375 mg/m^2 IV day 1, weekly
CHOP (as above)	Beginning day 3
Chemotherapy with autologous marrow support	
BCNU	112 mg/m^2 IV days 1–4
Cyclophosphamide	900 mg/m^2 IV q12h days 1–4
Etoposide (VP-16)	250 mg/m^2 IV q12h days 1–4
Infusion of autologous marrow cells	At least 2 × 10^6 CD34 cells/kg IV day 7

the treatment of CLL (see Chapter 22) and are now being used in the treatment of low-grade lymphomas. One downside is that these agents are highly immunosuppressive, especially in combination with corticosteroids, and their use increases the risk of opportunistic infections. Other drugs now under development include **bendamustine**, which combines alkylating and purine analog compounds; **bortezomib**, a proteasome inhibitor that has shown efficacy in mantle cell lymphoma and myeloma, and the **Bcl-2 inhibitors**.

At the same time, the most significant progress has been in the area of **immunotherapy**, using recombinant monoclonal antibodies against B-cell markers, especially CD20, or markers shared by B and T cells such as CD52. **Rituximab**, a chimeric anti-CD20 monoclonal antibody with specificity for the late pre–B stage to plasma cell differentiation, is now being used either alone or in various combinations with chemotherapy against all $CD20^+$ B-NHL. Patients with follicular lymphomas show the best response; 80% of patients who fail to respond to chemotherapy alone will show a response to rituximab with minimal toxicity. Although the best use of this agent is still a matter of study, it is typically given in doses of 375 mg/m^2 as a weekly infusion for up to 8 weeks. The incorporation of **rituximab in a combined immunochemotherapy regimen** as initial therapy is now under study.

Another approach to immunotherapy involves coupling a radionuclide, such as ^{131}I or ^{90}Y, to an anti-CD20 antibody (^{131}I tositumomab and ^{90}Y ibritumomab). When given in myeloablative doses followed by stem cell rescue, this approach is well tolerated and can produce prolonged remissions in more than 50% of relapsed patients. **Alemtuzumab** is a chimeric anti-CD52 monoclonal antibody that has proven to be highly effective in CLL and T-cell prolymphocytic leukemia (see Chapter 22). It has also demonstrated efficacy in disseminated forms of cutaneous T-cell lymphomas.

Some patients with low- or intermediate-grade lymphoma will show a pattern of continued slow growth of the disease despite therapy **(unresponsive disease)** or will have **brief responses followed by rapid resumption of growth**. These patients have a markedly poorer prognosis. In this case more aggressive chemotherapy protocols are justified in an attempt to achieve longer remissions. Such protocols include chemotherapy capable of crossing into the CNS, such as high-dose methotrexate with leucovorin rescue, cytosine arabinoside, or both. Such protocols involve a high level of treatment-related morbidity and mortality (up to 5%–10%) but do result in prolonged disease-free survival in up to 50% of patients. Because of a tendency to see late relapses, it is unclear what proportion of these may be considered cures.

Hematopoietic stem cell transplantation (see discussion at the end of this chapter) in follicular NHL has been extensively studied as a component of the treatment regimen for relapsing patients. Patients with treatment-sensitive relapse have the best outcome. However, a recent trial has shown no survival advantage when comparing autologous transplantation to immunochemotherapy (rituximab, cyclophosphamide, adriamycin, vincristine, prednisone [R-CHOP]). Patients receiving allogeneic transplants show lower relapse rates when compared with autologous transplant patients, but have severe transplant-related toxicity (graft-versus-host disease [GVHD]) and mortality. Reduced conditioning regimens in the setting of non-myeloablative allogeneic transplantation have recently shown very encouraging results with short-term disease-free survival rates up to 85%.

Mantle cell lymphoma deserves special consideration for therapy. The treatments recommended above are usually of limited efficacy and most MCL patients quickly progress to refractory disease. Front-line high-dose immunochemotherapy (a CHOP-like regimen—cyclophosphamide, vincristine, adriamycin, and dexamethasone [CVAD]—reinforced with alternating rituximab and methotrexate/cytarabine sequences) appears to produce superior results, but has little influence on overall survival. Recent trials have looked at bortezomib, alone or combined with other therapies; anti-angiogenic drugs such as thalidomide or lenalidomide; and myeloablative or non-myeloablative hematopoietic stem cell transplantation.

Lymphoma vaccine therapy is an interesting research approach for patients with low-burden residual disease. Typically the "vaccine" is custom made using a sample of the patient's own tumor cells to derive an idiotype protein, which is unique to the patient's lymphoma. This tumor-derived protein is then combined with an immunostimulant, such as keyhole limpet hemocyanin, and injected subcutaneously on a monthly schedule for up to 2 years. Simultaneous treatment with granulocyte colony-stimulating factor (G-CSF) may help magnify the immune response. Other current vaccine strategies are based on reinfusion of antigen-presenting cells (such as dendritic cells) primed ex vivo with the patient's own tumor B cells, with or without anti-CD20, or T cells transfected with immune response modifiers. Patients with the lowest tumor burden appear to do the best; therefore, candidate patients should be pretreated with combination chemotherapy.

Treatment of High-Grade Lymphomas

Patients with high-grade lymphomas have a poor prognosis when left untreated and should receive aggressive chemotherapy without waiting to see how the disease responds to milder therapy. In B-cell NHL, the best long-term results are currently observed with a high-dose, multidrug protocol, such as cyclophosphamide, adriamycin, vincristine, prednisone (CHOP) combined with the monoclonal antibody rituximab (R-CHOP), which is now the gold standard of large B-cell lymphoma treatment. According to the international index of prognostic factors (see Table 23–5), 5-year survival averages 80% in low-risk patients, whereas patients with 4 or more risk factors have survivals of 50%.

Based on these results, intensive treatment including autologous hematopoietic stem cell transplantation (see discussion at the end of this chapter), which was proven to be better than CHOP alone in a controlled trial, is no longer recommended as first-line therapy for patients with low- to intermediate-risk disease. High-risk patients, however, may get some benefit from this procedure based on a recent meta-analysis of randomized trials. This question is currently being evaluated in a prospective trial assessing consolidation with an autologous stem cell transplant rescue after R-CHOP in intermediate- to high-risk patients. Attempts to improve the dose intensity of the R-CHOP regimen are also currently under way.

Patients with high-grade lymphomas who relapse after chemotherapy are routinely treated with very high-dose chemotherapy regimens, sometimes including total body irradiation, followed by peripheral stem cell transplantation, either autologous or allogeneic. Here again, comparison of these approaches shows that patients receiving allogeneic transplants have lower relapse rates but more severe transplant-related toxicity and mortality when compared with patients treated with autologous transplants. However, reduced conditioning regimens offer very encouraging results with 3-year survival rates ranging from 52% up to 88%. Radio-immunotherapy is another promising approach for relapsed high-grade lymphomas.

Burkitt lymphoma deserves special treatment consideration. This lymphoma displays a high sensitivity to chemotherapy. Optimal treatment consists of intensive chemotherapy based on drugs such as cyclophosphamide, vincristine, methotrexate, doxorubicin, cytarabine, and etoposide administered sequentially over short periods of time in parallel with intrathecal infusions of methotrexate, cytarabine, and hydrocortisone. These treatments provide a high percentage of complete responses, ranging from 50%–80% long-term overall survival. CNS prophylaxis with irradiation, and intensification with autologous stem cell support are no longer recommended.

Treatment Regimens for T-Cell Lymphomas

For patients with nodal T-cell lymphomas, treatments are very similar to those described above. In the early stages of cutaneous T-cell lymphomas, the malignant T cells appear to be dependent on stimulation by epidermal Langerhans cells, and therapy directed entirely to the skin can be highly effective, even though it may be possible to demonstrate malignant T cells in other sites as well. Topical **chemotherapeutic agents** such as corticosteroids, mechlorethamine, or carmustine can be used on localized lesions. More extensive involvement responds to **electron beam irradiation**, if available. **Phototherapy**, with oral psoralen and ultraviolet UVA or UVB irradiation, is often used as first-line therapy and has the advantage of also treating unrecognized subclinical lesions. Because T cells circulate relatively more than B cells, they sometimes respond to repeated **leukapheresis** with decreased skin infiltration and adenopathy as well as decreased cell count. **Photopheresis**, in which the circulating T cells are exposed to UV radiation in an extracorporeal circuit, can achieve complete remissions, even though only a small fraction of the total T-cell pool is being treated. **Systemic chemotherapy** with single alkylating agents such as chlorambucil, cyclophosphamide, or BCNU can be beneficial with or without the addition of glucocorticoids. In more aggressive situations, **combination chemotherapy** including such drugs as methotrexate, bleomycin, and adriamycin is used. With most treatments, the initial response rate is high (50%–70%), but long-term responses are difficult to achieve.

Treatment of AIDS-Related Lymphomas

The treatment of **AIDS-related lymphomas** has been influenced more by the availability of highly active antiretroviral therapy (HAART, see Chapter 21) than by progress in chemotherapy regimens. HAART has made standard-dose chemotherapy, such as CHOP or CHOP-like regimens, feasible in AIDS patients. With this strategy, 3-year overall survival rates range from 22%–60%, depending on the International Prognostic Index, histopathology, and, of course, the HIV status of the patient. In order to minimize drug interactions and toxicity when combining the 2 regimens (HAART and chemotherapy) while still maximizing the dose intensity of the chemotherapy, it has been shown that interruption of HAART until completion of chemotherapy does not result in progression of AIDS and provides 5-year overall survival rates up to 87% for patients with $CD4^+$ counts higher than 0.1×10^9/L. However, patients with lower $CD4^+$ counts have a poor outcome. Trials with R-CHOP are currently in progress. Patients with AIDS-related CNS or Burkitt lymphoma should be treated with regimens similarly to HIV-negative patients.

Hematopoietic Stem Cell Transplantation

Hematopoietic stem cell transplant (HSCT) can be performed using stem cells harvested from the patient (autologous HSCT) or from an HLA-matched donor (allogeneic HSCT). There are advantages and disadvantages for each approach. **Allogeneic HSCT** has had great success in leukemia/lymphoma patients where the graft-versus-host reaction has been heralded for its ability to suppress the original malignant cells. **Autologous HSCT** is most useful in the treatment of lymphoma as a rescue maneuver in patients receiving ablative chemotherapy.

A. Allogeneic HSCT

Allogeneic HSCT is not for everyone. Only a minority of patients will be candidates based on age, stage of disease, complicating illness, and, most importantly, the availability of an HLA-matched donor. The latter is a function of family size (number of siblings) and HLA type, but it can be roughly estimated that fewer than 25% of patients will have access to a related HLA-matched donor. For patients with a common HLA type, an unrelated HLA-matched donor may be available from the international registry of marrow donors. However, this will still leave a majority of patients without a suitable donor.

The decision to undertake an allogeneic transplant must not be made without recognizing the difficulties involved. There is a double barrier to overcome in allogeneic HSCT. The first one is the immediate rejection of the graft by the recipient's immune system. Engraftment is only possible if the recipient's immune system is suppressed using conditioning regimens based on total body irradiation, high-dose alkylating agents such as cyclophosphamide, or other immunosuppressive drugs. As a consequence, recipients experience severe induction-related toxicities and remain immunodeficient for long periods of time with a high risk of infectious complications. The second barrier relates to the transplantation of donor immune-competent cells. With the exception of identical twin transplants (syngeneic HSCT), all allogeneic HSCT patients develop GVHD, the severity of which depends on the age of the patient and the level of HLA match between donor and recipient. GVHD, when severe and poorly controlled, is responsible for a high morbidity and mortality during the first months following the procedure. The short-term mortality resulting from the combination of graft rejection, complicating infection with organ failure, and acute GVHD is 20%–30% on average. Chronic GVHD, leukemia/lymphoma relapse, and both infections and malignancies secondary to prolonged immunodeficiency contribute to long-term morbidity and mortality.

Still, there is a major role for allogeneic HSCT in younger patients with leukemia or aggressive lymphomas, especially those that are unresponsive to chemotherapy. The disadvantage of long-term GVHD is offset by the graft-versus-malignant cell component of allogeneic HSCT. This has led to the purposeful grafting of relatively HLA-incompatible stem cells and immunocompetent cells. It is possible, by reducing the intensity of the conditioning regimen, to attain a **partial transplant**, that is, a stable mixed chimera of donor and recipient immunocompetent cells. Repeated infusions of donor lymphocytes have also been used to magnify the anti-leukemia/lymphoma effect in patients with little or no post-transplant GVHD. In both cases, relapse can be prevented or at least delayed by encouraging moderate long-term GVHD.

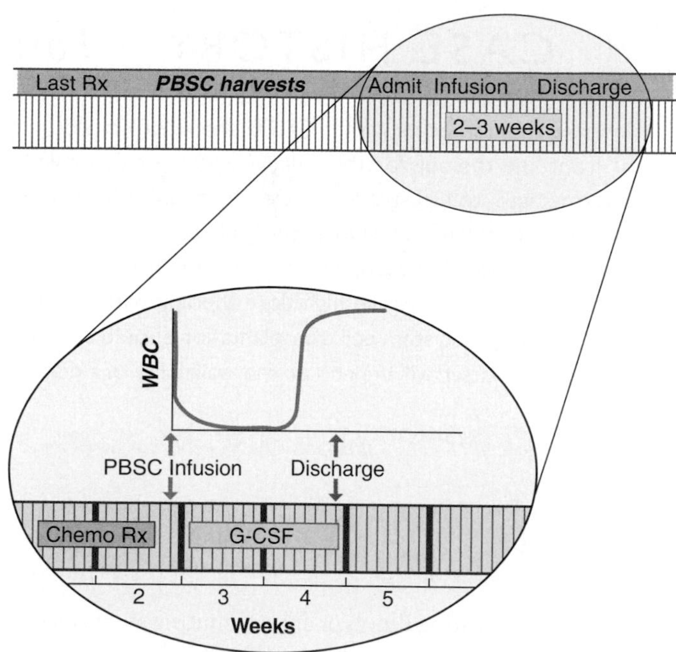

FIGURE 23–7. **Autologous hematopoietic stem cell transplantation protocol.** The sequence of autologous HSCT involves collecting an adequate number of peripheral blood stem cells (PBSC), usually over several days. Following high-dose marrow ablative chemotherapy, the harvested PBSC are used to rescue (reimplantation of) the patient's marrow. Supportive transfusions and G-CSF are needed during the aplastic interim until the white count recovers.

B. Autologous HSCT

Autologous stem cell transplantation (ASCT) is a technique designed to rescue the patient from the major hematopoietic toxicity resulting from high-dose chemotherapy/irradiation. The major advantage of ASCT is to allow very intensive treatment for diseases that are sensitive to chemoradiotherapy.

1. ASCT procedure—Peripheral blood stem cells (PBSCs) are collected from the patient by repeated leukapheresis, usually 1–5 times over as many days (Figure 23–7). The timing of these collections is critical. To obtain adequate numbers of stem cells, it is necessary to increase the proportion of circulating progenitor cells in the blood (priming). This may be done by collecting the cells either during the period that the patient is recovering from conventional chemotherapy or when the granulocyte count is rising in response to granulocyte colony-stimulating factor (G-CSF). In either case it is preferable to begin collections when the count is rising sharply, either at the level of 1,000–2,000/μL following chemotherapy or after 4–5 days of daily G-CSF injections. Usually between 1 and 10×10^{10} cells are collected and frozen until needed by the patient. Between 2 and 5×10^6 $CD34^+$ cells/kg are adequate for engraftment, and in some patients this goal may be reached in a single apheresis session.

The patient is then admitted for high-dose chemotherapy, which may contain any of a number of different combinations of drugs according to specific protocols. One of the most widely used, especially for lymphomas, is the BEAM combination (BCNU, etoposide, aracytine [or cytosine-arabinoside], melphalan). High-dose melphalan is also used as a conditioning regimen for myeloma. The object of the high-dose chemotherapy is to totally ablate the hematopoietic cells of the marrow while avoiding lethal toxicity to other organs such as lung, liver, and heart.

Within 1–4 days of completion of chemotherapy, patients receive intravenous infusions of their PBSC and begin receiving daily injections of G-CSF. Following reinfusion of the progenitor cells, there is a period of 5–10 days in which the patient is absolutely pancytopenic, with essentially no leukocyte or platelet production. After this latent period, there is, under the influence of the myeloid growth factors, a rapid rise in the leukocyte count. Platelet recovery usually lags behind the white cells, and the patients may require platelet support for weeks to months, although the use of PBSC hastens platelet recovery.

The management of these patients is essentially the same as that of any patient receiving high-dose, marrow-ablative chemotherapy. They are at high risk for severe infections and must receive intensive antibiotic coverage (see Chapter 18). In addition, the chemotherapy may result in reversible toxicity to other organs that would not be seen with lower doses.

2. ASCT outcome—The success rate of autologous HSCT therapy depends on 3 factors. First is keeping the treatment-related mortality low. Generally, the autologous HSCT procedure mortality is less than 1%–2%, which contrasts with the 20%–30% mortality observed in allogeneic HSCT. However, not all patients are candidates, especially older patients and

CASE HISTORY • Part 4

Immunochemotherapy with R-CHOP should be considered as front-line therapy for this relatively young patient with intermediate- to high-grade disease, no complicating illness, and good performance status. It is likely to induce a complete remission. If a complete remission is not promptly obtained, more aggressive high-dose therapy with autologous or allogeneic stem cell transplantation should be considered. The latter will depend on the availability of a donor.

With achievement of complete remission, only time will tell what the ultimate outcome will be. Based on his FLIPI score, the probability of long-term survival is approximately 50%. However, the up-front use of rituximab in combination with CHOP and, if necessary, transplantation may improve his survival. Of course, the patient will have to be followed carefully with laboratory and imaging studies for any signs or symptoms of relapse.

those with complicating illness or aplasia limiting stem cell collection. Second, and the most likely cause of failure, is the possibility that the patient's tumor was not ablated completely by the chemotherapy and irradiation. Whatever the NHL subtype, a fairly high percentage of patients relapse within the first 1–2 years after ASCT. Third, there is the real possibility that the PBSC collections contain small numbers of tumor cells that will regrow.

Since autologous HSCT therapy involves the reinfusion of more than 10^{10} cells, and since even the most sensitive detection methods permit the identification of only about 1 tumor cell in 10^6 cells, it is possible that the patient can receive as many as 10^4 tumor cells even if they are undetectable. Strategies for depleting these tumor cells, which involve treating the graft with monoclonal antibodies, in vitro chemotherapy, or immunotoxins ("purging"), have yet to offer a consistently clear improvement in outcome. Recently, devices for positive purification of the $CD34^+$ stem cells using immunoabsorptive columns based on the ability of monoclonal antibodies to bind to the CD34 antigen have become available. Although this procedure will simultaneously enrich for the desired stem cells and deplete unwanted tumor cells, it requires larger collections of PBSC since many cells are lost during the selection procedure. Moreover, even improved $CD34^+$ selection cannot be expected to greatly modify the long-term outcome and risk of relapse. Tumor regrowth after autologous HSCT is more often due to failure to eradicate residual tumor cells than reinfusion of malignant cells.

3. ASCT clinical applications—Although not curative, autologous HSCT represents a significant improvement over conventional chemotherapy for selected patients with non-Hodgkin lymphoma. However, with the emergence of drugs that have improved the results of non-intensive treatments, the best role for autologous HSCT is a subject of continued study. Therefore, future trials are needed to clarify the place of HSCT in light of these recent advances in treatment.

POINTS TO REMEMBER

Patients presenting with rapidly enlarging, non-tender lymph nodes in 1 or more sites should be biopsied without delay; watchful waiting is not an option.

Staging a lymphoma includes large-volume node biopsy for histology and cell markers/genotyping; cell marker and genotype studies of bone marrow and blood; total body scans to detect node and organ involvement; and CBC, liver chemistries, and LDH (tumor mass indicator).

Patients with follicular or nodular (small cell) lymphomas almost always have stage IV disease from the onset due to widespread nodal and both marrow and blood involvement. These lymphomas are relatively indolent (low grade), progressing slowly over several years.

Patients with diffuse (large cell) lymphomas may present with localized disease (stage I), but generally have an aggressive course (high grade, evolving rapidly to stage IV) with a very poor prognosis if not aggressively treated.

The most important prognostic factor in NHL is the presence of nodular versus diffuse histology. However, the International Prognostic Index scoring system denotes other clinical factors important to predicting outcome.

The treatment of low-grade NHL is tailored to the rate of disease progression, patient age, presence of complicating illness, and performance status.

The treatment of high-grade NHL is aggressive with immunochemotherapy and, if necessary, transplantation. Long-term survival, even cure, is possible.

As more sophisticated assays of cell markers and genotype have been introduced, the classification of non-Hodgkin lymphomas has become increasingly complex. Many subtypes of B- and T-cell NHL, although less common, can now be defined by their unique clinical presentations, histology, cell markers, and gene mutations.

Some NHL subtypes respond to targeted therapies that differ significantly from the immunochemotherapy approach. Therefore, accurate diagnosis is essential.

Effective treatment of NHL requires the specialized and long-term care of immunocompromised patients; a sophisticated clinical pathology laboratory that offers immunophenotyping, immunohistochemistry, and molecular diagnostics/genetic assays; expert imaging facilities; and a robust transfusion service.

BIBLIOGRAPHY

Diagnosis

Al-Saleem T, Al-Mondhiry H: Immunoproliferative small intestinal disease (IPSID): a model for mature B-cell neoplasms. Blood 2005;105:2274.

Blum KA, Lozanski G, Byrd JC: Adult Burkitt leukemia and lymphoma. Blood 2004;104:3009.

Catovsky D, Matutes E: Splenic lymphoma with circulating villous lymphocytes/splenic marginal-zone lymphoma. Semin Hematol 1999;36:184.

Chen YB, Rahemtullah A, Hochberg E: Primary effusion lymphoma. Oncologist 2007;12:569.

Craig FE, Foon KA: Flow cytometric immunophenotyping for hematologic neoplasms. Blood 2008;111:3941.

Dave SS, Wright G, Tan B, et al: Prediction of survival in follicular lymphoma based on molecular features of tumor infiltrating immune cells. N Engl J Med 2004;351:2159.

Girardi M, Heald PW, Wilson LD: The pathogenesis of mycosis fungoides. N Engl J Med 2004;350:1978.

Hans CP et al: Confirmation of the molecular classification of diffuse large B-cell lymphoma by immunohistochemistry using tissue microarray. Blood 2004;103:275.

Jaffe H, Harris NL, Stein H, Vardiman JW (eds): *World Health Organization Classification of Tumors. Pathology and Genetics of Tumors of the Hematopoietic and Lymphoid Tissues*. IARC Press, 2001.

Jorgensen JL: State of the Art Symposium: flow cytometry in the diagnosis of lymphoproliferative disorders by fine-needle aspiration. Cancer 2005;105:443.

Kim YH, Willemze R, Pimpinelli N, et al: TNM classification system for primary cutaneous lymphomas other than mycosis fungoides and Sézary syndrome: a proposal of the International Society for Cutaneous Lymphomas (ISCL) and the Cutaneous Lymphoma Task Force of the European Organization of Research and Treatment of Cancer (EORTC). Blood 2007; 110:479.

Küppers R: Mechanisms of B-cell lymphoma pathogenesis. Nat Rev Cancer 2005;5:251.

Kwee TC, Kwee RM, Nievelstein RAJ: Imaging in staging of malignant lymphoma: a systematic review. Blood 2008;111:504.

Leich E, Hartmann EM, Burek C, Ott G, Rosenwald A: Diagnostic and prognostic significance of gene expression profiling in lymphomas. APMIS 2007;115:1135.

Lossos IS, Czerwinski DK, Alizadeh AA, et al: Prediction of survival in diffuse large–B-cell lymphoma based on the gene expression of six genes. N Engl J Med 2004;350:1828.

Meyer GS, Hales CA, Amrein PC, Sharma S, Kradin RL: Case 26-2007: a 61-year-old man with recurrent fevers (case records of the Massachusetts General Hospital: intravascular lymphoma). New Engl J Med 2007;357:807.

Navarro WH, Kaplan LD: AIDS-related lymphoproliferative disease. Blood 2006;107:13.

Pals ST, de Gorter DJJ, Spaargaren M: Lymphoma dissemination: the other face of lymphocyte homing. Blood 2007;110:3102.

Parsonnet J, Isaacson PJ: Bacterial infection and MALT lymphoma. New Engl J Med 2004;350:213.

Ponzoni M, Ferreri AJM, Campo E: Definition, diagnosis, and management of intravascular large B-cell lymphoma: proposals and perspectives from an international consensus meeting. J Clin Oncol 2007;25:3168.

Rizvi MA, Evens AM, Tallman MS, Nelson BP, Rosen ST: T-cell non-Hodgkin lymphoma. Blood 2006;107:1255.

Rosenwald A, Wright G, Chan WC, et al: The use of molecular profiling to predict survival after chemotherapy for diffuse large-B-cell lymphoma. N Engl J Med 2002;346:1937.

Sánchez-Beato M, Sánchez-Aguilera A, Piris MA: Cell cycle deregulation in B-cell lymphomas. Blood 2003;101:1220.

Savage KJ: Primary mediastinal, intravascular, and primary effusion lymphoma. In: Ansell SM (ed). Rare B-Cell Lymphomas. Cancer Treat Res 2008;142:243.

Seam P, Juweid ME, Cheson BD: The role of FDG-PET scans in patients with lymphoma. Blood 2007;110:3507.

Solal-Céligny P, Roy P, Colombat P, et al: Follicular lymphoma international prognostic index. Blood 2004;104:1258.

Suarez F, Lortholary O, Hermine O, Lecuit M: Infection-associated lymphomas derived from marginal zone B cells: a model of antigen-driven lymphoproliferation. Blood 2006; 107:3034.

Thieblemont C, Nasser V, Felman P, et al: Small lymphocytic lymphoma, marginal zone B-cell lymphoma, and mantle cell lymphoma exhibit distinct gene-expression profiles allowing molecular diagnosis. Blood 2004;103:2727.

Tsao L, Hsi ED: The clinicopathologic spectrum of posttransplantation lymphoproliferative disorders. Arch Pathol Lab Med 2007;131:1209.

Tsimberidou AM , Wen S, O'Brien S, et al: Assessment of chronic lymphocytic leukemia and small lymphocytic lymphoma by absolute lymphocyte counts in 2,126 patients: 20 years of experience at the University of Texas M.D. Anderson Cancer Center. J Clin Oncol 2007;25:4648.

Tsukamoto N, Kojima M, Hasegawa M, et al: The usefulness of (18)F-fluorodeoxyglucose positron emission tomography (^{18}F-FDG-PET) and a comparison of (18)F-FDG-pet with (67)gallium scintigraphy in the evaluation of lymphoma: relation to histologic subtypes based on the World Health Organization classification. Cancer 2007;110:652.

Vega F, Medeiros LJ, Gaulard P: Hepatosplenic and other gamma-delta T-cell lymphomas. Am J Clin Pathol 2007;127:869.

Young KH, Leroy K, Moller MB, et al: Structural profiles of TP53 gene mutations predict clinical outcome in diffuse large B-cell lymphoma: an international collaborative study. Blood 2008;112:3088.

Therapy

Appelbaum FR: Hematopoietic cell transplantation for non-Hodgkin's lymphoma: yesterday, today, and tomorrow. J Clin Oncol 2008;26:2927.

Brice P, Bastion Y, Lepage E, et al: Comparison in low-tumor-burden follicular lymphomas between an initial no-treatment policy, prednimustine, or interferon alfa: a randomized study from the Groupe D'Etude des Lymphomes Folliculaires. J Clin Oncol 1997;15:1110.

Chen LT, Lin JT, Tai JJ, et al: Long-term results of anti–*Helicobacter pylori* therapy in early-stage gastric high-grade transformed MALT lymphoma. J Natl Cancer Inst 2005;97:1345.

Cheson BD: Radioimmunotherapy of non-Hodgkin's lymphomas. Blood 2003;101:391.

Cheson BD, Leonard JP: Monoclonal antibody therapy for B-cell non-Hodgkin's lymphoma. N Engl J Med 2008;359:613.

Cheson BD, Pfistner B, Juweid ME, et al: Revised response criteria for malignant lymphoma. J Clin Oncol 2007;25:579.

Coiffier B: Standard treatment of advanced-stage diffuse large B-cell lymphoma. Semin Hematol 2006;43:213.

Coiffier B, Lepage E, Briere J, et al: CHOP chemotherapy plus rituximab compared with CHOP alone in elderly patients with diffuse large-B-cell lymphoma. N Engl J Med 2002;346:235.

Fisher RI, LeBlanc M, Press OW, Maloney DG, Unger JM, Miller TP: New treatment options have changed the survival of patients with follicular lymphoma. J Clin Oncol 2005;23:8447.

Ghielmini M et al: Prolonged treatment with rituximab in patients with follicular lymphoma significantly increases event-free survival and response duration compared with the standard weekly X 4 schedule. Blood 2004;103:4416.

Greb A, Bohlius J, Schiefer D, Schwarzer G, Schulz H, Engert A: High-dose chemotherapy with autologous stem cell transplantation in the first-line treatment of aggressive non-Hodgkin lymphoma (NHL) in adults (review). Cochrane Database Syst Rev 2008 Jan 23;(1):CD004024.

Miller TP, Spier CM, Rimza L: Diffuse aggressive histologies of non-Hodgkin lymphoma: treatment and biology of limited disease. Semin Hematol 2006;43:207.

Milpied N, Deconinck E, Gaillard F, et al: Initial treatment of aggressive lymphoma with high-dose chemotherapy and autologous stem-cell support. N Engl J Med 2004;350:1287.

Mounier N, Spina M, Gisselbrecht C: Modern management of non-Hodgkin lymphoma in HIV-infected patients. Brit J Haematol 2007;136:685.

Mounier N, Spina M, Gisselbrecht C: Modern management of non-Hodgkin lymphoma in HIV-infected patients. Brit J Haematol 2007;136:685.

Nadermanee A, Forman SJ: Role of hematopoietic stem cell transplantation for advanced-stage diffuse large B-cell lymphoma. Semin Hematol 2006;43:240.

Sebban C, Brice P, Delarue R, et al: Impact of rituximab and/or high-dose therapy with autotransplant at time of relapse in patients with follicular lymphoma: a GELA study. J Clin Oncol 2008;26:3614.

Senff NJ, Noordijk EM, Kim YH, et al: European Organization for Research and Treatment of Cancer and International Society for Cutaneous Lymphoma consensus recommendations for the management of cutaneous B-cell lymphomas. Blood 2008;112:1600.

HODGKIN LYMPHOMA • 24

CASE HISTORY • *Part I*

A 26-year-old man presents with a lump in his neck that he discovered while shaving. He had noted this several months ago but it regressed and he ignored it until it reappeared several weeks ago. In the past few weeks, he has awakened during the night with drenching sweats and has had an unexplained 5-lb weight loss.

His past medical history and family history are unremarkable. He reports that 2 unrelated friends have been diagnosed with Hodgkin lymphoma in the past 5 years, prompting his concern.

Examination reveals a 3-cm anterior cervical lymph node that is non-tender, rubbery, and freely moveable. The remainder of his examination is normal.

Question

- What procedures and laboratory testing are indicated?

Hodgkin lymphoma is a distinct type of lymphoma that in many ways offers a paradigm for the diagnosis and treatment of all hematologic malignancies. Although the causes of Hodgkin lymphoma still remain largely unknown, advances in chemo- and radiotherapy have converted this previously lethal disease to one that is highly curable. The first major advance resulted from an understanding of its radiosensitivity and unique mode of anatomic spread, step by step, within the lymphoid system. This in turn led to the successful design of radiation therapy strategies with large fields encompassing not only involved lymph nodes, but also adjacent nodal areas; thus, accurate staging was shown to be of paramount importance. Subsequently, chemotherapy regimens have proven to be curative even in cases of extensive disease. Moreover, combining these 2 treatment modalities has allowed reduction in the toxicity of each. Before these treatment regimens were available, 90% of patients with Hodgkin lymphoma died within 2–5 years, whereas 85%–90% are now curable with modern therapy. Therefore, Hodgkin lymphoma is one of the best examples of a strategic approach to malignancy leading to cure.

Now that most patients with Hodgkin lymphoma can be cured, the long-term toxicity of the treatments has come into sharp focus, especially long-term vascular/cardiotoxicity and the development of secondary malignancies. Overall, these sequelae have prompted a search for new regimens that are able to combine high efficacy with low toxicity, and to preserve fertility in young adults. The major caveat of this search, of course, is to not reduce curability.

The incidence of Hodgkin lymphoma (HL) has been linked to several factors, including environmental, social status, infectious agents, and genetic propensity. HL is slightly more common in men and has occurred as clustered cases in families, communities, and schools, suggesting an infectious component. It is also more common in developed countries. Patients who have had infectious mononucleosis or have a positive test for prior Epstein-Barr virus (EBV) infection have a 3-fold increased risk for developing the disease. There is also an increased incidence in individuals with occupational chemical exposures or immune deficiency states. There is also a component of genetic susceptibility; studies of identical twins have suggested a genetic propensity to HL with some as-yet-undefined environmental or infectious processes superimposed.

DIAGNOSIS AND CLASSIFICATION

Hodgkin lymphoma usually presents in an adolescent or young adult as an enlargement of an isolated cervical or mediastinal lymph node, less frequently axillary or inguinal nodes. Systemic, constitutional symptoms (so-called **B symptoms**) such as fever, weight loss, night sweats, and fatigue can occur but are less common in the early presentation of HL. When the lymph node is superficial, the diagnosis can be confirmed by fine needle aspiration showing the presence of classic Reed-Sternberg cells among a population of small lymphocytes or within a granulomatous reaction (Figure 24–1). In general, however, a surgical lymph node biopsy is far preferable.

REED-STERNBERG CELLS AND LYMPHOCYTIC/HISTIOCYTIC CELLS

The putative malignant cell in HL is the **Reed-Sternberg cell**, a large, frequently binucleate cell that more closely resembles a macrophage-like cell than a lymphocyte (see Figure 24–1). The relative number of Reed-Sternberg cells may vary, but they should always comprise less than 2% of the apparent tumor load. In some cases, only a very careful search will reveal the presence of these cells, without which the diagnosis cannot be made with certainty. The majority of cells found in the lesion are a diverse population of lymphocytes, eosinophils, and other reactive cells that, although they may represent the majority of cells within the lesion, are thought to be passive or only secondary to the actual malignant process.

Reed-Sternberg cells have been difficult to study because they are present in such small numbers and are difficult to separate from the surrounding infiltrate of reactive cells. Therefore, only a few cell lines have been established. Immunophenotyping studies of isolated Reed-Sternberg cells suggest that they are monoclonal B cells derived from germinal center cells, although a small percentage (<2%) appears to be from T-cell precursors. At the same time, they lack many of the surface antigens typical of B and T cells, expressing instead a number of unusual antigens (eg, CD30, CD15, CD70, TARC, and IRF4). In addition, despite immunoglobulin (Ig) gene arrangements compatible with B-cell origin, Reed-Sternberg cells do not transcribe Ig. Overexpression of CCR7 is of interest as a possible reason behind the localization of Reed-Sternberg cells to lymph nodes and spleen. The elaboration of several cytokines and their receptors (tumor necrosis factor, nuclear factor-κB, Th2 cytokines, and interleukin [IL]-13) appear to be responsible for many of the clinical characteristics, including the B symptoms, fibroblast proliferation in the nodular sclerosis subtype, eosinophil infiltration, and abnormal immune response typical of Hodgkin lymphoma.

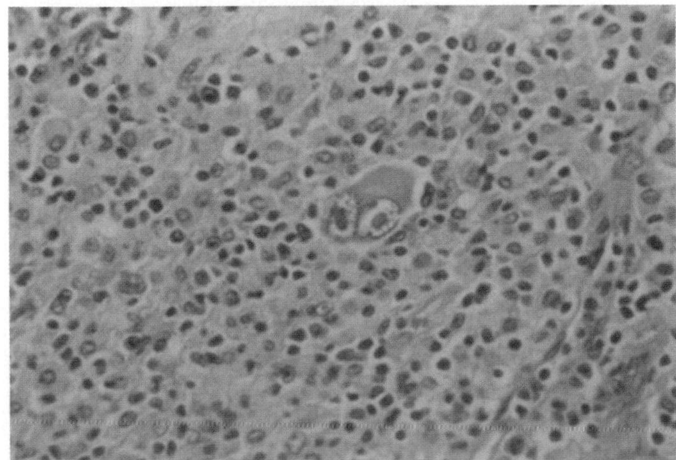

FIGURE 24–1. **Hodgkin lymphoma lymph node histopathology.** Lymph node section from a patient with Hodgkin lymphoma showing a classic Reed-Sternberg cell (binucleate giant cell with prominent red-staining nucleoli) surrounded by reactive lymphocytes.

Despite many years of study, the mechanism by which Reed-Sternberg cells arise and their precise role in the malignant process remain obscure. As with other lymphomas, there appears to be a primary failure in the normal apoptotic process, not an increase in proliferation. In classical Hodgkin lymphomas, **Epstein-Barr virus (EBV)** can be isolated from the Reed-Sternberg cell in approximately 50% of cases, and the incidence of Hodgkin lymphoma in patients with a past history of infectious mononucleosis is higher than in EBV-naive subjects. However, although there is evidence for early integration of EBV DNA in the malignant process (supported by the clonality of the EBV integrated genome in Reed-Sternberg cells), an etiologic role for EBV infection has not been proven.

Because of the limitations of immunologic and genetic studies, diagnosis of Hodgkin lymphoma is heavily reliant on the pathologic interpretation of biopsy material. Diagnostic certainty requires the identification of (a) Reed-Sternberg cells or (b) in the case of nodular lymphocyte-predominant disease, **"popcorn" or L&H cells (lymphocytic or histiocytic cells [or both] of Lukes-Butler classification)**, and (c) the presence of these cells within a diverse population of B and T lymphocytes, eosinophils, and other reactive cells (see Figure 24–1). The predominant infiltrating cell in Hodgkin nodes is a $CD4^+$ regulatory T cell that is present in 2 forms—one that secretes IL-10 (an immunosuppressive cytokine), and a second that suppresses immune cells through cell-cell contact. The presence of these cells has implications for protecting Reed-Sternberg cells from immune destruction and producing a generalized immunosuppression. The overall histologic pattern of the tumor has a strong association with clinical course and falls into one of 5 categories (Table 24–1).

Histopathologic Types of Hodgkin Lymphoma

Nodular lymphocyte-predominant Hodgkin lymphoma (NLPHL, 5%), also referred to as Poppema paragranuloma, is characterized histologically by a vague nodular pattern, rich in lymphocytes, containing a distinctive morphologic variant of the Reed-Sternberg cell, the so-called **L&H, or "popcorn" cell** (Figure 24–2). A collar of $CD57^+$ T cells and large numbers of small polyclonal B cells surround these cells. The phenotype of the "popcorn" cell resembles that of a B lymphocyte ($CD19/20/22/45^+$ and $CD15/CD30^-$). Other distinctive features of these cells are

TABLE 24–1 • Histologic classification of Hodgkin lymphoma

WHO Histologic Classification	Description	Frequency
Nodular/ lymphocyte predominant HL	Nodular pattern with "popcorn" cells	4%–5%
Classical HL		
Lymphocyte-rich	Abundant mature lymphocytes, a few classical Reed-Sternberg cells	5%–10%
Nodular sclerosis	Prominent fibrosis, mature lymphocytes, and Reed-Sternberg cells present	60%–80%
Mixed cellularity	Both mature lymphocytes and Reed-Sternberg cells	15%–30%
Lymphocyte-depleted	Predominantly large, poorly differentiated cells	<1%

functional Ig gene rearrangements and somatic Ig hypermutations, absence of integrated EBV genome, and overexpression of BCL6. This form is relatively indolent and slow to spread, often resembling a low-grade non-Hodgkin lymphoma.

The more common histologic types (classical Hodgkin lymphoma) are **nodular sclerosis** (60%), **mixed cellularity** (30%), **lymphocyte-depleted** (1%), and the newly proposed **lymphocyte-rich classical Hodgkin lymphoma** (5%). Histologically, **nodular sclerosis** Hodgkin disease is characterized by variable amounts of collagenous connective tissue separating nodules of lymphocytes containing lacunar-type Reed-Sternberg cells. Depending on the number and degree of atypia of the Reed-Sternberg cells, nodular sclerosis Hodgkin lymphomas can be subclassified as grade 1 or 2. Grade 1 disease, which makes up 75%–85% of cases, has the best prognosis. **Mixed cellularity and lymphocyte-depleted** Hodgkin disease, the other 2 histopathologic forms, carry the worst prognosis. They are characterized by fewer lymphocytes and relatively more classical bilobed Reed-Sternberg cells with prominent eosinophilic nucleoli. In some cases of mixed cellularity and lymphocyte-depleted HD, the predominant cells are difficult to distinguish from poorly differentiated NHL or even sarcomas.

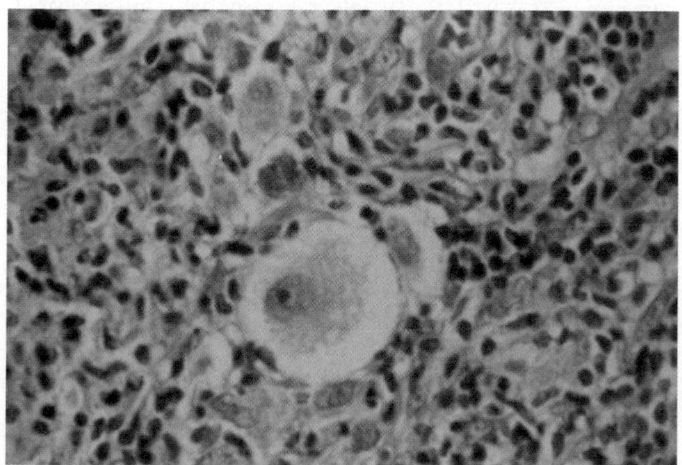

FIGURE 24–2. **L&H or popcorn cell.** High-power view of a single L&H/popcorn cell.

CLINICAL FEATURES

Hodgkin lymphoma has a **bimodal age-dependent incidence** with a peak in young adults and another peak in the fifth to sixth decades. The most common presentation is the appearance of a painless or only slightly tender, rubbery swelling of a superficial lymph node or group of nodes in a young adult. The tendency of Hodgkin lymphoma to first appear in a single node group in an otherwise healthy individual can make it difficult to distinguish from lymphadenopathy associated with an infectious or reactive process. Nodes that are slightly tender are even more of a problem because tender nodes often accompany acute infections. In addition, Hodgkin nodes can wax and wane in the same way as those associated with an infectious process. The diagnosis is more obvious when the mass is large, presents in more than 1 area, and is associated with B symptoms such as night sweats, fever, weight loss, pruritus, or fatigue. Nevertheless, in a patient with lymph node enlargement, waiting for the development of further node enlargement or B symptoms is a mistake, since early diagnosis is the best way to improve prognosis in HD.

The most common areas of involvement in young patients are the **cervical, axillary, and mediastinal nodes**. Extension to subdiaphragmatic nodes is seen in less than one-quarter of these patients if they seek medical attention without delay. Systemic symptoms are present in less than one-third of patients. Unusual presentations, such as disease limited to the spleen or an extranodal site, are more common in the elderly. Moreover, whereas lymphocyte-predominant and nodular sclerosis Hodgkin disease are common in the younger age group, mixed cellularity and lymphocyte-depleted Hodgkin disease are more often seen in patients 30 years or older. The presence of hepatomegaly suggests extension of the disease outside of the lymphatic system. Infiltration of the skin can result in generalized pruritus, appearance of subcutaneous nodular tumors, or in its most severe form, exfoliative dermatitis.

BIOPSY

A biopsy of the principal tumor mass or accessible enlarged node should be done, and the results reviewed with an experienced hematopathologist. It is not uncommon for the diagnosis of Hodgkin disease to be confused or delayed by an inadequate biopsy or too casual examination of a biopsy specimen, especially in the lymphocyte-rich and nodular variants. It is also common to find lymph nodes containing overt Hodgkin lymphoma located adjacent to nodes that show only reactive hyperplasia. Therefore, biopsy specimens of more than 1 node should be taken if available.

STAGING

Even though treatment strategies currently distinguish 2 categories of presentation, that is, limited (early) and advanced-stage Hodgkin lymphoma, accurate staging remains extremely important. The natural history of the disease suggests that it arises in a single site and then spreads in an orderly and more or less predictable pattern from 1 lymphoid (usually nodal) site to contiguous lymphoid sites and into contiguous non-lymphoid sites. This is not always the case (for instance, with involvement of the spleen, which has no afferent lymphatics), but it is a useful concept that has led to a very successful strategy of staging and treatment. Thus, the primary objective of staging is to determine the current location of all disease in order to plan a treatment that will address each of the involved areas and all contiguous sites of possible spread.

The **staging of Hodgkin lymphoma** is conceptually simple. One determines the location and extent of the disease, which then assigns a stage as outlined in Table 24–2. This staging requires a careful evaluation of the patient, including a full history, detailed physical examination, and several imaging and laboratory studies. The same staging strategy has been adapted for use in non-Hodgkin lymphoma (NHL), but it was originally developed, and remains most useful, in the setting of HL.

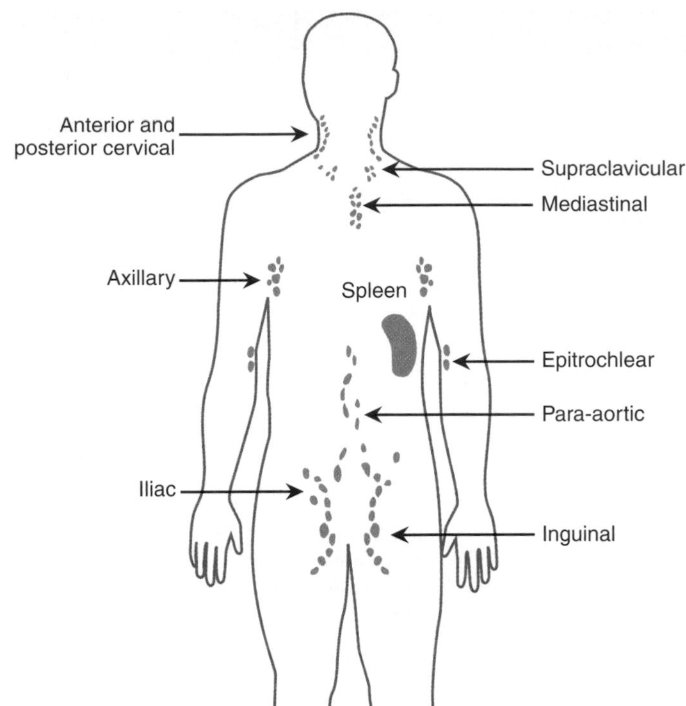

FIGURE 24–3. **The major sites of palpable lymph nodes.** Because Hodgkin lymphoma usually spreads to contiguous node regions, it is important to define which regions are involved as a part of the staging process.

History and Physical Examination

The history should document the timing and characteristics of the onset of the disease and the presence of B symptoms. On physical examination, all portions of the lymphoid organs should be carefully examined (Figure 24–3). Special attention should be paid to the lymphoid regions of the oral pharynx (Waldeyer ring), the popliteal and epitrochlear regions, the subclavicular regions, as well as the more common axillary, anterior and posterior cervical, and inguinal regions.

TABLE 24–2 • Staging system for Hodgkin lymphoma

Stage	Description	Example
I	Involvement of a single lymphoid region or a single non-lymphoid site (I_E)	Nodes on one side of the neck only
II	Involvement of 2 or more regions on the same side of the diaphragm	Nodes in the neck and chest
III	Involvement of 2 or more regions on both sides of the diaphragm	Nodes in the neck and retroperitoneum or the spleen
IV	Spread of disease from lymphoid sites to non-lymphoid organs, involvement of more than 1 non-lymphoid organ	Nodes in the chest and infiltration of the marrow and lung
B	Each stage is further modified as B by the presence of fever, weight loss, night sweats, or other B symptoms	Nodes in the retroperitoneum and groin with fever and night sweats (IIB)

Radiologic Studies

Radiologic studies are important to accurate staging. A routine chest study will reveal bulky mediastinal disease. To more accurately detect lymph node involvement, computed tomography (CT) scans are sensitive to node enlargement or tissue invasion within the mediastinum, lung, and abdomen, including the retroperitoneum, spleen, and liver. Recently, 18-fluorodeoxyglucose (FDG) positron emission tomography (PET) has proven to be even more sensitive as it can detect disease that is missed by CT scans, which results in upstaging for 15%–20% of patients. Since upstaging is of little relevance for treatment strategies, pretreatment PET is useful but not a prerequisite. However, since the PET-scan is considered the best method for assessment of response because of its ability to distinguish between active and inactive residual masses, it may be useful as initial imaging. In addition, PET documentation of an early response to therapy allows one to quickly evaluate the sensitivity of the tumor to the chosen treatment. Risk-adapted treatment modifications guided by this early result are currently under investigation.

Laboratory Studies

The laboratory evaluation of the patient with Hodgkin lymphoma should include a complete blood count (CBC), tests of renal and liver function (including alkaline phosphatase and lactate dehydrogenase [LDH]), a serum calcium, and bilateral

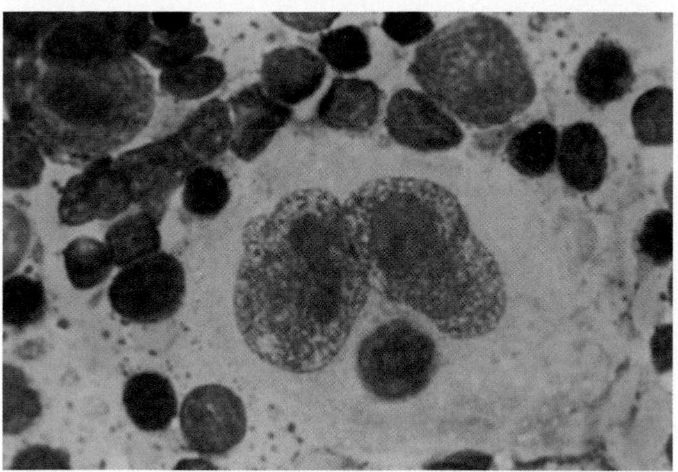

FIGURE 24–4. **Reed-Sternberg cell in a marrow aspirate.** High-power view of a single Reed-Sternberg cell in a marrow aspirate (Wright stain).

iliac crest bone marrow aspirates and biopsies. These tests are especially important in evaluating disease extension outside of the lymphatic system. When anemia is present, studies of iron supply should be ordered to determine whether it is secondary to the inflammatory nature of the disease or results from another mechanism. A marrow biopsy may be helpful in the latter. Even though the classic histologic patterns seen in lymph node biopsies are not reproduced in the marrow, it may be possible to identify Reed-Sternberg cells. Typically these cells are the size of a small megakaryocyte and contain 2 bean-shaped nuclei, each with a single large nucleolus (Figure 24–4). In some cases, Reed-Sternberg cells cannot be identified, but the normal marrow structure is disrupted by small noncaseating granulomata or patchy fibrous tissue.

Abnormalities of the granulocyte and lymphocyte counts may be observed. Some patients present with a mild eosinophilia, whereas others have an absolute lymphopenia. The latter is a bad prognostic sign and may be associated with lymphocyte-depleted Hodgkin disease and a loss in skin test responsiveness (anergy). Older patients presenting with splenic disease can demonstrate thrombocytopenia or an autoimmune hemolytic anemia. All of the peripheral blood changes are reactive in nature.

Patients with abnormal liver chemistries or a suspicious lesion on imaging should have a guided needle biopsy of the lesion or laparoscopic liver biopsy.

Prognosis

When radiotherapy was the main treatment for Hodgkin lymphoma, the patient's prognosis and subsequent management were determined largely by the stage of the disease, the number of node sites involved, and the spread to non-lymphoid organs. However, now that systemic chemotherapy has been recognized as highly effective, the exact anatomical extension of the disease is no longer the only relevant factor, and other observations that do have an impact on prognosis have been recognized. The most important of these is the presence of B symptoms, especially when fever and significant weight loss are both present. Other factors that suggest a poor prognosis include male sex, age greater than 40–50 years, Hb less than 10 g/dL, lymphocytopenia less than 600/μL, white blood cell (WBC) count greater than 15,000/μL, and albumin less than 4g/dL. A scoring system accounting for these factors predicts a probability of freedom from progression ranging from 84% (no adverse factors) to 42% (5 or more adverse factors) at 5 years.

Current definitions of prognostic subgroups in sponsored clinical trials (Eastern Cooperative Oncology Group [ECOG], German Hodgkin Study Group [GHSG], and European Organization for Research and Treatment of Cancer/Groupe d'Etude des Lymphomes de l'Adulte [EORTC/GELA]) are summarized in Table 24–3. Age, bulky mediastinal tumor, an elevated sedimentation rate, non-lymphoid organ involvement, severe marrow disease, and a poor response to initial radiotherapy or chemotherapy are considered the major adverse factors. These factors help distinguish a standard risk group with favorable and unfavorable features from an advanced-stage, high-risk group for distinct therapies.

TABLE 24–3 • Current definitions of prognostic subgroups in Hodgkin lymphoma

Prognostic Group	ECOG	GHSG	EORTC/GELA
Standard risk group/ early stage: favorable	Stages I/II, no risk factor	Stages I/II, no risk factor	Supradiaphragmatic stages I/II, no risk factor
Standard risk group/early stage: unfavorable	Stages I/II, ≥1 risk factor	Stages I/IIA, ≥1 risk factor; stage IIB with C/D but without A/B risk factors	Supradiaphragmatic stages I/II, ≥1 risk factor
Advanced stage	Stages I/II with bulky disease, subdiaphragmatic disease, stages III/IV	Stages IIB with A/B risk factors, stages III/IV	Stages III/IV
Risk factors	A. Age >40 y B. Not Nod or NS C. ESR >50 mm/h D. ≥4 involved areas	A. Large mediastinal B. Extranodal disease C. ESR >50 mm/h D. ≥3 involved areas	A. Large mediastinal B. Age >50 y C. ESR >50 mm/h D. ≥4 involved areas

CASE HISTORY • *Part 2*

The patient has a normal CBC and all blood chemistries are normal. The chest x-ray suggests mediastinal adenopathy, which is confirmed on CT scan. CT of the abdomen shows no abnormality. A bone marrow aspirate and biopsy prove normal.

Biopsy of the cervical lymph node shows the presence of extensive fibrosis, normal-appearing lymphocytes, increased eosinophils, and a very small number of cells suggestive of Reed-Sternberg cells after a careful search by an experienced hematopathologist. A diagnosis of nodular sclerosing Hodgkin lymphoma is made.

Questions

- What is the provisional stage of this patient?
- What further staging procedures, if any, should be performed?

THERAPY AND CLINICAL COURSE

The several possible combinations of histology, B symptoms, location of disease, and prognostic factors together with varying regimens of either radiotherapy or chemotherapy make it difficult to propose a rigid logic tree for the treatment of Hodgkin lymphoma. The current state of the art is derived from trials designed more than 10 years ago, while recent progress in management will not be evaluable for several more years. Nevertheless, there are some clear basic principles that guide the choice of therapy. It is well established that both radiotherapy and chemotherapy, when skillfully administered, can cure Hodgkin disease. The therapeutic goal, therefore, is to provide the highest cure rate in the shortest period with the least morbidity. This goal should be achievable in almost all patients with localized disease and in a sizable majority of those with more advanced disease. Treatment failure most often results from either inaccurate staging or a suboptimal radiotherapy/chemotherapy regimen.

Radiotherapy

Following the pioneering work of Henry Kaplan at Stanford in the 1960s, radiotherapy became the first curative treatment for patients with HD. The principles of effective radiation therapy are based on a dose of 40 Gy to involved nodes and 36 Gy to adjacent ones (extended field), delivered in fractions of 2.5 Gy 4 times a week for 4 weeks, according to the techniques of large, so-called mantle and inverted-Y ports (Figure 24–5). Application of these principles has proven to be curative in most patients with limited upper diaphragmatic or subdiaphragmatic (stage I/II) disease, and in some patients with limited-stage IIIa when mantle and upper abdominal ports are combined. However, up to 20% of patients treated in this fashion will relapse outside the irradiated fields.

Side Effects and Complications of Radiation Therapy

Side effects of radiation therapy include nausea and fatigue, especially in patients receiving abdominal radiation. Transient hair loss over the areas of radiation is expected. Patients who receive mantle radiation may develop parotitis after the first or second treatment. When multiple areas are irradiated, marrow depression can occur, generally near the end of a prolonged course of therapy; this is relatively mild with WBC counts of 1,000–2,000/μL and platelet counts not below 50,000/μL. Neutropenia leading to sepsis is very unusual, and recovery from marrow depression occurs spontaneously without the need for

CASE HISTORY • *Part 3*

This patient has nodular sclerosing Hodgkin lymphoma involving the neck and very likely the chest. There is no evidence of involvement below the diaphragm, but he has clear B symptoms. The provisional staging is IIB due to the presence of 2 sites of disease on the same side of the diaphragm and with chest involvement that is not bulky. If there is any question about the chest abnormality, a PET scan could be used to confirm the presence and extent of active disease.

Question

- What is the prognosis and what therapy is indicated?

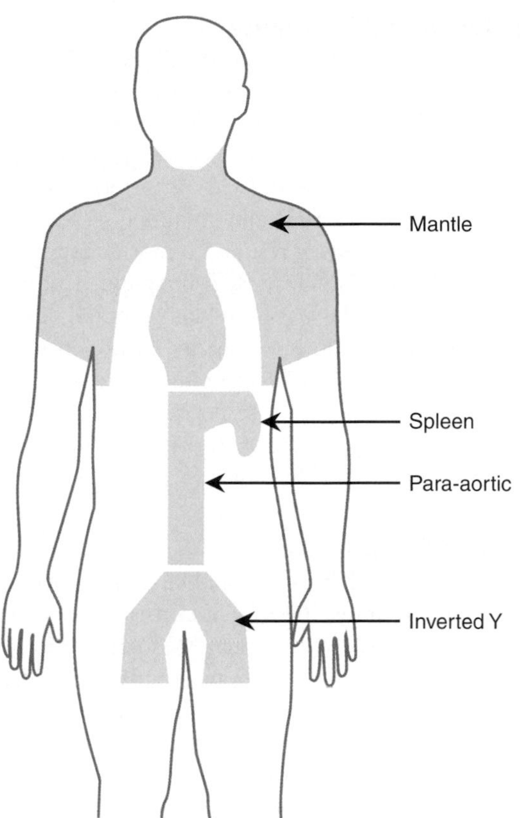

FIGURE 24–5. **Radiotherapy ports used in treating Hodgkin lymphoma.** These shaded ports are designed to deliver targeted radiation to both involved and contiguous nodal sites, while avoiding uninvolved regions and organs such as the lung, marrow, spine, and gonads.

TABLE 24–4 • Typical chemotherapeutic regimens for Hodgkin disease

Regimen	Dose and Schedule
MOPP	Repeat every 28 d for 6 mo
Nitrogen mustard	6 mg/m^2 IV, days 1 and 8
Vincristine	1.4 mg/m^2 IV, days 1 and 8
Procarbazine	100 mg/m^2 PO, days 1–14
Prednisone	40 mg/m^2 PO, days 1–14
ABVD	Repeat every 28 d for 6 mo
Adriamycin	25 mg/m^2 IV, days 1 and 15
Bleomycin	10 mg/m^2 IV, days 1 and 15
Vinblastine	10 mg/m^2 IV, days 1 and 15
DTIC	375 mg/m^2 IV, days 1 and 15
Stanford V	Repeat every 28 days × 3 cycles
Mechlorethamine	6 mg/m^2 IV, day 1 of each cycle
Adriamycin	25 mg/m^2 IV, days 1 and 15 of each cycle
Vinblastine	6 mg/m^2 IV, days 1 and 15 of each cycle
Bleomycin	5 mg/m^2 IV, days 8 and 22 of each cycle
Etoposide	60 mg/m^2 IV, days 15 and 16 of each cycle
Prednisone	40 mg/d PO, days 1–28
G-CSF	As required
BEACOPP	Repeat every 21 d
Bleomycin	10 mg/m^2 IV, day 8
Etoposide	100 mg/m^2 IV, days 1–3
Adriamycin	25 mg/m^2 IV, day 1
Cyclophosphamide	650 mg/m^2 IV, day 1
Oncovin (vincristine)	1.4 mg/m^2 IV, day 8
Procarbazine	100 mg/m^2 PO, days 1–7
Prednisone	40 mg PO, days 1–14
G-CSF	As required

growth factor treatment. Patients should be counseled to avoid sun exposure and to use ultraviolet (UV) protective measures for several months after radiation therapy.

Long-term complications of radiation therapy include decreased salivary flow, hypothyroidism, mediastinal fibrosis in patients who have received mantle therapy, and loss of marrow reserve in those patients who receive extensive irradiation. The most serious late complications are early atherosclerotic and fibrotic stenosing changes in irradiated arteries, cardiac complications resulting in coronary artery disease, valvular dysfunction, cardiomyopathy, and secondary malignancies. The risk of post-therapy leukemia, which is 20- to 70-fold increased during the 10 years after completion of HD radiotherapy, is unlikely to be due only to radiation. However, the 2- to 5-fold increase in other secondary malignancies such as NHL, and tumors of the breast, lung, gastrointestinal (GI) tract, skin, or colon during the first decade after treatment are clearly due to radiation exposure. For younger, prepubescent patients, irradiation of bones can result in early closure of growth plates, leading to deformity.

Chemotherapy

The chemotherapy of Hodgkin lymphoma was the first successful application of multiagent chemotherapy where several different drugs were chosen for their partial effectiveness against the disease and for their non-overlapping toxicities. The MOPP protocol (nitrogen mustard–vincristine-procarbazine-prednisone) was the first highly effective regimen but is no longer used by itself. Table 24–4 outlines some of the chemotherapeutic regimens currently used for Hodgkin disease. Newer drug combinations have a similar or better response rate with less toxicity. In particular, the ABVD regimen (adriamycin-bleomycin-vinblastine-DTIC) is at least as effective and does not appear to carry the increased risk of secondary leukemia associated with MOPP. The combination of MOPP with ABVD has been used to provide non–cross-resistant regimens for patients who relapse after

MOPP or whose disease is resistant to initial therapy. Stanford V and BEACOPP have been developed as shorter-duration protocols. However, they substantially increase short-term hematologic toxicity, and the long-term risk of myelodysplastic syndromes is a concern, especially with BEACOPP.

The key to effective chemotherapy is to give full doses on a tight schedule, according to the concept of maximizing dose intensity. Dose reductions and delays must be avoided if at all possible. In those patients who develop myelosuppression after each cycle of drugs, it is important to try to continue with the maximum dose of drug and to use a growth factor such as granulocyte colony-stimulating factor (G-CSF) to overcome myelosuppression.

Side Effects and Complications of Chemotherapy

Complications of chemotherapy differ from those observed with radiation therapy but are no less a concern. The most frequent immediate or early complications are alopecia, hematologic toxicity, neuritis with *Vinca* alkaloids, and amenorrhea. Nausea and emesis can be overcome, and even prevented with anti-H3 medications.

The most serious complications of chemotherapy are late toxicities. Even a few treatment cycles with MOPP or MOPP/ABVD will result in azoospermia in males secondary to irreversible damage to the testes. ABVD has been recommended in young males because of its lower incidence of testicular damage. Men should be offered sperm storage prior to beginning chemotherapy if they wish to father children. Young women have less difficulty with ovarian failure, but there is an increased risk of early menopause after 35 years of age. The cumulative dose–threshold of adriamycin cardiotoxicity is 550 mg/m^2, but only 200–250 mg/m^2 when combined with radiation heart exposure. The risk of a secondary malignancy, especially hematologic, is also increased. Radiation pneumonitis and pericarditis, together with drug-induced chronic restrictive pulmonary disease and myocardiopathy, increase in frequency with exposure to intensive chemo/radiotherapy. None of the treatments of HL in young women have been associated with teratogenicity.

Treatment Strategies

The goal of HL treatment is cure. Treatment is most likely to succeed in patients with early-stage I/II disease, but cure is still possible in many patients with advanced disease. The challenge is to use treatment modalities that are highly effective, while engendering as little long-term toxicity as possible.

A. Early Favorable Disease

Currently, the recommended strategy for this low-risk group of patients is for 2 or 3 cycles of ABVD, together with irradiation limited to involved nodes. However, ABVD or a similar chemotherapy regimen without irradiation has been reported to be as effective but with less long-term morbidity and mortality from cardiovascular events and secondary cancers. Given the current long-term, disease-free, and overall survival rates of 90%–95%, ongoing trials will require years and a large number of accrued patients to demonstrate the true advantage of one approach over the other.

B. Early Unfavorable Disease

Currently, 4 courses of ABVD (or MOPP/ABVD) followed by radiation (30 Gy) to involved fields provides an 85% progression-free and 90% overall survival at 5–7 years. The presence of a large mediastinal tumor represents a special challenge. Even with combined modality therapy with radiation to the mediastinal mass, a residual mediastinal abnormality is seen in 60%–90% of patients. Whether this is residual tumor or unresolved scar tissue can be distinguished by PET imaging. If there is avid uptake of the tracer by the mass, it is likely that the disease is still active. However, false-positive results, although infrequent, are observed especially early after mediastinal irradiation. Therefore, PET assessment for response should be delayed for 2–3 months after completion of therapy and should be compared with simultaneous CT scans.

C. Advanced Disease

Patients with advanced disease should be treated with intensive multidrug chemotherapy. Treatment consisting of 6–8 courses of ABVD, MOPP/ABVD, or similar regimens with or without involved field irradiation will yield a complete response rate of 60% on average, with a 45%–62% disease-free survival at 5 years and 79%–95% 5-year overall survival. Stanford V and BEACOPP protocols combined with targeted radiation therapy give response rates approaching 100% with 75%–94% disease-free survival at 5 years, depending on the number of individual risk factors. However, long-term toxicity is still an issue with these regimens. Maintenance chemotherapy is not recommended because it does not improve disease-free survival and can lead to secondary malignancy.

Treatment of the nodular form (Poppema paragranuloma) of HL deserves special mention. Patients with advanced disease should be treated with the same regimens as classical HL. For early-stage patients, reduced intensity regimens are recommended. Patients for whom there are no apparent remaining pathological lymph nodes after surgical biopsy can actually be managed with watchful waiting. As this variant of HL expresses CD20, monoclonal anti-CD20 antibody (ritumixab) is also an option either in combination with chemotherapy, or alone for limited-stage disease in children or for late relapse.

D. Salvage Therapy

Patients must be carefully monitored after successful initial treatment. Relapse can occur at any time, even in patients treated at an early/favorable stage, including late relapses in up to 15% of such patients. Patients with more advanced disease will relapse sooner and more frequently (Figure 24–6). There is still an excellent chance, however, to achieve a second remission and prolonged periods of disease-free survival.

Many salvage treatments can be offered, depending on the initial therapy. For patients relapsing after radiation treatment alone, combination chemotherapy retains high efficacy. Those relapsing after ABVD are likely to benefit from non–cross-resistant second-line combinations, which includes drugs such as platinum, gemcitabine, alkylating agents, high-dose cytarabine, and the epipodophyllotoxins.

CASE HISTORY • *Part 4*

With stage IIB disease, the treatment decision for this young patient is one of balancing the promise of cure versus the risk of long-term side effects. He should be offered the option of sperm storage prior to treatment. Faced with an early-stage unfavorable disease, he should be treated with 4–6 cycles of ABVD or MOPP/ABVD hybrid, possibly followed by radiation therapy to involved areas (the mantle port). If the response to chemotherapy alone is excellent, the decision can be made to avoid additional lymphoma therapy, which will significantly decrease the risk of long-term side effects such as cardiovascular disease and secondary malignancies.

A PET scan following initial chemotherapy would allow early assessment of the responsiveness of his disease. The PET scan is also the best way to detect residual mediastinal tumor or relapse, since biopsy at this site is impractical.

High-dose chemotherapy followed by autologous hematopoietic stem cell transplant (HSCT) rescue has provided better results when compared with non-intensive regimens for patients in relapse. Those with more responsive disease, lack of B symptoms, and a longer duration of remission are more likely to achieve long-term survival after this form of salvage therapy, but even patients with an unfavorable prognosis can benefit. High-dose chemotherapy regimens commonly used to prepare HL patients for transplant include some combination of BCNU, etoposide, cytarabine, and melphalan (BEAM). Total body irradiation is no longer used as part of the preparative regimen since it provides no benefit when compared to chemotherapy-only preparative regimens and increases the risk of secondary malignancies and myelodysplastic syndromes.

A majority of relapsing patients can be put into remission with this approach with a disease-free survival of 55%–65% after 5+ years. The success rate is greatly influenced by patient selection, however. Older patients, patients who have been exposed to a large number of chemotherapy drugs with or without irradiation, and those who have poorly responsive tumor from the onset more often fail to respond to high-dose chemotherapy/autologous HSCT. Another drawback of an autologous transplant is a reported incidence of secondary acute myeloid leukemia/myelodysplasia of 9%–15% after 5–7 years. Alternative salvage therapies for patients who are not candidates or who fail autologous HSCT include single-agent vinblastine; combination chemotherapy with drugs such as etoposide, ifosfamide, and cisplatin; or immunotherapy.

Allogeneic HSCT, especially partial transplants with reduced conditioning regimens, has provided interesting results in relapsing patients with Hodgkin lymphoma. However, this procedure is currently experimental.

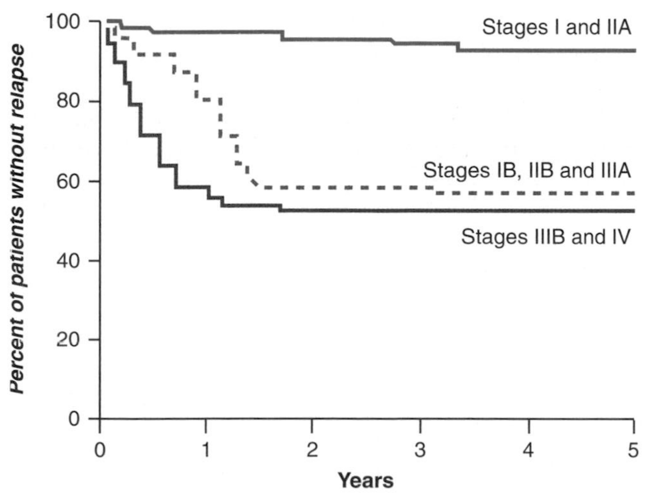

FIGURE 24–6. **Clinical stage and survival.** The influence of stage on the long-term survival of patients with Hodgkin lymphoma is greater than any other single prognostic factor.

POINTS TO REMEMBER

Despite considerable circumstantial evidence for a transmissible or infectious element in the etiology of Hodgkin lymphoma, the exact cause is still unknown.

Hodgkin lymphoma is categorized based on histopathology as lymphocyte-rich, nodular sclerosis, mixed cellularity, lymphocyte depleted, or nodular/lymphocytic-predominant disease.

In younger patients, nodular sclerosis Hodgkin lymphoma, presenting with some combination of lymphadenopathy in the neck, axilla, and/or mediastinum, is by far the most common disease type.

Hodgkin lymphoma patients generally present after discovering an easily palpable node or nodal mass in the neck or axilla. However, some patients will experience B symptoms including fever, night sweats, fatigue, weight loss, and pruritus, which convey a worse stage.

Older patients generally present with more advanced lymphocyte-depleted Hodgkin lymphoma, often involving subdiaphragmatic/inguinal nodes and the spleen. They can also exhibit autoimmune complications, such as hemolytic anemia or thrombocytopenia.

Accurate assessment of the extent of disease (staging) is critical to assessing prognosis and planning optimal treatment of Hodgkin lymphoma. Four stages of nodal disease are recognized (stages I–IV) with the addition of B for "B" symptoms or the addition of E for extension to adjacent tissues/organs.

Other factors adversely influencing prognosis include male sex, age above 40, elevated sedimentation rate, severe marrow disease with anemia/leukopenia, and a decreased absolute lymphocyte count.

Hodgkin lymphoma is a great success story for the use of chemotherapy and targeted radiation, based on an understanding of how the disease spreads and the principle of non-overlapping chemotherapy toxicities. The goal is to induce long-term disease control, even cure, in all patients.

Due to the high probability of cure, Hodgkin lymphoma is a perfect example of the need to balance an optimal treatment regimen against the probability of long-term complications. Few other hematologic malignancies offer the opportunity to be concerned about over-treatment.

BIBLIOGRAPHY

Brepoels L, Stroobants S: Is [^{18}F]fluorodeoxyglucose positron emission tomography the ultimate tool for response and prognosis assessment? Hematol Oncol Clin N Am 2007;21:855.

Canellos GP: Relapsed and refractory Hodgkin's lymphoma: new avenues? Hematol Oncol Clin N Am 2007;21:927.

Connors JM: State-of-the-art therapeutics: Hodgkin's lymphoma. J Clin Oncol 2005;23:6400.

Diehl V: Hodgkin's disease—from pathology specimen to cure. N Engl J Med 2007;357:1968.

Diehl VD, Engert A, Re D: New strategies for the treatment of advanced-stage Hodgkin's lymphoma. Hematol Oncol Clin N Am 2007;21:897.

Diehl W, Thomas RK, Re D: Part II: Hodgkin's lymphoma—diagnosis and treatment. Lancet Oncol 2004;5:19.

Fermé C, Eghbali H, Meerwaldt JH, et al: Chemotherapy plus involved-field radiation in early-stage Hodgkin's disease. N Engl J Med 2007;357:1916.

Feugier P, Labouyrie E, Djeridane M, et al: Comparison of initial characteristics and long-term outcome of patients with lymphocyte-predominant Hodgkin lymphoma and classical Hodgkin lymphoma at clinical stages IA and IIA prospectively treated by brief anthracycline-based chemotherapies plus extended high-dose irradiation. Blood 2004;104:2675.

Hjalgrim H, Askling J, Rostgaard K, et al: Characteristics of Hodgkin's lymphoma after infectious mononucleosis. N Engl J Med 2003;349:1324.

Juweid ME, Cheson BD: Role of positron emission tomography in lymphoma. J Clin Oncol 2005;23:4577.

Landgren O, Caporaso NE: New aspects in descriptive, etiologic and molecular epidemiology of Hodgkin's lymphoma. Hematol Oncol Clin N Am 2007;21:825.

Macdonald DA, O'Connors JM: New strategies for the treatment of early stages of Hodgkin's lymphoma. Hematol Oncol Clin N Am 2007;21:871.

Murphy SB, Morgan ER, Katzenstein HM, Kletzel M: Results of little or no treatment for lymphocyte-predominant Hodgkin disease in children and adolescents. J Pediatr Hematol Oncol 2003;25:684.

Stein H, Mann R, Delsol G, et al: Classical Hodgkin lymphoma. In: Jaffe H, Harris NL, Stein H, Vardiman JW (eds): *World Health Organization Classification of Tumors. Pathology and Genetics of Tumors of the Hematopoietic and Lymphoid Tissues*. IARC Press, 2001; 244–253.

Stein H, Mann R, Delsol G, et al: Nodular lymphocyte predominant Hodgkin lymphoma. In: Jaffe H, Harris NL, Stein H, Vardiman JW (eds): *World Health Organization Classification of Tumors. Pathology and Genetics of Tumors of the Hematopoietic and Lymphoid Tissues*. IARC Press, 2001; 240–243.

Thomas RK, Re D, Wolf J, Diehl W: Part I: Hodgkin's lymphoma—molecular biology of Hodgkin and Reed-Sternberg cells. Lancet Oncol 2004;5:11.

Yahalom J: Don't throw out the baby with the bathwater: on optimizing cure and reducing toxicity in Hodgkin's lymphoma. J Clin Oncol 2006;24:544.

ACUTE LYMPHOCYTIC LEUKEMIA • 25

CASE HISTORY • *Part I*

A 16-year-old female presents with the recent onset of fatigue, headache, and repeated, difficult to control, epistaxis over the past week. She has been in excellent health and has no personal or family history of serious illness. She has 4 siblings.

Examination reveals pale conjunctiva and multiple petechiae on her lower legs. Abdominal examination suggests a slightly enlarged spleen. The remainder of her examination, including a neurological examination is normal.

CBC: Hematocrit/hemoglobin 25%/8 g/dL
MCV - 90 fL MCH - 32 pg MCHC - 31 g/dL
WBC count - 110,000/μL
Differential count: Neutrophils 10%
Mature lymphocytes 3%
Immature blasts 85%
Monocytes/eosinophils/basophils <1%
Platelet count - 45,000/μL

• SMEAR MORPHOLOGY

Normocytic, normochromic red blood cells with the occasional shift cell (polychromasia). Dominant population of blasts—moderately large cells with little cytoplasm and prominent nucleoli surrounded by an abnormal nuclear chromatin pattern; the few remaining neutrophils and lymphocytes appear normal. Platelets are reduced in number.

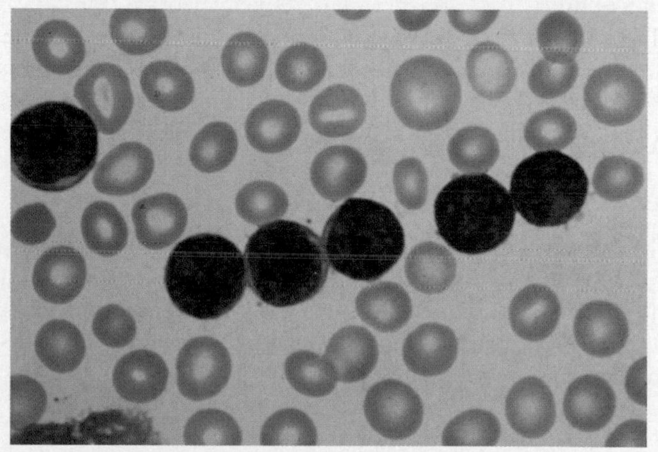

Questions

- What abnormality is apparent from the CBC?
- What further studies are indicated?

Acute lymphocytic leukemia (ALL) is a disease that primarily affects children. B-cell ALL is the most common malignancy in children under 15 years of age. The diagnosis and treatment of B-ALL in children constitutes one of the great success stories of hematology. Like Hodgkin disease, ALL has been approached with a combination of science and clinical insights that has produced a high frequency of true cures. An understanding of the principles of diagnosis and treatment of ALL serves as a model for the approach to all leukemias. Although the application of these principles to treat adult ALL is less likely to produce a cure, it is still the best approach to diagnosis and management.

CLASSIFICATION

The classification of ALL is based on a combination of morphologic (French-American-British [FAB]), immunophenotypic, and molecular/genetic characteristics.

Morphologic Characteristics

Similar to the FAB classification of the acute myelogenous leukemias, ALL can be divided into 3 classes—L1, L2, and L3—from the morphologic appearance of lymphocytes in the peripheral blood and marrow (Figure 25–1).

With **L1 disease** the lymphocytes are uniformly small with round nuclei, little cytoplasm, and inconspicuous nucleoli. **L2 disease** consists of large, heterogeneous cells with more cytoplasm, irregular nuclei, and prominent nucleoli, whereas **L3 disease** is characterized by large cells with abundant, deeply basophilic cytoplasm, round nuclei, and prominent nucleoli. As regards the **special stains** used in the FAB classification, ALL lymphoblasts generally show positive staining for periodic acid–Schiff (PAS) and terminal deoxynucleotide transferase (TdT) but are negative for esterase and peroxidase. The L1 form of ALL is more commonly seen in children, whereas the L2 form is more common in adults. These morphologic distinctions do not reliably differentiate between T- and B-cell ALL.

Immunophenotypic Classification

This classification divides ALL into those cells derived from very early T- and B-cell precursors (eg, pre–B cells) and those from the more mature B and T cells. The surface markers used in making this distinction as well as the relative frequency of the various subtypes are summarized in Table 25–1. A subset of ALL showing unclear lineage (previously termed "linage infidelity") can also be defined by antibodies to CD antigens. Another group of ALL patients may show aberrant expression of 1 or more myeloid markers, such as CD13 or CD33, together with the expected B/T lineage markers for ALL. This subgroup is more common in adults (perhaps 10%–20% of cases) than in children (5%–10%). In adults, it may carry a poorer prognosis.

TABLE 25–1 • Immunologic markers in ALL

		Frequency (%)	
Phenotype	**Characteristic Markers**	**Children**	**Adults**
B-cell ALL	CD19$^+$, CD22$^+$, CD79a$^+$, HLADR$^+$	87%	76%
B1 (pro-B)	TdT$^+$, CD10$^-$, CD34$^+$	5%	11%
B2 (common)	CD10$^+$, cIg$^-$, CD34$^+$	63%	52%
B3 (pre-B)	CD10^{++}, CD20$^+$, cIgM$^+$, CD34$^-$	16%	9%
B4 (B-cell)	sIgM$^+$	3%	4%
T-cell ALL	CD7$^+$, cCD3$^+$, sCD3$^-$	13%	24%
T1 (pro-T)	CD7$^+$		1%
T2 (pre-T)	CD7$^+$, CD2$^+$, CD5$^+$, CD8$^+$		11%
T3 (cortical)	CD1a$^+$		9%
T4 (mature)	sCD3$^+$, CD1a$^+$		3%

The classification of ALL may also be made genetically by studying the cells' **immunoglobulin or T cell–receptor (TCR) gene rearrangements**. It is the most definitive method for determining whether the cell is of B- or T-cell origin, but is often unnecessary because of the clear expression of a single lineage of surface antigens. Rearrangement of immunoglobulin heavy-chain genes, and to a lesser extent light-chain genes, is seen in the vast majority of B-cell and pre–B cell ALL. However, B-cell ALL can also show rearrangement of the TCR genes. In contrast, T-cell ALL rarely has concomitant rearrangement of the immunoglobulin genes.

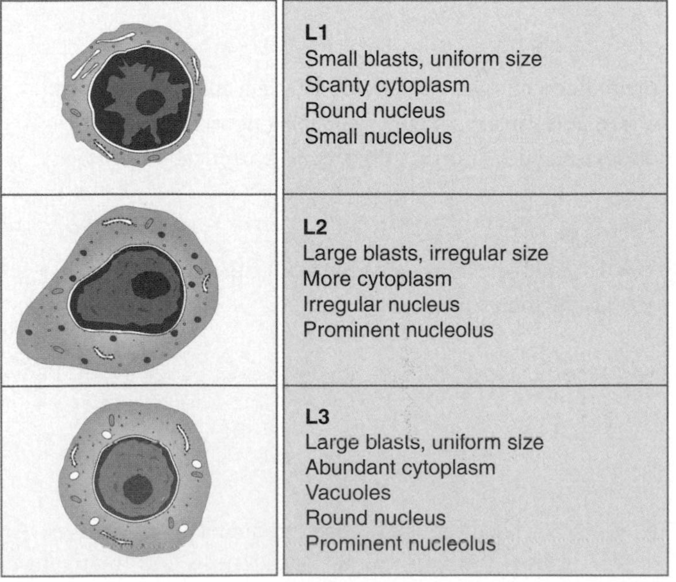

FIGURE 25–1. **Morphologic types of ALL.** There are 3 major morphologic types of ALL. The small cell type L1 is most common in children but also occurs in adults. The L2 and L3 forms are more common in adults and have a significantly worse prognosis.

Genetic Classification

Another basis for the classification of ALL is the presence of a molecular or cytogenetic abnormality. These occur in a nonrandom fashion and are known to have considerable prognostic significance. The presence of cytogenetic abnormalities may be defined on 2 different levels. The first level is the presence of an abnormal amount of DNA in each cell. This condition is referred to as **DNA aneuploidy** and is easily quantitated by flow cytometry as the amount of DNA per cell (DNA index). **Hyperdiploidy** (the presence of an increased number of chromosomes per cell, DNA index greater than 1.0) is more common in children, where an index greater than 1.15 defines a group with better prognosis. **Hypodiploidy** is more rare. Most cases present with a normal cellular DNA content. In these patients, however, karyotypic or molecular studies will frequently demonstrate a structural abnormality.

Most of the cytogenetic abnormalities involve translocations or **mutations of proto-oncogenes, active kinases, or transcription**

TABLE 25–2 • Some molecular/cytogenetic abnormalities in ALL

Genetic Abnormality	Cell Type	Frequency: Children	Frequency: Adults	Implications for Therapy
Hyperdiploidy >50 chromosomes	B	25%	7%	Sensitive to methotrexate
TEL-AML1 t(12;21)	B	22%	2%	Sensitive to asparaginase
MLL t(4;11) t(11;19) t(9;11)	B	8%	10%	Sensitive to high-dose cytarabine
BCR-ABL t(9;22)	B	3%	25%	Include TK inhibitor
E2A-PBX1 t(1;19)	B	5%	3%	Requires high-dose therapy
TAL1 1p32	T	7%	12%	Resistant to methotrexate
HOX11 10q24	T	0.7%	8%	Confers a more favorable prognosis in children

factors. Non-random translocations are the most common in children with ALL. They fall into several distinct subgroups. The t(8;14) translocation is highly correlated with B-cell ALL of the L3 morphology. The t(4;11) translocation has been associated with B-ALL with aberrant myeloid marker subgroup and a poorer prognosis, whereas B-ALL with t(12;21) in children has a better prognosis. Approximately 5% of children and up to 30% of adults with B-ALL will have a t(9;22) translocation similar to the Philadelphia chromosome (Ph^1) defect of chronic myelogenous leukemia (CML). Detailed mapping of the breakpoint cluster region (BCR) locus most often shows the p190 tyrosine kinase RNA of Ph^1-positive ALL versus the p210 product of CML. Both children and adults with B-ALL and t(9;22) have a very poor prognosis. Finally, the t(1;19) translocation is associated with pre–B cell, whereas the t(11;14) translocation is seen with T-cell ALL. Table 25–2 summarizes the most common genetic findings in adult and childhood ALL as well as some of their therapeutic implications.

CLINICAL FEATURES

There are actually 2 peaks in the incidence of ALL: one below 10 years of age and another, much smaller peak above 50 years. In childhood, ALL is most frequently seen between 3 and 7 years of age, although the disease can occur in infants. Although the middle-aged adult is more likely to present with acute myeloid leukemia (AML), detailed immunophenotypic and cytogenetic studies are necessary so as not to miss the occasional ALL patient.

The presenting symptoms and signs of ALL are similar in children and adults and do not differ significantly from those of any form of acute leukemia. The onset is usually abrupt with little or no history of prodromal symptoms. The **predominant signs and symptoms** are the consequence of both bone marrow failure and immature (blastic) cell growth, a moderate to severe anemia, neutropenia, and thrombocytopenia. Patients report increasing weakness and easy fatigability. If the anemia is severe, they may experience shortness of breath and congestive heart failure. Severe thrombocytopenia is associated with the appearance of petechiae, especially over the lower extremities; bruising; and epistaxis. Bacterial infections such as otitis media, pharyngitis, or pneumonia may result from the granulocytopenia.

Some patients, especially children, complain of bone pain or have pain with bony pressure or symptoms that simulate osteomyelitis. Sternal tenderness is common. Asymptomatic **central nervous system (CNS)** involvement is likely to be present in most patients and is a major issue in the treatment of ALL. At the same time, symptoms and signs of CNS involvement are unusual; only the occasional patient with advanced meningeal involvement will complain of headache and/or vomiting. Most patients will have diffuse adenopathy and splenomegaly on physical examination, although it is rarely so prominent as to be a presenting complaint. Both adenopathy and meningeal involvement are more typical of the mature B- and T-cell ALL phenotypes. Uncommon but not-to-miss symptoms at presentation are testicular swelling, retinal infiltrates with blurred vision, and polyuria due to pituitary infiltration.

Laboratory Studies

The **key laboratory studies for diagnosing ALL** are the complete blood count (CBC), blood film and marrow aspirate for cell morphology, and both immunophenotyping and molecular/cytogenetic analyses. In addition, since the initial tumor burden is a significant factor in a patient's response to therapy and prognosis, specific laboratory and imaging studies are important.

A. Complete Blood Count

The CBC is invariably abnormal in patients who present with ALL. The most striking finding is a high white blood cell (WBC) count, consisting primarily of lymphoblasts and lymphocytic

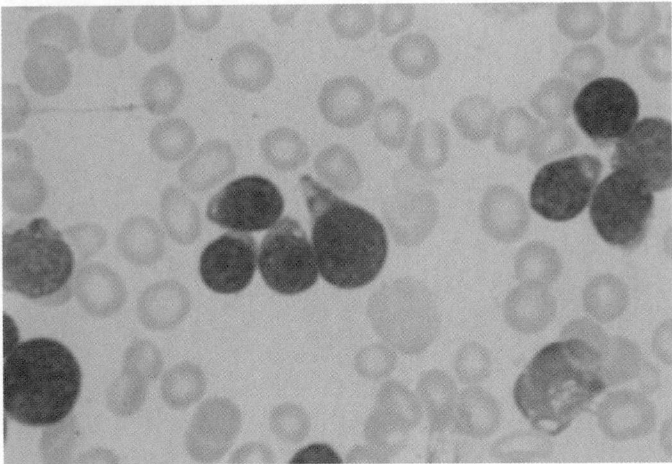

A

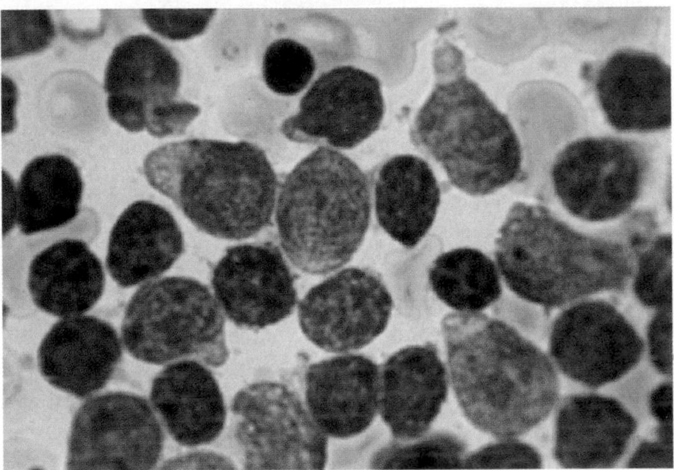

B

FIGURE 25–2. **Lymphoblasts in ALL. A:** Lymphoblasts in a patient with T-cell ALL; note the characteristic "hand-mirror" shape. **B:** Lymphoblasts in the marrow of a B-ALL patient; note the prominent nucleoli in many of the cells.

TABLE 25–3 • Risk factors for acute lymphocytic leukemia

Standard Risk	High Risk
Risk linearly related to WBC count	WBC >100,000/μL[a]
Age 1–10 y	Less than 1 y or >10 y
Females	Males[a]
No or asymptomatic CNS	Overt CNS involvement[a]
	Mediastinal mass[a]
Pre–B cell phenotype	T-cell phenotype (children)[a]
	Non-Caucasian
Hyperdiploidy, t(12;21), t(1;19), t(8;14) *HOX11* overexpression	Hypodiploidy, t(9;22), t(4;11)

[a]*These factors are probably not independent because they tend to be seen together.*
Note: Of the risk factors listed, WBC count and age are clearly independent and are by far the most significant.

cells, some of which may have the distinctive "hand-mirror" shape of a T-cell ALL (Figure 25–2A). Counts in excess of 100,000/μL, which are most often associated with T-cell ALL, can be seen (Table 25–3). At the same time, up to 30% of cases present with a normal or low total WBC count, again with a differential comprised mostly of lymphocytic morphology. Neutropenia is usually present and, in patients with very high lymphoblast counts, granulocytes may be undetectable. Anemia and thrombocytopenia are variable in degree but are nearly always present.

B. Blood Film and Marrow Aspirate

The marrow aspirate is usually diagnostic, showing massive replacement of normal marrow by a uniform population of lymphoblasts (Figure 25–2B). The marrow can be so packed that aspiration is unsuccessful and a biopsy is required. Rarely, the initial marrow may show hypoplasia or aplasia, suggesting an aplastic anemia. Usually, these patients will respond to glucocorticoid therapy with rising counts, thereby declaring themselves as having ALL.

Even the best hematologist or hematopathologist cannot always distinguish ALL from AML by cellular morphology alone. **Histochemical stains** (ie, peroxidase, combined esterase, PAS, and TdT stains) can be very helpful. The ALL blast should be peroxidase and esterase negative; PAS positivity is constant only in the L3 subtype. Primitive blasts will show positive TdT staining. Histochemistry can be confusing or equivocal, however, especially in adults. Currently, a reliable distinction between ALL and AML depends much more on immunophenotyping and cytogenetics than on morphology or histochemistry.

C. Immunophenotyping and Genetic Analyses

Immunogenetic studies are absolutely essential in distinguishing B- and T-cell ALL and in classifying the subtypes of ALL (see Tables 25–1 and 25–2). Cytogenetics and immunophenotyping must be obtained early in the diagnostic workup when blasts are abundant. Once therapy is initiated, these studies may be difficult to perform or impossible to interpret. Initial phenotypic and genotypic characterization of the malignant clone is also likely to be critical for the subsequent detection of minimal residual disease and possible relapse after induction and maintenance therapy.

Residual malignant cells can be detected with all of these highly sensitive procedures, including immunophenotyping and ploidy analysis, detection of fusion gene transcripts (eg, t[4;11]), karyotyping, and immunoglobulin or TCR gene rearrangement.

D. Other Laboratory Abnormalities

The other laboratory abnormalities that are associated with ALL include hypogammaglobulinemia, elevated lactic dehydrogenase (LDH) and uric acid levels, and a variety of electrolyte abnormalities such as hyperphosphatemia, hypocalcemia, and hyperkalemia.

Both the hyperphosphatemia and hyperkalemia can worsen dramatically during initiation of therapy when large numbers of leukemic blasts are lysed (tumor lysis syndrome).

E. Studies to Detect Tumor Growth

Although the level of the peripheral WBC count and the height of the LDH level provide a sense of the patient's tumor burden, a careful search should be made for node-based tumor masses. This search should include an **examination of the patient for lymphadenopathy and splenomegaly** and a **chest x-ray** to look for a mediastinal mass.

Any ALL may demonstrate significant adenopathy, and in fact, most ALL is now classified (both B- and T-cell) as acute lymphoblastic leukemia/lymphoma since either presentation is considered to be similar in terms of management and prognosis. A large mediastinal mass is seen in up to 50% of cases of T-cell ALL. If a **biopsy** is done, it usually shows the presence of lymphocytes identical to those found in marrow and blood and most typical of the cell type seen in primary lymphoblastic lymphomas. In fact, some children will present initially with a mediastinal tumor, without evidence of leukemia in the blood or marrow. However, such patients will usually demonstrate overt ALL within a short period.

Cerebrospinal fluid examination is usually performed as soon as the blast cells have disappeared from the peripheral blood, usually a week after starting the induction therapy. Although infrequent at presentation, CNS infiltration is more likely when patients display cranial nerve palsies or retinal infiltrates, whatever the results of cerebrospinal fluid examination. On the other hand, CNS infiltration can be found even in asymptomatic patients, when blast cells and/or elevated protein are observed in the cerebrospinal fluid. Recently, overexpression of IL-15 has been shown to be predictive of CNS infiltration.

DIAGNOSIS

A diagnosis of ALL is usually **easily made in children**. It is the dominant form of acute leukemia. When children present with a very high peripheral lymphoblast count, coupled with modest lymphadenopathy and splenomegaly, there is almost no chance that it can be confused with AML. If there is a question, histochemical stains and immunophenotyping studies will confirm the diagnosis.

In adults where ALL is an unlikely diagnosis, it can be more difficult to distinguish ALL from AML. Immunophenotypic marker studies are essential because morphology and histochemistry frequently do not clearly make the distinction. Some ALL cases will express a single aberrant myeloid antigen, and the occasional case of AML will have blasts that aberrantly express at least 1 lymphoid marker, usually CD7. The predominant antigenic markers will usually serve to classify the leukemia, but in the occasional case, the final diagnosis will require molecular or gene rearrangement studies. In addition, cytogenetic studies will often reveal abnormalities typical of either ALL or AML.

Other forms of lymphoma, particularly hairy cell leukemia, prolymphocytic leukemia, and Sézary cell leukemia, are unlikely to be confused with ALL. When the overall clinical picture of these diseases is considered, the morphology, clinical characteristics, and the presence of mature lymphoid markers should make the distinction (see Chapter 22). A few **non-lymphoid tumors** may be confused with ALL. Neuroblastoma and rhabdomyosarcoma in children and Ewing sarcoma and small cell lung cancer in adults can have the morphologic appearance of ALL. In each case, however, immunophenotypic markers should clearly show that these cells do not belong to either the lymphoid or myeloid lineages. Moreover, gene rearrangements typical of lymphoid cells will not be present.

CASE HISTORY • *Part 2*

This patient clearly has a leukemic process. The important decision to be made is the nature of the leukemia. Flow cytometric phenotyping of both blood and marrow is indicated and a marrow sample should be collected for cytogenetics and molecular studies. Radiological examination should include evaluation of both the chest and abdomen by computed tomography (CT). The possibility of CNS involvement should be addressed by examination of cerebrospinal fluid (CSF), including phenotyping any cells found.

In this patient, the bone marrow aspirate shows nearly total replacement of the marrow by a uniform population of blast cells (see Figure 25–2B), which when phenotyped are clearly early pre–B cells ($CD34^+$, $CD19^+$, $CD10^+$, $CD22^+$, $CD20^-$, $CD79a^+$, $HLADR^+$, and negative for all T-cell markers). Malignant pre-B cells may also demonstrate an abnormal $CD38^+/CD58^+$ phenotype that differs from normal hematogones. Cytogenetics shows hyperdiploidy (DNA index = 1.21 by flow cytometry) but with no specific translocation identified. The chest CT is normal. The abdominal CT confirms the presence of mild splenomegaly and suggests retroperitoneal adenopathy.

The CSF shows increased numbers of large lymphocytes with the identical phenotype as the marrow blasts with normal protein and negative cultures.

Questions

- What risk category does this patient fit into?
- What initial therapeutic interventions are indicated?

Activated normal lymphoid cells can closely resemble leukemic lymphoblasts morphologically. Reactive lymphocytosis, as seen in conditions such as infectious mononucleosis, can present with large numbers of atypical lymphocytes and, to the less sophisticated eye, be mistaken for ALL. If confusion arises, bone marrow examination and immunophenotyping will also show that reactive lymphoblasts consist of different cell types and have a mature phenotype. For example, the atypical lymphocytes of infectious mononucleosis are predominantly mature CD8 T cells. If necessary, genetic studies will confirm that the gene rearrangements present in reactive lymphocytes are polyclonal, not monoclonal, thus ruling out leukemia.

THERAPY AND CLINICAL COURSE

Soon after diagnosis, ALL must be treated with an intensive multidrug regimen that has a high probability of inducing remission. Several drugs have activity in this disease, and they are used in various combinations. Most institutions have treatment protocols that use varying drug combinations, doses, and treatment schedules based on internationally accepted risk factors. Currently, the Children's Oncology Group recognizes **4 initial treatment groups** based on age, WBC, and immunophenotype. They are T cell; infant; high-risk B precursor; and standard-risk B precursor. Treatment regimens specific to these groups are being studied. For example, T-cell ALL shows greater sensitivity to asparaginase and relative resistance to methotrexate, compared with B-ALL. The drugs commonly used to treat ALL are listed in Table 25–4.

Remission Induction

Remission induction needs to be preceded by steps to avoid **tumor lysis syndrome (hyperphosphatemia, hypocalcemia, and hyperuricemia)**, resulting from the rapid destruction of a very large blast population. Hyperuricemia can result in acute renal failure, while hyperphosphatemia induces calcium precipitation with a risk of hypocalcemia and tetany. Prevention of hyperuricemia is accomplished by aggressive diuresis, alkalinization of urine, and allopurinol (5mg/kg/d) usually for 8–10 days. Rasburicase (0.20 mg/kg/d) can help to reduce a threatening hyperuricemia even more quickly. The threat of hyperphosphatemia is reduced by hydration with large amounts of intravenous fluids.

Treatment protocols often start with prednisone alone for a week. This will allow one to assess prednisone sensitivity, which is an important prognostic factor. For induction, the most potent chemotherapy agents are vincristine, daunorubicin, asparaginase, cytosine-arabinoside, and cyclophosphamide (see Table 25–4). Induction therapy results in myelosuppression with a prolonged period of pancytopenia, requiring intensive support (see Chapter 18). Recovery of normal hematopoiesis cannot be expected for 3–4 weeks.

Follow-up examination of marrow should be done at 2 weeks with careful evaluation of immunophenotypic markers, ploidy, and genetics to confirm the disappearance of malignant cells. Persistence of lymphoblasts in the bone marrow 1–2 weeks after starting chemotherapy generally predicts a treatment failure, and is an indication to initiate salvage therapy without waiting for recovery of normal hematopoiesis. Hematologic remission is defined by full recovery of a normal blood and bone marrow. It is frequently difficult to assess remission in the bone marrow during the early recovery phase because of the hypocellularity and the presence of variable numbers of immature but reactive normal cells. Therefore, the detection of even a few remaining blast cells by immunophenotyping is now considered of paramount importance in predicting long-term survival. Current induction treatments provide complete remission rates as high as 95% in children and 85% in adults.

TABLE 25–4 • Chemotherapeutic regimens for ALL

	Usual Dose and Route	Major Toxicities
Vincristine	2 mg/m^2 IV weekly	Neuropathy
Prednisone	40 mg/m^2 PO daily	Psychosis, hypertension, ulcer
Asparaginase	500 IU/m^2 IV daily × 10 d	Allergic reaction
Daunorubicin	30–60 mg/m^2 IV daily × 3 d	Myelosuppression, cardiotoxicity
Methotrexate	15–25 mg/m^2 various schedules	Myelosuppression
6-Mercaptopurine	90 mg/m^2 PO daily	Myelosuppression
Cyclophosphamide	100 mg/m^2 PO daily	Myelosuppression
Cytosine arabinoside	100 mg/m^2 IV or SC daily	Myelosuppression

Prophylactic Treatment of the Central Nervous System

Once remission has been achieved, it is important to treat **sites potentially harboring previously undetected leukemic cells** that may have escaped eradication. The most common site is the CNS. Although overt CNS involvement is unusual at presentation, about 50% of patients will relapse in the CNS within 2 years if not specifically treated. Other sites include the testes and the ovary, although these are much less common. Therefore, a second requirement of therapy is the prophylactic treatment of the CNS.

Prophylactic CNS **irradiation** delivering 18 Gy for standard-risk patients and 25–28 Gy for high-risk patients has been proven to be very effective. However, irradiation has been associated with early and late CNS toxicity, such as leukoencephalopathy, meningioma, and neurocognitive defects. Thus, **intrathecal therapy**, most commonly with methotrexate, cytarabine, and hydrocortisone, is currently used with limited irradiation aiming at a reduction of the CNS radiation dose. Boys must be followed with careful physical examination of the testes to detect any masses that may indicate relapse. If masses are suspected, this should be confirmed with biopsy and then treated with local irradiation followed by reinduction chemotherapy.

Post-Induction Therapy

Further treatment once remission is obtained depends on the individual prognosis of the ALL subtype (see Table 25–3). Usually, patients receive an early intensification with high-dose treatments. For patients with very high risk of early relapse and failure, for instance, t(9;22), t(4;11), hypodiploidy, inadequate early response to steroids in adults, and induction failure whatever the age, allogeneic hematopoietic stem cell (HSC) transplantation is an option provided that a histocompatible sibling or unrelated donor can be found, but its place will probably need to be redefined according to the results of ongoing trials. Incorporation of tyrosine kinase inhibitors in t(9;22) ALL as part of first-line therapy is currently being evaluated with encouraging results. Minimal residual disease assessment can help to tailor post-induction therapy and monitor patients for the earliest signs of relapse.

Maintenance Chemotherapy

After completion of induction, prophylactic CNS treatment, and early intensification, a phase of maintenance chemotherapy is started for those patients with low-risk characteristics. The details of this phase vary depending on the protocol. They may consist of continued administration of relatively low doses of agents such as 6-mercaptopurine and methotrexate or periodic "consolidation" treatments with higher doses of multiple agents. The total duration of treatment is usually 2–3 years.

Prognosis

More than 80% of children who achieve complete remission and finish 2–3 years of maintenance therapy will be **cured** of their disease. The prognosis in adults treated with the conventional ALL protocol is much worse, with only a 30%–40% chance of long-term survival.

Patients who relapse 12 or more months following first remission will frequently achieve a second remission with a repeated course of conventional chemotherapy. However, second remissions are usually shorter with a poor long-term survival. Patients who relapse during chemotherapy or within 6 months of first remission have a very poor prognosis. An improved outcome in adults, 40%–50% survival rates, has been reported with aggressive chemotherapy, including CNS treatment, based on childhood protocols. The up-front CNS treatment reduced the rate of CNS relapse to less than 20%, versus 50% in conventionally treated patients.

The genetic array profile of the malignant cell line may also help predict outcome. A limited set of genes has been shown to be expressed differently and correlates with sensitivity to prednisolone, vincristine, asparaginase, and daunorubicin. It is anticipated that this approach to predicting outcome, and thereby modifying therapy, will be used more and more in the future.

Patients achieving long-term disease-free survival face some risk of a secondary malignancy, particularly gliomas in children. In addition, many patients will have decreased fertility, and this risk dictates offering male patients sperm preservation before treatment. There does not appear to be an increased incidence of birth defects in the offspring of ALL survivors.

Marrow/Stem Cell Transplantation

Hematopoietic stem cell transplantation is of benefit in first remission for adults with high-risk features, and in children after induction failure. All patients who relapse should be considered candidates for marrow transplantation as soon as they achieve second remission. In these situations, **allogeneic transplantation** offers the best chance of long-term disease control.

CASE HISTORY • *Part 3*

This patient falls into an indeterminate risk category. Young children with early pre–B cell ALL have an excellent chance of cure. Adults, on the other hand, may achieve an initial complete remission but are rarely cured. When presented with a case such as this, it is often difficult to determine whether the patient fits into the childhood or adult category of ALL.

Positive factors in this patient include the B-cell ALL phenotype, hyperdiploidy, and female gender. Negative factors include her age, the high blast count, and evidence of CNS involvement. Cytogenetics, while predictive of long-term survival, are not as yet useful in planning induction therapy.

Due to the presence of several negative factors, this patient should probably be intensively treated with remission induction chemotherapy, including intrathecal chemotherapy, followed by consolidation and maintenance. She and her siblings should be tested for histocompatibility in anticipation of the need for an allogeneic HSC transplant, especially if remission is not immediately achieved or if early relapse occurs.

POINTS TO REMEMBER

Acute lymphocytic leukemia (ALL) typically presents in childhood as an acute illness, characterized by the sudden onset of some combination of fatigue, bone pain, abnormal bleeding, and fever.

The bone marrow will usually show overwhelming infiltration by "blasts" and peripheral blast counts can be greater than 100,000/μL. Adenopathy can also be a presentation, confirming this disease's current World Health Organization (WHO) designation as acute lymphoblastic leukemia/lymphoma.

Immunophenotyping and cytogenetics are essential to the accurate diagnosis of the cell type and as a guide to therapy and overall prognosis. ALL can result from malignant transformation of either B-cell or T-cell precursors.

Due to the fact that lymphocytes are highly mobile, the concept of sanctuary disease in the CNS or testes has become an important concept in the treatment of ALL. Even in the absence of overt involvement, prophylactic treatment of sanctuary sites has greatly improved outcomes.

ALL (especially B-cell ALL) in young children is highly curable by modern combination chemotherapy, but still requires therapy tailored to the risk of relapse. In addition, laboratory studies for monitoring relapse or residual disease are standard for guiding therapy.

ALL in adults is uncommon but has a much poorer outcome than that seen in children, warranting an aggressive approach in adults who can tolerate intensive therapy and transplantation.

BIBLIOGRAPHY

Brüggemann M, Raff T, Flohr T, et al: Clinical significance of minimal residual disease quantification in adult patients with standard-risk acute lymphoblastic leukemia. Blood 2006; 107:1116.

Holleman A, Cheok MH, den Boer ML, et al: Gene-expression patterns in drug-resistant acute lymphoblastic leukemia cells and response to treatment. N Engl J Med 2004;351:533.

Lazarus HM, Luger S: Which patients with adult acute lymphoblastic leukemia should undergo a hematopoietic stem cell transplantation? Case-based discussion. Hematology (Am Soc Hem Educ Program) 2007:444.

Pui CH: Central nervous system disease in acute lymphoblastic leukemia: prophylaxis and treatment. Hematology (Am Soc Hem Educ Program) 2006:142.

Pui CH, Behm FG, Crist WM: Clinical and biologic relevance of immunologic marker studies in childhood acute lymphoblastic leukemia. Blood 1993;82:343.

Pui CH, Evans WE: Treatment of acute lymphoblastic leukemia. N Engl J Med 2006;354:166.

Pui CH, Reilling MV, Downing JR: Acute lymphoblastic leukemia. N Engl J Med 2004;350:1535.

Raff T, Gökbuget N, Lüschen S, et al: Molecular relapse in adult standard-risk ALL patients detected by prospective MRD monitoring during and after maintenance treatment: data from the GMALL 06/99 and 07/03 trials. Blood 2007;109:910.

Szczepanski SZ: Why and how to quantify minimal residual disease in acute lymphoblastic leukemia? Leukemia 2007; 21:622.

Thomas DA: Philadelphia chromosome–positive acute lymphocytic leukemia: a new era of challenges. Hematology (Am Soc Hem Educ Program) 2007:436.

Willemze R, Labar B: Post-remission treatment for adult patients with acute lymphoblastic leukemia in first remission: is there a role for autologous stem cell transplantation? Semin Hematol 2007;44:267.

PLASMA CELL DISORDERS • 26

CASE HISTORY • *Part I*

A 65-year-old man presents with a 1-month history of lower back pain, which began after he strained his back stacking fire wood. Despite rest and aspirin therapy it has not improved. He has not had similar back pain in the past and has been in good health. There are no neurological signs or symptoms on examination and he has no other complaints except possibly increased fatigability, which he attributed to his age. The remainder of his examination is normal with the exception of some conjunctival pallor.

CBC: Hematocrit/hemoglobin - 31%/10.1 gm/dL
MCV - 90 fL   MCH - 32 pg   MCHC - 31 g/dL
WBC - 8,500/μL
Differential - normal
Platelet count - 230,000/μL

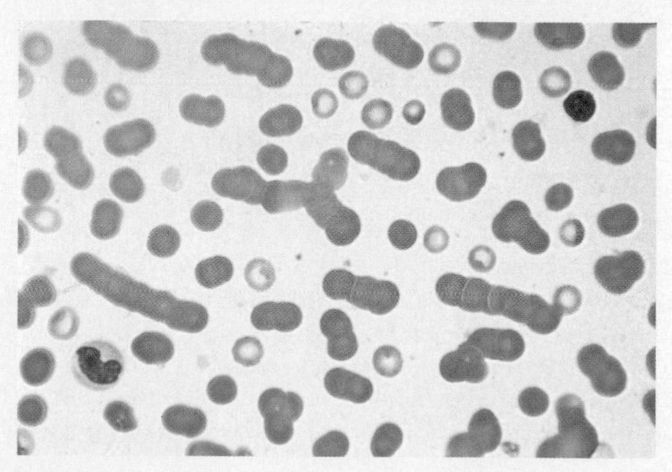

• SMEAR MORPHOLOGY

Normochromic, normocytic red blood cells with prominent rouleaux formation (stacking) and a vague bluish background on the slide.

Questions

- What feature(s) of this case might distinguish it from a routine lower back pain evaluation?
- What further evaluation is indicated?

Plasma cells are terminally differentiated cells of the B lymphocyte lineage. They are thought of as cellular factories whose entire energy and synthetic capacity is devoted to producing a single antibody protein. They are normally incapable of dividing and are thought to have a relatively short lifespan of perhaps several weeks. Plasma cells develop both in the lymph nodes, where they are found predominantly in the medullary cords, and in the marrow, although they represent a minority of cells in these tissues. They have a distinctive morphology and are easily identified in the marrow (Figure 26–1).

Plasma cell disorders, sometimes referred to as plasma cell dyscrasias, encompass several entities including monoclonal gammopathy of unknown significance (MGUS), Waldenström macroglobulinemia (WM), amyloidosis, and multiple myeloma (MM). The most common malignancy involving plasma cells is multiple myeloma, a multifaceted disease in which malignant plasma cells develop in bone marrow where they induce osteolytic lesions and produce monoclonal immunoglobulin components with humoral blood and urine repercussions.

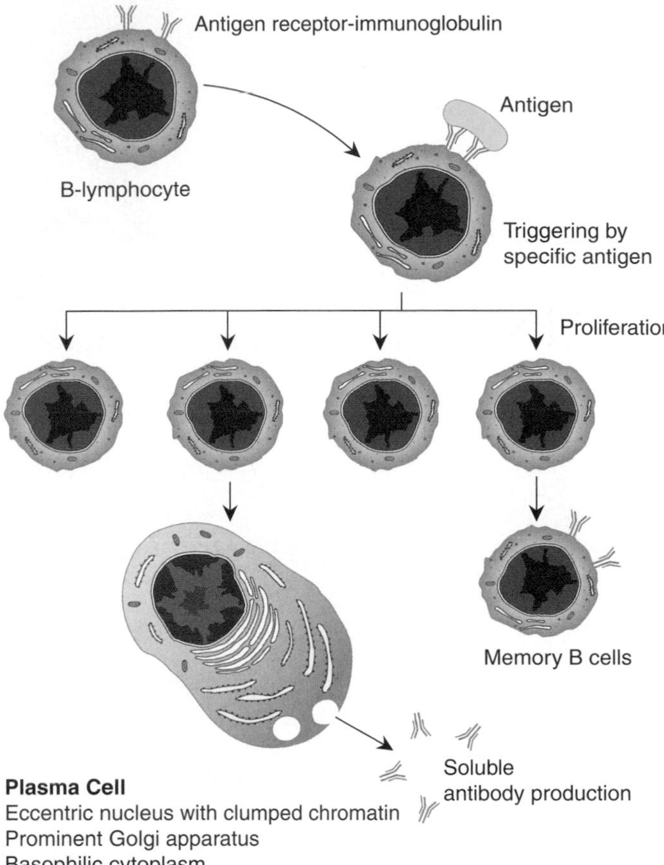

FIGURE 26–1. **Plasma cell differentiation and morphology.** Mature B lymphocytes express on their surface the antibody that serves as the receptor for specific antigen. When they encounter this antigen, they are stimulated to proliferate and differentiate, which leads to development of memory B cells and plasma cells. The plasma cell is highly specialized to produce and secrete large amounts of the same antibody.

THE BIOLOGY OF PLASMA CELL DISORDERS

After stimulation by specific antigen, the germinal center B cells differentiate to generate long-lived memory B cells on the one hand and plasma cells on the other (see Chapter 20). After then moving to the bone marrow, the plasma cell stops proliferating and manufactures large amounts (1 ng or more per cell per day) of the same antibody that was initially displayed on the surface of the B cell. The normal plasma cell lives only for several weeks or months. Two cellular substances have been shown to play key roles in the regulation of apoptosis in plasma cells. These are the **bcl-2 family** of mitochondrial proteins (bcl-2, bcl-XL, and mcl-1) and **interleukin [IL]-6**. The level of expression of bcl-2 and mcl-1 on the mitochondrial membrane determines the response of the plasma cell to apoptotic stimuli, whereas IL-6 is an important regulator of bcl-2 activity. Therefore, to normally maintain the continued production of any antibody, new plasma cells need to be regenerated from programmed B-cell precursors. The development of a plasma cell malignancy is marked by loss of apoptosis, and thus involves the "piling up" of a clone of plasma cells with marked overproduction of a single antibody that appears in the plasma as an M-component (also termed monoclonal immunoglobulin or **M-protein**).

Multiple myeloma (MM) is a classic example of a malignant disorder that results primarily from the failure of mature cells to respond to apoptotic stimuli and die rather than from excessive proliferation of precursors. Nearly 1 billion (10^9) plasma cells need to accumulate before sufficient M-protein is produced to be detected clinically. **Secondary mutations** are seen later in the disease process and are associated with chemoresistance and tumor growth independent of IL-6. The most important of these are mutations of the ***ras*** oncogene on chromosome 13 and **p53**.

As illustrated by animal models of multiple myeloma in mice and in human disease, clonal plasma cells develop preferentially in bones. The **cause of the bone disease in MM** is the local activation of osteoclasts (Figure 26–2A) by the clonal plasma cells. This involves the release of chemokines such as IL-1β, tumor necrosis factor-α, IL-6, and, most importantly, macrophage

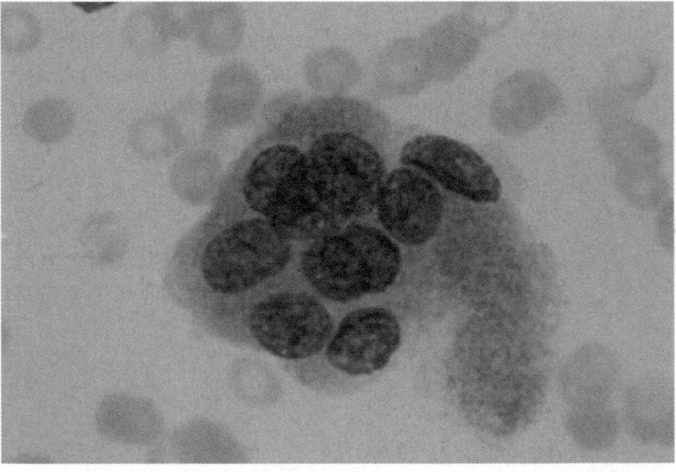

A

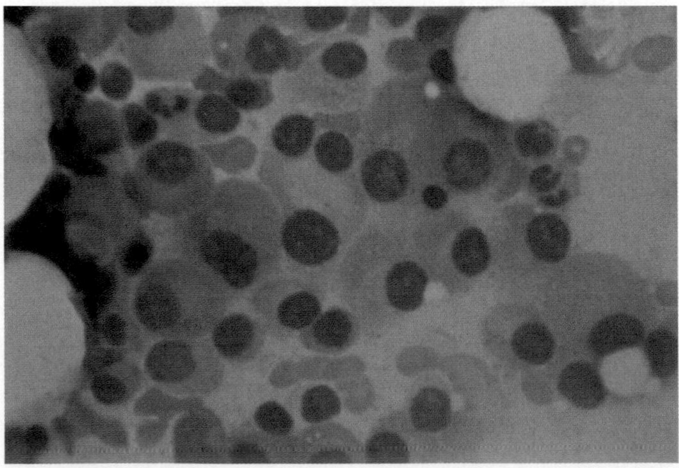

B

FIGURE 26–2. **Marrow osteoclasts versus a diffuse plasma cell infiltrate.** **A:** A solitary osteoclast (multinucleated cell that lacks the typical cytoplasm of a megakaryocyte). **B:** Diffuse plasma cell infiltrate in the marrow of a myeloma patient (marrow aspirate, Wright stain).

inflammatory protein (MIP)-1α and -1β. The latter are associated with an upregulation of RANKL (receptor activation of NF-κβ ligand) and a downregulation of OPG (osteoprotegerin, a natural antagonist of RANKL). Overexpression of RANKL is associated with increased generation of osteoclasts from monocyte precursors.

It is an apparent paradox for a malignant clone to retain mature functionality together with a capacity for self-renewal. However, recent data have shown that myeloma stem cells exist and demonstrate self-renewal and transplantability properties. The challenge in this disease is to eradicate not only plasma cell progeny but also the myeloma stem cells.

Use of M-Component in Diagnosis and Staging

The M-component is a readily measured, quantifiable tumor marker and as such has been used extensively to diagnose, stage, and follow plasma cell disorders. By measuring the level of M-component in serum and estimating the turnover rate of immunoglobulin, it is possible to use the M-component to estimate the total body burden of malignant plasma cells. In addition, by making some assumptions about the rate of accumulation of plasma cells, it is possible to estimate the amount of time that they have been accumulating and thus estimate the time of onset of the malignant process. These calculations have shown that the malignant transformation occurs at least 5 years before the onset of symptoms.

Cell Lineage and Immunologic Abnormalities

Since the M-component is a highly specific marker, the lineage of cells belonging to the clone has been traced from malignant B cells at the germinal center stage through the entire B-cell differentiation pathway to the plasma cell. One important **clue to the possible etiology** of plasma cell disorders comes from observations in the BALB/c mouse, which has a markedly increased propensity to develop myeloma after chronic antigenic stimulation. In humans, M-components have been recognized in some patients to display specific antibody activity for an antigen known to have been encountered by the patient, such as human immunodeficiency virus (HIV), bacterial polysaccharides, or natural self-antigens. It is likely, therefore, that clonal plasma cell proliferation results from the combination of a chronic B-cell antigenic stimulation and other cellular oncogenic events that lead to clonal plasma cell disorders. The resulting clone fails to apoptose and reveals itself years later with clinical symptoms due to an accumulation of plasma cells and M-component.

In addition to the clonal B and stem cells that lead to multiple myeloma, many patients with MM will also have abnormalities in the T-cell compartment. CD4 T cells are decreased and there is a concomitant increase in CD8 T cells and sometimes natural killer (NK) cells. These changes may serve as additional explanations for the immunodeficiency state that accompanies myeloma. Intriguing recent observations, however, of increased numbers of isotype- and idiotype-specific T cells in myeloma suggest a more active role for T cells in modulating B-cell function. There is some interest in the possible therapeutic exploitation of this by immunizing the patient (or a prospective marrow donor) with the patient's M-component in the hope of augmenting T-cell function against the malignant B cells.

The role of the bone marrow microenvironment in MM has also been emphasized. The **growth of myeloma cells** appears to be highly dependent on **exogenous IL-6** produced by bone marrow stromal cells. The production of IL-6 by these cells is stimulated by myeloma cells, perhaps mediated by transforming growth factor-β. This paracrine role for IL-6 has generated interest in designing therapies with antibodies against IL-6 and its receptor. Another factor produced by marrow stem cells that appears to be important in the growth of myeloma cells is **vascular endothelial growth factor (VEGF)**. Increased angiogenesis may play a role in promoting myeloma growth and anti-angiogenic therapies may have a role. Trials of **thalidomide** in MM have been very successful, supporting this proposition.

LABORATORY DIAGNOSIS OF MONOCLONAL GAMMOPATHY

All plasma cell dyscrasias are characterized by an accumulation of a clone of plasma cells producing a unique homogeneous immunoglobulin product. This monoclonality can be demonstrated either at the level of the soluble product, M-component, in serum/urine, or at the cellular level.

M-Components

An M-component is detected in serum as a discrete single band on electrophoresis (narrow spike on the electrophoretic pattern), and reaction of that band with specific antibodies to a single immunoglobulin heavy- (most commonly IgM, IgA, IgG, and rarely IgD or IgE) and light-chain forms: lambda (λ) or kappa (κ) (Figure 26–3). As these M-components modify the physical interactions between red cells and plasma, their presence increases the erythrocyte sedimentation rate (ESR), which can reach more than 100 mm/h. Physicians should keep in mind that patients with unexplained rouleaux or high sedimentation rates require an electrophoresis to rule out an M-component. An inflammatory process, especially in non-febrile patients, should not be assumed as the cause of the increased ESR without a negative electrophoresis (serum protein and/or immunofixation).

The special physical properties of the M-component protein also play an important physiologic role in the disease process. For example, monoclonal IgM components, because they are pentameric, and IgA, which frequently dimerize, are much more likely to lead to **hyperviscosity syndromes** at lower concentrations than IgG M-components. Monoclonal antibodies sometimes also have unusual binding properties, for example, **cold agglutinin hemolytic anemia** resulting from anti–I antibody specificity, and **peripheral neuropathy** resulting from anti-myelin activity.

The M-component may not be an intact immunoglobulin in a significant number of plasma cell disorders (Table 26–1).

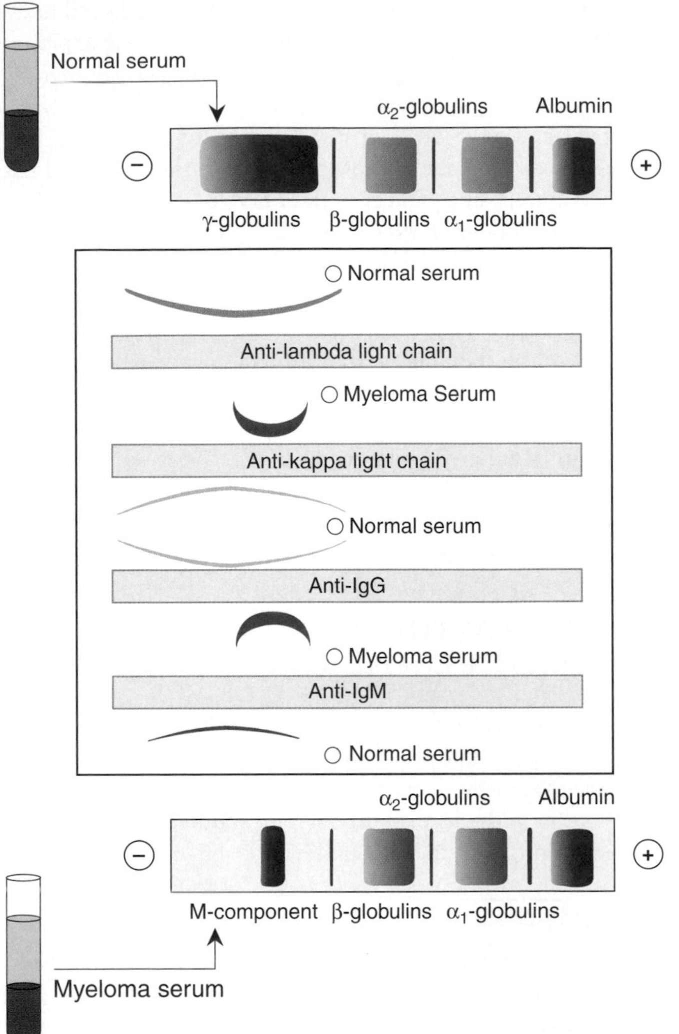

FIGURE 26–3. **Identification of an M-component.** Electrophoresis of normal serum results in a diffuse "gamma" region of polyclonal immunoglobulins containing a large spread of individual antibodies. Electrophoresis of a serum containing an M-component shows decreased levels of the polyclonal immunoglobulin and a prominent, electrophoretically homogeneous band. When tested with specific antibodies against light and heavy chains (immunoelectrophoresis), the M-component reacts with only one heavy chain (IgG) and one light chain (κ) antibody, demonstrating monoclonality. The immunoelectrophoresis technique illustrated here has been largely replaced by automated immunofixation electrophoresis systems.

Abnormal plasma cells can produce excess free light chains and, less frequently, free heavy chains or other immunoglobulin fragments. The different molecular weights of these proteins and their different solubilities can lead to various clinical syndromes. For example, lower molecular weight fragments such as free light chains will pass though the glomerular basement membrane and accumulate in the kidney parenchyma, resulting in renal dysfunction or failure due to **light-chain deposition disease**. Furthermore, some light chains have the property to accumulate as **amyloid deposits** in various organs, which can present as either the main feature of the disease or as a complication of the MM process.

TABLE 26–1 • Monoclonal proteins produced by plasma cell tumors

Type	%
IgG	52
IgA	21
IgD	2
IgE	<0.01
IgM (Waldenström)	12
Light chain only	11
Heavy chain only	<1
2 or more	0.5
None	1

Clonal Plasma Cells

Malignant plasma cells may be recognized on a marrow aspirate or biopsy specimen by their increased numbers and/or abnormal morphology, even to the point of complete infiltration and loss of all normal cellular elements (Figure 26–2B). Morphologic abnormalities, such as multiple nuclei and globules or crystals of immunoglobulin in the cytoplasm are another tip-off to multiple myeloma. At the same time, the distribution of clonal plasma cells throughout the marrow is not uniform, resulting in variations in the density of the plasma cell infiltrate in different areas of the marrow. Therefore, the estimation of the percentage of plasma cells in any marrow specimen can only approximate the size of the tumor load. This latter point is especially true for the aspirate sample, which often

TABLE 26–2 • Diagnostic criteria for multiple myeloma

Major criteria

Marrow plasmacytosis (>10%) with monoclonal immunoglobulin expression in serum or urine
Serum M-component >35 g/L of IgG or >20 g/L of IgA
A biopsy-proven plasmacytoma

Minor criteria

A. <10% plasma cells in the marrow but with monoclonal immunoglobulin expression
B. An M-component quantitatively less than specified above
Lytic bone lesions or unexplained osteopenia
Depressed normal (polyclonal) immunoglobulins
Unexplained normochromic, normocytic anemia
Serum β_2-microglobulin level of >3.5 mg/L
Unexplained renal dysfunction
Unexplained hypercalcemia

Note: The diagnosis of myeloma requires at least 1 major and 1 minor criterion or at least 3 minor criteria including both A and B.

underestimates the percentage of plasma cells as compared with the marrow biopsy specimen.

When the percentage of plasma cells in the marrow aspirate or biopsy is not greatly increased, it is diagnostically useful to determine if the cells are clonal using histochemistry or flow cytometry. This approach is especially important when a serum M-component cannot be demonstrated or is present in low concentration. Plasma cells can be specifically identified by their reactivity with **monoclonal antibodies to CD138 (immunohistochemistry) and CD38 (flow cytometry)**. Because the plasma cell produces large amounts of cytoplasmic immunoglobulin, it is possible to label the individual cells with antibodies directed against specific immunoglobulin heavy- and light-chain classes. Each plasma cell produces only one antibody, and therefore will label with only one heavy chain and/or one light chain reagent. The normal marrow contains plasma cells from many clones, and therefore cells will be found that label with antibodies to IgG, IgA, and IgM, in order of decreasing frequency, and the normal ratio of κ light chain to λ light chain expressing plasma cells will be about 2:1. In the case of a monoclonal gammopathy, plasma cells that express only a single heavy chain and a single light chain will predominate using immunohistochemistry on the biopsy specimen. Similarly, flow cytometry of the marrow aspirate can identify monoclonal plasma cells; the plasma cells can be distinguished from other marrow cells by their low level (or absence) of the leukocyte antigen CD45 and high expression of CD38. The plasma cells are permeabilized to permit entry of monoclonal antibodies directed against κ and λ light chain and, similar to detection of B-cell non-Hodgkin lymphoma, a predominance of one antibody's labeling makes the diagnosis of a plasma cell dyscrasia.

Detection of a chromosomal abnormality is also proof of a clonal disorder. Even though plasma cell dyscrasias have a low proliferative potential, making convential cytogenetics difficult, the advent of interphase FISH (fluorescence in-situ hybridization) methodology makes it possible to identify karyotypic abnormalities in nondividing cells. Using metaphase and FISH cytogenetics, it has now been shown that primary translocations involving either the IgH or IgL locus, including 11q13 (cyclin *D1*), 4p16, 6p21 (cyclin *D3*), 16q23, and 20q11, are present in 40%–50% of myeloma and monoclonal gammopathy patients. Other translocations—t(4;14), t(14;16), and t(11;14), and chromosomal abnormalities of 3, 5, 7, 9, 11, 13, 15, 19, and 21—occur but are less specific and may reflect disease progression. The most frequent chromosomal abnormalities are del 13, found in nearly half of myeloma patients, and translocations that dysregulate *c-myc*, which are seen in up to 20% of all MGUS and MM cases.

With evolution of plasma cell disease, **other cellular abnormalities** can be appreciated. Early on, the growth fraction of the malignant clone is low; generally less than 1% of the plasmablasts are dividing at any one time. This can increase dramatically to levels greater than 20% with disease progression, especially when a patient relapses after chemotherapy. The latter is associated with **point mutations of the *N-ras* and *K-ras* oncogenes,** as well as a **point mutation of p53** in patients with extramedullary disease. **Plasma cell phenotypic changes** include the initial loss of CD19 expression with CD56 overexpression, as detected by flow cytometry. Flow cytometric CD117 expression is associated with a more favorable prognosis, while CD28 positivity is associated with a less favorable outcome.

MULTIPLE MYELOMA (PLASMA CELL MYELOMA)

Multiple myeloma accounts for 10%–15% of hematologic neoplasms and about 1% of all cancer deaths.

Clinical Features

The manifestations of multiple myeloma are produced both by the tumor itself and the humoral factors it produces, as well as the spread of plasma cells throughout the skeleton. The most common clinical presentation of multiple myeloma is the recent onset of **unexplained back pain; normochromic, normocytic anemia; or renal insufficiency/failure** in an older patient. In recent times, however, up to 60% of new patients are first diagnosed when a **serum or urine M-component** is detected on routine laboratory testing, mainly because of an unexplained **increased sedimentation rate or excess globulin fraction**. Approximately 70% of myeloma patients are over 60 years of age and 90% are over 50 years old.

The diagnosis of multiple myeloma can easily be missed if the physician does not have a high degree of suspicion. In fact, the diagnosis is frequently missed on the first evaluation of a patient with back pain or anemia. This is even more of a problem in patients who have another disease, such as postmenopausal osteoporosis or rheumatoid arthritis, which may cause bone pain, anemia, or both. Therefore, it is important to **include myeloma in the differential diagnosis** of any older patient presenting with back pain or anemia, even when the history suggests a possible cause for the pain such as recent stress or trauma.

Up to 80% of myeloma patients present with bone pain as the first clue and more than 70% of myeloma patients develop 1 or more pathologic fractures during the course of their disease. Spinal cord compression is the most serious complication. It should be anticipated when the patient presents with fixed, progressive back pain, most frequently in the dorsal region. This presentation should be quickly explored by magnetic resonance imaging (MRI), even if there is no evidence of any neurological deficit or paraparesis, because spinal cord compression with paraplegia can be abrupt and irreversible. This complication is often the consequence of infiltration of the extradural space and compression by the plasma cell tumor itself; pure mechanical compression by a collapsed vertebra is another frequent etiology.

Less commonly, myeloma may present not as a bony or marrow-based process but rather as an isolated extramedullary mass lesion, the so-called **solitary plasmacytoma**. These lesions may be found in the skin, the gastrointestinal (GI) tract, the nasopharynx, and elsewhere. They are not clinically distinctive and can only be defined as plasmacytomas by biopsy. Most patients presenting with isolated plasmacytomas will also be found to have multiple myeloma on marrow examination; however, some patients will have an isolated tumor without significant marrow disease and can be treated with local radiotherapy.

A. Renal Manifestations and Hypercalcemia

Occasionally the myeloma patient will present with **acute renal insufficiency/failure** or sudden, symptomatic hypercalcemia. The cause of the **hypercalcemia** is primarily the rapid destruction of bone by osteoclast-activating factors secreted by plasma cells and/or bone marrow stromal cells. The cause of renal failure in MM is usually multifactorial, mainly related to acute tubular lesions resulting from light-chain deposition, dehydration, and hypercalcemia. Such tubular lesions are further exacerbated by nonsteroidal anti-inflammatory drug (NSAID) use; such drugs, therefore, are contraindicated in MM patients. Less common as a presenting symptom is **amyloid nephropathy**, which presents as glomerular dysfunction. The patient with resistant disease, however, is at risk for all of these problems. An episode of back pain requiring bed rest may result in hypercalcemia; similarly, an acute infection with fever may result in dehydration, which precipitates renal failure. With disease progression, renal failure can become a limiting factor in the design of an effective chemotherapy regimen.

B. Hematologic Manifestations

Myeloma patients have an **increased susceptibility to infection** secondary to decreased production of normal immunoglobulins, possibly because of dendritic cell dysfunction or other abnormality induced by the M-component. The major hematologic manifestation of myeloma is **anemia**, owing to decreased erythropoiesis. The degree of anemia is not related to the degree of marrow involvement by plasma cells. In addition, patients who have begun chemotherapy may have severe myelosuppression. Less commonly, the M-component may interfere with platelet function or coagulation factor X, leading to bleeding, or with phagocytic cell function, leading to recurrent infection.

Hyperviscosity of the blood, owing to large concentrations of IgG or dimerization of IgA at lower concentrations, is sometimes seen in myeloma, although it is much more common in macroglobulinemia with lesser concentrations of IgM. It is markedly worsened by dehydration. The clinical manifestations are fatigue and neurologic symptoms, including headache, blurring or loss of vision, confusion, and ischemia. Serum viscosity will be at least 3 times normal before symptoms can be attributed to hyperviscosity. Treatment of this complication must be undertaken promptly with hydration, plasmapheresis, and initiation of chemotherapy.

C. Laboratory Studies

Any patient suspected of having a plasma cell disorder should have a **serum protein electrophoresis (SPEP) and immunofixation electrophoresis (IFE)** for quantifying and typing the M-component, respectively, as well as quantitative measurement of albumin and polyclonal serum immunoglobulins. Additional important tests for staging and prognosis include electrophoresis of urine for light chains; a marrow aspirate and biopsy for morphology, flow cytometry, and karyotyping; a complete blood count (CBC); tests of kidney function, serum Ca^{2+}, albumin, and β_2-microglobulin; as well as x-rays of the skull and pelvis with careful inspection for excessive osteopenia or lytic lesions. Any area of localized bone pain should also be imaged.

D. Hematologic Studies

The CBC can provide important clues to the diagnosis of myeloma. As the disease advances, the patient will almost certainly develop a normocytic, normochromic anemia secondary to inhibition of erythropoiesis by plasma cell cytokines or renal damage. Since the distinction is important for managing the patient, any anemia should be fully evaluated with marrow, iron studies, and renal function measurements. Differential diagnosis of a marrow damage anemia is discussed in Chapters 3 and 4. In contrast to the early appearance of anemia, changes in granulocyte and platelet count occur much later and are usually associated with chemotherapy. It is impossible to identify the malignant plasma cell line from routine studies of the peripheral blood since the circulating B cells are polyclonal. Plasma cells or their progenitors are usually found in the circulation only with advanced disease. Rarely, patients will progress to plasma cell leukemia with circulating plasmablasts.

Another important clue from the CBC relates to the **amount and class of the patient's M-component**. As the level of this monoclonal protein increases, there is an increased tendency for red blood cell rouleaux formation. This tendency can be visually appreciated on the peripheral blood film, and when pronounced, can produce a false elevation in the mean cell volume (MCV) secondary to red blood cell agglutination. An **elevation of the sedimentation rate** to levels above 100 mm/h (Westergren method) in an otherwise healthy individual is also suggestive of the presence of an M-component. With older populations, where the incidence of plasma cell disorders is increased, a sedimentation rate can be a low-cost, high-yield screening test. At the same time, not all sedimentation rates above 100 mm/h turn out to be myeloma, and 10% of myeloma patients have only light chains in urine, without detectable M-component in blood. Vasculitis, arthritis, infections, and other malignancies are also associated with very high sedimentation rates. A golden rule is to consider every adult patient with a persistent unexplained elevated sedimentation rate for SPEP/IFE.

E. Immunoglobulin Studies

Eighty-five to ninety percent of patients will have an M-component in serum, the most common being IgG. About 25% of patients will have an IgA or rarely an IgD or IgE M-component, whereas 10%–15% of patients have only light chain detectable (see Table 26–1). Both the amount and class of the protein are important in diagnosing myeloma (Table 26–2). The presence of a high level of serum or urine M-component (or both) or light chains, together with a significant plasma cell infiltration of the marrow, provide the major criteria for MM diagnosis. Even without evidence of other organ damage, the level of the patient's M-component generally correlates with tumor burden and will guide management decisions.

The M-component may be first detected on routine serum protein electrophoresis as a narrow peak that deforms the normal symmetry of immunoglobulin electrophoresis pattern (see Figure 26–3). Depending on the class of protein, the peak can appear at any point in the distribution of the immunoglobulins, from $\alpha 2$ to γ migration zones. The quantity of M-component is

TABLE 26–3 • Risk stratification of patients with multiple myeloma

High Risk (25%)	Standard Risk (75%)
FISH studies: del 17p, t(4;14), t(14;16) **Karyotype:** Monosomy or del 13, hypodiploidy **Plasma cell labeling index:** ≥3%	All others. However, patients within this category and β_2-microglobulin >5.5 mg/L without renal failure or elevated LDH are likely to be considered as high risk.

better derived from the serum protein electrophoretic pattern than by direct quantitation with an anti-immunoglobulin antibody such as radial immunodiffusion or nephelometry. Although IFE cannot quantitate the M-component, it will type the monoclonal immunoglobulin as to heavy- and light-chain classes. IFE is more sensitive than SPEP for detecting very small M-components or for those M-components which migrate aberrantly outside the immunoglobulin zone, especially at the β-γ interface.

Although the level of M-component provides the most important measure of tumor burden, serial measurements of the β_2-microglobulin level have also been used clinically to follow the progression of myeloma. **β_2-microglobulin** is a protein that is shed as a part of the life cycle of all lymphocytes, including plasma cells. Levels above 3.5 mg/L suggest a major increase in the number of plasma cells, even when the M-component is not dramatically increased. In established MM patients, when measured serially during chemotherapy, a rise in the β_2-microglobulin level may precede a rise in the M-component with relapse. The relationship of tumor aggressiveness and serum β_2-microgloulin has been confirmed in large patient series, and serum β_2-microglobulin is now recognized as a powerful and independent prognostic indicator in multiple myeloma.

Free light chains and the κ/λ ratio in serum reflect the unbalanced production of either κ or λ light chains by the clonal process. The normal κ/λ ratio reference range in serum is 0.25–1.65. This test is of critical interest for monitoring patients when M-components are undetectable in serum, for example, after treatment. Given their short half-life, free light chain levels or ratios are also the earliest indicators of response to treatment but must be interpreted with caution when renal failure affects light chain clearance.

In research centers, the **plasma cell–labeling index** (the number of plasma cells with active DNA synthesis) has also been used to predict the rate of progression. Patients who demonstrate a low labeling index and a normal β_2-microglobulin in the past have demonstrated good survival (median 6 years) when treated with conventional chemotherapy.

F. Organ Function Studies

Although involvement of other organs is considered as part of the minor criteria in the diagnosis of myeloma (see Table 26–2), evidence of organ damage is integral to both the assessment and management of the patient. It is essential, therefore, that the patient be carefully evaluated for structural and functional defects of bone, kidney, and, to a lesser extent, other solid organs.

G. Cytogenetic Studies

With the advent of better methods for determining the molecular phenotype of the tumor, specific translocations are found to have biologic and prognostic significance. The main cytogenetic abnormalities in patients with multiple myeloma are translocations involving the IgH locus on 14q32 with various gene partners such as 11q13, 4p16, 16q23, 6p21, and 20q11. These translocations are observed in 60% of patients. Other significant cytogenetic abnormalities are hyperdiploidy (50%– 60%), loss of 13q (50%–60%), additional material in chromosome 1, and del 17p. Overall, the prognostic impact of

CASE HISTORY • *Part 2*

While this patient presents with the common complaint of lower back pain following stress, he also has a moderate anemia with prominent rouleaux formation on his blood smear. Given the high incidence of multiple myeloma in patients over age 50, this combination of findings should trigger a broader evaluation of this patient including plain films of the pelvis, lower spine, and skull; serum and urine electrophoresis; a full anemia workup panel; and blood chemistries, especially BUN, serum creatinine, and serum calcium.

These studies show the following:

Plain films - osteopenia of the vertebral bodies without compression and several lytic lesions in the skull and pelvis

Monoclonal IgG κ (M-component) of 45 g/L; monoclonal free κ light chain in the urine

Marrow aspirate/biopsy - Infiltration of the marrow by a uniform population of $CD138^+$ (by immunohistochemistry) plasma cells (>60%), which stain for IgG κ; other blood laboratories: reticulocyte index less than 1; normal serum iron, total iron-binding capacity (TIBC), and serum ferritin; negative stool guaiac; normal chemistries except for a modestly elevated BUN and serum calcium.

Questions

- What diagnosis can be made from these results?
- Is treatment indicated and, if so, what strategy should be used?
- Are there other tests that can help guide management?

these abnormalities is difficult to appreciate since they can overlap in a single patient or appear during the course of the disease. Nevertheless, patients with a t(4;14), t(14;16), $13q^-$, 1q+, del 17p do worse than patients with a t(11;14) or hyperdiploidy. Patients with 11q13 and 6p21 translocations have a better prognosis. These cytogenetic abnormalities are currently used in the risk stratification of multiple myeloma (Table 26–3).

Therapy and Clinical Course

The course of multiple myeloma is very heterogeneous. Some patients who present with a low tumor burden and stable or slowly growing disease are referred to as smoldering myeloma, whereas others evolve rapidly to full-blown symptomatic disease. Two staging methods of use in planning therapy and predicting survival have been described and validated in the last decades. The first, the **Durie-Salmon Staging System**, involves the calculation of tumor burden (number of plasma cells) based on the daily synthesis and turnover of the M-component. Together with the presence of anemia, the level of the M-component in blood or urine, calcium and creatinine blood levels, and number of osteolytic bone lesions on skeletal x-rays, patients can be stratified (Table 26–4) according to a 3-stage system—low, intermediate, and high tumor burden. The second and more recent staging method focuses on the albumin and β_2-microglobulin concentrations in serum. This **International Staging System** also appears to be highly predictive of overall survival (Table 26–5).

TABLE 26–5 • The International Staging System for multiple myeloma

Stage	Criteria	Overall Survival
1	β2m[a] <3.5 mg/L and albumin >3.5 g/dL	62 mo
2	β2m <3.5 mg/L and albumin <3.5 g/dL or β2m >3.5 mg/L but <5.5 mg/L and albumin >3.5 g/dL	44 mo
3	β2m >5.5 mg/L	29 mo

[a]*β2m, β_2-microglobulin.*

A. Traditional Therapy

Unlike the lymphomas and leukemias, **multiple myeloma responds poorly to traditional multidrug chemotherapy**. As a result, chemotherapy results in, at best, a 1–2 log reduction in the plasma cell-mass but never leads to cure. Because of this and depending on patient and MM characteristics, it may make sense to delay treatment as long as the disease remains stable and until the patient is at risk of progressive disease or organ damage. When myeloma is diagnosed before onset of symptoms, it may be years before the disease becomes symptomatic and early chemotherapy does not lengthen the time to progression. At the same time, asymptomatic patients should be followed carefully with quantitative serum immunoglobulins, CBC, and tests of renal function and serum calcium every 3–6 months, as well as periodic imaging to determine the rate of progression of bone disease. Early detection of complications is key; patients who are allowed to develop renal failure or severe marrow damage may not respond to subsequent treatment.

Until the past few years, the combination of **melphalan** (6–9 mg/m^2 daily) together with **prednisone** (40–60 mg/d for 4–7 days) cycled every 4–6 weeks was the gold standard for treatment of myeloma. Although this regimen (which began being used in the 1960s) provides a response as judged by a gradual decrease in the quantity of the M-component in about 50%–60% of patients, few will achieve a "complete" remission as judged by disappearance of the M-component. Moreover, the duration of the response is usually less than 1 year, and the median overall survival is about 3 years in clinically overt multiple myeloma. Attempts to improve these results with multidrug and high-dose regimens in the 1980s and 1990s, including combinations of vincristine, doxorubicin, and dexamethasone **(VAD)** or the **M^2** and C-VAMP protocols (vincristine, adriamycin, BCNU, melphalan, cyclophosphamide, and prednisone) have been of little benefit. Although these combinations can provide a more rapid induction response, they do not significantly prolong overall survival.

However, new treatment regimens have been introduced that demonstrate significant improvements in survival and even hold promise for complete remission in some patient subgroups.

TABLE 26–4 • The Durie-Salmon Staging System for multiple myeloma

	Stage I	Stage II	Stage III
Plasma cell concentration (10^{12}/m^2)	<0.6	0.6–1.2	>1.2
Hemoglobin g/dL	>12	10–12	<10
Calcium	85–105 mg/L	106–120 mg/L	>120 mg/L
M-component (g/L)	IgA <30; IgG <50	IgA 30–50; IgG 50–70	IgA >50; IgG >70
Bence Jones proteinuria	<4 g/24 h	4–12 g/24 h	>12 g/24 h
Osteolytic lesions	0–1 visible lesion	2 visible lesions	≥3 visible lesions
Median overall survival[a]	60 mo	45 mo	25 mo

[a]*With standard (eg, melphalan/prednisone) treatment.*

B. Newer Therapies

The efficacy of multiple myeloma treatment has been greatly improved during the last 2 decades by several major advances, including intensive chemotherapy with autologous stem cell support, and new drugs including thalidomide, lenalidomide (Revlimid), bortezomib (Velcade), and bisphosphonates.

1. Intensive treatment with autologous stem cell rescue—Patients receiving intensive chemotherapy, mainly high-dose melphalan (140–200 mg/m^2) with or without total body irradiation, followed by autologous stem cell rescue (ASCR) have a 12- to 18-month gain in overall survival when compared with less intensive chemotherapy regimens. Subsequent trials have attempted to define the best intensive regimen schedule and timing of the ASCR. All of these trials have confirmed a clear-cut benefit regarding overall survival for patients eligible for this procedure.

The failure of these regimens to cure the patient are due to the persistence of monoclonal plasma cells after induction chemotherapy, and possibly also because of the inevitable reinfusion of some tumor cells harvested from the patient as part of the ASCR procedure. Despite attempts to purge plasma cell precursors from **peripheral blood collections of CD34$^+$ progenitor cells**, a constant relapse rate is observed, suggesting that the failure to eradicate myeloma cells by chemotherapy is the primary cause for relapse. Nevertheless, the increase in median overall survival to 42–66 months makes this procedure the best choice for MM patients under age 65.

Allogeneic transplantation has also been evaluated in selected patients, mostly those with relapsing or refractory disease. This procedure is of limited feasibility given the older age and general status of most MM patients, and the frequent lack of availability of a compatible HLA-matched donor. The few studies so far available show that some patients escaping the lethal complications of the procedure may expect to be cured. Non-myeloablative allogeneic transplantation following a single autologous transplantation has also been studied with some benefit in selected patients.

2. Newer chemotherapy drugs for MM—Three drugs have demonstrated major efficacy in myeloma patients during the last decade. The first one is thalidomide, an immunomodulatory drug, which has shown impressive results in myeloma patients when given alone or in combination with dexamethasone and/or traditional chemotherapy. The treatment-limiting toxicity is the development of a sensory neuropathy, and there is also an increased risk of thromboembolic episodes, but myelosuppression does not occur. A large, controlled trial has established that the addition of thalidomide 200 g/d to the classical melphalan/prednisone regimen (MPT) can improve the response rate and, more importantly, extend the median overall survival to 51.6 months as compared to 33 months with melphalan/prednisone alone. Given these results, the MPT regimen is now considered the new gold standard first-line treatment for elderly patients not eligible for intensive chemotherapy/ASCR.

Lenalidomide, an analog of thalidomide, and bortezomib, a proteasome inhibitor, have also shown significant efficacy in association with high-dose dexamethasone in advanced-stage myeloma patients. Based on current studies, lenalidomide (Revlimid) is administered orally (25 mg/d on days 1–21 each month) together with sequential dexamethasone (40 mg/m^2/d on days 1–4, 9–12, and 17–20). Compared with thalidomide, lenalidomide displays less neurotoxicity but a comparable risk of thromboembolic events. Both drug dosages should be reduced in patients with renal failure. Bortezomib (Velcade) can be administered at a dose of 1.3 mg/m^2/d intravenously on days 1, 4, 8, and 11, in association with dexamethasone 40 mg/d on days 1–2, 4–5, 8–9, and 11–12, for 2–8 three-week courses. Peripheral neuropathy and myelosuppression are the main limiting toxicities. Both regimens display high efficacy in both relapsing/refractory and previously untreated patients. In the latter setting, current results with these regimens compare well with intensive treatments including autologous stem cell transplantation.

C. Management of Complications

Among the hematologic malignancies, multiple myeloma stands out for its destructive action on bone resulting in severe pain and disability. During the course of their disease, most patients will have severe and sometimes intractable pain secondary to progressive osteolysis and pathologic fractures. **Adequate pain relief** should therefore be a very important aspect in caring for these patients. At the same time, the prevention, or at the very least inhibition, of lytic bone lesions is becoming more of a reality. The bisphosphonates are potent inhibitors of osteolysis and are now widely used in the control of myeloma bone disease. The bisphosphonate, **pamidronate**, given in a dose of 90 mg as a 4-hour intravenous infusion every 4 weeks for 6 or more cycles, can reduce the incidence of bone fractures, prevent hypercalcemia, and decrease the patient's bone pain. The mechanism of action is unclear but may involve OPG stimulation and inhibition of RANKL activity. This has led to a search for other RANKL and MIP-1 inhibitors for use as therapeutic agents.

Fractures heal normally, and therefore their management does not differ from standard orthopedic procedures. Vertebral collapse should be treated as an emergency. In the absence of spinal cord or nerve root compression, high-dose steroid and local irradiation should be started immediately. However, any neurologic symptoms of spinal or nerve compression require a surgical consult for laminectomy or decompression.

Hypercalcemia and acute renal failure usually improve rapidly with treatment. Patients with **mild hypercalcemia (≤120 mg/L)** can usually be managed with hydration, steroids, and antimyeloma chemotherapy. More **severe hypercalcemia**, levels of 120–140 mg/L or higher, need to be treated as an emergency. Following aggressive hydration (3 or more liters of 0.9% saline over 12–24 hours) and a loop diuretic (furosemide 20–40 mg every 12 hours), pamidronate or calcitonin or both should be administered.

The **dose of the bisphosphonate pamidronate** is 60–90 mg and can be administered intravenously over 4–24 hours. The onset of effect is apparent within 3–4 days, with a maximal effect at about 10 days. The duration of effect can persist for 7–30 days. Repeated doses are effective for intractable hypercalcemic conditions. Recent data suggest that pamidronate may also slow the progression of the underlying myeloma and increase survival. **Calcitonin** is a peptide hormone that rapidly inhibits bone resorption and decreases renal calcium reabsorption, perhaps through its effect on parathormone secretion. It is administered in a dose of 4 IU/kg body weight, subcutaneously every 12 hours.

CASE HISTORY • Part 3

The patient clearly has multiple myeloma with osteolytic lesions, a significant M-component in both serum and urine, a marrow damage anemia, hypercalcemia, and mild renal dysfunction. Based on these findings, he fits into the Durie-Salmon intermediate-stage II (see Table 26–4). A measurement of the β_2-microglobulin level is indicated as another guide to staging and management. This was reported as 5.2 mg/L, a level indicating stage 2 disease, according to the International Staging System (see Table 26–5).

Given his age, disease stage, and evidence of organ damage, he should be treated aggressively. Immediate hydration and diuretic therapy should correct his modest hypercalcemia as well as lower his BUN. He should then be treated with lenalidomide/dexamethasone or MPT. His management should include careful monitoring for any progression of his bone disease, changes in renal function, infection, or neurological complication. If his back pain becomes localized and is the major complaint, it should respond well to targeted radiation therapy.

MPT or lenalidomide/dexamethasone therapy should give him an expected median survival of 4–5 years. Because of his age and renal function, high-dose chemotherapy with ASCR carries a considerable risk of early morbidity and mortality and does not offer a promise of longer survival.

The dosage can be increased to 8 IU/kg every 6–12 hours after a day or two if the response is unsatisfactory. Since tachyphylaxis is expected, calcitonin is only used to stabilize the hypercalcemic patient until pamidronate takes effect.

Most myeloma patients develop a **symptomatic anemia** as their disease progresses. The underlying mechanism is multifactorial, involving both marrow damage and a relative failure of the erythropoietin response to the anemia. Both renal compromise and overexpression of cytokines, especially IL-6 and tumor necrosis factor (TNF)-related apoptosis-inducing ligand (TRAIL), inhibit hepcidin and suppress the erythropoietin response (see Chapters 3 and 4). Stem cell damage from chemotherapy only makes the situation worse. Fortunately, the anemia of myeloma will usually respond to pharmacologic doses of erythropoietin. Anemic patients should be treated with recombinant erythropoietin (Epogen) 40,000 U once a week subcutaneously (SC), or darbopoietin 200 μg every 2 weeks until the hematocrit rises above 36%.

Symptomatic **hyperviscosity** with mucocutaneous bleeding, and ocular (retinal hemorrhages and papilledema), neurologic (headache, dizziness, and somnolence), and cardiovascular (high-output cardiac failure) manifestations may be seen in 2%–6% of myeloma patients, invariably those with higher levels of serum immunoglobulin: greater than 40 g/L of IgG or greater than 60 g/L of IgA. These symptoms and signs resolve rapidly with a reduction in the level of serum paraprotein by plasmapheresis and chemotherapy.

D. Treatment of Plasmacytomas

Patients with a solitary plasmacytoma involving soft tissue can be effectively cured with a minimum of 4.5 Gy of local irradiation. This is not true for solitary plasmacytomas of bone, most likely because the disease is already more widespread, although not detectable by standard staging procedures (bone imaging and marrow sampling). These patients will eventually go on to develop full-blown multiple myeloma and should be managed as such.

SECONDARY MONOCLONAL GAMMOPATHY

A **secondary monoclonal gammopathy** is occasionally observed as an incidental laboratory finding in patients who have another disorder such as autoimmune disease; immunodeficiency, either primary or acquired; AIDS; chronic infections; carcinoma; and lymphoma. Approximately 2%–5% of patients with B-cell non-Hodgkin lymphoma (NHL) or lymphocytic leukemia will have a detectable M-component. The **important clinical issue** is to determine if the patient has occult NHL, carcinoma, or multiple myeloma, and if the patient is likely to develop overt myeloma in the future. These patients should undergo the same diagnostic evaluation as the patient suspected of myeloma, including CBC, marrow examination for clonal plasma cells or NHL, renal function studies, and examination for lytic bone lesions. In addition, such patients should be followed at close intervals with quantitation of their M-component.

It is unusual for the M-component to increase in cases of secondary gammopathy. Although these patients may have increased plasma cells in their marrow, they are usually polyclonal or oligoclonal by flow cytometry, and karyotypic abnormalities are rare. Anemia or osteopenia that cannot be explained on the basis of the underlying disorder should increase the level of suspicion that the patient may have myeloma rather than secondary gammopathy.

MONOCLONAL GAMMOPATHY OF UNKNOWN SIGNIFICANCE

Many older patients with a small M-component will, on complete evaluation, be found to not fit the criteria for multiple myeloma, nor to have any underlying disorder associated with secondary gammopathy. They usually have less than 10% marrow plasmacytosis, no anemia, and no bone lesions, hypercalcemia, or renal dysfunction.

Monoclonal gammopathy of unknown significance (MGUS) is a common finding in adults; its frequency increases from 2% in the fifth decade to more than 6% beyond 80 years of age. When this group of patients was first recognized it was questioned whether they had a different disease, perhaps one that was not malignant because they frequently remain free from progression for many years. Cytogenetic studies have shown, however, that translocations are common findings in MGUS, as they are in multiple myeloma. They typically involve 14q32 (46%) with most frequent gene partners being 11q13 (25%), 4p16 (9%), and 16q23 (5%). Other genetic abnormalities are hyperdiploidy and 13q deletions, the frequency of which is similar in MGUS and multiple myeloma.

Long-term follow-up of MGUS patients has shown that up to 26% of patients will progress to overt multiple myeloma, amyloidosis, Waldenström macroglobulinemia, or other B-cell lymphoproliferative disorders at a rate of about 1% per year. Interestingly, the M-component disappears spontaneously in 2% of patients. Since it is not possible to predict which patients will convert to MM, all MGUS patients should be followed with yearly measurements of serum and urine M-component. No treatment is advised until the onset of symptoms or clear progression in terms of increased M-component or organ damage.

POEMS SYNDROME

The acronym POEMS refers to a monoclonal plasma cell disorder characterized by Polyneuropathy, Organomegaly, Endocrinopathy, an M protein, and Skin changes. Less frequent symptoms are erythrocytosis or lymph node hyperplasia reminiscent of Castleman disease. POEMS patients, by definition, must have a serum (and urine) M-component, usually of modest amount: 1–2 g/L of an IgG or IgA protein containing almost always a monoclonal λ light chain. Most of these patients also present with a single sclerotic bone lesion or a mixture of several sclerotic and lytic lesions; plasma cells in the marrow rarely exceed 20%.

Treatment of POEMS syndrome is based on focal radiation therapy for localized osteosclerotic bone lesions; systemic therapy similar to myeloma treatment is proposed for widespread disease. The median overall survival was 13.8 years in the largest cohort so far studied.

AMYLOIDOSIS

One dreaded complication of plasma cell dyscrasias is amyloidosis (AL). This clinical syndrome is caused by the tissue accumulation of large amounts of insoluble glycoproteins. The glycoprotein is usually a degradation product of larger proteins that have in common the ability to form β-pleated sheets. Several such proteins can give rise to amyloid deposits in a variety of clinical settings. The one most likely to cause amyloidosis in a patient with a plasma cell disorder is the immunoglobulin light chain (AL). Patients with **overproduction of immunoglobulin light chains**, especially λ light chain, are at risk for the gradual accumulation of amyloid deposits that can cause a variety of signs and symptoms.

Clinical Features

In some cases, AL is discovered during the workup of a patient with a known plasma cell dyscrasia. The more difficult diagnostic situation is when a patient with no previous plasma cell disease presents with symptoms related to amyloidosis. It requires a high degree of suspicion to make the correct diagnosis. Any patient found to have amyloid pathology should have a **thorough workup for a plasma cell disorder**. The patient may have asymptomatic myeloma with a small M-component or only free light chains. Common clinical presentations and/or symptoms of amyloidosis are listed in Table 26–6. A severe bleeding tendency

TABLE 26–6 • Diseases frequently associated with amyloidosis

Classification	Diseases	Common Clinical Manifestations
AL amyloidosis (primary or Ig light chain associated)	Multiple myeloma and other monoclonal gammopathy Lymphoma	Macroglossia, cardiomyopathy, hepatosplenomegaly, nephrotic syndrome, carpal tunnel syndrome, peripheral neuropathy, purpura, and ecchymoses
AA amyloidosis	Tuberculosis Hansen disease Bronchiectasis Chronic osteomyelitis Inflammatory bowel disease Rheumatoid arthritis Carcinoma	Usually: hepatosplenomegaly, nephrotic syndrome, adrenal insufficiency Less frequently: AL manifestations
	Familial Mediterranean fever	Recurrent fever, arthritis, pleuritis, and abdominal pain; glomerulonephritis, renal failure
Aβ2m amyloidosis	Long-term hemodialysis	Hepatosplenomegaly, nephrotic syndrome, adrenal insufficiency
ATTR (transthyretin) amyloidosis	Senile systemic or familial amyloidosis	Neuropathy, cardiomyopathy, nephropathy, vitreous opacities
Other amyloid proteins (Apo AI/II, gelsolin, lysozyme fibrinogen, cystatin C, Aβ, AprP, ABri)	Hereditary amyloidosis	Peripheral neuropathy, autonomic dysfunction, nephropathy, cardiomyopathy, dementia
Aβ amyloid (cerebral)	Alzheimer disease	Dementia

is seen in up to 10% of patients with AL amyloid disease as a result of acquired factor X deficiency, secondary to absorption of factor X onto amyloid fibrils.

Diagnosis

The best diagnostic amyloid test is a blind **biopsy of subcutaneous fat** that should be stained with **Congo red** and examined under a polarizing microscope. Amyloid deposits give a birefringent, green staining pattern that is diagnostic and can be observed in every tissue involved. If a patient has signs or symptoms in a region amenable to needle biopsy, it may be wiser to seek the diagnosis there. On echocardiogram, an interventricular septum thicker than 15 mm and with bright echogenicity is highly suggestive of amyloid cardiomyopathy.

Amyloidosis can also arise from the deposition of proteins unrelated to a clone of plasma cells. **AA amyloidosis** is seen with chronic infections (especially tuberculosis and Hansen disease), chronic inflammatory diseases, and carcinomas, though rarely to an extent that results in major organ damage, unlike AL. AA patients present with hepatosplenomegaly, nephrotic syndrome, or adrenal insufficiency (see Table 26–6). A family history may reveal evidence of one of the familial forms of amyloid, especially in persons of Mediterranean heritage. A number of other proteins have been implicated in small numbers of patients with amyloidosis (see Table 26–6) and, infrequently, no underlying cause for the amyloid is found. In cases such as renal amyloidosis, it may be difficult to tell if the amyloid deposits are the cause or the result of chronic renal failure.

Therapy and Clinical Course

Because of their insoluble nature, it is very difficult to remove amyloid deposits or to reverse their formation. Treatment of the underlying disease may slow or stop amyloid deposition with very slow improvement in symptoms. Thus, patients with amyloid related to a **plasma cell disorder** should be treated with high-dose melphalan and autologous transplantation, if cardiac status permits. Otherwise, they should receive lower dose melphalan, together with high-dose dexamethasone. This is a reasonably effective regimen with partial responses in more than 60% of patients. Patients with **cardiac involvement** or orthostatic hypotension have a very poor prognosis, with median survival on the order of 6 months. By contrast, amyloid glomerulopathy, when isolated, is not associated with a poor prognosis and is amenable to treatment. Combination therapy using steroids with thalidomide (and also bortezomib) have recently demonstrated impressive efficacy in overt AL amyloidosis, including cardiac disease.

HEAVY AND LIGHT CHAIN DISEASES

As mentioned earlier, about 20% of patients with plasma cell disorders produce only monoclonal **light chains**. Such patients may have deposits of intact light chains, usually in the kidneys and other organs. These deposits are not amyloid and do not stain with Congo red. **Light-chain deposition disease** (LCDD) can present with renal failure or nephrotic syndrome as the major clinical manifestation, but it may be difficult to demonstrate monoclonal light chains in either serum or urine by electrophoresis. However, light-chain analysis (including ratio) in serum is usually diagnostic. Other organs are also vulnerable to LCDD, including the pulmonary and cerebral parenchyma. Increased numbers of plasma cells with the appropriate light-chain expression can be demonstrated in the marrow by flow cytometry. The approach to diagnosis and treatment is the same as for MM.

Much less commonly, patients may produce only free **heavy chains** or fragments of heavy chains. The production of α chains is most commonly reported, although free λ and μ chains have also been found. These abnormal proteins may be difficult to demonstrate in the serum or urine and may accumulate in the tissues in a manner analogous to light chains. α-Heavy chain disease most often affects the GI tract and is now referred to as *I*mmuno-*P*roliferative *S*mall *I*ntestine *D*isease (IPSID). This disease follows a course that closely resembles a malabsorption syndrome evolving to a lymphoma affecting gut-associated lymphoid tissue, rather than a plasma cell dyscrasia.

WALDENSTRÖM MACROGLOBULINEMIA

Although usually discussed in connection with plasma cell disorders, Waldenström macroglobulinemia is more accurately classified as a lymphoplasmacytic lymphoma. The only feature that it shares with the plasma cell disorders is the presence of an M-component. Unlike myeloma, this component is always of the IgM class. The presentation, diagnosis, staging, clinical course, and therapy of macroglobulinemia are similar to the non-Hodgkin B-cell lymphomas (see Chapter 23). Unlike myeloma, it does not present with bone pain, renal failure, lytic lesions, or hypercalcemia. The major organ involvement in macroglobulinemia is the marrow, spleen, and other lymphoid tissues.

Clinical Features

Macroglobulinemia is more common in older patients (median age 60 years). Many patients remain asymptomatic, even with an M-component as high as 30–40 g/L. However, most patients present with fatigue, weight loss, anemia, mucocutaneous bleeding, lymphadenopathy, hepatosplenomegaly, or symptoms related to hyperviscosity (Table 26–7). Because of the higher molecular weight of IgM, the M-component is primarily confined to the vascular space and does not cause renal failure. However, neuropathy and hyperviscosity are common complications of macroglobulinemia; up to one-third of patients will develop symptoms and signs of hyperviscosity as their serum M component rises to levels above 30 g/L.

Some specific clinical presentations depend on the physical properties of the IgM antibody. **Cold agglutinin disease** is the consequence of anti-I specificity (see Chapter 11), with some patients developing hemolytic anemia, often intravascular on exposure to cold. Antibody specificity against **myelin-associated glycoprotein** (MAG) is associated with neuropathy, including

TABLE 26–7 • Symptoms and signs of hyperviscosity

Organ System	Symptoms and Signs
Ocular	Retinal hemorrhage
	Papilledema
	Dilated retinal veins (boxcar changes)
Neurologic (central)	Headache
	Tinnitus
	Vertigo/dizziness
	Mental status changes
Neurologic (peripheral)	Neuropathy
Cardiac	High-output congestive failure

distal symmetric paresthesia, paresia, and tremor. Nerve conduction velocity is reduced, similar to demyelinating neuropathies. Some monoclonal IgM antibodies behave as **cryoglobulins** that precipitate when exposed to temperatures lower than 36°C. These cryoglobulins are classified as monoclonal IgM without (type 1) or with anti-rheumatoid factor activity (type 2). Type 3 cryoglobulin is a separate entity of polyclonal IgM with rheumatoid activity. These cryoglobulins can present as vasculitis following cold exposure, with vascular purpura, urticaria, Raynaud syndrome, glomerulonephritis, peripheral neuropathy, and arthritis. Interference of M-components with platelet adhesion or fibrin formation can induce bleeding.

Diagnosis

Patients with Waldenström macroglobulinemia will invariably have an IgM M-component, although it may not be quantitatively large. The pentameric nature of IgM may give rise to hyperviscosity phenomena at much lower concentrations than IgG or IgA. The typical IgM M-component in this disorder is between 10 and 30 g/L. The marrow is infiltrated by small lymphocytes with variable degrees of "plasmacytoid" features such as eccentric nuclei, basophilic cytoplasm, and prominent Golgi, and there is an increased number of mast cells. These plasmacytoid lymphocytes invariably express surface IgM, more often κ, and unlike typical plasma cells they express the monoclonal immunoglobulin both on their surface and in their cytoplasm. Abnormal, clonal lymphocytes are usually demonstrable in blood, in contrast with myeloma, where blood lymphocytes are polyclonal, and plasma cells are only observed in blood in the terminal phase.

The CBC is usually normal as long as the M-component remains below 20 g/L. Above this value, a dilutional normocytic, normochromic anemia due to plasma volume increase is frequent. Patients suspected of macroglobulinemia should have a marrow examination or biopsy of involved lymphoid tissues, and an evaluation identical to that performed in patients with other B-cell non-Hodgkin lymphomas (see Chapter 23).

Hyperviscosity can be suspected when the fundoscopic examination shows clumping of red blood cells in the retinal veins (so-called sausage or boxcar segmentation), papilledema, or retinal hemorrhages (see Table 26–7). The serum viscosity level can confirm the diagnosis of hyperviscosity. Compared to water (1.4–1.8 cp), a serum viscosity that exceeds 4–5 cp is almost invariably associated with symptomatic hyperviscosity. However, this assay is not required for the diagnosis when symptoms of hyperviscosity are present, especially if the M-component is greater than 30–40 g/L.

Therapy

Hyperviscosity should be treated promptly as it is life threatening. Hydration, with careful attention to the possibility of congestive heart failure, plasmapheresis, and institution of chemotherapy, will usually control the syndrome. Because the IgM protein is confined to the intravascular space, plasmapheresis can rapidly lower the concentration of M-component. For long-term control, cytotoxic chemotherapy must be added.

Patients who have relatively small M-components and mild or no symptoms should be observed closely with repeated quantitation in order to determine the rate of disease progression. Some patients may be asymptomatic for several years. Patients with a progressive increase in their M-component or the onset of anemia or other symptoms should be treated with a single alkylating agent, usually chlorambucil or cyclophosphamide, or in combination with prednisone or the purine analog fludarabine—therapies appropriate for NHL. The goal of therapy is to control disease progression and decrease the M-component. The additional toxicity of multiagent chemotherapy is problematic in most older patients, and the outcomes for aggressive therapy have not justified its use.

The median survival of patients with full-blown macroglobulinemia is 5–10 years, but is worse in patients older than 65 or with the presence of lymphadenopathy or organomegaly.

POINTS TO REMEMBER

Plasma cells are the end product of stepwise differentiation of B-cell progenitors. Each plasma cell is programmed to produce approximately 1 ng/d of a single antibody with either λ or κ light chain, but never both. This fact is useful in identifying clonal populations of plasma cells where all of the cells show either λ or κ light chains instead of the normal 40:60 mix.

Plasma cell dyscrasia is defined as a clonal proliferation of plasma cells, with multiple myeloma being the most common malignancy, especially in older age groups where the incidence greatly exceeds that of other hematopoietic malignancies.

Patients with multiple myeloma often present with common and/or minor complaints of back pain, fatigue, or anemia that have other ready explanations. Because of this, the diagnosis is often missed until the patient presents with major organ damage. Therefore, a high degree of suspicion and careful investigation are necessary to reach a correct diagnosis.

Accurate diagnosis and staging requires a panel of tests including CBC; bone marrow aspirate and biopsy for morphology, flow cytometry, and karyotyping; imaging of the skull, long bones, and spine; measurement of the M-component in blood and urine; studies of renal function; serum calcium; and β_2-microglobulin level.

Two staging systems can help in planning therapy. The Durie-Salmon system uses the major and minor diagnostic criteria (see Table 26–4) to classify patients as stage I, II, or III, while the International Staging System (see Table 26–5) relies on the β_2-microglobulin and albumin levels to derive a similar 3-level stage.

Plasma cells are relatively resistant to standard chemotherapy. However, combinations of chemotherapy and autologous stem cell rescue plus the use of newer drugs—thalidomide, lenalidomide, and bortezomib—have shown the ability to diminish or even eliminate the M-component and to significantly increase survival times in MM.

The complications of myeloma are related to the effect of the disease on the marrow, especially with replacement of normal medullary elements; bony changes with expansion of tumor mass; and the properties of the monoclonal immunoglobulin itself.

In the marrow, erythropoiesis is most commonly affected, producing a normochromic, normocytic anemia. Studies to rule out iron deficiency are warranted, and the anemia of myeloma generally responds to erythropoietin until very late stages. Leukocyte and platelet production are not usually affected until chemotherapy.

Bone disease is a frequent complication of multiple myeloma. Patients may present with widespread lytic lesions, hypercalcemia, or osteopenia, or a single large bony lesion, including plasmacytoma of bone. Bone pain may be caused by pathologic fractures or by heavy invasion of the bone by the malignancy without fracture. Neurologic signs indicating nerve entrapment is a medical emergency. Bone disease and hypercalcemia can be significantly ameliorated by bisphosphonate therapy.

The monoclonal paraprotein may cause pathology because of its specificity (causing hemolytic anemia or neuropathy) or because of its predilection to organ involvement. The kidneys are commonly affected by myeloma, with both tubular and glomerular involvement. Light-chain deposition disease may occur in the parenchyma of the kidneys, brain, heart, and lungs.

Large concentrations of IgG and IgA paraprotein may cause hyperviscosity, similar to smaller concentrations of the pentameric-capable IgM in Waldenström macroglobulinemia. Some light-chain paraproteins with β-pleated sheet confirmation can precipitate in tissue parenchyma as amyloid, causing irreversible cardiac, mucosal, and renal damage.

Patients often have a small M-component without evidence of organ damage, thereby not meeting the diagnostic criteria for myeloma, so-called monoclonal gammopathy of unknown significance (MGUS). This early-stage plasma cell dyscrasia progresses to myeloma at about 1% per year and should be followed for organ damage or an increase in the paraprotein.

Waldenström macroglobulinemia is a lymphoplasmacytic lymphoproliferative disease characterized by an IgM M-component but without the MM features of bony disease, hypercalcemia, and renal failure. It clinically resembles a B-cell non-Hodgkin lymphoma (NHL).

Waldenström macroglobulinemia is sensitive to NHL chemotherapy. Periods of remission can be suddenly interrupted by a dramatic increase in serum viscosity secondary to a rising IgM level. This is a medical emergency, requiring aggressive plasmapheresis and subsequent chemotherapy.

BIBLIOGRAPHY

Diagnosis

Al-Saleem T, Al-Mondhiry H: Immunoproliferative small intestinal disease (IPSID): a model for mature B-cell neoplasms. Blood 2005;105:2274.

Bladé J, Rosiñol L: Complications of multiple myeloma. Hematol Oncol Clin N Am 2007;21:1231.

Dispenzieri A, Kyle RA, Lacy MQ, et al: POEMS syndrome: definitions and long-term outcome. Blood 2003;101:2496.

Greipp PR, San Miguel J, Duric BGM, et al: International Staging System for multiple myeloma. J Clin Oncol 2005;23:1.

Guidelines Working Group of UK Myeloma Forum; British Committee for Standards in Haematology, British Society for Haematology. Guidelines on the diagnosis and management of AL amyloidosis. Br J Haematol 2004;125:681.

Huff CA, Matsui W: Multiple myeloma cancer stem cells. J Clin Oncol 2008;26:2895.

Kyle RA, Rajkumar SV: Monoclonal gammopathy of undetermined significance and smoldering multiple myeloma. Hematol Oncol Clin N Am 2007;21:1093.

Kyle RA, Rajkumar SV: Multiple myeloma. Blood 2008; 111:2962.

Kyle RA, Remstein ED, Therneau TM, et al: Clinical course and prognosis of smoldering (asymptomatic) multiple myeloma. N Engl J Med 2007;356:2582.

Lentzsch S, Ehrlich LA, G. Roodman D: Pathophysiology of multiple myeloma bone disease. Hematol Oncol Clin N Am 2007;21:1035.

Mehta J, Singhal S: Hyperviscosity syndrome in plasma cell dyscrasia syndromes. Semin Thromb and Hemost 2003;29:467.

Merlini G, Bellotti V: Molecular mechanisms of amyloidosis. N Engl J Med 2003;349:583.

Mitsiades CS, McMillin DW, Klippel S, et al: The role of the bone marrow microenvironment in the pathophysiology of myeloma and its significance in the development of more effective therapies. Hematol Oncol Clin N Am 2007;21:1007.

Stewart AK, Fonseca R: Prognostic and therapeutic significance of myeloma genetics and gene expression profiling. J Clin Oncol 2005;23:6339.

Tonon G: Molecular pathogenesis of multiple myeloma. Hematol Oncol Clin N Am 2007;21:985.

Therapy

Dispenzieri A: Complications of myeloma therapy. Hematol Oncol Clin N Am 2007;21:1247.

Facon T, Mary JY, Hulin C, et al: Melphalan and prednisone plus thalidomide vs melphalan and prednisone alone or reduced-intensity autologous stem cell transplantation in elderly patients with multiple myeloma (IFM 99-06): a randomised trial. Lancet 2007;370:1209.

Kastritis E, Mitsiades CS, Dimopoulos MA, Richardson PG: Management of relapsed and relapsed refractory myeloma. Hematol Oncol Clin N Am 2007;21:1175.

Rajkumar SV, Palumbo A: Management of newly diagnosed myeloma. Hematol Oncol Clin N Am 2007;21:1141.

San-Miguel J, Harousseau JL, D Joshua D, Anderson KC: Individualizing treatment of patients with myeloma in the era of novel agents. J Clin Oncol 2008;26:2761.

Soutar R, Lucraft H, Jackson G, et al: Guidelines on the diagnosis and management of solitary plasmacytoma of bone and solitary extramedullary plasmacytoma. Brit J Haematol 2004; 124:717.

Treon SP, Gertz MA, Dimopoulos M, et al: Update on treatment recommendations from the Third International Workshop on Waldenström's Macroglobulinemia. Blood 2006;107:3442.

van Rhee F, Dhodapkar M, Shaughnessy JD, et al: First thalidomide clinical trial in multiple myeloma: a decade. Blood 2008;112:1035.

MONOCYTE-MACROPHAGE DISORDERS • 27

CASE HISTORY • *Part I*

A 45-year-old man is referred by his orthopedic surgeon following the development of a pathological fracture of the neck of the femur after a fall on ice. X-rays taken at the time of the fracture show an abnormality of the ends of the long bones resembling an inverted Erlenmeyer flask.

The patient has otherwise been in good health. He is of Ashkenazi Jewish descent with a small family and is unaware of any genetic disorders in his family.

Examination is notable for an enlarged spleen, which is easily palpable several centimeters below the costal margin, and hepatomegaly. The remainder of his physical examination is normal.

His complete blood count (CBC) is normal with the exception of a moderately reduced platelet count of 80,000/μL.

Questions

- Given this limited amount of information, what diagnoses come to mind?
- What additional tests and procedures are necessary to evaluate this patient?

The mature cells that comprise the **monocyte-macrophage system** function both as phagocytes and as antigen-presenting cells. Disorders of the monocyte/macrophage lineage are quite heterogeneous and include "benign" disorders such as Langerhans-cell histiocytosis, reactive histiocytosis, and the lysosomal storage diseases, as well as monocytic and histiocytic malignant proliferations. In naming these disorders, the term "histiocyte" is used interchangeably with "macrophage" to describe the tissue-bound phagocytic cells found throughout the body.

The morphologic appearance of the tissue macrophage is key to the differential diagnosis of these disorders. For example, **reactive histiocytosis** is characterized by prominent monocytosis and a tissue granulomatous reaction typical of the normal role of macrophages in host defense against infection. The so-called **storage diseases** are a manifestation of genetic deficiencies of certain enzymes responsible for the degradation of carbohydrates and lipids. Even though these enzyme deficiencies presumably affect all the cells in the body, the characteristic abnormality is an accumulation of degraded cellular debris within tissue macrophages. Primary **malignancies of the tissue macrophages** are quite rare; marrow and tissue invasion by erythrophagocytic histiocytes is a primary distinguishing feature of such malignancies.

THE NORMAL MONOCYTE-MACROPHAGE SYSTEM

As with the other hematopoietic cell lines, the monocyte-macrophage cell lineage arises from the common hematopoietic stem cell. Cell differentiation and maturation to form mature circulating monocytes is under the control of **granulocyte macrophage colony-stimulating factor (GM-CSF), granulocyte colony-stimulating factor (G-CSF),** and **monocytic colony-stimulating factor (M-CSF)**. Two distinct categories of blood monocytes are recognized according to their phenotypic expression. All monocytes display CD14, and the majority are CD16$^-$, whereas 10% are more mature and express CD16$^+$ together with class II major histocompatibility complex (MHC) molecules and adhesion molecules such as CCR2 and CX3CL1 (see Chemokines and Their Receptors in Chapter 16). These "mature" monocytes synthesize proinflammatory cytokines such as interleukin [IL]-1, IL-6, tumor necrosis factor [TNF]-α and IL-12. When activated, monocytes also play a role in coagulation and fibrin deposition at inflammatory sites, through expression of tissue factor and binding to activated platelets via P-selectin glycoprotein ligand-1 (PSGL-1) (see Chapter 28).

Monocytes migrate into tissues and transform into tissue macrophages/histiocytes, which are then named based on their distinctive morphology within individual tissues. These are then specifically referred to as alveolar macrophages, hepatic Kupffer cells, dermal Langerhans cells, and marrow reticuloendothelial cells. These tissue macrophages display many distinct membrane receptors. **Pattern recognition receptors, also called toll-like receptors**, are able to recognize highly conserved pathogen-associated molecular patterns (PAMP), which are highly conserved motifs involved in innate immunity. Monocyte **Fc receptors** (see also Chapter 17) interact with the Fc portion of the immunoglobulin molecules, the best characterized being receptors for IgG referred to as FcγRI (CD64), II (CD32), and III (CD16). These monocyte receptors differ according to their immunoglobulin (Ig) affinity and the specific nature of subsequent signal transduction. Through this Fc-receptor binding, monocytes recognize immune complexes, as well as opsonized particles and pathogens. **Complement receptors** CR1 (CD35) and CR3 (CD11b/CD18) on monocytes bind respectively to the C3b/C4b and C3b complexes fixed on opsonized pathogens. Monocytes are also involved in other complement pathways through their **mannose receptors** recognizing mannose oligosaccharides on pathogens. Other important receptors are **"scavenger" receptors** for bacterial lipopolysaccharides and cholesterol from lipoproteins and atherosclerotic plaques; **cytokine receptors** for γ-interferon, M-CSF, and TNF-α; and **transferrin receptor** (CD71).

Using the above receptors, the monocyte-macrophage system has **4 principal functions**: bacterial phagocytosis and killing, antigen presentation to T lymphocytes to initiate the immune reaction, modulation of the inflammatory response, and incorporation of monocytes into clots, where they play a role in fibrinolysis. Only the first 3 functions are clearly associated with clinical disease entities and will be discussed here.

Phagocytosis and Bacterial Killing

Together with neutrophils, monocytes and macrophages actively phagocytize bacteria. With activation, these cells are then able to kill the ingested bacteria by superoxide generation. There are clear similarities and differences in the antimicrobial abilities of the monocyte and macrophage as compared with the neutrophil. For example, the tissue-based macrophage contains much less myeloperoxidase than either the circulating neutrophil or monocyte. These differences are partly responsible for the clinical manifestations of some infections. The formation of granulomas in patients with certain infections, such as tuberculosis, reflects the inability of the tissue macrophage to lyse the mycobacterium. Patients with chronic granulomatous disease have an inherited defect in the ability of the monocyte-macrophages to generate superoxide.

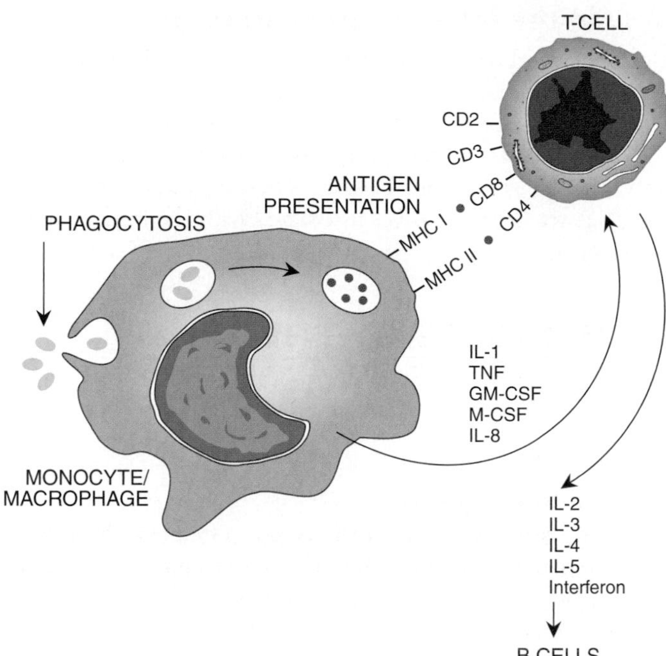

FIGURE 27–1. **Monocyte-macrophage function.** The normal monocyte-macrophage is capable of phagocytosis, ie, the killing of pathogens, and presentation of digested antigen to T cells to eventually promote the full immune response. Monocytes also release several cytokines to stimulate the T-cell response and promote the generalized inflammatory response.

Role in Immunity

Monocytes and tissue macrophages play a key role in both the innate and adaptative immune systems. They process antigen and present it to T lymphocytes (Figure 27–1) in a complex manner. The presentation of antigen involves a shared characteristic of the macrophage and T cell, the expression of both class I and class II MHC molecules. The **class I MHC molecules** are involved in CD8 T-cell interactions, whereas the **class II MHC molecules** play a role in CD4 T-cell interactions (see Chapter 20). According to the type of pathogen and the balance of secreted cytokines, macrophages and dendritic cells can elicit 2 types of T-cell responses. The T_H1 response is associated with stimulation of IL-2, γ-interferon, and TNF-α secretion, which in turn results in activation of the cellular effectors of cytotoxicity. The T_H2 response is associated with IL-4, IL-5, IL-10, and IL-13 secretion, which trigger mostly humoral responses.

Role in the Inflammatory Response

Monocytes and tissue macrophages also play a role in the generalized inflammatory response by the release of cytokines such as GM-CSF, G-CSF, M-CSF, IL-1, IL-8, TNF, and the interferons. They can also secrete proteases such as tissue plasminogen activator, collagenase, and elastase. These enzymes play a role in the tissue structural changes associated with the inflammatory reaction.

DISORDERS OF THE MONOCYTE-MACROPHAGE SYSTEM

Clinical Features

A. Blood Monocytosis

Benign or reactive monocytosis is most often associated with impaired neutrophil production. Classical examples of reactive monocytosis are seen during the recovery phase of a drug-induced agranulocytosis or cyclic neutropenia. In these cases, blood monocytosis is transient and usually mild, and is limited to the days immediately preceding the rebound increase in neutrophils. Chronic, mild monocytosis can be the first manifestation of myelodysplastic or myeloproliferative syndromes (see Chapters 9 and 19), but reactive causes must first be ruled out. Severe, prolonged inflammatory responses (subacute bacterial endocarditis, tuberculosis), lymphoproliferative disease states (Hodgkin disease), and collagen vascular diseases are frequently accompanied by a modest monocytosis, with counts of 500–1,000/μL. In any of these situations, the dominant clinical features are those of the primary illness, not the monocytosis.

B. Tissue Histiocytosis

1. Langerhans cell histiocytic disorders—Langerhans cell histiocytic disorders are non-malignant diseases characterized by histiocytic infiltrates of tissue but with a wide spectrum of clinical presentation. **Hand-Schüller-Christian disease** presents in adolescents or young adults with diabetes insipidus, exophthalmia, and cranial bone defects. **Letterer-Siwe disease** affects children under 5 years of age and presents as a severe life-threatening hepatosplenomegaly with skin infiltrates and pancytopenia. **Eosinophilic bone granuloma** is usually localized to flat bones, mainly the skull, as well-circumscribed single or multiple osteolytic lesions.

2. Non-Langerhans histiocytic disorders—Non-Langerhans **histiocytic disorders** usually present as non-malignant, although severe, histiocytic proliferations. The most striking feature in these disorders is hemophagocytosis by histiocytes in spleen, liver, or bone marrow, so that they are also referred to as **hemophagocytic syndromes**. Common presentations include fever, hepatosplenomegaly, pancytopenia, hepatic dysfunction, and hypofibrinogenemia, all usually severe. However, the hemophagocytic syndromes display a wide clinical heterogeneity. Reactive or secondary **hemophagocytic histiocytosis**, also referred to as **Risdall syndrome**, is often observed as a complication of severe infection in patients with immune defects, systemic diseases, or malignancies (Table 27–1). This complication is usually life threatening, depending on the underlying disease.

TABLE 27–1 • Underlying conditions and agents involved in secondary hemophagocytic histiocytosis

Underlying Diseases	Triggering Agents
Malignant	**Virus**
Non-Hodgkin and Hodgkin lymphoma cancers	HSV/VZV
	Adenovirus
Immunosuppression	HHV6, HHV8
Transplantation	Hep A, B, C
Chemotherapy	Dengue virus
AIDS	Epstein-Barr virus
Liver cirrhosis	Cytomegalovirus
Asplenia	Parvovirus B19
Sysemic diseases	**Bacteria**
Lupus erythematosus	Gram-negative bacillus
Still disease	Gram-positive cocci
Rheumatoid arthritis	*Mycobacterium tuberculosis*
Ulcerative colitis	Intracellular pathogens
Kawasaki disease	**Parasites**
Autoimmune thyroiditis	*Leishmania donovani*
Sarcoidosis	**Protozoans**
Pyoderma gangrenosum	Toxoplasma, Pneumocystis
Systemic sclerosis	**Fungal agents**
	Candida, Aspergillus, Cryptococcus

3. Malignant proliferations of monocyte-histiocyte lineage cells—Patients with **malignancies of the monocyte-macrophage lineage** can present either as a leukemic state or as a wasting illness with marked fever, weight loss, and pancytopenia secondary to organ infiltration with malignant histiocytes. A small percentage of **adult leukemias** demonstrate pure monocyte (M5) morphology (see Chapter 18). Chronic myelomonocytic leukemia is classified on the basis of the chronic monocytosis in blood and marrow (see Chapter 19). Patients who present with a myelodysplastic syndrome may also have an increase in their absolute monocyte count, although patients with myelodysplasia (MDS) with prominent monocytosis do not differ significantly from those with normal monocyte counts (see Chapter 9).

True **malignant histiocytosis** is a very infrequent disease. Formerly, it had been confounded with T-cell non-Hodgkin lymphoma (NHL), especially anaplastic large cell lymphoma, which can now be definitively defined by immunophenotyping and T cell–receptor (TCR) gene rearrangement. However, true malignant histiocytosis, although extremely rare, is a definite entity. It usually presents in adults or elderly patients with hepatosplenomegaly, pancytopenia, lung infiltrates, and liver abnormalities. The diagnosis is made on biopsy, and the prognosis is poor.

4. Lipid-storage disorders—The storage diseases are typically diagnosed during childhood or early adult life based on distinctive abnormalities of the liver, spleen, bone, and central nervous system, including blindness, deafness, and marked motor weakness or spasticity. Dramatic expansion of tissue macrophages is responsible for the hepatosplenomegaly typically seen in patients with Gaucher and Niemann-Pick disease.

Basic Laboratory Studies

A. Complete Blood Count

Diagnosis of a reactive monocytosis or leukemia may be made from the complete blood count (CBC). The normal absolute monocyte count is less than 500/μL. Reactive monocytosis is associated with modest increases in the absolute count to 500–1,500/μL. Very high monocyte counts suggest an acute leukemia, myeloproliferative disorder, or leukemoid reaction.

B. Marrow Aspirate, Biopsy, and Other Tests

Diagnosis of **malignant histiocytosis** or a **lipid-storage disease** can usually be made from the marrow aspirate and biopsy. The key finding is invasion of the marrow structure by morphologically abnormal macrophages. In patients with **Gaucher disease**, the marrow is infiltrated with large macrophages whose cytoplasm is filled with a characteristic pinkish, striated material (crinkled-paper appearance) and a few vacuoles (Figure 27–2). This material is actually an insoluble glycolipid, **glucocerebroside**. Patients with Gaucher disease also show increases in **acid phosphatase activity, serum ferritin, and serum chitotriosidase**, which parallel the disease activity. With increasing splenomegaly, most patients develop a normocytic, normochromic anemia; thrombocytopenia; or pancytopenia secondary to hypersplenism. In a small percentage of patients with Gaucher disease, serum electrophoresis discloses an M-component. It is now recognized that the risk of multiple myeloma is increased in this population.

Patients with **Niemann-Pick disease** can also be diagnosed from the appearance of large, foamy macrophages in the marrow. The droplet-like material in these cells is **sphingomyelin**. Any confusion with Gaucher cells can be eliminated based on the pinkish staining quality with **periodic acid–Schiff stain** and by examining an unstained preparation by phase microscopy. The sphingomyelin droplets within the cells are birefringent under polarized light. The diagnosis is definitively confirmed by the amount of sphingomyelinase in peripheral blood leukocytes.

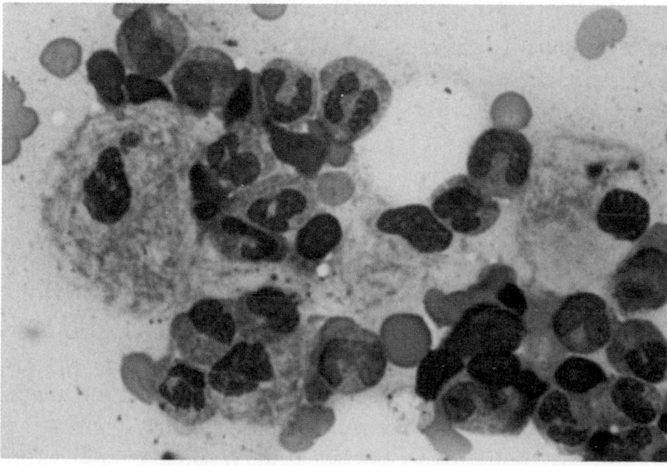

FIGURE 27–2. **Gaucher cells.** Giant histiocytes are noted to contain large amounts of glucocerebroside. Note the abundant cytoplasm with a crinkled-paper or so-called onion-skin appearance.

DIFFERENTIAL DIAGNOSIS

Lipid/Lysosomal-Storage Disorders

A. Gaucher Disease

Gaucher disease is the most common of the lipid-storage disorders. It is an autosomal recessive disease caused by a defect in the production of the enzyme β-glucocerebrosidase, which is encoded by chromosome 1q21. This enzyme is required for the terminal step digestion of glycolipids in the lysosomes of all macrophages. When the enzyme is missing or defective, the extremely insoluble compound glucocerebroside accumulates within the cell's cytoplasm (Table 27–2).

Gaucher disease is most **common in the Ashkenazi Jewish population** where carrier frequency is 8.9% and incidence of clinical disease is 1 in 450. The prevalence of homozygotes or composite heterozygotes in non-Jewish populations is estimated at approximately 1/60,000. More than 200 mutations of the glucocerebrosidase gene have been described. The 4 most common mutations encompass 94% of the Ashkenazi and 52% of the non-Ashkenazi cases. The type of mutation affects the severity of the clinical manifestations, which range from severe disease presenting at infancy to almost asymptomatic forms diagnosed only in adults or the elderly. For instance, the presence of the *N370S* mutation, either as a homozygote or in combination with another mutation, is associated with mild forms of the disease, whereas mutations *L444P*, *84gg*, or *IVS2(+1)* are predictive of severe disease except when combined with *N370S*.

1. Clinical subtypes—Three clinical subtypes of Gaucher disease have been identified (Table 27–3). **Type 1** is the most common, representing more than 99% of cases. It also has the less severe presentation, with disease limited to the macrophages of the spleen, marrow, and liver. **Type 2** disease is much more severe, presenting in early infancy with fulminating neurologic symptoms and early death, usually within 18 months of life.

TABLE 27–2 • Most frequent mutations in Gaucher disease and their phenotypic counterpart

Mutation	*N370S*	*L444P*	*84gg*	*IVS2(+1)*
Type of disease	1	1, 2, 3	1, 3	1, 3
Severity	Mild	Severe	Severe	Severe
Frequency (%)				
Ashkenazi	75	4	12	3
Non-Ashkenazi	18	32	1	1

TABLE 27–3 • Characteristics of Gaucher disease subtypes

	Type 1	Type 2	Type 3
Age at diagnosis	1–70 years	<1 year	2–20 years
Hepatosplenomegaly	++++	±	+
Bone lesions	+++	—	±
Lung disease	±	±	±
Encephalopathy	—	++++	±
Ocular apraxia	—	+	±
Corneal opacities	—	±	±
Life expectancy (years)	60–90	<5	<30

Type 3 disease also presents during childhood with neurologic symptoms. It has a much longer natural history, but its prognosis is as severe as type 2. Heterozygotes for Gaucher disease have one-half the normal enzyme levels and can be accurately diagnosed by genetic analysis. They do not have Gaucher cells in the marrow and are clinically normal.

Patients with type 1 Gaucher disease commonly present at any age with hepatosplenomegaly, bony abnormalities, thrombocytopenia, and progressive liver dysfunction. Establishing the diagnosis is usually easy, providing that every patient presenting with unexplained splenomegaly or thrombocytopenia should have a bone marrow aspiration. The presence in marrow of large numbers of the characteristic Gaucher cells is a strong diagnostic feature (see Figure 27–2). These are very large macrophages filled with glucocerebroside, giving the cytoplasm a crinkled paper or onion-skin appearance. Other unique clinical findings are the development of the Erlenmeyer flask deformity of the ends of long bones, pathologic fractures, and aseptic necrosis of the femoral heads. Patients can also experience episodes of bone pain and swelling without clear radiologic findings.

Gaucher-like cells may be seen in the elderly patient or individual who has a myeloproliferative or lymphoproliferative disorder. On occasion, Gaucher-like cells may be observed in the marrow of patients with mycobacterium infection due to AIDS or other immunosuppression. This presence is not owing to a deficiency of β-glucocerebrosidase, but rather reflects a marked increased uptake of cellular debris by the macrophages, producing an over-stuffed cytoplasm. Gaucher disease activity can be assessed by several biologic markers. Increased serum acid phosphatase, ferritinemia, angiotensin converting enzyme, and chitotriosidase assays are helpful to document disease progression or the efficacy of treatment. Nevertheless, the amount of peripheral blood leukocyte β-glucocerebrosidase is now the gold standard of diagnosis and for following response to therapy. Genotyping for the most prevalent mutations is also necessary for genetic counseling when both parents are heterozygotes.

2. Prenatal and genetic diagnosis—For couples at risk of transmitting a severe form of the disease, that is, when there is a risk of a non-*N370S* mutation, prenatal diagnosis by amniocentesis is possible by measuring β-glucocerebrosidase activity in harvested cells or, better yet, by testing amniotic material for the parental mutations. There is a characteristic restriction length polymorphism associated with each of the most common mutations.

B. Niemann-Pick Disease

Niemann-Pick disease is a less common lysosomal storage disease, but also with a higher incidence in the Ashkenazi Jewish population. The disease transmission is autosomal recessive. The disease encompasses different subtypes, all characterized by the accumulation of sphingomyelin in the macrophage to produce the typical foam cells in marrow, lymph nodes, and other organs. The sphingomyelinase abnormality can also be assessed in peripheral blood leukocytes, skin fibroblasts, and amniotic fluid cells for prenatal diagnosis.

The most frequent types, A and B, result from a sphingomyelinase deficiency, resulting from gene mutations on 11p15.4–p15.1. Type A disease presents in early infancy with hepatosplenomegaly and neurological defects, leading to cachexia and death before 3 years of age. Type B disease has a similar presentation with milder or absent neurologic symptoms, and a chronic course lasting into adulthood. Type C and D disease, due to mutations in the *NPC-1* gene on 18q11–12, are characterized by normal sphingomyelinase activity but display abnormal intracellular cholesterol esterification. The presentation and course of type C and D disease fall between that seen with types A and B, with the disease evolving to death during adolescence. A subtype E has been recently described.

Marrow histiocytes with a pale bluish cytoplasm **(sea-blue histiocytes)** are seen in **Niemann-Pick disease**, but similar cells are observed in patients with **chronic myelogenous leukemia, myeloproliferative disorders, and idiopathic thrombocytopenic purpura**. It is hypothesized that some of the latter could represent partial defects of sphingomyelinase activity leading to increased cell membrane turnover and formation of these morphologically unique foam cells.

Reactive and Leukemic Monocytosis

Any patient who presents with an absolute chronic monocyte count greater than 500/μL must be considered a candidate for a leukemic monocytosis or a myeloproliferative/myelodysplastic syndrome. A full study of the hematopoietic profile with special stains, immunophenotyping, and chromosomal analysis will usually identify those patients who have a hematopoietic malignancy. This malignancy can take the form of an acute or subacute leukemia where the predominant cell form in circulation can range from an immature **(promonocyte)** cell to mature monocytes; marrow examination is nearly always warranted to make the diagnosis. True leukemic patients generally have leukocyte counts well in excess of 10,000/μL, while those with myeloproliferative or myelodysplastic disorders may demonstrate an absolute monocytosis but with much lower overall white counts. In addition to characteristic marrow findings, most of these patients will show distinctive chromosomal abnormalities (see Chapters 9 and 19).

CASE HISTORY • Part 2

The combination of hepatosplenomegaly and modest thrombocytopenia is suggestive of a number of disorders, including liver disease, a myeloproliferative or myelodysplastic disorder, or a lymphoma. A bone marrow aspirate and biopsy are clearly indicated, as well as liver function tests and a careful search for lymphadenopathy. The results of these tests are as follows.

The liver function tests are all normal and no lymphadenopathy is detected. The bone marrow aspirate shows normal hematopoiesis with adequate megakaryocytes and large numbers of histiocytes with abundant crinkled-paper (onion-skinning) cytoplasm, typical of Gaucher cells.

Questions

- What additional tests are available to confirm the diagnosis and guide therapy?
- How should the patient be managed?

Patients who have cyclic neutropenia, drug-induced agranulocytosis or are made neutropenic with chemotherapy can also demonstrate a significant monocytosis in the recovery phase. A mild monocytosis (<1,000/ μL) is also seen in a wide spectrum of diseases, where this finding itself is of little diagnostic value. Following the counts is clearly the first order of investigation, with marrow examination the next step.

Hemophagocytic Syndromes

The diagnosis is usually made based on unique macrophage morphology—hemophagocytosis of red blood cells by tissue (especially marrow) macrophages. These cells are found in bone marrow in most of these disorders, such as familial lymphohistiocytosis or Risdall syndrome. Diagnosis of **sinus histiocytosis with massive lymphadenopathy** (Destombes-Rosai-Dorfman syndrome) **is based on examination of a lymph node biopsy**; the lymph node sinuses are distended by plasma cells and histiocytes showing hemophagocytosis.

Malignant Histiocytosis

Malignant histiocytosis (a malignancy of the monocyte-macrophage line) presents with severe anemia, pancytopenia, hepatosplenomegaly, and lymphadenopathy. The course of the disease process is usually rapid with dramatic wasting, recurrent fevers, bone pain, and in some cases skin and soft-tissue tumor infiltrates. The most common form of malignant histiocytosis is **histiocytic medullary reticulosis (HMR)**, which also presents with prominent hemophagocytosis by marrow macrophages. However, these cells are quite pleomorphic with immature nuclei containing 1 or more nucleoli. Malignant histiocytes typically display CD68, CD1c, and S100 positivity by immunohistochemistry.

THERAPY

Effective management obviously is dictated by the specific abnormality of the monocyte-macrophage system. Reactive monocytosis is usually self-limited or transient. Acute and subacute monocytic leukemia is treated like other acute leukemias with ablative chemotherapy (see Chapter 18). Malignant histiocytosis (HMR) is usually a rapidly progressive disease that responds poorly to chemotherapy, which is, at best, palliative.

Gaucher Disease

For a long period of time, the management of patients with Gaucher disease was limited to splenectomy for marked hypersplenism and **orthopedic procedures** such as hip replacements to provide symptomatic relief and maintain mobility. Although splenectomy may improve the patient's hematologic picture, it can be associated with a rapid worsening of liver and bone involvement, as macrophages in those sites take on the increased burden of dealing with the extra amounts of glucocerebroside.

This management situation has changed dramatically since the pharmacologic availability of the missing enzyme, β-glucocerebrosidase, which was produced first as a placental extract in the beginning of the 1990s **(Ceredase)**, and subsequently as a recombinant enzyme **(Cerezyme)**. Moreover, added mannose residues on the molecule have improved its uptake and internalization by deficient macrophages, thereby magnifying its effectiveness. Intravenous infusion of 60 U/kg of the enzyme every other week will result in a gradual regression of the signs and symptoms of Gaucher type 1 disease when given over a long period. Although it is safe, long-term use is very expensive.

Cerezyme treatment is ineffective or much less effective in Gaucher types 2 and 3 disease. Reducing the substrate of β-glucocerebrosidase with Miglustat is also much less effective but can be somewhat helpful for patients who cannot tolerate enzyme therapy. Attempts to use gene implant therapy to correct the enzyme deficiency have not succeeded as yet. Bone marrow transplantation has provided improvement of both storage disease and neurologic symptoms in type 3 patients. This procedure has no place in the treatment of type 1 patients given the efficacy of enzyme therapy.

CASE HISTORY • *Part 3*

The management of the patient with Gaucher disease depends on confirmation of the genetic defect and placement in 1 of the 3 major subtypes. In this case, genetic analysis shows the patient to be homozygous for the *N370S* mutation of β-glucocerebrosidase, placing him in the mild or type I category of Gaucher disease. His presentation late in life with bone disease and hepatosplenomegaly are also consistent with this diagnosis and subtype.

Although he has been well up to this point in his life, he is at risk for recurrent fractures and bone pain, as well as slowly progressive hepatosplenomegaly, worsening thrombocytopenia, and bone marrow failure. Therefore, he is a candidate for lifelong replacement therapy with recombinant β-glucocerebrosidase. The dose can eventually be adjusted according to the response in his spleen, and liver size, liver function, and skeletal changes. Although this patient has a mild form of this disease, he should also receive genetic counseling regarding the possibility of his passing the disorder to his offspring.

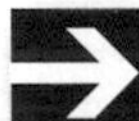

POINTS TO REMEMBER

Reactive monocytosis is often seen as part of inflammatory, autoimmune, and hematopoietic disorders. It is also characteristic of the early stages of recovery from myelosuppression of any cause.

Many myeloproliferative disorders and myeloid leukemias include cells with varying degrees of monocytic differentiation.

True malignant transformation of tissue macrophages (histiocytes) is very rare and is often characterized by phagocytosis of erythrocytes documented by tissue or marrow hemophagocytosis.

There are a number of lipid and carbohydrate storage diseases resulting from the genetic inability to metabolize various substances. The major manifestation of these disorders is hepatosplenomegaly and the appearance of macrophages filled with the offending substance in the bone marrow. The most common of the lipid-storage disorders is Gaucher disease.

Type I Gaucher disease is amenable to recombinant enzyme therapy, whereas the more severe subtypes do not respond to this therapy.

BIBLIOGRAPHY

Dale DC, Boxer L, Liles WC: The phagocytes: neutrophils and monocytes. Blood 2008;112:935.

Henter JI, Horne AC, Aricó M, et al: HLH-2004: diagnostic and therapeutic guidelines for hemophagocytic lymphohistiocytosis. Pediatric Blood & Cancer 2004;48:124.

Jaffe ES: Histiocytic and dendritic cell neoplasms: introduction. In: Jaffe H, Harris NL, Stein H, Vardiman JW (eds): *World Health Organization Classification of Tumors. Pathology and Genetics of Tumors of the Hematopoietic and Lymphoid Tissues*. IARC Press, 2001.

Janka GE: Hemophagocytic syndromes. Blood Reviews 2007;21:245.

Lipton JM, Westra S, Haverty CE, Roberts D, Harris NL: Case records of the Massachussets General Hospital. Case 28-2004: newborn twins with thrombocytopenia, coagulation defects, and hepatosplenomegaly. N Engl J Med 2004;351:1120.

McClain KL, Natkunam Y, Swerdlow SH: Atypical cellular disorders (Destombes-Rosai-Dorfmann disease). Hematology Am Soc Hematol Educ Program 2004:283.

Medzhitov R, Janeway C Jr: Innate immunity. N Engl J Med 2000;343:338.

Pastores GM, Weinreb NJ, Aerts N, et al: Therapeutic goals in the treatment of Gaucher disease. Semin Hematol 2004;41(Suppl 5):5.

Rosenbloom BE, Weinreb NJ, Zimran A, Kacena KA, Charrow J, Ward E: Gaucher disease and cancer incidence: a study from the Gaucher Registry. Blood 2005;105:4569.

Schmidt D: Malignant histiocytosis. Curr Opin Hematol 2001;8:1.

Trinchieri G, Sher A: Cooperation of toll-like receptor signals in innate immune defence. Nat Rev Immunol 2007;7:179.

Weinreb NJ, Agio MC, Andersson HC, et al: Gaucher disease type 1: revised recommendations on evaluations and monitoring for adult patients. Semin Hematol 2004;41(Suppl 5):5.

Worth RG, Jones BA, Schreiber AD: Fcγ receptor structure/function and role in immune complex mediated autoimmune disease. Hematology (ASH Education program book) 2004;54.

SECTION III
Disorders of Hemostasis

NORMAL HEMOSTASIS • 28

Normal hemostasis is best conceptualized according to its major components—vessel wall, platelet function, coagulation factor cascade, and clot inhibition/fibrinolysis. These components work together to prevent prolonged bleeding or thrombosis under normal physiologic conditions. Disruption of the vascular endothelium is a potent stimulus to clot formation. As a localized process, hemostasis by cellular and protein components acts to seal the break in vascular continuity, limit blood loss, and begin the process of wound healing. Prevention of an exuberant response that would result in pathologic thrombosis involves counterbalancing mechanisms, including anticoagulant properties of intact endothelial cells, circulating inhibitors of activated coagulation factors, and localized fibrinolytic enzymes. Most abnormalities in hemostasis involve a defect in 1 or more of the integrated steps in this coagulation process. It is important, therefore, to understand the physiology of hemostasis.

VESSEL WALL

The intact endothelial cell lining of the vessel wall plays an **essential role in preventing thrombus formation**. First and foremost, it provides a physical barrier between circulating platelets and highly thrombogenic subendothelial connective tissue. In addition, endothelial cells are active metabolically in the regulation of blood flow, platelet aggregation, and the coagulation cascade. Endothelial cells are a primary source for production of nitric oxide and prostacyclin, both of which are important in promoting smooth muscle relaxation and vessel dilatation. Disruption of the endothelial cell surface results in unopposed smooth muscle contraction and vessel spasm. This is an effective reflex to stem blood loss and sets the stage for thrombus formation. When damaged, endothelial cells are capable of encouraging platelet adhesion, activation, and aggregation. Endothelial cells are also the primary source of **von Willebrand factor (vWF) multimers**, the essential cofactor for platelet adhesion to sites of vessel disruption.

Normal endothelial cells adjacent to an injury site are simultaneously crucial to **limiting clot formation**. Thrombin in the microenvironment causes normal endothelial cells to dramatically increase secretion of prostacyclin, which inhibits downstream platelet activation and aggregation. Thrombin also binds to endothelial cell thrombomodulin, which promotes protein C activation and subsequently downregulates further thrombin generation. Since thrombomodulin is found in greater amounts in smaller vessels, the latter function may be especially critical to the integrity of the microvasculature. Finally, endothelial cells are the primary source of **tissue plasminogen activator (t-PA)**, the principal physiologic fibrinolytic enzyme.

PLATELET FUNCTION

Normal circulating platelets resemble an oblong disk, measuring 2–4 μm on the long axis with a volume of 5–12 fL. They are essentially fragments of megakaryocyte cytoplasm. Although lacking a nucleus, the cytoplasm contains mitochondria for aerobic metabolism, glycogen stores for anaerobic glycolysis, and specific granules whose contents are important for coagulation (Figure 28–1). Almost 20% of the platelet volume comprises these granules, whereas 25% of the protein in the platelet is actin and myosin needed for platelet contraction.

Platelets provide the cell-based platform for hemostasis. When circulating platelets contact subendothelial tissue in a damaged vessel, they adhere to the exposed collagen via the integrin receptor, GPIa/IIa, and to vWF bound to collagen via

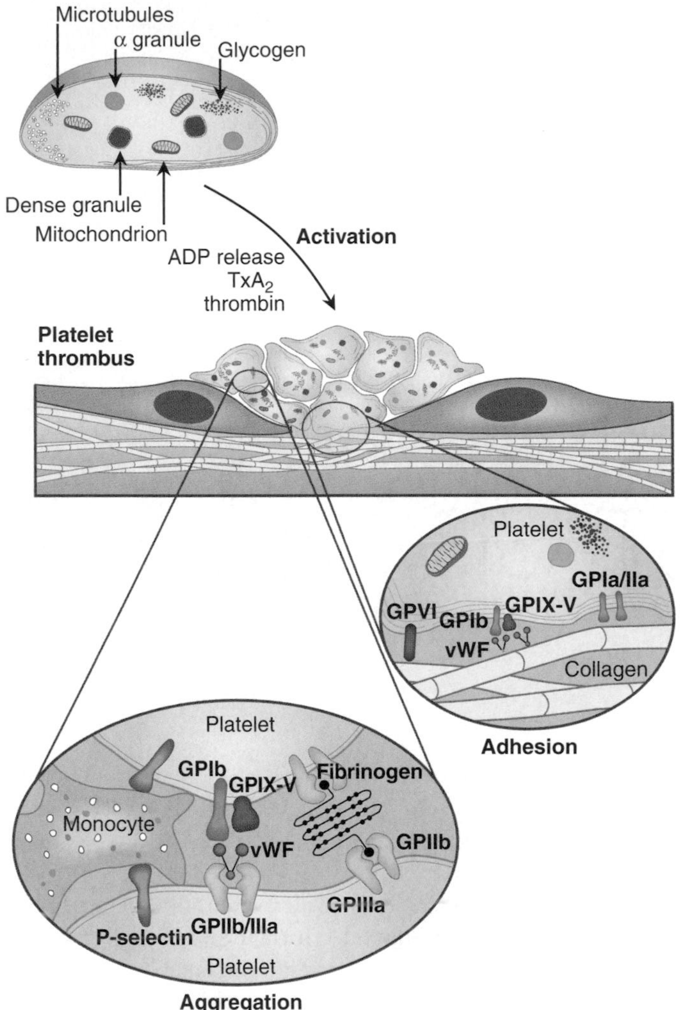

FIGURE 28–1. **Platelet adhesion, activation, and aggregation.** Platelet adhesion and activation initially involves shape change with extension of pseudopods and subsequently a release reaction where the contents of intracellular granules are expelled into the extracellular milieu to stimulate and recruit circulating platelets into the clot. Formation of a platelet thrombus at the site of injury requires both platelet adhesion and aggregation. Platelet GPIa/IIa receptors bind directly to exposed collagen, while GPIb/IX-V and GPIIb/IIIa receptors interact with von Willebrand factor (vWF) to adhere to the subendothelial tissue. Aggregation also involves the GPIIb/IIIa receptor with fibrinogen as its essential cofactor. Activation-induced expression of the α-granule receptor P-selectin binds monocytes and neutrophils to platelets and incorporates them within the clot where they enhance fibrin formation.

a second receptor, GPIb/IX-V. As platelets first adhere to vWF, they begin to tumble and slide over the damaged surface and undergo shape change with extension of pseudopods. This helps maintain close proximity between platelets and enhances platelet-platelet adhesion and activation. GPIb/IX-V binding to vWF also induces a conformational change in the GPIIb/IIIa receptor, which results in firmer adhesion to vWF.

Thrombin activation of platelets also plays a role. Platelet GPIb is the cofactor for this reaction via the membrane-associated receptors—GPV and PAR (protease activated receptor). This helps recruit more platelets to the growing platelet plug. Collagen also helps guide platelet adhesion and activation. It can anchor platelets to 1 locus via the GPIa/IIa receptor, while activating platelets at a second locus via the GPVI receptor. GPVI binding to collagen is also a key mediator of subsequent intracellular signaling of the kinase-family proteins, including HS1 (hematopoietic lineage cell-specific protein 1). The importance of these adhesion and activation receptors is illustrated clinically by the significant defect in hemostasis observed in patients deficient in GPIIb/IIa, GPIb/IX-V, GPVI, and GPIa/IIa.

Platelet adhesion is also influenced by blood shear rates (the velocity of blood flow over the endothelial surface). At low shear rates (<1,000 sec^{-1}), typical for the microvasculature, platelets rely almost entirely on the GPIIb/IIIa receptor to activate and bind to fibrinogen. By contrast, at very high shear rates (>10,000 sec^{-1}), as seen in the arterial system, adhesion and aggregation is mediated primarily via GPIb/IX-V without prior platelet activation. At intermediate shear rates, both pathways are active, platelet activation is required, and fibronectin plays a significant role.

The initial adhesion of platelets to one another can be measured in the laboratory as the aggregation of platelets in plasma. The first wave of in vitro aggregation is reversible, and may be sustained only briefly, less than 1–2 minutes, when the aggregatory stimulus is weak, such as seen with epinephrine or lower doses of adenosine 5′-diphosphate (ADP). High-dose ADP, thrombin, and thromboxane A_2 (through arachadonic acid stimulation) provide a **stronger stimulus for platelet activation**, resulting in a second wave of irreversible aggregation. This second wave is associated with platelet degranulation and release of dense granule contents (ADP and serotonin), α-granule contents (platelet factor 4 and β-thromboglobulin), and further generation of thromboxane A_2 through the platelet cyclooxygenase (COX-1 isoform) pathway (Table 28–1). ADP activates platelets through the G protein–linked $P2Y_{12}$ receptor and through GPIIb/IIIa to stabilize platelet-platelet adhesion.

The activated platelet also provides a surface to facilitate thrombin generation through specific surface receptors for clotting factors V, XI, and VII; through binding of IXa, Xa, and the VIII-vWF complex; and via membrane expression of the negatively charged phospholipid, phosphatidylserine. This platelet-localized burst of thrombin generation recruits additional activated platelets into the clot and stimulates fibrinogen conversion to fibrin to stabilize the platelet aggregate-fibrin clot. Thrombin also indirectly promotes platelet adhesion by proteolysis of ADAMTS13, the protease that cleaves large vWF multimers into less active subunits. The availability of large vWF multimers enhances GPIb/IX-V binding. Runaway platelet aggregation, resulting in pathologic thrombus, is naturally inhibited by release of t-PA, prostacyclin, and nitric oxide by the adjacent normal endothelial cells, blockade of thrombin activity by circulating antithrombin, and degradation of ADP by a membrane-associated ADPase.

Several **other substances are released by platelet degranulation** (see Figure 28–1). In addition to ADP and serotonin,

TABLE 28–1 • Platelet coagulant factors

Adhesive platelet antigens
GPIa/IIa: collagen receptor
GPIb/IX-V: vWF receptor
GPIIb/IIIa: fibrinogen receptor
P-selectin
Platelet-associated proteins
Specific (synthesized by megakaryocytes)
Platelet factors 3 and 4
β-thromboglobulin
Platelet-derived growth factor
Nonspecific (endocytosed from plasma)
Fibrinogen
Proteins (albumin, IgG)
vWF, other coagulation factors (V, VIII)
Plasminogen
Reactive compounds
Biogenic amines
Serotonin
Histamine
Catecholamines
Adenine nucleotides (ADP, cyclic AMP)
Cations (Ca^{+2})
Thromboxane A_2

dense granules release **ionized calcium**, an essential cofactor in both platelet aggregation and thrombin generation, as well as subsequent clot retraction. Platelet factor 4 from the α-granule binds to and neutralizes both pharmacologic heparin and endogenous heparan sulfates. Other α-granule contents include the clotting proteins fibrinogen, factors V and VIII, thrombospondin, and fibronectin, and possibly factor XI as well. Once activated, platelet surface expression of the integral α-granule membrane protein, P-selectin, mediates binding of monocytes and neutrophils (via the leukocyte-expressed P-selectin glycoprotein ligand) to activated platelets, incorporating these inflammatory cells into the clot where they promote fibrin formation. Released platelet factor XIII is activated by thrombin and converts the soluble fibrin-platelet clot into an insoluble polymer; XIIIa also binds α_2-antiplasmin to fibrin to further protect the clot from dissolution by circulating plasmin.

COAGULATION CASCADE

The cascade of interactions of the circulating clotting factors is shown from a laboratory testing perspective in Figure 28–2, in which the soluble protein factors are divided into intrinsic and extrinsic pathways. This schema fits the commonly used laboratory tests of plasma-dependent clotting, the prothrombin time (PT) measurement for the extrinsic pathway, and the partial thromboplastin time (PTT) for the intrinsic pathway. Initiation of the intrinsic pathway, as measured in the laboratory by the PTT, involves activation of factor XII (Hageman factor) to XIIa, which then catalyzes the activation of factor XI. Essential cofactors for this reaction include the presence of a contact surface (eg, kaolin for the PTT), prekallikrein, and high-molecular-weight kininogen (HMWK). Although contact activation is a well-defined reaction for monitoring the PTT in the laboratory, its physiologic relevance is unclear. Deficiencies in factor XII, prekallikrein, and HMWK prolong the PTT but are not associated with clinical bleeding.

From a physiologic standpoint, the coagulation cascade may best be thought of as a continuous process with distinct but interrelated components including exposure of tissue factor (TF) to the blood; TF-mediated activation of Xa and generation of small amounts of thrombin; feedback activation of XI, V, IX, and VIII by thrombin to produce large amounts of Xa and a subsequent burst of thrombin generation; and finally, production of large amounts of fibrin monomers by thrombin, which are stabilized in polymer form after covalently crosslinking by XIIIa.

Tissue Factor

When the endothelial cell barrier is lost, TF is exposed to the blood by constitutive expression in subendothelial tissues. TF can also be induced on the surface of circulating monocytes by endotoxin stimulation during sepsis. TF is the initiator of physiologic coagulation. TF binds to small amounts of circulating activated factor VII (VIIa) that is thought to be generated by basal levels of thrombin activity. Once formed, the TF-VIIa complex activates factors X and IX, causing generation of Xa and small amounts of thrombin (see Figure 28–2). This TF-VIIa stimulus, however, is not sustained; it is rapidly downregulated by **tissue factor pathway inhibitor (TFPI)**, which forms a quaternary complex with TF-VIIa-X and inactivates the enzymes. Sustained factor X activation, sufficient to generate enough thrombin to form a stable clot, is dependent on activation of factors IX and VIII and, at least partially, through activation of XI.

Activation of the Common Pathway

Factors IXa and VIIa are both highly active serine proteases. They are closely allied in the subsequent activation of the common pathway factors X and V (see Figure 28–2). The action of each requires the presence of a cofactor. Factor VIIIa is the essential cofactor for IXa, whereas the microsomal lipoprotein TF is the cofactor for VIIa.

Rather than existing as 2 distinct physiologic systems, the factor IXa-VIIIa intrinsic pathway and the tissue factor-VIIa extrinsic pathway are highly integrated in vivo. The sequence of events for the common pathway activation of factor X is illustrated in Figure 28–3. TF, the most potent activator of factor VII, initiates clotting by directly activating X to Xa, which in turn generates small amounts of thrombin. TF-VIIa also activates IX. Moreover, although the initial thrombin formation is limited, it serves to activate multiple factors, including XI, IX, VIII, and V. At the same time, common pathway activation through the

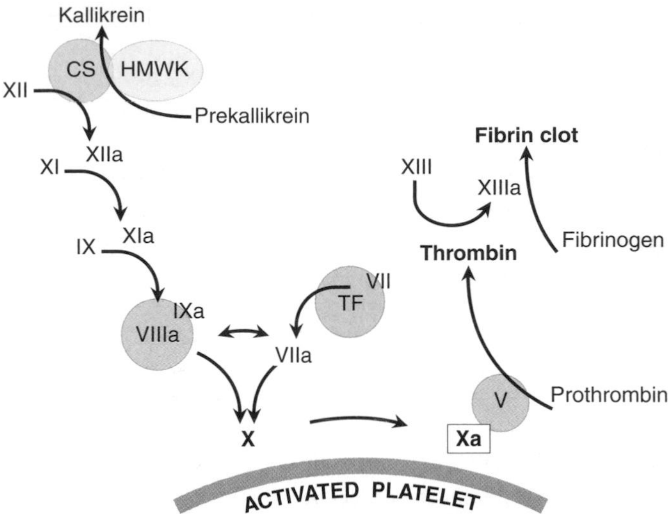

FIGURE 28–2. **The coagulation cascade.** From the laboratory viewpoint, the coagulation cascade is characterized by intrinsic and extrinsic pathways. The intrinsic pathway is initiated by activation of factor XII (Hageman factor) by surface contact (CS), whereas the extrinsic pathway begins with the activation of factor VII by tissue factor (TF). Physiologically, the 2 pathways work together to accelerate production of activated factor X (Xa), which, in the presence of factor V, activates factor II (prothrombin) to thrombin. The last step in the cascade is thrombin-induced activation of fibrinogen to fibrin clot with incorporation of factor XIII to further stabilize the clot.

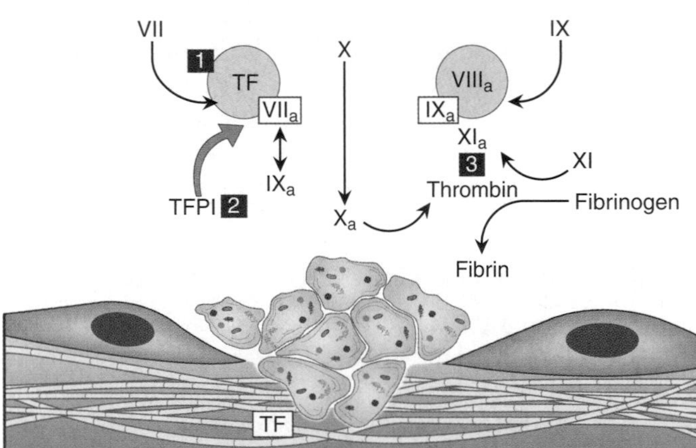

FIGURE 28–3. **Common pathway activation in vivo.** Coagulation factors are activated on the platelet surface to generate a fibrin-platelet clot. Subendothelial tissue factor (TF) in combination with small amounts of circulating factor VIIa is the physiologic initiator of factor X activation (1), which generates small amounts of thrombin. Further VIIa-TF action on X is inhibited, however, by tissue factor pathway inhibitor (TFPI), which rapidly binds to and inactivates the TF-VIIa-X complex (2). Therefore, continued formation of factor Xa depends on an intact factor IX-VIIIa (intrinsic) pathway, which is activated by factor XIa and in a feedback manner by thrombin (3). Activation of X through the intrinsic pathway generates explosive amounts of thrombin, which produces full generation of fibrin polymers and stable clot formation.

TF-factor VIIa-Xa complex is rapidly downregulated by TFPI, limiting the extent of factor X activation by TF. Sustained Xa formation depends on an intact factor IXa-VIIIa pathway in part activated by factor XIa with thrombin as a primary stimulus. Because of this essential interaction, mature clot formation depends on an intact factor IXa pathway and adequate amounts of factor VIII. This helps explain why patients with hemophilia (factor VIII or IX deficiency) demonstrate a bleeding diathesis. The concomitant role of XI is postulated because XI deficiency results in a bleeding disorder of variable, but usually mild, intensity that often does not present until late adulthood.

The final steps of the common pathway involve both the **platelet membrane surface** to support the reaction and **factor V** as an essential cofactor. Factor V bound to its platelet receptor greatly enhances activation of Xa, and a marked deficiency in factor V or a defect in the membrane binding of the factor Xa-Va complex usually results in a significant bleeding tendency. Therefore, the importance of the platelet membrane both as a localizing site for binding clotting factors and as a facilitator of activation of the common pathway cannot be overemphasized.

Clot Formation

The Xa-Va complex enzymatically cleaves prothrombin to form thrombin. The amount of prothrombin in circulation is relatively large compared with other factors, providing an amplification of the final step of thrombin generation and cleavage of fibrinogen to produce fibrin monomers. Thrombin further amplifies the coagulation sequence by stimulating platelet activation to provide additional membrane surface for activation of factors X and V, by activating VIII to VIIIa, and finally, by activating factors XI and XIII. Factor XIIIa is an active transamidase, which in the presence of calcium converts the gel-like fibrin monomers to an insoluble fibrin polymer clot.

CLOT INHIBITION/LYSIS

The type of vessel and its location influences the character of the thrombus. In major arteries, high blood flow rates limit the growth of a thrombus on the vessel wall. As platelets attempt to aggregate on the disrupted arterial surface, those platelets that are not tightly bound, as well as other blood cells, are dislodged by the arterial flow. Similarly, locally released factors such as ADP, thromboxane A_2, and thrombin, which stimulate aggregation and clot formation, are also subject to be swept downstream and rapidly dissipated from the area of injury. This aspect of arterial clotting naturally limits the thrombus to the site of the initial platelet aggregate, producing the so-called **"white thrombus"** in which platelets predominate, and there are very few red cells present. By contrast, clotting in smaller or severely atherosclerotic arteries or in the venous circulation is often characterized by more static blood flow. In this situation, platelet aggregates incorporate other blood cells, including red blood cells, into the final fibrin clot producing the characteristic **"red thrombus."**

Several inhibitors of coagulation and the fibrinolytic system also influence the size and stability of a newly formed clot. Inhibitors of platelet activation and aggregation are described in Chapter 37. **Direct inhibitors of the coagulation cascade** include protein C, protein S, antithrombin, and TFPI. They are essential to downregulation of thrombin generation and the control of thrombus formation. A deficiency in any of these can trigger a hypercoagulable state and predispose the patient to thromboembolic (especially venous) disease.

Thrombin binds to the endothelial cell membrane surface protein, **thrombomodulin** (Figure 28–4). This binding activates circulating protein C, which then inhibits further thrombin formation by enzymatically cleaving factors Va and VIIIa. Activated protein C, besides this anticoagulant effect, has distinct cytoprotective functions, which are linked to anti-inflammatory and anti-apoptotic activity. **Protein S** acts as an anticoagulant cofactor for **activated protein C** by helping to overcome the inhibition of protein C. In contrast to its effect on activated protein C, the thrombin-thrombomodulin complex actually can enhance clot formation by inducing thrombin-activated fibrinolysis inhibitor (TAFI). TAFI interferes with plasmin activity. **Antithrombin** is an inhibitor of serine protease enzymes with activity against thrombin and activated factors Xa, IXa, and XIa. Activity of antithrombin is dramatically enhanced by the presence of exogenous heparin and endogenous endothelial cell heparan sulfates.

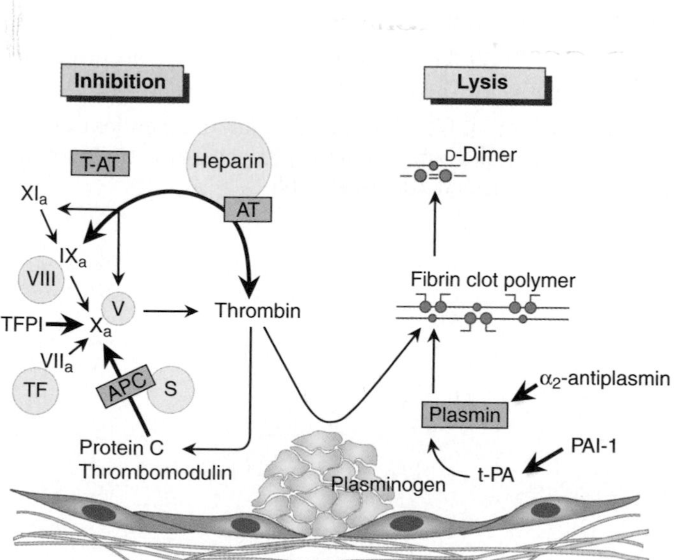

FIGURE 28–4. **Clot inhibition and lysis.** Clot size is controlled by inhibitors of platelet function and coagulation and by the fibrinolytic system. One inhibitor of the coagulation cascade is thrombin-initiated activation of protein C (APC), which enzymatically cleaves factors V and VIII in the presence of free protein S. Antithrombin (AT) is a direct circulating inhibitor of thrombin and factors Xa, IXa, and XIa, and heparin enhances AT activity by more than 1,000-fold. Tissue factor pathway inhibitor (TFPI) is a plasma and endothelial cell–bound inhibitor of Xa and the VIIa-TF-X complex. When the fibrinolytic system is activated by clot formation, adjacent healthy endothelial cells release tissue plasminogen activator (t-PA), which activates clot-bound plasminogen to plasmin. Plasmin breaks down the fibrin polymer, releasing crosslinked fibrin fragments, such as D-dimer.

As noted, TFPI binds Xa and the VIIa-TF in a complex that inhibits further VIIa-TF activation of X. **TFPI** is found both in plasma and bound to the surface of the vascular endothelium. It is unclear whether TFPI deficiency can result in a hypercoagulable state. **α_2-macroglobulin** is another protease inhibitor capable of complexing with enzymes such as trypsin, plasmin, and kallikrein, but its clinical role is still unclear.

The fibrinolytic system is key to localizing the thrombus to the site of injury and eventually dissolving the thrombus as part of vessel healing to re-establish normal blood flow. With thrombus formation, circulating plasminogen is incorporated within the newly formed clot, bound to fibrin. Normal endothelial cells adjacent to the injury site release tissue plasminogen activator (t-PA), which activates clot-bound plasminogen to plasmin.

Limiting lysis to the surface of the clot and preventing destruction of circulating fibrinogen occurs, in part, through the specificity of t-PA binding to the plasminogen-fibrin complex. At least 4 other inhibitors of fibrinolysis also play a role. **Plasminogen activator inhibitor-1 (PAI-1)** is present in plasma at a concentration greater than the physiologic concentrations of t-PA released by endothelial cells. PAI-1 has a high affinity for and binds to any t-PA in circulation. In addition, any plasmin that escapes into the circulation is bound and inactivated by **α_2-antiplasmin**, an extremely rapid reaction that prevents generalized fibrinogenolysis. Activation of XI and XIII then further stabilizes the clot. **XIIIa** inhibits fibrinolysis by crosslinking fibrin chains and by binding α_2-antiplasmin to fibrin.

Thrombin, generated by the exposure of collagen and the release of tissue factor, plays a central role in the formation and maintenance of the platelet-fibrin clot. As a **procoagulant**, it generates additional thrombin by the activation of factors XI, V, and VIII, and helps recruit platelets to the injury site. Thrombin induces fibrin formation and stabilizes the fibrin clot by inactivating ADAMTS13 (inhibiting the breakdown of vWF multimers) and activating factor XIII to crosslink fibrin molecules. Thrombin simultaneously acts as an **anticoagulant** to limit clot formation to the area of injury. Together with thrombomodulin and heparan sulfates released by surrounding normal endothelial cells, thrombin serves to block uncontrolled platelet plug expansion beyond the damage site. A natural inhibitor of thrombin, anti-thrombin (AT), serves to scavenge any excess thrombin released into the general circulation, which is essential to preventing disseminated intravascular coagulation.

By nature of the crosslinking process of fibrin clot formation, degradation/fibrinolysis results in specific fibrin fragments, which has led to the development of laboratory tests to identify fibrinolysis. The most unique and clinically useful product currently is the **D-dimer** fragment, which consists of 2 crosslinked D moieties originating from 2 different fibrin molecules. Appearance of the D-dimer fragment in circulation has been shown to be an indication of active clot turnover, and its absence can be used to exclude the presence of venous thromboembolism in select patient groups.

POINTS TO REMEMBER

Normal hemostasis requires a complex interaction of endothelial cells, platelets, and circulating coagulation factors to prevent bleeding due to injury, yet still preserve liquid blood flow. Endothelial cells play a key role by secreting numerous proteins that both encourage and limit platelet adhesion/activation and clot formation.

Platelet adhesion and activation is the first step in clot formation. Von Willebrand factor released by damaged endothelial cells is the primary ligand for platelet adhesion to subendothelial collagen. Subsequent activation and formation of a platelet clot involves the expression of platelet surface receptors and active secretion of several activation factors. The surface of activated platelets also serves as a platform for subsequent fibrin clot formation.

The coagulation cascade (intrinsic, extrinsic, and common pathways) responds to "tissue factor" to promote thrombin generation, which catalyzes the fibrinogen to fibrin reaction necessary for formation of a stable fibrin clot. Deficiencies in any of the key factors can result in a bleeding disorder, as exemplified by the hemophilias.

Simultaneous with fibrin generation, thrombin promotes natural anticoagulant factors to regulate thrombus formation and prevent spread of the fibrin clot beyond the immediate area of injury. Anticoagulant and fibrinolytic factors also serve to limit systemic activation of clotting, and thereby decrease the risk of pathologic thromboembolism.

The hemostatic system functions differently in the high flow (high shear) arterial circuit as compared to the lower flow (low shear) venous circuit. The platelet–von Willebrand interaction and formation of a platelet (white) clot is the typical response to arterial wall injury, whereas thrombin generation and formation of a fibrin (red) clot is seen in the venous circuit. Therefore, prophylaxis and treatment of thrombotic disease will differ according to the location and nature of the clot, either platelet inhibition or coagulation factor-directed anticoagulation.

BIBLIOGRAPHY

Hoffman M: Remodeling the blood coagulation cascade. J Thrombos Thrombolys 2003;16:17.

Jackson SP: The growing complexity of platelet aggregation. Blood 2007;109:5087.

Kahner BN et al: Hematopoietic lineage cell-specific protein 1 (HS1) is a functionally important signaling molecule in platelet activation. Blood 2007;110:2449.

Lane DA, Phillippou H, Huntington JA: Directing thrombin. Blood 2005;106:2605.

Mann KG et al: Models of blood coagulation. Blood Cells Mol Dis 2006;36:108.

Mosnier LO, Zlokovic BV, Griffin JH: The cytoprotective protein C pathway. Blood 2007;109:3161.

Sarratt KL et al: GPVI and $\alpha2\beta1$ play independent critical roles during platelet adhesion and aggregate formation to collagen under flow. Blood 2005;106:1268.

CLINICAL APPROACH TO BLEEDING DISORDERS • 29

Evaluation of a patient for a bleeding tendency or excessive hemorrhage is common in clinical medicine. It requires identification of key elements in the patient's history and physical examination and integration of these data with laboratory measurements and therapeutic maneuvers. Often the evaluation is part of the diagnosis and management of another illness as, for example, the patient who bleeds excessively during or after surgery or who develops a coagulopathy as part of a systemic illness. Therefore, successful diagnosis of a bleeding disorder very much depends on the skills of the clinician at the bedside.

CLINICAL EVALUATION

Important diagnostic information is provided by the clinical setting because of the clear associations between bleeding abnormalities and certain disease states. To uncover these relationships, the clinician needs to collect the following data:

- **Who:** The patient's age, sex, racial background, and family history of abnormal bleeding all are important.
- **When:** Any association with a disease state, trauma, surgery, or drug ingestion should be identified. In addition, details of the time of onset and course of the bleeding event are important.
- **Where:** The site or sites of bleeding, whether skin, mucous membranes, gastrointestinal (GI) tract, solid organ, joint, or muscle, need to be identified.
- **What:** The physical characteristics of the bleeding, especially the distinction between petechial (capillary) hemorrhage and the purpura, ecchymoses, and hematoma formation seen with larger vessel bleeding, need to be described.

Based on these data, it is often possible to target the **nature of the bleeding disorder**. Patients who have a hematologic malignancy or are undergoing high-dose chemotherapy are at risk for severe thrombocytopenia and mucosal bleeding. Platelet dysfunction can also cause mucosal bleeding, as seen in patients with acquired von Willebrand disease (vWD) or essential thrombocythemia. In contrast, patients receiving warfarin can be expected to show an abnormality in the production of the vitamin K–dependent coagulation factors. Liver disease patients are at risk for developing a multifactor deficiency state and, at times, a defect in fibrinogen structure and function. Finally, patients with severe sepsis can develop a consumptive coagulopathy affecting all coagulation factors.

As for the detection of a **congenital coagulopathy**, the absence of any complicating illness or anticoagulant drug exposure obviously directs the clinician's attention to the possibility of an inherited defect. In this situation, the patient's age, sex, race, family history, and the characteristics of the onset and course of the bleeding can be major clues to the diagnosis.

LABORATORY STUDIES

Several laboratory tests are available to evaluate the coagulation pathways. Some of these tests, such as platelet function, require the expertise of a consultant hematologist and a reference laboratory. Others are available through the routine laboratory. It is the routine tests that every clinician should be able to use in evaluating a coagulation defect (Table 29–1). These tests include the platelet count, bleeding time (BT), whole blood platelet function analysis (PFA), prothrombin time (PT), activated partial thromboplastin time (aPTT), thrombin time (TT), assays (including mixing studies) for specific factor and factor inhibitor levels, fibrinogen concentration and breakdown products, and measurements of proteins that regulate thrombolysis, such as α_2-antiplasmin levels.

Platelet Count

The platelet count is accurately measured, even at extremely low levels, by modern cell counting instruments, which use either optical or impedance methodologies. Cell counters also

TABLE 29–1 • Routine coagulation tests to assess bleeding

Test	Normal Values[a]
Platelet count	150,000–450,000/μL
Bleeding time (BT) (template)	3–8 min
PFA-100 (collagen/epinephrine)	82–150 sec
PFA-100 (collagen/ADP)	60–100 sec
Prothrombin time (PT)	10–14 sec
International normalized ratio (INR)	0.80–1.30
Partial thromboplastin time (aPTT)	22–35 sec
Thrombin time (TT)	9–25 sec
Fibrinogen assay	
Healthy individuals	200–400 mg/dL
With severe illness	400–800 mg/dL
Fibrin/fibrinogen fragments	
Latex agglutination	0–1+ (<10 μg/mL)
D-dimer assay	<2.5 μg/mL
α_2-Antiplasmin level	80%–120%

[a]*Note that the reference ranges included in Table 29–1 are specified either by the manufacturer or a single institution. All laboratories must establish their own reference ranges.*

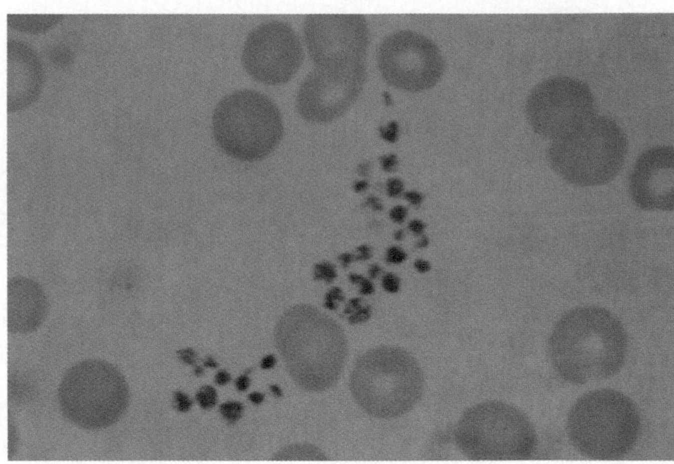

FIGURE 29–2. **Platelet clumping on the peripheral blood smear.** Microscopic examination of the blood smear to confirm thrombocytopenia demonstrated platelet aggregates in this EDTA-anticoagulated specimen. A subsequent blood drawn into heparin anticoagulant demonstrated a normal platelet count without aggregates, suggesting that an EDTA-dependent antibody was the cause of this laboratory artifact.

use immunologic techniques to confirm severe thrombocytopenia. Of course, the platelet count can be estimated by inspecting a Wright stained peripheral smear. Normally, at least 1 platelet is seen for every 20 red blood cells (Figure 29–1). When the count is severely depressed to levels below 20,000/μL, it can be difficult to identify by microscopy even a single platelet per high-power field.

The normal platelet count should fall between 150,000 and 450,000/μL of whole blood. Falsely low levels can occur when platelets aggregate because of poor anticoagulation of the specimen leading to clotting or, more rarely, when the presence of an ethylenediaminetetraacetic acid (EDTA)-sensitive antibody causes either platelet agglutination or platelet satellitism. Inspection of the blood tube for clot or detection of platelet aggregates or satellitism around leukocytes on a stained blood smear (Figures 29–2 and 29–3) will usually reveal these respective causes of pseudothrombocytopenia.

Template Bleeding Time and Platelet Function Analysis

The BT is used clinically to detect a significant defect in platelet function. A template apparatus (eg, Simplate) should always be employed. To perform the technique, a blood pressure cuff is

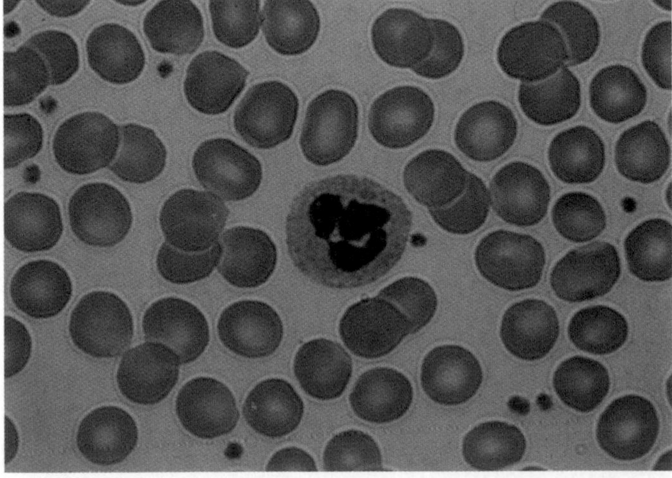

FIGURE 29–1. **Normal blood smear.** Single platelets can be identified on the routine blood smear as 2–4 μm, slightly granulated, anucleate cells. When present in normal numbers (150,000–450,000/μL), at least 1–2 platelets should be seen for every 20 red blood cells.

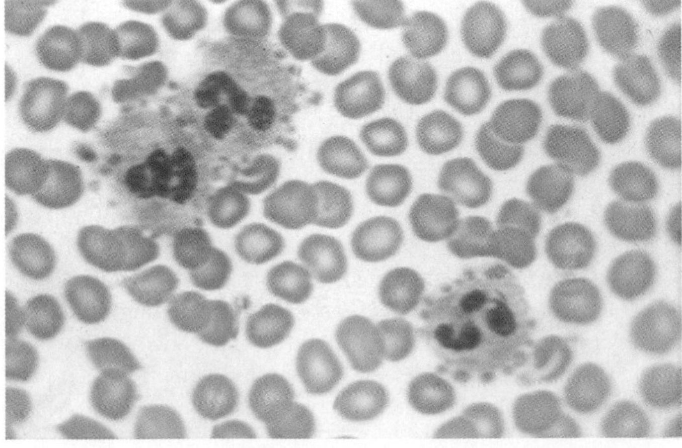

FIGURE 29–3. **Platelet satellitism.** Microscopic examination of a blood smear to confirm thrombocytopenia demonstrated multiple platelets binding to neutrophils (platelet satellitism). Although rare, this in vitro, EDTA-dependent phenomenon can be noted in patients with clinical conditions causing extreme platelet activation (sepsis, microangiopathy) and an artificially low platelet count.

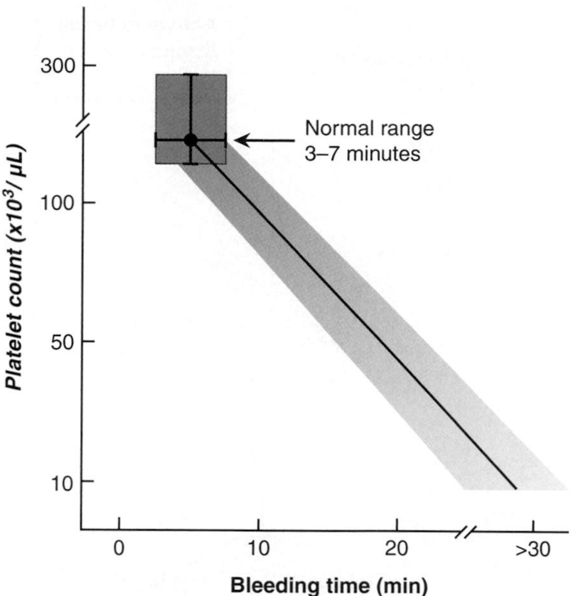

FIGURE 29–4. **The effect of thrombocytopenia on the bleeding time (BT).** Normal patients with platelet counts greater than 100,000/μL have a BT between 3 and 7 minutes. As the platelet count falls below 100,000/μL, the BT becomes progressively longer, reaching values in excess of 25–30 minutes once the count falls below 10,000/μL.

placed around the patient's upper arm and inflated to 40 mm Hg. The volar surface of the forearm is cleaned with alcohol and air dried. The template is then firmly apposed to the skin (without indentation and avoiding superficial veins) and the template is activated; for the Simplate, two 1-mm deep, 10-mm long incisions are made. A stopwatch is started, and at 30-second intervals, the blood from each of the wounds is carefully blotted with filter paper without interfering with the wound itself. A normal BT should range from 3–8 minutes.

There is a **direct relationship between the platelet count and the BT** (Figure 29–4). With counts above 100,000/μL and normal platelet function, the BT should be less than 8 minutes. As the count falls below 100,000/μL, the BT lengthens, reaching levels of 20–30 minutes as it approaches 10,000/μL. This predictable relationship makes the BT determination unnecessary (and inappropriate) in the evaluation of thrombocytopenic patients.

The true value of the BT is to detect a platelet functional defect in a bleeding patient with a normal platelet count. Both uremia and aspirin therapy prolong the BT to values of up to 15 minutes or longer. These results can be highly variable, however, since some individuals are more sensitive to aspirin than others, and platelet dysfunction may still not be detectable unless the BT is very carefully done. At the same time, the BT can also detect patients with clinically significant von Willebrand disease (vWD), a congenital defect in the synthesis of von Willebrand factor (vWF) or assembly of vWF multimers. In this situation, the BT is often longer than 10 minutes.

Although some institutions continue to use the in vivo bleeding time, many have chosen to substitute an "in vitro bleeding time" test using venous whole blood samples. This in vitro platelet function analysis (PFA) can be performed on fresh (within 4 hours of blood drawing) citrate anticoagulated whole blood using any one of several types of instrumentation. The assay generally involves perfusion at moderate shear rates of a membrane channel impregnated with platelet activating compounds such as collagen, epinephrine, and adenosine 5′-diphosphate (ADP). The time required for activation of the platelets and aggregation leading to occlusion of the perfusion channel is recorded as the in vitro bleeding time, more commonly referred to as "closure time." The assay is now widely available and easily performed in general laboratories. The PFA test offers several advantages over the BT. Closure times are more reproducible than BT, with coefficients of variation (CVs) generally less than 10%, and the PFA is a rapid, automated assay of low technical difficulty. Because the test is done on blood drawn by venipuncture, the patient avoids the incision (and possible scarring) associated with the BT.

Prolonged closure times are reliably seen with platelet dysfunction induced by aspirin or other drugs and in patients with vWD. Collagen/epinephrine closure times appear to be more sensitive to platelet dysfunction than collagen/ADP values; hence, many laboratories have chosen to screen blood samples first with the collagen/epinephrine assay, and then follow with the collagen/ADP if the former is abnormally prolonged. Collagen/epinephrine closure time is more sensitive to aspirin than the collagen/ADP, but both are equally sensitive to such disorders as vWD, Glanzmann thrombasthenia, and both Bernard-Soulier and Hermansky-Pudlak syndromes. Thus, if only the collagen/epinephrine closure time is prolonged (and not the collagen/ADP), this result appears to be more specific for drug-induced platelet dysfunction due to aspirin, nonsteroidal anti-inflammatory drugs (NSAIDs), or platelet receptor blockade.

Prothrombin Time and International Normalized Ratio

The PT provides a measure of the extrinsic and common pathways. Compared with the PTT, it is more sensitive to deficiencies of the vitamin K–dependent liver factors (II, VII, IX, and X). The assay is performed by adding back to citrated plasma both calcium ion and either a purified or recombinant thromboplastin/tissue factor, for example, Innovin (Figure 29–5). This provides a strong stimulus to the activation of factor VII and the common pathway.

The PT can vary significantly depending on the **type of thromboplastin used**. Purified thromboplastins generally give normal values of 10–14 seconds, which is somewhat shorter than results for the recombinant tissue factor. When the PT is used to monitor a patient receiving an oral warfarin, the sensitivity of the thromboplastin on the particular clotting instrument must be taken into account in interpreting the prolongation of the PT. This laboratory situation has led to the development of a standardized method of expressing the PT prolongation as an **international normalized ratio** (INR; see Chapter 37).

As a screen for any single factor deficiency, the PT is most sensitive to a reduced level of factor VII. In patients with liver

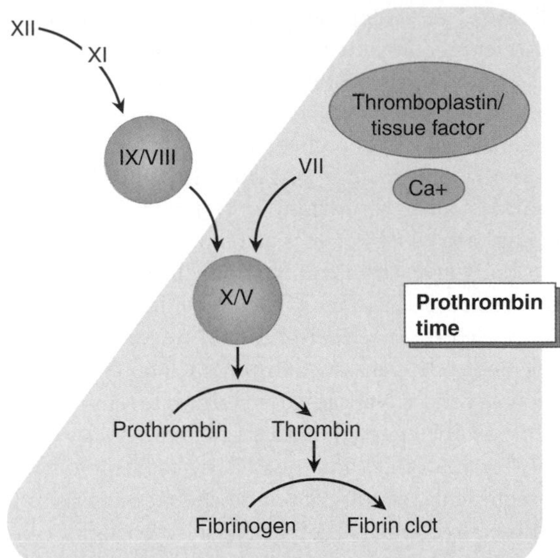

FIGURE 29–5. **The prothrombin time (PT).** Laboratory measurement of the PT is performed by adding a purified or recombinant thromboplastin/tissue factor and calcium ion to citrated plasma to activate the extrinsic pathway. The test detects deficiencies of factors VII, X, V, II (prothrombin), and fibrinogen but is insensitive to deficiencies of factors in the intrinsic pathway (XI, IX, VIII).

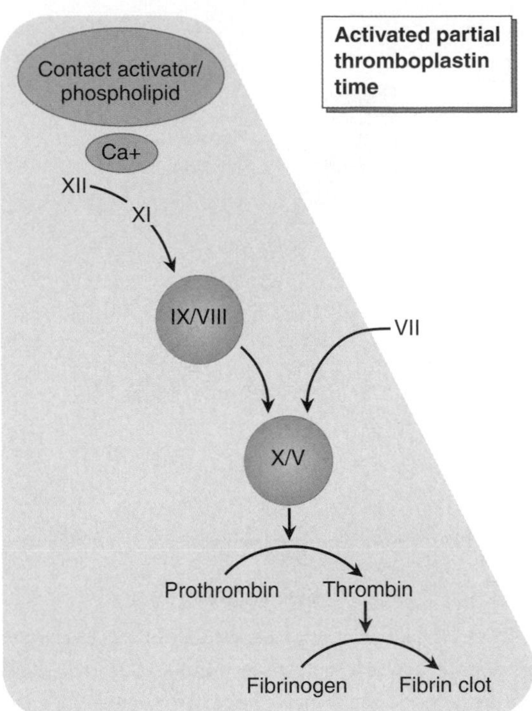

FIGURE 29–6. **The activated partial thromboplastin time (aPTT).** Laboratory measurement of the aPTT is performed by adding a contact activating factor such as kaolin, plus phospholipid, and calcium ion to citrated plasma to activate the intrinsic pathway. This test can detect significant deficiencies in factors XII, XI, IX, VIII, X, V, II (prothrombin), and fibrinogen but is insensitive to factor VII deficiency. The aPTT is generally more sensitive than the PT to the presence of a circulating anticoagulant (eg, heparin, lupus anticoagulant, or an acquired antibody to factor VIII or IX).

disease, the levels of the vitamin K–dependent factors must be reduced by more than 50%–60% to prolong the PT. As a general rule, a prolonged PT that is 1.5–2 times the control value suggests reduced levels of VII and other vitamin K–dependent factors to below 30% of normal. When the PT is greater than twice the control, factor levels are most likely below 20% of normal.

The **PT can also be slightly prolonged** by large amounts of heparin in circulation; more rarely by a circulating inhibitor; and either a reduced level of fibrinogen (<100 mg/dL) or the appearance of large amounts of abnormal fibrinogen molecules or fibrin fragments in circulation. Finally, the PT may be prolonged if the whole blood specimen is stored too long prior to plasma separation, owing to degradation of coagulation proteins in whole blood.

Activated Partial Thromboplastin Time

The aPTT (synonymous with PTT) measures both the intrinsic and common coagulation pathways (factors XII, XI, IX, VIII, X, V, and II). For this assay, citrated plasma is activated with a contact surface material such as kaolin, together with calcium ion and phospholipid (Figure 29–6). Depending on the reagents, the normal aPTT generally ranges from 22–35 seconds, but unlike the INR, this PTT normal range may vary widely between laboratories. Thus, the clinician must be familiar with the normal range of clotting times in different laboratories.

The **aPTT can be prolonged** by a deficiency of any of the factors in the intrinsic or common pathway, by the presence of a circulating inhibitor, or because of a fibrinogen abnormality, with the latter due to either a reduced level or function. In order to significantly prolong the aPTT, single factor deficiencies must be relatively severe, that is, levels below 30%–40% of normal. Multiple factor deficiencies of somewhat lesser severity will also prolong the aPTT.

Although the aPTT is much less sensitive than the PT to low levels of vitamin K–dependent factors, the aPTT is more sensitive to the presence of circulating anticoagulants such as heparin and the lupus anticoagulant. To identify a circulating anticoagulant, the laboratory can repeat the aPTT with a 1:1 mix of patient and normal plasma. Although the admixture of normal plasma will completely correct a prolonged aPTT secondary to a factor deficiency (ie, factor VIII or IX deficiency), it will not fully correct (ie, shorten) the aPTT that is prolonged because of a high titer antibody, also known as a "circulating anticoagulant." A prolonged aPTT resulting from unfractionated heparin in the sample, either because of therapeutic anticoagulation or inadvertent contamination by drawing the sample through an indwelling line, can be determined by mixing the patient plasma with a substance such as heparinase or polybrene; this procedure will neutralize the heparin and correct the aPTT to within or near the normal reference range. Thus, a prolonged aPTT in a hospitalized patient should be investigated first with heparin neutralization, followed by a mixing study if there is no evidence for heparin in the sample. Failure to correct the prolonged aPTT with plasma mixing requires subsequent evaluation for a lupus anticoagulant (see Chapter 36) or a factor inhibitor such as seen with hemophilia patients (see Chapter 33).

Thrombin Time

The thrombin time (TT) measures the last step in the common pathway; that is, conversion of fibrinogen to fibrin. It is performed by adding a dilute solution of bovine thrombin to citrated plasma. The normal control is generally adjusted to give a TT of between 9 and 25 seconds, depending on the thrombin dilution. The TT is prolonged in patients with decreased fibrinogen amounts or abnormal fibrinogen function, or more rarely because of high levels of inhibitory fibrin degradation products. Therefore, the thrombin time is a relatively sensitive (but nonspecific) indicator of disorders such as disseminated intravascular coagulation (DIC) and liver disease. In addition, even very small amounts of heparin in circulation can dramatically prolong the TT by directly inhibiting the function of the added thrombin. If the TT is prolonged and heparin is thought to be present (eg, prolonged aPTT that corrects with polybrene), the heparin-insensitive reptilase time should be used to determine if fibrinogen concentration and function are normal. The reptilase time uses a snake venom from *Bothrops atrox* to cleave the α-chain of fibrinogen. This initiates the polymerization of fibrin independent of the action of thrombin, and thus the reptilase time is unaffected by circulating heparin. The reptilase time is prolonged by hypofibrinogenemia, elevated fibrin split products, and some dysfibrinogenemias. It is most useful when a hospitalized patient has both a prolonged TT and aPTT; heparin as a cause of the prolonged TT is confirmed if the reptilase time is normal.

Fibrinogen (Quantitative) Assays

The concentration of fibrinogen in plasma can be measured by chemical or immunologic methods where the ability of the fibrinogen to clot does not influence the assay. The normal fibrinogen concentration is 200–400 mg/dL. Fibrinogen is an acute phase reactant, however, and levels of 400–800 mg/dL are common in patients with acute, severe illness.

The level of functional fibrinogen can also be assayed, and most laboratories prefer screening for fibrinogen levels by activity. The **von Clauss kinetic assay** employs a dilute solution of patient plasma with an excess of exogenous thrombin to make fibrinogen the rate-limiting factor in the clotting reaction. The resulting clotting time in seconds is compared with a standard dilution curve to determine the concentration of clottable fibrinogen. This assay is very sensitive to the presence of inhibitors of fibrin formation, such as dysfibrinogenemia or the presence in high titer of fibrin degradation products.

The presence of fibrin split products or fibrinogen fragments in serum can be measured directly by a **latex particle agglutination method**. Using latex particles coated with an antiserum to various fragments of fibrin or fibrinogen, it is also possible to semiquantitatively estimate the presence of these fragments, also known as fibrin split-products. Although a normal individual will show 0–1+ agglutination (corresponding to a quantitative value <10 μg/mL), a patient with DIC and marked breakdown of fibrin will be strongly positive for fibrin split-products, 3–4+ agglutination (>40 μg/mL). A false-negative test may be observed, however, in some patients with consumptive coagulopathies if the antiserum is not sensitive to the smaller D and E fragments of degraded fibrin. Moreover, positive agglutination reactions are often seen in patients with liver disease because of the production of abnormal fibrinogen molecules and elevated levels of immunoglobulins.

D-dimer tests for fibrin fragments generally use a monoclonal antibody to the crosslinked D regions of degraded fibrin. This test is more specific for the appearance of split-products secondary to fibrinolysis and should not detect abnormal fibrinogen molecules or fibrinogen fragments. Normal patients without DIC or ongoing clotting/fibrinolysis generally have D-dimer levels below 2.5 μg/mL (2,500 ng/mL), whereas DIC patients can have levels up to 10 times the upper limit of the reference range (and occasionally higher), according to the severity of their illness and underlying organ function. The D-dimer assay is also sufficiently sensitive to fibrinolysis that the assay can also be used to exclude the diagnosis of venous thromboembolic (VTE) disease in certain low-risk patient subsets (see Chapter 36). Each laboratory must establish its own D-dimer range for VTE exclusion, but in general, values less than 1,500 ng/mL indicate the likely absence of VTE in selected patient subsets.

Tests of Fibrinolysis

The **euglobulin lysis time** has been used in many research studies as a diagnostic test for excessive fibrinolysis, but this test has not easily translated to a clinically useful assay. It is performed using the plasma euglobulin fraction prepared from fresh, citrated platelet-poor plasma. After clot formation, the time for spontaneous lysis is measured; the normal euglobulin lysis time is from 60–300 minutes. In research studies, the euglobulin lysis time is shortened in conditions characterized by increased fibrinolysis—liver disease, after administration of tissue-type plasminogen activator, α_2-antiplasmin deficiency, plasminogen activator inhibitor (PAI-1) deficiency, or systemic hyperfibrinolysis. However, it is rarely shortened in patients with DIC, even when such patients have significantly elevated D-dimer levels. The barriers to a clinically useful euglobulin lysis time include difficulties with standardization and control materials, variability of the assay with fluctuating levels of fibrinogen and immunoglobulin, and poor correlation with concentrations of known fibrinolysis-associated proteins, such as α_2-antiplasmin. Thus, it is currently unclear if the euglobulin lysis assay has sufficiently high negative or positive predictive values to justify its clinical use.

Plasminogen activator inhibitor type 1 (PAI-1) is the naturally occurring inactivator of fibrinolysis and blocks plasminogen conversion to its active plasmin form. Elevated levels of PAI-1 activity are associated with the presence of atherosclerotic coronary artery and thromboembolic disease. Metabolic panels for atherosclerotic risk generally include both PAI-1 activity and, if PAI-1 is abnormally elevated, the 4G/5G polymorphisms of PAI-1. The 4G/4G genotype is associated with higher activity and thrombotic risk. A rare deficiency of PAI-1 activity has been reported in patients with bleeding diatheses whose previous laboratory testing failed to show any abnormalities of platelet function or other factor deficiency. These reports, however, must be viewed in light of the fact that normal individuals without a bleeding tendency have also demonstrated absent PAI-1 activity in routine assays; thus, the clinical utility of PAI-1 for the evaluation of bleeding is not justified.

α_2-Antiplasmin is the natural inhibitor of plasmin. As plasminogen is activated to plasmin, α_2-antiplasmin binds to plasmin and removes it from circulation. Thus, low levels of α_2-antiplasmin in plasma can be used to evaluate the rate of plasmin generation in fibrinolysis, either de novo or following pharmacologic thrombolytic therapy. Like most factor assays, α_2-antiplasmin levels are measured as a percentage of normal (range 80%–120%). Individuals with dramatically increased levels of fibrin turnover as a part of ongoing DIC will generally have α_2-antiplasmin levels well below 60% of normal. However, both plasminogen activator inhibitor-1 and α_2-antiplasmin are produced by the liver, and severe liver disease is associated with reduced levels of both proteins. This can cause confusion in clinical circumstances when distinguishing between low-grade DIC and concomitant liver disease. Hence, serial measurement of the D-dimer (increasing over time) and factor VIII levels (decreasing with consumption) are more valuable at distinguishing DIC from liver disease and associated coagulopathies.

TABLE 29–2 • Evaluation of the bleeding patient

Step 1:	**Platelet problem?** Thrombocytopenia or a platelet functional defect	Platelet count PFA, Bleeding time
Step 2:	**Single factor deficiency?** Factor VII, VIII, IX, X, V, XI, fibrinogen	PT, aPTT Factor assays
Step 3:	**Multiple factor deficiency?** Vitamin K deficiency, liver disease, warfarin	PT, aPTT, TT Factor assays
Step 4:	**Circulating anticoagulant?** Heparin, factor VIII or IX antibody, lupus anticoagulant	aPTT with polybrene/heparinase aPTT with 1:1 mix, aPTT with excess phospholipid TT Reptilase time
Step 5:	**Consumptive coagulopathy?** TTP, HUS, vasculitis, sepsis, obstetrical complication, trauma, liver disease	DIC screen: Platelet count PT, aPTT, TT, fibrinogen, D-dimer, blood smear review

APPROACH TO THE PATIENT

Clinical evaluation of a bleeding patient can be defined as a 5-step algorithm (Table 29–2). This also provides a basis for planning management, including the initial decisions regarding administration of blood components.

Step 1: Is There a Problem With the Patient's Platelets?

Often as not, a platelet problem can be anticipated because of an **associated disease process**. Patients with damaged marrows secondary to aplastic anemia, a hematologic malignancy, or drug exposure (especially chemotherapy for malignant disease) can be expected to present with thrombocytopenia secondary to decreased platelet production. Severe thrombocytopenia secondary to increased destruction can accompany autoimmune and, more rarely, lymphoproliferative disorders (see Chapter 31). Abnormalities in platelet function can be inherited but more commonly result from drug exposure (see Chapter 32).

One clinical tip-off to a platelet abnormality is the appearance of **petechial hemorrhage**. Depending on the severity of the thrombocytopenia, they may be limited to the legs or arms (see Chapter 31) or become widespread, involving virtually every organ. Severe thrombocytopenia and platelet functional defects also result in easy bruisability, mucous membrane bleeding, epistaxis, menometrorrhagia, and a tendency for small vessel oozing during surgery.

Screening laboratory tests for a suspected platelet defect include the platelet count and, in those patients with a normal platelet count, a BT or PFA to evaluate function. The tendency for abnormal bleeding in patients who are thrombocytopenic is not a simple reflection of the severity of the thrombocytopenia. Although an otherwise normal individual may show little in the way of bleeding until the platelet count falls to below 10,000/μL, patients with a malignancy, an obstetrical complication, or ongoing sepsis can demonstrate severe bleeding when the platelet count falls below 20,000/μL. This drop may reflect a combination of thrombocytopenia and platelet dysfunction or an increased requirement for platelets because of endothelial cell damage. The latter possibility is most dramatically illustrated when thrombocytopenic patients undergo surgery or experience trauma. In this setting, abnormal bleeding can occur when the platelet count falls to below 50,000 or even 100,000/μL.

Clinically significant platelet dysfunction can be detected using the **PFA** or **BT**. The BT is at best a crude test, however, and should not be used as a routine screening test. This situation is especially true for preoperative patients without a bleeding history where modest prolongations of the BT do not predict surgical bleeding. It is also difficult to get an accurate BT measurement when the patient is seriously ill. Patients who are septic, uremic, or receiving a drug that inhibits platelet function can be assumed to have some degree of platelet dysfunction. An attempt to quantitate this by doing a BT can be frustrating and can provide such conflicting data that it is useless. Therefore, the BT (or better yet, the PFA in vitro "bleeding" time) should be reserved for patients who have a bleeding history suggestive of aspirin or other anti-platelet therapy, an inherited defect in platelet function, or a defect in platelet-dependent clotting such as clinically significant von Willebrand disease.

Step 2: Does the Patient Have an Inherited Coagulopathy, for example, a Single-Factor Deficiency?

An inherited coagulopathy may be suspected because of the clinical presentation. The patient with a severe factor deficiency as, for example, factor VIII or factor IX deficiency (hemophilia A or B, respectively), will usually present with a history of repeated bleeding episodes beginning as an infant and extending throughout childhood and adult life (see Chapter 33). When the deficiency is less severe, the patient may report abnormal bleeding following trauma or surgery, an unexplained hemarthrosis, or muscle hematoma. In contrast to patients with platelet defects, factor-deficient individuals have complaints of purpura, hemarthrosis, muscle hematomas, and large vessel bleeding, as opposed to petechial and mucosal hemorrhage with platelet abnormalities.

The **PT and aPTT** are the most valuable screening tests for detecting a single factor deficiency. They must be interpreted as a matched pair. If the PT is significantly prolonged and the aPTT is normal, the patient may have factor VII deficiency. If the aPTT is prolonged and the PT is normal, an intrinsic pathway defect, especially factor VIII, IX, or XI deficiency, is suspected.

This interpretation of PT and aPTT values is generally valid in patients with an appropriate clinical history who are not receiving an anticoagulant drug, and who do not have either liver disease or a consumptive coagulopathy such as DIC. The PT is very sensitive to even modest depletion of common pathway factors. Therefore, a long PT with a normal aPTT is typical of patients receiving warfarin therapy or who have early liver disease. In contrast, the aPTT is more sensitive to heparin and circulating anticoagulants (anti-factor VIII is most common) that seldom prolong the PT. These possibilities need to be excluded before concluding that a single-factor deficiency is present.

Step 3: Does the Patient Have a Deficiency of Several of the Vitamin K–Dependent Coagulation Factors?

Both **warfarin therapy** and **liver disease** typically produce multiple factor deficiencies involving the extrinsic and common pathways (see Chapter 34). Patients with severe liver disease can also demonstrate defects in the production of fibrinogen in terms of both the total amount and its functional characteristics. Therefore, it is important to look for any history of poor nutrition, vitamin K malabsorption, warfarin ingestion, or the symptoms and signs that would indicate worsening liver disease.

The **type of bleeding** may also be a clue. As with a single coagulation factor–deficiency state, petechial hemorrhages are not expected in multiple factor deficiency; patients usually show a combination of easy bruisability and widespread purpura, as well as mucous membrane/GI tract bleeding. The patient with severe liver disease frequently presents with a dramatic upper GI bleed due to varices or Mallory-Weiss tears, which compound the factor deficit.

The **PT, aPTT, TT, and fibrinogen assays** are key laboratory tests for the identification of a multiple factor–deficiency state. As mentioned, the PT is very sensitive to modest reductions in the vitamin K–dependent factors, factors VII, IX, X, and II (prothrombin). The vitamin K–deficient patient would be expected to have a prolonged PT with a normal or only slightly prolonged aPTT. Similarly, patients receiving warfarin or with early liver disease would be expected to have a prolonged PT (generally INR <5) and normal aPTT. In contrast, the patient with more severe liver disease or warfarin overdose/poisoning can show prolongations of the PT, aPTT, and TT. Prolongation of the aPTT occurs more frequently when the PT is extremely prolonged (INR >5–10). The prolonged TT in end-stage liver disease also reflects the dysfibrinogenemia and buildup of fibrinogen and fibrin breakdown products that act as inhibitors of the TT. Finally, the very severe liver disease patient may also show a discrepancy between the von Clauss fibrinogen assay that detects clottable fibrinogen and immunologic assays of total fibrinogen.

Step 4: Is There a Circulating Anticoagulant Present?

A circulating anticoagulant may explain the patient's bleeding tendency. Administration of heparin to prevent venous thrombosis or maintain catheter patency is almost universal in severely ill patients, and over-anticoagulation with heparin is a common cause of abnormal bleeding. Much more rare is the spontaneous appearance of a circulating antibody (inhibitor) to factor VIII or IX, which will also lead to severe and abnormal bleeding. In both circumstances, the aPTT is preferentially prolonged over the PT, but rare inhibitors to factor VII that prolong the PT have been described.

A prolonged aPTT also can be the result of a lupus anticoagulant (sometimes seen in lupus erythematous patients or those with primary antiphospholipid syndrome). However, lupus anticoagulants rarely cause bleeding; instead, they are frequently associated with venous or arterial thrombosis. When present, the lupus anticoagulant will usually prolong the aPTT to a greater extent than the PT, although exceptions have been noted.

Once considered, it is not difficult to confirm the **presence of a circulating anticoagulant**. Prolongation of the aPTT by heparin can be corrected by neutralizing agents such as heparinase or polybrene. When heparin has been ruled out, **the presence of a lupus anticoagulant or factor VIII inhibitor** can be confirmed by demonstrating failure of the aPTT to correct after a 1:1 mix of the patient's plasma and normal plasma, in contrast to coagulation factor deficiency states where the addition of normal plasma will completely correct the aPTT. A lupus anticoagulant can then be specifically detected by correction of the aPTT by addition of excess phospholipid to correct the aPTT and other confirmatory tests (see Chapter 36). The specificity of a circulating inhibitor to factor VIII, or less commonly factor IX, can be determined by demonstrating decreased factor activity (which is usually severe) and then mixing patient plasma with normal plasma at various dilutions to quantitate the inhibitor titer.

Step 5: Does the Patient Have a Consumptive Coagulopathy?

Depending on the disease process, patients can exhibit a high rate of platelet consumption and/or activation of the entire coagulation cascade. Platelet microthrombi with symptoms and signs of multiple organ damage, especially to the kidney, brain, and skin, are seen in microangiopathic hemolytic conditions such as thrombotic thrombocytopenic purpura (TTP), hemolytic uremic syndrome (HUS), and in some vasculitides. Thrombocytopenia secondary to the consumption of platelets is most severe in patients with TTP and less prominent in individuals with HUS or vasculitis. Red blood cell fragmentation (**schistocytosis** and an elevated lactic dehydrogenase [LDH] with anemia) are tip-offs to the presence of these microangiopathic conditions, which generally do not involve the soluble coagulation factors, unlike DIC.

Full-blown **disseminated intravascular coagulation (DIC)** is a more common disorder (see Chapter 35) than microangiopathic hemolytic anemia. DIC is most often seen in patients after major trauma, with sepsis, or an obstetric complication. It is the coagulopathy of the critically ill patient. Clinically, these patients present with widespread bleeding, including purpura, oozing from needle puncture and catheter insertion sites, mucous membrane and GI bleeding, and severe bleeding with surgery.

Hospital laboratories usually offer a battery of coagulation **tests to screen for DIC**. This battery should include a platelet count, PT, aPTT, TT, fibrinogen assay, D-dimer or fibrin split-product tests for fibrin fragments, and a blood film examination for red blood cell fragmentation (schistocytes) to determine the presence of microangiopathy. Together, these tests provide an overview of the major components of the coagulation cascade. The PT and aPTT measure the coagulation factor pathways. The TT, fibrinogen, and D-dimer assays provide information as to fibrinogen consumption, clot formation, and fibrinolysis. Clinical scoring systems for the likelihood of DIC use both the clinical scenario and lab testing; if a patient has a disorder known to be associated with overt DIC, then the platelet count, D-dimer, fibrin split-products, PT, and fibrinogen values can be used to score the probability that DIC is present.

DIC can be **confused with severe liver disease**, especially when the DIC is relatively low grade. This situation reflects the fact that the liver is the major site of production of most coagulation factors, including fibrinogen and α_2-antiplasmin. The liver also plays a role in the removal of fibrin degradation products. It is important, therefore, to exclude significant liver disease when making the diagnosis of DIC. This should not be difficult in patients with advanced cirrhosis where liver synthetic function is poor (decreased albumin, prolonged PT) and the serum bilirubin and other liver enzymes are clearly elevated. It can be more difficult in the critically ill or septic patient, when both DIC and acute liver failure may be present. The presence of an elevated factor VIII level may help. Typically, factor VIII levels are high in patients with liver disease, reflecting the ability of reticuloendothelial cells and megakaryocytes to produce factor VIII as an acute phase reactant. By contrast, factor VIII levels are normal or decreased with DIC.

THE BLEEDING PATIENT: DEFINITIVE DIAGNOSIS AND MANAGEMENT

Early and repeated assays of coagulation pathways are essential in the management of the acutely bleeding patient. This is especially true for life-threatening bleeds in critically ill patients. For example, severe thrombocytopenia or a platelet functional defect or both should be treated with platelet transfusions (see Chapter 38). Similarly, a single-factor deficiency can be effectively reversed by administering the appropriate purified factor or fresh frozen plasma. Treatment with vitamin K and/or fresh frozen plasma can also be effective in the patient with multiple deficiencies of vitamin K–dependent factors resulting from warfarin or other causes.

As for the DIC patient, stepwise replacement of platelets, fibrinogen, and coagulation factors are temporizing measures to lessen the bleeding; effective therapy and survival depend on the clinician's ability to gain control of the underlying clinical disorder that initiated the consumptive coagulopathy. Once that condition is controlled, the DIC patient will better respond to transfusions. The pharmacologic use of activated protein C in sepsis has been shown to ameliorate DIC and improve survival in a small percentage of patients, but this effect may not be entirely mediated by its anticoagulant function.

Long-term management of a bleeding diathesis obviously requires a definitive diagnosis of the patient's condition. This diagnosis may require the expertise of a consultant hematologist and a hemostasis reference laboratory to define platelet functional abnormalities and/or deficiencies in specific factors. When the latter are acquired, the reference laboratory must also identify and quantitate the presence of specific factor inhibitors.

POINTS TO REMEMBER

Evaluation of a patient with a possible coagulopathy requires a detailed assessment of the patient's presentation, past medical history, family history, and the physical characteristics of the bleeding diathesis. The association of bleeding with an illness, surgery, a traumatic event, or drug ingestion, and the sites of hemorrhage (eg, mucosa, skin, joint, or muscle) can point to a diagnosis.

Petechial and mucosal bleeding suggests a platelet-based etiology (thrombocytopenia or platelet dysfunction), whereas muscle hematomas and bleeding into joints or closed spaces suggests a coagulation factor deficiency, most often an inherited defect, such as hemophilia.

A number of tests of coagulation are available to evaluate the patient with a suspected coagulopathy. A routine battery includes the platelet count, measurement of platelet function, PT, aPTT, and TT. Accurate assessment of any single test abnormality requires that all of these tests be performed at the same time.

The risk of platelet-based bleeding increases progressively as the platelet count falls below 50,000/μL, and/or the patient has a significant functional defect, as measured by the bleeding time or in vitro platelet function assay (PFA).

The PT (prothrombin time) measures the extrinsic and common pathways—factors VII, X, V, thrombin generation, and fibrin clot formation. It is exquisitely sensitive to the presence of vitamin K inhibitors (warfarin) and liver dysfunction.

The aPTT (activated partial thromboplastin time) measures the intrinsic and common pathways—factors XI, VIII, IX, X, V, thrombin generation, and fibrin clot formation. It is especially sensitive to deficiencies in factors VIII and IX (the hemophilias), circulating anticoagulants, heparin, and multiple factor deficiencies.

The TT (thrombin time) measures the last step in the common pathway, the rate of conversion of fibrinogen to fibrin clot. It is especially sensitive to the presence of hypofibrinogenemia, heparin, and degraded fibrin fragments.

Consumption of multiple coagulation factors and platelets can be seen with liver disease and disseminated intravascular coagulation (DIC). An additional battery of tests, including measures of fibrinogen quantity and function, D-dimer level (presence of crosslinked fibrin fragments), and, in some cases, α_2-antiplasmin level (natural inhibitor of plasmin) are used to evaluate the presence and severity of these conditions.

Finally, it is important for clinicians to know the methodologies and normal values particular to their coagulation laboratory. Without this knowledge, the interpretation of individual test results is impossible.

BIBLIOGRAPHY

Hess JR, Lawson JH: The coagulopathy of trauma versus disseminated intravascular coagulation. J Trauma-Injury Infect Crit Care 2006;60:S12.

Levi M: Disseminated intravascular coagulation. Crit Care Med 2007;35:2191.

Levi M, Peters M, Buller HR: Efficacy and safety of recombinant factor VIIa for treatment of severe bleeding: a systematic review. Crit Care Med 2005;33:883.

Levy JH, Tanaka KA, Dietrich W: Perioperative hemostatic management of patients treated with vitamin K antagonists. Anesthesiology 2008;109:918.

Mencin AA: Severe gastrointestinal bleeding. Clin Pediatr 2006;45:683.

Oyelese Y, Smulian JC: Placenta previa, placenta accreta, and vasa previa. Obstet Gynecol 2006;107:927.

Spinella PC: Warm fresh whole blood transfusion for severe hemorrhage: U.S. military and potential civilian applications. Crit Care Med 2008;36:S340.

St Andre AC, DelRossi A: Hemodynamic management of patients in the first 24 hours after cardiac surgery. Crit Care Med 2005;33:2082.

Toh CH, Downey C: Back to the future: testing in disseminated intravascular coagulation. Blood Coagulation & Fibrinolysis 2005;16:535.

VASCULAR PURPURA · 30

CASE HISTORY • Part I

A 46-year-old woman presents with a complaint of more than 3 months of fatigue and dyspnea on exertion. Her history is notable for lifelong recurring epistaxis, requiring repeated nasal packing, septal dermoplasty, and laser therapy. Her father also had repeated epistaxis; he died at age 60 from a brain abscess. Examination is notable for pallor and multiple blue-red lesions involving the lips and fingers. The remainder of the examination is benign except for a positive test for occult blood in the stool.

CBC: Hemoglobin/hematocrit - 7 g/dL/22%
MCV - 64 fL MCH - 24 pg MCHC - 24 g/dL
RDW-CV - 24% WBC count - 6,500/μL
Platelet count - 410,000/μL

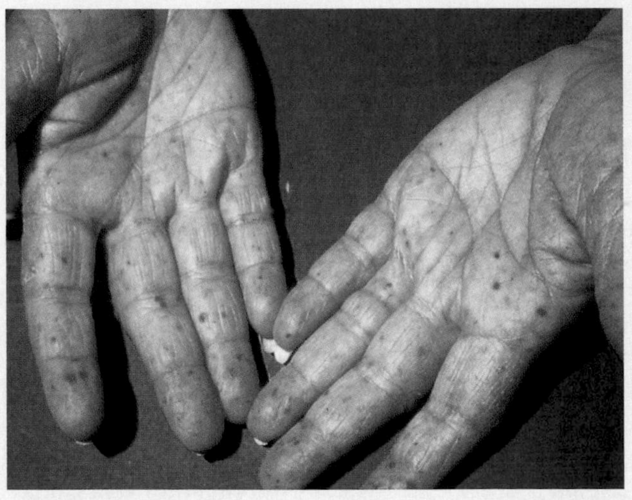

• SMEAR MORPHOLOGY

Microcytic, hypochromic with marked aniso- and poikilocytosis, polychromasia, and the occasional cigar-shaped cell. White blood cells and platelets are both normal.

Reticulocyte count/index - 1.3%/<1.0

Questions

- How should the anemia be described and does the history suggest a specific etiology?
- What additional tests should be ordered to confirm the cause of the anemia?

A vessel wall defect, either intrinsic or induced by trauma or inflammatory changes, can result in abnormal bleeding despite an otherwise normal coagulation system. Since there are no reliable clinical tests of vascular integrity, the diagnosis of an abnormality in vascular structure often depends on keen observation. For example, multiple small telangiectases on the lips can be a tip-off to the diagnosis of hereditary hemorrhagic telangiectasia. In patients with a normal platelet count, normal coagulation studies, and normal platelet function, the presence of petechiae, purpura, or excessive bleeding after minor trauma or surgery also must raise the question of an underlying vascular defect.

NORMAL VESSEL FUNCTION

Blood vessels provide a critical balancing act to contain and promote liquid blood flow, and at the same time resist thrombus

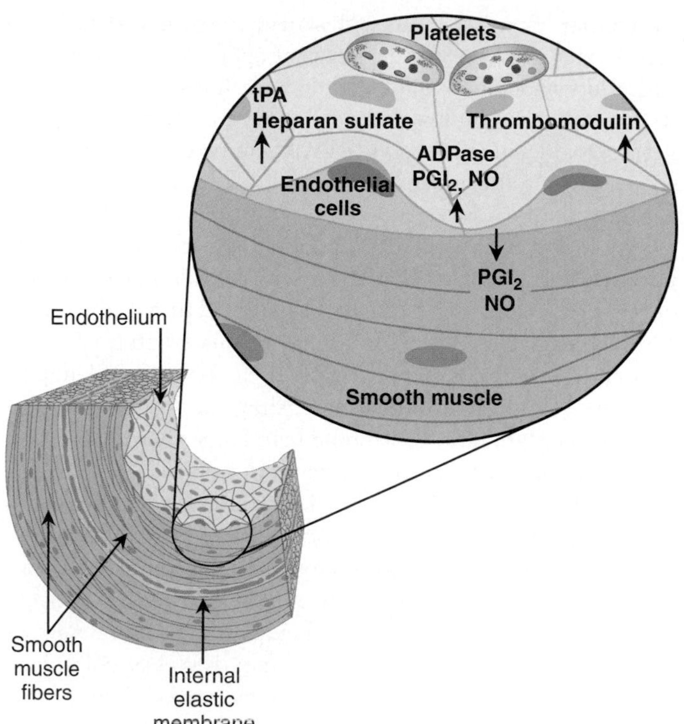

FIGURE 30–1. **Vessel wall structure and function.** Endothelial cells of the vessel wall play an important role in hemostasis. They produce inhibitors of platelet activation, including ADPase, prostacyclin, and nitric oxide. They also play a role in counteracting clot formation by providing thrombomodulin, heparan sulfates, and tissue plasminogen activator. Nitric oxide and prostacyclin produced by the endothelial cell are also important in determining vessel wall tone. When endothelial cells are damaged, the loss of nitric oxide production results in vasospasm secondary to unopposed smooth muscle contraction.

formation. As illustrated in Figure 30–1, there is an organized structure to the blood vessel wall that serves these functions. Endothelial cells that line the blood vessels provide much more than a simple barrier to prevent the escape of blood cells. The endothelial cell is very active metabolically, synthesizing **mediators of the interaction between blood components and the vessel wall.** Some of these, such as prostacyclin (PGI_2), nitric oxide, heparan sulfate, tissue plasminogen activator (t-PA), thrombomodulin, tissue factor pathway inhibitor (TFPI), and ADPase act to maintain blood in its fluid state by counter-acting platelet activation, aggregation, and clot formation, whereas others are primed and positioned to enhance blood procoagulant function should trauma or some other event produce bleeding (Table 30–1).

Important intracellular organelles responsible for the supply of pro- and anticoagulant factors are the Weibel-Palade (WP) bodies, which contain and secrete ultra-large von Willebrand factor (vWF) multimers, the vasoconstrictor endothelin, t-PA, and angiopoietin-2, a protein active in vascular remodeling and inflammation. The balance of these secreted factors helps to maintain hemostasis, clot remodeling, and vascular integrity. Endothelial cell function is also modulated by feedback

TABLE 30–1 • Endothelial cell factors regulating coagulation

Procoagulant	Anticoagulant
Vessel contraction	**Platelet inhibition**
Endothelin	ADPase
Coagulation factor production	Nitric oxide
Factor C inhibitor	Prostacyclin
Factor VIII	**Clot inhibition/lysis**
Von Willebrand multimers	Heparan sulfates
Fibronectin	Thrombomodulin
Adhesive antigen expression	Tissue factor pathway inhibitor
Selectins (CD62P, CD62E)	Plasminogen activator inhibitor-1
PECAM-1	t-Plasminogen activator
Integrins (β_1 and β_2)	
Vascular remodeling	
Angiopoietin-2	

mechanisms inherent in the cells, especially the release of nitric oxide, which can block WP fusion with the cellular membrane and release of procoagulants.

Another important function of endothelial cells is their contribution to the regulation of the **migration of leukocytes out of the blood, through the vessel wall, and into tissues** (see Chapter 16). P-selectin expressed by endothelial cells encourages loose adhesion of leukocytes to the vessel wall and initiates the sequence of rolling, margination, and migration. Endothelial cell factors including the β_1- and β_2-integrins, and the immunoglobulin (Ig)-like receptor PECAM-1, all play a role. They also interact with hemostatic mechanisms as a part of the inflammatory response. Erythrocytes are affected in this cycle of inflammation and hemostasis as well, since tethering of red cells to adherent leukocytes can influence vasoocclusion in diseases such as sickle cell anemia.

Endothelial cells also play a major role in **determining the structure and function of the subendothelium**, including production of components of the subendothelial matrix (ie, elastin, laminin, thrombospondin, vWF, fibronectin, and several types of collagen). In addition, endothelial cells control vessel wall tone by continuously secreting prostacyclin and nitric oxide, which diffuse into the vessel wall and act as potent smooth muscle relaxants.

Vessel Structure

Vessel structure **varies according to the location** in the circulatory system. Although most vessels are lined by a continuous layer of tightly opposed endothelial cells, fenestrated endothelium is seen in the sinusoids of the liver and spleen, reflecting the special transport needs of these organs.

The subendothelial structure of the vessel **also varies according to functional needs**. For example, larger arteries that must resist high intraluminal pressures have thick muscular walls with a well-defined internal elastic lamina. In the lower-pressure venous circuit, the concentration of smooth muscle cells, elastic tissue, and collagen fibers decreases proportionately. Arterial endothelial cells tightly regulate vascular smooth muscle tone by their production of nitric oxide, prostacyclin, and endothelin, whereas venous endothelial cells are not major producers of these vasoactive mediators.

The **reaction to injury also varies** according to the structure of the vessel. Larger vessels with thick muscular walls rapidly contract when injured to slow or stop blood flow, and the high shear rate in arteries encourages platelet adhesion and thrombus formation. Veins and venules are more easily damaged and rely to a greater extent on activation of the coagulation cascade to generate thrombin and stop bleeding. In contrast, capillary disruption is associated with much less extensive bleeding, and repair may occur with little involvement of the coagulation system.

Shear rates also determine specific interactions between platelets and endothelial cells. At high shear, ultra-large vWF multimers are secreted from the WP bodies that have immediate affinity for circulating platelets. This adhesive function of secreted vWF is enhanced if the endothelial cells are disrupted, exposing subendothelial collagen, which avidly binds vWF, allowing the shear force to further unfold these string-like multimers and expose platelet binding sites. Platelets roll along these multimers and adhere to the vWF multimers like beads on a string (if the procoagulant balance fosters platelet activation). Alternatively, if there is no additional platelet stimulation, the platelets gradually disengage and return to the circulation. If there is no committed vWF-platelet interaction, these ultra-large multimers are promptly cleaved by the metalloproteinase ADAMTS13 into large multimers that coil up around hydrophobic regions, obscuring the platelet-binding site and protecting bound factor VIII, thereby increasing its half-life. When these mechanisms are acutely disrupted, for example, by inflammation associated with vasculitis, bleeding symptoms and purpuric lesions can result. Chronic alterations in these homeostatic mechanisms may be crucial in the development of atherosclerosis.

CLINICAL FEATURES

The clinical presentation of the patient may be sufficient to make the diagnosis. Clues to look for in the **history** include the clinical pattern of bleeding, the relationship to minor trauma or drug ingestion, dietary habits, and symptoms or signs of systemic illness. Often, the patient is aware of specific factors that contribute to the abnormal bleeding and the characteristics of past bleeding episodes and can convey that critical information if specifically asked about such factors.

The **physical examination** by itself may be diagnostic. For example, an elderly patient with marked skin atrophy and multiple bluish-colored ecchymoses on the forearms and back of the hands almost certainly has senile purpura. In the case of a congenital disorder of subcutaneous collagen, **Ehlers-Danlos syndrome**, the patient's skin lacks its normal resistance to traction and can be easily pulled away from underlying structures. This condition places blood vessels at great risk for disruption even with minor trauma. Patients with **scurvy** (vitamin C deficiency) can be identified from their physical appearance; the patient with scurvy and abnormal bleeding will almost always demonstrate marked weight loss and a gait disturbance. Bleeding manifestations include the unique trio of gum bleeding, widespread ecchymoses on the inner upper thighs (saddle distribution), and perifollicular hemorrhages.

Another clue to a vascular abnormality is the **nature of the purpuric lesion**. In patients with vasculitis, individual petechial or purpuric lesions may be slightly raised and firm to the touch, so-called **palpable purpura**. This may be immediately preceded by an urticarial lesion in patients with Henoch-Schönlein purpura. As vasculitic lesions resolve, they can leave an area of hyperpigmentation or an atrophic scar. Larger purpuric tumors of the skin are seen in AIDS patients who develop Kaposi sarcoma and in patients with amyloid deposition in the skin. With amyloidosis, purpura is usually associated with plaques or papules of waxy-appearing skin. Furthermore, skin bleeding can be easily induced in the patient with amyloidosis by pinching or stroking the skin. Finally, a careful examination of the mucous membranes of the nasal passages and mouth is essential to look for the telangiectasia that characterizes patients with hereditary hemorrhagic telangiectasia.

Laboratory Studies

By definition, a patient with vascular purpura should have normal coagulation studies. Routine screening tests should be performed, including a measurement of the platelet count, prothrombin time (PT), and activated partial thromboplastin time (aPTT). More in-depth studies of platelet function may need to be ordered if the diagnosis is not clear from the patient's history and physical examination. Since the diagnosis of vascular purpura is one of exclusion, the general algorithm to follow for a bleeding patient with normal platelet count, PT, and aPTT is as follows: (1) rule out primary hemostatic disorders such as von Willebrand disease (vWD) and platelet dysfunction; (2) subsequently examine for more uncommon abnormalities in secondary hemostasis, including factor XIII deficiency and dysfibrinogenemias; and (3) rule out fibrinolytic disorders such as α_2-antiplasmin deficiency. Provocative tests of vascular fragility, such as the tourniquet test, are not recommended. First of all, the tourniquet test does not discriminate between vascular bleeding and defects in platelet function and, more importantly, even a few moments of compression of venous return from an extremity can result in severe purpura in patients with a major vascular abnormality. Generally, it is the history and presentation of the vascular purpura patient, as well as the lack of abnormal coagulation studies, that help to guide the diagnosis.

DIFFERENTIAL DIAGNOSIS

Simple bruising of exposed areas of the skin without other signs of abnormal bleeding is a very common complaint. It is seen frequently in fair-skinned women and may be worsened by aspirin ingestion. Some of these individuals may have mild vWD. Many

CASE HISTORY • *Part 2*

Based on smear morphology and the red blood cell indices (mean cell volume [MCV], mean cell hemoglobin [MCH], mean corpuscular hemoglobin concentration [MCHC]), the patient has a severe microcytic, hypochromic anemia most likely caused by iron deficiency (see Chapter 5). This was confirmed by iron studies showing:

Serum iron - 10 μg/dL, TIBC - 460 μg/dL, % saturation - 2%
Serum ferritin - 3 μg/L

The history of repeated epistaxis and the positive test for blood in the stool strongly suggest chronic blood loss as the etiology of the iron deficiency. This obviously will require a careful workup of the gastrointestinal (GI) tract for a bleeding site and any correctable anatomic lesion. At the same time, a search for a coagulation defect is in order. Therefore, additional screening laboratory studies of importance include PT/international normalized ratio (INR), aPTT, platelet function studies, and vWF antigen and activity (see Chapter 29). The following results were obtained in this patient:

PT/INR - 13.1 sec (<14.0 sec)/1.10 (<1.30)
aPTT - 28.9 sec (<35.0 sec)
Platelet function analysis (PFA) closure time - 99 sec (80–110 sec)
vWF antigen - 95% (50%–150%)
Ristocetin cofactor activity - 89% (50%–150%)

Questions

- Based on these results, does the patient have a coagulopathy?
- If not, what is the most likely cause of her bleeding?

more appear, however, to have no identifiable defect in platelet or vWF function; they simply bruise very easily. In a similar fashion, the appearance of a conjunctival hemorrhage brought on by coughing or development in the elderly of purpuric lesions over the lower extremities is best classified as **mechanical purpura**, that is, purpura resulting from increased mechanical stress to a vessel. It does not suggest an underlying vascular or coagulation factor defect.

STRUCTURAL ABNORMALITIES

Abnormalities in structure of the subcutaneous tissue are commonly associated with vascular purpura (Table 30–2). Senile purpura in the elderly patient is a direct result of atrophy of the skin and subcutaneous tissues. Purpura can also be seen in patients receiving prolonged steroid therapy which causes collagen breakdown. Chronic venous stasis of the lower extremity is another common cause of purpura.

Pseudoxanthoma elasticum, an inherited defect in the elastic fibers of the vessel wall, is associated with skin purpura, severe bleeding from the GI and genitourinary tracts, excessive menstrual bleeding, and spontaneous retinal hemorrhages. The characteristic elastic fiber calcification is caused by mutations in the *ABC-C6* gene which encodes the transmembrane transporter protein. These patients can be recognized from the characteristic yellowish xanthoma-like skin lesions over the neck and axillae (and other flexural sites) and angioid streaks in the retina. Patients with **Ehlers-Danlos** syndrome demonstrate abnormalities in the various types of collagen in vessels and subcutaneous tissue. Because of this structural defect, the skin is so fragile that it bruises with the slightest trauma. These patients are easily identified because of their velvety, hyperelastic skin and hyperextensible joints.

Severe bleeding from several sites is more typical of patients with **vitamin C deficiency** or anatomic defects of vessels. The importance of vitamin C in collagen biosynthesis is dramatically

TABLE 30–2 • Causes (and features) of vascular purpura

Structural abnormalities
Senile/steroid purpura (thinned subcutaneous tissue, flat bruising)
Pseudoxanthoma elasticum (leathery skin, flexural plaques)
Ehlers-Danlos syndrome (skin hyperelasticity, hyperextensible joints)
Scurvy (perifollicular hemorrhage)
Hereditary hemorrhagic telangiectasia (telangiectases on lips, nose, mouth)
Vasculitis
Henoch-Schönlein purpura (urticaria preceding purpura)
Bacterial sepsis (fever and thrombocytopenia)
Polyarteritis (temporal arteritis symptoms)
Dysproteinemias
Mixed cryoglobulinemia (purpura with skin breakdown)
Multiple myeloma (monoclonal paraprotein)
Waldenström macroglobulinemia (monoclonal IgM paraprotein)
Benign hyperglobulinemic purpura (rheumatoid factor positive)
Cryofibrinogenemia (purpura with vascular compromise)
Amyloidosis (waxy plaques)

illustrated in the patient with scurvy. The pathognomonic lesion of scurvy has the appearance of perifollicular hemorrhages surrounding individual deformed, corkscrew-shaped hairs. Easy bruisability and the formation of widespread ecchymoses over the lower extremities, particularly the inner upper thigh (saddle distribution), are also seen. Bleeding gums (when teeth are present) and deep intramuscular and subperiosteal hemorrhages also may occur.

Congenital defects of blood vessels will also result in an abnormal bleeding tendency. The autosomal dominant disorder **hereditary hemorrhagic telangiectasia (HHT)** is the best example of such an abnormality. This relatively common (>1:10,000 incidence) genetic disorder is characterized by vascular dysplasia presenting most often as telangiectases in the mucosa of the oropharynx and upper GI tract, and lesions on the tongue, lips, and fingers. HHT patients also demonstrate arteriovenous malformations (AVM), which are mostly pulmonary, central nervous system (CNS), upper GI, or hepatic. More than 80% of HHT cases have been found by sequencing to have mutations in either the endoglin gene (chromosome 9, *HHT1*) or the activin receptor-like kinase 1 gene (chromosome 12, *HHT2*). These 2 genes encode members of the transforming growth factor-β superfamily of receptor proteins, suggesting that HHT is presumably linked to disruption of this particular signaling pathway in vascular tissue. Genetic diagnosis should include analysis for mutations in both genes; clinically, however, no specific mutations have been associated with HHT severity.

Almost all individuals with HHT have frequent epistaxis, with some having dozens of bleeding events each month. GI bleeding commonly results in iron deficiency. Pulmonary AVM occur in about 30% of patients with HHT. Because pulmonary and other AVM have direct artery-vein connections, HHT symptoms of respiratory AVM may present either gradually, as a shunt (dyspnea on exertion, polycythemia, or cyanosis), or suddenly, as CNS thromboembolism. The latter must be differentiated from CNS AVM (10% of individuals with HHT), which can similarly present as intracranial hemorrhage or ischemic stroke. CNS symptoms can also occur as a result of brain abscess caused by paradoxical shunting of septic emboli. The diagnosis of HHT is solid if at least 3 of the following criteria are met and likely when only 2 are seen: (a) recurrent epistaxis, especially without trauma, for example, while sleeping; (b) telangiectases; (c) AVM; and (d) relatives with HHT manifestations (a–c). Screening studies recommended in patients with HHT and in their relatives who are found to have an endoglin or *ALK1* mutation should include brain magnetic resonance imaging (MRI; with and without gadolinium) to detect CNS AVM and contrast echocardiography to examine for pulmonary shunting.

Vasculitis

Petechial and purpuric eruptions accompany several bacterial, viral, rickettsial, fungal, and parasitic infections (Table 30–3). A variety of lesions may be seen, including petechiae, discrete purpuric macules and papules, diffuse purpura, hemorrhagic bullae, and marked, widespread purpura with infarction of the skin **(purpura fulminans)**. The mechanism involved is not simply damage to the endothelial cell lining. Often as not, there are multiple, simultaneous abnormalities of hemostasis, including thrombocytopenia, disseminated intravascular coagulation, immune-complex vasculitis, and septic emboli. For example, bacterial endocarditis patients will present with a mixture of lesions from simple petechiae to purpuric papules on palms and fingertips **(Osler nodes)**, hemorrhagic lesions of the retina **(Roth spots)**, and evidence of immune vasculitis (proteinuria and red cells in the urine).

TABLE 30–3 • Infectious purpura

Bacterial
Endocarditis (acute and subacute)
Meningococcemia purpura fulminans
Gram-negative sepsis
Henoch-Schönlein purpura
Viral
Parvovirus
Rubella, varicella, roseola
Cytomegalovirus
Coxsackie B6
Herpes (HHV-6)
Hanta virus
Hemorrhagic fevers
Rickettsial
Rocky mountain spotted fever

Sudden appearance of palpable purpura, often preceded by an urticarial rash, suggests a septic or aseptic vasculitis. When a purpuric rash is associated with fever, malaise, polyarthralgia, and colicky abdominal pain, a diagnosis of **Henoch-Schönlein purpura** can be made. This syndrome is most common in childhood and early adolescence, although it can also affect young adults. There is often a history of a recent upper respiratory infection suggesting a hypersensitivity reaction to a bacterium such as β-hemolytic streptococcus. The role of an autoimmune reaction is further supported by the appearance of an IgA-immune complex in the serum during the first weeks of the illness. The vasculitis is not limited to the skin but involves other organs, such as the bowel and kidney. Hemorrhage into the bowel wall is responsible for the abdominal tenderness and colic and can produce intussusception as hemorrhagic segments of bowel are invaginated into normal segments. Bleeding from the GI tract can be significant, and in severe cases bowel necrosis can occur. Renal involvement can also be significant, with hematuria, proteinuria, and transient renal failure. The histologic lesion resembles IgA nephropathy.

Dysproteinemias

Several of the dysproteinemias may be associated with abnormal bleeding (see Table 30–1). **Mixed cryoglobulinemia** can produce a syndrome resembling Henoch-Schönlein purpura

CASE HISTORY • Part 3

The patient's history and physical examination (telangiectasia involving the lips, tongue, and palms) are consistent with a diagnosis of hereditary hemorrhagic telangiectasia (HHT). Three diagnostic criteria are met: multiple telangiectases, recurrent epistaxis, and a positive family history (father's history of epistaxis and a brain abscess, which can occur in 5%–10% of patients with HHT). The diagnosis of HHT can be confirmed by screening for mutations in the endoglin and *ALK1* genes, which are present in more than 80% of patients fulfilling HHT clinical criteria.

As for the evaluation of the patient's ongoing blood loss, upper endoscopy revealed multiple telangiectases in the mucosa of the stomach and duodenum, while colonoscopy was unremarkable. Because of the marked dyspnea, she was also screened for the presence of arteriovenous malformations in the lung and central nervous system (both common sites of major prognostic significance in patients with HHT). No malformations were found.

Questions

- Given the diagnosis of HHT, how should this patient be managed?

with nonthrombocytopenic vascular purpura, vasculitis, polyarthralgia, and nephritis. In patients with **multiple myeloma** or **Waldenström macroglobulinemia**, the development of bleeding may be multifactorial. When the disease is severe, thrombocytopenia is usually the dominant problem. Other mechanisms may be involved, however, including coagulation factor deficiencies, interference with platelet function **(acquired vWD)**, interference with fibrin monomer aggregation, and the development of a vessel wall abnormality. Episodic purpura has also been reported in patients with **diffuse polyclonal hypergammaglobulinemia**, a rare condition that is typically seen in adult females. Most often, development of purpuric lesions over the lower extremities is preceded by localized tenderness or a burning sensation with or without an urticarial eruption. **Aseptic vasculitis** may be detected by biopsy and is often associated with collagen vascular disorders such as lupus erythematosus, rheumatoid arthritis, or sarcoidosis. However, patients can have no other apparent abnormality and are carried under the diagnosis of **benign hyperglobulinemic purpura**.

Patients with **amyloidosis** can demonstrate a significant bleeding tendency. Systemic amyloidosis has been associated with factor X deficiency on the basis of selective binding of X to the monoclonal paraprotein and rapid clearance of the complex from the circulation. Amyloidosis of the skin is associated with vascular purpura. Typically, purpuric lesions are easily induced by gently pinching or stroking the involved skin areas. Moreover, these patients report the appearance of widespread purpura following minor trauma. Coughing or straining at stool can result in periorbital purpura by increasing hydrostatic pressure.

THERAPY AND CLINICAL COURSE

For those patients who complain of lifelong easy bruisability without an identifiable coagulation defect, there is little to offer in the way of treatment. They should be assured of the benign nature of the condition and cautioned against the use of aspirin and nonsteroidal analgesics that are not cyclooxygenase-2 (COX-2) selective. The same is true for the elderly patient with senile purpura. The patient should be counseled as to the cause of the purpura and should be urged to try to avoid minor trauma to the hands, lower arms, and legs.

Conditions that do respond to therapy include scurvy (vitamin C deficiency) and, in some instances, the aseptic vasculitis of Henoch-Schönlein purpura. In the first case, just a few days of **oral ascorbic acid (vitamin C)** will correct the abnormal bleeding tendency. Patients with vasculitis can respond to **corticosteroid therapy** or, in the case of severe multiorgan disease, full **immunosuppressive therapy**.

Patients with hereditary hemorrhagic telangiectasia represent a major management dilemma. As the patient with HHT ages, the severity of the blood loss increases and the patient will often develop arteriovenous malformations in the lungs, liver, and central nervous system. Treatment of the recurrent episodes of epistaxis is ever more problematic, even with surgical and laser therapy to eradicate visible telangiectasia. Gastrointestinal blood loss becomes intractable with ever-increasing amounts of blood loss in stool. Studies have shown that oral contraceptives (estrogen-progesterone) can halt bleeding in symptomatic premenopausal women, but it is unknown if doses commonly used for hormone replacement therapy are effective in postmenopausal women. Case reports in the latter have shown efficacy of several drugs, including Tamoxifen. Anti-fibrinolytics such as ε-aminocaproic acid (Amicar) have also been used with some success. As the disease progresses, it is impossible, however, to prevent continuous and worsening blood loss.

Patients with HHT with ongoing blood loss invariably become iron deficient and can develop a severe iron-deficient anemia. This presents a major therapeutic challenge, especially as the amount of blood loss increases. As discussed in Chapter 5,

CASE HISTORY • Part 4

As this patient with HHT grows older, her bleeding tendency will likely become progressively more difficult to manage. If she were premenopausal, oral contraceptives would be an option, but in this patient, she may respond instead to tamoxifen. She must also be carefully followed for any symptoms of arteriovenous malformations, which need to be immediately treated by catheter-directed embolization.

The management of this patient's iron deficiency will also become a significant problem. She should receive maximum oral iron therapy in combination with repeated doses of parenteral iron (see Chapter 5). If this regimen fails to correct her anemia, she will eventually require increasingly frequent red cell transfusions to maintain a stable hematocrit around 30%.

there are limits to the amount of iron that can be derived from any single route of iron administration. **Oral iron**, given to the point of GI intolerance, will provide only 40–60 mg of iron per day, an amount sufficient to support a marrow production level of only 2–3 times normal (40–60 mL of new red cell production per day). This is often not enough to make up for the amount of blood being lost from the oral mucosa and GI tract. Administering intravenous iron dextran can attain somewhat higher marrow production (5–6 times basal). To promote maximum marrow production, the **iron dextran** should be given in doses of 1–2 g intravenously at monthly intervals together with full oral iron therapy. When tolerated, the combined therapy should provide from 100–120 mL of new red blood cells per day—the equivalent of a transfusion of red cells every 2 days. If this does not make up for the blood loss, repeated red blood cell transfusion will be necessary.

POINTS TO REMEMBER

The diagnosis of "vascular" purpura is one of exclusion, made after a full evaluation of the patient's coagulation profile. Most often, the etiology of the vascular defect is clear from the clinical presentation, past medical history, and physical examination.

Elderly individuals with scattered purpuric lesions over the back of the hands and on the forearms, and in some cases the shins, as a result of atrophy of the subcutaneous tissues, are said to have senile purpura. They require no further workup. Unique physical findings can provide clues to specific etiologies, for example, hyperelastic skin and hyperextensible joints in Ehlers-Danlos syndrome, and perifollicular hemorrhages and gingivitis in scurvy (vitamin C deficiency).

The presence of distinctive, often palpable purpuric lesions can be an important clue to the presence of disorders such as Henoch-Schönlein purpura (palpable purpura often preceded by urticaria), amyloidosis (waxy, plaque-like structures), and hereditary hemorrhagic telangiectasia (HHT; readily visible telangiectasia involving the oropharynx, lips, tongue, nose, and fingers).

HHT is the most common inherited cause of vascular bleeding (>1:10,000). Better than 80% of patients with HHT have dominant mutations in the endoglin and *ALK1* genes. Therefore, genetic testing can be used to confirm the diagnosis in the patient and determine at-risk first-degree relatives. Since there is a high frequency of arteriovenous malformations in HHT, screening should be done for those organs most affected—lungs, brain, liver, and GI tract.

Therapy in HHT includes avoidance of inhibitors of platelet function (as in all vascular purpuras), replenishment of iron stores because of the constant depletion due to bleeding, and hormonal therapy in some cases to decrease the incidence of epistaxis and GI bleeding. As patients with HHT grow older the severity of their blood loss can increase dramatically, requiring aggressive oral and parenteral iron therapy and frequent transfusion.

The sudden onset of purpuric lesions in patients with a number of viral, fungal, and rickettsial diseases is an indicator of small vessel vasculitis. These acute lesions can progress rapidly, sometimes leading to infarction of the skin (purpura fulminans) and are often accompanied by thrombocytopenia and disseminated intravascular coagulation (DIC). The skin lesions will respond to therapy of the specific infection but may require transfusion of blood products for replacement of cells and factors consumed during DIC.

Abnormal globulins and dysproteinemias predispose to purpura and, on occasion, bleeding. Cryoglobulins associated with Waldenström macroglobulinemia and multiple myeloma, especially of the IgM subtype, can be treated with plasmapheresis and chemotherapy of the primary disorder. Collagen vascular disorders such as lupus erythematosus, rheumatoid arthritis, and sarcoidosis are often associated with vasculitis and require treatment of the underlying disorder.

BIBLIOGRAPHY

Baxter BT: Heritable diseases of the blood vessels. Cardiovasc Pathol 2004;14:185.

Bayrak-Toydemir P et al: Hereditary hemorrhagic telangiectasia: an overview of diagnosis and management in the molecular era for clinicians. Genet Med 2004;6:175.

Jameson JJ, Cave DR: Hormonal and antihormonal therapy for epistaxis in hereditary hemorrhagic telangiectasia. Laryngoscope 2004;114:705.

Wagner DD, Frenette PS: The vessel wall and its interactions. Blood 2008;111:5271.

Zumberg M, Kitchens CS: Purpura and other hemovascular disorders. In: Kitchens CS, Alving BM, Kessler CM (eds): Consultative Hemostasis and Thrombosis, 2nd ed. Saunders, 2007; 159.

THROMBOCYTOPENIA · 31

CASE HISTORY • *Part I*

A 56-year-old man presents with a complaint of rash and bleeding from the nose and mouth for the past week. His history is notable for non-Hodgkin lymphoma (NHL; follicular center cell) treated with chemotherapy and radiation therapy 10 years prior. He has been taking cholesterol-lowering medication for 3 years; no new drugs have been prescribed. Examination is notable for a petechial rash, which is prominent on the feet and shins, and multiple blood blisters in the mouth. The remainder of the examination is benign.

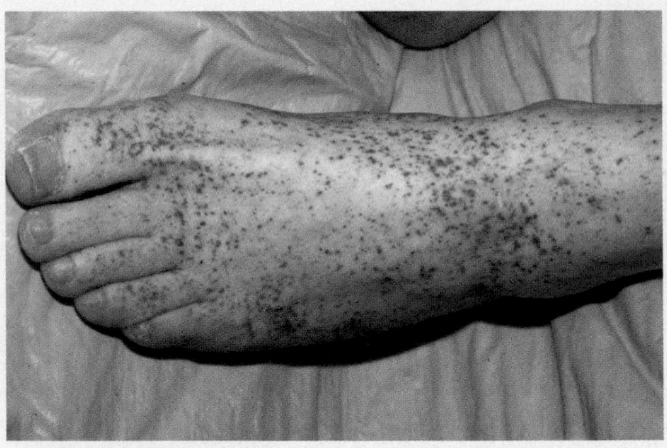

CBC: Hemoglobin/hematocrit - 12 g/dL/36%
MCV - 84 fL WBC count - 7,500/μL
Platelet count - 10,000/μL

• SMEAR MORPHOLOGY

Normocytic, normochromic; no abnormal red cell morphology. White blood cells are normal. There are very few platelets; giant platelets are noted.

Questions

- What abnormality is apparent from the complete blood count (CBC)?
- What additional workup/tests are indicated?

Normal hemostasis requires an adequate number of well-functioning platelets in circulation. Chances of bleeding increase as the platelet count falls. The overall risk of thrombocytopenia to the patient depends, however, on the presence of other disease states. Although a normal individual can tolerate a platelet count less than 10,000/μL, an acutely ill patient is at risk for bleeding with platelet counts of 20,000–30,000/μL or even as high as 100,000/μL if surgical hemostasis is required. Thus, clinical evaluation must match the degree of thrombocytopenia to the disease state. This is also true in planning management.

NORMAL PLATELET KINETICS

The normal circulating platelet count is maintained within relatively narrow limits (150,000–450,000 platelets/μL in Northern Europeans and 90,000–300,000 platelets/μL in people of Mediterranean descent). This difference is related to an inherited slight variation in individual platelet volume (size). The platelet volume is inversely related to the platelet count, so the mass of circulating platelets is the same for these 2 populations. Approximately one-third of platelets are sequestered in the spleen at any one time. Splenic sequestration of platelets can increase dramatically with splenomegaly. Since a platelet has a lifespan of approximately 9–10 days, some 15,000–45,000 platelets/μL must be produced each day to maintain a steady state. New platelet production is the responsibility of the **megakaryocyte**, a very large multinucleated cell (10,750 fL) found in relatively small numbers in the marrow (0.1% of marrow cells) (Figure 31–1). As with other hematopoietic cells, megakaryocytes are derived from the pluripotent stem cell under the control of growth factors such as interleukin (IL)-3, IL-6, granulocyte macrophage colony-stimulating factor (GM-CSF), IL-11, and thrombopoietin (c-Mpl ligand).

Thrombopoietin (TPO) is by far the most important regulatory protein in the production of platelets. The gene for TPO is located on chromosome 3 (3q26-27). TPO mRNA is expressed in the liver, kidneys, and marrow stroma. It translates a 38-kDa protein that is heavily glycosylated to give a 90-kDa glycoprotein with a plasma half-life of 20–30 hours. The receptor for TPO is **c-Mpl**, which is present on both megakaryocytes and platelets. The normal plasma TPO level averages 100 pg/mL. Levels rise exponentially as the platelet count falls, and then they decline as both the megakaryocyte and platelet mass increase (not just the platelet count). This helps explain why TPO levels and platelet production are not increased in patients with hypersplenism, since splenic pooling does not decrease the megakaryocyte/platelet mass. When TPO is absent, the marrow megakaryocyte mass is reduced by more than 80%.

Endogenous TPO is capable of stimulating megakaryocyte growth (proliferation and endomitosis), cytoplasmic maturation, and platelet release. Stimulation of the marrow by recombinant TPO or TPO-mimetics/agonist antibodies results in visible increases in both the number of megakaryocytes and the size and ploidy of individual megakaryocytes, followed by a rise in the platelet count. TPO stimulation normally results in the release of young, reticulated platelets that are larger than normal and contain increased RNA, similar to the release of marrow reticulocytes in response to erythropoietin. Platelet production generally can increase by 6- to 8-fold within 10 days when there is a normal physiologic response to increased platelet destruction. Feedback regulation involves uptake and catabolism of TPO by platelets. Therefore, patients with idiopathic thrombocytopenic purpura (ITP) with maximum levels of platelet production will show normal TPO levels as the growth factor is cleared along with the platelets. The effect of TPO on platelet production can also be altered by abnormalities in the megakaryocyte receptor, post-receptor signaling, and TPO clearance.

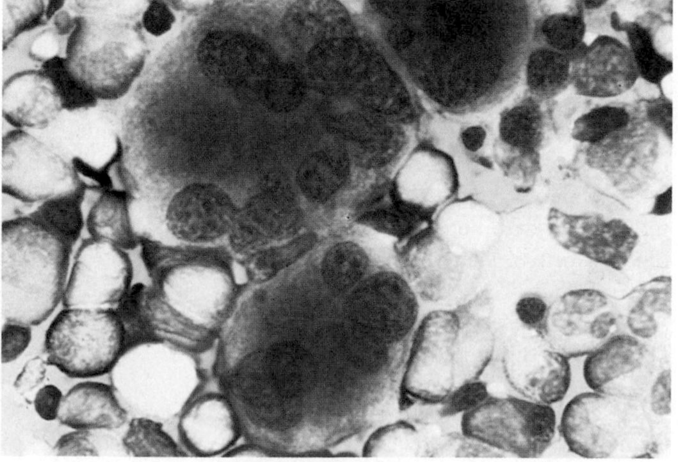

FIGURE 31–1. **Megakaryocytes.** Megakaryocytes (very large cells with multi-lobed nuclei) are easily identified in a marrow aspirate specimen.

CLINICAL FEATURES

There are no specific symptoms or unique clinical features that unerringly point to the presence of thrombocytopenia. Patients with very low platelet counts demonstrate significant bleeding from multiple sites including the nose, mucous membranes, gastrointestinal (GI) tract, skin, and vessel puncture sites. One sign that strongly suggests thrombocytopenia is the appearance of a **petechial rash** involving the skin, conjunctiva, and/or mucous membranes. This condition is usually most pronounced over the lower extremities (increased hydrostatic pressure). Hemarthrosis and hematoma formation are not typical and usually indicate a coagulation factor defect (eg, hemophilia).

The diagnosis of thrombocytopenia is made from **laboratory measurement of the platelet count**. With automated cell counters, even very low counts can be measured rapidly and accurately. Errors leading to spuriously low counts are generally limited to undercounting based on sample clotting or because of spontaneous platelet agglutination or binding to circulating white blood cells. Pseudothrombocytopenia is usually detected by the laboratory technologist on inspection of the blood film. There are 3 principal causes of pseudothrombocytopenia: ethylenediaminetetraacetic acid (EDTA)-antibody–induced agglutination, cold agglutinins, and platelet satellitism (platelet-leukocyte rosette formation; Figure 31–2).

The clinician may often anticipate development of thrombocytopenia. For example, chemotherapy patients and patients with hematopoietic malignancies are at high risk for impaired platelet production. Thrombocytopenia is also commonly associated with chronic viral infections such as hepatitis C and human immunodeficiency virus (HIV). Septic (bacterial infection) patients can develop a consumptive thrombocytopenia

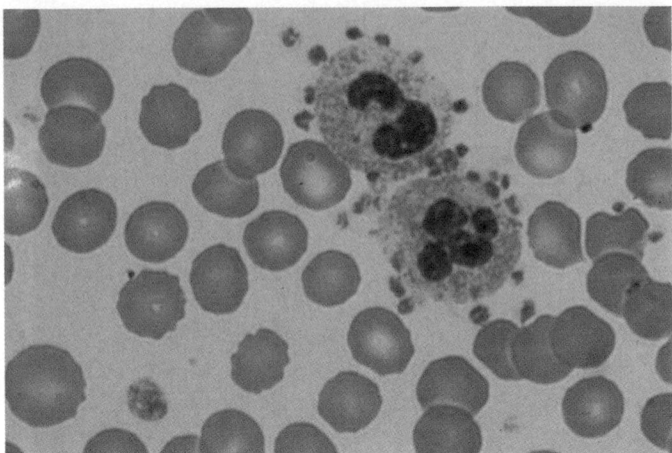

FIGURE 31–2. **Platelet satellitism.** One etiology of artifactual thrombocytopenia is rosetting of platelets around leukocytes; instrument-based platelet counting will miss leukocyte-associated platelets.

secondary to activation of the coagulation cascade (see DIC in Chapter 35). Therefore, a careful evaluation of the overall clinical situation to look for an etiologic connection is essential. It is also important in judging the severity of the thrombocytopenia and the need for replacement (platelet transfusion) therapy.

Laboratory Studies

Whenever the etiology of thrombocytopenia is unclear, studies should be carried out to assess platelet production and destruction. A **marrow aspirate** and **biopsy** should be performed to look for a hematopoietic disease process, especially infiltration by malignant cells, and to evaluate the number and appearance of megakaryocytes. Platelet production can also be assessed using an assay of the number of reticulated platelets in the peripheral blood, similar to using the red cell reticulocyte count to assess red cell production. Defects in platelet production are associated with low reticulated platelet percentages, whereas the megakaryocyte proliferation typically seen with platelet destructive disorders (eg, ITP or thrombotic thrombocytopenic purpura [TTP]) is accompanied by a high reticulated platelet percentage. Although measuring reticulated platelets by flow cytometry is a specialty assay, its adaptation to automated cell counters is now routine and is reported as the immature platelet fraction.

In the evaluation of platelet destruction, autoimmune-related thrombocytopenia (autoimmune idiopathic thrombocytopenia purpura [AITP]) is primarily a diagnosis of exclusion. The clinical diagnosis of AITP can be entertained, however, when thrombocytopenia is the sole finding in an otherwise normal patient. This means that all other cell lines are intact—no anemia, no abnormalities in white blood cell morphology, and no evidence of splenomegaly or lymphadenopathy secondary to a myelo- or lymphoproliferative disorder. Direct testing for platelet surface antibodies (the platelet version of the Coombs test) is offered by some laboratories, but its reliability is open to question. The platelet-associated (antiplatelet) antibody assay **(PAIg assay)** detects the presence of IgG, IgM, and complement on the platelet surface. A positive test does not, however, prove the presence of AITP. In fact, the PAIg test may be positive in thrombocytopenia associated with malignancies and with liver disease, sepsis, and HIV infection. **Assays that measure serum antibodies to specific platelet epitopes (eg, GPIa, GPIIbIIIa, GPIbIX)** are more specific (positive predictive value approximately 90%) but relatively insensitive for diagnosing AITP. An increased percentage of circulating reticulated platelets will be noted with AITP, but is not specific for this particular cause of destructive thrombocytopenia. The clinical diagnosis of AITP, thus, does not rely on laboratory testing.

A specific test is available to identify patients with **thrombotic thrombocytopenic purpura** (TTP). The assay involves quantitating ADAMTS13 activity and, if low, subsequently detecting antibody (by enzyme-linked immunosorbent assay [ELISA] or mixing study) to ADAMTS13 itself. ADAMTS13 is an obligate enzyme in circulation responsible for the metabolic breakdown of ultralarge von Willebrand multimers. In its absence (congenital or acquired), widespread formation of platelet thrombi results in thrombocytopenia and severe organ damage. In patients with undetectable (<10%) ADAMTS13 activity levels, antibodies (mostly IgG but some IgM) to ADAMTS13 are ubiquitous. The value of this test is limited, however, by the need for urgent intervention in TTP patients. At best, it can be used to confirm that TTP-directed therapy is appropriate, usually after the clinical situation has resolved (see later discussion).

Another useful assay in the workup for thrombocytopenia is the test for the **antibody associated with heparin-induced thrombocytopenia (HIT)**. The HIT antibody occurs in patients exposed to either unfractionated or, less frequently, low-molecular-weight heparin and is directed at the complex of heparin and platelet factor 4 (PF4). Antibody can be detected using a functional assay **(serotonin release assay or heparin-induced platelet aggregation)** or an **immunoassay (usually an ELISA) for the antibody-heparin-PF4 complex**. The serotonin assay measures the release from serotonin-loaded normal platelets exposed to patient plasma and varying amounts of heparin. The aggregation method, which is simpler but much less sensitive, can be performed by a routine laboratory using a standard aggregometer or flow cytometer. The ELISA immunoassay method is highly sensitive, detecting the presence of the antibody in more than 95% of affected patients. The serotonin release assay is somewhat less sensitive but may be more specific for detecting clinically significant HIT.

DIFFERENTIAL DIAGNOSIS

The diagnosis of thrombocytopenia is best organized according to the normal physiology of platelet production, distribution in circulation, and destruction. This protocol provides an overall

CASE HISTORY • Part 2

Based on the CBC and smear morphology, the patient has an isolated thrombocytopenia, which is almost certainly the cause of the petechial lesions noted on examination. The history of NHL is important; recurrent disease involving the bone marrow may interfere with platelet production. NHL is also associated with autoimmune thrombocytopenia. The absence of splenomegaly and any evidence of organ damage (TTP) make increased platelet sequestration or organ-based consumption unlikely.

To evaluate platelet production, a bone marrow aspirate and biopsy are performed, revealing a normocellular marrow with no evidence of lymphomatous infiltration, but a clear increase in the number of megakaryocytes and the percentage of hyperlobulated megakaryocytes. This finding supports the diagnosis of a destructive thrombocytopenia, most likely an immune thrombocytopenia. A reticulated platelet count of 42% (normal 7%–15%) is further evidence of a platelet destruction defect with a major compensatory increase in production.

Questions

- Based on these findings, are additional studies required to make the diagnosis?
- What initial therapies are appropriate?

classification that helps guide the differential diagnosis of specific disease states (Figure 31–3).

Production Disorders

A failure in platelet production can result from **marrow damage** where all aspects of normal hematopoiesis are depressed, even to the point of marrow aplasia **(aplastic anemia)**. Reductions specifically in marrow megakaryocyte mass are also seen in individuals receiving radiation therapy or cancer chemotherapy, as a result of exposure to toxic chemicals such as benzene and insecticides, or as a complication of viral hepatitis. An effort should always be made to look for a reversible cause, especially whenever there is recent exposure to common drugs such as thiazide diuretics, alcohol, or estrogens. Infiltration of the marrow by a malignant process, such as metastatic carcinoma, or a "benign" hematologic disorder, such as Gaucher disease, will infrequently disrupt thrombopoiesis. By contrast, hematopoietic malignancies, including multiple myeloma, acute leukemia, Hodgkin or non-Hodgkin lymphoma, and myeloproliferative disorders, frequently produce a platelet production defect.

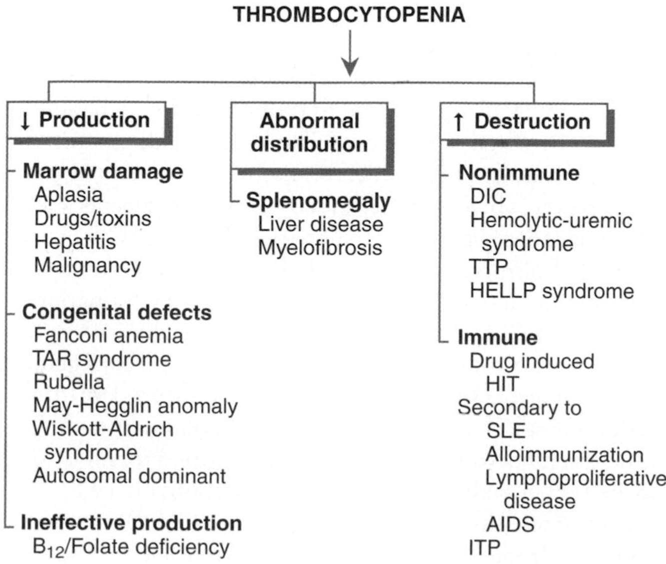

FIGURE 31–3. **Differential diagnosis of thrombocytopenia.** Evaluation of thrombocytopenia is best organized according to the apparent defect in platelet production, distribution, or destruction.

In the newborn, megakaryocytic hypoplasia can be a complication of rubella infection or the use of thiazide diuretics during the pregnancy. Congenital hypoplastic thrombocytopenia with absent radii **(TAR syndrome)** and Fanconi syndrome are much more rare causes of megakaryocyte hypoplasia. Otherwise unexplained thrombocytopenia due to megakaryocytic hypoplasia may initially be confused clinically with ITP because of the severity of the thrombocytopenia. However, a failed response to standard ITP therapy, marrow morphology, low reticulated platelet percentage in blood, and progression to pancytopenia, aplastic anemia, or leukemia will confirm the diagnosis.

Reduced production of platelets can also result from an intrinsic **abnormality of the megakaryocyte**. In this situation, the marrow megakaryocyte mass is increased but formation of new platelets is reduced **(ineffective thrombopoiesis)**. Several hereditary thrombocytopenias are characterized by ineffective platelet production, including May-Hegglin anomaly, Wiskott-Aldrich syndrome, and autosomal dominant thrombocytopenia. The patient with **May-Hegglin anomaly** typically has bizarre, giant platelets in circulation and **Döhle bodies** (basophilic inclusions) in white blood cells (Figure 31–4) and platelets.

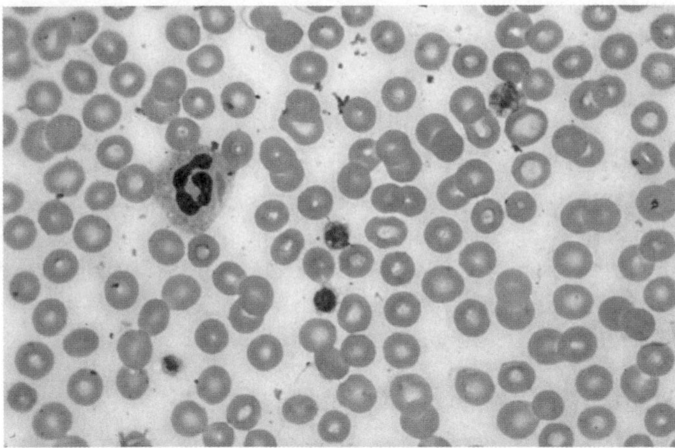

FIGURE 31–4. **May-Hegglin anomaly.** Patients with this disorder display macrothrombocytopenia (mildly low platelet count with giant platelets) and neutrophils with prominent Döhle bodies.

Platelet production is variably ineffective; one-third of patients are significantly thrombocytopenic and at risk for bleeding. **Wiskott-Aldrich syndrome** is an X-linked disorder that presents with a combination of eczema, immune deficiency, and thrombocytopenia. Circulating platelets are smaller than normal, function poorly because of granule defects, and have a reduced survival. The latter, however, is not enough to explain the severity of the thrombocytopenia; ineffective thrombopoiesis is the principal abnormality. Finally, patients with **autosomal dominant thrombocytopenia** generally show increased megakaryocyte mass with ineffective production, and in some cases the release of macrocytic platelets into circulation. Many of these patients have nerve deafness and nephritis **(Alport syndrome)**.

Ineffective thrombopoiesis is also seen in patients with vitamin B_{12} or folate deficiency, including patients with alcoholism and defective folate metabolism. The defect is identical to the maturation defect seen in the red blood cell and white blood cell lines. Marrow megakaryocyte mass is increased, but effective platelet production is reduced. This failure in platelet production is rapidly reversed by appropriate vitamin therapy.

Disorders of Distribution

The total number of platelets available for hemostasis includes those in circulation and the exchangeable pool of platelets in the spleen. Normally, up to one-third of platelets are held within the spleen. With conditions that produce splenomegaly, the percentage of trapped platelets can increase significantly in proportion to the size of the spleen. However, since platelets in the splenic pool continue to be in equilibrium with those in circulation, platelet survival is relatively normal and there is little risk of thrombocytopenia-related bleeding.

Splenomegaly by itself should not reduce the platelet count to below 40,000–50,000/μL. With lower counts, it is important to look for a concomitant defect in platelet production or destruction. For example, patients with lymphoma or autoimmune disease can demonstrate both increased splenic pooling and a reduced platelet survival secondary to an autoantibody. In this situation, splenectomy can be an effective therapy. In contrast, patients with advanced liver disease who demonstrate congestive splenomegaly without a reduction in platelet lifespan do not benefit from splenectomy. The bleeding tendency of the cirrhotic patient is a multifactorial problem where deficiencies in coagulation factors and abnormal fibrinolysis are more significant issues than the moderate thrombocytopenia commonly seen in cirrhosis.

Patients with **advanced myelofibrosis due to clonal myeloproliferative disorders** develop marked splenomegaly late in their course with extramedullary hematopoiesis. In this circumstance, the spleen is both producing and sequestering platelets, so it can be extremely difficult to determine the balance between the two. Patients may present with thrombocytopenia, suggesting a marked pooling/destruction defect, or a very high platelet count indicating excessive production. Furthermore, splenectomy for the thrombocytopenia associated with myelofibosis can dramatically upset the balance, either by converting the thrombocytopenic patient with massive sequestration to one with marked thrombocytosis or by further crippling extramedullary platelet production to accentuate an already severe thrombocytopenia.

Nonimmune Destruction Disorders

Platelet consumption as a part of intravascular coagulation is seen in several clinical settings. When the entire coagulation pathway is activated, the process is referred to as **disseminated intravascular coagulation (DIC)**. It can be dramatic, with severe thrombocytopenia and marked prolongations of coagulation factor assays leading to bleeding, or more of a "low-grade" DIC picture, with minimal thrombocytopenia and less tendency for bleeding (see Chapter 35).

Platelet consumption can also occur as an isolated process **(so-called platelet DIC)**. Viral infections, bacteremia, malignancy, high-dose chemotherapy, and vasculitis can result in sufficient endothelial cell damage that dramatically increases the rate of platelet clearance without full activation of the coagulation pathway. Basically, this is an accentuation of the normal vessel repair process, where platelets adhere to exposed subendothelial surfaces and then aggregate with fibrinogen binding. With marked endothelial disruption, enough platelets will be consumed to result in thrombocytopenia. Vessel occlusion by formation of platelet thrombi is rare but can occur occasionally with severe vasculitis. AIDS patients, for example, can develop a consumptive thrombocytopenia with resultant organ damage secondary to arterial thrombosis. The various disorders that result in a microangiopathic thrombocytopenia are briefly summarized in Table 31–1 and are further outlined in the following sections on TTP.

Thrombotic thrombocytopenic purpura (TTP), hemolytic uremic syndrome (HUS), and **HELLP syndrome** are the most important examples of nonimmune, microangiopathic destruction of platelets. Although the underlying pathophysiologies are distinctly different, these entities can lead to thrombus formation and organ damage.

TABLE 31–1 • Features of microangiopathic thrombocytopenic syndromes

Disease	Possible Causes	Clinical Features	Therapy
Congenital TTP	*ADAMTS 13* mutations	Relapsing, cyclical episodes, often in children	FFP infusions at regular intervals
Sporadic TTP	Deficiency of ADAMTS13, often due to inhibitor	Sporadic but may chronically relapse, sometimes associated with pregnancy	Plasma exchange, ie, plasmapheresis with FFP replacement
HUS	Shiga-like toxin from *E. coli* O157:H7, factor H deficiency	Bloody diarrhea prodrome, renal failure more severe than TTP	Hemodialysis; plasma exchange in adults or for atypical HUS in children
Quinine type-mediated acute TTP	Drug-dependent antibodies, may occur with ticlopidine, clopidogrel, and other drugs	Acute onset, often with fever, diarrhea neutropenia, and acute renal failure	Plasma exchange drug cessation for others
Chronic TTP due to chemotherapeutic and immunosuppressive agents	Mitomycin, gemcitabine, cyclosporine, tacrolimus, among others	Insidious presentation, often with progressive renal failure	Discontinue etiologic agent
Stem cell (allogeneic only) transplantation and TTP	Higher risk with unrelated or HLA mismatched and graft-versus-host disease (GVHD)	Renal failure	Supportive care; no clear value to plasma exchange

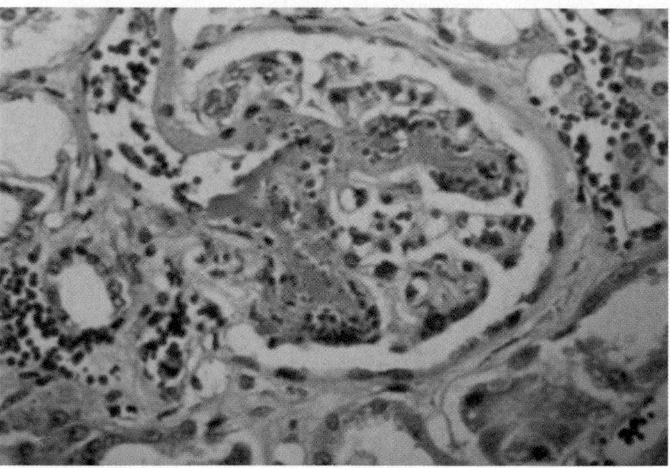

FIGURE 31–5. **Platelet thrombi in TTP.** Renal glomerulus partially obstructed by platelet aggregates/thrombi (solid reddish material) in a patient with TTP.

A. Thrombotic Thrombocytopenic Purpura

TTP may present as a symptom complex that includes low-grade fever, microangiopathic hemolytic anemia with fragmented red cells (schistocytes), thrombocytopenia with an otherwise negative DIC screen (normal prothrombin time [PT], partial thromboplastin time [PTT], and fibrinogen levels), and multiple small vessel occlusions (platelet thrombi) involving the kidney (Figure 31–5), central nervous system, and on occasion, the skin and distal extremities. However, the triad of **thrombocytopenia, schistocytosis, and an elevated lactic dehydrogenase (LDH)** (the latter 2 evidence of microangiopathic hemolysis) is more common and considered sufficient for diagnosis. Presenting symptoms are usually nonspecific and include abdominal pain, weakness, nausea, and vomiting. About half of patients present with neurologic abnormalities, while perhaps one-third have renal insufficiency. Schistocytosis results from mechanical fragmentation of red blood cells flowing past intravascular platelet thrombi.

TTP can occur as a congenital disease; a sporadic illness without apparent cause (idiopathic), which can evolve into a chronic relapsing condition; or a complication of marrow transplantation or drug therapy (quinine, ticlopidine, α-interferon, pentostatin, gemcitabine, tacrolimus, or cyclosporine). Preeclamptic women with HELLP syndrome also can evolve to full-blown TTP peripartum or postpartum. As reported by the Oklahoma TTP-HUS Registry, one-third to one-half of patients present with **idiopathic TTP**, whereas most of the remainder are evenly divided among post-transplantation, pregnancy-related, and drug-associated disease.

TTP is perhaps the purest example of increased platelet destruction secondary to platelet activation, aggregation, and thrombus formation resulting in organ damage. The underlying mechanism with familial or cyclic disease involves a deficiency of **von Willebrand factor (vWF)**—cleaving protease activity (ADAMTS13 deficiency) secondary to an inherited mutation of the *ADAMTS13* gene. In sporadic TTP cases, the decrease in protease activity is associated with a **circulating inhibitor (antibody)**. As a result of the decrease in protease activity in both conditions, ultra-large multimers of vWF (ULvWF) normally released by endothelial cells persist in the circulation and promote uncontrolled platelet adhesion and aggregation leading to characteristic disseminated platelet thrombi.

Congenital TTP (Upshaw-Schulman syndrome) is inherited as an autosomal recessive trait. More than 50 different mutations involving the chromosome 9q34 locus and *ADAMTS13* gene have been identified, most of which abrogate cleaving activity. However, the phenotypic presentation can vary widely. About half of these patients present with their first TTP episode before age 5; the others remain asymptomatic until adulthood. Regardless of the age of onset, most patients experience cyclical disease with multiple relapses, which typically respond to **fresh frozen plasma (FFP) therapy** as a source of vWF-cleaving protease activity. Prophylactic FFP infusions every 2–4 weeks can be used to prevent episodes and decrease the frequency of relapse.

Drug-induced TTP has been associated, in many instances, with an inhibitor-mediated cleaving protease deficiency. Quinine is perhaps the best example of a drug causing an immune-mediated TTP. Patients present with the sudden onset of nausea, vomiting, diarrhea, fever, and chills within hours of quinine ingestion. Renal failure also may be a prominent feature of quinine-induced TTP, thereby raising the possibility of HUS as the diagnosis. However, the severity of the illness and the incidence of neurologic symptoms, including coma, is no different from that seen with sporadic TTP. These patients usually respond well to **plasma exchange**. Ticlopidine (and much less often another adenosine 5′-diphosphate [ADP] receptor antagonist, clopidogrel) has been reported to cause drug-induced TTP, but the mechanism involved, whether immune related or not, is unclear. TTP usually occurs within the first 1–2 months of exposure to the offending drug.

In patients receiving chemotherapeutic or immunosuppressive agents (gemcitabine, cyclosporine, tacrolimus), the onset is generally insidious and not immune mediated. Simply stopping the drug will often reverse the process. Although infrequently used, **mitomycin C–associated TTP-HUS** is typically seen when patients receive cumulative doses greater than 40 mg. The most common presentation in such patients is severe dyspnea and progressive renal failure; the prognosis is very poor and plasmapheresis is ineffective. Severe inflammatory diseases (systemic lupus erythematosis, catastrophic antiphospholipid syndrome) can demonstrate TTP-like features secondary to high levels of IL-6 blocking the vWF cleavage site for ADAMTS13. Plasmapheresis is recommended, but its efficacy is not established.

Sporadic or idiopathic TTP is a diagnosis of exclusion. The full pentad of diagnostic criteria is present far less often than previously thought. Thus, the diagnostic criteria are now based solely on the combination of **thrombocytopenia** and a **microangiopathic hemolytic anemia** without an apparent alternative cause. Early diagnosis and treatment are very important because the mortality in untreated patients can reach 90%. **Plasmapheresis with FFP** (or cryopoor plasma) replacement reduces the mortality to about 10%, but only if plasma exchange is begun before signs of significant organ damage appear. The urgency of starting treatment is further underscored by reports that at least 25% of patients have symptoms for several weeks before diagnosis.

Anemia and thrombocytopenia with a normal leukocyte count are suggestive of and consistent with the diagnosis of TTP; additional supportive lab evidence for TTP includes schistocytosis and increased reticulocytes on the peripheral smear; normal PT and activated partial thromboplastin time (aPTT); elevated serum LDH and indirect bilirubin; and a negative Coombs test. Assays for **vWF-cleaving protease activity** (ADAMTS13 level) are available in reference laboratories, but the results from several series of TTP patients suggest an uncertain clinical relevance. The level of protease activity is often less than 5% in congenital TTP, but the overall sensitivity with sporadic TTP and TTP associated with other illness or chemotherapy/transplantation is much lower. Patients with normal cleaving protease activity have been shown to have characteristic TTP features, while some patients with autoimmune platelet destruction (idiopathic thrombocytopenic purpura, see below) have been reported with severe deficiency of protease activity. Thus, treatment decisions should not wait on the ADAMTS13 level. A clinical picture suggesting sporadic TTP mandates the use of plasma exchange, in contrast to congenital ADAMST13-deficient patients who can be managed with FFP infusions alone. Ongoing evaluation of TTP patients treated with plasma exchange is equally critical; the Oklahoma TTP-HUS Registry reported that 10% of patients treated for sporadic TTP were eventually shown to have cancer or septicemia as the primary cause of their microangiopathy.

B. Hemolytic Uremic Syndrome

Although the diagnostic criteria for **hemolytic uremic syndrome (HUS)** and TTP are similar, TTP is primarily a disease of adults. By contrast, HUS is seen most often in children below the age of 5 who present with bloody diarrhea secondary to *Escherichia coli* (0157:H7) or related bacteria that produce the Shiga-like toxin. Unlike TTP, children with HUS do not demonstrate deficiency of ADAMTS13 activity. Acute renal failure dominates the presentation of HUS; thrombocytopenia and anemia are generally less pronounced than seen with TTP, and neurologic signs are rare. Typical patients with HUS do not need plasmapheresis or FFP therapy. Most children spontaneously recover with hemodialysis support, and mortality is less than 5%. However, about 10% of children presenting with HUS have an atypical and severe disease, especially those with concomitant *Streptococcus pneumoniae* infection. In these atypical pediatric cases, and in adults infected with *E. coli* 0157:H7, a combination of features characteristic of both HUS and TTP are present. Such patients should be treated with both plasma exchange and hemodialysis. Despite this aggressive approach, the morbidity and mortality in this group is higher than for typical patients with HUS, and chronic renal failure is much more common.

Adults with an atypical (no diarrhea or toxin) and/or chronic HUS presentation have frequently been determined to have ongoing complement activation due to mutations in regulatory genes for factors H, I, or B, or membrane cofactor protein-1 (MCP-1). This pathology resembles the complement activation leading to thrombocytopenia or thrombosis in paroxysmal nocturnal hemoglobinuria; hence, experimental anti-complement drug trials are currently ongoing in this subset of patients with HUS. Renal transplants for chronic renal failure in these patients may fail because of the ongoing complement activation, whereas combined liver-renal transplants have been successful.

C. HELLP Syndrome

Thrombocytopenia is a frequent complication of pregnancy. Mild so-called gestational thrombocytopenia (platelet count 70,000–150,000/μL) is seen in 6%–7% of women nearing gestation and represents a physiologic change similar to the dilutional anemia of pregnancy. Thrombocytopenia in association with hypertension is observed in 1%–2% of pregnancies, and as

TABLE 31–2 • Types of autoimmune thrombocytopenia

Neonatal thrombocytopenia
Alloimmune Associated with maternal ITP Drug related
Drug induced (immunologic)
Drug dependent (haptens)—quinidine, quinine, sedormid Drug related—sulfonamides, gold salts, antibiotics, cyclosporin, tacrolimus Heparin induced
Lymphoma/leukemia
Non-Hodgkin lymphomas Chronic lymphocytic leukemia
Autoimmune disorders
Lupus erythematosus Thyroiditis Colitis/ileitis
Infectious disease
HIV infection Rubella, rubeola, and chickenpox in children Infectious mononucleosis Viral hepatitis Cytomegalovirus Lyme disease Sarcoidosis/histoplasmosis
Post-transfusion purpura **Idiopathic thrombocytopenic purpura (ITP)**
Acute autoimmune ITP (AITP, ?viral-induced in children) Transplantation of solid organ or hematopoietic stem cells Chronic AITP (adults mostly)

many as 50% of preeclamptic mothers develop a DIC-like picture with severe thrombocytopenia, platelet counts of 20,000–40,000/μL, at the time of delivery. This is referred to as **HELLP syndrome** when the combination of red cell hemolysis (H), elevated liver enzymes (EL), and low platelet count (LP) is present. Physiologically, HELLP very much resembles TTP. Control of the patient's hypertension and completion of the delivery is usually enough to bring this process to a halt. However, a few patients go on to full-blown TTP-HUS after delivery. Postpartum TTP is a life-threatening illness with a poor prognosis. Treatment with both plasma exchange and intravenous immunoglobulin has given variable results.

Autoimmune Thrombocytopenia

Thrombocytopenia is a common manifestation of autoimmune disease. A list of conditions associated with autoimmune destruction of platelets can be found in Table 31–2. The severity of the thrombocytopenia is highly variable. With some conditions the patient's platelet count falls to as low as 1,000–2,000/μL. In other patients, the ability of the megakaryocytes to increase platelet production results in a compensated state with platelet counts ranging from 20,000/μL to near normal levels.

Diagnosis of immune platelet destruction can usually be made from the clinical presentation, an increase in the reticulated platelets in blood, or demonstration of an **increase in marrow megakaryocyte number and ploidy**.

Expansion of the megakaryocyte mass is taken as prima facie evidence that a high rate of platelet production is trying to compensate for a shortened survival of platelets in circulation. The more severe the thrombocytopenia, the easier the diagnosis, since the disparity between marrow megakaryocyte proliferation and platelet count is most pronounced. Diagnosis is more difficult when the thrombocytopenia is less severe and there is no obvious clinical condition to explain the finding. In this situation, an **assay for reticulated platelets and/or research measurements of platelet lifespan** may be necessary to make the diagnosis.

A. Neonatal Thrombocytopenia

Neonates are at risk for thrombocytopenia resulting from maternal alloimmune sensitization during pregnancy or maternal autoimmune thrombocytopenia (Figure 31–6). Alloimmune thrombocytopenia has been associated with intracranial hemorrhage. Mothers who lack the HPA-1a (Pl^{A-1}) platelet antigen are at risk for alloimmunization when the fetus is positive for HPA-1a. Other, less common alloantigens absent in the mother (Pen, Bak, Ko, and Br) or class I HLA antigens also are targets for allosensitization. Most affected children are delivered without difficulty but soon after develop petechiae and purpuric lesions. The thrombocytopenia can be severe and, if left untreated, can persist for several weeks. If available, measurement of antibody in the mother's plasma and its specificity for the newborn's (or father's) platelets can be diagnostic.

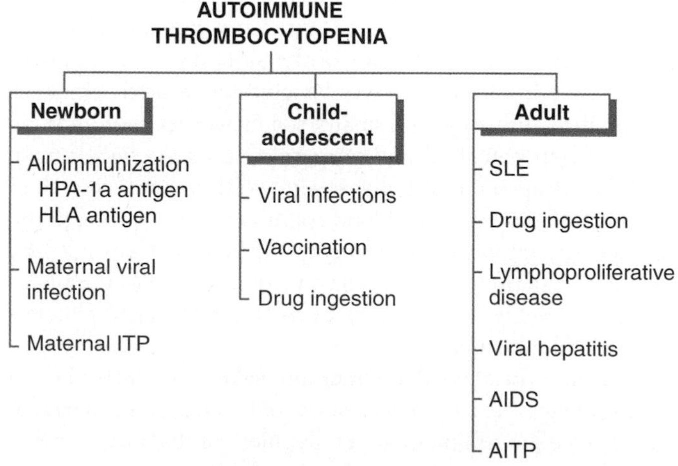

FIGURE 31–6. **Diagnosis of autoimmune thrombocytopenia.** The patient's age and clinical presentation provide a basis for evaluating autoimmune thrombocytopenia. The differential diagnosis for each age group is distinctly different.

Measurements of in utero fetal platelet counts by cordocentesis in women who are known to be HPA-1a negative have shown counts below 20,000/μL before 24 weeks' gestation in 50% of affected children. Furthermore, even when counts are above 80,000/μL, repeated measurement demonstrated a fall of approximately 10,000/μL per gestation week, resulting in severe thrombocytopenia by the time of birth in most children. This is associated with a 10%–20% chance of intracranial hemorrhage, a quarter of which occur while in utero. When there is a history of a previous birth complicated by alloimmunization and intracranial hemorrhage, the chances of severe thrombocytopenia with hemorrhage are even higher. This has led to the recommendation to treat such mothers with intravenous immunoglobulin with or without steroids.

Children born to mothers with chronic autoimmune idiopathic thrombocytopenic purpura (AITP) are a different story, although there is still some risk for neonatal immune thrombocytopenia, since the mother's IgG antibody crosses the placenta. However, the incidence of severe neonatal thrombocytopenia complicating maternal ITP is very low. Fewer than 12% of newborns of ITP mothers will have platelet counts below 50,000/μL and 5% or less has platelet counts below 20,000/μL. Intracranial hemorrhage or a life-threatening bleed is very uncommon, with a reported incidence of less than 1%. The chance of being affected correlates to some degree with the severity of the mother's illness; very high levels of maternal platelet-associated IgG place the fetus at greatest risk. Such mothers need to be monitored during pregnancy and treated according to the severity of their thrombocytopenia to suppress antibody production. A history of severe neonatal thrombocytopenia in a sibling is an inconsistent indicator of a greater chance of more severe disease in the next newborn.

B. Postviral Thrombocytopenia in Children

During childhood and adolescence, an abrupt onset of severe autoimmune thrombocytopenia most often is related to a recent viral infection. The incidence is highest before 10 years of age. The affected child presents 1–2 weeks after an infection such as rubella, rubeola, chickenpox, or a respiratory viral infection with petechial and purpuric lesions of the skin and mucous membranes. Immunization with live vaccine for measles, chickenpox, mumps, influenza, and smallpox can also act as an inciting event. When petechial and purpuric lesions are widespread, thrombocytopenia is usually severe, with counts less than 10,000/μL. The rest of the blood count is normal, although the number of activated lymphocytes in circulation may be increased. Examination of a marrow aspirate reveals normal to increased numbers of megakaryocytes, and reticulated platelets in blood are increased.

Generally, the clinical presentation makes diagnosis of ITP in children relatively easy. The absence of fever, organ damage, or abnormal cell morphology generally rules out diagnoses such as sepsis (especially meningococcemia), TTP or HUS, or acute leukemia. When there is no evidence for a complicating etiology, bone marrow studies need not be performed; a rapid rise in the platelet count in response to intravenous immune globulin will confirm the diagnosis. Additional testing can then be reserved only for those children who have failed therapy and are being considered for splenectomy. Drug-induced thrombocytopenia must be considered in any child taking a medication in the weeks preceding the fall in the platelet count, even when there is a preceding viral illness. A good rule is to stop all medications immediately, even if the association is unlikely.

C. Thrombocytopenic Purpura in Adults

Differential diagnosis of autoimmune thrombocytopenia in the adult begins with a careful history to identify any exposure to drugs, blood products, or viral infections (see Figure 31–6). As a corollary to neonatal thrombocytopenia, HPA-1a–negative adults can develop **post-transfusion purpura** following exposure to a blood product, most often red blood cells or platelets. In this situation, the antigen contributed by the transfusion product in a soluble form is adsorbed by the patient's antigen-negative platelets, resulting in the generation of antibodies. The patient's own HPA-1a–negative platelets are destroyed as innocent bystanders. Like neonatal alloimmune thrombocytopenia, any of the platelet polymorphisms can cause post-transfusion purpura, although HPA-1a is the most frequently associated. Although multiparous antigen-negative women are at greatest risk, post-transfusion purpura has been reported in both men and women. Usually, a potent alloantibody with specificity for HPA-1a can be readily detected in the patient's plasma; this test is performed only in reference laboratories.

1. Association with drugs—Several drugs can produce immune thrombocytopenia. **Quinine, quinidine, and sedormid** are the best known and have been studied extensively. Clinically, patients present with severe thrombocytopenia, with platelet counts below 20,000/μL. These drugs act as haptens to trigger antibody formation and then serve as obligate molecules for antibody binding to the platelet surface. Drug-specific antibodies can be detected using drug coupled to a carrier protein, and reference laboratories offer this test as a surrogate measure for detecting drug-induced immune thrombocytopenia. Drug binding results in a conformational change in the receptor and the exposure of a neoepitope, leading to antibody formation. The antibodies then reversibly bind by their Fab regions to these epitopes of GPIb/IX or GPIIb/IIIa. Thrombocytopenia can also occur within hours of the first exposure to a drug because of preformed antibodies. This has been reported with varying frequency (0%–13%) with abciximab (Reo-Pro) and other GPIIb/IIIa inhibitors. Other drugs, such as α-methyldopa, sulfonamides, and gold salts, also stimulate autoantibodies. They are not, however, obligate haptens in the resultant platelet destruction.

2. Association with heparin—The association of heparin with thrombocytopenia deserves special emphasis. **Heparin-induced thrombocytopenia (HIT)** can take one of several forms. A modest fall in the platelet count, HIT type I (nonimmune HIT), is observed in the majority of patients within the first day of full-dose unfractionated heparin therapy. This relates to passive heparin binding to platelets, resulting in a modest shortening of platelet lifespan. It is transient and clinically insignificant.

A second form of HIT, **HIT type II or immune-mediated HIT**, demands more attention. In patients typically receiving heparin for more than 5 days, antibodies to the heparin-platelet factor 4 (PF4) complex can form that are capable of binding to platelet Fc receptors and inducing platelet activation and aggregation. Platelet activation results in further release of PF4 and the appearance of platelet microparticles in circulation, both of which magnify the procoagulant state of HIT. Furthermore, PF4 complex binding to endothelial cells stimulates thrombin release. In vivo, HIT pathophysiology leads to an increased clearance of platelets with resultant thrombocytopenia and venous and/or arterial thrombus formation, with the potential for severe organ damage (loss of limbs, stroke, myocardial infarction) and unusual sites of thrombosis (adrenal, portal vein, skin). Such thromboses can masquerade as hemorrhage into an end organ (eg, adrenal) following infarction.

The pretest probability of heparin-induced thrombocytopenia can help in determining both the need for intervention and the relative utility of testing for the antibody to the heparin-PF4 complex. Events that lend to a high probability score include: a greater than 50% decrease in platelet count but with an absolute count above 20,000/μL; the onset of thrombocytopenia within 5–10 days of heparin institution; new thrombosis or skin necrosis (especially if the latter occurs at the site of heparin injection); and no other explanation for thrombocytopenia. Of course, the many clinical scenarios of inpatient heparin use often suggest multiple possible causes for thrombocytopenia, and the onset of a thrombosis may be difficult to gauge in patients already being treated with anticoagulation.

The incidence of HIT type II varies with the type and dose of heparin used and the duration of therapy. Although 10%–15% of patients receiving bovine unfractionated heparin develop an antibody, fewer than 6% of patients receiving porcine heparin do so. The risk of heparin-induced thrombosis is far lower than the incidence of antibody formation. Fewer than 10% of those who develop an antibody to the heparin-PF4 complex will exhibit a thrombotic event. However, the risk varies considerably with the clinical situation and can reach 40% or more in the postoperative setting of peripheral vascular or orthopedic surgery, when high circulating levels of both activated platelets and thrombin are present. The risk of a thromboembolic event in general is magnified by HIT and is thought to be 10–30 times the rate for patients under similar circumstances without HIT. Patients with HIT are equally likely to develop a thromboembolic event prior to, following, or concurrent with the appearance of thrombocytopenia.

The association of heparin with significant thrombocytopenia should not be taken lightly. Patients placed on full-dose unfractionated heparin for more than 5 days, or who have previously received heparin, should be routinely monitored with every-other-day platelet counts. A 50% or greater decrease in platelet count, even if the absolute platelet count is within the normal range, or a decline in platelets to less than 100,000/μL can signal the appearance of HIT type II, and therefore mandates stopping the heparin and substituting a direct thrombin inhibitor, such as lepirudin or argatroban. If heparin is continued, and this includes even low-dose subcutaneous heparin or low-molecular-weight heparin, there is a significant increased risk of a major thromboembolic event and prolongation of the duration of HIT. Fondaparinux has not been associated with HIT. Danaparoid is used to treat HIT in some countries, but caution is required since danaparoid has some cross-reactivity (3%) with the antibody to heparin-PF4.

An **acute form of HIT type II** can occur in patients who are restarted on heparin within 20 days of a prior exposure. When an HIT antibody is already present, a patient restarted on heparin can exhibit an acute drug reaction with a sudden onset of severe dyspnea, shaking chills, diaphoresis, hypertension, and tachycardia. Such patients are at extreme risk of fatal thromboembolic events if heparin is continued.

Finally, patients with a history of HIT may subsequently require a procedure that is best accomplished using heparin anticoagulation. One example would be cardiac surgery using cardiopulmonary bypass. Unfortunately, direct thrombin inhibitors for bypass surgery have resulted in severe bleeding that is not reversible. For this reason, such patients with a history of HIT have been briefly re-exposed to unfractionated heparin during bypass. This procedure appears to be safe if they had been previously positive for the antibody to heparin-PF4 and have been documented to have turned negative (using the highly sensitive ELISA assay) or if they are greater than 100 days from their last dose of heparin.

3. AIDS/HIV infection—Thrombocytopenia is a common complication of HIV infection and may be the first manifestation of the disease. Early in the course of HIV infection, immune destruction of platelets is common, presumably secondary to immune complex binding to platelets. Megakaryocytes can be increased in number, and platelet survival is significantly reduced. Although 10%–20% of HIV patients may experience a spontaneous remission, most behave like chronic ITP patients (see below) and require therapy with some combination of zidovudine (AZT), steroids, and immune globulin. As HIV disease progresses, however, platelet production gradually fails, and patients become resistant to standard ITP therapy. This latter condition may relate to infection of the marrow with mycobacterium avium intracellulare or even direct infection of megakaryocytes by HIV. Many end-stage AIDS patients show severe thrombocytopenia with an associated tendency for bleeding that can only be ameliorated by platelet transfusion.

4. Lymphoproliferative and autoimmune disorders—Immune destruction of platelets is a common component of several lymphoproliferative and autoimmune disorders. Hodgkin and non-Hodgkin lymphoma and chronic lymphocytic leukemia are associated with production of autoantibodies with platelet specificity. Autoimmune thrombocytopenia can also complicate organ or hematopoietic stem cell transplantation. ITP can also occur with nonmalignant diseases associated with immune stimulation, for example, with infectious mononucleosis, histoplasmosis, sarcoidosis, viral infections, viral hepatitis, and Lyme disease.

Thrombocytopenia can be an early manifestation of autoimmune disease, especially systemic lupus erythematosus (SLE), and may precede other symptoms and signs. It is important, therefore, to look for a history of arthralgia, arthritis, skin disease, unexplained pleurisy, hepatitis, or inflammatory bowel disease. Antiphospholipid syndrome, either by itself or in association with SLE, should be considered when thrombocytopenia is associated with a history of thrombosis or recurrent miscarriage/fetal loss. Laboratory evaluation of any patient with autoimmune thrombocytopenia should include tests for rheumatoid factor, complement levels, and antinuclear antibodies including single- and double-stranded DNA. A search should also be made for other autoantibodies including red blood cell antibodies (Coombs test) when there is hemolytic anemia, a lupus anticoagulant if there is a history of thrombosis, and anti-leukocyte antibodies in patients with white blood cell counts below 4,000/μL.

D. Idiopathic Thrombocytopenic Purpura

Thrombocytopenia unrelated to a drug, infection, or autoimmune disease is generally classified as **autoimmune** ITP (AITP). This diagnosis can only be made by excluding all other causes of non-immune and immune destruction. Similar to immune thrombocytopenia in children, it can be an acute disease in adults. However, most adult cases proceed to a chronic form of AITP where a continued high level of marrow platelet production is required to maintain a chronically low to near-normal platelet count in the face of a shortened platelet lifespan.

AITP patients usually present because of **bleeding**. The site of the bleeding may vary, although petechial and purpuric lesions of the skin and mucous membranes are most typical. Some patients report increased bruising, recurrent epistaxis, or menorrhagia for some weeks or months prior to diagnosis. Typically, thrombocytopenia is severe (<10,000/μL) before bleeding becomes a problem. This condition reflects the fact that increased platelet production in ITP is associated with an output of reticulated platelets that demonstrate greater than normal function, providing some protection. Thus, ITP patients are usually not at great risk for a major organ or intracerebral bleed.

The initial presentation of mild, often chronic AITP can be very difficult to diagnose. Whereas severe autoimmune thrombocytopenia typically shows a normal or increased number of megakaryocytes with increased ploidy in the marrow, the least severe of the chronic ITP patients may have little or no expansion of the marrow megakaryocyte mass together with a relatively modest shortening of platelet lifespan. In this situation, reticulated platelet values, direct measurements of platelet lifespan, or response to therapy after excluding all other likely causes may be the only way to make the diagnosis.

Assays for **anti-platelet-antibodies** in ITP patients can show specificity for the platelet glycoproteins GPIb, IIb, and IIIa, as well as the GPIIb/IIIa complex. Interaction of the antibody with one of these sites rarely produces a functional aggregation abnormality. The principal effect is rapid removal and destruction of involved platelets via opsonization. Measurements of platelet-associated antibody are usually not necessary to make the diagnosis of AITP, nor do the results have any prognostic or therapeutic value. Antibody detection methods are highly variable in their sensitivity and specificity, and studies in thrombocytopenic patients have failed to show a unique AITP pattern. Because of this, clinical recommendations are that antibody assays not be done, and the diagnosis of AITP should be made by exclusion of other causes.

AITP patients can have unbound **antibody in their plasma**. Classic studies of the effect of infusing plasma from AITP patients into normal subjects have demonstrated the destructive effect of this antibody on platelets (Figure 31–7). Transfused platelet lifespan is also dramatically shortened, with destruction mainly in the spleen. In fact, platelet survival in the most severely affected patients can be measured in hours rather than days. With less severe ITP, radiolabeled homologous and autologous platelet survivals show a more variable picture. Some patients demonstrate only modest shortening in platelet survival, suggesting a subnormal rate of platelet production, perhaps caused by antibody-specific suppression of megakaryocyte proliferation and platelet production. In support of this, thrombopoietin receptor activating drugs have shown significant efficacy at increasing the platelet count to levels greater than 50,000/μL in refractory ITP. Two such drugs, romiplostim and eltrombopag, have been approved by the Food and Drug Administration (FDA) for use in chronic AITP. The inconsistency in the balance of destructive versus hypoproliferative pathophysiology of ITP is also reflected in the variable responses to platelet transfusions. Although most ITP patients receiving

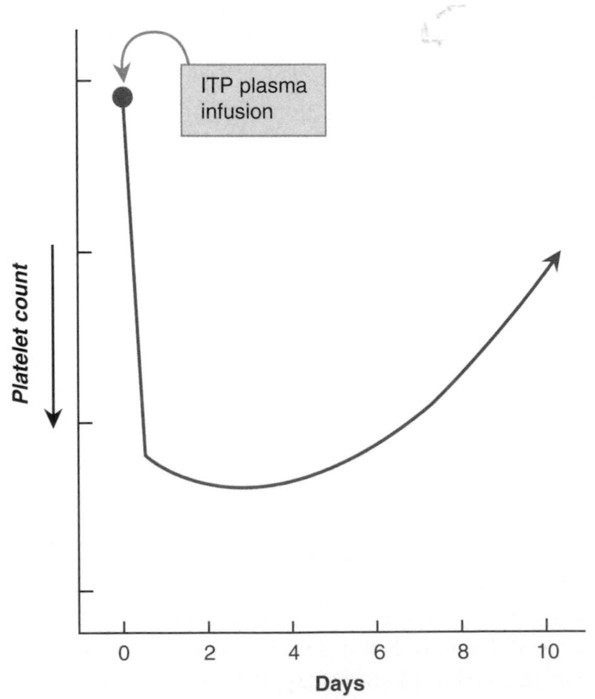

FIGURE 31–7. **Thrombocytopenia in response to an infusion of plasma from a patient with ITP.** Patients with ITP often have unbound antibody in their plasma that when infused into a normal subject will cause a sudden and dramatic thrombocytopenia. Platelets are rapidly cleared by reticuloendothelial cells of the spleen and liver. Over the next several days, antibody is cleared from circulation and new platelet production overtakes destruction, resulting in a rise in platelet count.

platelet transfusions rapidly destroy the infused platelets, up to 30% of patients demonstrate near-normal post-transfusion platelet increments and survival.

THERAPY AND CLINICAL COURSE

As with the diagnosis of thrombocytopenia, therapy should be planned according to the likely pathophysiologic defect, whether an abnormality of platelet production, distribution in circulation, or destruction. Management decisions may need to be made before the full workup is completed. In this case, they must be based on the clinician's best estimate of the disease process. Regardless of the cause of thrombocytopenia, platelet transfusions are appropriate if the patient is experiencing life-threatening bleeding, for example, intracranial hemorrhage. Long-term management usually requires other therapeutic maneuvers to either improve platelet production or decrease high levels of platelet destruction.

Production Disorders

A. Platelet Transfusion

Platelet transfusions are a mainstay in the management of patients with platelet production disorders. Random donor platelets are prepared from units of donated whole blood by centrifugation or directly from a single donor by cytapheresis (see Chapter 38). One unit of apheresis platelets is equivalent to a random donor pool of 4–6 units. For patients who become alloimmunized to random donor platelets, blood banks can provide HLA-matched single-donor platelets. Based on the patient's HLA type, donors can be selected for the best fit for HLA identity. The more closely HLA-matched the platelets, the better chance they have of surviving after transfusion in an alloimmunized patient. Platelet crossmatching has also been used in some blood centers to predict compatibility and at times may be better than HLA matching.

1. Tailoring therapy to the patient—Platelet transfusion therapy must be adjusted to the severity of the thrombocytopenia, the presence of bleeding complications, and the patient's underlying disorder (Table 31–3). A normal individual can tolerate a

TABLE 31–3 • Recommended platelet counts (per μL) to avoid bleeding

Platelet Count	Clinical Condition
>100,000	Major abdominal, chest, or neurosurgery
>50,000	Trauma, surgery other than above types
>30,000	Minor surgical procedures
>20,000	Prevention/treatment of bleeding in patients with sepsis, leukemia, malignancy
>10,000	Uncomplicated malignancy, leukemia, aplastic anemia
>5,000–10,000	Normal individuals
>5,000	ITP patients at low risk

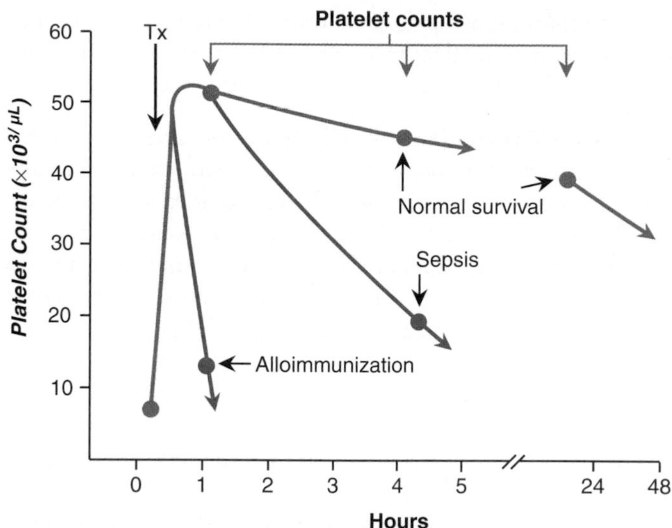

FIGURE 31–8. **Platelet transfusion therapy.** Transfusion (Tx) of a single unit of pheresed platelets or a 6-pack of random donor platelets should increase the platelet count by 60,000/μL. Post-transfusion platelet counts should be measured at 1 hour to determine recovery and at 4 and 24 hours for survival. Alloimmunized and septic patients generally show dramatically reduced recovery and survival, respectively.

platelet count of 5,000–10,000/μL without difficulty. The uncomplicated patient undergoing chemotherapy for malignancy, or even leukemia, does not require prophylactic transfusion until the platelet count falls below 10,000/μL. However, patients with similarly low counts who have complications of sepsis, fever, splenomegaly, or pregnancy are at risk for bleeding with platelet counts of 10,000–30,000/μL. Even higher platelet counts are needed for invasive procedures or surgery. For relatively minor procedures such as catheter insertions, biopsies, or lumbar puncture, efforts should be made to increase the platelet count to at least 30,000/μL. If major surgery is required, the platelet count should, if possible, be increased to 50,000–100,000/μL to control bleeding. Maintenance transfusions of platelets during and after surgery may also be necessary if there is considerable platelet consumption. Therefore, platelet counts within 1 hour after transfusion and at frequent intervals are important in planning for further platelet transfusion needs (Figure 31–8).

The **usual platelet transfusion order** is for a single unit of apheresis platelets or a pool of between 4 and 6 units of random donor platelets. Hospitalized, uncomplicated chemotherapy patients requiring prophylactic platelet transfusions can be given fewer units (3-unit pools) at more frequent time intervals without increased bleeding risk and with a significant savings in the total number of units transfused. Unlike red cell transfusions, random and single-donor platelets do not need to be "type specific." In fact, because platelet units contain very few red blood cells, they do not need to be ABO compatible. However, when multiply transfused patients demonstrate poor post-transfusion platelet count increments, ABO-compatible platelets should be used to try to improve the response. In Rh– women of childbearing age, sufficient red blood cells are transfused in the platelet pool to raise the risk of sensitizing the mother. Therefore, such women should receive platelets from Rh– donors or be treated with RhoGAM following transfusion of Rh+ product.

2. HLA alloimmunization—Each unit of apheresis platelets or 6 units of random donor platelets (6-pack) should raise the platelet count in a normal-sized (70-kg) adult by approximately 60,000/μL (see Figure 31–8). This condition assumes, of course, no problems with alloimmunization or an increased rate of destruction secondary to a complicating illness. If a patient is repeatedly exposed to platelet transfusions, HLA alloantibodies can develop that will effectively shorten the lifespan of transfused platelets. Usually, such antibodies will not appear until 1–2 months after significant exposure to blood products and are less likely to occur in immunosuppressed patients and patients receiving leukocyte-depleted platelets.

To detect HLA alloimmunization, a platelet count should be measured within 1 hour after an ABO-compatible platelet transfusion. If it is repeatedly below the expected increment, HLA sensitization is possible. The first step in such patients is to provide platelets that lack the target antigen(s); this is done by using patient serum to crossmatch for compatible donor platelets. If these crossmatched platelets repeatedly fail to yield adequate platelet increments, the patient should be HLA-typed and transfused only with single-donor HLA-matched platelets (see Chapter 38). However, when HLA-matched or crossmatched platelets do not give an adequate platelet increase, a careful evaluation should be made to look for other causes of platelet destruction (eg, splenomegaly). Finally, to plan subsequent platelet transfusions, serial platelet counts post-transfusion, usually at 4 and 24 hours, should be performed (see Figure 31–8). More frequent measurements may be needed in the massively transfused trauma victim or acutely ill patient who is consuming large amounts of platelets because of vasculitis or DIC related to sepsis.

3. Adverse reactions—Adverse reactions associated with platelet transfusion are similar to those of other blood products. Immediate febrile reactions are most often the result of leukocyte-related cytokines in the platelet supernatant and have been ameliorated by the increased use of leukodepleted platelet concentrates (either double spun or filtered pre-storage) and by premedicating the patient. Bacterial contamination resulting in sepsis is somewhat more common than that seen with red cell transfusion, since platelets are stored at room temperature rather than in the cold. Despite routine testing, there is a small risk of transmission of non-A, non-B, and non-C hepatitis, and transfusion-transmitted variant Creutzfeldt-Jakob disease is a rare consideration (especially in the United Kingdom). Routine testing for HIV and human T-cell leukemia virus-1 (HTLV-1) largely eliminates the risk for transmission of these viruses. Testing for cytomegalovirus (CMV) can be very important in patients undergoing any form of transplantation. The CMV-negative transplant patient should receive CMV-negative platelet products.

4. Long-term management—Long-term management of the patient with a platelet production defect depends on the cause and the ability to reverse the production abnormality. For example, thrombocytopenia in the leukemic patient should reverse with effective control of the leukemia. In this situation, platelet transfusion support is only required during periods of ablative chemotherapy. By contrast, patients with irreversible marrow damage or aplastic anemia require chronic platelet transfusions. Although this is technically feasible, the risk of alloimmunization over the long term is very high and strategies should be used to reduce the number of transfusions, including establishing a lower platelet count trigger when the patient is asymptomatic and using antifibrinolytic drugs as an alternative to platelet transfusion for minor bleeding.

Patients with ineffective thrombopoiesis secondary to an intrinsic abnormality of megakaryocytes may be treated similarly to those with a production disorder when there is a bleeding episode. Ineffective thrombopoiesis associated with either vitamin B_{12} or folate deficiency should be immediately treated with appropriate vitamin therapy. Recovery of the platelet count to normal occurs within a matter of days, making platelet transfusion unnecessary in all but the most acute situations.

B. Platelet Growth Factors

Theoretically, platelet growth factors should decrease the severity of thrombocytopenia and/or platelet transfusion requirements in patients with thrombocytopenia caused by cancer chemotherapy. IL-11 (Neumega) is used to reduce platelet transfusion requirements in cancer patients undergoing non-myeloablative chemotherapy, but it has a risk for anaphylaxis, as well as an inflammatory reaction that accompanies treatment.

Drugs with homology to thrombopoietin (TPO) were promising until they were found to stimulate neutralizing antibodies with cross-reactivity to native TPO, resulting in refractory thrombocytopenia. Several alternative production-stimulating drugs, TPO peptide mimetics, and TPO agonist antibodies that don't have sequence homology to TPO are in development or have been approved for chronic ITP. They are also under study in patients with myelodysplasia or following myelosuppressive chemotherapy. Unfortunately, when marrow cellularity is severely compromised, production-stimulating drugs are less effective than in patients with refractory ITP. One exception (although not in malignancy) is that eltrombopag has shown promise at improving platelet counts in thrombocytopenic hepatitis C patients, thereby allowing institution of interferon therapy.

Disorders of Distribution

Low platelet counts secondary to splenomegaly are generally not associated with abnormal bleeding. Therefore, platelet transfusions are not recommended. If the count falls to below 20,000–30,000/μL, the patient with splenomegaly needs to be evaluated for a concomitant platelet production or destruction defect. The presence of one or the other of these will dictate therapy. If a production abnormality appears to be present, a trial of platelet transfusions can be attempted. Measurements of the platelet count 4 and 24 hours after transfusion can help predict the effectiveness of further transfusion therapy (see Figure 31–8). Patients with very large spleens will show a lower than normal increment following transfusion owing to the pooling of platelets in the spleen. Unless there is a significant component of increased destruction, however, the platelet count should remain relatively stable for the next 24 hours. When an immune destruction defect is present, little in the way of post-transfusion increment is observed, and the count quickly falls back to pretransfusion levels.

Patients with myelofibrosis and massive splenomegaly can be a therapeutic dilemma. In the thrombocytopenic myelofibrotic patient, it can be very difficult to predict whether splenectomy will improve or worsen the patient's thrombocytopenia. In addition, in some patients, the spleen is actually controlling a tendency to overproduction. A splenectomy in this type of patient will result in a rise in platelet counts in excess of 1 million/μL, along with the possibility of thromboembolic complications.

Destruction Disorders

Proper management of patients with platelet destruction disorders depends on the diagnosis. In those individuals who have non-immune destruction as a part of DIC, the only effective therapy is the treatment of the underlying cause of the DIC (see Chapter 35). If the primary condition can be corrected, coagulation factors and platelet count will recover on their own. Similar to patients with DIC, patients with TTP or HUS should only receive platelet transfusions for life-threatening bleeding. With these conditions, potential harm from platelet transfusions is of even greater concern; **platelet transfusions in TTP have directly led to increased thrombosis** and organ damage (including sudden cardiac death) secondary to marked platelet aggregation and activation.

A. Management of Patients With TTP, HUS, or HELLP

Children and adults with **relapsing congenital TTP** may be managed with infusions of FFP as a source of vWF-cleaving protease. The recommended therapy for sporadic TTP and adults with a mixed **TTP-HUS** picture is plasmapheresis with plasma exchange to remove the vWF protease-inhibitor complex and supply a new source of protease. Suitable plasma products include FFP, cryopoor FFP, and SD FFP; it has not been proven that one plasma product is superior to the others for TTP therapy. Plasmapheresis should be initiated without delay and repeated at least daily with exchange of at least 1 plasma volume (~3,000 mL). Plasma infusion alone is appropriate only when plasma exchange is delayed, for example, by the need to transport the patient to a plasmapheresis-capable facility. High-dose steroid therapy may also be given acutely, although evidence for its effectiveness is lacking, and similarly, there is little evidence for an effect of corticosteroids in chronic relapsing TTP. Speed is essential in the management of TTP. The sooner the plasma exchange is initiated, the better the response. Patients who have progressed to coma and severe renal failure have a very poor prognosis. Other parameters of disease activity, including the severity of the anemia and thrombocytopenia, or the elevation of the lactic dehydrogenase (LDH) level, are poor initial predictors of outcome. However, a rapid fall in the LDH within the first 3 days of plasma exchange generally predicts recovery.

The response of **TTP** patients to plasma exchange can be distressingly slow, requiring frequent, even daily, treatments over several weeks. Furthermore, the duration of therapy must be determined by trial and error. Once a response is attained (normal platelet count and LDH level), the frequency of the treatments should be gradually decreased and the patient closely observed for exacerbation/relapse of disease. As long as plasma exchange appears to have a beneficial effect, it should be continued, even if the patient shows only a partial response. Addition of Rituxan therapy has induced remission of TTP in some patients who either failed to respond to plasma exchange or who relapsed soon after discontinuation of plasmapheresis. Some patients may evolve into a chronic, smoldering form of the disease with continued thrombocytopenia but without progressive organ damage. In this case, they may be indistinguishable from chronic ITP patients, but obviously, their primary treatment (repeated plasma exchange) is much different.

Plasmapheresis and plasma infusions have had a major positive impact on overall prognosis in TTP. More than 90% of patients with idiopathic TTP and very low ADAMTS13 levels (<5%) who are treated early in their disease now survive, whereas in the past TTP was a fatal illness in more than 80%–90% of patients. Severe deficiency of ADAMTS13 in the TTP presentation, though, is not a prerequisite for a successful response; plasma exchange restored normal platelet counts in 75% of TTP patients without significant ADAMTS13 deficiency. At the same time, 20% or more of idiopathic TTP patients relapse at least once within 5 years, and another 25% demonstrate chronic renal insufficiency (creatinine clearance <40 mL/min). The presence of an ADAMTS13 inhibitor does not appear to affect the outcome, unless the inhibitor levels are very high; for the latter, plasmapheresis does little to improve the ADAMTS13 levels, and early relapse occurs in 50% of these high inhibitor patients. When TTP is associated with chemotherapy (gemcitabine, ticlopidine), HIV, immunosuppressive agents, sepsis, lupus, or stem cell transplantation, the mortality is greater than 50% in this subset.

HUS and HELLP syndrome present a somewhat different therapeutic challenge. Typical HUS in children usually can be managed without plasmapheresis, although acute dialysis is often necessary when renal failure is severe. By contrast, atypical HUS, seen with streptococcal infections and complement (eg, factor H) deficiency, generally requires both plasma exchange and hemodialysis and has a poor long-term prognosis. HELLP syndrome, like preeclampsia, usually resolves with delivery of the fetus. However, a small number of women convert to a TTP-like syndrome postpartum. They should undergo aggressive pheresis with plasma exchange. The response to therapy, however, is generally poor once there is organ damage in postpartum TTP. Women who develop TTP during or after pregnancy are likely to have successful future pregnancies, but TTP recurs in at least 10%–20% of subsequent pregnancies. If the decision is made to go ahead with a pregnancy, aspirin and persantine have been used successfully as prophylaxis.

B. Neonatal Thrombocytopenia

Treatment of autoimmune thrombocytopenia must be disease specific. Mild, neonatal thrombocytopenia, whether isoimmune or associated with maternal ITP, does not require therapy. For severe thrombocytopenia, an infusion of immunoglobulin in a dose of 400 mg/kg body weight, given daily for up to 5 days, is the therapy of choice. Its immediate effects are thought to increase fractional excretion of the antibody and to form an idiotype–anti-idiotype dimer, preventing antibody binding to its antigen. Platelet transfusions for neonatal thrombocytopenia should be reserved for children with evidence of intracranial hemorrhage. HPA-1a–negative platelets can be highly effective in treating alloimmune thrombocytopenia. Such platelets are generally obtained from reference blood banks and not from the mother, in part because of her postpartum condition but also because maternal platelets contain anti–HPA-1a antibody in the plasma.

Newborns of mothers with autoimmune thrombocytopenia should have daily platelet counts for the first 4 days after birth. In addition, any newborn with a platelet count below 50,000/μL should have brain imaging to rule out intracranial hemorrhage. Newborns with platelet counts below 20,000/μL should be treated with intravenous immunoglobulin. If there is evidence of intracranial hemorrhage, combined immunoglobulin/prednisone therapy with platelet transfusion is indicated.

C. Autoimmune Thrombocytopenia in Children

In children who develop an autoimmune thrombocytopenia following viral illness, severe thrombocytopenia is usually self-limited, lasting less than 1–2 weeks. If the platelet count is above 30,000/μL and there is little in the way of mucocutaneous bleeding, the child can simply be observed. More than 90% of these children will recover completely. Any child with a count below 10,000/μL or below 20,000/μL with mucous membrane or life-threatening bleeding should be hospitalized and treated with intravenous immune globulin, 1 g/kg on day 1 and 400 mg/kg per day for the next 2–5 days, together with high-dose oral or parenteral glucocorticoids. The prolonged effect of immunoglobulin therapy is presumably related to induction of T-cell suppression and downregulation of B-cell autoantibody production. About 30% of children with refractory ITP will respond to Rituxan. Splenectomy for chronic disease should only be considered for the child who continues to have marked thrombocytopenia with abnormal bleeding for more than a year. Emergency splenectomy and platelet transfusion are only appropriate if a child is experiencing a life-threatening hemorrhage. More than 70% will achieve a sustained remission after splenectomy, but not without a future risk of fatal bacterial sepsis.

D. Drug-Induced Thrombocytopenia

In patients with autoimmune thrombocytopenia secondary to drug ingestion, the most important management step is to discontinue the drug. Corticosteroid therapy may speed recovery in patients with an ITP-like picture, such as may be seen in patients reacting to sulfamethoxazole. The rate of recovery will then depend both on the clearance rate of the drug and the ability of marrow megakaryocytes to proliferate and increase platelet production. Even when the platelet count is very low, bleeding is unlikely, and patients can be allowed to recover without specific therapy.

The **management of HIT** is a different matter. Once there is a strong clinical suspicion of HIT, all unfractionated and low-molecular-weight heparin forms, including the small amounts used in intravenous (IV) line maintenance, must be stopped immediately. Any delay, such as waiting for an assay result or a further fall in the platelet count, can prolong the duration of HIT, putting the patient at further risk of thrombosis. Thrombosis risk in HIT is already high; most studies note a minimum 30% incidence of thromboembolic events in both medical and surgical HIT patients out to 1 month following HIT diagnosis. Substitution of low-molecular-weight heparin (and to a lesser extent, danaparoid) is not an option inasmuch as there is significant antibody cross-reactivity. Because HIT is a highly prothrombotic state that is not immediately diminished by discontinuing heparin, HIT patients should be started on a direct thrombin inhibitor, such as lepirudin or argatroban (see Chapter 37), and anticoagulation is monitored based on changes from the baseline PTT. Lepirudin is recommended as an intravenous bolus of 0.4 mg/kg, followed by a continuous infusion at 0.15 mg/kg/h. The infusion is adjusted to keep the PTT between 1.5 and 2.5 times the baseline PTT. However, high bleeding rates have been noted for lepirudin at these doses; alternative dosing has suggested that lepirudin be given as an infusion (without a bolus) at 0.06 mg/kg/h. In either dosing regimen, it is most critical that the PTT be maintained above 1.5 times the baseline.

Argatroban is given as an infusion of 2.0 μg/kg/min, titrated to keep the PTT between 1.5 and 3 times baseline. Oral anticoagulants should never be started until there is continuous coverage with a direct thrombin inhibitor, and the platelet count has risen to near-normal levels. The immediate reduction in protein C levels with the initiation of warfarin therapy can lead to worsening thrombosis in HIT, including massive skin necrosis and venous limb gangrene. Because factor VII levels may mirror the decrease in protein C, venous limb gangrene can be associated with an inappropriately high and rapid rise in the international normalized ratio (INR; INR >3.5 after a single dose is the hallmark) after initiating warfarin. If this occurs, warfarin should be discontinued and vitamin K given to reverse the effect.

Lepirudin for HIT in the face of renal insufficiency is associated with increased bleeding risk, and the dose should be adjusted to target the PTT increase to just above 1.5 times baseline, usually less than 65 seconds. However, trying to titrate this dosage adjustment can compromise its efficacy in preventing thrombotic complications of HIT; for this reason, argatroban may be preferred for HIT with renal insufficiency. Another drawback for lepirudin therapy is the 40% incidence of developing anti-lepirudin antibodies, and anaphylaxis to reinstitution of lepirudin has occurred. Thus, lepirudin cannot be given twice to any patient.

If HIT is present without thrombosis, the direct thrombin inhibitor (DTI) should be continued until the platelet count is above 150,000/μL; depending on the clinical situation, the DTI can be continued or changed to warfarin for up to 4 weeks of additional therapy. If thrombosis is present with HIT, the DTI should similarly be continued until the platelet count normalizes. Warfarin is then added but should overlap with DTI therapy for at least 5 days. Because the PT will already be prolonged by DTI therapy, one must resist the impulse to decrease DTI dosing as the INR increases after warfarin addition. When the INR is in the therapeutic range for at least 48 hours, the DTI can be stopped; warfarin is then continued for at least 3–6 months.

E. AIDS-Associated Thrombocytopenia

HIV-infected patients who develop thrombocytopenia early in their disease can be treated with AZT. Approximately 60% of patients will show a response, and up to 50% will have a long-lasting improvement in their platelet counts. The effect is not immediate; it can take up to 1–2 months before the platelet count improves. In those patients who do not respond, splenectomy can help in more than 85% of the cases. Splenectomy is only effective, however, if done early in the course of disease, when the marrow megakaryocyte mass can still compensate for the increased rate of platelet destruction.

Corticosteroids, intravenous immune globulin, and intravenous anti-D (WinRho) have also been used in AIDS patients. Although corticosteroids have a positive effect, long-term treatment runs the risk of encouraging opportunistic infection. Intravenous immune globulin can give a good response, but the relapse rate is high and thus requires repeated treatment. In patients who are Rh+, anti-D therapy seems to be more effective but is limited by how low the hemoglobin can be permitted to fall. With disease progression, HIV-infected patients develop a platelet production defect that only responds to platelet transfusion therapy. AIDS patients who develop a microangiopathic thrombocytopenia with schistocytes and organ damage should be treated with plasmapheresis and plasma exchange, similar to HIV-negative TTP patients, but HIV-associated TTP has a worse prognosis.

F. Adult Autoimmune Thrombocytopenia

Thrombocytopenia secondary to a definitive autoimmune disease is best treated by controlling the systemic illness. For patients with autoimmune thrombocytopenia associated with either **Hodgkin or non-Hodgkin lymphoma**, successful **radiation therapy, chemotherapy, and/or marrow transplantation** for the lymphoma will eventually ameliorate the immune-related platelet destruction. The immune destruction of platelets that occurs as a complication of an infectious disease will usually resolve as the infection is controlled. Corticosteroids may be used occasionally on a short-term basis to treat patients with very low platelet counts, such as patients with infectious mononucleosis who develop severe thrombocytopenia.

Severe de novo AITP with bleeding manifestations in adults should be treated as a medical emergency with methylprednisolone by intravenous infusion, 1 g given daily for the first 3 days (Figure 31–9). High-dose dexamethasone (40 mg daily for

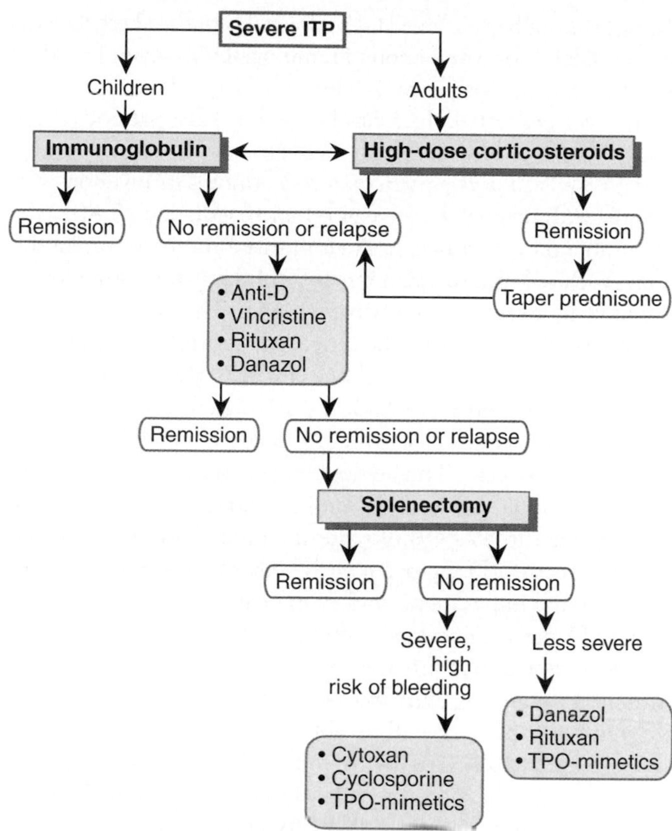

FIGURE 31–9. **Treatment of severe autoimmune thrombocytopenia.** Management of the patient with ITP begins with high-dose corticosteroids, immune globulin therapy, or both. If these modalities fail, anti-D, vincristine, rituxan, and danazol should be attempted to avoid splenectomy. Should disease recur following splenectomy, more intensive chemotherapy (cytoxan, cyclosporine) and the newly approved TPO mimetics, romiplostim and eltrombopag, are indicated for chronic therapy.

4 days every 2–4 weeks) has also been used effectively as initial therapy for adult AITP. If there is clinical evidence of intracranial or other serious hemorrhage, the patient should also be given intravenous immunoglobulin (1 g/kg/d for 2–3 days) and platelet transfusions at least every 8–12 hours, regardless of the effect on the platelet count. Some patients who receive platelet transfusions will show a relatively normal post-transfusion increment and reasonable platelet survival over the next 24 hours. However, even when there is no post-transfusion increment, sufficient numbers of the transfused platelets may survive to improve hemostasis. Other therapies to consider for emergent treatment of ITP bleeding include intravenous anti-D (75 μg/kg) in Rh+ patients, IV vincristine (1–2 mg), and even recombinant factor VIIa.

When patients present with less urgent ITP, high-dose corticosteroid therapy (either prednisone 1 mg/kg/d continuously or as pulse dexamethasone 40 mg/d × 4 days monthly) is the mainstay of treatment. Corticosteroids should be continued until the platelet count rises to levels above 50,000/μL. It can then be tapered rapidly as the platelet count enters the normal range. Some adults do not respond optimally to corticosteroids and remain thrombocytopenic. In this circumstance, high-dose corticosteroid therapy cannot be continued for prolonged periods. These patients are candidates for **intravenous immunoglobulin** given in a dose of 1 g/kg intravenously over 6–8 hours over 1–3 days.

Intravenous anti-D IgG can be used in Rh+ patients, especially those who have not had splenectomy. The recommended initial dose is 75 μg/kg given over 3–5 minutes intravenously in patients with hemoglobins greater than 10 g/dL and 25–40 μg/kg when anemia is a concern. A substantial increase in platelet count within 1–3 days, peaking at 7–14 days and lasting for up to a month, is seen in responsive patients. The dosage and timing of subsequent treatments, if needed, depend on the clinical response to the first dose. Since anti-D's therapeutic effect involves Fc receptor blockade by sensitized red blood cells, extravascular hemolysis with a fall in the hemoglobin level is an anticipated event. The hemoglobin decrease by 2 weeks after treatment should be around 2 g/dL, although decreases of 4–6 g/dL are seen in 3%–4% of patients. Immediate intravascular hemolysis to anti-D can occur with hemoglobinemia, hemoglobinuria, renal impairment, and even death.

If AITP persists or relapses after initial therapy with corticosteroids and/or either intravenous immunoglobulin (IVIG) or anti-D, it is extremely unlikely that the patient will spontaneously recover. Some patients will be able to maintain platelet counts above 30,000–50,000/μL with minimal or no therapy; such patients need to be monitored closely since worsening of thrombocytopenia with viral illnesses is common, with an attendant risk of hemorrhage. However, many patients will have persistently low counts that require therapy (<20,000–30,000/μL). Options for these patients include low-dose prednisone (generally up to 10 mg/d), anti-D (50–75 μg/kg/dose), Rituxan (375 mg/m^2 weekly × 4 wks), and Danazol (10–15 mg/kg/d). These therapies should be re-evaluated over several months, and if the platelet count remains below 20,000–30,000/μL, splenectomy should be strongly considered. Approximately 75%–80% of patients will achieve a permanent remission after splenectomy. However, the platelet count is maintained by a continued increased level of marrow production that compensates for the shortened platelet lifespan. These patients are at risk for thrombocytopenic episodes later in life, for example, with significant viral illness. If splenectomy is recommended for a patient with chronic ITP, it is extremely important to immunize with pneumococcal, meningococcal, and *Haemophilus influenzae* vaccines prior to surgery to reduce the risk of postsplenectomy sepsis. In children less than 5 years of age, postsplenectomy prophylactic antibiotic therapy is also advisable.

Refractory immune thrombocytopenia after therapeutic trials of prednisone, IVIG, and splenectomy is not uncommon. The decision as to when and how to treat such patients depends on the chronic platelet count and the associated risk for hemorrhage. Sustained thrombocytopenia with counts below 20,000/μL should be treated since such patients are at risk for severe, life-threatening bleeding. Initial therapies mainly recapitulate pre-splenectomy strategies, including Rituxan, Danazol, corticosteroids, and IVIG. **Intravenous cyclophosphamide and oral cyclosporine** may be effective fallback therapies.

Several new drugs are now available for treating chronic ITP, which is refractory to corticosteroids, IVIG, and/or splenectomy. **Romiplostim and eltrombopag** act by binding to and activating the thrombopoietin receptor, thereby stimulating platelet production. Although antibody-mediated platelet destruction is thought to be the primary pathology in ITP there also appears to be a component of impaired platelet production in many, if not most, patients. These drugs, therefore, can ameliorate the severity of the thrombocytopenia without addressing the rate of destruction.

Romiplostim is given IV at between 1 and 10 μg/kg/wk, while eltrombopag is administered orally at 25–75 mg/d. The goal for both drugs is to maintain platelet counts above 50,000/μL and to reduce the dosage of or discontinue other ITP therapies, especially corticosteroids. Most patients will respond with increased platelet counts, and sustained counts (>50,000/μL) are seen in between 20% and 40% of responders. Marrow reticulin deposition and hepatic toxicity have been reported as adverse effects and should be monitored. Importantly, these drugs have no sequence homology to thrombopoietin, and thus no apparent risk for antibody production to the autologous growth factor.

Management of **chronic ITP in pregnancy** deserves special attention. Most women can be managed throughout their pregnancy with no medication, modest amounts of **prednisone**, or intermittent use of **intravenous immunoglobulin**. To avoid the side effects of prednisone therapy (gestational diabetes, hypertension, and even abruption), high-dose IVIG, 1 g/kg (prepartum weight) given once per month or, in severe cases, as often as every week, is effective in two-thirds of women. In those cases where the thrombocytopenia is severe, higher-dose steroid therapy, 0.5–1 mg/kg prednisone per day together with weekly intravenous immunoglobulin, during the last 2–3 weeks of pregnancy may be needed to prevent maternal bleeding. Even with severe ITP in the mother, most children are born with normal platelet counts. Less than 4% will have a platelet count below 20,000/μL and less than 1% will exhibit a bleeding complication. Neonatal platelet counts may fall in a delayed fashion or continue to fall for 7 or more days following delivery. Therefore, children at risk should have their platelet counts checked at delivery (cord blood) and every 2–3 days thereafter until the count rises.

Despite the low incidence of bleeding complications in children born to ITP mothers, prophylactic cesarean section is still recommended by some obstetricians to decrease the chance of intracranial hemorrhage. There is no good evidence that cesarean section is significantly better at protecting the child. Moreover, this approach actually increases the risk of serious maternal bleeding and often requires platelet transfusion support. The risk for the fetus does not reflect the severity of the mother's ITP, nor is it predicted by prior pregnancy outcomes. A child with severe thrombocytopenia and bleeding complications may be born to a mother with apparently mild disease, while neonates with minimal bleeding complications can follow severely affected pregnancies. These outcomes, moreover, cannot be predicted by assays of maternal platelet-associated antibody. In addition, attempts to anticipate the problem by measuring a percutaneous umbilical vein platelet count carry a risk that is likely greater than the risk of intracranial hemorrhage.

CASE HISTORY • Part 3

The patient's history, physical examination, and smear/marrow studies are consistent with a diagnosis of autoimmune idiopathic thrombocytopenic purpura (AITP). ITP secondary to a relapse of his lymphoproliferative disorder needs to be ruled out by additional studies, including thoracic and abdominal scans for lymphadenopathy and flow cytometry of blood and marrow to detect re-emergence of clonal disease (see Chapter 22). Assays for anti-platelet or platelet glycoprotein-specific antibodies are not routinely recommended to confirm AITP, due to their poor sensitivity and specificity. The diagnosis is primarily made by exclusion of other causes of thrombocytopenia and response to immunosuppressive therapies.

Because of the patient's very low platelet count, he was hospitalized and started on IV methylprednisolone, 1 g/d × 3 days. By day 4, the platelet count had increased to 25,000/μL, but he continued to have epistaxis and bleeding from the gums. He was subsequently begun on IV immune globulin, 1 g/kg/d × 2 days. His platelet count increased to greater than 150,000/μL by hospital day 7, and he was discharged on oral prednisone (1 mg/kg/d) with outpatient follow-up.

The patient was counseled in the need for careful, long-term follow-up, since adult AITP patients are highly likely to develop chronic or relapsing disease, the latter especially when attempting to decrease or discontinue corticosteroids. Many adult AITP patients will require additional courses of therapy, including immunosuppressive agents such as Rituxan. Splenectomy may also be considered in refractory and corticosteroid-dependent patients. As for the new thrombopoietin-mimetic drugs, their role in managing chronic ITP remains to be defined.

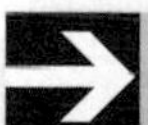

POINTS TO REMEMBER

Petechial hemorrhages, usually most evident over the lower extremities, are most often associated with severe thrombocytopenia, that is, platelet counts below 10,000–20,000/μL. An accurate platelet count is available as a routine part of the automated CBC.

The diagnostic approach to thrombocytopenia is best organized according to the functional defect—a disorder of platelet production, increased peripheral destruction, or abnormal distribution. Examination of the bone marrow (frequency and appearance of megakaryocytes) and the abdomen for splenomegaly (platelet sequestration) are critical components in this differential.

A production disorder is often apparent from the patient's clinical presentation. A history of a hematopoietic malignancy or other primary hematopoietic disorder (aplastic anemia, myelofibrosis, etc), myelosuppressive chemotherapy, or widespread bone metastases should point to a production defect. A number of drugs, chemicals, and radiation can also interfere with megakaryocyte proliferation. A simple bone marrow aspiration/biopsy generally should confirm low numbers or absence of megakaryocytes.

Destruction disorders, regardless of etiology/mechanism, demonstrate a normal marrow response with megakaryocyte proliferation and hyperploidy; reticulated platelets in blood are also increased. Platelet transfusions and radiolabeled survival studies typically show rapid platelet destruction.

Disorders of distribution are all associated with splenomegaly, the degree of thrombocytopenia correlating with the size of the spleen. Severe thrombocytopenia (platelet counts <40,000/μL) can't be explained by splenomegaly alone. In this situation, increased platelet destruction and/or abnormal production must also be playing a role.

Thrombocytopenia secondary to increased platelet destruction can be caused by non-immune or immune mechanisms. Non-immune destruction is seen with disseminated intravascular coagulation, sepsis, vasculitis, and TTP. Immune thrombocytopenia is associated with a number of drugs, lymphoproliferative disorders, certain infectious diseases, and as a component of autoimmune disorders such as SLE. Idiopathic autoimmune thrombocytopenia (AITP), by definition, presents as immune platelet destruction in the absence of concurrent disease.

ITP is common, especially in children as the aftermath of a viral infection or immunization. Unlike adults with AITP, children generally recover without therapy or, when severe, a limited course of immunoglobulin therapy. AITP in adults is usually a chronic disease, which responds erratically to immunosuppression and, even when controlled, can relapse on more than one occasion.

The rapid diagnosis and treatment of thrombotic thrombocytopenic purpura (TTP) can be lifesaving. TTP should be considered when a patient presents with thrombocytopenia and hemolytic anemia. Microangiopathy (schistocytosis), fever, and organ damage from platelet thrombi further confirm the diagnosis. Therapy of the sporadic form of TTP requires plasma exchange to remove antibodies to ADAMTS13 and plasma infusion of normal ADAMTS13. Congenital TTP will respond to plasma infusions alone.

Hemolytic uremic syndrome (HUS) is most often seen in children in association with *E. coli* infection (0157:H7 strain) and has a lesser incidence of thrombocytopenia and organ damage other than the kidneys. HUS generally resolves on its own, though short-term dialysis support may be required.

HELLP syndrome in pregnancy falls within the TTP-HUS spectrum of thrombocytopenic disorders. If delivery of the fetus fails to resolve the illness, a TTP-like regimen of plasma exchange must be instituted.

Heparin-induced thrombocytopenia (HIT) is a highly procoagulant state caused by antibodies to the heparin-PF4 complex and platelet activation. Removal of all forms of heparin and treatment with a direct thrombin inhibitor must be instituted immediately to prevent new or recurrent thromboembolic disease.

Platelet transfusions play a major role in controlling life-threatening bleeding, especially in patients with production defects. Prophylactic platelet transfusions are routinely used in association with ablative chemotherapy. At the same time, platelet transfusions should not be overused because of the risk of alloimmunization and subsequent refractoriness.

Platelet transfusions are not indicated in patients with TTP or HIT. The addition of fresh platelets can lead to an exacerbation of platelet thrombotic damage to organs, especially the brain and kidneys.

Platelet transfusions will generally fail to significantly increase the platelet count (post-transfusion increment) in patients who are alloimmunized or suffer from AITP (rapid destruction) or have significant splenomegaly (increased sequestration and/or destruction). Alloimmunized patients may respond to HLA-matched platelets. ITP patients with uncontrolled, life-threatening hemorrhage may respond to platelet transfusions even in the absence of a measurable increase in the platelet count.

BIBLIOGRAPHY

Pathophysiology

Kenney B, Stack G: Drug-induced thrombocytopenia. Arch Pathol Lab Med 2009;133:309.

Martel N, Lee J, Wells PS: Risk for heparin-induced thrombocytopenia with unfractionated and low-molecular-weight heparin thromboporphylaxis: a meta-analysis. Blood 2005;106:2710.

Ono T et al: Severe secondary deficiency of von Willebrand factor-cleaving protease (ADAMTS13) in patients with sepsis-induced disseminated intravascular coagulation: its correlation with development of renal failure. Blood 2006;107:528.

Prandoni P et al: The incidence of heparin-induced thrombocytopenia in medical patients treated with low-molecular-weight heparin: a prospective cohort study. Blood 2005;106:3049.

Ruaova L et al: Role of platelet surface PF4 antigenic complexes in heparin-induced thrombocytopenia pathogenesis: diagnostic and therapeutic implications. Blood 2006;107:2346.

Stahl A et al: Factor H dysfunction in patients with atypical hemolytic uremic syndrome contributes to complement deposition on platelets and their activation. Blood 2008;111:5307.

Tardy B et al: Predictive factors for thrombosis and major bleeding in an observational study in 181 patients with heparin-induced thrombocytopenia treated with lepirudin. Blood 2006;108:492.

Autoimmune and Heparin-Induced Thrombocytopenia

Areaplly GM, Ortel TL: Heparin-induced thrombocytopenia. N Engl J Med 1006;355:809.

Bougie DW, Wilker PR, Aster RH: Patients with quinine-induced thrombocytopenia have both "drug-dependent" and "drug-specific" antibodies. Blood 2006;108:922.

Warkentin TE. Heparin-induced thrombocytopenia. Hematol Oncol Clin N Am 2007;21:589.

TTP

Fakhouri F et al: Efficiency of curative and prophylactic treatment with rituximab in ADAMTS13-deficient thrombotic thrombocytopenic purpura: a study of 11 cases. Blood 2005;106:1932.

Ferrari S et al: Prognostic value of anti-ADAMTS13 antibody features (Ig isotype, titer, and inhibitory effect) in a cohort of 35 adult French patients undergoing a first episode of thrombotic microangiopathy with undetectable ADAMTS13 activity. Blood 2007;109:2815.

George JN: Thrombotic thrombocytopenic purpura. N Engl J Med 2006;354:1927.

Levy GG, Motto DG, Ginsburg D: ADAMTS13 turns 3. Blood 2005;106:11.

Rieger M et al: ADAMTS13 autoantibodies in patients with thrombotic thrombocytopenic microangiopathies and other immunomediated diseases. Blood 2005;106:1262.

Therapy

Bennett CM et al: Prospective phase 1/2 study of rituximab in childhood and adolescent chronic immune thrombocytopenic purpura. Blood 2006;107:2639.

Boruchov DM et al: Multiagent induction and maintenance therapy for patients with refractory immune thrombocytopenic purpura (ITP). Blood 2007;110:3526.

Bromberg ME: Immune thrombocytopenic purpura—the changing landscape. N Engl J Med 2006;355:1643.

Bussel JB et al: AMG 531, a thrombopoiesis-stimulating protein, for chronic ITP. N Engl J Med 2006;355:1672.

Bussel JB et al: Eltrombopag for the treatment of chronic idiopathic thrombocytopenic purpura. N Engl J Med 2007;357:2237.

Cines DB, Bussel JB: How I treat idiopathic thrombocytopenic purpura. Blood 2005;106:2244.

Gaines AR: Disseminated intravascular coagulation associated with acute hemoglobinemia or hemoglobinuria following Rh_0(D) immune globulin intravenous administration for immune thrombocytopenic purpura. Blood 2005;106:1532.

George JN et al: The Oklahoma Thrombotic Thrombocytopenic Purpura-Hemolytic Uremic Syndrome (TTP-HUS) Registry: a community perspective of patients with clinically diagnosed TTP-HUS. Semin Hematol 2004;41:60.

Godeau B et al: Rituximab efficacy and safety in adult splenectomy candidates with chronic immune thrombocytopenic purpura—results of a prospective multicenter phase 2 study. Blood 2008;112:999.

Kuter DJ: New thrombopoietic growth factors. Blood 2007;109:4607.

Kuter DJ et al: Efficacy of romiplostin in patients with chronic immune thrombocytopenic purpura: a double-blind randomised controlled trial. Lancet 2008;371:1672.

Lubenow N et al: Lepirudin for prophylaxis of thrombosis in patients with acute isolated heparin-induced thrombocytopenia: an analysis of 3 prospective studies. Blood 2004;104:3072.

Mazzucconi MG et al: Therapy with high-dose dexamethasone (HD-DXM) in previously untreated patients affected by idiopathic thrombocytopenic purpura: a GIMEMA experience. Blood 2007;109:1401.

Stasi R et al: Idiopathic thrombocytopenic purpura: current concepts in pathophysiology and management. Thromb Haemost 2008;99:4.

Vesely SK et al: Management of adult patients with peristent idiopathic thrombocytopenic purpura following splenectomy. Ann Intern Med 2004;140:112.

Webster ML et al: Relative efficacy of intravenous immunoglobulin G in ameliorating thrombocytopenia induced by antiplatelet GPIIbIIIa versus GPIbα antibodies. Blood 2006;108:943.

Zheng XL et al: Effect of plasma exchange on plasma ADAMTS13 metalloproteinase activity, inhibitor level, and clinical outcome in patients with idiopathic and nonidiopathic thrombotic thrombocytopenic purpura. Blood 2004;103:4043.

PLATELET DYSFUNCTION AND VON WILLEBRAND DISEASE · 32

CASE HISTORY • *Part 1*

A 76-year-old man presents with a complaint of headache, which began several hours after a fall and has steadily worsened. His history is notable for hypertension and coronary artery disease, status post-bypass grafting 4 years prior. He denies any history of bleeding or thrombosis other than his previous coronary symptoms. Medications include a cholesterol-lowering agent, beta-blocker, and a daily aspirin. Examination is notable for a tender bruise over the left occipital region. The remainder of the examination is benign.

CBC: Hemoglobin/hematocrit - 13 g/dL/39%
MCV - 94 fL MCH - 31 pg MCHC - 32 g/dL
RDW-CV - 11% White blood cell count - 8,500/μL
Platelet count - 310,000/μL

BLOOD SMEAR MORPHOLOGY

Normocytic, normochromic with no aniso- or poikilocytosis or polychromasia. White blood cells are normal and platelets are numerous with normal morphology.

PT = 12.6 seconds (<14 seconds)
INR = 1.1 (<1.3)
PTT = 31 seconds (22–35 seconds)

Questions

- Given the risk of an intracranial hemorrhage, do these laboratory results rule out a coagulopathy?
- What other test(s) might be in order?

An abnormality in platelet function can result in bleeding despite the platelet count being normal. Disordered platelet function occurs when there is an abnormality of either the platelet itself or its primary adhesive ligands, for example, von Willebrand factor. Therapeutic inhibition of platelet function is very common in the developed world, and although most platelet function disorders are associated with a relatively mild bleeding tendency, awareness of these conditions can be important in the overall clinical management of these patients.

NORMAL PLATELET FUNCTION

The steps involved in platelet adhesion, aggregation, and subsequent clot formation are illustrated in Figure 32–1. Important elements of the system include the vessel wall, functional components of the platelet, and both **von Willebrand factor (vWF)** and fibrinogen. The ability of the vessel to contract and the condition of the subendothelial connective tissue are both important elements. Reflex contraction of the injured vessel reduces flow and

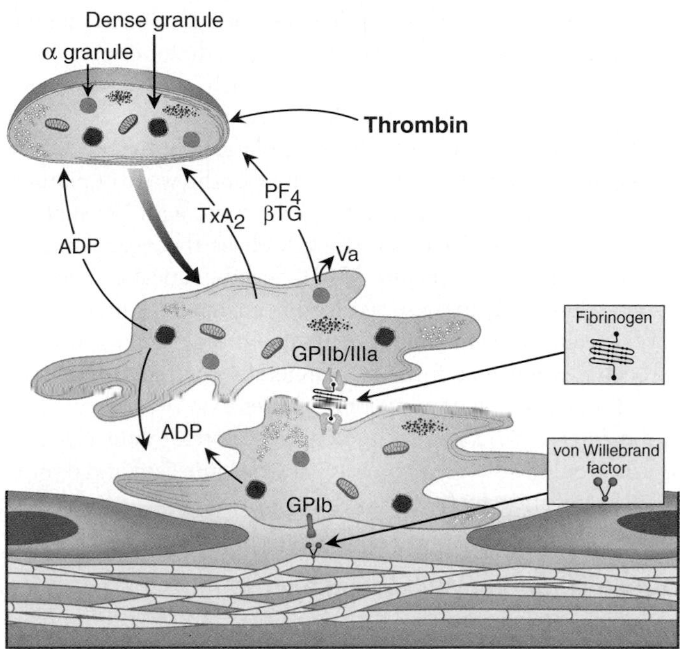

FIGURE 32–1. **Normal platelet function.** Important elements in platelet adhesion and aggregation include platelet shape change; adhesion to subendothelial collagen; aggregation of activated platelets; and release of ADP, thromboxane A_2 (TxA_2), platelet factor 4 (PF4), and β-thromboglobulin (βTG) to stimulate further platelet activation and recruit additional platelets into the aggregate. Thrombin acts as the most potent physiologic platelet activator to accelerate the process. von Willebrand factor bound to subendothelial collagen is essential for platelet adhesion via the GPIb receptor, whereas fibrinogen is the essential cofactor in the GPIIb/IIIa-mediated platelet-platelet aggregation process.

encourages adhesion of platelets to exposed collagen. Loss of this reflex because of a distortion in vessel anatomy or an underlying collagen defect will interfere with normal platelet thrombus formation.

Platelet adhesion, activation, and aggregation play pivotal roles in platelet thrombus formation. A defect in any of these components, including the expression of the GPIb or GPIIb/IIIa receptor, release of α-granule or dense granule contents, thromboxane A_2 synthesis, nucleotide metabolism, or the expression of factor V receptors, will result in a functional defect. In addition, both vWF and fibrinogen are essential to platelet adhesion, aggregation, and clot formation; vWF is required for the initial adhesion of the GPIb surface receptor of the platelets to the bridging collagen of the subendothelial connective tissue. Both fibrinogen and vWF act as cofactors in the subsequent platelet-platelet aggregation by interacting with GPIIb/IIIa receptors.

Endothelial cells appear to be the primary source of plasma vWF. Initially, a propolypeptide is produced and stored as a dimer in the Weibel-Palade bodies of the endothelial cells. A portion of the peptide is then removed, and dimers are linked by disulfide bonds to form **multimers** of varying sizes. These multimeric forms are released into circulation, where they serve both as a cofactor in platelet adhesion/aggregation and as a carrier for factor VIII. The latter is important in determining the clearance rate of factor VIII from circulation. The largest circulating plasma vWF multimers are cut into smaller multimers by the vWF-cleaving protease, ADAMTS13 (see Chapter 31 discussion of thrombotic thrombocytopenic purpura [TTP]). The size distribution of multimeric forms of vWF is an important determinant of platelet function; larger multimeric vWF is associated with increased platelet adhesion and function.

Megakaryocytes also manufacture vWF, which is then incorporated into the α-granules of the released platelets. The multimers within α-granules are larger than those seen in circulation and are referred to as **ultra-large vWF (ULvWF)**. This platelet vWF appears on the surface as platelets change shape and release their α-granule contents. Platelet surface vWF then binds to the GPIIb/IIIa complex on other platelets to recruit additional platelet aggregation in collaboration with fibrinogen.

CLINICAL FEATURES

As with thrombocytopenia, there are no specific symptoms or signs that always indicate a platelet functional defect. Inherited defects are rare and are generally characterized by a relatively mild bleeding tendency. Von Willebrand disease (vWD) is an exception to this rule, since certain vWD subtypes can be associated with severe bleeding.

Patients with platelet functional defects generally present with easy bruisability, mucocutaneous bleeding of a purpuric nature, and bleeding from the gastrointestinal (GI) and genitourinary tracts (women may have severe menorrhagia) rather than the petechial bleeding that characterizes thrombocytopenia. It is not unusual for the bleeding tendency to escape detection until aggravated by another abnormality. For example, the defect may first be suspected because of excessive bleeding following minor surgery or a dental extraction, or unusual mucocutaneous bleeding following the administration of anticoagulants or a platelet inhibitor such as aspirin or clopidogrel. Therefore, a history of unusual bleeding, a family history suggestive of a congenital abnormality, and the clinical picture can provide important clues.

Laboratory Studies

A. Platelet Function Analysis (In Vitro Bleeding Time)

The in vivo template bleeding time (BT) had traditionally been used as a screening test for the presence of a platelet functional defect. However, over time this assay has been recognized to be a relatively poor screening tool for hemostasis disorders and has been discontinued in most centers. An automated "in vitro bleeding time" test, **platelet function analysis (PFA)**, has largely replaced the template bleeding time performed in vivo; the PFA measures the time required for whole blood to clot, so-called "closure time," after introduction of a platelet agonist (see Chapter 29) and can be used to detect inhibition of platelet function by aspirin or the presence of vWD (Table 32–1). Closure times less than 180 seconds (for the collagen/epinephrine cartridge) and less than 120 seconds (for collagen/adenosine 5′-diphosphate [ADP]) are consistent with normal platelet function.

TABLE 32–1 • Platelet function analysis (PFA—closure time) in bleeding disorders

Clinical Entity	Collagen/ Epinephrine PFA	Collagen/ADP PFA
No bleeding disorder	Normal	Normal
Aspirin therapy	Prolonged	Normal
von Willebrand disease	Prolonged	Prolonged
Glanzmann thrombasthenia	Prolonged	Prolonged

The PFA has obvious advantages over the template bleeding time. Not only is it more easily standardized and not subject to operator variability, but it also avoids the time-consuming bedside procedure of the template bleeding time, inasmuch as the test is performed on an anticoagulated sample of blood in the laboratory. The PFA-100 (Siemens) has been employed in the assessment of bleeding risk and transfusion therapy in cardiac surgery, platelet dysfunction in uremia, screening and follow-up for patients with vWD, and evaluating the efficacy of anti-platelet agents such as aspirin and clopidogrel. The PFA assay does have its limits; adhesion and aggregation within the PFA test are dependent upon the underlying platelet and red cell counts, such that significant anemia (hematocrit <20%) and/or thrombocytopenia (platelets <100,000/μL) may artifactually prolong closure times. Additionally, as with other assays of vWD, blood group O may correlate with prolonged closure times in normal individuals.

B. Complete Blood Count and Review of the Blood Film

A complete blood count (CBC) with examination of the blood film can also be helpful. The CBC can provide evidence of hematopoietic disease, especially a myeloproliferative disorder where high numbers of circulating platelets are associated with abnormal function, which can result in bleeding. Platelet morphology on the smear can help in diagnosing disorders such as Bernard-Soulier syndrome and α-granule deficiency (gray platelet syndrome).

C. Measurements of Platelet Activation/Aggregation

Direct optical measurements of platelet aggregation are possible with an aggregometer using either whole blood or purified platelet-rich plasma. **Whole blood aggregation** is available as a point-of-care (POC) test utilizing specific platelet agonists including arachidonic acid (for aspirin-related dysfunction), ADP (for clopidogrel), and thrombin-receptor activating peptide (TRAP, for GPIIb-IIIa inhibitors like abciximab). However, studies of whole blood aggregation have concentrated on monitoring the efficacy of anti-platelet therapy, for example, in patients with acute coronary syndromes, and there is little data, as yet, on patients with acute bleeding episodes due to platelet inhibition (by therapy) or intrinsic platelet dysfunction.

Platelet-rich plasma aggregation, although more time-consuming and cumbersome, has been used more than the whole blood POC devices to diagnose platelet dysfunction. The **aggregometer** provides a graphic display of the wave of platelet aggregation seen in response to physiologic agonists such as ADP, epinephrine, or collagen, as well as the agglutination response to ristocetin (Figure 32–2). Specific functional defects respond differently to these agonists. For example, patients with vWD specifically show decreased or absent agglutination only to ristocetin, whereas an intrinsic platelet disorder, such as storage pool disease, demonstrates poor responses to ADP, epinephrine, and collagen. By contrast, an acquired platelet defect due to aspirin would show no response to arachidonic acid and diminished aggregation to ADP and epinephrine.

D. Assays for von Willebrand Factor

Full evaluation of the patient with vWD requires an array of tests, including assays for factor VIII activity, vWF antigen, vWF activity, and vWF multimer pattern by agarose gel electrophoresis. In addition, because of the functional interaction of platelets and vWF, some diagnoses may require mixing various combinations of platelets and plasma from the patient and normal controls in order to pinpoint the adhesive lesion. Together with the patient's bleeding history, family history, and the PFA analysis, these assays will generally diagnose and classify vWD into one of several clinically important subtypes.

E. Research Assays

Several research assays have been used to identify platelet structural and functional abnormalities. **Flow cytometry** employs fluorescent tagged monoclonal antibodies that can accurately detect levels and conformational changes of key platelet activation/aggregation antigens, including GPIb, GPIIb/IIIa, P-selectin, and both fibrinogen and factor Va binding. Such assays are employed in research laboratories to diagnose rare congenital deficiencies of surface antigens. However, flow-cytometry-based assays that detect storage pool disease or platelet dysfunction, for example, following extracorporeal circulation, have proven difficult to standardize and interpret. Other research platforms have been utilized for detection of platelet-based bleeding disorders, for example, **electron microscopy** to demonstrate the absence of dense or α-granules. Platelet α-granule deficiency can also be confirmed by direct **measurement of platelet factor 4 and β-thromboglobulin by radioimmunoassay**. Similarly, thromboxane B_2, the end-product of thromboxane metabolism, can be measured to assess the platelet cyclooxygenase pathway (and platelet inhibition by aspirin or nonsteroidal anti-inflammatory drugs [NSAIDs]). In conjunction with direct measurements of **dense granule ADP and adenosine triphosphate (ATP)**, these latter assays may further differentiate storage pool deficiency from aspirin-induced platelet dysfunction.

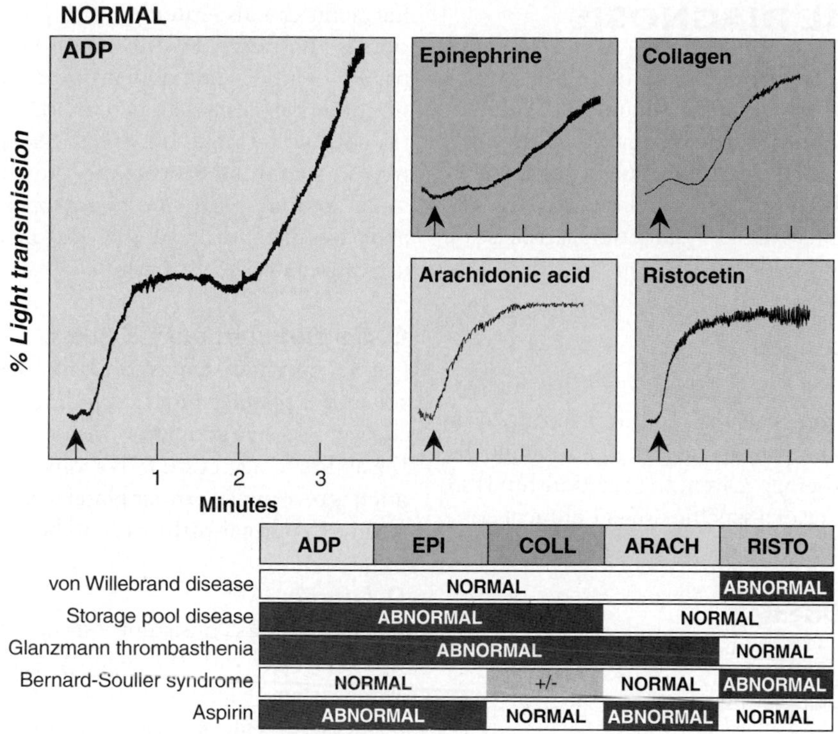

FIGURE 32–2. **Aggregometry studies in patients with congenital and acquired disorders of platelet function. Upper panels:** The normal pattern of aggregation to ADP, epinephrine, collagen, arachidonic acid, and ristocetin. **Lower panels:** von Willebrand disease can be identified because of an abnormal ristocetin aggregation pattern. This condition is distinctly different from patterns seen with storage pool disease, aspirin inhibition, and Glanzmann thrombasthenia, but may be difficult to distinguish from the pattern in Bernard-Soulier syndrome.

CASE HISTORY • *Part 2*

The platelet count, prothrombin time (PT), and partial thromboplastin time (PTT) are all normal, ruling out thrombocytopenia or a factor deficiency, but this is not surprising given the patient's age and lack of bleeding history or liver disease. Neither cholesterol-lowering agents nor beta-blockers are strong inhibitors of platelet function, but daily aspirin use can significantly inhibit platelet function through its blockade of cyclooxygenase-dependent activation. Furthermore, von Willebrand disease, a common inherited platelet functional defect, must be considered in any patient with uncontrolled bleeding after trauma or with surgery.

To look at these possibilities, a PFA screening test is ordered, the results of which are as follows:

PFA collagen/ADP closure time = 95 seconds (80–120 seconds)

PFA collagen/epinephrine closure time = 245 seconds (110–180 seconds)

In addition, a computed tomography (CT) scan of the head with contrast demonstrates a subdural hematoma. The neurosurgeon recommends immediate surgery, but because of the aspirin use and the PFA result, the neurosurgeon requests a consult for medical management of bleeding risk prior to the operation.

Questions

- Based on these results, does the patient have a coagulopathy?
- If so, does he require immediate treatment prior to surgery?

DIFFERENTIAL DIAGNOSIS

Diagnosis of a platelet abnormality requires a high level of suspicion and a lot of detective work. Acquired functional abnormalities, especially due to anti-platelet therapy, are clearly the most common abnormality; vWD leads the category of congenital disorders, in terms of both incidence and severity. Therefore, an initial evaluation into platelet dysfunction as a cause of bleeding should look for a disorder in these 2 areas.

Acquired Abnormalities of Platelet Function

Acquired platelet dysfunction occurs in 3 clinical settings—in association with hematopoietic disease, as part of a systemic illness, or as a result of drug therapy. Often, the relationship is so strong that the mere presence of a specific drug or clinical condition is enough to make the diagnosis.

A. Myeloproliferative Disease

Patients with myeloproliferative disorders (ie, polycythemia vera, primary myelofibrosis [previously termed myeloid metaplasia], essential thrombocythemia, and chronic myelogenous leukemia) frequently exhibit abnormal platelet function. Some of these patients have very high platelet counts and demonstrate either abnormal bleeding or a tendency for arterial or venous thrombosis, or even both. Although the height of the platelet count alone does not correlate with the bleeding or thrombotic tendency, thrombocytosis in excess of 1 million/μL is considered to be a risk factor. At the same time, increased platelet turnover, as measured by the reticulated platelet count, may correlate with thrombotic risk. In patients with polycythemia vera, expansion of the total blood volume and an increase in blood viscosity also contribute to thrombotic risk.

Other laboratory findings related to platelet function with myeloproliferative disorders can be quite variable. In the past, a prolonged bleeding time proved to be a poor predictor of abnormal bleeding. Perhaps the most consistent laboratory abnormalities in bleeding patients are defects in epinephrine-induced platelet aggregation and other abnormalities of dense and α-granule function; however, these findings in advance of bleeding or thrombosis have little predictive value. The demonstration of decreased vWF activity in myeloproliferative disease is an important finding since bleeding caused by an acquired form of vWD also may be observed in these disorders, secondary to increased clearance of higher-molecular-weight vWF multimers.

B. Dysproteinemia

Abnormal platelet function, including defects in adhesion, aggregation, and procoagulant activity, are observed in patients with dysproteinemias. Almost one-third of patients with Waldenström macroglobulinemia or IgA myeloma will have a demonstrable defect; IgG multiple myeloma patients are less commonly affected. The level (concentration) of the monoclonal (M)-protein spike appears to correlate with the abnormalities in platelet function. Normal fibrinogen breakdown fragments can also interfere with platelet function. This condition is illustrated by the functional defect that appears in patients with disseminated intravascular coagulation (DIC) and fibrin/fibrinogen breakdown. Fibrin fragments impair both fibrin polymerization and platelet aggregation. Of course, failure of platelet thrombus formation in the DIC patient is usually multifactorial, with thrombocytopenia, hypofibrinogenemia, and a loss of dense and α-granule function secondary to platelet activation all playing a role.

C. Cardiopulmonary Bypass

Cardiopulmonary bypass and, to a lesser degree, hemodialysis produce a platelet functional defect. During bypass, platelets show progressive activation with loss of α-granule contents, and the ability to aggregate in response to ADP declines. This situation is reversible without platelet transfusion; platelet function returns to normal within 12–36 hours after surgery.

D. Uremia

Uremic patients consistently show a defect in platelet function that correlates with the severity of the uremia and anemia. It appears that at least 1 uncleared metabolic product, **guanidinosuccinic acid**, acts as an inhibitor of platelet function by inducing endothelial cell nitric oxide (NO) release. Platelet adhesion, activation, and aggregation are abnormal, and thromboxane A_2 generation is decreased.

In patients with severe uremia, platelet dysfunction is corrected by hemodialysis. Abnormal platelet function may also be related to the severity of the patient's anemia, since bleeding can also be prevented with either transfusion or erythropoietin therapy. For acute bleeding episodes, desmopressin (DDAVP) therapy (0.3 μg/kg) can improve platelet function transiently. Infusion of conjugated estrogens (0.6 mg/kg/d) for 5 days will also correct platelet function; this improvement takes several days to appear and can last for up to 2 weeks. The mechanism of the conjugated estrogen effect appears to be the normalization of plasma levels of NO metabolites.

E. Liver Disease

In general, the most likely cause of hemorrhage in a patient with liver disease is a discrete defect, such as bleeding varices or a gastric/duodenal ulcer. If, however, the patient has widespread bleeding, including ecchymoses and oozing from intravenous sites, a coagulopathy should be considered. Patients with liver disease have a multifaceted defect in coagulation. Thrombocytopenia related to hypersplenism and a failed thrombopoietin response is common. Platelet dysfunction, secondary to high levels of circulating fibrin degradation products, further increases the bleeding tendency. In addition, reduced production of factor VII (principal cause of the prolonged PT in mild liver disease patients) and low-grade, chronic DIC with increased fibrinolysis can add to the coagulopathy. Severe liver disease, on the other hand, involves deficiency of all of the liver-synthesized factors and markedly reduced clearance of activated factors and fibrin fragments; management of the patient with liver disease must address each of these abnormalities (see Chapter 34).

F. Drug Inhibition

Several classes of drugs also affect platelet function (Table 32–2). **Aspirin and the nonsteroidal anti-inflammatory (NSAID)** drugs have a well-recognized impact on platelet function. Aspirin is a powerful inhibitor of platelet thromboxane A_2 synthesis through its irreversible inhibition of cyclooxygenase function. Patients on aspirin show a decrease in total platelet contents released after stimulation with ADP or epinephrine, the agonists used in aggregation testing; this result parallels the inhibition of thromboxane A_2–dependent second-wave aggregation to those agonists (see Figure 32–2). The aspirin effect on platelet function is reliably detected either by the complete absence of platelet aggregation to arachidonic acid or by the prolongation of the PFA closure time with collagen/epinephrine (together with a normal collagen/ADP closure time; see Table 32–1). By contrast, the collagen/ADP closure time is prolonged by treatment with clopidogrel (Plavix), whose active thienopyridine metabolite blocks the ADP ($P2Y_{12}$) receptor.

NSAID drugs (eg, indomethacin, ibuprofen, sulfinpyrazone) also inhibit platelet cyclooxygenase, but the effect is reversible and lasts only as long as the drug is in circulation. From the clinical viewpoint, these agents are weak inhibitors of platelet function and are usually not associated with severe clinical bleeding. However, they will contribute to bleeding when other aggravating factors, such as other anticoagulants, a GI disorder, or surgery, are present. Certain **foods and food additives** (vitamins C and E, omega-3 fatty acids, Chinese black tree fungus) can also reversibly inhibit platelet function (usually to only a mild degree) through the cyclooxygenase pathway.

The impact of **antibiotics** on platelet function can be a major contributor to hemorrhage in critically ill patients. The **penicillins**, including carbenicillin, penicillin G, ticarcillin, ampicillin, nafcillin, and to a lesser extent mezlocillin, interfere with both platelet adhesion and platelet activation/aggregation. These drugs bind to the platelet membrane and interfere with vWF binding and the response of platelets to agonists such as ADP and epinephrine. Significant clinical bleeding can occur in the critically ill patient receiving one of these antibiotics in very high doses. The presence of aggravating factors of the critical illness itself is important because abnormal bleeding is rarely seen when antibiotics are used in generally healthy patients. Platelet dysfunction has also been reported with selected **cephalosporins**, including moxalactam and cefotaxime. Most other antibiotics in this class do not produce a defect.

Volume expanders, such as the neutral polysaccharide dextran, can interfere with platelet aggregation and procoagulant activity when infused in large amounts. This result can be a significant disadvantage in the trauma or surgical setting when a dextran solution is being used for volume support. At the same time, dextran is used in the vascular surgery setting to prevent platelet thrombosis. Hydroxyethyl starch, also a popular volume expander, is less likely to interfere with platelet function, but will cause a detectable defect in von Willebrand function if given in doses in excess of 2 L of the 6% solution. This is generally manifest as continued postoperative mucosal bleeding associated with low levels of ristocetin cofactor activity; this interference can last for days to weeks if high doses of the volume expander have been given. Many other drugs have been reported to cause platelet dysfunction occasionally. This list includes several cardiovascular drugs, alcohol, and several of the oncologic drugs (see Table 32–2). The mechanisms involved have not been clearly defined.

TABLE 32–2 • Drugs that inhibit platelet function

Strong association
Aspirin (aspirin-containing compounds)
Clopidogel/ticlopidine
Abciximab (ReoPro)
Nonsteroidal anti-inflammatory drugs including naproxen, ibuprofen, indomethacin, phenylbutazone, piroxicam, sulfipyrazone
Penicillins—carbenicillin, penicillin G, ampicillin, ticarcillin, nafcillin, azlocillin, mezlocillin
Cephalosporins—moxalactam, cefotaxime
Nitrofurantoin
Volume expanders: dextran, hydroxyethyl starch
Heparin; fibrinolytic agents
Weak association
Oncologic drugs
BCNU, daunorubicin, mithramycin
Cardiovascular drugs
Beta-blockers, calcium-channel blockers, nitroglycerin, nitroprusside, quinidine
Alcohol

Congenital Disorders of Platelet Function

vWD is the most common inherited abnormality affecting platelet function. All other intrinsic platelet disorders, including Bernard-Soulier syndrome, Glanzmann thrombasthenia, dense and α-granule deficiencies, and disorders of secretory and procoagulant activities, are rare. These defects can be grouped according to the in vitro functional defect. **Bernard-Soulier syndrome** is a disorder of adhesion, whereas **Glanzmann thrombasthenia** is characterized by defective aggregation. The other defects are classified as disorders of granule secretion and platelet metabolism.

A. Bernard-Soulier Syndrome

Bernard-Soulier syndrome is an autosomal recessive defect in the expression of the GPIb-IX-V platelet membrane receptor. This defect effectively interferes with the platelet's ability to bind vWF and adhere at high shear rates to subendothelial connective tissue. It is characterized by abnormal ristocetin aggregation (see Figure 32–2). Although this finding is similar to vWD, the abnormal aggregation response is not corrected by the addition of normal vWF to patient platelets.

Clinically, patients with Bernard-Soulier syndrome present in childhood with epistaxis, mucocutaneous bleeding, and purpura, although the severity varies. The collagen/epinephrine closure time on the PFA is typically prolonged in the presence of a normal to slightly reduced platelet count. Platelets are large,

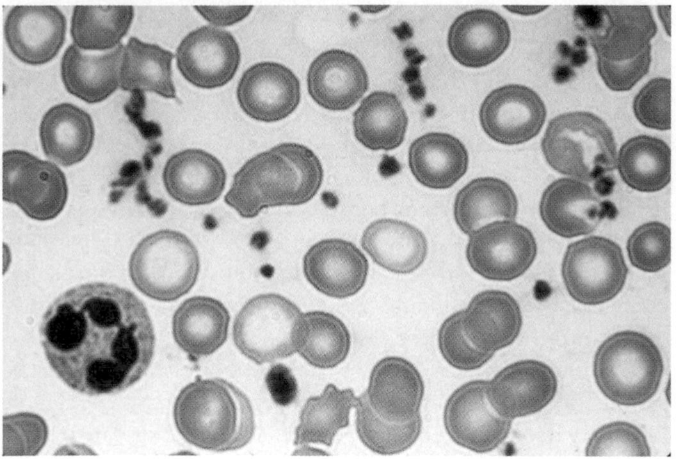

FIGURE 32–3. **Peripheral blood smear from a patient with congenital platelet dysfunction due to Bernard-Soulier syndrome.** This autosomal recessive defect in the GPIb-IX-V receptor interferes with platelet-vWF binding and is characterized by abnormal ristocetin aggregation. Children present with epistaxis and mucocutaneous bleeding. On smear, platelets are large, with some forms greater than 20 μm in diameter; the absence of Döhle bodies and the abnormal aggregation response to ristocetin distinguishes this from May-Hegglin anomaly.

with some forms greater than 20 μm in diameter (Figure 32–3). However, the absence of Döhle bodies and the abnormal aggregation response to ristocetin clearly distinguishes Bernard-Soulier syndrome from May-Hegglin anomaly (see Figure 31–4).

B. Glanzmann Thrombasthenia

Glanzmann thrombasthenia is a very rare, autosomal recessive, qualitative or quantitative deficiency in platelet surface GPIIb/IIIa, the receptor required for fibrinogen-dependent platelet-platelet interaction. This bleeding disorder usually presents in infancy with mucocutaneous bleeding. Platelet count and morphology are both normal. However, platelets fail to aggregate with any of the standard agonists—ADP, collagen, epinephrine, or thrombin in platelet aggregometry (see Figure 32–2). The response to ristocetin is normal or only slightly impaired. Glanzmann platelets prolong the collagen/epinephrine closure time on the PFA.

Abnormal platelet function with clinical bleeding is also seen in patients with inherited defects in dense and α-granules (storage pool deficiencies). **α-Granule deficiency (gray platelet syndrome)** imparts a relatively mild bleeding tendency. The presence of the abnormality is often first recognized from the gray appearance (lack of azurophilic granules) of the patient's platelets on the Wright stained blood film; the platelets are also larger than normal. Patients with dense granule deficiency present with a more severe bleeding tendency, often associated with a congenital developmental defect, such as Chédiak-Higashi, Hermansky-Pudlak, or Wiskott-Aldrich syndrome, or congenital hypoplastic thrombocytopenia with absent radii. The characteristic laboratory abnormality is a failure in the second wave of platelet aggregation (see Figure 32–2); Hermansky-Pudlak patients have been tested with the PFA, and as expected, the collagen/epinephrine closure time is increased. These results reflect the inability of the platelet to release granule contents critical to secondary platelet-platelet interaction.

Poor platelet function owing to **abnormal arachidonic acid metabolism** has also been described, independent of aspirin or NSAID use. This may involve a defect in thromboxane A_2 generation or in the aggregation response to thromboxane A_2 or other platelet agonists. Rare patients have a deficiency in cyclooxygenase similar to that acquired with aspirin therapy. Platelet morphology and granule content are normal in these conditions, and the bleeding tendency tends to be mild unless the patient is exposed to a platelet-inhibitory drug such as clopidogrel or aspirin.

Several conditions in patients with defects in the second wave of platelet aggregation but normal dense granule morphology are classified together as **"platelet secretion/release defects."** Many of these appear to have Ca^{2+} signaling abnormalities or defective protein kinase C activation despite a normal signaling process. Finally, a very uncommon **defect in platelet procoagulant activity**, specifically the ability of the platelet surface to translocate membrane phospholipids and to bind factor Va, can result in a bleeding diathesis. In this situation, routine studies of platelet function, including platelet aggregation studies, may be within normal limits. This condition is an exceedingly rare cause of platelet dysfunction and can only be diagnosed by studying the role of platelets in generating thrombin activity.

C. von Willebrand Disease

vWD is **inherited as either an autosomal dominant or an autosomal recessive trait** with an estimated prevalence ranging from 1 in 100 to 3 in 100,000 individuals. However, severe vWD with a history of life-threatening bleeding is seen in fewer than 5 individuals per million in Western countries. In the case of type 1 vWD, 40% of involved family members carry the allele for vWD but have normal or only slightly reduced vWF levels, both functional and antigenic. Even though autosomal dominant parents transmit the abnormal gene to 50% of their children, symptomatic disease is seen in only 30%–40% of offspring. Patients with a single recessive gene are typically asymptomatic but can show abnormal vWF antigen and activity levels. Patients with type 2 vWD are generally thought to have more severe bleeding symptoms; these patients have qualitative abnormalities that may be reflected in their pattern of vWF multimers. Rarely, acquired type 2 vWD, secondary to autoantibodies directed at vWF, can be seen in patients with lympho/myeloproliferative disorders or immunologic disease states. Double heterozygote offspring, born to parents who each carry one defective gene, usually a nonsense or frameshift mutation, exhibit severe disease (type 3 vWD).

As with the other platelet functional defects, symptomatic vWD patients usually present with mucocutaneous bleeding, especially epistaxis, easy bruising, menorrhagia, and gingival and GI bleeding. vWD patients with very low factor VIII levels can exhibit hemarthroses and deep tissue bleeds. From a population perspective, however, the number of patients with slight to moderate reductions in vWF activity far exceeds the number with overt clinical bleeding. This can lead to a gross over-diagnosis of vWD, if the vWF level is the sole criteria for diagnosis. Therefore, the diagnosis of "clinically important" vWD, especially type 1 vWD, should be limited to those patients who demonstrate abnormal bleeding, typically in association with an aggravating factor such as drugs, trauma, or surgery.

1. Diagnosis—Diagnosis of vWD requires a high level of clinical suspicion and the skilled use of the laboratory. When the patient is critically ill and receiving several drugs and blood products, it is virtually impossible to make an accurate diagnosis. If vWD is considered to be a contributing factor to such a patient's bleeding, it should be empirically treated and the laboratory evaluation postponed until the patient is clinically stable and has not received either blood products or drugs for several weeks.

2. Screening laboratory tests and other tests—Screening laboratory evaluation for vWD should include measurements of platelet count, PFA, PT, and PTT. Patients with very mild type 1 vWD will generally have near-normal studies and may even have normal PFA closure times. With moderate or more severe vWD, the PFA is uniformly prolonged for both the collagen/epinephrine and collagen/ADP values. Patients with severe deficiencies of vWF or defective binding of factor VIII to vWF will also have a prolonged PTT secondary to low levels of factor VIII in plasma. Specific assay of vWF antigen level and ristocetin cofactor activity (function) are then necessary to confirm the diagnosis.

Full evaluation for vWD requires measurements of factor VIII coagulant activity (VIII:C), von Willebrand factor antigen (vWF:Ag), vWF activity (ristocetin cofactor or collagen binding activity), and vWF multimer distribution by agarose gel electrophoresis. Factor VIII activity is measured against a curve derived from dilutions of normal plasma (defined as 100% activity) using either the PTT or a chromogenic assay. VWF:Ag can be quantitated by rapid immunologic-based methods such as the immuno-turbidimetric **Liatest** using latex microparticles coated with antibody to vWF. By contrast, **ristocetin cofactor (RcoF) activity** measures vWF function. RcoF activity can be quantitated by mixing patient plasma and normal platelets in the presence of ristocetin and then assaying for agglutination using either an aggregometer or other turbidimetric instrument. Activity is also reflected in a direct assay of vWF collagen-binding ability by enzyme-linked immunosorbent assay (ELISA). The vWF activity level will usually be proportional to the vWF:Ag level in type 1 vWD and will often be lower (by 50% or more) than the antigen with type 2 vWD disease, especially subtypes 2A and 2B. vWF multimer analysis is of diagnostic importance in the classification of type 2 vWD variants (Table 32–3). The classification of vWD is important in planning clinical management.

3. Type 1 disease—Type 1 vWD is the most common variant, accounting for 80% of observed cases. It represents a quantitative defect in plasma vWF levels. Clinical severity of the disease is quite variable, but generally correlates with the overall reduction in the plasma levels of vWF antigen and activity, as well as factor VIII activity. Most patients with type 1 vWD have concordant decreases in vWF antigen and activity, and the ratio of RcoF activity to vWF antigen is 1.0–2.0. Because vWF is the carrier protein for factor VIII in circulation, factor VIII levels will be reduced in proportion to the severity of type 1 disease, resulting in a prolongation of the PTT. Analysis of vWF multimers shows a mild to moderate, but otherwise balanced reduction in all multimer forms. In patients and families with histories of repeated and severe bleeding episodes, vWF:Ag and vWF activity are usually reduced to below 15%–20% of normal. These patients can be said to truly have highly penetrant, dominant type 1 vWD and should be treated aggressively for any bleeding episode and given prophylaxis for even minor surgical procedures; the etiology for severe type 1 vWD is thought to be abnormal intracellular secretion/transport.

At the same time, a moderately low vWF level (<50%), by itself, does not make the diagnosis. The majority of such individuals will not suffer from an increased bleeding tendency, and therefore should not be labeled as having vWD. Similarly, healthy blood group O patients normally demonstrate lower vWF levels than non–group O individuals, but do not have a bleeding diathesis and should not be automatically diagnosed as mild type 1 vWD.

TABLE 32–3 • Characteristics of von Willebrand disease subtypes

	Type 1	Type 2A	2B 2M	2N	Type 3
RCoF[a]	Decreased	Markedly decreased	Normal to slightly decreased	Normal	Absent
vWF:Ag	Decreased	Decreased	Normal to slightly decreased	Normal	Absent
Factor VIII	Decreased	Decreased	Normal to decreased	Markedly decreased	Absent
RIPA[b]	Slightly decreased	Decreased	Normal/increased	Slightly decreased	Absent
Multimeric analysis	Normal	Larger multimers absent	Larger multimers absent	Normal	Absent

[a]*Ristocetin cofactor activity = patient's vWF activity with control platelets.*
[b]*Ristocetin-induced platelet agglutination = patient's vWF activity with patient platelets.*

Type 1 vWD appears to result from a **defect in vWF release from the Weibel-Palade bodies of endothelial cells**; platelet and endothelial stores of vWF are normal in most patients. This is supported clinically by the observation that type 1 vWD patients demonstrate a release of vWF from endothelial cells with administration of desmopressin (DDAVP). Furthermore, vWF levels continue to behave as an acute phase reactant in type 1 vWD. Pregnancy, estrogen use, and inflammatory states can acutely increase vWF levels, even to the point of masking the diagnosis of mild type 1 vWD.

4. Type 2 disease—Type 2 vWD is characterized by a qualitative defect in plasma vWF. This can involve a reduction in the larger vWF multimers (types 2A and 2B vWD) or variable changes in vWF:Ag and factor VIII binding (types 2M and 2N vWD). The absence of the larger multimers results in a disproportionate decrease in the vWF activity (ristocetin cofactor activity) when compared with vWF:Ag. Factor VIII activity is less likely to be significantly reduced in types 2A, 2B, and 2M vWD, but is severely affected with type 2N disease.

Type 2A vWD patients have an absence of high- and intermediate-molecular-weight vWF multimers in plasma. This defect is considered to be caused by at least 2 mechanisms: (1) mutations in the vWF A2 domain that increase multimer sensitivity to proteolysis by the cleaving protease, ADAMTS13; and (2) abnormal assembly/secretion of the intracellular protein. This heterogeneity is reflected in the fact that some patients release larger multimers into circulation when stimulated by DDAVP, whereas others show little or no response. Type 2A patients have a moderately severe bleeding tendency.

Type 2B vWD patients have a gain-of-function mutation in vWF that results in increased affinity for platelet GPIb. The increased binding of vWF to platelets results in selective clearance and degradation of the larger multimers, resulting in a reduction in the plasma levels of high and intermediate vWF multimers, similar to type 2A vWD. The abnormal vWF molecule on the platelet surface may also interfere with adhesion, further promoting a bleeding diathesis. Because of the higher affinity of vWF for platelets, there is an abnormal increased agglutination of platelets at low concentrations of ristocetin on ristocetin-induced platelet agglutination (RIPA) that is not seen in type 1 or type 2A vWD. Clinically, excessive vWF-platelet binding can lead to platelet clearance and resultant thrombocytopenia. Pregnancy, inflammation, or DDAVP administration can, by increasing vWF release, actually worsen the thrombocytopenia. Despite the gain-of-function mutation leading to platelet-vWF binding and clearance, these patients do not present with thrombotic disease; instead, the lack of higher-molecular-weight multimers causes a bleeding tendency.

Platelet-type (pseudo-) vWD deserves special comment at this point because it presents with many of the characteristics of type 2B vWD. However, increased platelet binding (and clearance) of vWF multimers in platelet-type vWD is caused by a mutation in the platelet GPIb receptor, not vWF. This is an important distinction when it comes to therapy. Platelet-type vWD patients require platelet transfusions, and possibly vWF replacement as well, to correct the bleeding diathesis.

Type 2M vWD is characterized by a normal pattern of vWF multimers in plasma but a disproportionate decrease in vWF activity as compared with vWF:Ag levels. This is the result of mutations in the A1 domain (the GPIb binding site of vWF) that decrease its affinity for the platelet receptor. Many of these patients, though, will respond to DDAVP, whereas others require vWF replacement.

Type 2N vWD results from mutations in the factor VIII binding site of vWF, such that factor VIII is poorly bound and subject to increased clearance. Factor VIII activity levels are decreased, similar to a mild hemophilia A. Measurements of vWF activity and antigen are both normal, however, as is the analysis of vWF multimers. Type 2N disease should be considered in the differential whenever a female patient presents with a low factor VIII level, when female relatives of a "hemophiliac" male appear to be affected, or when the pattern of "hemophilia" inheritance is autosomal dominant.

5. Type 3 disease—Type 3 vWD is characterized by a virtual absence of both vWF:Ag and vWF activity and very low levels of factor VIII (1%–10% of normal). These patients experience severe bleeding with mucosal hemorrhage, hemarthroses, and muscle hematomas reminiscent of hemophilia. However, unlike classical hemophilia, tests of platelet-vWF–dependent bleeding are also abnormal. The genotype of type 3 disease is varied. Most mutations are specific to the family in which they were identified, and these mutations can include both nonsense and frameshift mutations. Patients may be complex heterozygotes with 2 distinct abnormal vWD mutations or homozygous for a single gene defect. In some cases, neither of the parents of a child with type 3 vWD will have a bleeding diathesis, suggesting an autosomal recessive pattern of inheritance. A subset of type 3 vWD patients may develop inhibitors to vWF after infusion therapy.

Finally, **acquired forms** of vWD have been described in association with myeloproliferative diseases (especially essential thrombocytosis), non-Hodgkin B-cell lymphomas, plasma cell dyscrasias, autoimmune disorders (systemic lupus erythematosis), hypothyroidism, solid tumors, inherited connective tissue diseases such as Ehlers-Danlos syndrome, and congenital or acquired cardiac defects (aortic stenosis). Low vWF antigen and disproportionately low vWF activity are seen in affected patients who had previously not exhibited any bleeding tendency. About one-third of reported cases are associated with a monoclonal gammopathy of unknown significance (MGUS). Most of these conditions reflect an increase in vWF clearance and a decrease in larger vWF multimers, leading to a type 2 vWD phenotype. This clearance of larger vWF multimers can occur via several mechanisms: (1) through autoantibody binding to vWF and subsequent antigen-antibody complex removal from the circulation, (2) secondary to increased adherence of vWF multimers to platelets or tumor cells, and (3) with increased shear from aortic stenosis leading to enhanced cleavage by ADAMTS13.

Less often, there is direct inhibition of vWF function secondary to a circulating inhibitor or a general depression in the levels of both vWF and factor VIII.

THERAPY AND CLINICAL COURSE

Abnormalities in platelet function are often first appreciated as a complication of an acute illness or surgery, and multiple aggravating factors may play a role in determining the severity of the bleeding tendency. Consequently, this is not a time when an accurate diagnosis is easily made. A minimal number of laboratory tests should be performed, and treatment should address as many potential contributing factors as possible. This list includes discontinuing drugs that inhibit platelet function, empirically replacing vWF or treating with DDAVP, and, according to the severity of the patient's bleeding, transfusing normal platelets. Although this approach lacks precision, it is effective. Both acquired and congenital disorders of platelet function can be acutely reversed in order to control severe clinical bleeding.

Long-term management of a platelet functional defect, by contrast, should be based on an accurate diagnosis. Patients with congenital defects should be counselled to avoid drugs that can aggravate the functional abnormality and cause bleeding. Obviously, aspirin and nonsteroidal analgesics are prime offenders in this regard; patients with vWD or Glanzmann thrombasthenia are similarly at greater risk for clinical bleeding with aspirin ingestion. These patients should also be educated regarding the nature of their abnormality and should carry identification or wear a medical alert bracelet. This information can be invaluable as a guide to appropriate transfusion therapy in an emergency situation.

As a general principle, the **nature of the functional abnormality** will guide the choice of therapy. For example, the patient with vWD who lacks normal amounts of vWF will respond to agents that increase plasma vWF levels. In this situation, the platelets will function normally once the vWF abnormality is corrected. In contrast, patients with congenital defects of platelet receptor expression, granule content, or platelet metabolism will generally require platelet transfusion. As for the acquired abnormalities of platelet function, the best approach to therapy lies somewhere in between. There is clinical evidence that patients with acquired defects secondary to drug ingestion, uremia, and liver disease will respond to DDAVP, vWF replacement, or both. These data suggest that an increase in plasma vWF levels may partially compensate for a platelet-based defect.

Platelet Transfusion

For the acutely bleeding patient with congenital or acquired platelet dysfunction, the most direct therapy to restore platelet function is to transfuse platelets. Platelet transfusions are generally reserved for serious bleeding in patients with Glanzmann thrombasthenia, since these patients may develop alloantibodies to platelets following transfusion; this phenomenon has not been reported in other congenital platelet disorders such as Hermansky-Pudlak and Bernard-Soulier syndrome.

Patients with significant bleeding who have taken an antiplatelet drug, such as aspirin, will benefit from platelet transfusion regardless of their baseline platelet count. In vitro studies with aspirin have suggested that addition of only 20% new platelets will adequately reverse the aggregation defect, translating into an in vivo practice of transfusing a single platelet pool for aspirin-related bleeding, for example, adding 50,000–60,000 normal platelets/μL for a platelet count of 250,000–300,000/μL. More recent studies suggest that a higher percentage of normal functioning platelets may be required to reverse significant drug-induced platelet dysfunction. Many patients with coronary or cerebrovascular disease are treated with the combination of 2 potent anti-platelet drugs, aspirin and clopidogrel, which respectively block the cyclooxygenase pathway of activation and the platelet ADP ($P2Y_{12}$) receptor. With both drugs blocking platelet function, transfusion of 2 platelet pools (40%–50% of circulating platelets) appears to be necessary to adequately reverse the aggregation defect for perioperative hemostasis. For patients with drug-induced platelet dysfunction but only mild bleeding, platelet transfusion can be avoided by using local measures or other alternatives such as DDAVP.

Desmopressin

Desmopressin (DDAVP) is a synthetic analogue of the antidiuretic hormone vasopressin, which when given parenterally (either intravenous or intranasal) stimulates a release of vWF from endothelial cell Weibel-Palade bodies to produce an immediate rise in plasma vWF and factor VIII activity and correct the bleeding defect in vWD. This rise in vWF activity enhances platelet function and shortens the PFA closure times. The PFA is efficacious in monitoring response to DDAVP in type 1 vWD. Because of its impact on factor VIII levels, DDAVP also has been used to manage patients with mild hemophilia A who are undergoing minor surgery. Platelet functional abnormalities caused by aspirin, GPIIb/IIIa inhibitors, uremia, or liver disease are only partially corrected by DDAVP-induced release of very large vWF multimers, but this may be sufficient when bleeding symptoms are mild. However, efficient dialysis and erythropoietin therapy in uremic patients have significantly decreased their bleeding tendency, obviating the need for chronic DDAVP therapy.

Success in treating vWD patients with DDAVP depends mostly on the disease type. Patients with type 1 vWD show the best response, with a shortening of the closure times and a rise in vWF and factor VIII levels. If a successful response is defined as at least a 2-fold increase in vWF and factor VIII levels over baseline, more than 80%–90% of type 1 vWD patients will respond to DDAVP, although children younger than 2 years do not respond as well as older children.

The value of treatment with DDAVP in type 2 vWD is less certain, but a trial of DDAVP in most vWD patients is warranted since individual responses vary widely. Although the overall response in all type 2 vWD is about 20%, only type 2N vWD patients who carry the *R854Q* mutation will reliably respond (but the half-life of increased factor VIII activity after DDAVP is about 3 hours); type 2A or 2M vWD patients generally show a poor, if any, response. Type 3 vWD patients will not respond to DDAVP because they lack endothelial stores of vWF. Both vWF and factor VIII must be provided together to reliably treat bleeding in type 3 vWD. Patients with acquired vWD may respond to DDAVP, so that a trial of this agent is worthwhile.

DDAVP, once considered to be **contraindicated** in patients with type 2B and platelet-type vWD, can be used with caution. With both defects, stimulation of vWF release can cause an increase in vWF-platelet binding and a worsening (or development) of thrombocytopenia. However, few patients have been reported to bleed or thrombose in association with thrombocytopenia after DDAVP, and vWF levels may be transiently increased. In most type 2B patients, both the abnormality in platelet function and the thrombocytopenia are related to the production of an abnormal vWF molecule, leading to depletion of larger multimers, while in platelet-type (pseudo-) vWD, the abnormal platelet GPIb is the underlying cause. Therefore, the reliably effective treatment for such patients includes vWF replacement and platelet transfusion, respectively.

DDAVP formulations include both **intravenous and intranasal preparations**. DDAVP is administered intravenously in a dose of 0.3 μg/kg. It should be diluted in 30–50 mL of saline and infused over 10–20 minutes to minimize side effects, especially the tachycardia and hypotension. Like its parent compound, DDAVP will cause headache, light-headedness, nausea, and facial flushing, especially when given rapidly. The drug also has an antidiuretic effect that can lead to hyponatremia, especially if the patient receives multiple treatments and/or large volumes of parenteral fluids.

A highly **concentrated nasal spray** can be used in children and be self-administered in women with type 1 vWD for the management of menorrhagia. It can also be effective in controlling the bleeding associated with tooth extractions or minor surgery in vWD and patients with mild hemophilia A. Intranasal DDAVP (Stimate nasal spray) contains a 150-μg dose of DDAVP (100 μL of a 1.5 mg/mL solution); 1 dose to each nostril (300 μg total) will usually increase the vWF level 3- to 5-fold in persons weighing more than 50 kg; for smaller individuals, a single 150-μg dose is recommended.

DDAVP therapy is most effective in treating mild bleeding episodes or in preventing bleeding during minor surgery. Patients with baseline vWF and factor VIII levels of greater than 10–20 IU/dL also seem to do the best, demonstrating 3- to 5-fold increases in vWF levels. However, even when the patient's response to DDAVP is suboptimal (less than 2-fold increase), bleeding may be partially contained or, in the case of surgical prophylaxis, both blood loss and the need for transfusion are reduced. A **drawback** of DDAVP is the short-lived nature of its effect. The improvement in the bleeding time and vWF level is limited to 12–24 hours. The response to repeated doses can decrease over time because of depletion of vWF multimers from Weibel-Palade bodies, although this is much less of an issue than that seen in patients with hemophilia A. In those situations where control of the vWD patient's bleeding tendency is critical, such as following major surgery, DDAVP alone will be inadequate, and additional vWF replacement is recommended.

TABLE 32–4 • Guidelines for VIII-vWF concentrate and cryoprecipitate dosing in von Willebrand disease

Patients with severe vWD (vWF-VIII <20%)	Major Bleed/Major Surgery	Less Severe Bleed/ Dental Procedure
VIII-vWF (Humate P)	40–75 IU/kg, once a day[a]	20–30 IU/kg, one time
Cryoprecipitate	30–40 U/kg[b]	20 U/kg
Milder, type I patients		
VIII-vWF	30–40 IU/kg, once a day[c]	10–20 IU/kg, one time
Cryoprecipitate	20–30 U/kg	10 U/kg

[a]*After loading doses on day one (see text), maintain plasma vWF:Ag level above 50% of normal until healing complete.*
[b]*Cryoprecipitate (the precipitate harvested from a unit of whole blood) should have at least 80 U of vWF and VIII activity in each single unit. Therefore, a 70-kg patient with type I vWD and a major bleed would receive 20–30 "units" of cryoprecipitate per day (70 kg × 30–40 U/kg = 20–30 "units" of cryoprecipitate). This is usually given as 10 U at any one time, 2–3 times a day.*
[c]*Maintain plasma vWF:Ag level above 30% of normal until healing complete.*

von Willebrand Factor

vWF replacement is considered the more reliable therapy for severe bleeding and surgical prophylaxis and can be achieved by the transfusion of cryoprecipitate or purified concentrates containing the vWF-VIII complex. Cryoprecipitate is a readily available and effective blood product that contains concentrated fibrinogen, vWF, and factors VIII and XIII. The **dosage schedule for cryoprecipitate** is highly empiric (Table 32–4). Patients with severe type 1 or 3 disease are managed like patients with severe hemophilia A, by increasing factor VIII levels to 50%–70% for a major surgical operation and 30%–50% for minor surgery or less severe bleeding.

Because there is still a small risk of transfusion-transmitted infection with cryoprecipitate, purified commercial preparations of factor **VIII/vWF concentrate** are preferred. Not all purified factor VIII preparations used in the treatment of hemophilia A are suitable for the treatment of vWD. The concentrate must contain the larger vWF multimers to be effective. One preparation rich in vWF and approved for use in the United States is Humate P. The recommended guidelines (expressed in IU of both vWF and factor VIII) for bleeding management and surgical prophylaxis are summarized in Table 32–4. The initial loading dose of Humate P in the treatment of severe vWD is 40–75 IU/kg intravenously (IV), followed by repeat doses of 30–60 IU/kg at 8- to 24-hour intervals. Therapy should be guided by the degree of bleeding and/or the extent of surgery needed, as well as the likely duration needed for wound healing. Once bleeding is controlled, a single daily dose of concentrate is usually sufficient, since the half-life of the VIII-vWF complex in vWD patients is 24–26 hours. Type 2N vWD patients may be diagnosed by the fact that a "hemophiliac" responds poorly to recombinant factor VIII but well to Humate P because it contains normal vWF.

Type 3 vWD patients, because of their very low levels of vWF, are capable of developing antibodies to vWF after transfusion of any replacement product. Once this has occurred, the patient is at risk for an anaphylactic reaction with re-exposure to vWF concentrate or cryoprecipitate. Moreover, subsequent vWF infusions are much less effective. **Antihistamines and steroids** can blunt the anaphylactoid reaction; **intravenous immunoglobulin** given at doses of 1 g/kg/d for 2–3 days may transiently decrease the level of the anti-vWF antibody. Platelet transfusions can be used to treat patients with type 3 vWD who have developed alloantibodies because platelets themselves contain very large vWF multimers (about 10%–15% of total body vWF). Patients with acquired vWD may respond to concentrate infusions, but the effect may be short-lived because of antibody-induced vWF clearance or inhibition. Treatment of the underlying disorder is most efficacious for long-term control of bleeding in acquired vWD.

Other Agents

Other drugs of value in managing patients with vWD include **estrogens** and the fibrinolytic inhibitor **ε aminocaproic acid (EACA)**. Estrogens appear to increase plasma vWF levels in most patients, but the response is highly variable. During pregnancy, patients with vWD (especially type 1) can even normalize their vWF and factor VIII levels. A positive direct effect on platelet function also has been observed in uremic patients given Premarin. The use of oral contraceptives containing synthetic estrogen and progesterone has been noted to decrease menorrhagia in women with all types of vWD, probably by its impact on the endometrium, rather than on vWF-VIII levels. EACA (Amicar) has been used in both hemophiliacs and patients with vWD to prevent bleeding associated with minor surgery, especially dental extractions. It is given to adults in a dose of 3–4 g every 4–6 hours either intravenously or as a mouth wash beginning just prior to the procedure and continuing for up to 5–7 days (see Chapter 33). By decreasing autoantibody-mediated vWF clearance, **intravenous IgG** has been shown to provide a sustained therapeutic effect on the bleeding tendency in patients with MGUS and acquired vWD.

CASE HISTORY • *Part 3*

The prolonged collagen/epinephrine PFA closure time, together with a normal collagen/ADP PFA closure time, is indicative of a platelet-based coagulopathy, namely inhibition by aspirin. However, concurrent type I von Willebrand disease, worsened by aspirin therapy, cannot be fully excluded given the setting of acute trauma causing an acute phase reaction. A diagnostic workup for vWD (including ristocetin cofactor activity, vWF antigen, and factor VIII activity) must wait until the patient is fully convalescent.

Since aspirin irreversibly blocks platelet cyclooxygenase function, and the patient has been taking aspirin on a daily basis, nearly all of the platelets in circulation can be assumed to be affected. Depending on the severity of the defect in platelet function, this can lead to excessive bleeding with surgery or trauma and may have exacerbated the subdural hemorrhage. Moreover, the aspirin effect on platelets is irreversible, so that platelet function will only normalize as new platelets, not exposed to aspirin, enter the circulation. This will obviously take several days—a delay which is not tolerable in this patient. The aspirin inhibition must be overcome by increasing the general procoagulant platelet function. This can, in part, be accomplished by increasing the von Willebrand factor concentration in blood through transfusion of vWF product or administration of DDAVP. However, complications of DDAVP include hyponatremia and hypertension, both of which may be problematic in a patient with subdural hematoma.

The best option in this patient is the transfusion of normal platelets. Complete replacement of circulating platelets is not necessary. For most surgeries or mild to moderate trauma, a single platelet transfusion will supply at least 10% of circulating platelets, which is enough to normalize the PFA and restore adequate platelet function. For neurosurgery, where bleeding into a closed space can be devastating, transfusion of 2 U of pooled platelets should provide extra insurance against postoperative bleeding. In this case, the patient received 2 U of pooled platelets prior to surgery; the hematoma was successfully evacuated, and there was no further bleeding.

POINTS TO REMEMBER

Patients with platelet dysfunction generally present with mucosal bleeding, petechiae, and purpuric lesions, similar to thrombocytopenia, but unlike the hemarthroses and muscle hematomas typical of hemophilia.

The diagnostic approach to platelet dysfunction, especially to von Willebrand disease (vWD), requires a high degree of suspicion and a careful history of any abnormal bleeding in the patient and family. Patients with vWD may give a history of recurrent epistaxis, menorrhagia, prolonged bleeding following a tooth extraction, or be completely asymptomatic until challenged with surgery/trauma or platelet inhibition by drugs.

Rare congenital causes of platelet dysfunction include loss of the critical platelet glycoprotein receptors, GPIIb/IIIa (Glanzmann thrombasthenia), and GPIb (Bernard-Soulier); defects in platelet granule function (Chédiak-Higashi, Hermansky-Pudlak), and abnormalities in granule content (gray platelet, storage pool disease).

For rapid laboratory diagnosis of platelet dysfunction or vWD, the in vivo bleeding time test has been replaced with an in vitro bleeding time—platelet function analysis (PFA). The PFA measures the time for platelet-vWF–dependent clotting (closure time) after exposure to collagen/epinephrine or collagen/ADP. The former is most sensitive to aspirin inhibition, while a prolongation of both times is seen with clopidogrel or vWD.

Besides specific anti-platelet therapy like aspirin, clopidogrel, and ReoPro, platelet function is inhibited by many different classes of drugs. The most common culprits in the hospital setting are high-dose penicillin antibiotics and volume expanders, while outpatients on NSAID therapy can present with GI bleeding partially due to platelet dysfunction.

Platelet aggregometry is useful in sorting out the causes of platelet dysfunction, but cannot be done in real time and, like the PFA, requires an adequate platelet count for valid interpretation. Responses to specific agonists like ristocetin and arachidonic acid assist in pinpointing the etiology of platelet-dependent bleeding.

Other conditions that inhibit platelet function include recent cardiopulmonary bypass surgery, uremia, disseminated intravascular coagulation, and severe liver disease. Hemodialysis, correction of anemia, and platelet transfusion are the mainstays for treating platelet-based bleeding due to these disorders.

When vWD is suspected, laboratory testing for vWF antigen and activity (ristocetin cofactor), and factor VIII activity serve to diagnose and characterize the subtype of disorder. The majority of vWD patients will have quantitative type I deficiency, which can range from relatively asymptomatic to severe bleeding with a strong family history.

In patients with marked platelet dysfunction secondary to aspirin therapy, platelet transfusion can be used to restore adequate hemostasis. Depending upon the degree of platelet dysfunction, transfusion of 1 or at the most 2 U of pooled platelets (or pheresis units) should be sufficient to guarantee normal hemostasis during surgery.

Treatment of vWD must be tailored to its characteristic type. DDAVP successfully induces endothelial cell release of vWF in most patients with type 1 vWD and in some patients with type 2, but is rarely, if ever, efficacious in type 3 disease. Transfusion of vWF concentrate (Humate P or with cryoprecipitate) will reliably raise vWF to hemostatic levels.

BIBLIOGRAPHY

Acquired and Congenital Platelet Function Defects

Bailey AL, Scantlebury DC, Smyth SS: Thrombosis and antithrombotic therapy in women. Arterioscler Thromb Vasc Biol 2009;29(3):284.

Coppinger JA et al: Moderation of the platelet releasate response by aspirin. Blood 2007;109:4786.

Harrison P: The role of PFA-100 testing in the investigation and management of haemostatic defects in children and adults. Br J Haematol 2005;130:3.

Nurden AT, Nurden P: Inherited disorders of platelets: an update. Curr Opin Hematol 2006;13(3):157.

Ruggeri ZM, Mendolicchio GL: Adhesion mechanisms in platelet function. Circ Res 2007;100(12):1673.

Shah U, Ma AD: Tests of platelet function. Curr Opin Hematol 2007;14(5):432.

Zimmerman GA, Weyrich AS: Signal-dependent protein synthesis by activated platelets: new pathways to altered phenotype and function. Arterioscler Thromb Vasc Biol 2008; 28(3):s17.

von Willebrand Disease

Cariappa R et al: Comparison of PFA-100 and bleeding time testing in pediatric patients with suspected hemorrhagic problems. J Pediatr Hematol Oncol 2003;25:474.

Das P, Carcao M, Hitzler J: DDAVP-induced hyponatremia in young children. J Pediatr Hematol Oncol 2005;27:330.

James A, Matchar DB, Myers ER: Testing for von Willebrand disease in women with menorrhagia: a systematic review. Obstet Gynecol 2004;104(2):381.

Kujovich JL: von Willebrand disease and pregnancy. J Thromb Haemost 2005;3:246.

Kumar S, Pruthi RK, Nichols WL: Acquired von Willebrand disease. Mayo Clinic Proceedings 2002;77(2):181.

Pruthi RK: A practical approach to genetic testing for von Willebrand disease. Mayo Clinic Proceedings 2006;81(5):679.

Rodeghiero F et al: The discriminant power of bleeding history for the diagnosis of type 1 von Willebrand disease: an international, multicenter study. J Thromb Haemost 225;3:2619.

Sadler JE: New concepts in von Willebrand disease. Annu Rev Med 2005;56:173.

Therapy

Amesse LS et al: Oral contraceptives and DDAVP nasal spray: patterns of use in managing vWD-associated menorrhagia: a single-institution study. J Pediatr Hematol Oncol 2005; 27:357.

Berntorp E, Petrini P: Long-term prophylaxis in von Willebrand disease. Blood Coagul Fibrinolysis 2005;16 Suppl 1:S23.

Federici AB: Management of von Willebrand disease with factor VIII/von Willebrand factor concentrates: results from current studies and surveys. Blood Coagul Fibrinolysis 2005;16 Suppl 1:S17.

Federici AB, Mannucci PM: Advances in the genetics and treatment of von Willebrand disease. Curr Opin Pediatr 2002;14(1):23.

Vilahur G et al: Normalization of platelet reactivity in clopidogrel-treated subjects. J Thromb Haemost 2007;5:82.

HEMOPHILIA AND OTHER INTRINSIC PATHWAY DEFECTS · 33

CASE HISTORY • *Part I*

A 66-year-old man presents with a complaint of bruising and severe pain in the right arm and forearm after painting a wall yesterday. His history is notable for osteoarthritis, hypertension, and non–insulin-dependent diabetes mellitus; he denies any prior history of bleeding. His medications include hydrochlorothiazide and glyburide (a sulfonylurea), and he took ibuprofen for the pain last night. Examination is notable for large ecchymoses over the right shoulder and triceps, with swelling and tenderness of the right forearm and wrist. The remainder of the examination is benign.

CBC: Hemoglobin/hematocrit - 13 g/dL/39%
MCV - 94 fL MCH - 29 pg MCHC - 28 g/dL
RDW-CV - 11% WBC count - 13,500/μL

Differential: Neutrophils - 45%
Lymphocytes - 50%
Monocytes - 5%
Platelet count - 300,000/μL
PT = 12.1 seconds (<14 seconds)
INR = 1.0 (<1.3)
PTT = 77 seconds (22–35 seconds)

Questions

- Do the CBC and screening coagulation test results point to a specific cause for a bleeding tendency in this patient?
- Are additional studies warranted for diagnosis or determining therapy?

Defects in the intrinsic pathway coagulation factors (factors VIII, IX, and XI) are associated with a significant bleeding tendency. The X-linked recessive disorders, hemophilia A (factor VIII) and B (factor IX), are the principal examples of this type of abnormality. A marked reduction in either factor VIII or IX is associated with spontaneous and excessive hemorrhage, especially hemarthroses and muscle hematomas. A deficiency in factor XI, which is encoded by a gene on chromosome 4, generally results in a less severe, but still significant, bleeding tendency.

THE NORMAL INTRINSIC PATHWAY

Laboratory-based interactions of the coagulation factors of the intrinsic pathway are illustrated in Figure 33–1. The initial activation stimulus is surface contact activation of **factor XII (Hageman factor)** to produce XIIa. This reaction is facilitated by the presence of high-molecular-weight kininogen (HMWK) and the conversion of prekallikrein (PK) to the active protease,

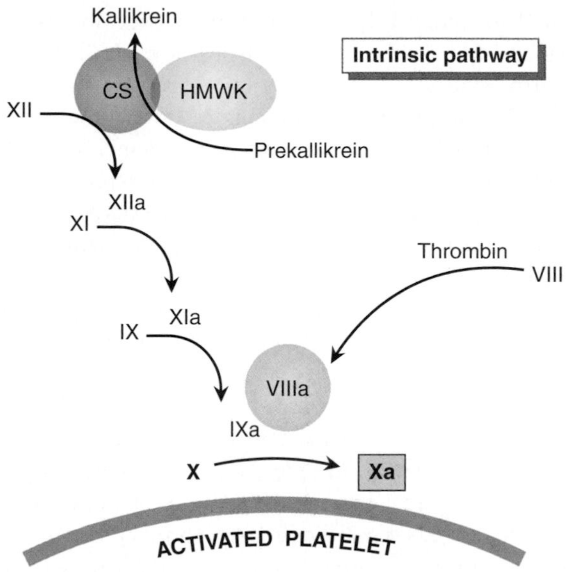

FIGURE 33–1. **The intrinsic pathway.** The intrinsic pathway as measured by the PTT assay is initiated by surface contact (CS) (often via kaolin) with facilitation by high-molecular-weight kininogen (HMWK) and its conversion of prekallikrein to the active protease, kallikrein. This stimulus converts factor XII to XIIa, which in turn activates factor XI to XIa and factor IX to IXa. Factor IXa then catalyzes cleavage of factor X. In normal physiologic clotting, the Xase reaction is facilitated by binding of factor X to the activated platelet surface together with the critical cofactor VIIIa, which is generated in response to thrombin. Once Xa appears, there is further thrombin generation and formation of clot.

kallikrein. Although this contact activation step is required in the measurement of the partial thromboplastin time (PTT), deficiencies of factor XII, HMWK, and PK are not associated with clinical bleeding.

Factor XIIa in the laboratory PTT activates factor XI to XIa, which in turn activates **factor IX (Christmas factor).** Factor IXa then catalyzes the cleavage of factor X to Xa to begin the reaction of the common pathway of coagulation. The reaction between factors IXa and X is facilitated by binding, in the presence of calcium, to phospholipid; in the PTT, phospholipid is included in the proprietary activating reagent. In normal physiology, the phospholipid surface is supplied by platelets, especially when they are activated. The conversion of X to Xa by IXa also requires activated factor VIII as a cofactor to achieve a maximum reaction rate.

Factor IX is a single-chain, vitamin K–dependent glycoprotein produced in the liver. Its activation by factor XIa involves a cleavage of 2 successive internal peptide bonds to form a 2-chain serine protease. Factor VIII is synthesized by the liver and also by megakaryocytes and reticuloendothelial tissues throughout the body. The small factor VIII protein circulates bound to von Willebrand factor (vWF), a much larger carrier protein. This relationship is extremely important. When the vWF level is reduced in patients with von Willebrand disease (see Chapter 32), unbound factor VIII is more rapidly cleared from plasma, effectively reducing the activity level. In order to participate as a cofactor in the activation of factor X, factor VIII must first be cleaved by thrombin to form factor VIIIa.

CLINICAL FEATURES

A severe deficiency of either factor VIII or IX results in a major bleeding disorder, clinically known as **hemophilia A (VIII deficiency)** or **hemophilia B (IX deficiency)**. Even though hemophilia is a relatively rare disorder (1 per 5,000 male births for hemophilia A and 1 per 30,000 male births for hemophilia B), descriptions of hemophilia as a sex-linked familial bleeding disorder can be traced back to biblical times. In part, this reflects the fact that the severe hemophiliac patient experiences major bleeds that start soon after birth and recur at frequent intervals during childhood. Moreover, once the hemophilia mutation appears in a family, it can be sustained through successive generations with little variation in expression. At the same time, hemophilia can present as a new spontaneous mutation, usually in the maternal gamete, in approximately one-third of cases.

Hemophilia A

The molecular basis of hemophilia A is defined. The factor VIII gene is a very large, 186-kb gene on the X chromosome. Almost half of the patients with hemophilia A exhibit an inversion of a major portion of the VIII gene (intron 22) with a resultant failure in factor VIII production. The remainder show various point mutations, insertions, and deletions that may involve as little as 1 base pair to the entire gene. The most severe hemophiliacs generally have an inversion or a deletion of major portions of the X chromosome genome, resulting in very low levels of factor VIII antigen and activity, usually less than 1% of normal activity. Missense mutations also can be associated with severe disease. Other mutations, including stop codon and point mutations and minor deletions, generally result in milder disease with factor VIII levels greater than 1%. In some patients, a functionally abnormal protein is produced, which can be demonstrated by showing a discrepancy between the immunologic measurement of factor VIII antigen (protein level is normal) and the coagulation assay of factor VIII activity (low activity).

As a rule of thumb, the **clinical severity** of hemophilia A is best **correlated with the factor VIII activity level.** The range of factor VIII activity is between 50% and 150% in normal individuals, with 100% activity defined by the level in pooled normal plasma. Severe hemophiliacs have factor VIII activity levels less than 1% of normal (<1.0 IU/mL) and are usually diagnosed during childhood because of frequent, spontaneous hemorrhages into joints, muscles, and vital organs. They require frequent treatment with factor VIII replacement and even then are at risk of developing a progressive, deforming arthropathy.

Even a level of detectable factor VIII activity of 1%–5% of normal is enough to reduce the severity of the disease. These patients are still at increased risk of hemorrhage with surgery or trauma, but have much less difficulty with spontaneous hemarthroses or hematomas. Patients with factor levels 6%–30%

are only mildly affected and may go undiagnosed well into adult life. They are at risk, however, for excessive bleeding with a major surgical procedure.

Female carriers of hemophilia A can also be at risk of bleeding, especially with surgery. Women who are not carriers for hemophilia A have a median factor level of 102%, with a range from 45% to greater than 300%; female carriers have a much lower median at 60% and levels ranging from 5% to greater than 200%. Extremely low factor VIII activity is explained by nonrandom lyonization of the X chromosome; indeed 10% of female carriers have factor VIII activity levels of less than 30%. Female carriers with levels less than 60% have increased bleeding risk in association with wounds; ear, nose, and throat (ENT) and dental procedures; and major surgery. They also have a significantly greater frequency of menorrhagia. Thus, women with menorrhagia should be evaluated for carrier status (see Clinical Genetic Testing section below) if the factor VIII activity is less than 60%, and a trial of therapy directed at mild hemophilia A is warranted.

An inherited **combined deficiency of factors V and VIII,** due in most cases to a single mutation on the long arm of chromosome 18, is associated with a moderate bleeding defect. Factor V and VIII levels are 5%–30% of normal. The gene mutation appears to result in a defect in the transport of V and VIII from the endoplasmic reticulum through the Golgi complex.

Hemophilia B

Hemophilia B patients have a similar clinical spectrum of disease. Factor IX levels of less than 1% are associated with severe bleeding, whereas more moderate disease is seen in patients with levels of 1%–5%. Patients with factor IX levels of 5%–40% generally have very mild disease. This situation reflects the need for both factor VIII and IX in the critical Xase activity of the intrinsic pathway. Hemophilia B can result from several genetic mutations including deletions, point mutations, and frameshift defects involving the factor IX gene on the long arm of the X chromosome. Most patients show an absence of factor IX activity because of a functionally abnormal protein; less commonly there is absence of both factor IX antigen and activity. One rare mutation (FIX Leyden) produces a hemophilia B picture in children that resolves at puberty as factor IX production increases.

Hemophilia in General

The most characteristic clinical manifestation of the hemophilias is **bleeding into large joints of upper and lower extremities.** This condition usually begins once the affected child reaches the toddler stage and increases in frequency as the child becomes more active. Often, 1 or 2 joints become the principal targets of repeated hemarthroses. With time, this situation can result in a chronic synovitis, destruction of cartilage and bone, and a progressive flexion contracture at the **target joint**. Bleeding into muscle (iliopsoas, gastrocnemius, and flexor muscles of the arm) or soft tissues with the formation of large spreading hematomas is also common. Damage to muscle results in further muscle atrophy and contractures. Wound healing is also abnormal in hemophilia, demonstrating excessive persistent angiogenesis and increased iron deposition, similar to hemophilic arthropathy.

Other less common bleeding manifestations include hematuria, intracranial hemorrhage, and mucous membrane bleeding, and prolonged bleeding following minor trauma or surgery. Milder hemophiliacs (>5% factor VIII or IX activity) may not be detected until surgery is performed or the patient has a dental extraction. Usually, the procedure is completed without evidence of unusual bleeding because of normal primary (platelet-based) hemostasis. However, within a few hours, the surgical wound or tooth socket begins to ooze, wound healing is disrupted, and blood seeps into surrounding tissues. Hematoma formation in the pharyngeal and retropharyngeal areas can threaten airway patency and present a medical emergency.

Large subperiosteal or muscle bleeds can on occasion lead to the formation of a **hemophilic pseudotumor**. These are cyst-like structures containing serosanguinous or dark brown viscous material bound to a fibrous membrane. Over time, pseudotumors expand and impinge on adjacent structures. Those that arise from a subperiosteal bleed, usually involving the pelvis or femurs, can eventually erode adjacent bone to form large cystic lesions.

Acquired Factor VIII or IX Inhibitors

Hemophilia A patients are at significant risk for developing circulating inhibitors (alloantibodies) to factor VIII, usually within the first 20–30 exposures to replacement therapy. The overall incidence of inhibitors is about 25%, with the majority of these being high-titer antibodies. Severe mutations (inversions, large sequence deletions, and nonsense mutations) that lead to a complete failure of production or the release of a severely truncated factor VIII protein are associated with the highest incidence of acquired inhibitors, 30%–40% overall and 55% in patients with inversion. Hemophilia B patients are less likely to develop an inhibitor to factor IX; only 3%–5% of patients will become affected during their lifetime.

Historically, up to 20% of all children with hemophilia A receiving fresh frozen plasma (FFP) and cryoprecipitate developed an inhibitor by age 10 years. Unfortunately, this problem has not been solved by the arrival of the high-purity concentrates and recombinant factor VIII. The development of inhibitors is still a major issue, and there is no difference in inhibitor rates (and no benefit in switching) between patients receiving plasma-based and recombinant products. It is possible (but not yet confirmed) that some plasma-derived VIII products may have a lower inhibitor risk in previously untreated severe hemophilia A. In general, factor VIII inhibitor patients fall equally into one of 2 groups according to the level of inhibitor. **High responders** demonstrate a marked inhibitor response after any factor infusion, reaching levels that cannot be neutralized by high-dose replacement therapy. The response is typical of induction of an alloantibody, and the patient is constantly at risk for an anamnestic response when re-exposed to factor antigen. In contrast, **low responders** develop and maintain relatively low levels of inhibitor that are constant despite repeated exposure to factor VIII replacement. The vWF content of the plasma-derived products does not appear to influence inhibitor development.

The risk of a hemophiliac, especially those with high-risk mutations, developing a factor VIII inhibitor is related to early and intensive therapy, particularly if infusions are related to surgery or very high post-infusion peak levels. Therapy within the first month of life is a clear risk factor, but this category also generally includes high treatment intensity (consecutive days of treatment with minimal intervals between infusion). By contrast, early and regular prophylaxis is not associated with an increased inhibitor risk. Thus, it is important to attempt to delay intensive therapy as long as possible, circumstances permitting, in children with high-risk mutations and/or a family history of hemophilia inhibitors. The tumor necrosis factor α *308A/A* genotype may also be used as a marker for increased inhibitor risk.

A **severe hemophilia-like syndrome** can occur in genetically normal individuals secondary to the appearance of an acquired autoantibody to either factor VIII or, very rarely, to factor IX. These antibodies are in effect circulating anticoagulants. They bind to factor VIII at the A2 and/or C2 domains of the protein and result in a loss of coagulant activity. Inactivation of factor VIII is rapid and non-linear (second-order kinetics), such that the laboratory assay may falsely detect some residual activity. These patients are usually middle-aged or older (median age 60–67) with no personal or family history of abnormal bleeding; men and women are equally affected. They present with a sudden onset of severe, spontaneous purpura or soft tissue hemorrhage involving skin, mucous membranes (gastrointestinal [GI] or hematuria), muscles, central nervous system (CNS), and vital organs. As a rule, hemarthroses are less common as compared to the congenital hemophilias. Bleeding into the tongue and retropharynx can threaten the airway, whereas severe muscle bleeding can be highly destructive.

Inhibitor development can coincide with drug therapy, especially penicillin and related antibiotics. Even though the inhibitor is an autoantibody against factor VIII or IX, there is only occasionally (5%–10%) other evidence of autoimmune disease. A similar percentage of these patients will demonstrate a lymphoproliferative disorder such as chronic lymphocytic leukemia or non-Hodgkin lymphoma, but two-thirds of patients with spontaneous inhibitors have no underlying causative condition. About 7% of patients develop their inhibitor in the peripartum period.

Viral Infections in the Hemophiliac

Viral hepatitis and human immunodeficiency virus (HIV) infection progressing to AIDS in hemophiliacs resulted from repeated exposure to virally contaminated clotting factor concentrates. It is estimated that 80% or more of severe hemophiliacs over age 10 years were infected with HIV, hepatitis B virus (HBV), or hepatitis C virus (HCV) during the early 1980s. With the advent of highly purified factor VIII products, younger patients are now at far lower, even negligible risk. The use of second-generation recombinant products, which eliminate exposure to human or animal source protein, also lowers the risk of both virus and nonviral pathogens, such as Creutzfeldt-Jakob disease. Coinfection with HIV and HCV promotes viral replication and progression of the patient's liver disease. The presence of HIV increases the risk of liver failure in HCV-infected hemophiliacs; end-stage liver disease occurred in 12% of patients with HIV and 35% of HIV-positive, HCV-infected hemophiliacs. There is also a higher incidence of hepatocellular carcinoma in the latter group.

HIV transmission to sexual partners is a major concern. Safe sex practices are essential and, if an HIV-positive hemophiliac chooses to have children, the couple should be counseled regarding adoption or the use of sperm from a healthy donor. Even so, up to 15% of female sexual partners of HIV-positive hemophiliacs will become infected. Once this occurs, there is a significant risk of transmission to the newborn.

Factor XI Deficiency

The only other intrinsic pathway defect associated with a bleeding tendency is **factor XI deficiency (Rosenthal disease).** It is inherited as an autosomal recessive trait, and therefore affects males and females equally. It is much more rare than either hemophilia A or B, but does affect up to 5% of Jews of Ashkenazi descent from Eastern Europe. Generally, the bleeding tendency, if present at all, is quite mild and may only be apparent following a surgical procedure. Hematomas and hemarthroses are very unusual, even in those patients with factor XI levels of less than 5%. However, patients homozygous for the type II mutation (*Glu117Stop*) have very low levels of factor XI and can develop a factor XI inhibitor when exposed to plasma therapy.

Laboratory Studies

A. Partial Thromboplastin Time and Prothrombin Time

Severe hemophilia A or B patients present with bleeding and a prolonged PTT. With milder disease, the PTT may be only a few seconds longer than normal. Since the tissue factor (TF)-VIIa–dependent (extrinsic) pathway of laboratory clotting is intact, the prothrombin time (PT) is normal. Thus, a **prolonged PTT together with a normal PT** should focus attention on an abnormality of the intrinsic pathway, that is, a deficiency of factor VIII, IX, or XI.

B. Tests for Factor Deficiencies

As a part of the initial workup, it is also important to distinguish a factor deficiency from the presence of an inhibitor. This process is routinely done by performing a 1:1 mix of patient plasma and normal plasma to determine whether the prolonged PTT shortens. The mixing study of a patient with classic hemophilia A with a deficiency in factor VIII activity but no circulating VIII inhibitor will usually show a shortening of the PTT to within 4 seconds or less of the normal PTT control or PTT reference range. In contrast, a patient with a factor VIII inhibitor will not correct the PTT to that extent, if at all. It is also important to quantitate the factor VIII activity level and, using a modification of the PTT called the **Bethesda assay method,** measure the inhibitor titer (units of inhibitor/mL of plasma). One Bethesda unit is the amount of antibody that inactivates 50% of factor VIII activity in normal plasma. Patients who develop spontaneous factor VIII inhibitors can be a diagnostic challenge, not only because the inhibitor titer may underestimate antibody potency, but also because the occasionally weak antibody may require up to 60 minutes for binding. Therefore, all mixing studies should routinely incorporate both an immediate and a 60-minute clotting time for antibody detection. It is also essential that **nonspecific inhibitors of the PTT, heparin and lupus anticoagulants,** be quickly excluded. This can be accomplished in the laboratory by demonstrating correction of the PTT with polybrene, protamine, or heparinase (heparin) or with excess phospholipid (lupus anticoagulants).

Full characterization of factor VIII or IX deficiency requires both an **immunologic measurement of the level of factor antigen** (VIII:Ag) and an **assay of coagulant activity** (VIII:C), but in most clinical labs, only coagulant activity is measured. The measurement of the activity level as a percent of normal provides a guide to the severity of the patient's illness. In the evaluation of the patient with less severe hemophilia A, a measurement of vWF antigen and activity is important to distinguish classic hemophilia from von Willebrand disease (vWD) (see Chapter 32). Type 1 and type 2N vWD patients demonstrate factor VIII levels between 10% and 50% of normal. Type 2N vWD should be considered whenever a female shows factor VIII levels below 50% or the pattern of inheritance is unusual, or both. For factor XI deficiency, demonstration of low XI activity is sufficient; inhibitor assays with XI deficiency are identical to those performed for hemophilia. It is important to note that false-positive tests for low XI activity with evidence of a mild inhibitor can occur as an artifact of a lupus anticoagulant; the latter will be evident by the prolonged PTT correction with phospholipid.

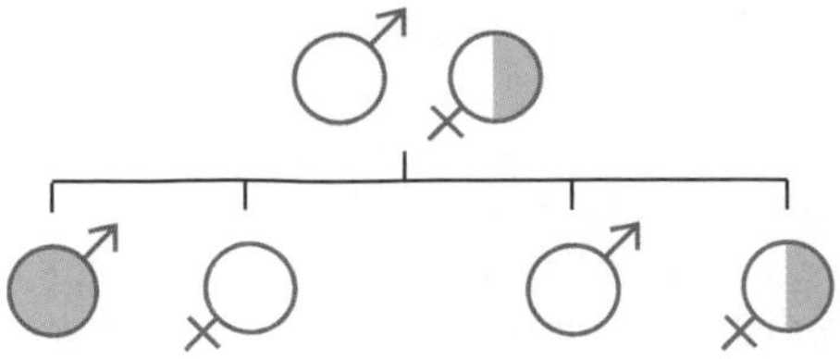

FIGURE 33–2. **The sex-linked inheritance pattern of hemophilia.** Children of a female hemophilia A or B carrier will have a 50-50 chance of inheriting the abnormal gene. The male children who inherit the abnormal X chromosome will have clinical disease; the female children who inherit the abnormal X chromosome will be carriers, most likely asymptomatic.

C. Tests to Detect Carriers of Hemophilia A or B

Accurate detection of carriers of hemophilia A or B in a family is required for genetic counseling and prenatal diagnosis. A detailed family history is essential. All of the female children of a father with hemophilia will be obligate carriers. The same is true for the mother of more than 1 hemophiliac son. These individuals do not need to be tested for carrier status. On the other hand, as illustrated in Figure 33–2, sisters of a patient with hemophilia have a 50-50 chance of carrying the abnormal gene. Carrier status for hemophilia A may be identified by **measuring the ratio of factor VIII activity to vWF antigen;** a 1:1 stoichiometry normally exists between these. Because of the random (lyonization) inactivation of the X chromosome, female carriers may express from 1%–100% factor VIII activity, whereas the vWF antigen level is unaffected. Thus, a factor VIII/vWF ratio of less than 1 can identify more than 90% of hemophilia A carriers. Identification of hemophilia B carriers is generally based on the detection of abnormally low factor IX activity or by DNA analysis.

CASE HISTORY • *Part 2*

The patient's platelet count is normal, ruling out thrombocytopenia, and a single dose of ibuprofen would not be expected to result in a severe tissue hemorrhage, even with trauma. The PTT is prolonged, suggesting an abnormality of the "intrinsic" coagulation factors XI, IX, or VIII. Since this patient has no history of hemophilia A or B, a "mixing study" using a 1:1 dilution of patient plasma with pooled normal plasma to exclude an inhibitor is in order. A platelet function assay for von Willebrand disease is also indicated. The results in this patient are as follows:

Inhibitor mixing assay - PTT (@ time 0) = 34 seconds (control = 32 seconds)
PTT (@ 60 minutes) = 56 seconds (control = 34 seconds)
Platelet function assay - PFA collagen/ADP closure time = 95 seconds (80–120 seconds); PFA collagen/epinephrine closure time = 145 seconds (110–180 seconds)

At the same time, a computed tomography (CT) scan of the right shoulder and arm demonstrates a large hematoma within and surrounding the muscles of the upper arm and extending from the axilla through the brachial plexus and into the forearm. The vascular surgeon recommends immediate surgery to relieve the compartment syndrome, but because of the coagulation results, the surgeon requests a consult for management of the coagulopathy.

Questions

- Based on these results, what is the most likely cause of the coagulopathy and how can this be confirmed?
- Does the patient require treatment prior to surgery and, if so, what treatment?

D. Clinical Genetic Testing

Clinical genetic testing is becoming more available. **A DNA test for the intron 22 inversion,** which is found in 40%–50% of severe factor VIII hemophiliacs, is now offered commercially. This test should only be performed in patients who have factor VIII activities of less than 1% or to detect carriers in families with severe hemophilia A. Alternative DNA screening methods (eg, Southern blot, sequencing after polymerase chain reaction [PCR] amplification) are required to detect carriers in families with moderate or mild disease or intron 22–negative disease, in whom point mutations or deletions are likely. In the occasional patient where a point mutation cannot be identified, potential female carriers can still be identified by linkage analysis, that is, demonstration of gene sequence differences between the subject's 2 X chromosomes. The same is true for factor IX deficiency diagnosis. **Direct DNA testing** or linkage analysis performed on chorionic villus biopsy material can then be used for prenatal diagnosis. This will not, of course, identify a proband with a new mutation, which is true for up to one-third of children born with hemophilia A or B.

THERAPY AND CLINICAL COURSE

Appropriate treatment obviously depends on knowing whether the patient has hemophilia A or B, or XI deficiency and the severity of the factor deficiency. It is also of great value to know the details of the patient's past clinical course. This knowledge not only provides another measure of disease severity and the response to therapy, but also produces a wealth of information as to the patient's and family's understanding of the illness and its management.

General Principles

When a hemophiliac A or B, or XI-deficient family is identified, every attempt should be made to develop an ongoing relationship with a regional hemophilia center, where teams of experienced nurses, social workers, physical therapists, dentists, genetic counselors, and orthopedic surgeons under the leadership of pediatric and adult hematologists provide a comprehensive approach to the medical and social needs of the patient and their family. Most centers offer a semiannual clinic visit for the patient to meet with the comprehensive care team to review their disease and for screening for evidence of transfusion-transmitted viral infections such as HIV, HBV, and HCV, and for the appearance of a factor inhibitor. A comprehensive center can also assist the primary care physician in the day-to-day management of a hemophilia patient and provide up-to-date information on available therapeutic products.

Guidelines for Bleeding Management

The overriding principle of good management of a hemophilia or factor XI–deficient bleed is **rapid and effective factor replacement**. With the exception of minor lacerations, which can be controlled locally, factor should be given for any episode of bleeding, regardless of location. Factor should also be given prior to any procedure, including routine intramuscular injections, such as a tetanus shot. The increased safety provided by purified and recombinant factor preparations also has made long-term prophylaxis in hemophilia feasible. **Prophylactic therapy**, which in the past was reserved for situations of anticipated bleeding, including surgery, invasive procedures, and high-risk physical activities, is now being used to convert the phenotype of patients with severe hemophilia to more moderate disease. Administration of recombinant factor VIII, 20–40 U/kg 3 times weekly, or in the case of hemophilia B, 25–40 U/kg twice a week, will increase basal factor levels to 1% or greater, enough to prevent spontaneous hemarthroses.

The adult hemophiliac patient is usually very sensitive to the **onset of a bleed**. Often there is an aura of mild discomfort localized to the muscle or target joint that becomes increasingly painful over the next hour. This stage is followed by progressive swelling, constant severe pain, and limitation of motion of the muscle or joint. However, the severity of the bleed can be significantly reduced if factor treatment is begun immediately. To prevent tissue damage, any bleed into a muscle or joint must be stopped as soon as possible. If bleeding is not stopped, the structure of the muscle will be disrupted, resulting in severe scarring and loss of function. Recurrent hemarthroses lead to destruction of cartilage and bone, synovial proliferation, and with time, a loss of joint function and crippling deformity. Therefore, as soon as a bleeding episode is suspected, the best management is **self-infusion of factor.** This will minimize the extent of the bleed and will also reduce the amount of factor needed for treatment (Tables 33–1 and 33–2). If a hemarthrosis goes untreated for several hours or a large muscle hematoma forms, the initial dose of factor must be increased significantly and replacement maintained for several days or even longer, followed by extensive rehabilitation.

A. Central Nervous System Bleeding After Head Trauma

Central nervous system bleeding following head trauma is another situation where treatment must begin immediately. The home-treatment patient should administer sufficient factor to increase the level to 100% of normal as soon as possible after an injury to the head or face. Patients with hemophilia presenting to the emergency room with head trauma should be treated with factor immediately, even if there are no clear signs of bleeding and certainly before proceeding with the diagnostic workup. This strategy will prevent a fatal bleeding episode during the time required for history, physical examination, and CT/magnetic resonance imaging (MRI) scanning. Furthermore, no attempt should be made to perform a lumbar puncture without prior treatment with factor. Tables 33–1 and 33–2 summarize the dosage recommendations for replacement therapy.

B. Internal Bleeding of the Chest and Abdomen

Bleeding internally in the chest or abdomen can be difficult to diagnose. In the young child, the only indication of a bleed into a large muscle group such as the iliopsoas may be vague

TABLE 33–1 • Factor VIII replacement therapy

	Initial Dose (U/kg)	Maintenance (U/kg)
Hemarthrosis	10–20	10–20 q 12 h
Muscle hematoma	20–30	20 q 12 h
Mouth bleeds (if tongue laceration; postdental procedure)	20–30	20 q 12 h Add antifibrinolytics[a]
Major surgery/tissue damage (eg, major trauma; possible intracranial bleed; potential airway obstruction; severe abdominal pain; GI bleeding)	50	20–30 q 8 h
Dental prophylaxis		
Severe hemophiliac	20	10–20 q 12 h
Milder hemophiliac		Antifibrinolytics plus DDAVP

[a]*Antifibrinolytics include ε aminocaproic acid (EACA; Amicar) or tranexamic acid.*

abdominal pain or a decrease in physical activity. To avoid severe destruction of muscle or the development of a pseudotumor, the patient should be rapidly evaluated with diagnostic imaging. Watchful waiting or suboptimal factor replacement is not recommended.

C. Mucous Membrane Bleeding

Mucous membrane bleeding can be a recurrent problem with hemophiliacs. Treatment varies according to the site and cause. Epistaxis can be controlled by packing or cautery. However, the clot that forms is often very friable and unstable, leading to recurrent bleeding when the pack is removed. In this situation, factor replacement may be necessary. Any tongue or mouth laceration in the young child must be treated immediately with appropriate factor, and therapy will need to be continued over several days to avoid rebleeding. Uncontrolled bleeding into the soft tissues of the mouth can result in airway obstruction if blood tracks into the retropharyngeal area.

TABLE 33–2 • Factor IX replacement therapy

	Initial Dose (U/kg)	Maintenance (U/kg)
Hemarthrosis	30–60	20 q 24 h
Muscle hematoma	30–50	30 q 24 h
Major surgery/ tissue damage	60–100	40–80 q 24 h
Intracranial bleed	80–100	60–80 q 24 h
Dental prophylaxis	10–20	20 q 12 h

D. Bleeding After a Dental Extraction

Bleeding following a dental extraction can be prevented with prophylactic therapy, or in the less severe hemophiliac, by pretreatment with DDAVP, or an antifibrinolytic agent such as tranexamic acid or ε aminocaproic acid (EACA). Antifibrinolytics will stabilize the clot that normally forms immediately following extraction. If the original clot can be maintained long enough to permit normal healing, high-dose factor therapy is usually unnecessary with mild hemophilia. This strategy also can be effective for very minor surgical procedures in a moderate hemophiliac. However, most hemophilia patients undergoing even minor surgery should be prepared with appropriate factor therapy.

E. Hematuria and Gastrointestinal Bleeding

Hematuria, either microscopic or macroscopic, occurs in nearly all patients with moderate and severe hemophilia. The course is usually self-limited and the bleeding source rarely identified. However, gross or persistent hematuria should provoke evaluation for a renal papillary hematoma or underlying urinary tract infection. Hematuria is best managed with bed rest, increased fluid intake, and a short course of prednisone (1 mg/kg/d for 3 days). Factor therapy for several days may be needed in patients with gross or persistent genitourinary bleeding. GI bleeding is much less common. If it occurs, the patient should be fully evaluated for GI disease. The assumption that the bleed is the result of "stress gastritis" should be avoided. Bleeding from hemorrhoids or proctitis can usually be controlled with local measures, unless symptoms are severe or protracted. If any surgical procedure is needed, factor therapy is indicated to achieve levels greater than 50%.

F. Major Surgery in Patients With Hemophilia A

Whenever major surgery is necessary in a patient with hemophilia A, the factor VIII level must be brought to near normal (100%) for the procedure. In addition, repeat doses should be given postoperatively every 8–12 hours to avoid any significant period of low factor VIII levels. Peak and trough factor VIII levels should be measured once to confirm the appropriate dosing level and dosing interval. Therapy is often continued for up to 2 weeks to avoid postoperative bleeding that disrupts wound healing. Even longer periods of therapy may be required in patients who undergo bone or joint surgery or who have a pseudotumor excised. In this situation, 4–6 weeks of replacement therapy may be needed.

G. Treatment of Hemophilia B

Recommended dosage schedules for the treatment of hemophilia B are summarized in Table 33–2. Guidelines for managing patients with hemophilia B do not differ significantly from those for patients with hemophilia A. Recombinant/purified product or **factor IX–prothrombin complex concentrate (FIX-PCC)** is used to treat mild bleeding episodes or as prophylaxis with minor procedures. However, a note of caution is needed when using FIX-PCC preparations, which can contain activated clotting factors, at higher doses. When given in amounts sufficient to increase factor IX levels to 50% or greater, there is an increased risk of thromboembolic complications, especially in patients undergoing orthopedic procedures. Therefore, it is essential to use only recombinant factor IX in treating patients undergoing major orthopedic surgery and those with severe traumatic injuries or liver disease.

H. Treatment of Factor XI Deficiency

For patients with factor XI deficiency, the most widely used product for replacement is **fresh frozen plasma** (FFP). This product from healthy blood donors is frozen within a few hours of collection. As such, it contains normal (ie, therapeutic) levels of all coagulation factors necessary to maintain hemostasis. FFP is the best choice for replacement of coagulation factors for a number of conditions besides XI deficiency, including liver failure and deficiencies of factors II, V, and X. Appropriate dosing of FFP should be weight based and not dependent on the extent of prolongation of the PTT. Dosing of FFP at 10–15 mL/kg should be sufficient to replace deficient coagulation factors and correct abnormal coagulation studies. Thus, assuming a volume of approximately 200 mL per unit of FFP, a reasonable dose for a 70-kg individual would be 3–4 U of FFP. It is also important to recognize that dosing is time sensitive in that coagulation factors will degrade at standard half-lives upon infusion. Therefore, appropriate dosing of FFP also includes providing this product immediately before an intended procedure to ensure adequate hemostasis.

Acquired Inhibitors

Management of the patient with hemophilia A with an inhibitor will vary according to whether the patient is a high or low responder. The factor VIII inhibitor should always be titered. Using a modification of the PTT called the **Bethesda assay**, it is possible to measure units of inhibitor/mL of plasma. Low responders generally have titers less than 5 Bethesda U/mL and do not show anamnestic responses to factor VIII concentrates, whereas the high responders can have titers of several thousand Bethesda units and dramatic anamnestic responses to therapy.

Patients in the low-responder category can usually be managed with **factor VIII concentrates**, occasionally with DDAVP. Larger initial and maintenance doses of factor VIII are required, and assays of peak and 1–2 hours post-infusion factor VIII levels are essential to guide therapy. When the titer of the factor VIII inhibitor exceeds 5–10 U/mL (high-responder category), treatment with factor VIII concentrates alone is not feasible. Faced with this dilemma, it is best to try to manage the patient conservatively without replacement therapy for minor bleeding episodes. Major, life-threatening bleeds can be treated with bypass products such as **activated prothrombin complex concentrate** (Autoplex T, FEIBA in the United States), or **recombinant factor VIIa** (rVIIa; Novo-Seven). Both therapies have associated risks that must be taken into account.

FEIBA showed an 86% response rate when given at 75 U/kg q 8–12 hours, but treatment with this activated prothrombin complex concentrate (PCC) runs a risk of initiating disseminated intravascular coagulation (DIC) or widespread thromboembolism when more than 200 U/kg is given in a 24-hour period. Despite up to a 5% incidence of thromboembolic (TE) complications in off-label use, recombinant factor VIIa has a much lower incidence of TE events (<1 in 10,000) in hemophilia, and therefore may well be the treatment of choice for acquired inhibitors. Although hemophiliacs can generate Xa via factor VIIa binding to TF-expressing monocytes and smooth muscle cells, they are unable to generate enough Xa and the subsequent thrombin burst on the platelet surface in the absence of factor VIII or IX. Recombinant factor VIIa in pharmacologic concentrations directly activates factor X on the platelet, leading to formation of the Xase complex and the thrombin burst. Tissue-factor-bearing cells are required for this response to rVIIa. Although the fibrin clots formed via rVIIa may not be as strong as that seen with factor VIII therapy, rVIIa does effectively reduce bleeding with inhibitors (75% response rate to 90–120 μg/kg q 3 hours). A parallel approach to inhibitor management is to induce immune tolerance using large daily doses of **factor VIII** given for up to a year or more. Although this is extremely expensive; it is actually more cost-effective over the long run for the 60%–80% of children with inhibitors who successfully develop tolerance.

Patients with severe hemophilia B are also at risk for developing a factor IX inhibitor, but the incidence is far less than in hemophilia A. They need to be evaluated in the same manner as the patients with factor VIII inhibitor. A **modified Bethesda assay** is similarly used to quantitate the inhibitor level. Usually, factor IX inhibitor patients can be managed acutely using the bypass products noted above. Attempts to induce immune tolerance in patients with hemophilia B have been problematic, because many of these patients can experience anaphylactic reactions with the subsequent administration of FIX-PCC or develop nephrotic syndrome as a complication of PCC. Therefore, hemophilia B inhibitors should preferentially be treated with recombinant VIIa.

Patients who develop an autoantibody to factor VIII or IX without a past history of hemophilia can present with life-threatening hemorrhage (9% mortality rate) and exhibit very high inhibitor levels in excess of several thousand Bethesda units. Treatment with **recombinant factor VIIa** or an **activated prothrombin concentrate** is required; factor VIII or IX alone will not be effective. However, not all patients with inhibitors have high titers, and up to 30% will not even require hemostatic therapy. Immunosuppression is generally needed to suppress autoantibody production. Only 30% of patients will respond to intravenous immunoglobulin (IVIG) or prednisone (50–80 mg/d), while 60%–70% remit with the combination of prednisone and oral cyclophosphamide (100–200 mg/d). However, this response may take months to reduce inhibitor-associated bleeding and is associated with other significant morbidity. Studies have now shown successful control of spontaneous inhibitors as quickly as within 2 weeks after starting anti-CD20 (rituximab) therapy, using a standard 375 mg/m^2 weekly dose for 4 weeks. Other therapies, 2-chlorodeoxyadenosine, azathioprine, vincristine, and cyclosporin A, may be used when initial treatment fails or relapses (about 20% for the latter). Spontaneous improvement with a decrease (or complete remission) in the antibody level and a recovery of factor activity occurs in the majority of women with postpartum factor VIII inhibitors.

THERAPEUTIC PREPARATIONS

Major progress is being made in developing safe, effective products for treating hemophilia A and B, especially in the development of third-generation recombinant products. It is important, therefore, to be aware of the various products available and to check on whether a new agent has been released. Patients with hemophilia and their families follow the development and availability of new products very closely and will want to be treated with the safest product regardless of cost.

Hemophilia A

Products available for treating hemophilia A include DDAVP, antifibrinolytics (tranexamic acid and EACA), fresh frozen plasma (FFP), cryoprecipitate, purified/recombinant factor VIII, FEIBA, and recombinant VIIa. For patients with a high titer spontaneous inhibitor, recombinant VIIa is preferred.

A. DDAVP

DDAVP is an arginine vasopressin analogue that rapidly releases von Willebrand factor (vWF) from endothelial cells. Since vWF is the carrier protein for factor VIII, DDAVP can increase the circulating level of factor VIII by 2- to 10-fold in the milder hemophiliac. Severe hemophiliacs will not respond, so DDAVP's effectiveness must be defined for each patient by measuring the factor VIII level 60 minutes after administration (peak effect). If the factor VIII level increases significantly, DDAVP can be used to manage minor bleeding episodes or for preparing the patient for minor surgery or dental work, especially if used in conjunction with antifibrinolytics (see section B below).

An intravenous dose of 0.3 μg/kg (up to 20 μg) of DDAVP infused slowly over 20–30 minutes is the same as recommended for the treatment of type 1 vWD. Alternatively, DDAVP can be given as an **intranasal spray (Stimate)** in doses of 150 μg (1 metered dose) for individuals less than 50 kg in weight or 300 μg (2 doses) for heavier patients. Peak effect is observed 60–90 minutes after administration. DDAVP treatments can then be repeated at 12- to 24-hour intervals, although there is a significant risk of tachyphylaxis after the first few doses. Side effects include flushing, headache, tachycardia, nausea, and abdominal cramping. In patients who are receiving hyponatremic intravenous fluids, there is a risk of water intoxication secondary to the antidiuretic effect of repeated injections.

B. Antifibrinolytics

Antifibrinolytic agents can be helpful in controlling milder bleeding episodes, especially those associated with dental procedures. In effect, these agents enhance hemostasis by stabilizing the clot and discouraging rebleeding. The adult dose for ε aminocaproic acid (EACA; Amicar) is 5 g every 6 hours orally or the same dose by slow intravenous infusion, whereas the dose in children is 100–200 mg/kg initially, followed by 50–100 mg/kg every 6 hours. The other available antifibrinolytic, tranexamic acid, is given in doses of 1.5 g orally (oral preparation not available in the United States) or 1 g intravenously every 8 hours to adults and 10 mg/kg intravenously to children.

C. Fresh Frozen Plasma

FFP contains the same factor VIII and IX concentrations as normal plasma, that is, 1 U of VIII or IX activity per milliliter of plasma. Therefore, the normal FFP unit contains 200–250 U of factors VIII, IX, and XI. When transfused, each unit of FFP can be expected to increase a patient's factor VIII level by only 5%–10%. Since very large volumes of FFP would be needed to achieve factor levels better than 50% of normal for hemophiliac patients, FFP has a very limited use in emergency situations where other factor products are not readily available. However, for factor XI deficiency, FFP will raise levels to greater than 30%, which appears to be sufficient for treatment of bleeding.

D. Cryoprecipitate

Another product that can be used in a directed-donor program for the emergent treatment of bleeding when purified VIII concentrates are unavailable is cryoprecipitate. Cryoprecipitate is prepared from FFP and contains high levels of factors VIII and XIII, vWF, and fibrinogen. One cryoprecipitate "unit" prepared from a single unit of donated blood will contain from 80–150 U of factor VIII in a small volume (30-fold concentrated compared with FFP). In a 75-kg patient who needs an initial treatment dose of 20 U/kg (total dose 1,500 U), infusion of 10–15 cryoprecipitate "units" should provide an adequate treatment dose. A post-infusion measurement of factor VIII will help confirm the success of the treatment.

Complications of FFP and cryoprecipitate therapy include allergic reactions, immunosuppression, and transmission of viral infections. Allergic reactions include urticaria, bronchospasm, and anaphylaxis. Before the development of purified and recombinant products, most severe hemophiliacs became infected with hepatitis B or C. Prior to the introduction of HIV testing in 1985, most patients were also exposed to HIV. The combination of HCV and HIV in hemophilia can result in severe hepatitis that is poorly responsive to interferon therapy. Up to 20% of HBV-infected hemophiliacs are chronic antigen carriers. Thus, cryoprecipitate should only be used when purified factor concentrates or recombinant factors are not available in a life-threatening bleeding emergency.

E. Purified Factor VIII

Purified factor VIII concentrates are easy to store and prepare for infusion, and are therefore preferred by most patients. Dosing is

TABLE 33–3 • Factor VIII concentrates

Brand Name	Preparation Method to Inactivate Viruses
Factor VIII: ultrapure recombinant	
Recombinate	Pasteurization of albumin stabilizer
Kogenate FS	Solvent detergent
Xyntha	Solvent detergent/nanofiltration
Helixate FS	Solvent detergent
Bioclate	None
Refacto	None
Factor VIII: high purity from human plasma	
Monoclate P	Pasteurization
Hemofil M	Solvent detergent
Monarc M	Solvent detergent
Factor VIII: intermediate/high purity from plasma	
Alphanate	Solvent-detergent, dry heat
Koate DVI	Solvent-detergent, dry heat
Humate-P	Pasteurization

straightforward because each product is assayed for the concentration of factor VIII activity. Several purification processes are used to eliminate the risk of viral transmission, including pasteurization, dry heat treatment, solvent-detergent treatment, and immunoaffinity purification using mouse monoclonal antibodies (Table 33–3). Manufacturers test product for HIV, HCV, HBV, hepatitis A virus (HAV), and B19 parvovirus using PCR amplification assays. To date, no assay for spongiform encephalopathy pathogen or Creutzfeldt-Jakob disease is available. Current products that have been tested for purity include the very high purity (immunoaffinity purified) products (Hemophil M, Monarc-M, and Monoclate P) and the intermediate/high-purity products (Alphanate, Koate DVI, and Humate-P). The latter group also contains high-molecular-weight multimers of vWF, making them more effective for the treatment of types 2 and 3 vWD patients. Affinity-purified VIII is capable of initiating an allergic reaction secondary to small amounts of mouse protein in the final product.

F. Recombinant Factor VIII

Recombinant factor VIII is commercially produced using mammalian cells transfected with factor VIII complementary DNA. It appears to be biologically identical to human factor VIII and has proved both safe and effective in clinical trials. Compared with cryoprecipitate or purified concentrates, **recombinant products (Recombinate and Kogenate)** are equally efficacious, although considerably more expensive. Despite the costs, recombinant factor VIII is recommended for mild hemophiliacs who are HIV negative and have only the occasional need for factor therapy. Severe adult hemophiliacs can be given either recombinant or, to reduce the cost, purified product, recognizing that the latter may still carry a risk of transmitting an as yet unrecognized infectious agent. First-generation recombinant products may be contaminated with small amounts of human or animal source protein, thereby posing a theoretical risk of transmitting a nonviral pathogen such as the prions responsible for spongiform encephalopathy (Creutzfeldt-Jakob disease). Second-generation concentrates are manufactured without protein exposure.

An understanding of the pharmacokinetics of a factor VIII infusion is important. Dosage recommendations in Table 33–1 are general guidelines that need to be modified according to the character of the bleed and the patient's measured response. Replacement of factor VIII to achieve a 100% plasma factor level will require an initial infusion of 50–60 U/kg (3,500–4,000 U in a 70-kg patient). Since the half-life of factor VIII is approximately 12 hours in adults, repeated infusions of 25–30 U/kg every 12 hours will be needed to keep the plasma factor VIII level above 50%. When lower doses (20–30 U/kg) are used, mean post-infusion plasma levels will fall to between 30% and 50% (the plasma VIII level will rise ~2% for each unit per kilogram infused). In children the half-life of factor VIII may be as short as 6 hours, necessitating more frequent infusions and laboratory assays to confirm efficacy.

Up to 30% of patients with severe hemophilia A exposed to factor VIII concentrate or recombinant product will eventually develop **inhibitor alloantibodies**, some within 10–12 days of first exposure. Approximately a third or more are low responders (<5 Bethesda units), and some of these will disappear spontaneously. In the management of patients with high-titer inhibitors, it is possible to reduce inhibitor levels by inducing immune tolerance. This strategy involves desensitizing the patient's immune system to factor VIII by administering large, frequent doses of factor VIII product (100 U/kg twice a day) over a prolonged period. Lower-dose regimens (25–50 U/kg) given daily or every other day have also been successful. Immunosuppressive agents also have been used as adjuncts to high-dose therapy. Lower-titer inhibitors generally respond within 6 months, while higher-titer antibodies may take 12–40 months to respond, if at all. **Newer recombinant preparations** have not resulted in a reduction in the incidence of inhibitor formation.

G. Prothrombin Complex Concentrate

Prothrombin complex concentrate (PCC) can be used to treat life-threatening bleeding in severe hemophiliacs with high-titer inhibitors. Dosing (Autoplex or FEIBA) is on the order of 50–75 U/kg every 8–12 hours. Because of the risk of thromboembolic complications, PCC is relatively contraindicated in postoperative or septic patients and those with other risk factors for thromboembolic disease.

H. Recombinant Factor VIIa

At pharmacologic concentrations, **factor VIIa** (when complexed with tissue factor bearing cells) binds activated platelets and facilitates the direct activation of factor X to Xa which, in concert with Va and prothrombin, generates thrombin on the platelet surface, even when factors VIII or IX or both are absent or a high-titer inhibitor is present. Tissue-factor-bearing cells must be present for the initial platelet activation to occur.

Recombinant VIIa (NovoSeven) is markedly less effective when thrombocytopenia, acidosis, or hypothermia are present, probably because of inhibition of the conversion of X to Xa. NovoSeven is currently recommended in the United States for the treatment of patients with bleeding caused by inhibitors to factor VIII or IX; surgery in patients with hemophilia A or B and inhibitors; and bleeding in patients with factor VII deficiency. In the European Union, rVIIa is additionally approved for bleeding in the postoperative setting (up to 90 μg/kg) and with Glanzmann thrombasthenia (70–100 μg/kg). For hemophilia and inhibitors, it is recommended to give a dose of 90–120 μg/kg intravenously every 2–3 hours until hemostasis is achieved; the half-life and dosing frequency are shorter in children. There is also evidence that a single high-dose regimen (270 μg/kg) can be effective in hemophilia with inhibitors (recently approved in Europe). Factor VII-deficient patients can be managed with a lower dose, 15–20 μg/kg, with re-dosing according to prothrombin time (PT) results. By contrast, anecdotal rVIIa use (80–100 μg/kg) in liver disease patients does not demonstrate a correlation between lesser bleeding and normalization of the PT.

Continuous infusions of factor VIIa have been used to manage hemophilia inhibitor patients undergoing surgery. Laboratory monitoring of rVIIa therapy in inhibitor patients will demonstrate a shortening of the PT, but the degree of shortening or absolute PT value does not appear to correlate with the clinical control of hemostasis. Recombinant VIIa therapy is successful in controlling bleeding in greater than 80% of inhibitor patients. The risk of widespread thrombosis or DIC appears to be very low. However, significant thromboembolic adverse events have been reported with recombinant VIIa, most often when employed for off-label use, but also during therapy for hemophilia inhibitors. Recombinant VIIa has been preliminarily reported to decrease mortality in non-hemophiliac patients presenting with intracranial hemorrhage, but this study has not been confirmed. Thromboembolic complications include both arterial (myocardial infarction/stroke) and venous thromboemboli and device occlusion; approximately two-thirds of the reported deaths with rVIIa are thought to result from thromboembolism.

Hemophilia B

Several products are also available for treating patients with hemophilia B. Purified factor IX preparations are preferable and include AlphaNine and Mononine and the recombinant product Benefix. Benefix and Mononine have no detectable factor II or X activity, whereas AlphaNine has minimal activity of both factor II and X. **Factor IX-prothrombin complex concentrates (FIX-PCC)** including Proplex T, Profilnine, and Bebulin VH, are also available for treatment (Table 33–4).

Like factor VIII replacement, purified factor IX concentrates or recombinant IX is used over several days to treat bleeding in hemophilia B. **Dosing recommendations** are approximately double those for factor VIII concentrates (see Table 33–2). Because of absorption to collagen sites in the vasculature, recovery of factor IX is about half that of factor VIII. Therefore, in order to achieve a 100% plasma level in a severe hemophiliac, a dose of 100 U/kg (7,000 U in a 70-kg patient) needs to be administered. At the same time, factor IX has a half-life of 18–24 hours, so repeated infusions at 50% of the original dose every 12–24 hours are sufficient to keep the factor IX plasma level above 50%. Like factor VIII recommendations, doses of 30–50 U/kg will generally give mean IX levels of 20%–40%, which is adequate for less severe bleeds. As for factor VIII inhibitors, recombinant factor VIIa is the therapy of choice for factor IX inhibitor patients.

TABLE 33–4 • Factor IX concentrates

Brand Name	Preparation Method to Inactivate Viruses
Factor IX: recombinant	
Benefix	Membrane filtration
Factor IX: purified concentration	
AlphaNine SD	Solvent-detergent, nanofiltered
Mononine	Affinity purified, ultrafiltration
Factor IX: complex concentrates (factors IX, II, and X)	
Proplex T	Dry heat
Profilnine SD	Solvent-detergent
Bebulin VH	Vapor heated
Factor IX: activated complex (factors IX, II, X, and activated VII)	
Autoplex T	Dry heat
Konyne	Dry heat
FEIBA VH	Vapor heated

Gene Therapy

Hemophilia is the ideal disease for gene therapy since stable expression of even a small number of gene-transfected cells would convey a significant clinical benefit. An increase in the factor VIII or IX level of only a few percent in severe hemophilia would change the clinical classification to moderate or even mild disease. This hypothesis has been successfully modeled in animals such that there is hope for a strategy some day in human hemophilia. Hematopoietic stem cells transduced with recombinant retrovirus containing porcine factor VIII (B-domain deleted) have been used to achieve curative VIII activity in murine models; the retrovirus itself and the pretransplant conditioning with targeted immunosuppression appear to have low toxicity.

CASE HISTORY • *Part 3*

The PTT mixing study is consistent with an inhibitor, and the pattern of immediate correction followed by prolongation after incubation for 60 minutes is characteristic of a factor VIII inhibitor. PFA closure times rule out platelet dysfunction, either ibuprofen induced or von Willebrand disease. Further workup of the "inhibitor" requires measurements of factor levels and inhibitor titer. The results in this patient are as follows:

Factor XI activity = 85%
Factor IX activity = 91%
Factor VIII activity = 2%; non-linear pattern with dilutions
Factor VIII inhibitor titer = 23 Bethesda U/mL

These results confirm a factor VIII deficiency–based coagulopathy consistent with an acquired "strong" autoantibody to factor VIII (a factor VIII of 2% with non-linear dilutions and a titer of 23 Bethesda U/mL).

In order to undergo surgery to relieve the hematoma and save the forearm from ischemic injury, the coagulopathy must be reversed. Since the high titer inhibitor will overwhelm any factor VIII infusions, an alternative "bypass" strategy must be employed—infusion of 120 μg/kg of recombinant VIIa every 3 hours prior to and following surgery. The frequency of infusions can then be gradually decreased once hemostasis is attained.

Most acquired factor VIII inhibitors are not associated with an underlying disease. However, given the modest lymphocytosis in this patient, a search for a lymphoproliferative disease is in order. In this case, immunophenotyping reveals a CD5+ B-cell clone consistent with the diagnosis of CLL (see Chapter 22). Moreover, subsequent treatment with rituximab results in eradication of the inhibitor and return of the PTT to normal.

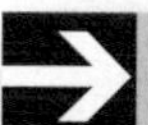

POINTS TO REMEMBER

The "intrinsic" pathway involves the interaction of factors XI, IX, and VIII to activate factor X for subsequent thrombin/fibrin generation. Factors VIII and IX are absolutely required for this process; hence, absence of either factor produces severe hemophilia (A and B, respectively). Deficiency of factor XI does not produce as severe a bleeding disorder in general.

The partial thromboplastin time (PTT) is the preferred screening test for intrinsic pathway defects (factor VIII, IX, and XI deficiencies). At the same time, a prolonged PTT can result from deficiency of factors (XII, prekallikrein) that are not associated with any clinical bleeding.

A PTT "mixing" study (1:1 mix of patient and normal plasma) is used to identify an inhibitor of either factor VIII or IX, including a factor-specific antibody, a lupus anticoagulant, or heparin. Measurements of the PTT with heparinase neutralization and addition of excess phospholipid will serve to exclude the latter two.

Hemophilia A and B are X-linked disorders—half of the sons of a maternal carrier will be affected, and half of her daughters will be carriers. A family history of bleeding in maternal uncles is one clue to the presence of hemophilia, but up to one-third of new hemophiliacs are de novo mutations and thus will not have a family history.

Most patients with hemophilia A have large deletions, nonsense mutations, or inversions (specifically intron 22) that result in complete absence of factor VIII protein. By contrast, most hemophilia B gene defects are point mutations, frameshift, and small deletions that result in nonfunctional factor IX. Factor XI is encoded on chromosome 4; defects in this gene are especially frequent in persons of Ashkenazi Jewish descent.

The severity of hemophilia A is directly proportional to the activity level of the coagulant factor. Absent activity (<1%) results in the most severe disease with spontaneous bleeding. Activity levels of 1%–5% are associated with procedure-related bleeding, and only rarely with spontaneous hemorrhage. Finally, patients with levels greater than 5% may go undetected for years until they are challenged with major surgery or trauma. Women carriers with levels between 5% and 60% have a slight increased risk of bleeding, most often detected during the workup for menorrhagia.

Unlike platelet dysfunction defects, hemophiliacs demonstrate good primary hemostasis, but unstable clots, and delayed hemorrhage, for example, bleeding hours after a dental procedure. Bleeding into joints, large and small muscles, and soft tissue is also the rule.

Because many patients with hemophilia A lack factor VIII protein (especially with the intron 22 inversion), they have a high incidence of inhibitor development (about one-quarter) that will block the function of transfused factor VIII. Inhibitors can occur in hemophilia B but to a lesser incidence (<5%).

Factor VIII inhibitor titers (Bethesda U/mL) can be measured in the laboratory by a mixing assay using dilutions of patient plasma. Patients with inhibitor titers greater than 5 U/mL generally do not respond to factor infusions and will have anamnestic responses to repeated therapy.

Older patients with no genetic hemophilia defect can develop an acquired inhibitor, most commonly to factor VIII, occasionally in association with autoimmune disease or malignancy. These acquired hemophiliacs can have severe disease with a high mortality.

Hemophilia treatment employs a team approach to prevent and treat hemorrhage and to deal with the long-term sequelae of bleeding. Older generations that were exposed to transfusion-transmitted infections still pose a challenge for simultaneous therapy of hepatitis (B and C) and HIV infection. The current use of recombinant and viral-inactivated purified factor products has made infection much less of a concern today.

Like the classification of hemophilia, treatment depends on the severity. Patients with severe disease often use prophylactic and home infusion at the first indication of bleeding, while those with more moderate disease deserve less intense therapy. The level of therapy is also dictated by the severity and location of hemorrhage, with intracranial bleeding one of the most feared complications.

Both plasma-derived and recombinant factors are used for treatment; the incidence of inhibitor development is similar between the 2 product types. The more severe the bleed, the higher the level of factor needed after infusion, with 100% activity required for severe trauma, major surgery, or neurosurgical intervention. Factor VIII is given roughly every 8–12 hours, while factor IX can be infused daily because of its increased half-life.

When inhibitors are present in low titer, factor infusions may overcome the inhibitor and result in effective levels. However, high titers rarely respond and require treatment using bypass activity agents such as FEIBA and recombinant VIIa. Both agents have a relatively short half-life and require frequent infusion. FEIBA's daily dose is limited by the risk of DIC and systemic thrombosis, whereas rVIIa appears to have a more constant low-level risk of thromboembolism (5% incidence at most). These bypass agents are also effective in acquired hemophilia.

For patients with hemophilia with high-titer inhibitors, long-term immune tolerance regimens may be effective with about two-thirds of patients responding to the combination of frequent high-dose infusions and immunosuppression. For acquired hemophilia, early institution of immunosuppression, starting with rituximab, appears efficacious. Gene therapy using factor transduced into stem cells is one strategy that holds promise for converting severe hemophilia to a more benign phenotype.

BIBLIOGRAPHY

Diagnosis

Astermark J et al: Polymorphisms in the *TNFA* gene and the risk of inhibitor development in patients with hemophilia A. Blood 2006;108:3739.

Collins PW et al: Acquired hemophilia A in the United Kingdom: a 2-year national surveillance study by the United Kingdom Haemophilia Center Doctors' Organisation. Blood 2007;109:1870.

Goudemand J et al: Influence of the type of factor VIII concentrate in the incidence of factor VIII inhibitors in previously untreated patients with severe hemophilia A. Blood 2006;107:46.

Hoffman M et al: Cutaneous wound healing is impaired in hemophilia B. Blood 2006;108:3053.

O'Connell KA et al: Thromboembolic adverse events after use of recombinant human coagulation factor VIIa. JAMA 2006;295:293.

Plug I et al: Bleeding in carriers of hemophilia. Blood 2006;108:52.

Posthouwer D et al: Progression to end-stage liver disease in patients with inherited bleeding disorders and hepatitis C: an international multicenter cohort study. Blood 2007;109:3667.

Sadler JE: New concepts in von Willebrand disease. Ann Rev Med 2005;173.

Therapy

Abshire T, Kenet G: Safety update on the use of recombinant factor VIIa and the treatment of congenital and acquired deficiency of factor VIII or IX with inhibitors. Haemophilia 2008;14:898.

Gomperts ED et al. From theory to practice: applying current clinical knowledge and treatment strategies to the care of hemophilia A patients with inhibitors. Blood Rev 2008;22:S1.

Gouw SC et al: Recombinant versus plasma-derived factor VIII products and the development of inhibitors in previously untreated patients with severe hemophilia A: the CANAL cohort study. Blood 2007;109:4693.

Gouw SC et al: Treatment-related risk factors of inhibitor development in previously untreated patients with hemophilia A: the CANAL cohort study. Blood 2007;109:4648.

Ide LM et al: Hematopoietic stem cell gene therapy of hemophilia A incorporating a porcine factor VIII transgene and nonmyeloablative conditioning regimens. Blood 2007;110:2855.

Kenet G, Martinowitz U: Single-dose recombinant activated factor VII therapy in hemophilia patients with inhibitors. Semin Hematol 2008;45:S38.

Mayer SA et al: Recombinant activated factor VII for acute intracerebral hemorrhage. N Engl J Med 2005;353:777.

Pabinger I et al: Prothrombin complex concentrate (Beriplex P/N) for emergency anticoagulation reversal: a prospective multi-national clinical trial. J Thromb Haemost 2008;6:622.

Roberts HR, Monroe DM, White GC: The use of recombinant factor VIIa in the treatment of bleeding disorders. Blood 2004;104:3858.

Spence RK: Clinical use of plasma and plasma-fractions. Best Pract Red Clin Haematol 2006;19:83.

EXTRINSIC AND COMMON PATHWAY COAGULOPATHIES · 34

CASE HISTORY • *Part I*

A 71-year-old woman presents with 1 day of headache and left-sided weakness after complaining for several days of dyspnea and confusion. Her history is notable for non-valvular atrial fibrillation and hypertension; she denies any prior history of thrombosis or bleeding. Her medications include a beta-blocker and warfarin (coumadin). Examination is notable for partial left hemiplegia; ecchymoses are noted over both forearms. The remainder of the examination demonstrates rales over both lung bases, an irregularly irregular heart rhythm, and a heave at the left sternal border.

CBC: Hemoglobin/hematocrit - 12 g/dL/35%
MCV - 89 fL MCH - 30 pg MCHC - 27 g/dL
RDW-CV - 10% WBC count 6,500/μL
Platelet count - 225,000/μL
PT = 55.1 seconds (<14 seconds)
INR = 7.1 (<1.3)
PTT = 39 seconds (22–35 seconds)

Questions

- Do the screening coagulation test results point to a specific cause for a bleeding tendency in this patient?
- Are additional studies warranted for diagnosis or determining therapy?

An abnormality in the extrinsic or common pathways can result in a significant bleeding tendency. Inherited deficiencies of a single coagulation factor, including factors VII, V, X, and prothrombin, are rare. More commonly, bleeding results from acquired deficiencies in several factors. This reflects the fact that most vitamin K–dependent factors are produced by the liver, so liver disease or vitamin K deficiency (from any of multiple causes) can be expected to produce a multifactor abnormality.

THE NORMAL EXTRINSIC AND COMMON PATHWAYS

Interactions of the factors involved in the extrinsic and common pathways are illustrated in Figures 34–1 and 34–2. The extrinsic pathway begins with circulating activated factor VII (VIIa) combining with tissue factor (TF) that is derived from damaged tissues or expressed on activated monocytes. In the presence of tissue factor, VIIa provides a potent stimulus for the activation of factor X to Xa. This is the pathway that initiates physiologic hemostasis, generating small amounts of thrombin, which then feeds back to activate the intrinsic coagulation factors and subsequently generate higher thrombin levels. The tissue factor-VIIa-Xa complex is rapidly inhibited by tissue factor pathway inhibitor (TFPI); thus, further factor X activation and adhesive fibrin formation depend on the intrinsic pathway, which explains the severity of hemophilia A (factor VIII deficiency) and hemophilia B (IX deficiency; see Chapter 33).

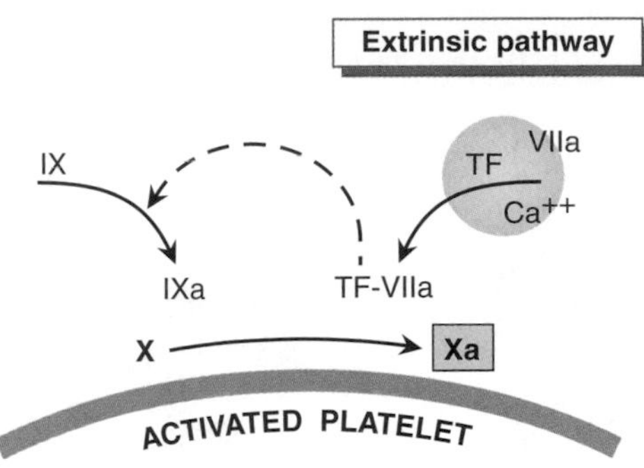

FIGURE 34–1. **The extrinsic pathway.** The extrinsic pathway (and physiologic hemostasis) is initiated by release of microsomal lipoproteins (tissue factor) from damaged tissue. This tissue factor (TF) combines with the normal small amounts of circulating activated factor VII (VIIa) to activate factors X and IX.

The common pathway (see Figure 34–2) involves Xa activation of prothrombin to form thrombin and the subsequent thrombin conversion of fibrinogen to fibrin clot. The formation of the prothrombin complex also requires the presence of surface membrane phospholipid and factor V. A major deficiency in any one of these elements can impair clotting and result in a bleeding tendency.

CLINICAL FEATURES

A single deficiency in any of these coagulation factors can be asymptomatic if it is a mild decrease, or if more severe, can produce a bleeding tendency ranging from easy bruising, epistaxis, and menorrhagia to severe hemophilia-type bleeding with major mucous membrane bleeding, hemarthroses, and hematoma formation. The latter is only seen in patients who have factor levels below 1%–2%.

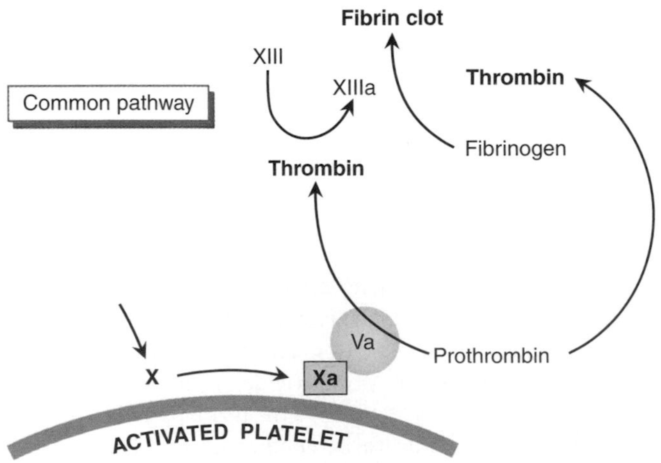

FIGURE 34–2. **The common pathway.** Both the intrinsic and extrinsic pathways lead to activation of the common pathway. Factor X is activated to Xa, which then stimulates the conversion of prothrombin to thrombin, facilitated by the presence of phospholipid in the platelet surface membrane and activated factor V (Va). Generation of thrombin and its subsequent action on fibrinogen amplify the formation of a fibrin clot. The fibrin polymer is further stabilized by activated factor XIII (XIIIa) crosslinking.

CONGENITAL ABNORMALITIES

Hereditary deficiency of factor VII is a very rare autosomal recessive disease with highly variable clinical severity. Only homozygous-deficient patients have factor VII levels low enough (<15%) to have symptomatic bleeding. These patients are easily recognized from their unique laboratory pattern of a prolonged prothrombin time (PT) but normal partial thromboplastin time (PTT) (Table 34–1) and isolated deficiency of factor VII, which does not respond to vitamin K repletion.

Congenital deficiencies in factors X, V, and prothrombin are also inherited as autosomal recessive traits, and severe deficiencies are quite rare, on the order of 1 in a million live births. Since all of these factors are part of the common pathway, patients with severe deficiencies demonstrate prolongations of both the PT and PTT. Patients with congenital factor V deficiency may also have a prolonged platelet function analysis (PFA) closure time because of the relationship between factor V and platelet function in supporting clot formation.

Congenital abnormalities in fibrinogen production will obviously interfere with the final step in the common pathway. Decreased levels of fibrinogen, either hypofibrinogenemia or afibrinogenemia, are relatively rare conditions inherited as autosomal recessive traits. Patients with afibrinogenemia have a severe bleeding diathesis with both spontaneous and post-traumatic bleeding. Since the bleeding can begin during the first few days of life, this condition may be initially confused with hemophilia. Hypofibrinogenemic patients usually do not have spontaneous bleeding but may have difficulty with surgery or trauma. Severe bleeding can be anticipated in patients with plasma fibrinogen levels below 50–100 mg/dL.

Dysfibrinogenemia

A more common defect than hypofibrinogenemia or afibrinogenemia is the **production of an abnormal fibrinogen**. The normal fibrinogen molecule is a 340-kDa glycoprotein composed of 3 pairs of polypeptide chains referred to as α, β, and γ. Fibrinogen is synthesized in the liver under the control of 3 genes, one for each chain, on chromosome 4. Mutations in one or another of these genes can impair the normal polymerization of the fibrinopeptides to form insoluble fibrin, resulting in a dysfibrinogenemia. More than 300 different mutations producing dysfunctional and, at times, reduced amounts of fibrinogen have been reported. Many of these mutations are inherited as autosomal dominant traits.

The clinical presentation of dysfibrinogenemia is highly variable. Patients who demonstrate both a reduced amount and a dysfunctional fibrinogen (hypodysfibrinogenemia) usually exhibit excessive bleeding. This is also true for a few families who are homozygous for dysfibrinogenemia. Most dysfibrinogenemic patients, however, appear to be heterozygous for the trait

TABLE 34–1 • Prothrombin (PT) and partial thromboplastin time (PTT) patterns with different diseases

Defect	PT	PTT	PTT 1:1 Mix
Extrinsic pathway			
Factor VII deficiency	Prolonged	Normal	—
Intrinsic pathway			
Factor VIII, IX, or XI deficiency	Normal	Prolonged	Shortens
Lupus anticoagulant	Usually normal	Prolonged	No correction
Antibody to factor VIII or factor IX	Normal	Prolonged	No correction
Common pathway			
Congenital deficiencies			
Factor X, V, or prothrombin (II)	Prolonged	Prolonged	Shortens
Hypofibrinogenemia/dysfibrinogenemia	Prolonged	Prolonged	Shortens
Liver disease/vitamin K deficiency			
Mild	Prolonged	Normal	PT mix shortens
Severe	Prolonged	Prolonged	Shortens
Anticoagulants			
Heparin therapy	Normal	Prolonged	No correction
Warfarin therapy	Prolonged	Normal	—
Heparin overdose	Mildly Prolonged	Prolonged	No correction
Coumadin overdose	Prolonged	Mildly Prolonged	Correction

and, although they have abnormal coagulation tests, most do not have a bleeding tendency. Overall, roughly 60% of dysfibrinogenemias are clinically silent, whereas the remainder can present with either a bleeding diathesis or a thrombotic tendency, in equal measure. A small number of dysfibrinogenemias have been associated with spontaneous abortion and poor wound healing.

Factor XIII Deficiency

Stability of the fibrin clot is hemostatically important. **Factor XIII (fibrin-stabilizing factor) deficiency** is a rare autosomal recessive disorder with an estimated prevalence of 1 in 5 million for the homozygous deficiency. Patients present at birth with persistent umbilical or circumcision bleeding. Adult patients demonstrate a severe bleeding diathesis, characterized by recurrent soft tissue bleeding, poor wound healing, and a high incidence (25%–40%) of intracranial hemorrhage. Typically, the bleeding is somewhat delayed based on the role of factor XIII in stabilizing the fibrin clot. Blood clots form but are weak and unable to maintain hemostasis. Fetal loss in women with factor XIII deficiency can approach 100%, suggesting a critical role for this factor in maintaining pregnancy.

Laboratory Studies

The first step in evaluating the extrinsic and common pathways is the measurement of the **PT** and **PTT**, and these assays are discussed in Chapter 29. As summarized in Table 34–1, comparison of these 2 measurements can separate a congenital factor VII deficiency from a factor deficiency in the common pathway. Since both tests require normal fibrinogen function, hypofibrinogenemia or dysfibrinogenemia will prolong both the PT and PTT. Definitive diagnosis of a single coagulation factor deficiency requires specific factor assays for VII, X, V, and prothrombin. Diagnosis of hypofibrinogenemia or dysfibrinogenemia requires **assays of fibrinogen concentration and function**.

The most accurate measurement of total fibrinogen protein is provided by **immunoassay** or a **protein precipitation technique**. Although this approach will give a good measure of total fibrinogen, it does not provide information regarding the ability of the fibrinogen to polymerize to form fibrin. Functional assays, such as the von Clauss method, provide a measure of clottable fibrinogen. This method uses thrombin to convert fibrinogen to fibrin, followed by measurement of the amount of fibrin in the clot. A dysfibrinogenemia should be suspected whenever there is a significant difference between the amount of fibrinogen measured immunochemically (normal antigenic or precipitant levels) versus that measured by the thrombin clot (decreased von Clauss activity) technique. **Other screening tests for fibrinogen dysfunction** include the thrombin time (TT) and reptilase time. Both are sensitive to fibrinogen dysfunction, but only the **reptilase time is not inhibited by heparin**. Definitive diagnosis and subclassification of a dysfibrinogenemia **requires fibrinopeptide chain analysis by sodium dodecyl sulfate (SDS) polyacrylamide gel electrophoresis and amino acid sequencing**.

Factor XIII deficiency should be considered in a patient with a severe bleeding diathesis who has otherwise normal coagulation screening tests, including PT, PTT, fibrinogen level, platelet count, and PFA closure time. Clot dissolution in 5M urea can be used as a screening assay for complete deficiency. Definitive diagnosis after an abnormal urea screen can be accomplished by enzyme-linked immunosorbent assay (ELISA). Patients at risk for severe hemorrhage generally have factor XIII levels near 1% of normal. Heterozygotes (factor XIII levels of around 50%) usually exhibit no bleeding tendency.

ACQUIRED ABNORMALITIES

Differential diagnosis of an acquired coagulation defect involving the extrinsic or common pathway has to be done at the bedside. The patient's disease history, nutritional status, and drug history must be carefully defined and integrated with the laboratory studies. If the PT is very prolonged but the PTT is normal, a congenital deficiency in factor VII is most likely (see Table 34–1). More often, however, the discordance between the 2 measurements is less marked. This situation is compatible with a multiple factor deficiency state secondary to hepatocellular disease, deficiency of vitamin K, or treatment with warfarin. Basically, the PT is a more sensitive measure of modest reductions in multiple common pathway factors than the PTT.

A more balanced prolongation of the PT and PTT is seen in patients with **severe liver disease**. In addition to greater reductions in the vitamin K–dependent factors produced by the liver, abnormal fibrinogen molecules and fibrin degradation products circulate in greater amount and act as inhibitors of the 2 assays. In this circumstance, the PTT and the TT are especially sensitive to the fibrinogen abnormalities. Prolongations of the PT and PTT are also seen in patients with **disseminated intravascular coagulation (DIC)**. This condition results from a combination of factor consumption, severe hypofibrinogenemia, and fibrinolysis with the appearance of fibrin degradation products.

The clinician must always be alert to the potential impact of **anticoagulant drugs** on these pathways. Warfarin (coumadin) inhibits vitamin K reductase and interferes with carboxylation of glutamyl residues of prothrombin (II) and factors VII, IX, and X. Because of its short half-life, factor VII is the most sensitive to warfarin, which generally results in a prolongation of the PT with little or no effect on the PTT. Heparin, by contrast, also interferes with the common pathway by blocking the activation of fibrinogen by thrombin; heparin at therapeutic levels prolongs the PTT with little effect on the PT.

Less common causes of a defect in the common pathway are listed in Table 34–2. Vitamin K–dependent factor deficiencies can result from the ingestion of drugs that interfere with vitamin K absorption. Cholestyramine binds bile acids and interrupts the absorption of fat-soluble vitamins like vitamin K. Excessive doses of vitamins E or A can also interfere with the absorption or metabolism of vitamin K. Salicylate overdose affects vitamin K metabolism and prolongs the PT. Cephalosporins, especially cefamandole and cefoperazone, will directly interfere with the intrahepatic metabolism of vitamin K. Severe malabsorption can result in a rapid depletion of vitamin K over a matter of days. Finally, vitamin K deficiency is often seen in patients with small bowel disease such as bacterial overgrowth, short bowel syndrome, sprue, and regional enteritis.

TABLE 34–2 • Acquired deficiencies of common and extrinsic pathway factors

Vitamin K deficiency
Hemorrhagic disease of newborn
Poor diet (lack of leafy vegetables)
Malabsorption
Pancreatitis
Small bowel disease (eg, sprue, regional enteritis)
Biliary obstruction
Vitamin A or E excess
Drug ingestion
Cholestyramine
Mineral oil
Antibiotics
Abnormal metabolism
Hepatocellular disease
Protein-calorie malnutrition
Drug ingestion
Salicylates
Hydantoins
Antibiotics
Superwarfarins (rodenticides)
Other mechanisms
Amyloidosis: factor X binding
Homocystinuria: factor VII deficiency

Acquired deficiencies of single factors are rare. A deficiency in factor VII has been described in patients with homocystinuria, whereas low prothrombin levels have been reported in some patients with lupus anticoagulant. Patients with amyloidosis can develop a factor X deficiency owing to binding of factor X to amyloid protein. Finally, factor IX as well as antithrombin levels can fall because of urinary protein loss in patients with nephrotic syndrome, but this only affects the intrinsic (PTT) pathway.

Laboratory Studies

The laboratory evaluation of a possible acquired defect must be guided by the clinical picture. If a patient obviously has liver disease or is receiving an anticoagulant drug, the **PT** and **PTT** results may be satisfactory for diagnosis. Since the PT is the most sensitive measure of a common pathway abnormality, this test is frequently used as a screening test to rule out disease or drug effects. In fact, many clinicians include the PT as a routine part of their evaluation of liver function.

In severely ill patients who demonstrate an abnormal bleeding tendency or who are at risk for bleeding, a **full evaluation of the extrinsic and common pathways**, together with measurements of fibrinogen concentration and fibrin turnover **(fibrinolysis)**, is in order. Most laboratories offer a panel of tests for this evaluation. At a minimum, this panel should include a PT, PTT, TT, an assay of fibrinogen concentration, and a

CASE HISTORY • *Part 2*

The patient's normal platelet count rules out thrombocytopenia but not necessarily platelet dysfunction; a platelet function assay (PFA) is required to exclude the latter. The PT (international normalized ratio [INR]) is markedly prolonged, while the PTT is only slightly prolonged, suggesting an abnormality of the vitamin K–dependent coagulation factors, including II, VII, and X, of the extrinsic/common pathways. This strongly implicates warfarin, since the PT is much more sensitive to warfarin inhibition. To confirm a warfarin-induced prolongation of the PT and the absence of an inhibitor, a "mixing study" using a 1:1 dilution of patient plasma with pooled normal plasma is indicated. The results in this patient are as follows:

Mixing study - PT (@ time 0) = 11.4 seconds (control = 11.1 seconds)
PT (@ 60 minutes) = 11.6 seconds (control 11.4 seconds)
Platelet function assay:
PFA collagen/ADP closure time = 95 seconds (80–120 seconds)
PFA collagen/epinephrine closure time = 145 seconds (110–180 seconds)

At the same time, a computed tomography (CT) scan with contrast of the head demonstrates a large right intracerebral hemorrhage with extension into the lateral ventricle. The neurosurgeon recommends immediate evacuation to relieve intracranial pressure, but because of the coagulation results, the neurosurgeon requests consultation for management of the coagulopathy.

Questions

- Based on these results, does the patient require treatment prior to surgery and, if so, what treatments should be considered?
- Are any additional laboratory studies needed? Does her overall condition favor one treatment over another?

measurement of fibrin degradation products (D-dimer, split-products, or both). Other valuable tests for evaluating the rate of clot formation and dissolution are the **antithrombin** and **α_2-antiplasmin levels**; the interpretation of these tests is discussed in Chapters 35 and 36.

THERAPY

The treatment of a single-factor–deficiency state depends on the severity of the bleeding. The therapeutic objective is to replace enough of the missing factor to maintain a level sufficient to control bleeding and permit healing. This approach is similar to that for treating the patient with hemophilia.

Congenital Abnormalities

Most patients with factor VII deficiency can be treated with infusions of **fresh frozen plasma (FFP)**. Patients with factor VII levels less than 1% require treatment with **prothrombin complex concentrate (PCC)** or, better yet, with **recombinant activated factor VII (Novoseven)**.

Deficiencies in factors X, V, and prothrombin are generally treated with FFP. FFP is basically the frozen plasma harvested from a single unit of donated blood (1 donor). The concentration of the vitamin K–dependent factors in FFP is approximately the same as that of normal plasma in vivo. Therefore, to obtain a significant increase in the level of any factor, a considerable volume of FFP must be infused. As a rule of thumb, at least 4–6 U of FFP (200–250 mL per unit) are needed to attain a 20%–30% increase in any missing factor level in an average-sized adult. This level represents a considerable volume of plasma (800–1,500 mL) and may present a significant cardiovascular challenge to the patient. Moreover, the duration of effectiveness of this replacement therapy depends on the turnover time of each factor (Figure 34–3), which then dictates how often repeated infusions of FFP will be needed to maintain a factor level. Factor V deficiency can also be treated with platelet transfusion, especially for prophylaxis of late bleeding postoperatively and following successful FFP treatment.

For a severe bleeder, several PCCs are commercially available (Table 34–3). The advantage of these products is that factor levels of 50% or higher can be achieved without the risk of volume overload. The disadvantages of PCCs are the risk of transmission of hepatitis B and C and the risk of induction of thromboembolism or widespread thrombosis leading to DIC. It is also important to recognize the variation in factor levels in the several PCC products. The preferred PCC product to treat patients with factor VII deficiency in the United States is **Proplex T** because of its high level of factor VII. However, rVIIa (NovoSeven) is now approved by the US Food and Drug Administration (FDA) for the treatment of factor VII deficiency and is probably the therapy of choice.

Most patients with **congenital dysfibrinogenemia** have no clinical disease and therefore do not require therapy. For those

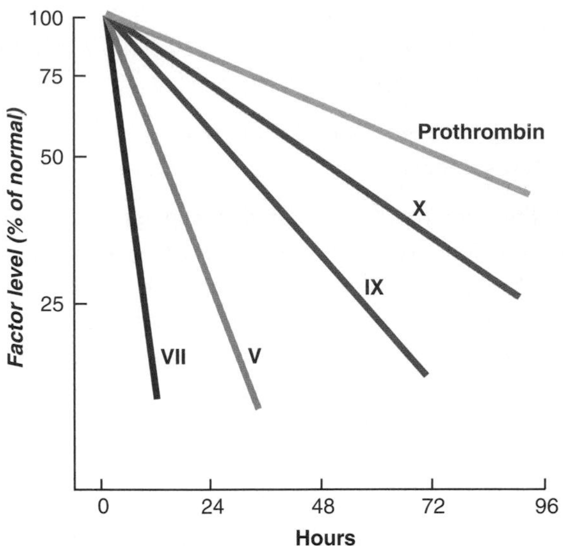

FIGURE 34–3. **Coagulation factor turnover.** Factors IX, X, and prothrombin have circulating half-lives after transfusion of 24–72 hours. In contrast, factor V has a half-life of approximately 12 hours and factor VII a very short half-life of 2–5 hours. The shorter the turnover time of a factor, the more frequently the factor-deficient patient will need repeated infusion of FFP.

who are symptomatic or are at risk for bleeding with surgery, **cryoprecipitate therapy** is warranted. To increase the fibrinogen level by at least 100 mg/dL in the average-sized adult, 10–12 U of cryoprecipitate should be infused, followed by 2–3 U each day (fibrinogen is catabolized at a rate of 25% per day). By contrast, dysfibrinogenemia patients with a thrombotic tendency will require long-term anticoagulation.

Factor XIII–deficient patients can be treated with FFP, cryoprecipitate, or a plasma-derived factor XIII concentrate—**Fibrogammin P**. Acute hemorrhage should be treated with an infusion of 50–75 U/kg body weight; prophylaxis is possible using intravenous injections of 10–20 U/kg at 4- to 6-week intervals depending on the patient's preinfusion plasma factor XIII level. Factor XIII has a long circulating half-life of 7–12 days, and adequate hemostasis is achieved with even very low plasma concentrations (1%–3%). A recombinant factor XIII-A homodimer (rXIII-A2) holds promise for therapy since most deficient patients lack the A unit of factor XIII. After infusion, rXIII-A2 complexes with the endogenous B units in plasma to form active factor with a half-life of 8.5 days; each recombinant unit per kilogram dose yields a 2%–3% increase in XIII activity. Laboratory measures also show efficacy of the rXIII product with normalization of the urea lysis tests and increased clot strength by thromboelastography.

Acquired Abnormalities

A. Vitamin K Deficiency

Patients with vitamin K deficiency should be treated with oral or parenteral vitamin K according to the cause of the deficiency state. Simple dietary deficiency can easily be corrected with a daily oral supplement of 5–10 mg. Patients with severe malabsorption or a defect in vitamin K metabolism should receive 5–10 mg of vitamin K subcutaneously daily.

In the case of the patient on well-adjusted warfarin therapy, vitamin K administration (vitamin K_1 at a dose of 1–2 mg intravenously or 5–10 mg subcutaneously) can reverse the warfarin effect within 6–12 hours, that is, the time required for renewed synthesis of vitamin K–dependent factors. If the effect must be reversed more rapidly, as in the case of a severe bleeding episode or emergency surgery, the patient should be given 4–6 U of FFP every 6–12 hours until the PT normalizes.

The INR value, together with the bleeding history, can also be used as a guideline to treatment (Table 34–4). Since warfarin is a competitive inhibitor of vitamin K, the amount of vitamin K required to reverse the effect will depend on the blood warfarin level. Patients suffering from a major overdose of the drug with very high INR will need much larger doses of vitamin K

TABLE 34–3 • Prothrombin complex concentrates

	Factor Levels (U/100 Units Factor IX)		
	Prothrombin	***Factor VII***	***Factor X***
Proplex T (Baxter Hyland)	50	400	50
Konyne-HT (Cutter)	100	20	140
Profilnine-HT (Alpha)	150	11	60
Bebulin VH	120	13	140

TABLE 34–4 • Interventions for elevated INR caused by vitamin K antagonists (VKA), eg, Warfarin

Situation	Intervention
INR 3.0–4.9; no bleeding	Lower or omit VKA dose until INR therapeutic; resume at lower VKA dose
INR 5.0–8.9; no bleeding	Omit VKA doses until INR therapeutic and/or give vitamin K 1–2.5 mg PO; resume at lower VKA dose. If ↑ bleed risk or urgent surgery pending, give vitamin K 2.5–5 mg PO
INR ≥9.0; no bleeding	Hold VKA; give vitamin K 2.5–5 mg PO
INR >1.5; major bleeding	Hold VKA; give vitamin K 10 mg IV and supplement with FFP, PCC, or rVIIa as needed based on clinical severity
INR >1.5; life-threatening hemorrhage	Hold VKA; immediately administer FFP, PCC, or rVIIa, plus vitamin K 10 mg IV

and immediate factor replacement (FFP, PCC) or treatment with rVIIa if they are bleeding.

When patients are on long-term warfarin therapy because of an increased risk of thromboembolic disease (atrial fibrillation, recurrent venous thrombosis with pulmonary emboli, etc.), it can be important to return the INR to within the therapeutic range, but without normalizing the PT, and thereby avoid putting the patient at increased thromboembolic risk for some period of time. Some randomized controlled studies have found that simply holding the warfarin dose for non-bleeding patients with INR elevations up to 9–10 is as effective and safe as giving low-dose (1.25 mg) oral vitamin K; both regimens have less risk of over-correction and induction of a prothrombotic state. Unlike the patient with short-acting vitamin K antagonist (VKA) prolongation of the INR, the patient who has ingested a rodenticide containing one of the long-acting warfarin congeners will require daily 50–100 mg doses of vitamin K or more by mouth for extended periods. FFP or rVIIa will also be required if the patient is acutely bleeding.

Recombinant activated factor VII (rVIIa; NovoSeven) is now approved for use by the FDA in several clinical situations other than for its originally designated bypass activity for congenital hemophilia with development of inhibitors. These indications include acquired hemophilia (no congenital disorder), factor VII deficiency, and liver disease; in addition, rVIIa is in widespread use for other situations of uncontrolled bleeding (off-label in the United States but approved in other countries). These latter may include trauma bleeding that is unresponsive to transfusion of multiple hemostatic blood products and unprovoked intracranial hemorrhage. Dosing for both approved and off-label indications is somewhat problematic, but consensus recommendations exist (Table 34–5). Since controlled studies examining rVIIa efficacy and incidence of thromboembolic complications are not always available, use of rVIIa for off-label indications must balance the severity of the hemorrhage with possible risk of thrombosis.

TABLE 34–5 • Broad dosing recommendations for rVIIa in bleeding patients

Indication for rVIIa	Dosing Range Recommended for rVIIa
Hemophilia inhibitor (congenital/acquired)	80–120 μg/kg
Intracranial hemorrhage with ↑ INR	40–80 μg/kg
Surgery/trauma hemorrhage	40–80 μg/kg
Reversal of elevated INR	10–40 μg/kg
Factor VII deficiency	10–40 μg/kg
Liver disease	10–40 μg/kg

The incidence of thromboembolic complications with rVIIa use is estimated to be approximately 5% in off-label uses; this frequency in adults is likely higher than the incidence in children with hemophilia. Thrombosis can occur in venous or arterial systems, and fatal thromboembolism or thrombosis has been reported, including myocardial infarction and pulmonary embolism.

B. Liver Disease

Treatment of a patient with liver disease can be very difficult, since bleeding is usually multifactorial. There is often a specific lesion associated with the bleeding, such as varices, gastritis, or peptic ulcer, which must be controlled locally. If the liver dysfunction is mild and associated with a poor diet, vitamin K supplementation may improve factor production and shorten the PT and PTT. More often, however, it will be ineffective or have a short-lived effect.

The results of the **coagulation test profile should drive the approach to therapy of bleeding caused by liver disease**. First, the platelet count should be maintained above 50,000/μL by repeated transfusions of random donor platelets. The higher count is necessary to counteract both the mild platelet function defect and the more severe thrombocytopenia seen with advanced liver disease and associated DIC. This can be difficult, however, since patients with advanced liver disease respond poorly to platelet transfusions, especially in those with portal hypertension who will trap transfused platelets in their enlarged spleens.

Next, if the fibrinogen level is less than 125 mg/dL, the patient should be transfused with 10 U of cryoprecipitate, and the fibrinogen level should be monitored to determine the need for additional cryoprecipitate. Third, if the PT and PTT are both prolonged, the patient should receive FFP. Since the principal defect may be a reduced production of factor VII, a transfusion of 2 U of FFP, raising the factor VII level by 5%–10%, will shorten the PT and may have a positive clinical effect. Attempts to normalize the PT and PTT must be discouraged, since this would require the repeated infusion of large volumes of FFP, resulting in marked fluid overload. If the INR is being used as a crude monitor of efficacy in liver disease, it is highly unlikely that any volume of FFP transfusion will lower the INR below 1.5–1.7. Most recently, infusions of rVIIa (NovoSeven) have been used with some success in coagulopathic liver disease patients, and selected patients have successfully undergone plasma exchange as an acute bridge to liver transplantation. Finally, red blood cell transfusions should be given as required to maintain a hematocrit of approximately 30%.

Since abnormal fibrinolysis can be a significant factor in the bleeding diathesis of the liver disease patient, a trial of an antifibrinolytic, such as **ε aminocaproic acid (EACA)** or tranexamic acid, may be beneficial. EACA should be given as a bolus intravenously, 4–5 g in the first hour, followed by a continuous infusion of 1 g per hour for 8 hours. Maintenance is possible using an oral dose of 4 g of EACA every 4 hours. **Tranexamic acid** is initiated with a 10 mg/kg intravenous bolus, followed by 10 mg/kg intravenously, every 6–8 hours.

CASE HISTORY • Part 3

Complete correction of the PT mixing study at 0 and 60 minutes is consistent with factor deficiency, not the presence of an inhibitor. Given the history of warfarin use, together with the greatly prolonged INR and only slightly elevated PTT, warfarin overdose is almost certainly the cause of the coagulopathy. PFA closure times rule out platelet dysfunction and von Willebrand disease.

Further workup for a single factor deficiency is unwarranted. The role(s) of new drug use (especially antibiotics) which interfere with warfarin metabolism and the worsening of the patient's cardiac failure do need to be explored. It is also essential to review the patient's recent warfarin dosage schedule, since unintended overdose is of major concern.

In order to undergo lifesaving surgery for her intracerebral bleed, the coagulopathy must be reversed as quickly as possible. Fresh frozen plasma (FFP) can be used, but a volume of 4–6 U of FFP may well exacerbate heart failure in this patient. Alternatively, prothrombin complex concentrates could be used, but these are relatively contraindicated in a patient who may have had a thromboembolic event (atrial fibrillation). A single dose of recombinant VIIa is likely the therapy of choice, even though it too carries thrombotic risk. The patient should also receive 10 mg of vitamin K by slow intravenous infusion. This dose is likely to result in normalization of the PT/INR, but the risk of further intracerebral hemorrhage far outweighs that of thromboembolism. In fact, the neurosurgeon recommends no further anticoagulation, at least until the intracerebral hemorrhage is completely healed, and perhaps permanently.

POINTS TO REMEMBER

The extrinsic pathway is the first to react to tissue injury (tissue factor activates factor VII, which in turn activates factor X). This activates the common pathway (factor Xa forms the prothrombinase complex with factors V and II to generate thrombin and subsequent fibrin). Factors II, V, VII, and X are absolutely required; hence, the complete absence of any of these factors produces a severe bleeding diathesis. Factors II, VII, and X are also dependent on vitamin K for the hepatic synthesis of functional protein.

The prothrombin time (PT) is the preferred screening test for an extrinsic pathway defect. A greatly prolonged PT with a normal PTT is typical of congenital factor VII deficiency. Since VII has the shortest half-life of all vitamin K–dependent factors, the PT is also the most sensitive test for detecting vitamin K deficiency, inhibition (warfarin therapy), and poor factor production (liver disease). The international normalized ratio (INR) is employed to standardize for the different sensitivities of PT reagents in monitoring anticoagulation therapy.

A PT "mixing" study (1:1 mix of patient and normal plasma) can be used to distinguish between extrinsic/common pathway factor deficiencies and the rare inhibitor. Since factor V is not vitamin K dependent, measurement of factors V and VII levels can help distinguish between liver disease and vitamin K deficiency.

Both the PT and PTT are prolonged with deficiency of 1 or several of the common pathway factors (X, V, and II). They are also prolonged with severe fibrinogen deficiency or dysfunction (dysfibrinogenemia). Homozygous congenital deficiencies of factors VII, X, V, and II have a very low incidence of about 1 in 1 million. By contrast, congenital hypo- or afibrinogenemia (levels <100 mg/dL) or dysfibrinogenemia are much more common. Since factor V is found in platelets, this rare single-factor deficiency can also prolong the PFA closure time.

Fibrinogen defects can be confirmed by an elevated thrombin time, unlike the factor deficiencies which only prolong the PT and PTT. Heparin in the sample will also yield a long thrombin time, but heparin can be ruled out by a normal reptilase time, unlike the fibrinogen disorders, which prolong the reptilase time.

Factor XIII homozygous deficiency should be suspected when bleeding is associated with normal laboratory screening results (PT, PTT, platelet count and function, thrombin time) and especially with a history of pregnancy loss or intracranial hemorrhage. The urea clot dissolution test is an effective screening assay for complete XIII absence; the actual level can then be confirmed by ELISA.

Acquired abnormalities of the extrinsic and common pathway factors are much more frequent than congenital disorders. Liver disease will prolong the PT but not the PTT when liver synthetic dysfunction is mildly to moderately impaired; the PTT additionally prolongs once severe liver disease is present. Similarly, mild-moderate vitamin K deficiency or therapeutic levels of vitamin K antagonists (eg, warfarin) preferentially elevate the PT first, and only prolong the PTT when severe deficiency or overdosing is present.

Vitamin K deficiency is extremely common among hospitalized patients for multiple reasons. Poor diet (lack of leafy vegetables) often results in the hospital because of clinical illness; antibiotics interfere with gut metabolism that normally produces vitamin K or directly block hepatic uptake of vitamin K.

Rare acquired single-factor deficiencies include factor X, which can be adsorbed by the amyloid protein in systemic amyloidosis, and factor II, which can become deficient due to antibody-mediated clearance with a lupus anticoagulant. The latter condition paradoxically demonstrates bleeding with a prothrombotic lupus anticoagulant.

Therapy for congenital deficiency of factors X, V, and II is straightforward; fresh frozen plasma (FFP) contains all of these factors at physiologic concentration. A single unit of FFP (250 mL) contains about 5% activity; thus, infusion of 4–6 U will yield an increase of 20%–30% factor activity, enough to restore hemostasis. The difficulty with FFP is the need for repeated infusion based on the half-lives of the specific factors. Since factor VII has the shortest half-life of 2–6 hours, repeated FFP infusion for congenital VII deficiency or acquired liver disease may result in fluid overload.

Treatment of congenital or acquired factor VII deficiency can be accomplished with prothrombin complex concentrates (PCC), which also contain common pathway factors; thus, PCC is effective for bleeding due to liver disease or vitamin K deficiency. The PCC dose is limited by thromboembolic risk since the factors within PCC are pre-activated.

Recombinant activated factor VII (rVIIa) is yet another option for congenital factor VII deficiency, liver disease, and warfarin excess, and is approved in several countries for generalized bleeding disorders unresponsive to blood product transfusion. Like PCC, rVIIa carries a thromboembolic risk but is often effective with a single dose. Whether off-label uses of rVIIa prove efficacious remains to be seen.

Vitamin K deficiency or excess vitamin K antagonist can be reversed with vitamin K itself, either oral or parenteral; this effect occurs within 12–18 hours. When bleeding is not present, vitamin K alone can be used even when the PT (and INR) are substantially prolonged; if any bleeding is present, FFP, PCC, and rVIIa must be considered in addition to vitamin K replacement.

Therapy for specific deficiencies/abnormalities of fibrinogen includes cryoprecipitate and other derived-fibrinogen products. These should be transfused to maintain levels greater than 100 mg/dL when there is deficiency or to restore a normal thrombin time with dysfibrinogenemia. Factor XIII deficiency can also be treated with cryoprecipitate infusion, but derived and recombinant products are becoming more widely available for treatment.

BIBLIOGRAPHY

Aguilar MI et al: Treatment of warfarin-associated intracerebral hemorrhage: literature review and expert opinion. Mayo Clin Proc 2007;82:82.

Ansell J et al: Pharmacology and management of the vitamin K antagonists. Chest 2008;133:160S.

Crowther MA et al: Oral vitamin K versus placebo to correct excessive anticoagulation in patients receiving warfarin. Ann Intern Med 2009;150:293.

Lovejoy AE et al: Safety and pharmacokinetics of recombinant factor XIII-A2 administration in patients with congenital factor XIII deficiency. Blood 2006;108:57.

Marsh S et al: Population variation in VKORC1 haplotype structure. J Thromb Haemost 2006;4:473.

Sconce E et al: Vitamin K supplementation can improve stability of anticoagulation for patients with unexplained variability in response to warfarin. Blood 2007;109:2419.

Shander A et al: Consensus recommendations for the off-label use of recombinant human factor VIIa (NovoSeven) therapy. P&T 2005;30:11.

CONSUMPTIVE COAGULOPATHIES · 35

CASE HISTORY • *Part I*

A 37-year-old man is admitted to the hospital intensive care unit for his third episode of acute pancreatitis. Other than a history of chronic alcoholism without evidence of cirrhosis, his past medical history is unremarkable. Examination reveals an anxious white male with a diffusely tender, somewhat rigid abdomen; few if any bowel sounds; and a positive Turner sign. Vital signs: BP - 110/60 mm Hg, P - 110 bpm, R - 16 bpm, temp - 38°C.

CBC: Hemoglobin/hematocrit - 11 g/dL/33%
MCV - 90 fL MCH - 30 pg MCHC - 33 g/dL
WBC count - 16,000/μL
Platelet count - 110,000/μL
Serum amylase and lipase - both elevated
Serum LDH - 1,000 IU/mL
Coagulation studies:
  PT = 15.1 seconds (<14 seconds)
  PTT = 42 seconds (22–35 seconds)

Questions

- What abnormalities are apparent from the initial laboratory work?
- In a patient with acute (hemorrhagic) pancreatitis, what additional coagulation studies are in order?

Widespread activation of the coagulation pathways can occur as a part of a systemic illness. When severe, it presents as **disseminated intravascular coagulation (DIC)** with life-threatening intravascular clotting and fibrinolysis. This can result in sufficient platelet and coagulation factor depletion to cause severe bleeding. Other conditions are associated with lower-grade DIC or a process that is limited to platelet thrombus formation (**so-called platelet DIC**). In the latter case, organ damage can be the dominant abnormality. Therefore, it is important to be able to recognize the presence and nature of DIC because it will help to speed the diagnosis, prevent organ damage, and manage the patient's bleeding tendency.

THROMBOSIS AND THROMBOLYSIS

Thrombus formation is a highly controlled process, where platelet activation and aggregation, thrombin generation, and subsequent clot formation are under delicate control. Normal endothelial cells adjacent to a site of injury are responsible for limiting platelet activation and aggregation by releasing prostacyclin and nitric oxide and by degradation of adenosine 5′-diphosphate (ADP) by a membrane-associated ADPase (Figure 35–1). **Tissue factor pathway inhibitor (TFPI)** limits activation of factor X by binding to the TF-VIIa-Xa complex.

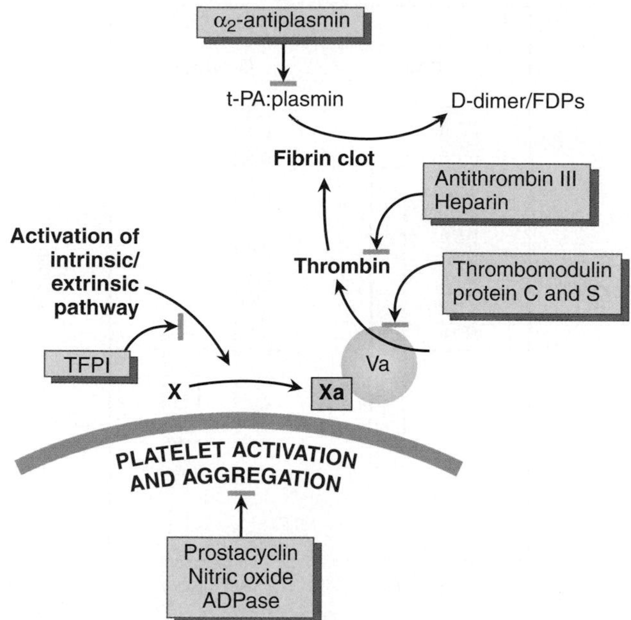

FIGURE 35–1. **Thrombosis and thrombolysis.** The rush to fibrin clot formation in a consumptive coagulopathy is counteracted by several inhibitors. Endothelial cells release prostacyclin, nitric oxide, and ADPase to inhibit platelet activation and aggregation. Tissue factor pathway inhibitor (TFPI) inhibits factor X activation by binding to the TF-VIIa-Xa complex. In addition, thrombomodulin is induced by endothelial cells after activation by thrombin, and thrombomodulin catalyzes conversion of protein C to its activated form, which then downregulates thrombin formation through cleavage of factors V and VIII. Protein S is a cofactor in this reaction. Antithrombin directly inhibits thrombin, and this reaction is accelerated by heparan sulfate molecules expressed on the surface of endothelial cells. Finally, fibrin clot can be dissolved by the t-PA–driven plasmin system. The rate of fibrinolysis is assessed from the levels of α_2-antiplasmin, the inhibitor of plasmin, and D-dimer.

At the same time, circulating thrombin is inactivated by **antithrombin**, a specific protease inhibitor. This reaction is facilitated by exogenous heparin and endogenous heparan sulfates, heparin-like molecules produced by endothelial cells. In addition, endothelial release of thrombomodulin after thrombin activation effectively downregulates thrombin activity by activating protein C, which then cleaves factors Va and VIIIa. Protein S is a cofactor in this latter reaction.

Formation of the fibrin clot is also carefully controlled. **Tissue plasminogen activator (t-PA)** produced by endothelial cells activates plasminogen incorporated within the clot to the active protease, plasmin. Plasmin facilitates fibrin clot degradation. The end result is localized fibrinolysis and remodeling of the clot. Runaway fibrinolysis and destruction of fibrinogen is prevented by a circulating inhibitor of plasmin, α_2-antiplasmin, blockade of t-PA by plasminogen activator inhibitor-1 (PAI-1), and thrombin activatable fibrinolysis inhibitor (TAFI).

An understanding of these interactions provides a framework for the diagnosis of a consumptive coagulopathy. Normal individuals maintain levels of platelets and coagulation factors within a relatively narrow normal range. When the coagulation pathways are strongly activated, the number of circulating platelets and the level of individual factors are maintained as long as marrow and liver synthetic capability, respectively, can compensate for consumption of cells and factors. Platelets and factor levels will decrease if there is compromised production or when the severity of the consumptive process outstrips production. In addition, increased fibrinolysis is a significant contributor to the consumptive coagulopathy.

CLINICAL FEATURES

A consumptive coagulopathy may present with symptoms and signs of organ damage secondary to microvascular thrombosis or as an abnormal bleeding tendency, or both. Often the pattern of the coagulopathy is characteristic of the underlying systemic illness. For example, patients with widespread malignancy are at increased risk for thromboembolic disease and chronic low-grade DIC. In contrast, septic patients or women with an abruptio placentae or amniotic fluid embolism will more often demonstrate acute, severe DIC and a bleeding diathesis. It is extremely important, therefore, to evaluate the patient for both thrombotic and hemorrhagic manifestations typical of DIC (Table 35–1).

Thrombosis of the microvasculature is characterized by multifocal neurologic signs, skin infarction, acute renal shutdown, acute respiratory distress syndrome, and bowel infarction. Marked reductions in coagulation factors and platelets result in a combination of petechial hemorrhages and widespread purpura, mucous membrane bleeding, oozing around central lines and venipuncture sites, gastrointestinal (GI) and genitourinary (GU) bleeding, and even intracerebral hemorrhage. In some patients, intravascular fibrin deposition results in red blood cell fragmentation and sufficient hemolysis to produce an anemia (microangiopathic hemolytic anemia); the peripheral smear may demonstrate schistocytes as a result of red cell fragmentation.

TABLE 35–1 • Signs and symptoms of consumptive coagulopathies

Microvascular thrombosis	
Neurologic	Seizures, delirium, coma, multifocal cortical infarction
Pulmonary	Hypoxemia, acute respiratory distress syndrome
Renal	Oliguria, renal insufficiency or failure
Gastrointestinal	Mucosal ulceration, bowel infarction
Skin	Skin infarction, digital gangrene
Bleeding manifestations	
Neurologic	Hemorrhagic infarction, intracerebral bleeding
Pulmonary	Pulmonary hemorrhage
Renal	Hematuria
Gastrointestinal	Mucous membrane and intestinal bleeding
Skin	Petechiae, purpura, epistaxis, generalized oozing from venipuncture sites and wounds

The importance of the clinical setting cannot be overemphasized. The common association of platelet consumption or DIC with severe, systemic illnesses should be enough to stimulate a full evaluation of the coagulation pathways as a part of the patient's management. This situation is certainly true if the patient exhibits any signs of unexplained organ failure or abnormal bleeding.

Laboratory Studies

To properly evaluate a patient for DIC, a battery of coagulation tests should be ordered including, at a minimum, a platelet count, prothrombin time (PT), partial thromboplastin time (PTT), fibrinogen, and test(s) for D-dimer or fibrin degradation products (FDP). At tertiary care centers, tests for both antithrombin and α_2-antiplasmin levels also can be obtained; there is some evidence that antithrombin levels may be prognostic for outcome in DIC, but it is unclear that low antithrombin may predict early phases of DIC. The blood film should be examined for red cell fragmentation and any abnormal cell forms. By performing these tests at one time, it is possible to get the truest picture of the balance between coagulation factor consumption and fibrinolysis. The DIC picture can change very rapidly. Therefore, when tests are drawn at separate times, it will be difficult to interpret the results.

The diagnosis of DIC cannot be made from any single observation or laboratory measurement. Rather, it is based on the concordance of the right clinical setting and repeated examination for laboratory evidence of aggressive coagulation and fibrinolysis. In patients with **high-grade DIC**, the consumption of platelets and coagulation factors exceeds production capacity, resulting in thrombocytopenia and a decline in the levels of key coagulation factors, including fibrinogen. This condition is assessed clinically with **measurements of platelet count, PT, PTT, and fibrinogen**. Usually there is a balanced simultaneous reduction in cells and coagulation factors in that the platelet count falls to below 50,000–100,000/μL, both the PT and PTT are modestly prolonged, and the fibrinogen falls below 100 mg/dL. The more severe the DIC, the lower the platelet count and fibrinogen level. In patients with **low-grade DIC**, increased production levels of platelets and coagulation factors may be sufficient to compensate for the consumption. This increase makes the diagnosis more difficult. In fact, chronic low-grade DIC may only be diagnosed at some tertiary centers with **radiolabeled turnover studies of platelets and/or fibrinogen**. Alternatively, empiric therapy for low-grade DIC (including systemic anticoagulation) may be required to actually make the diagnosis and relieve symptoms.

The **fibrinolytic component of DIC** is assessed by measurements of the thrombin time (TT), D-dimer or circulating FDP, and the antithrombin and α_2-antiplasmin levels. Fibrin split-products can be detected with the **latex agglutination measurement of fibrin(ogen) degradation products (FDPs)** while the **D-dimer assay measures a specific fibrin split-product**. The latex agglutination assay for FDP is sensitive, but it is a subjective assay that is poorly specific for fibrin breakdown. By

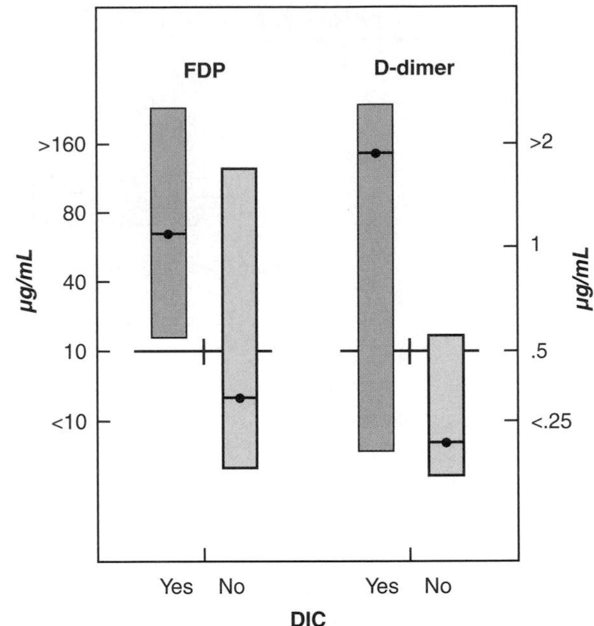

FIGURE 35–2. **FDP and D-dimer levels in patients with DIC.** Measurement of the FDP level is very sensitive to the presence of fibrinolysis in patients with DIC. It lacks specificity, however. Patients with liver disease and other systemic illnesses can have FDP levels well above 10 μg/mL (left-hand y-axis). However, the D-dimer assay is more specific but somewhat less sensitive. Levels greater than 1 μg/mL (1,000 ng/mL, right-hand y-axis) are only seen in patients with severe DIC. The D-dimer assay can fall within the normal range in patients with less severe disease.

contrast, the D-dimer test is quantitative and highly specific for fibrin clot lysis (Figure 35–2). The TT can be used as another indicator of active fibrinolysis; high levels of FDP in circulation will prolong the TT. When taken together, these readily available tests have been used in validated scoring systems to identify most patients with DIC who have known underlying risk factors (Table 35–2).

Assays for antithrombin and α_2-antiplasmin may also provide valuable information regarding **severity of the DIC**. As the specific inhibitor of thrombin, **antithrombin** is progressively depleted with high levels of thrombin activation. Similarly, **α_2-antiplasmin** as the inhibitor of plasmin is depleted with increased rates of fibrinolysis. Depressions of both antithrombin and α_2-antiplasmin to below 40%–50% of normal suggest severe, ongoing DIC. Normal levels of both inhibitors suggest consumption limited to platelets, low-grade DIC, or recovery from a time-limited episode of DIC. In the latter case, antithrombin and α_2-antiplasmin levels recover quickly once the stimulus for intravascular coagulation is removed and fibrinolysis ceases. Since α_2-antiplasmin has a somewhat faster recovery, a disparity can exist between the 2 levels, that is, an antithrombin level below 40%–50% and an α_2-antiplasmin level approaching normal. This situation typifies the patient who had a discrete DIC episode some 12–24 hours before the evaluation. By 48 hours after a limited DIC episode, both levels should be back to normal.

TABLE 35–2 • Modified scoring system for diagnosis of overt DIC[a]

Test	Score = 0	Score = 1	Score = 2
Platelet count	>100,000/μL	50–100,000/μL	<50,000/μL
FDP/D-dimer	Normal levels	Modest elevation	Highly elevated
Prothrombin time	<3 s above normal range	3–6 s above normal range	>6 s above normal range
Fibrinogen	>100 mg/dL	<100 mg/dL	

[a]*Total score ≥5 compatible with DIC.*

DIFFERENTIAL DIAGNOSIS

The differential diagnosis of a severe consumptive coagulopathy is relatively straightforward. **DIC resulting in abnormal bleeding** because of thrombocytopenia and hypofibrinogenemia is easily recognized from both the clinical setting and the pattern of laboratory abnormalities. It most often accompanies a severe systemic illness (Table 35–3). Sepsis, shock, crush injury or surgical trauma, widespread malignancy, hemorrhagic pancreatitis, or an obstetric complication such as eclampsia, intrauterine fetal death, amniotic fluid embolism, or abruptio placentae are **common clinical settings** where DIC occurs with some frequency. These situations generally involve massive exposure of tissue factor (endotoxin with hypotension; trypsin with pancreatitis; and cellular thromboplastin with trauma, surgery, or amniotic fluid embolism) to the blood and the attendant activation of circulating coagulation factors. The presence of any one of these conditions, therefore, should raise the possibility of DIC. Detection of the typical laboratory profile of DIC should then confirm the presence and severity of the illness.

TABLE 35–3 • Diseases associated with consumptive coagulopathies

Platelet consumption

- Vasculitis (antiphospholipid syndrome)
- Thrombotic thrombocytopenic purpura
- Hemolytic uremic syndrome
- Intravascular prosthetic devices
- Anti-neoplastic therapy/stem cell transplant

Disseminated intravascular coagulation

High-grade DIC
- Septicemia
- Acute promyelocytic leukemia
- Transfusion reaction (ABO mismatch)
- Crush injury
- Hemorrhagic pancreatitis
- Obstetric complications (eclampsia, abruptio placentae, amniotic fluid embolism)
- Snake venoms
- Prothrombin complex concentrate (PCC) administration

Low-grade DIC
- Metastatic and other malignancies (breast, lung, GI)
- Vasculitis
- Chronic inflammatory disorders
- Paroxysmal nocturnal hemoglobinuria (PNH)
- Giant hemangiomas (Kasabach-Merritt syndrome)
- Eclampsia (pregnancy-induced hypertension)
- Retained fetus

Isolated platelet consumption (so-called platelet DIC) is seen most often in patients with vascular disorders such as vasculitis, hemolytic uremic syndrome (HUS), and thrombotic thrombocytopenic purpura (TTP; see Chapter 31). Usually, these patients present with symptoms and signs of organ damage, including renal failure from glomerular thrombosis, skin necrosis, and multifocal microinfarcts in the brain. Red blood cell hemolysis owing to fragmentation by platelet and fibrin thrombi is common in platelet DIC and is most marked in patients with HUS/TTP. Platelet consumption resulting in thrombocytopenia has also been reported with adenoviral infection. This may be due to direct platelet activation by the virus or be mediated by endothelial release of ultralarge von Willebrand factor (vWF) multimers, similar to the pathophysiology of TTP. Platelet consumption could therefore complicate eventual gene therapy modalities that employ adenoviral gene transfer vectors. Importantly, platelet consumption under the above conditions almost never leads to bleeding as a major manifestation, even when the platelet count falls to less than 20,000/μL.

Association with Multidrug Chemotherapy or Stem Cell Transplantation

A high level of platelet consumption is also seen in patients who receive multidrug chemotherapy or undergo stem cell transplantation. In this situation, drug-related endothelial cell damage may well be responsible for increased platelet turnover. Add to that the megakaryocyte damage secondary to myeloablative chemotherapy and it is no wonder that platelet counts are the last to recover following transplantation. It can be difficult to attain good post-transfusion increments of platelets for several weeks; platelets are rapidly consumed in these patients even in the absence of sepsis or alloimmunization.

Organ Damage Versus an Atypical Clinical Presentation

When a patient presents with the constellation of symptoms typical of vasculitis (see Chapter 31), TTP, or HUS, it can be assumed that the thrombocytopenia is the result of vascular consumption, so-called platelet DIC. However, when the **clinical presentation is atypical**, the diagnosis of vascular platelet consumption can be difficult and only approached by ruling out other possible causes of thrombocytopenia, including defects in platelet production (loss of megakaryocytes from the marrow) and immune destruction (autoimmune disorders, such as idiopathic thrombocytopenic purpura). This situation requires a more extensive laboratory workup, including a marrow aspirate and biopsy for the presence of megakaryocytes and blood measurement of reticulated platelets. Besides TTP, the clinician must also consider the possibility of heparin-induced thrombocytopenia so laboratory studies for ADAMTS13 activity and antibody to the heparin-PF4 complex, respectively, may be warranted.

Association with Severe Sepsis

Severe sepsis is often accompanied by a consumptive coagulopathy. With septic shock, the onset and severity of the coagulation abnormalities can be dramatic, resulting in both a bleeding diathesis and life-threatening organ damage secondary to widespread thrombus formation. Bacteria are capable of activating coagulation factors in both the extrinsic and intrinsic pathways. Gram-negative bacteria release endotoxins that can induce tissue factor (TF) expression to drive factor VII and X activation, and TF levels in sepsis patients have been shown to be markedly elevated. Activation of the intrinsic pathway by direct binding of contact factors (kallikrein, high-molecular-weight kininogen, and factors XI and XII) to the surface of bacteria has also been implicated in both coagulation factor consumption and, because of release of bradykinin, septic shock. The marked fibrinolysis that accompanies activation of the coagulation pathways adds to the problem. Rapid depletion of fibrinogen, platelets, and coagulation factors contributes to the bleeding tendency, whereas eventual exhaustion of plasminogen and plasmin levels contributes to widespread fibrin deposition and further vascular/organ damage.

Low-Grade Disseminated Intravascular Coagulation

Low-grade DIC is even harder to diagnose. Although many patients with solid tumors can have some degree of DIC, this is rarely severe enough to lead to organ damage or abnormal bleeding. Moreover, routine coagulation tests do not show a pattern typical of platelet or coagulation factor consumption and fibrinolysis. Many patients have very mildly abnormal laboratory studies, including slight reductions in the platelet count; modest prolongations of PT, PTT, or TT; and a fibrinogen measurement that may be in the normal range but is lower than expected for the patient's disease state. It is important to remember that fibrinogen is an acute phase reactant and tends to increase to levels in excess of 600 mg/dL in patients with inflammatory illness or malignancy. A fibrinogen level of 200–300 mg/dL in such a patient must be regarded as a lower than expected level. The D-dimer assay provides perhaps the most sensitive and specific assay for low-grade DIC in these patients.

Some patients with occult visceral malignancies will have antecedent or concomitant thromboembolism (TE), generally referred to as Trousseau syndrome. These tumors often, but not exclusively, secrete mucins, which induce activation of the coagulation system; tissue factor activity within the tumor itself or induction of cellular tissue factor expression is another mechanism by which such tumors cause a consumptive coagulopathy. In those patients who present with idiopathic TE without evidence of a malignancy, aggressive evaluation to detect an occult cancer does not appear to be efficacious; malignancy is not detected at a greater rate, and most importantly, overall survival and morbidity are not improved by an exhaustive workup. For those patients who already have an established cancer, TE risk is clearly increased for carcinomas of the lung, breast, and GI tract, and with metastatic solid tumors or hematologic malignancies. Inherited risk factors (factor V [FV] Leiden and prothrombin *G20210A*) for thrombosis (see Chapter 36) double the TE risk in such patients.

Significant Liver Disease

Confusion about the diagnosis of DIC arises whenever significant liver disease is present. The production of many of the coagulation factors, including fibrinogen, antithrombin, and α_2-antiplasmin, depends on normal liver function. Moreover, clearance of FDP and D-dimer fragments is liver dependent. Therefore, even in the absence of DIC, it is possible to see thrombocytopenia (due to hypersplenism from portal hypertension); prolongation of the PT and PTT (decreased liver production of coagulation factors); hypofibrinogenemia and dysfibrinogenemia (decreased hepatic protein synthesis); TT prolongation, accumulation of FDP, and elevated D-dimer (decreased clearance of split-products); and modest depressions of antithrombin and α_2-antiplasmin (poor hepatocellular synthetic function). Patients with severe liver disease can also have a component of low-grade DIC that further complicates management by increasing factor and platelet clearance such that blood product transfusion is less effective.

THERAPY AND CLINICAL COURSE

The overriding principle in the treatment of DIC is targeting management to the underlying illness. For those conditions where there is rapid, effective therapy (eg, bacterial sepsis, acute promyelocytic leukemia) or an obstetric complication, immediate treatment of the cause is the most important first step. This treatment will remove the impetus to ongoing DIC and allow the normal production capacity of the marrow and liver to correct the deficiencies of individual coagulation factors. Any attempt to replace coagulation factors by blood component transfusion without treating the basic illness will, at best, simply maintain the status quo without clearly benefiting the patient, and at worst runs the risk of adding fuel to the DIC fire.

Transfusions for Severe Disseminated Intravascular Coagulation

If the patient presents with severe DIC and a life-threatening bleed, treatment of the basic illness and the replacement of coagulation factors and platelets go hand-in-hand. As soon as the therapy for the systemic illness is begun, these patients need to have aggressive transfusion with platelets, cryoprecipitate, and fresh

CASE HISTORY • Part 2

The patient presents with a clinical picture typical for recurrent acute pancreatitis, supported by elevations in both serum amylase and lipase. He also exhibits a moderate anemia and leukocytosis with an elevated serum lactic dehydrogenase (LDH) and positive Turner sign (hemorrhagic discoloration of both flanks), suggesting a major intra- and/or retroperitoneal hemorrhagic/hemolytic component. Screening coagulation tests reveal a low platelet count and slight elevations of the PT and PTT.

Hemorrhagic pancreatitis complicated by peritoneal bleeding is often associated with a marked consumption of platelets and coagulation factors. This is a life-threatening complication and demands immediate attention, starting with a full DIC coagulation panel.

The results in this patient are as follows:

Platelet count - 90,000/μL
Repeat PT with a mixing study - no evidence of a circulating anticoagulant
PTT = 46 seconds (22–35 seconds)
TT = 60 seconds (25–30 seconds)
Fibrinogen = 120 mg/dL
D-dimer = 980 ng/mL (<500 ng/mL)
Antithrombin = 40%
α_2-Antiplasmin = 25%

• BLOOD SMEAR MORPHOLOGY

Normocytic, normochromic with small numbers of fragmented red blood cells, polychromasia, and increased numbers of granulocytes.

Questions

- What coagulation defect is apparent from this panel of tests?
- Can you estimate the severity of the abnormality and recommend appropriate therapy?

frozen plasma (FFP), in that order of importance. Platelet transfusions offer the best chance of gaining control of the patient's microvascular bleeding, especially when it is manifest as widespread skin, mucous membrane, GI, and vital organ bleeding.

Replacement of fibrinogen by transfusing cryoprecipitate is also important. In the patient with a fibrinogen level below 50–100 mg/dL, bleeding is hard to control without transfusions of sufficient cryoprecipitate to raise the fibrinogen level to above 100–200 mg/dL. In a 70-kg patient with a total blood volume of 5 L (plasma volume of approximately 3 L), transfusion of 10–12 U of cryoprecipitate should raise the fibrinogen level above 100 mg/dL. However, since it is hard to predict the result of a single transfusion, repeated measurements of the plasma fibrinogen should be used to guide therapy. Correction of other factor deficiencies is less critical than ensuring adequate fibrinogen levels. If the PT and PTT are very long, the patient can be given 4–6 U of FFP, which is sufficient to increase the overall level of coagulation factors by more than 30%, but this treatment will need to be repeated every 4 hours in order to maintain levels of the factors with the shortest half-life in plasma (factor VII).

Treatment of Severe Sepsis and Septic Shock

Specific attempts to inhibit coagulation and fibrinolysis in severe sepsis and septic shock patients have met with limited success. Both TFPI and antithrombin have been shown to inhibit thrombin formation and ameliorate the coagulopathy, but it is unclear that either has a significant effect on overall survival. Activated protein C has been shown to convey a significant, albeit small, survival advantage in septic patients. Other potential inhibitors under investigation include C1 inhibitor, thrombomodulin, protein S, and C4b-binding protein, but none are ready for clinical use.

Treatment of Less Severe DIC

When the DIC is less severe and the patient does not demonstrate a severe bleeding tendency, therapy of the primary illness should be initiated and factor replacement can be withheld. Once the stimulus is removed, normal marrow and liver production capacities will usually correct the laboratory abnormalities within 24–48 hours. Anticoagulation with heparin is not recommended for treating general DIC, except in very specific hypercoagulable pathologies that lead to marked factor consumption, such as homozygous protein C–deficient children who develop widespread skin and digit necrosis (purpura fulminans; see Chapter 36) or patients with Trousseau syndrome. In the latter, treatment with unfractionated heparin appears to be more effective than low-molecular-weight heparins (LMWH), direct thrombin inhibitors, or warfarin. Some of the therapeutic effect of unfractionated heparin may be due to its longer glycosaminoglycan sequences, perhaps explaining why LMWH and fondaparinux may not be as effective.

CASE HISTORY • *Part 3*

The patient's coagulation panel results are typical for an acute consumptive coagulopathy, almost certainly secondary to pancreatic tissue necrosis and intra/retroperitoneal bleeding. The falling platelet count and low antithrombin and α_2-antiplasmin levels suggest the process is ongoing, and almost certainly is a threat to the patient's survival.

The ideal therapy for this patient is an immediate reversal of the inciting problem—his necrotizing pancreatitis. Unfortunately, gradual resolution over several days while receiving analgesics for pain, intravenous fluids/colloids/blood to prevent further hypovolemia and anemia, and nasogastric suction to decrease gastrin release is the best that can be expected.

His full coagulation panel needs, therefore, to be monitored frequently to guide blood component therapy—especially platelet and coagulation factor support. Platelet transfusions should be given to keep the platelet count above 100,000/μL and a combination of fresh frozen plasma and cryoprecipitate to keep the fibrinogen above 100 mg/dL and the PTT within the normal range.

Treatment of Platelet DIC

Treatment of patients with platelet DIC (vasculitis, TTP, or HUS) involves using several additional therapeutic modalities. For patients with vasculitis who present with thrombocytopenia without signs of organ damage, **prednisone** in a dose of 100–200 mg per day orally or **methylprednisolone** 0.75mg/kg intravenously (IV) every 12 hours may be effective as much as 50% of the time. Patients with TTP and symptoms and signs of organ damage should be treated with aggressive **plasmapheresis with plasma exchange** (see Chapter 31). High-dose methylprednisolone therapy has also been used empirically, assuming the presence of an antibody to ADAMTS13 protease activity.

Patients with HUS, especially children, have a somewhat better prognosis, including a high expectation for complete recovery of renal function. HUS patients with severe renal failure will require **acute hemodialysis** but not plasma exchange, since classic HUS is not related to ADAMTS13 deficiency or inhibition. Patients with a mixed TTP-HUS picture (usually adults or children with streptococcal infection or complement deficiency) are candidates for both plasma exchange and dialysis. **Platelet DIC** patients should not routinely receive platelet transfusions or anti-platelet agents; infusion of platelets can possibly lead to accelerated organ damage, and drugs that inhibit platelet function can lead to more severe bleeding. If there is clear evidence of a life-threatening bleed such as an intracerebral hemorrhage, platelet transfusions should be given.

POINTS TO REMEMBER

Increased consumption of platelets and coagulation factors is seen with a wide spectrum of illness, from acute sepsis or tissue necrosis to disorders of the vessel wall. When severe, the rate of consumption can easily exceed the capacity to regenerate factors and platelets, resulting in so-called disseminated intravascular coagulation (DIC).

Depending on the underlying disease process, the patient may demonstrate bleeding symptoms, thrombosis of vital organs, or both simultaneously. The most common presentation is microvascular and mucosal hemorrhage, including bleeding from the skin at puncture and around intravascular lines, from the oropharyngeal and respiratory mucosa, and from the gastrointestinal tract.

So-called platelet DIC is seen in patients with vascular injury (vasculitis, eclampsia, hemangiomas, TTP, HUS, etc) and is characterized by thrombotic events rather than hemorrhage. Thrombocytopenia without significant prolongation of the PTT or depletion of fibrinogen is the norm.

The laboratory evaluation for DIC requires a panel of tests, including blood smear inspection for red cell fragmentation (schistocytes), platelet count, PT, PTT, TT, fibrinogen level, D-dimer, and, if available, antithrombin and α_2-antiplasmin levels.

Thrombocytopenia (counts <100,000/μL) is one of the earliest signs of DIC, and eventual depletion of factors results in increases in the PT, PTT, and thrombin time (TT). In severe DIC, fibrinogen levels, which normally rise as an acute-phase reactant, will remain in the low-normal range (150–250 mg/dL) or become depleted (<100 mg/dL).

Consumption of factors due to clot formation is only one component of DIC. With runaway thrombin formation, activation of the anticoagulant and fibrinolytic pathways are in high gear. Fibrinolysis contributes to bleeding by rapidly degrading adhesive thrombi and releasing fibrin degradation products (FDP). Measurements of the TT, D-dimer, antithrombin, and α_2-antiplasmin levels are used to evaluate ongoing fibrinolysis.

Severe DIC is most often seen with sepsis, crush injuries, placenta previa, amniotic fluid embolism, ABO mismatched transfusion, and acute promyelocytic leukemia. Low-grade DIC is associated most often with metastatic malignancies.

The management of life-threatening DIC depends on the primary disease. As a rule, DIC cannot be reversed without effective treatment of the underlying disease, for example, antibiotics in the septic patient or evacuation of the uterus in the woman with placenta previa.

The same is true for so-called platelet-type DIC. TTP and HUS (see Chapter 31) are medical emergencies, requiring a high level of diagnostic suspicion and immediate therapy to prevent thromboembolism and major organ damage.

Transfusion of blood products is warranted for DIC, despite evidence that it may not affect outcome and may even fuel continuing DIC. However, it is difficult to withhold transfusion in a bleeding patient. Rational transfusion, emphasizing the order of need for platelets, cryoprecipitate, and fresh frozen plasma, as well as maintaining adequate red cell mass, is critical.

Certain vascular disorders, such as antiphospholipid syndrome or mural thrombus, leading to low-grade or chronic DIC, will respond to systemic anticoagulation. However, anticoagulation for severe DIC accompanied by significant factor depletion is almost always contraindicated since it may exacerbate bleeding and cause life-threatening hemorrhage.

BIBLIOGRAPHY

Blom JW et al: Malignancies, prothrombotic mutations, and the risk of venous thrombosis. JAMA 2005;293:715.

Othman M et al: Adenovirus-induced thrombocytopenia: the role of von Willebrand factor and P-selectin in mediating accelerated platelet clearance. Blood 2007;109:2832.

Rak J et al: Oncogenes, Trousseau syndrome, and cancer-related changes in the coagulome of mice and humans. Cancer Res 2006;66:10643.

Rickles FR: Mechanisms of cancer-induced thrombosis in cancer. Pathophysiol Haemost Thromb 2006;35:103.

Toh CT, Downey C: Back to the future: testing in disseminated intravascular coagulation. Blood Coagul Fibrinolysis 2005;16:535.

Varki A: Trousseau syndrome: multiple definitions and multiple mechanisms. Blood 2007;110:1723.

THROMBOTIC DISORDERS · 36

CASE HISTORY · *Part 1*

A 37-year-old woman presents to the emergency department with a swollen, tender left calf and dyspnea. She noted the development of symptoms 3 days ago, the day following her arrival on a plane trip from Australia to the United States. She admits to pleuritic chest pain but denies cough or fever, and has no significant past medical history. Her only medication is an oral contraceptive. She does not smoke cigarettes or use alcohol. Her parents are alive; her father takes a "blood thinner" medication for an unknown reason.

Examination reveals a diaphoretic white female with tachypnea; positive examination findings include an inspiratory friction rub on the left side of the chest, a swollen left calf with a circumference 50% greater than on the right, and a positive left Homans sign. Vital signs: BP - 100/60 mm Hg, pulse - 115 bpm, resp - 26/min, temp 38°C. Pulse oximetry shows O_2 saturation on room air of 92%.

CBC: Hemoglobin/hematocrit - 13 g/dL/39%
MCV - 88 fL MCH - 31 pg MCHC - 32 g/dL
WBC count - 11,000/μL with normal differential
Platelet count - 310,000/μL
Troponin I <0.04 ng/mL (<0.04 ng/mL)
Pregnancy test - negative
Coagulation studies:
PT = 12.1 seconds (<14 seconds)
PTT = 27 seconds (22–35 seconds)
D-dimer = 1,400 ng/mL (<500 ng/mL)

Questions

- Given this history and physical findings, what diagnosis must be considered?
- Do the screening laboratory tests confirm this diagnosis?
- If not, what further workup is indicated?

Abnormal thrombus formation and thromboembolism can occur secondary to a wide variety of diseases or as a primary hypercoagulable state. The pathophysiologic basis for thrombotic disease includes acquired abnormalities of blood vessels or blood flow, excessive production of thromboplastic substances as with localized tissue necrosis, and inherited abnormalities of coagulation factors. Thus, clinical evaluation of a patient with thrombotic disease involves both a search for a clinical condition that is known for its association with thrombosis or thromboembolism, and laboratory evaluation of the anticoagulant and fibrinolytic pathways.

NORMAL CONTROL OF THROMBUS FORMATION

Thrombus formation is normally limited by several physiologic systems. Excessive platelet aggregation is inhibited at the site of thrombosis by rapid dissipation of platelet stimulatory substances such as adenosine 5′-diphosphate (ADP), thromboxane A_2, and thrombin and direct platelet inhibition by ADPase, prostacyclin, and nitric oxide produced by adjacent normal endothelial cells. Together, these inhibitors limit the size of the platelet thrombus and further activation of coagulation by platelets.

Fibrin clot formation is also controlled by several mechanisms, including antithrombin (AT) inhibition of thrombin, endothelial protein receptor/thrombomodulin-driven protein C/S inactivation of factors Va and VIIIa, tissue factor pathway inhibition, protein Z–dependent protease inhibitor, and fibrinolysis. As shown in Figure 36–1, tissue factor pathway inhibitor (TFPI) stops factor Xa activation of prothrombin by binding to the tissue factor (TF)–factor VIIa-Xa complex. This process acts to limit the procoagulant effect of TF. Protein Z–dependent protease inhibitor, in the presence of protein Z, inhibits factor Xa, resulting in a reduction in thrombin generation. Endothelial cell activation by thrombin releases thrombomodulin, which feeds back in a negative manner to downregulate further prothrombotic effects; once thrombin is bound to thrombomodulin, it can no longer interact with fibrinogen or activate platelets. Circulating AT also avidly binds to thrombin and other serine proteases in the coagulation cascade to neutralize their activity. This reaction is facilitated by heparin-like substances on the endothelial surface, heparan sulfates, just as pharmacologic heparin therapy acts via the AT mechanism.

Protein C activation via its interaction with endothelial protein C receptor (EPCR) and the thrombin/thrombomodulin complex is another important natural anticoagulant pathway.

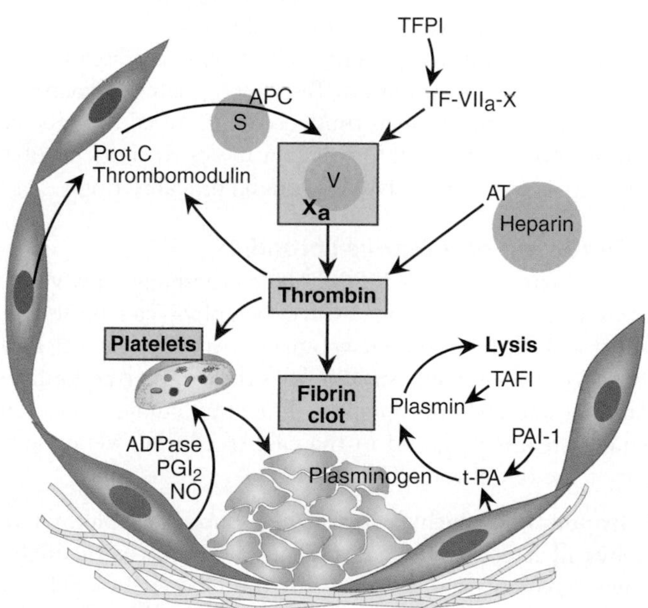

FIGURE 36–1. **Normal prevention of pathologic thrombosis.** Thrombus formation is controlled at several points. Platelet aggregation is inhibited by ADPase, prostacyclin (PGI2), and nitric oxide (NO) released by adjacent normal endothelial cells. Tissue factor pathway inhibitor (TFPI) binds to the TF-VIIa-Xa complex to suppress further TF-driven clotting. Fibrin clot formation is also downregulated by direct inhibition of thrombin by antithrombin (AT) and by activated protein C (APC) inactivation of factors V and VIII (not shown). APC is stimulated in a feedback loop by the interaction of thrombin with thrombomodulin and then facilitated by the cofactor protein S. Finally, the size of the fibrin clot is controlled by fibrinolysis. Endothelial cells release t-PA, which interacts with plasminogen incorporated within the clot to generate plasmin and break down fibrin polymers.

EPCR binding appears to play a role in larger vessels, whereas the thrombomodulin pathway is most active in the microcirculation. Activated protein C (APC), with protein S serving as a cofactor, cleaves factors Va and VIIIa to inhibit the further formation of thrombin. Another important clot-controlling mechanism is **fibrinolysis**. Tissue plasminogen activator (t-PA) produced by endothelial cells activates the plasminogen incorporated in the fibrin clot to form the serine protease, plasmin. This reaction is kept specific for fibrin clot by the high affinity of plasminogen activator for fibrin within the clot. Fibrinolysis is downregulated by the circulating plasminogen activator inhibitor (PAI-1), which counteracts the action of t-PA, and the plasmin inhibitors: α_2-antiplasmin and α_2-macroglobulin. Thrombin-activatable fibrinolysis inhibitor (TAFI) also tends to suppress fibrinolysis by removing carboxy-terminal lysine residues from fibrin to limit plasmin binding to fibrin clot.

A hypercoagulable state can occur because of a defect in any of these normal anticoagulant mechanisms. The most common genetic risk factors are APC resistance secondary to a point mutation of the factor V gene (V Leiden) and prothrombin gene mutation *G20210A*, resulting in increased levels of prothrombin (factor II). Natural anticoagulant (AT, protein C, and protein S) deficiency states, and hyperhomocysteinemia are similarly associated with an abnormal thrombotic tendency. Increased levels of factors VIII, XI, IX, and fibrinogen have also been implicated in both venous and arterial thrombosis. A decreased level of t-PA or increased level of TAFI or PAI-1 may result in a thrombotic tendency. At the same time, venous thrombosis and thromboembolism occur most frequently in association with acquired vessel injury and certain disease states. Coagulation defects responsible for arterial thrombosis include elevations in fibrinogen and levels of the t-PA (antigen)–PAI-1 complex, hyperhomocysteinemia, platelet function defects (the HPA-1b polymorphism of GPIIIa), and the appearance of an antiphospholipid antibody (eg, a lupus anticoagulant).

CLINICAL FEATURES

An abnormal thrombotic tendency can present with symptoms and signs of venous thromboembolism, pulmonary embolism (PE), or occlusion of an arterial vessel.

Deep Venous Thrombosis

Thrombosis involving the deep veins of the leg can be clinically silent, or present with pain and swelling of an extremity. Even when symptomatic, it can be difficult to diagnose. A deep venous thrombosis (DVT) can be accompanied by an inflammatory response with tenderness, warmth, and erythema of the extremity, which makes it difficult to distinguish from other inflammatory disorders such as cellulitis; inflammation of a muscle, tendon, or bone; or a traumatic rupture of a popliteal cyst or the muscle itself following trauma. Moreover, since the physical examination may not clearly separate these conditions, skilled use of tests such as impedance plethysmography, Doppler ultrasound, and contrast venography may be required to diagnose the condition.

Thrombotic disease is not limited to the deep vessels of the extremities and pelvis. Subclavian or external jugular vein thrombosis is not uncommon in patients with indwelling catheters. Spontaneous thrombosis of the subclavian, axillary, or brachial veins usually is the result of strenuous exercise with or without an anatomical defect such as thoracic outlet obstruction. Thrombosis of the renal, hepatic, or mesenteric veins can occur in specific clinical situations. Renal vein thrombosis is associated with nephrotic syndrome and may be in part related to interference with the AT or protein C pathways (or both). Hepatic vein thrombosis is seen with advanced cirrhosis or paroxysmal nocturnal hemoglobinuria (PNH), and after trauma or surgery. Acute mesenteric or portal vein thrombosis is seen in association with PNH, polycythemia vera, essential thrombocytosis, protein C and S deficiency, and antiphospholipid antibodies. Unlike mesenteric artery thrombosis, which presents as an acute abdomen in elderly patients with atherosclerotic disease, mesenteric vein thrombosis generally presents with the gradual onset of insidious abdominal pain and nausea over several weeks. Although mesenteric vein thrombosis usually can be managed effectively with anticoagulation, recurrence is common and mortality high; one-fourth of patients with mesenteric venous thromboembolism (VTE) die during an episode.

Venous Thromboembolism

The estimated incidence of VTE, including pulmonary embolism, is 1–3 per 1,000 individuals each year, although it increases markedly with age to more than 1 per 100 individuals age 85 or older (see Thromboembolism in the Elderly later in this chapter). This translates into 600,000 episodes in the United States each year with up to 200,000 deaths. A pulmonary embolism can occur with little warning, almost always in association with a thrombus in the deep venous system of the thigh or pelvis in response to trauma, surgery, bed rest, other immobilization, pregnancy, a malignancy, or an inherited susceptibility to thrombotic disease. Thrombosis in other locations is an infrequent cause of embolism. Superficial veins of the legs and arms can thrombose because of trauma, irritation by an intravenous infusion or infection, or as a complication of varicose veins, but as long as the deep venous system is not involved, there is little risk of thromboembolism.

Arterial Thrombosis or Thromboembolism

An arterial thrombosis or thromboembolism is easier to diagnose than VTE. Acute occlusion of an arterial vessel is recognized from the symptoms and signs of severe organ ischemia. In the case of the central nervous system, the patient manifests symptoms and signs of a stroke. With occlusion of a coronary artery, patients develop myocardial ischemia and infarction. Peripheral artery occlusions can also result from thrombosis or thromboembolism. Mural thrombi form in the heart in patients with atrial fibrillation or following anterior wall infarctions. These are innately unstable and will shed fragments of clot, which can occlude distal arterial vessels. The brain and kidney are at greatest risk of thromboembolic damage from a cardiac site; less frequently, a large fragment will occlude a major vessel to an extremity. Thromboembolism can also occur as a result of a severely diseased vessel. Platelet and fibrin thrombi form on the surface of atheromatous plaques, break loose, and embolize to the distal branches of the involved vessel. This scenario is common in patients with atherosclerosis of carotid and coronary artery vessels. In some patients, the embolus will actually consist of atheromatous material that breaks loose from the surface of the vessel, so-called cholesterol emboli. An arterial thrombus can also paradoxically originate from a DVT by way of a patent foramen ovale.

Importance of Rapid, Accurate Diagnosis

The importance of rapid and accurate diagnosis of thrombotic and thromboembolic disease cannot be overemphasized. Pulmonary embolism can be prevented in patients with DVT with appropriate anticoagulant therapy. Therefore, every effort should be made to be alert to and evaluate patients at risk for VTE and to take preventive steps in high-risk patients.

In patients with arterial thrombosis or thromboembolism, the speed of diagnosis is the most important component of good management. Fibrinolytic therapy of patients with coronary artery thrombosis can be extremely effective if delivered with minimal delay. Most patients treated with t-PA or streptokinase within 4 hours of the onset of their chest pain demonstrate clot lysis and reduced myocardial injury. Thrombolysis in patients with thrombotic strokes also can be effective if the decision to treat is made early, within the first 1–2 hours.

The evaluation of a patient with thrombotic disease varies according to the presentation. Tests appropriate for diagnosing a DVT are not the same as those used for arterial thromboembolism. Moreover, laboratory evaluation of the anticoagulant pathways is only appropriate in certain clinical settings.

A. Detection of a Venous Thrombus

Three diagnostic tests—impedance plethysmography, venous ultrasonography, and contrast venography—can be used to detect a DVT. From the viewpoints of necessary expertise and cost-effectiveness, plethysmography is the easiest to perform and interpret and also the cheapest. The other studies cost more, require greater skill, and in the case of contrast venography, carry some risk of complications.

1. Impedance plethysmography—Impedance plethysmography will detect occlusive thrombi in the vessels of the thigh or pelvis in patients with symptomatic thrombophlebitis. The test involves inducing temporary venous congestion by inflation and deflation of a thigh blood pressure cuff to look for an impairment of venous drainage from the affected leg. Sensitivity and specificity are improved by repeating the measurement over several days. The method is insensitive to venous thrombosis limited to the calf, and measurements are compromised when there is a defect in arterial flow, an anatomic abnormality of the deep venous system, or venous obstruction from a mass in the abdomen. It is the least invasive test for the detection of iliac vein thrombosis in pregnant women. However, a false-positive result is common during the third trimester owing to compression of the pelvic vessels by the gravid uterus. If this test is used, the pregnant patient should be tested in the lateral recumbent position.

2. Venous ultrasonography—Compression ultrasonography (B-mode and Doppler) can also be used to detect major thrombi in the thigh. It will accurately detect a total occlusion (noncompressible femoral vein) or major partial obstruction that produces a compensatory increase in flow rates around the obstruction. This method is as good as or better than impedance plethysmography for detecting major thrombi in the thigh and for documenting recanalization of veins after a DVT episode. Still, both tests detect DVT in less than 40% of patients with documented pulmonary emboli, reflecting both the accuracy of the method and the fact that not all emboli originate in the leg veins. Like plethysmography, ultrasound is insensitive at detecting thrombi in the calf. Ultrasound can be used to rule out external and common iliac vein thrombosis during the first 2 trimesters of pregnancy, and like plethysmography, the sensitivity of ultrasound is improved by repeating the study over several days. In patients suspected of having a first-episode DVT, a normal repeat ultrasound at 5–7 days effectively excluded a clinically important DVT.

Certain clinical features will increase the likelihood of an abnormal (DVT presence) ultrasound finding, including:

- A cancer diagnosis
- Paralysis or immobilization
- Lower leg cast
- Unilateral leg or calf swelling
- Unilateral pitting edema
- Tenderness along the distribution of the deep venous system

Patients with several of these features will test positive for DVT more than 60% of the time, and the positive predictive value of the test will approach 100%. By contrast, when the clinical probability is low, a negative ultrasound will virtually exclude a thigh DVT, similar to a D-dimer test result below the cutoff value.

Diagnosis of a recurrent DVT can be a problem since compression ultrasound can remain abnormal for up to 1 year in one-half of patients. When this occurs, serial ultrasonography or contrast venography may be necessary. However, persistent abnormal findings by compression ultrasound may also predict increased recurrence risk for VTE and necessitate continuing therapeutic anticoagulation.

3. Contrast venography—Contrast venography is the most definitive method for detecting deep venous thrombotic disease of the lower extremity. It involves the injection of contrast material into a superficial vein on the dorsal surface of the foot to visualize the deep venous system of the calf and thigh. When performed by an expert radiologist, thrombi can be detected as filling defects in major veins, often with evidence of abnormal collateral flow around the obstruction. Major distortions in the venous anatomy can also be defined in patients with chronic disease. When this method is done well, the entire venous anatomy of the leg is visualized. The technique is not without its complications, however; patients can develop phlebitis from the dye.

B. Diagnosis of a Pulmonary Embolism

A pulmonary embolism cannot always be reliably diagnosed from the history, physical examination, or routine studies of lung anatomy and function such as the chest x-ray and blood gas analysis. However, the presence of certain risk factors and physical findings can be used to estimate the clinical probability of an embolus (Table 36–1). This is a useful exercise because it provides a framework for interpreting the lung scan, specifically to analyze the probability of an embolus in the face of an equivocal or nondiagnostic lung scan. Patients are classified as having a low, intermediate, or high pretest clinical probability based on the number and weight of several risk factors (see Table 36–1).

1. Ventilation/perfusion lung scan—Whenever one suspects PE, it is essential to obtain a ventilation/perfusion lung scan. If one compares the distribution of an injected isotope to that of an inhaled isotope, it is possible to identify localized areas of perfusion/ventilation mismatch. If a section of lung appears to have an abnormality in blood flow but normal ventilation, there is a high probability of a pulmonary embolus. A matched perfusion/ventilation defect usually results from scarring or consolidation and is often seen in patients with preexisting lung disease. Lung scans can be safely performed during pregnancy. Radiation exposure to the fetus is minimal, but this can be further reduced by restricting ventilation scanning to those patients who have an abnormal perfusion scan.

Lung scans should be read by the radiologist as high probability, nondiagnostic (which includes older terms, such as intermediate, low probability, and indeterminate), or normal. Overall, the lung scan has a sensitivity of only 41% but a specificity of 97%.

TABLE 36–1 • Clinical probability of a pulmonary embolism

Risk factor		Points
Signs/symptoms of a DVT		3.0
Absence of an alternative diagnosis		3.0
Past history of DVT or PE		1.5
Recent surgery or prolonged bed rest		1.5
Cancer[a]		1.0
Pulse rate >100		1.5
Hemoptysis		1.0
Clinical probability score		**PE risk[b]**
Low	<2	5%–30%
Intermediate	2–6	20%–50%
High	>6	40%–70%

[a]The risk associated with a cancer diagnosis varies with the site and stage of the disease. Widespread malignancy, cancers under treatment, and certain cancer sites (pancreatic cancer, cystadenocarcinomas) are associated with a much higher incidence of thromboembolic complications.

[b]The risk of a pulmonary embolus (PE) in patients with an equivocal or nondiagnostic lung scan.

When the scan shows more than one wedge-shaped, segmental perfusion defect without a matched ventilation defect in a patient with a normal chest x-ray, the probability of PE is greater than 80% (positive predictive value). At the other extreme, a completely normal ventilation/perfusion lung scan virtually excludes a major pulmonary embolus. However, many scans are equivocal and should be read as nondiagnostic. In such patients, there is still a significant probability of a pulmonary embolus, depending on the pretest clinical probability (see Table 36–1).

2. Pulmonary angiography—Management of the patient with an equivocal scan requires judgment on the part of the clinician. If it is important to confirm the diagnosis, pulmonary angiography should be performed. However, this test requires the expertise of either a cardiopulmonary specialist with experience in right heart catheterization or a skilled radiologist. Therefore, the technique should be reserved for the patient who is a diagnostic dilemma or is at high risk of bleeding if exposed to anticoagulant therapy. Patients who have a documented DVT by ultrasound do not need angiography even if the lung scan is negative, since they will need to be treated regardless. At the same time, the sensitivity of compression ultrasonography in detecting a peripheral thrombus in patients without clinical leg findings is very low. Less than 30% of patients who exhibit an embolism following surgery or as a complication of their congestive heart failure or cancer will have a positive compression ultrasonography test if they have a negative physical examination.

3. Helical CT scan with contrast—Helical CT scan with contrast can be used as an alternative to angiography. However, its sensitivity is greatest for proximal emboli in the great vessels of the lung. If it is positive, it is definitive. If negative, angiography is better at detecting distal emboli. Pulmonary angiography can also be of great value in diagnosing patients with multiple small pulmonary emboli that result in pulmonary hypertension. In this situation, the lung scan will generally be indeterminate.

4. Echocardiography—Transthoracic echocardiography has been used as both a diagnostic and prognostic tool. Even when the patient shows no clinical symptoms/signs of hypotension, hypoxia, or congestive heart failure, a transthoracic echocardiogram can show signs of right heart hemodynamic strain. Findings include hypokinesis of the mid-right ventricular wall with normal contraction of the apex, and with massive emboli, right heart dilatation, tricuspid regurgitation, and bulging of the interventricular septum into the left ventricle. The mismatch of normal apex contraction and mid-right ventricular wall hypokinesis has been promoted as an indication for thrombolytic therapy because of its relatively poor prognosis. A high troponin level in patients with right ventricular strain suggests severe dysfunction and can be used as another reason for immediate thrombolysis.

5. Measurement of the D-dimer—Degradation of fibrin clot by plasmin generates specific breakdown products, the E and D-dimer fragments. The negative predictive value of the D-dimer test is its greatest strength. Since most patients with a DVT/PE show an increase in their D-dimer level, a "normal" D-dimer level in a low clinical probability patient rules strongly against clinically significant VTE. A D-dimer level less than 500 ng/mL (<0.5 μg/mL) by enzyme-linked immunosorbent assay (ELISA), together with a negative impedance plethysmography or ultrasound examination in patients who present with a low pretest probability for PE, has a negative predictive value between 96% and 99.6%, and therefore virtually rules out PE. Moreover, because the D-dimer level is elevated in patients with DVT, it can also be used to exclude a clinically significant DVT in relatively asymptomatic patients without VTE risk factors (again, low probability). Each laboratory must establish its own cutoff D-dimer assay value in order to exclude VTE in low probability patients; this threshold will often be within the normal range of the assay. For example, the reference range for D-dimer in healthy outpatients may be 0.5–2.5 μg/mL for a turbidometric assay, but the cutoff value for excluding VTE in low probability patients ranges from 1.3–1.6 μg/mL. A negative D-dimer result in hospitalized patients or cancer patients cannot be used to exclude DVT/PE, since by definition, these patients cannot be characterized as low probability.

Guidelines for the diagnostic workup of PE—Given this panoply of tests, the following is a list of proposed guidelines according to the clinical probability of a pulmonary embolus:

- **High Clinical Probability.** The prevalence of a PE in patients with a high clinical probability (score >6) is 70%–90%. A lung scan or helical computed tomography (CT) scan is the study of choice, and a positive (high probability or diagnostic) scan will confirm the diagnosis with greater than 95% certainty. If the scan is reported as nondiagnostic (intermediate or low probability), angiography should be considered to rule out small distal vessel emboli. When the scan shows clot involving more than one-third of the lungs or the patient is unstable, an echocardiogram should be performed to look for right ventricular hypokinesis. When strain is present, peripheral thrombolysis with recombinant tissue-type plasminogen activator (rt-PA) or urokinase should be considered to restore pulmonary blood flow.

  Because patients with a confirmed DVT by ultrasound need to be anticoagulated anyway, further workup may be considered optional in the otherwise stable, healthy patient, and if a scan is performed, a negative result does not justify discontinuing anticoagulation. The results of the scan may help, however, in making a decision as to hospitalization versus home therapy.
- **Intermediate Clinical Probability.** From 20%–45% of patents with an intermediate clinical probability (score 2–6) turn out to have a PE, and 90% of these have a high probability lung scan, thereby making the diagnosis. A positive ultrasound for DVT further supports the diagnosis. If the lung scan is reported to be nondiagnostic (intermediate or low probability) and the ultrasound is negative, there is still a 10%–20% chance of a PE. In this situation, a normal D-dimer test can be used to rule out either DVT or PE. A positive D-dimer does not, however, make the diagnosis because of the high rate of false positives. Pulmonary angiography is required if the risk of anticoagulation is very high.

- **Low Clinical Probability.** Less than 10% of low clinical probability patients (score <2) are diagnosed with a PE. A negative D-dimer test virtually rules out a PE or DVT. If the D-dimer is elevated, both ultrasound and a lung or helical CT scan should be performed. A positive result for DVT or PE makes the diagnosis and demands anticoagulation.

C. Diagnosis of an Arterial Thrombus

The evaluation of a patient with an arterial thrombus or thromboembolism includes studies of the occluded vessel and a search for a potential embolic source. A Doppler flow study can be used to locate and define the extent of blockage in patients with occlusions of extremity vessels. However, arteriography is almost always required to prepare the patient for surgery, whether thrombectomy or vessel bypass grafting.

Doppler flow studies can also be used to define patency of the carotid vessels and detect atherosclerotic narrowing in patients with cerebral artery thrombosis or thromboembolism. Common sites for atheromas are the junction of the vertebral and basilar arteries, the internal carotid arteries at the level of the carotid sinus, and the bifurcation in the middle cerebral artery. Atheromatous plaques promote thrombus formation at the site and can be a source for both cholesterol and platelet emboli. In patients with neurologic defects, a **CT scan** or magnetic resonance imaging **(MRI)** can help define the site and extent of disease. These studies are also important as guides to therapy by distinguishing between a cerebral infarction secondary to an embolus and a hemorrhagic stroke.

All patients with thromboembolic disease should be evaluated for a **cardiac source for the emboli** and whether or not a patent foramen ovale is present. Mitral valve disease and atrial fibrillation are associated with an increased risk for thrombus formation in the left atrium with subsequent embolization. Even without valvular disease, paroxysmal atrial fibrillation and atrial fibrillation associated with chamber dilatation and heart failure can result in thromboembolism. Mural thrombus formation in patients following acute anterior wall myocardial infarction is another potential source for emboli. If one of these is present, **echocardiography** can be used to document the mural thrombus. However, sensitivity of the measurement is poor and should not be used to rule out a cardiac source for emboli. The decision for anticoagulation must be based on the relative risk of embolization versus bleeding with each condition.

Coronary artery thrombosis is the most common clinical example of arterial thrombosis secondary to atherosclerosis and plaque rupture. Clinical presentation together with electrocardiographic signs of ischemia and infarction are enough to make the diagnosis and initiate thrombolytic therapy. The key role of platelets and coagulation in infarction has also been recognized in the recommendations for the use of aspirin and anticoagulants in management of patients with coronary artery disease. Since **anticoagulant therapy** cannot by itself prevent occlusion in a patient with a severe stenotic lesion, a full workup of the patient with coronary artery disease requires **coronary angiography leading to either angioplasty or bypass grafting.**

TABLE 36–2 • Laboratory testing in thromboembolic disease

Arterial	Venous
Fibrinogen level	Factor V Leiden/APCR
Factor VIII level	Prothrombin *G20210A*
vWF antigen level	Antithrombin deficiency
t-PA:antigen/PAI-I activity	Protein C and protein S deficiency
Platelet function	Dysfibrinogenemia
Lp (a) level	Increased levels of factors XI, IX, VIII, fibrinogen
Increased levels of factors XI, IX, VIII, fibrinogen	Homocysteine level
Homocysteine level	Antiphospholipid antibody/lupus anticoagulant
Antiphospholipid antibody/lupus anticoagulant	

D. Coagulation Studies

The standard laboratory coagulation tests are primarily designed to monitor anticoagulation and to detect the patient with a factor-deficient bleeding tendency. For example, the prothrombin time (PT) and partial thromboplastin time (PTT) are used to detect coagulation factor deficiencies. There are no comparable screening tests for a hypercoagulable state. Certainly, a shortening of the PT or PTT cannot be equated to a thrombotic tendency. Laboratory measurements that are important in the **evaluation of a patient with thrombotic disease** are listed in Table 36–2. They can be roughly divided into risk factors for arterial thrombosis versus those that lead to venous thrombotic disease. Elevated homocysteine levels are associated with both arterial and venous disease. Several markers of prothrombotic activity are available, including prothrombin fragment 1.2, thrombin antithrombin complex, D-dimer, and soluble fibrin polymer. Several studies have now shown elevated levels of these markers in thrombophilic patients. However, they are not yet acceptable for widespread clinical use.

The clinical setting is an important guide for evaluating a hypercoagulable state. Conditions commonly associated with an **increased thrombotic tendency** are listed in Table 36–3. This list includes conditions where there is an abnormality in platelet number or function, endothelial cell function, blood flow, or the activation of the coagulation pathways. Laboratory findings in most of these conditions are nonspecific and not diagnostic. Routine coagulation screening tests are generally normal. One exception to this rule is the patient with essential thrombocytosis and a platelet count greater than 1 million/μL. Thrombocytosis is associated with increased thrombosis risk, although the reverse is also true; these patients can present with an abnormal bleeding tendency owing to platelet dysfunction.

Assays used for detecting an inherited hypercoagulable state—Laboratory testing is of greater value in the diagnosis of patients with an inherited hypercoagulable state (Table 36–4). A deficiency in one of the inhibitors of coagulation can result in a thromboembolic tendency (see Figure 36–1). Therefore, when the clinical presentation is appropriate, specific assays can be ordered to screen for APC resistance (factor V Leiden by mutation

TABLE 36–3 • Conditions associated with a thrombotic tendency

Platelet abnormalities
Thrombocytosis/myeloproliferative disorders
Diabetes mellitus
Hyperlipidemia
Heparin-induced thrombocytopenia
Lupus anticoagulant
Blood vessel defects
Venous disease/stasis/immobilization
Atherosclerosis/myocardial infarction
Atrial fibrillation
Prosthetic surfaces
Hyperviscosity
TTP/HUS/vasculitis
Systemic illness/coagulopathies
Trauma/long-bone fractures
Orthopedic or major surgery
Malignancy
Pregnancy/oral contraceptives
Nephrotic syndrome
Infusion of prothrombin complex concentrates
Fat/marrow embolism after long-bone trauma
Sickle cell disease

TABLE 36–4 • Inherited hypercoagulable states

Factor V Leiden (APC resistance functionally)
Prothrombin *G20210A* gene mutation
Antithrombin deficiency
Protein C and protein S deficiency
Fibrinolytic system defects
Tissue plasminogen activator (t-PA) deficiency
Plasminogen activator inhibitor (PAI) excess
Low plasminogen activity
Dysfibrinogenemia
Hyperhomocysteinemia

analysis), the presence of an antiphospholipid antibody (eg, lupus anticoagulant), and deficiencies of AT, protein C, protein S, t-PA, plasminogen levels (and activity), and fibrinogen function.

Available assays vary in their ease of performance and accuracy. The presence of **factor V Leiden** can be measured indirectly using a functional modification of the PTT. This activated protein C resistance assay compares PTT times with and without the addition of a standardized amount of APC. A low ratio (PTT with APC divided by the PTT without APC) indicates the presence of the Leiden mutation, which is confirmed by a DNA-based assay.

The functional **assay for antithrombin (AT)** is based on heparin-dependent inhibition of either thrombin or factor Xa. The ranges of normal and heterozygote AT values do not overlap, making this a highly sensitive and specific test. In contrast, **assays for proteins C and S** are less accurate and there is considerable overlap of normal and heterozygote levels. To make matters worse, oral anticoagulants will give a false-positive result by lowering the synthesis of active protein C and S. Reference laboratories offer both antigenic and functional assays, with antigenic assays performed as a reflex when functional activity is low.

The **PTT and Russell viper venom time (RVVT)** can be used to screen for a **lupus anticoagulant** (a functionally defined

CASE HISTORY • *Part 2*

The patient presents with a high-probability clinical picture for venous thrombosis and pulmonary embolism (PE), given the swollen left calf, positive Homans sign (calf pain on simultaneous extension at the knee and flexion at the ankle), and several signs of PE including pleuritic pain, tachypnea, the friction rub, and a low oxygen saturation without fever or evidence of infection.

As for the screening laboratory tests, there is no troponin leak indicative of myocardial ischemia, and the D-dimer is significantly elevated, which is compatible with ongoing thrombosis. At the same time, the D-dimer never establishes a diagnosis of venous thrombosis; its principle value is to rule out thrombosis in low-risk patients. Therefore, the patient must undergo an immediate radiologic workup for VTE including chest radiograph, compression ultrasound of the lower extremities, and ventilation/perfusion (V/Q) scanning.

These study results are reported as follows: Chest radiograph shows a small left pleural effusion but no parenchymal abnormalities. Compression ultrasound reveals clot in the left popliteal and femoral veins with extension into the left iliac vein, as well as development of early collateral flow. The V/Q scan demonstrates 2 wedge-shaped areas of mismatch in the left lung and 1 mismatch in the right—read as high probability for PE. An electrocardiogram is also performed; there are no acute ST–T wave changes and no signs of right heart strain.

Questions

- What coagulation tests should be done at this point?
- Are there any tests that should be performed at a later date?
- How should the patient be managed?

type of **antiphospholipid antibody**). For both assays, the lupus anticoagulant (LA) prolongs the clotting time; addition of normal plasma in a 1:1 mixing study will not shorten the clotting time. Addition of excess phospholipid will significantly decrease the clotting time, expressed either as the difference between clotting time values (PTT) or a ratio (RVVT >1.20 is positive in LA). The lupus anticoagulant assays are functional tests for antiphospholipid antibodies; antigenic detection of antibodies can also be performed by **ELISA**. Both tests should be employed if antiphospholipid antibody syndrome is suspected.

DIFFERENTIAL DIAGNOSIS

The diagnostic workup begins with the evaluation of the disease state that is associated with the thrombotic tendency. Often, the clinical situation is enough to define the proximate cause of the thrombosis. When a patient presents with a coronary artery thrombosis, the relationship of the thrombosis to localized atherosclerosis is so strong that a workup of the coagulation pathways is unnecessary. Similarly, the elderly patient with a thrombotic stroke is almost certainly an example of either local vessel thrombosis or embolization from a cardiac source. This situation is not true, however, for a young patient with a stroke where a lupus anticoagulant may be the cause of the thrombosis. Recurrent venous thrombosis or a strong family history of thrombotic disease should also stimulate a more extensive coagulation workup.

The pathophysiology of the thrombotic tendency associated with a specific disease state can be quite complex (see Table 36–3 and Figure 36–1). Hypercoagulability can result from a defect in 1 or several components of hemostasis. A patient with severe venous stasis, or hyperviscosity, can develop a thrombotic tendency even when the coagulation system and inhibitor levels are normal. Paroxysmal nocturnal hemoglobinuria and myeloproliferative disorders, especially polycythemia vera and essential thrombocytosis, are associated with an increased incidence of thrombophlebitis, VTE/PE, and arterial occlusions. Patients with these conditions are also at risk for thrombosis of splenic, hepatic, portal, and mesenteric veins. A common cause of hepatic vein thrombosis (Budd-Chiari syndrome) is the myeloproliferative disorder polycythemia vera. The pathogenesis of the thrombosis in these patients is not clear. Both the thrombocytosis and an abnormality in platelet function may play a role. Increased activation and aggregation of platelets has been postulated as a cause for the hypercoagulable state. Other conditions where platelet function may contribute to both a thrombotic tendency and accelerated atherosclerosis are the hyperlipidemias, hyperhomocysteinemia, and diabetes mellitus.

Malignancy

Patients with certain malignancies can demonstrate a marked thrombotic tendency. Adenocarcinomas of the pancreas, colon, stomach, and ovaries are the leading tumors associated with thromboembolic events. In fact, these malignancies can first present with a single or multiple episodes of VTE or migratory superficial thrombophlebitis. Overall, patients who present with primary thrombophlebitis show a 25%–30% incidence of recurrence, and 20% of these will turn out to have cancer. The pathogenesis of the thrombotic tendency is multifactorial (see discussion of Trousseau syndrome in Chapter 35). Laboratory testing may show no abnormalities, or some combination of thrombocytosis, elevation of the fibrinogen level, and low-grade disseminated intravascular coagulation (DIC). In the latter case, it is assumed that the tumor must be a thromboplastic stimulus to coagulation. Chemotherapy and the placement of central venous catheters are also associated with an increased risk of thromboembolism.

Pregnancy or Oral Contraceptive Use

Pregnancy and oral contraceptive use have been reported to increase the risk of thrombosis. The overall incidence of thrombosis is approximately 1 in 1,500 pregnancies (a 5- to 6-fold increase in relative risk), but is higher in women with an inherited hypercoagulable state, a past personal history of VTE or PE, a positive family history of thromboembolic disease, obesity, those kept at bed rest for a prolonged period, or those who require cesarean section. The risk of VTE/PE is highest during the third trimester and immediate postpartum period, and is a leading cause of maternal death. Of the inherited hypercoagulable states, AT-deficient women are at the greatest risk and require anticoagulation throughout pregnancy. Factor V Leiden and the prothrombin *G20201A* mutation are also associated with thrombosis risk in the peripartum period, but may not be associated with thrombosis prior to that time period, and therefore do not need to be anticoagulated unless they have a history of VTE/PE.

The diagnosis of thromboembolic disease during pregnancy can be difficult. First of all, the clinical probability of a DVT or PE in a pregnant woman presenting with leg pain or swelling, chest pain, or dyspnea is much lower than that of nonpregnant women. In addition, uterine compression of iliac vessels in the third trimester can make impedance plethysmography and compression ultrasound unreliable. Serial testing, when feasible, can improve sensitivity and specificity. Otherwise, a venogram will be necessary in very high-risk patients. The approach to the diagnosis of PE in a pregnant patient does not differ from that of nonpregnant women; ventilation perfusion scans are safe and reliable. Helical CT scans are less desirable because of the higher levels of radiation exposure for the fetus.

The association of **oral contraceptives** with thrombosis and thromboembolism also appears to be multifactorial. Since low-dose estrogen contraceptive pills have been introduced, the incidence has decreased significantly. However, women who also smoke, have a history of migraine headaches, or carry an inherited hypercoagulable defect are at increased risk (up to 30-fold) for venous thrombosis, PE, and cerebrovascular (arterial) thrombosis. However, the relationship between the use of estrogen following menopause and the occurrence of venous or arterial thrombosis is much more complex and the object of ongoing investigation.

Nephrotic Syndrome

Patients with nephrotic syndrome are at risk for thromboembolic disease, including renal vein thrombosis. The explanation for this is unclear. It has been attributed to lower than normal levels of AT or protein C secondary to renal loss of the specific coagulation protein, platelet hyperactivity, abnormal fibrinolytic activity, and higher than normal levels of other coagulation factors. Hyperlipidemia and hypoalbuminemia have also been proposed as possible etiologic factors.

Primary Hypercoagulable States

Inherited defects in coagulation factors or the fibrinolytic system can set the stage for a thrombotic tendency (see Table 36–4). It is possible, furthermore, that all patients who develop a DVT or PE actually suffer from a genetic (but unidentified) predisposition, which varies according to the type of mutation and the coagulation factor involved. The mere presence of a genetic predisposition does not, however, predict that a thrombotic event will occur. This risk depends on the nature of the genetic defect and the presence of provocative factors such as surgery, pregnancy, estrogen use, and local anatomical factors, reflecting the need for a second insult to initiate a thrombotic event. A family history of thrombotic disease is a strong predictor of a genetic predisposition and recurrent thromboembolic disease in other family members. A primary hypercoagulable state can now be identified in up to 70% of patients with a strong family history of thromboembolic disease and in up to 50% of patients without such a history. The relative prevalences of the various congenital defects in VTE patients are shown in Table 36–5. Indications for a full evaluation for an inherited defect include the following:

- Presentation before age 50 without a predisposing factor
- Recurrent thrombotic events
- A strong family history of thromboembolic disease
- A life-threatening thromboembolic event
- Thromboembolism during pregnancy or while taking estrogen

Any testing for a primary hypercoagulable state must take into account the overall clinical picture. As a routine, patients should be tested for factor V Leiden; the *G20210A* prothrombin gene mutation; deficiencies in AT, and proteins C and S; and lupus anticoagulant or antiphospholipid antibodies. At the same time, a full battery of coagulation screening tests should be performed. This will avoid missing a coagulation abnormality that explains lower than normal levels of any of these factors. For example, a patient with liver disease or DIC will demonstrate deficiencies in AT, protein C, protein S, and abnormalities in the fibrinolytic system secondary to defects in coagulation factor production or excessive factor consumption (or both).

TABLE 36–5 • Prevalence of hypercoagulable states in DVT patients

Factor V Leiden	12%–40%
Hyperhomocysteinemia	10%–20%
Prothrombin *G20210A* gene mutation	6%–18%
AT, protein S, or protein C deficiency	5%–15%
Antiphospholipid antibody/lupus anticoagulant	10%–20%

A. Factor V Leiden

APC resistance secondary to the factor V *G1691A* mutation (*Arg506Gln* or Leiden mutation) on chromosome 1 has been detected in 20%–60% of adult patients with a strong family history of thromboembolic disease. The prevalence of the gene mutation in the general population is about 1%–7%, with a wide range for different ethnic groups. Allele prevalence can be as low as 0.5%–2% for Hispanic, African, and Asian populations to as high as 3%–5% in Northern Europeans and 14% in Greeks.

The lifelong risk of thrombosis with factor V Leiden depends on the patient's age; the presence of contributing factors such as surgery, trauma, or pregnancy; and whether the patient is heterozygous or homozygous for the abnormal gene. Leiden-positive individuals generally have a strong family history, and those who are homozygous are at risk for thromboembolism at a young age. Heterozygous factor V Leiden deficiency, by itself, increases the risk of a primary DVT by 4- to 6-fold, not enough to justify anticoagulation without a history of thromboembolic disease. This is not to say that the presence of the Leiden mutation does not confer increased risk. Cerebral vein thrombosis is more common in carriers of the Leiden mutation. Women with the factor V mutation run an increased risk of recurrent fetal loss. Coinheritance of AT, protein C, or protein S deficiency dramatically increases the risk of thrombosis. Once a thrombosis has occurred, the presence of the Leiden mutation helps to make management decisions (see Chapter 37). The risk of recurrent DVT is influenced by coinheritance of the factor V Leiden and *G20210A* prothrombin gene mutations, increasing the risk of recurrent DVT sufficient to consider lifelong anticoagulation. The same is true for other deficiency combinations with Leiden. The Leiden mutation does not appear to be a risk factor for arterial thrombosis.

B. Prothrombin Gene Mutation

Prothrombin is translated by a 21-kb gene located on chromosome 11. A point mutation in the 3′-untranslated region produces a genotype, *G20210A*, which is associated with higher than normal prothrombin levels and an increased incidence of recurrent thrombosis. This genotype can be detected in 18% of patients with strong family histories of thromboembolism. Furthermore, patients with recurrent DVT in the Leiden Thrombophilia Study showed a 6.2% frequency for the *G20210A* mutation, whereas the genotype is seen in only 1%–2% of normal individuals. Women with the mutation also appear to be more susceptible to cerebral vein thrombosis, especially if they use oral contraceptives.

C. Antithrombin Deficiency

Antithrombin (AT) deficiency is inherited as an autosomal dominant trait, with an estimated frequency of 1 per 1,000–5,000 individuals. Typically, a heterozygote patient has an AT level of between 40% and 70% of normal. Two types of AT deficiency can be defined from measurements of antigen and activity levels. **Type 1** patients have low levels of both antigen and activity, whereas **type 2** patients have low activity but normal antigen levels. AT-deficient individuals tend to have recurrent DVT and PE, although not all heterozygotes appear to have difficulty. Unusual sites, such as the cavernous sinus or brachial or mesenteric vein, may be involved. The onset of disease is often associated with factors that promote thrombosis in normal individuals, including venostasis, trauma, pregnancy, and the use of oral contraceptives. Although the trait increases the risk of thrombosis 20-fold, less than 4% of patients with a clinical diagnosis of primary hypercoagulable state will be AT deficient.

D. Protein C or S Deficiency

Proteins C and S deficiencies increase the risk of recurrent VTE usually beginning in the second or third decade of life. Approximately 50% of protein C heterozygotes will develop a thrombosis without a predisposing event by age 50 years. However, just like AT deficiency, the incidence of disease in any family can be highly variable and may require a contributing factor. Compared with factor V Leiden, protein C and S deficiencies are far less common. All together, hereditary deficiencies of AT, protein C, and protein S are responsible for no more than 10% of patients with a primary hypercoagulable state.

E. Hyperhomocysteinemia

Excess levels of homocysteine in plasma are clearly atherogenic and thrombogenic. **Marked hyperhomocysteinemia** (plasma homocysteine levels of >100 μmol/L) is observed in children who are homozygous for a deficiency in cystathionine β-synthase, a rare defect seen in only 1 in 200,000 births. These children demonstrate severe mental retardation, lens and skeletal defects, and a high incidence of both atherosclerotic and thromboembolic disease at an early age.

Moderately elevated levels of plasma homocysteine are seen in association with functional polymorphisms of cystathionine β-synthase, methylenetetrahydrofolate reductase, methionine synthase, and methionine synthase reductase in connection with deficiencies in folic acid, pyridoxine (vitamin B_6), and vitamin B_{12} intake. The normal pathways of homocysteine metabolism are shown in Figure 36–2. The key steps include the conversion of homocysteine to methionine by the acceptance of a methyl group from N^5-methyltetrahydrofolate via methylcobalamin and transulfuration to cystathionine and cysteine. The former reaction is folate and vitamin B_{12} dependent, whereas the conversion to cystathionine is pyridoxine dependent. Therefore, nutritional deficiencies, which are common in processed foods because of the removal of folic acid, vitamin B_6, and vitamin B_{12}, can result in slightly elevated plasma homocysteine levels, 10–16 μmol/L.

In addition, approximately 5% of the general population (38% of French-Canadians) exhibit a thermolabile methylenetetrahydrofolate reductase variant (*MTHFR 677TT* genotype) that is only 50% active. This genotype strongly interacts with low folate levels to produce mild to moderate hyperhomocysteinemia, especially in males. Using a cutoff point of 10 μmol/L, one-third or more of young men have an elevated plasma homocysteine level related to poor folate intake and this enzyme polymorphism. The **presence of an enzyme or vitamin defect** can be further revealed by oral methionine loading and pre-load and post-load plasma homocysteine measurements.

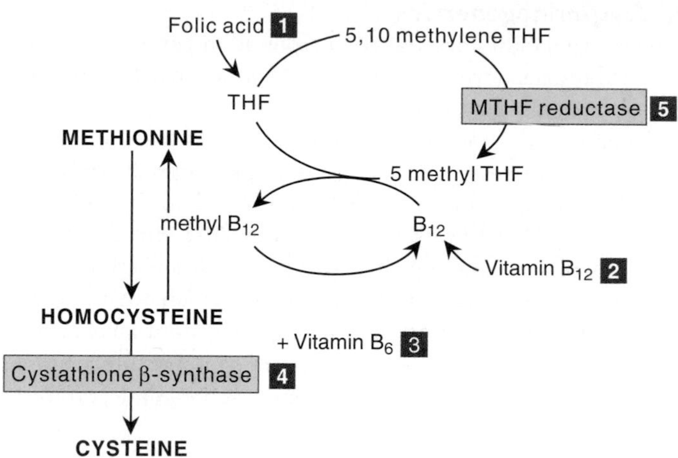

FIGURE 36–2. **The methionine-homocysteine metabolic pathway.** Deficiencies of folic acid (1), vitamin B_{12} (2), or vitamin B_6 (3) can result in elevations of plasma homocysteine, which are readily reversed with vitamin therapy. Patients can exhibit mild to marked hyperhomocysteinemia depending on specific enzyme genotypes and the levels of folate and vitamin B_{12} nutrition; elevated homocysteine occurs with genetic defects in cystathione β-synthase (4), MTHFR (5), or methionine synthase reductase [the latter is not shown here: this enzyme is responsible for the reduction of cob(II)alamin to methylcobalamin; see Figure 8 4].

Patients with an **underlying enzymatic defect** will show an exaggerated irreversible increase in plasma homocysteine levels with methionine loading, whereas the exaggerated response in purely folate-deficient patients can be corrected with folate supplementation.

Mild to moderate hyperhomocysteinemia is an independent risk factor for atherothrombosis, especially coronary artery disease and stroke. Patients with end-stage renal disease routinely show plasma homocysteine levels of 20–30 μmol/L, which are not correctable with folate supplementation, and this factor may play a role in the increased pace of atherosclerosis in these patients. The mechanism behind homocysteine toxicity that leads to atherogenesis is thought to be caused by direct damage to endothelial cells rather than a functional defect that would involve the nitric oxide pathway; this damage results in heightened platelet adhesion, loss of thrombolytic function, and smooth muscle proliferation. Endothelial dysfunction due to high homocysteine levels may also decrease activated protein C, further promoting thrombin generation. Hyperhomocysteinemia in an individual who is heterozygous for factor V Leiden may further increase the risk of thromboembolic disease and fetal loss secondary to placental infarction, although this is still somewhat controversial.

F. Coagulation Pathway Factors

A higher risk of thrombosis has been reported in patients with elevated levels of 1 or more coagulation factors, including factors XI, VIII, IX, and perhaps VII. The mechanism of action may involve the generation of higher than normal thrombin levels, leading to generation of TAFI and, as a result, fibrinolytic-resistant fibrin clot. Very low levels of TFPI also may be a weak risk factor for thromboembolism.

G. Dysfibrinogenemias

Hypercoagulability has also been reported in patients with elevated fibrinogen levels and functional fibrinogen defects (dysfibrinogenemias). The plasma fibrinogen level, by itself, is an independent risk factor for coronary artery disease and acute myocardial infarction. In fact, it is as good a predictor as the low-density lipoprotein (LDL) cholesterol or high-density lipoprotein (HDL) level. Approximately 20% of patients who present with a dysfibrinogenemia will demonstrate a thrombotic tendency and, less frequently, an increased incidence of spontaneous abortion or poor wound healing. Apparent mechanisms include defective plasminogen activation and impaired thrombin binding that allows excess thrombin to circulate and initiate clotting.

H. Impaired Fibrinolysis

Any defect in the functional capacity of plasminogen to be converted to plasmin or in endothelial cell release of t-PA can result in a tendency for arterial and venous thrombotic disease. Furthermore, an increase in the circulating inhibitors of the plasminogen pathway (PAI-1 and TAFI) may be associated with a thrombotic tendency. Both t-PA and PAI-1 are now felt to be markers for future cardiovascular disease in otherwise normal populations. High levels of PAI-1 increase the risk of myocardial infarction by 1.5- to 3-fold.

I. Antiphospholipid Antibodies

An increased tendency to both venous and arterial thrombosis is seen in patients who develop a circulating lupus anticoagulant (part of the spectrum of antiphospholipid antibodies) as a secondary disorder in association with systemic lupus erythematosus or, more often, as a primary syndrome without other manifestation of autoimmune disease. Besides thrombosis, antiphospholipid antibodies have also been associated with recurrent miscarriages. The term "anticoagulant" is, therefore, a clinical misnomer.

Antiphospholipid antibodies are a mix of several IgG, IgM, and less commonly IgA antibodies directed at phospholipid-associated proteins, particularly β_2-glycoprotein I, prothrombin, and annexin V. The antibodies are clinically defined by the method of detection. **Lupus anticoagulant** antibodies are detected by their prolongation of phospholipid-dependent clotting tests, including the PTT and dilute Russell viper venom time (dRVVT), whereas **antiphospholipid antibodies (APLAs)** are measured directly by immunoassay. Thrombotic risk appears to be associated with the presence of a lupus anticoagulant and/or APLA with IgG activity specifically directed at either β_2-glycoprotein I or prothrombin for thromboembolism, or at annexin V for spontaneous abortion.

There is no evidence to support testing for nonstandard APLAs, for example, against phosphatidylethanolamine, phosphatidylcholine, or phosphatidylserine. If the pre-test probability of APLAs is high, for example, recurrent fetal loss without other risk factors, but the laboratory diagnosis fails consensus criteria, retesting at an interval of ≥12 weeks for antibody to β_2-glycoprotein I is warranted. This may also eventually hold true for anti-prothrombin antibodies but requires confirmation.

The pathogenesis of thrombosis and/or recurrent fetal loss with APLAs appears to be multifactorial. Antibody binding to β_2-glycoprotein I may potentiate platelet adhesion and both platelet and endothelial cell activation; this procoagulant stimulus is tipped even further by antibody blocking activated protein C function, possibly through loss of protein S binding. APLAs also disrupt the anticoagulant function of annexin molecules and fibrinolysis in general. Antibodies that activate endothelial cells increase the expression of adhesion molecules to subsequently bind platelets to the endothelial surface, leading to thrombus formation.

The presence of an APLA should be considered in patients with lupus erythematosus, where the prevalence is as high as 30%, even in the absence of thromboembolic complications; in women with recurrent miscarriages; and in the differential diagnosis of both venous or arterial thrombosis, especially if unprovoked or in younger patients without other risk factors. The **initial tip-off to the presence of a lupus anticoagulant** is often a prolongation of the PTT or, much more rarely, the PT, neither of which corrects using a 1:1 mix with normal plasma. This reflects the fact that the antibody inhibits the activity of phospholipid/prothrombin complex in the PTT reaction.

Another commonly used phospholipid-dependent clotting assay for diagnosing a lupus anticoagulant is the Russell viper venom test (RVVT). Like the PTT, this snake venom clotting time is prolonged by the lupus anticoagulant then corrected with addition of excess phospholipid. The RVVT is often expressed as the ratio of the clotting time without phospholipid divided by the time with phospholipid; high ratios (eg, >1.20) are consistent with a lupus anticoagulant.

Up to 20% of patients presenting with VTE not associated with other disease, surgery, or trauma will demonstrate antiphospholipid antibodies. Therefore, along with factor V Leiden and the prothrombin gene mutation, the presence of an antiphospholipid antibody must be considered as one of the top causes of thromboembolic disease in younger individuals and when thrombosis is unprovoked. Patients with lupus anticoagulant (LA) have shown an **increased propensity to thrombosis**, with 30%–60% of patients experiencing one or more thrombotic events during their lifetime. However, without a prior thromboembolic history, the mere presence of APLA or lupus anticoagulant does not justify prophylactic anticoagulation. Thrombotic events are mostly isolated VTE with a lesser incidence of cerebral thrombosis. Coronary, renal, retinal, subclavian, and pedal artery occlusions occur but are uncommon. Patients can also present with "catastrophic antiphospholipid syndrome" characterized by multiorgan failure secondary to widespread small vessel thrombosis, thrombocytopenia, acute respiratory distress syndrome, DIC, and, on occasion, an autoimmune hemolytic anemia. This clinical picture is indistinguishable from that of thrombotic thrombocytopenic purpura (TTP). Bacterial infections often appear to be triggering events for this syndrome.

Women with antiphospholipid antibodies are susceptible to fetal death during the second or early third trimester, and repeated miscarriage is a major clue to the presence of APLAs. The incidence of pregnancy-associated hypertension (preeclampsia and HELLP syndrome) and premature delivery secondary to placental insufficiency is also increased with APLAs.

J. Coronary Artery Disease

Hypercoagulability plays a very limited role in coronary artery occlusion, especially since the relationship of genetic polymorphisms to arterial thrombosis is not as strong as that seen with venous thrombotic disease. Hyperhomocysteinemia has been cited as an independent risk factor for atherosclerosis. Increased fibrinogen levels have been associated with a higher risk for new coronary events, even in the absence of a lipidopathy. A genetic polymorphism in platelet function involving the glycoprotein IIIa polypeptide (HPA-1b) has been reported to increase the risk of coronary thrombosis 6-fold, but its clinical implication is unclear. Fibrinolytic impairment secondary to an increase in t-PA–PAI-1 complex has also been advanced as a risk factor. Finally, elevated levels of factor VIII, as well as the appearance of an antiphospholipid/lupus anticoagulant, may be associated with myocardial infarction or arterial thrombosis in general (see Table 36–2). The **hs–C-reactive protein (CRP)** (high sensitivity CRP—an assay that detects CRP levels in the normal range) predicts a higher incidence of coronary occlusion, and the combination of a high hs-CRP level and increased total cholesterol/HDL cholesterol ratio is associated with a 5- to 10-fold increased risk of a future coronary event, much greater than either risk factor alone. It is now standard practice to measure a metabolic risk panel in middle-aged individuals to gauge coronary artery risk and to recommend intervention for obesity, hypertension, high cholesterol, and high CRP.

PRINCIPLES OF MANAGEMENT

Good management depends on accurate diagnosis. Both the choice and duration of therapy differ greatly according to the nature of the thrombotic disease. As a general rule, patients with venous thrombosis or cardiac mural thrombi should immediately receive intravenous heparin and then change to full-dose warfarin therapy. In contrast, patients at risk for coronary artery or cerebrovascular thrombosis are best managed with a platelet inhibitor such as aspirin and/or clopidogrel (see Chapter 37).

Venous Thrombosis

The best management of venous thromboembolic disease (VTE) is prevention. This begins with a careful assessment of risk factors for DVT, including patient age, prior episodes of DVT or PE, paralysis, long-bone fractures, malignancy, obesity, congestive heart failure, estrogen use, and the presence of a primary hypercoagulable state. It also recognizes the thromboembolic potential of trauma and surgery, especially orthopedic and neurosurgery. Hip and knee replacement surgery in patients who do not receive prophylaxis is associated with a greater than 50% incidence of VTE and a 6% fatal PE rate. This is reduced to less than 10% for VTE and less than 0.2% for PE mortality by prophylaxis with low-molecular-weight heparin (LMWH) or low-dose coumadin. Elastic stockings or intermittent pneumatic compression of the lower legs can also help reduce the incidence of VTE. Patients with a history of prior episodes of VTE or PE, or a hypercoagulable state, must receive prophylaxis, preferably with LMWH.

A. Location and Extent of the Thrombotic Disease

In managing patients with a venous thrombosis, the location and extent of the thrombotic disease is a major guide to planning therapy. When the thrombus is limited to superficial veins of the leg or the deep veins of the calf, there is little risk of a pulmonary embolus. These patients can be managed with simple bed rest, a nonsteroidal anti-inflammatory drug, and support hose. At the same time, patients with symptomatic calf DVTs are at risk of developing chronic venous insufficiency, and it can therefore be of benefit to treat with anticoagulation. The availability of LMWH makes it feasible to give these patients 10–14 days of therapy at home, avoiding a costly hospitalization.

When the thrombus resides in the deep veins of the thigh, the patient is at risk for PE and should receive full-dose anticoagulation with heparin, either weight-adjusted LMWH, corresponding to an anti-Xa level of 0.6–1.0 IU/mL for Lovenox or Fragmin, or unfractionated heparin, adjusted to achieve a therapeutic PTT. This regimen is overlapped with beginning warfarin to achieve an international normalized ratio (INR) of 2.0–3.0, such that heparin may be discontinued once the INR is therapeutic for 48 hours. In general, warfarin is then continued for at least 3–6 months or longer, and this interval determination is becoming more of an individualized decision based on the relative risks of recurrent VTE versus major hemorrhage (see Chapter 37) rather than on a population-based recommendation. The incidence of recurrent VTE and/or PE is highest during the first 6–12 months after discontinuing anticoagulation, but the risk of a second VTE, depending on the patient's risk factors, can continue to be high for years. Population-based recommendations clearly favor prolonging anticoagulation; in trials comparing 6 weeks versus 6 months of warfarin, the rate of recurrence was reduced by 50% by the latter. For a first-episode idiopathic VTE, warfarin for more than a year resulted in a 95% reduction in recurrence compared with a 27% per patient year recurrence rate in those who stopped anticoagulation after 3 months. However, anticoagulation is continuously associated with the risk of a major bleeding episode of up to 3% per year.

Based on these studies, recommendations regarding the length of therapy can be modified according to the relative risk of recurrence, whether high, moderate, or low. Patients who develop VTE in association with trauma, surgery, a fracture, or bed rest generally have a low risk of long-term recurrence (<5%) and can be treated for only 3 months. Patients who develop VTE without a provocative factor or who have a weak risk factor (eg, estrogen use) still have a less than 10% incidence of recurrence and can be conservatively anticoagulated for 6 months. New studies have recently suggested modifying the interval of treatment for such patients based on individual assessments of D-dimer levels and imaging of venous patency and recanalization.

High-risk patients, however, are a different story. When a patient has had more than one VTE, a life-threatening PE, or suffers from VTE with an advanced malignancy, the risk of recurrence is greater than 10%–20%. These individuals deserve to be anticoagulated for an indefinite period unless they develop an increased risk for bleeding complications that clearly outweighs the thrombotic risk.

B. Ileofemoral Thrombosis

Thrombolytic therapy has been used in patients with ileofemoral venous thrombosis, where the risk of postphlebitic venous insufficiency is extremely high. Peripheral streptokinase use is effective less than 25% of the time, most likely because the thrombosis often completely occludes the vein, preventing the drug from reaching the clot surface. Catheter-delivered urokinase can be more effective in this situation. Even when lysis is successful and venous patency is restored, it may still not prevent chronic venous insufficiency. This may reflect deep vein valves being irreversibly damaged early in the course of the thrombosis. Since extension of this thrombosis retrograde, and also antegrade into the vena cava, is common, if catheter-delivered thrombolysis is not quickly successful, interventional radiologic consultation should be immediately sought for mechanical clot disruption and removal.

C. Vena Caval Filters

In patients who have an absolute contraindication to anticoagulation, or have had a major bleeding complication to therapeutic anticoagulation levels, the placement of a vena caval filter can be used to prevent recurrent PE. Available filters include the Greenfield filter, the bird's nest filter, the Simon nitinol filter, the Vena Tech filter, and the Gunther Tulip Retrievable Vena Caval Filter. The latter can be removed in 7–10 days if bleeding is controlled and anticoagulation can be reinstituted. The filters compare well in terms of efficacy, reducing the incidence of PE to less than 4% (median follow-up in most study series was 12–18 months), but are not more effective than long-term anticoagulation. In cancer patients who have recurrent VTE despite adequate anticoagulation, a vena caval filter combined with continued anticoagulation may provide greater protection. Complications include insertion site (20%–40%) and inferior vena caval thrombosis, tilting or migration of the filter, damage to the wall of the inferior vena cava, and filter fracture.

D. Disease-Related Thrombosis

Patients with malignancy and VTE can be a therapeutic challenge. Even with adequate warfarin to an INR of 2–3, malignancy is associated with a 15%–20% recurrence rate and a similarly high risk of major bleeding complications. Moreover, it can be difficult to maintain a therapeutic INR because of changes in diet, drug interactions, periodic thrombocytopenia, and associated liver disease. LMWH (eg, dalteparin 200 IU/kg once a day) has been shown to reduce the risk of both recurrence and bleeding by one-half, making it preferred over warfarin. Placement of a vena caval filter may be necessary in refractory patients or patients who are actively bleeding. However, although vena caval filters reduce the short-term risk of PE, they can increase the long-term risk of DVT, especially forming on the filter itself. The duration of anticoagulation depends on the clinical status of the patient. Anticoagulation must be continued indefinitely in the face of active or metastatic malignant disease leading to thromboembolism. Even if a solid remission is achieved, treatment should still be continued for at least 6 months.

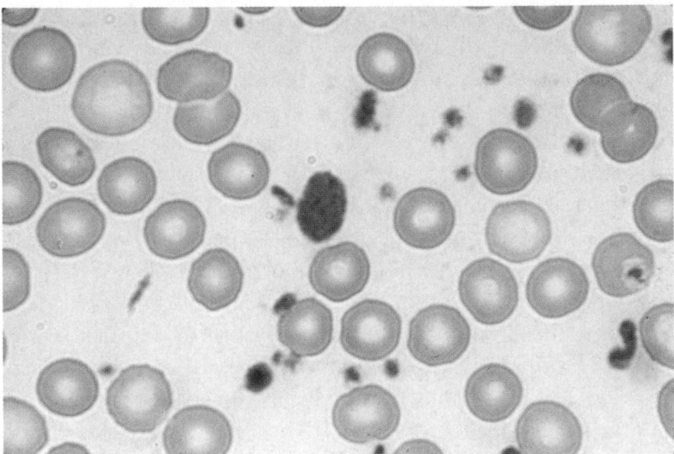

FIGURE 36–3. **Peripheral smear in essential thrombocythemia.** Giant platelets, together with a marked increase in the platelet count, are seen in myeloproliferative disorders like essential thrombocythemia that are associated with increased thrombotic risk.

Thrombosis associated with essential thrombocytosis (ET) can present as an arterial event (stroke), venous thromboembolism (VTE), or as microcirculatory insufficiency (erythromelalgia), the latter being especially noticeable in the distal extremities. The peripheral smear may demonstrate abnormal, giant platelets (Figure 36–3), or only an elevated platelet count; platelet aggregometry is often abnormal. Unfortunately, predicting thrombosis risk in ET using the platelet count or platelet function abnormalities has not succeeded; most patients are begun on anti-thrombotic therapy once they show signs or symptoms of thrombosis. Low-dose (81–162 mg) aspirin has usually been combined with hydroxyurea or anagrelide to decrease the incidence of thrombotic events. Recent randomized studies have shown that the combination of anagrelide with aspirin, although decreasing the incidence of VTE, actually increases the rates of both arterial thrombosis and marrow myelofibrosis, despite equivalent control of the platelet count. Thus, hydroxyurea and low-dose aspirin should be the standard therapy for ET. When ET occurs in pregnancy, hydroxyurea cannot be administered; unfortunately, low-dose aspirin alone is ineffective at preventing thrombosis or first-trimester fetal loss during pregnancy.

E. Pregnancy

Warfarin must be avoided in the treatment of venous thrombosis during pregnancy because of its teratogenic potential. Unfractionated heparin and LMWH are both safe for therapeutic anticoagulation since they do not cross the placenta. LMWH is preferred because it has reliable weight-based dosing and bioavailability such that it does not require constant monitoring. A weight-adjusted dose of enoxaparin (1–1.5 mg/kg), dalteparin (200 U/kg), or tinzaparin (175 U/kg) administered once daily subcutaneously is the most convenient and can be given safely throughout pregnancy. In women who gain considerable weight, a periodic measurement of the anti-Xa level can be used to adjust the dosage to achieve a therapeutic anti-Xa level of

0.5–1.0 U/mL measured 4–6 hours after dosing. Treatment with unfractionated heparin is a reasonable alternative, although monitoring (PTT every 1–2 weeks) is required.

To avoid excessive blood loss at delivery, heparin therapy should be discontinued 24 hours before elective induction, and restarted 12–24 hours postpartum. For those patients who need extended anticoagulation, warfarin can be initiated in a similar timeframe. In the case of spontaneous labor, the risk of bleeding depends on the time between the last LMWH dose and the time of delivery. If unfractionated heparin was used, protamine sulfate can be used to reverse anticoagulation, but protamine does not reverse the LMWH anticoagulant effect. Caution also must be exercised in the avoidance of epidural anesthesia at delivery when women are receiving any heparin therapy, including LMWH.

TABLE 36–6 • Risk stratification for pediatric VTE therapy

Risk Level	Low	Standard	High
Definition	No predisposing conditions; transient trigger	1–2 thrombophilic traits	Factor 8 >150%; persistently ↑ D-dimer; APLA; ≥3 thrombophilic traits
Therapy	Anticoagulation only	Anticoagulation ± thrombolysis	Anticoagulation + thrombolysis
Duration	6–12 weeks	3–12 months	≥12 months

F. Cerebral Vein/Sinus Thrombosis

Thrombosis of the cerebral veins or sinus thrombosis mostly occurs in children and young adults. Cerebral vein thrombosis causes intracerebral edema, venous infarcts, and hematoma formation, while sinus thrombosis often only demonstrates intracranial hypertension with no other signs. Similar to any venous thromboembolism, risk factors include oral contraceptives, an adjacent procedure or trauma, and thrombophilic mutations; nearby infection is a unique risk factor for sinus thrombosis. Neurologic symptoms may be nonspecific such as headache or seizures, but specific neurologic abnormalities occur, especially ocular. Diagnosis is best made using MRI with venography, but angiography may be required for definitive imaging.

Immediate therapy is aimed at decreasing intracranial pressures and anticoagulation, even if there is a hemorrhagic infarction; there is evidence that patients receiving unfractionated heparin prior to the transition to warfarin did no worse than those with warfarin alone. There are no data on the efficacy of thrombolysis. Warfarin should be adjusted to an INR of 2–3 for at least 6 months. Early mortality is about 6%, while long-term cumulative mortality reaches 9%. Nearly 90% of survivors make a full (or near-full) recovery; only 3% of treated survivors have a recurrence.

G. Pediatric Thromboembolism

The diagnosis of pediatric VTE relies on similar methods used in adults, including ultrasound, magnetic resonance angiography (MRA), and CT scans. Children with VTE have a similar rate (20%) of pulmonary embolism, and the diagnosis is made using the same techniques of helical CT or CT with angiography. Therapy for VTE in children, however, is somewhat different. For example, thrombolysis should always be considered in pediatric VTE because of its generally excellent outcome (exceeding 90% patency in some studies). Stratification of children with VTE into low-, standard-, and high-risk groups may help in their management (Table 36–6).

Unfractionated heparin anticoagulation in pediatric VTE is similar to that of adults and has the same complications, including heparin resistance. As in adults, LMWH in children is easier to dose because of its superior bioavailability. Heparin-induced thrombocytopenia has an incidence of about 1% in children and is treated identically with removal of heparin exposure and use of direct thrombin inhibitors. Warfarin dosing, as in adults, can be variable in children, but the bleeding risk with oral anticoagulation in children may be lower than in adults. As with adults, it is critical to monitor and maintain fibrinogen levels above 100 mg/dL and platelets above 50,000/μL in anticoagulated children.

Thrombolysis is recommended in high-risk children with VTE within 2 weeks of symptom onset, especially with an acute occlusive proximal DVT and an elevated factor VIII/D-dimer. Thrombolysis decreases the incidence of post-thrombotic syndrome at 18–24 months compared with anticoagulation alone.

As in adults, the duration of therapeutic anticoagulation in high-risk children may require modification based on the presence of underlying diseases and risk factors. Risk factors that indicate a need for prolonged duration of therapeutic anticoagulation include the presence of APLA syndrome or systemic inflammatory disorders (eg, systemic lupus erythematosus [SLE], juvenile rheumatoid arthritis). In the absence of specific risk guidelines, some studies suggest following levels of C-reactive protein, factor VIII, or D-dimer to determine if it is safe to discontinue anticoagulation.

H. Thromboembolism in the Elderly

The rate of VTE begins to steadily rise after age 55, and by age 80, the incidence of VTE is approximately 1 per 100 patient years, that is, 1% per year; the rate of pulmonary embolism (PE) rises even faster with advancing age (Figure 36–4). The causes of this increased VTE incidence are multi-factorial. Clearly, comorbid conditions will enhance the risk of VTE, as well as the mortality rate from VTE and PE. Besides older age itself as a mortality risk from VTE, chronic diseases of the cardiac, pulmonary, renal, and neurologic systems all promote the risk of death from VTE in older individuals.

The rise in levels of thrombosis-related proteins with aging appears to be a VTE risk factor. Factor VIII and fibrinogen are increased with age, and higher levels may contribute to thrombotic risk based on net thrombin generation. Interestingly, the regulation of plasminogen activator inhibitor-1 (PAI-1) is affected by aging itself, as well as several of the pathologic

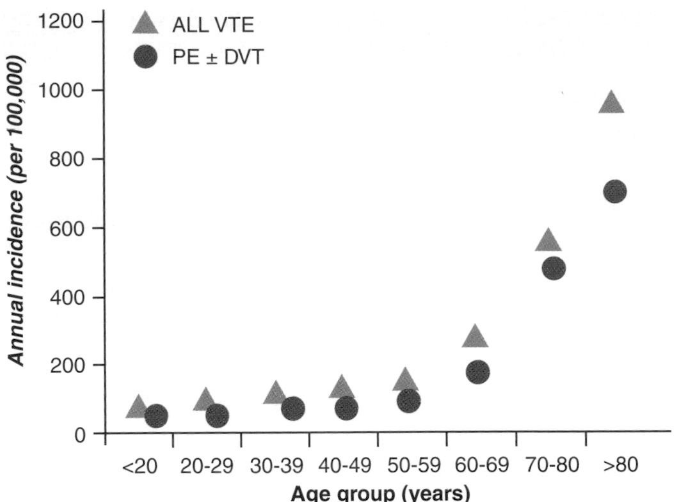

FIGURE 36–4. **Annual incidence of venous thromboembolism (VTE) and pulmonary embolism (PE) increases with age.** VTE and PE rates are shown for the different age groups (adapted from Silverstein et al: Blood 2007).

processes that accompany aging, such that PAI-1 activity is increased with age. This loss of fibrinolytic activity may promote thrombosis and vascular damage/atherosclerosis.

Elevated D-dimer values in the elderly are also associated with thrombotic risk, but because the D-dimer level in blood normally increases with aging, this may affect the workup of elderly patients presenting with symptoms of VTE or PE. A "negative" D-dimer result is used to definitively exclude the risk for VTE/PE in patients who are classified as low probability based on widely used clinical algorithms. Since older patients have higher de novo D-dimer levels, there may be a higher incidence of false positives and older patients unnecessarily undergoing further VTE workup. An age-specific D-dimer cutoff value is not currently available.

Other, perhaps independent causes of increased VTE incidence in the elderly include obesity and both acute and chronic inflammatory diseases. The pathologic link between inflammation and thrombosis is well established, especially for arterial thrombosis risk; the laboratory investigation of the latter includes the "metabolic panel" and C-reactive protein. However, there is little knowledge of how inflammatory stimuli affect thrombosis risk with increasing age. Certainly the markers of the thrombosis/inflammatory link are increased with age, including the levels of factor 8, D-dimer, and fibrin generation. Hopefully, future studies will demonstrate the use of such assays for predicting VTE risk.

Older individuals with VTE and/or PE show a higher morbidity and mortality. This fact alone necessitates appropriate prophylaxis and aggressive diagnostic measures to determine VTE/PE occurrence in the elderly. However, the 30-day case fatality rates are still very high in older individuals, at 5% for deep vein thrombosis alone and 33% when VTE is associated with PE. Prophylaxis is critical for the latter category since at least 25% of older PE patients present with sudden death. Besides the acute event, the morbidity and mortality risk of VTE do not abate with time in older patients; indeed, the risk of VTE recurrence increases by 15%–20% with each subsequent decade of age.

As more of the population lives longer, the difficulty in dealing with VTE in the elderly will become more critical, and specific studies are needed to determine risk and outcomes in order to make better-informed decisions. Currently, there are few data on the appropriate utilization of thrombolysis or inferior vena cava filters (temporary or permanent) in the elderly. However, studies on "personalized" medicine hold promise for individualizing therapy for older patients with VTE. For example, rather than discontinuing anticoagulation at a set interval (3 or 6 months) following a VTE episode, recent data suggest that following individual patients with ultrasonography to determine recanalization and venous patency will better determine if anticoagulation can be stopped. Patients followed by the latter method had lesser recurrence rates of VTE than those who discontinued anticoagulation at a set interval. This personalized approach may prove particularly useful in older patients with thrombosis.

Pulmonary Embolism

The initial therapeutic approach to a pulmonary embolus (PE) will depend on the patient's hemodynamic status. Hemodynamically unstable patients with massive or multiple pulmonary emboli should receive thrombolytic therapy (rt-PA 100 mg or urokinase infused over 2 hours) followed by full-dose unfractionated heparin for 10–14 days. Emergent thoracic surgery for embolectomy is dangerous but can be lifesaving in the patient with a large saddle embolus. Hemodynamically stable patients who demonstrate right ventricular hypokinesis on echocardiogram should also be considered for thrombolysis. The window of opportunity for thrombolysis is quite long, and patients will demonstrate a therapeutic response for up to 14 days. There is now good evidence that mortality is reduced and recovery is accelerated when thrombolytics are used in patients with large clot burdens. Otherwise, all patients who present with a high probability of PE, a positive lung scan, and/or ultrasound evidence of a DVT with PE symptoms should receive heparin for 10–14 days followed by oral anticoagulation to an INR of 2–3 for at least 6 months. If the patient is clinically stable, the hospitalization may be shortened by substituting LMWH, given as home therapy, after several days.

Cardiac Thromboembolic Disease

Patients with unexplained atrial fibrillation or, even more important, atrial fibrillation with valvular disease, a dilated atrium, and evidence of heart failure or a previous systemic embolus should receive warfarin indefinitely with an INR target of 2–3. Patients with acute anterior wall myocardial infarction who, because of a wall motion abnormality, are likely to form a mural thrombus need to receive warfarin for at least 2–3 months, after which anticoagulation should be guided by imaging results. Chronic anticoagulation is indicated in patients with artificial heart valves and dilated myocardiopathies, where valvular or mural thrombus formation, respectively, is likely. Acute anticoagulation of patients with unstable angina with heparin and aspirin can reduce the incidence of acute myocardial infarction and death by 33%. Recent studies show a slight advantage of LMWH over unfractionated heparin, as well as a lower cost and a reduction in bleeding complications.

Primary Hypercoagulable States

Management of the patient with a primary hypercoagulable state presents additional problems. First, the incidence of thromboembolic disease in patients with one of these conditions varies so much that therapy should only be considered for patients who exhibit a strong thrombotic tendency. Heterozygous factor V Leiden patients without a history of thromboembolism have a normal life expectancy and a low to normal risk of future thromboembolism. This is also true for family members of patients with clinical disease. They need not receive chronic anticoagulation therapy. High-risk patients, who should be considered for lifelong anticoagulation, include those who have had more than 1 spontaneous thrombosis or a life-threatening thromboembolism, and any individual who is a double heterozygote. Asymptomatic carriers of factor V Leiden, lupus anticoagulant or antiphospholipid antibody, or an AT, protein C, or protein S defect should, however, always receive vigorous prophylaxis in situations that predispose them to thrombosis.

In **high-risk patients** with the Leiden or *G20210A* prothrombin gene mutation or a deficiency of AT, protein S, or protein C, long-term anticoagulation with warfarin is recommended. Some caution must be taken in initiating warfarin therapy, especially in protein C– or S–deficient patients. These patients should receive full heparin anticoagulation prior to initiating the warfarin therapy, thereby preventing **warfarin-induced skin necrosis**. This rare complication is manifest by thrombosis of skin vessels within the first few days after beginning warfarin therapy. It is related to the rapid reduction of vitamin K–dependent protein C (and perhaps protein S) levels by warfarin. Similarly, in patients with **AT deficiency**, heparin therapy may be unpredictable. This situation reflects the lower than normal AT levels, or rarely, a defective AT protein. If full heparin anticoagulation is required, it may be necessary to provide the patient with exogenous AT by administration of purified AT (Thrombate III), recombinant AT, or transfusion of fresh frozen plasma. Prophylactic AT therapy can decrease the risk of thrombosis in deficient patients undergoing surgery or during childbirth.

Antiphospholipid Antibodies

Patients with antiphospholipid antibodies (APLA; especially lupus anticoagulants) and thromboembolic disease can represent a major therapeutic challenge. In women who have experienced recurrent fetal loss (but not other thromboembolic disease) secondary to APLA or a lupus anticoagulant, heparin plus low-dose (81–162 mg/d) aspirin are recommended during pregnancy to prevent thrombosis of the placenta and loss of the fetus. Dosing with unfractionated heparin is suggested at 10,000–15,000 U/d in divided doses, or daily LMWH can be substituted as prophylaxis (anti-Xa level of 0.1–0.3 U/mL) for the duration of the pregnancy. However, women with APLA and a history of thromboembolic complications require more aggressive therapy during pregnancy, including therapeutic LMWH (100 U/kg every 12 hours) subcutaneously (SC) or intravenous unfractionated heparin (aiming for a PTT 1.5–2.5 times normal). If the PTT is prolonged by the lupus anticoagulant and cannot be used to monitor heparin, the anti-Xa target level is 0.3–0.7 U/mL.

When the APLA is a complication of active systemic lupus erythematosus (SLE), aggressive treatment of the primary disease can reduce the antiphospholipid titer and perhaps reduce the likelihood of thromboembolic complications. Indeed, severe SLE patients aggressively treated with hematopoietic stem cell transplant were shown to become lupus anticoagulant negative, and 80% of those with recurrent VTE were able to have their anticoagulant therapy discontinued after transplant.

Patients with venous or arterial thrombosis with very clear laboratory evidence of APLA and without other manifestations of autoimmune disease should receive therapeutic heparin, and then switch to long-term warfarin therapy with a target INR of 2–3. Most INR reagents are insensitive to APLA, but if the INR appears to be artifactually increased for the level of warfarin dosing, functional monitoring of factor II or X activity (20%–25% is the target value) can be substituted. One exception to the use of warfarin in APLA syndrome is when stroke is the only thromboembolic complication; in this circumstance, anti-platelet therapy with aspirin ± clopidogrel appears to be the best therapy. Warfarin does not reduce the stroke recurrence rate more than aspirin.

Anticoagulation should be continued indefinitely in APLA patients with a history of thromboembolism because the recurrence rate in such patients reaches 50%–60% per year when off anticoagulant therapy. The response to this treatment is variable. Some patients seem to do very well, whereas others continue to demonstrate a thrombotic tendency despite therapeutic anticoagulation (ie, INR of 2–3 on warfarin). In refractory APLA patients, therapeutic options include increasing warfarin anticoagulation to a target INR of 3–4, with or without low-dose aspirin; substituting therapeutic LMWH dosing; or immunotherapy (eg, Rituxan or hematopoietic stem cell transplantion).

Arterial Thrombotic Disease

Platelet inhibitors are of proven value in the prevention of coronary artery and cerebrovascular thrombosis. Aspirin has been shown to decrease the incidence of myocardial infarction in patients with coronary artery disease, and the combination of clopidogrel and aspirin is routinely used for long-term treatment of ischemic cardiac disease. Dietary supplementation with folic acid, vitamin B_{12}, and vitamin B_6 to lower homocysteine levels has not been shown to be effective in reducing the incidence of either cardiovascular or cerebrovascular disease in at-risk patients, and therefore should not be recommended for anti-atherothrombosis therapy.

In the treatment of acute arterial thrombosis, immediate thrombolysis, whether administered peripherally (rt-PA) or by catheter (urokinase), is key to successful recanalization and prevention of end organ damage. As demonstrated in coronary angioplasty patients (see below), agents such as the GPIIb/IIIa inhibitors are effective in combination with clopidogrel and aspirin in the prevention of rethrombosis following thrombolysis. Institution of heparin therapy is also strongly recommended in acute peripheral arterial disease (PAD), while warfarin with aspirin is used for chronic PAD.

Antithrombotic Therapy During Percutaneous Coronary Artery Interventions

Successful revascularization of the patient undergoing angioplasty/stents depends on effective anticoagulation to prevent acute and subacute thrombosis. Antithrombins (heparin, bivalrudin) and anti-platelet agents (aspirin, clopidogrel, and the GPIIb/IIIa antagonists) are the mainstays of therapy during the procedure. All patients should be preloaded with aspirin (325 mg) and clopidogrel (75 mg/d for 3 days or, for urgent cases, a single dose of 300 or 600 mg). In the case of heparin, optimal dosing during angioplasty should increase the activated clotting time (ACT) to 250–300 seconds when used alone, or 200–250 seconds when used together with a GPIIb/IIIa antagonist. Once the procedure is over, the heparin can be discontinued and the sheath removed when the ACT falls below 170 seconds. Stent patients should then be maintained on both aspirin (81 mg/d) and clopidogrel (75 mg/d) for 4 weeks to 1 year after the procedure, to prevent subacute thrombosis until endothelialization of the stent has completed.

The prominent role of platelets in the pathogenesis of thrombosis during standalone balloon angioplasty or when a stent is placed to maintain vessel patency has led to multiple trials looking at the added effectiveness of a GPIIb/IIIa antagonist in combination with heparin during the procedure. Three agents have been tried: abciximab (ReoPro), eptifibatide, and tirofiban. Each has shown a decrease in thrombosis and myocardial infarction at 3 months. The impact on long-term mortality is less clear. ReoPro has the longest duration of action and may have a greater protective effect, especially in ST segment elevation patients with myocardial infarction (MI).

CASE HISTORY • *Part 3*

The patient demonstrates several risk factors for thrombosis, including oral contraceptive use, a recent long airplane trip (venous stasis), and a presumptive family history of an inherited thrombophilia (father is on anticoagulation therapy). This will require further testing but not as a prerequisite to beginning appropriate therapy.

Based on the radiological studies, the patient has a deep vein thrombosis and bilateral pulmonary emboli with significant clot burden in her lungs to lower her arterial O_2 saturation. She is therefore a potential candidate for thrombolysis, especially in light of her presenting within 3 days of developing symptoms and the absence of comorbid conditions that would increase her risk of bleeding. Following thrombolysis, she will need to be anticoagulated, beginning with heparin, and then transitioned to warfarin therapy with an INR target of 2–3 for a prolonged period (>6 months).

A search for other underlying thrombophilic defects is warranted in a young patient like this one. Without specific symptoms, an extensive workup for an occult malignancy is not efficacious. However, testing for an inherited/metabolic defect is in order. Therefore, a battery of coagulation tests needs to be sent from the emergency room, prior to thrombolysis/anticoagulation, including tests for APC resistance (APC-R/factor V Leiden), prothrombin *G20210A* mutation, a lupus anticoagulant, and AT, protein C, and protein S levels. This patient's results are as follows:

Prothrombin *G20210* mutation - not detected
AT = 65% (80%–120%)
Protein C = 60% (70%–140%)
Protein S = 35% (50%–150%)
APC-R = 1.80 (>2.20)
dRVVT = 1.22 (<1.20)

These coagulation panel results point out the difficulty in evaluating studies drawn during an acute thrombosis episode. All of the natural anticoagulants—AT, protein C, and protein S—are slightly lower than the normal range, a finding that is common due to consumption of factors with an acute clot. When repeated once the patient finished her anticoagulation, they are found to be normal. Similarly, testing for the lupus anticoagulant with the dilute RVVT can also be affected by acute stress or thrombosis.

The most common inherited causes of thrombophilia are the factor V Leiden and prothrombin *20210* mutations; the latter was not detected in this patient, but the screening APC-resistance test for Leiden was abnormal. Unlike the natural anticoagulant activities, APC-R is not affected by acute thrombosis or anticoagulation. When the APC-R result was confirmed by mutational analysis, the patient was found to be heterozygous for the V Leiden mutation, as was her father on subsequent analysis. The heterozygous V Leiden mutation, by itself, does not increase the incidence of recurrent thrombosis in otherwise healthy individuals. Therefore, the duration of her anticoagulation need not be extended and lifelong therapy is not indicated.

POINTS TO REMEMBER

Normal hemostasis and liquid blood flow reflect a physiological balance of procoagulant and anticoagulant mechanisms. When this balance is disrupted and tipped toward excessive procoagulant forces, thrombosis results. Procoagulant factors include blood stasis, vascular injury, and blood hypercoagulability.

A number of acquired and inherited defects in the coagulation pathways, both the factors involved in thrombin generation and the natural anticoagulant and thrombolytic mechanisms, can tip the balance to a hypercoagulable state and result in thromboembolic disease.

Venous and arterial thrombosis differs clinically in the mechanism of clot formation, and therefore are managed quite differently. Venous thrombosis is heavily dependent on excessive thrombin generation from soluble coagulation factors, while arterial thrombosis is dominated by platelets interacting with damaged endothelium.

Detection of clots in the arterial system is generally straightforward. End-organ arterial clots cause ischemia and infarction, which is readily diagnosed by tissue damage (eg, a cold, painful extremity with distal arterial occlusion), enzyme leak (eg, troponin I from a myocardial infarction), and specific symptoms (eg, hemiparesis from a stroke). Imaging with contrast will establish the diagnosis and the site of infarction.

Detection of deep venous thrombosis can be much more difficult, requiring a variety of studies. Ultrasound examination of the lower limbs, with Doppler or compression, can show the loss of patency of vessels, collateral flow, and recanalization.

Pulmonary embolism can be detected by scanning for a ventilation-perfusion mismatch, helical CT for wedge-shaped pulmonary infarction, or the gold standard, pulmonary angiography for direct visualization.

The approach to the workup of a patient with a suspected venous thrombosis depends on the pretest probability, based on clinical symptoms and signs suggesting thrombosis, provocative factors, and presence of other disease. High-risk patients need immediate imaging studies for both peripheral thrombosis and pulmonary embolus. The workup of a low-risk patient can be limited to a D-dimer assay, which, if normal, virtually excludes the presence of thromboembolic disease.

Inherited or acquired coagulation factor abnormalities (dysfibrinogenemia, factor V Leiden, prothrombin *G20210A*, hyperhomocysteinemia, and lower than normal levels of the natural anticoagulants—AT, and proteins C and S) are associated with varying degrees of thrombophilia.

There are a host of acquired conditions associated with venous thrombosis, including pregnancy and oral contraceptive use, solid and metastatic malignancies, inflammatory diseases such as lupus erythematosus, and primary hematologic disorders. Although underlying malignancy presents a significant thrombosis risk, studies do not justify an extensive search for occult cancer in patients with idiopathic venous thrombosis.

Antiphospholipid antibodies predispose to both venous and arterial clotting. The so-called "lupus anticoagulant" is one form of antibody associated with thrombosis. The most common presentations in otherwise healthy patients are thrombotic stroke or, in the case of pregnancy, recurrent miscarriage.

The primary hematologic malignancies associated with thrombosis affect both venous and arterial systems. Essential thrombocythemia is a myeloproliferative disorder with extremely high platelet counts and abnormal platelet function, including a propensity to platelet thrombus formation. Paroxysmal nocturnal hemoglobinuria (PNH) often presents with unusual venous clotting manifestations involving the portal and hepatic circulation.

The overall incidence of thrombotic disease and thrombosis-related mortality is increased in the elderly and rises progressively with age. This makes it an important comorbid factor in the management of other disease states, especially cardiopulmonary disease and cancer. At the same time, aggressive anticoagulation in elderly patients must be balanced with the higher bleeding risk at an advanced age.

Skilled management of a thrombosis is extremely important. Arterial thrombosis generally presents as an acute organ-threatening emergency and requires immediate thrombolysis, procedures such as angioplasty and stent placement, and specific anticoagulation including platelet inhibitors. By contrast, venous thrombosis may present in a distal vein with little or no threat to the patient or, alternatively, as a life-threatening thromboembolic event, requiring aggressive thrombolysis and prolonged anticoagulation.

Thrombolysis should be considered in venous thrombosis patients with appropriate indications, including all pediatric patients, adults with extensive venous or pulmonary thrombotic disease, or when there are indications of high mortality, such as right heart strain with pulmonary embolism. Thrombolysis can be performed either systemically or delivered on site with catheter-based interventions; intervention for mechanical clot removal should be considered when clot lysis is incomplete.

Anticoagulation is the key to effective treatment and long-term prevention of recurrent venous thrombosis. Rapid anticoagulation with heparin, either unfractionated or low-molecular-weight heparin, followed by long-term treatment with warfarin is required. The duration of therapy will depend on the resolution of the clot, any history of recurrent disease, and the presence of an acquired or inherited risk factor.

BIBLIOGRAPHY

Diagnosis of Thromboembolic Disease

Dayal S et al: Enhanced susceptibility to arterial thrombosis in a murine model of hyperhomocysteinemia. Blood 2006; 108:2237.

Dentali F, Crowther M, Ageno W: Thrombophilic abnormalities, oral contraceptives, and risk of cerebral vein thrombosis: a meta-analysis. Blood 2006;107:2766.

Garcia DA, Khamashta MA, Crowther MA: How we diagnose and treat thrombotic manifestations of the antiphospholipid syndrome: a case-based review. Blood 2007;110:3122.

Tebo AS et al: Diagnostic performance of phospholipid-specific assays for the evaluation of antiphospholipid syndrome. Am J Clin Pathol 2008;129:870.

Hypercoagulable Disorders

Caruso V et al: Thrombotic complications in childhood acute lymphoblastic leukemia: a meta-analysis of 17 prospective studies comprising 1752 patients. Blood 2006;108:2216.

Dentali F et al: Natural history of cerebral vein thrombosis: a systematic review. Blood 2006;108:1129.

Galli M et al: Clinical significance of different antiphospholipid antibodies in the WAPS (warfarin in the antiphospholipid syndrome) study. Blood 2007;110:1178.

Giannakopoulos B et al: Current concepts on the pathogenesis of the antiphospholipid syndrome. Blood 2007;109:422.

Potti A: Gene-expression patterns predict phenotypes of immune-mediated thrombosis. Blood 2006;107:1391.

Silverstein RL et al: Venous thrombosis in the elderly. Blood 2007;110:3097.

Stam J: Thrombosis of the cerebral veins and sinuses. N Engl J Med 2005;352:1791.

Yamamoto K et al: Aging and plasminogen activator inhibitor-1 (PAI-1) regulation: implication in the pathogenesis of thrombotic disorders in the elderly. Cardiovasc Res 2005;66:276.

Management

Barbui T, Finazzi G: When and how to treat essential thrombocythemia. N Engl J Med 2005;353:85.

Goldenberg NA et al: A thrombolytic regimen for high-risk deep venous thrombosis may substantially reduce the risk of post-thrombotic syndrome in children. Blood 2007;110:45.

Harrison CN et al: Hydroxyurea compared with anagrelide in high-risk essential thrombocythemia. N Engl J Med 2005; 353:33.

Hillmen P et al: Effect of the complement inhibitor eculizumab on thromboembolism in patients with paroxysmal nocturnal hemoglobinuria. Blood 2007;110:4123.

King CR et al: Performance of commercial platforms for rapid genotyping of polymorphisms affecting warfarin dose. Am J Clin Pathol 2008;129:876.

Loscalzo J: Homocysteine trials—clear outcomes for complex reasons. N Engl J Med 2006;354:1629.

Manco-Johnson MJ: How I treat venous thrombosis in children. Blood 2006;107:21.

Statkute L et al: Antiphospholipid syndrome in patients with systemic lupus erythrmatosus treated by autologous hematopoietic stem cell transplantation. Blood 2005;106:2700.

Wright CA, Tefferi A: A single institutional experience with 43 pregnancies in essential thrombocythemia. Eur J Haematol 2001;66:152.

ANTICOAGULATION IN THE MANAGEMENT OF THROMBOTIC DISORDERS · 37

CASE HISTORY • *Part I*

A 57-year-old woman, scheduled for an elective hysterectomy, is referred for management of her anticoagulation during the perioperative period. She is currently receiving warfarin 3 mg daily for a 5-year history of atrial fibrillation with past evidence of a single embolic event. Other medical problems include hypertension and diabetes, controlled with an angiotensin-converting enzyme (ACE) inhibitor and diet. She also takes a baby aspirin each day.

Examination reveals a healthy black female with no complaints. Positive findings on examination include an irregularly irregular heart rhythm and a faint diastolic murmur.

Vital signs: BP - 155/80 mm Hg, pulse - 75 bpm, resp - 16/min, T - 37°C.

Coagulation studies:
Platelet count = 210,000/μL
PT = 25.1 seconds (<14 seconds)
INR = 2.4 (0.8–1.3)
PTT = 29 seconds (22–35 seconds)

Question

- Given the potential for significant hemorrhage during surgery, how should this patient be managed?

Successful management of the patient with a thrombotic disorder requires evaluation of risk factors for thrombosis, a careful assessment of the site and extent of the thrombus, and a skilled choice and application of a number of anticoagulants. Diagnostic evaluation of the thromboembolic patient is discussed in Chapter 36. Treatment of the patient with a thrombus involves both dissolution of the clot and prevention of recurrence. Specific therapy will be dictated by the type of vessel involved, whether arterial or venous, and the clinical setting (Table 37–1). As a general rule, thrombotic disorders of arterial vessels are best managed using a combination of thrombolytic agents to rapidly dissolve the obstructing clot and anti-platelet drugs to prevent recurrence. In contrast, venous thromboembolism responds best to drugs such as heparin, fondaparinux, and warfarin that inhibit the function and formation of coagulation factors.

ANTI-PLATELET DRUGS

Anti-platelet drugs act by inhibiting platelet function. They are most useful in preventing recurrent arterial thrombosis in patients with advanced atherosclerosis. Aspirin and clopidogrel are used most extensively. Of these drugs, aspirin is the best studied, the most popular, and the cheapest. Other inhibitors of platelet aggregation include the integrin blockers: abciximab (ReoPro), eptifibatide, and tirofiban. Abciximab has been approved by the US Food and Drug Administration (FDA) for

TABLE 37–1 • Recommended therapy of thrombotic disorders[a]

Condition	Therapy
Coronary artery disease	
Stable angina/infarct prevention	Aspirin
Unstable angina	Aspirin ± clopidogrel for outpatients; aspirin plus LMWH or UFH for hospitalized patients
Acute myocardial infarction (<6 hours old)	Thrombolysis using intravenous streptokinase or t-PA plus full-dose heparin and aspirin
Anterior transmural infarcts (risk of mural thrombosis)	Full-dose heparin followed by warfarin therapy for 2–3 months
Reinfarction prevention	Long-term aspirin ± clopidogrel
Bypass graft patency	Aspirin/clopidogrel
Cerebral artery disease	
Transient ischemic attacks	Aspirin or clopidogrel or both
Recurring TIAs/evolving thrombotic stroke	LMWH or UFH followed by warfarin or aspirin alone (treatment debatable)
Completed thrombotic stroke	Aspirin or clopidogrel or both
Cerebral embolism	
Without hemorrhage on CT scan	LMWH or UFH followed by long-term warfarin therapy
With hemorrhage on CT scan	Postpone anticoagulation for 2 weeks
Valvular heart disease	
Valvular disease (especially mitral stenosis) with atrial fibrillation or history of embolism; recurrent episodes of paroxysmal atrial fibrillation	Long-term warfarin therapy
Atrial fibrillation cardioversion	Warfarin therapy for 2–3 weeks prior to and 4 weeks after cardioversion
Bioprosthetic mitral valves	Long-term moderate-dose warfarin therapy (INR 2.0–2.5)
Mechanical prosthetic valves	Long-term warfarin therapy (INR 3.0–4.0) with or without dipyridamole
Venous disease	
Deep venous thrombosis with pulmonary embolism	LMWH, fondaparinux, or full-dose UFH for 7 days followed by warfarin for 6 months or longer according to risk factors
Superficial phlebitis or limited to calf vessels	Anticoagulation not indicated unless extends proximally
Subclavian/superior vena cava thrombosis secondary to an indwelling catheter	Thrombolysis with streptokinase or t-PA followed by heparin, short-term warfarin, and line removal
Thromboembolism prevention	
Forced bed rest/general surgery	LMWH (30 mg SC bid) or fondaparinux (2.5 mg SC)
Orthopedic/elective hip surgery	LMWH, fondaparinux, or low-dose warfarin

[a]Recommendations for the use of newer anti-Xa and thrombin inhibitors (eg, fondaparinux) will change as the results of clinical trials become available. It is anticipated that oral agents will become the preferred therapy for most situations of thromboembolic risk based on their ease of use, comparable efficacy, and lower incidence of bleeding and thromboembolic complications.

use in patients undergoing percutaneous transluminal coronary angioplasty. Eptifibatide has been approved for the treatment of acute coronary events and for patients undergoing angioplasty or stenting. Tirofiban is also FDA approved for the treatment, in conjunction with heparin, of acute coronary events.

Pharmacokinetics

Aspirin acetylates prostaglandin G/H synthase, causing a loss of cyclooxygenase activity and an inhibition of thromboxane A_2 production and platelet aggregation. The effect is irreversible, so the impact on function is permanent for the 10-day lifespan of the affected platelet. A single dose of as little as 40–100 mg of aspirin is sufficient to inhibit the function of most platelets in circulation. Aspirin has no specific effect on platelet adhesion. **Dipyridamole** (Persantine) interferes with the platelet response to agonists by inhibiting phosphodiesterase and increasing cellular content of adenosine 3′,5′-cyclic monophosphate (cAMP). It is a far less effective inhibitor than aspirin.

Clopidogrel (Plavix) is a second-generation adenosine 5′-diphosphate (ADP) receptor blocker that has largely replaced ticlopidine because of the incidence of thrombotic thrombocytopenic purpura (TTP) with the latter. It is metabolized to an active thienopyrimidine compound that blocks ADP binding to its platelet receptor, thereby interfering with ADP-induced platelet aggregation.

Abciximab (ReoPro) is the Fab fragment of the monoclonal antibody 7E3. It binds irreversibly to the GPIIb/IIIa adhesion receptor, and by blocking fibrinogen and von Willebrand factor (vWF) binding, inhibits platelet aggregation. It is far more powerful than aspirin. When given in full dose, it can completely inhibit ADP-induced platelet aggregation. Moreover, the effect lasts for the lifespan of the platelet; platelet aggregation is inhibited for more than 24 hours after treatment. Similarly functioning inhibitors include eptifibatide and tirofiban. **Eptifibatide** (Integrilin) is a peptide antagonist of GPIIb/IIIa, whereas **tirofiban** (Aggrastat) is a "small molecule" tyrosine derivative (peptidomimetic) with high specificity for the GPIIb/IIIa receptor. Both drugs have short durations of action, 2–3 hours. Oral small molecule inhibitors are under study as long-term platelet inhibitors, although adverse effects, such as thrombocytopenia, have delayed clinical introduction.

Clinical Applications

A. Aspirin

Aspirin still enjoys the widest applicability. In general, aspirin therapy appears to work best in patients with distorted arterial anatomy, especially atherosclerotic vascular disease. This is a situation where a disruption in the endothelial surface provides a strong stimulus for platelet activation, aggregation, and subsequent clot formation.

Several clinical trials have supported the use of aspirin to prevent thrombosis in patients with cerebrovascular disease, coronary artery disease, and most recently, peripheral arterial disease. For the latter (defined as arterial disease in the extremities and including the carotid arteries), anti-platelet therapy alone was as effective at preventing vascular events/death as its combination with therapeutic warfarin (international normalized ratio [INR] 2.0–3.0). The incidence of nonfatal stroke is reduced by as much as 25%. The use of aspirin in patients with known coronary artery disease is clearly established; the incidence of nonfatal coronary occlusion is reduced by 30%–40%.

As for primary prevention in individuals without a prior vascular event, a single aspirin (325 mg) given every other day or a baby aspirin (81 mg) given daily has been shown to reduce the incidence of myocardial infarction by 44% in a 5-year study of 22,000 male physicians. Since platelet turnover rates vary between individuals, the daily baby aspirin dosing is preferable and may also reduce the risk of bleeding, but the risk for hemorrhagic stroke likely outweighs the benefit in patients without risk factors for coronary disease.

As with all drugs used to prevent atherothrombosis, vascular complications continue to occur despite aspirin therapy. This may reflect aspirin's inhibition (at higher doses) of vascular prostacyclins, leading to decreased vasodilatation. Treatment failure despite aspirin use has also been termed "aspirin resistance." However, this is a misleading term because it does not recognize the variable biochemical response between individuals to a fixed dose of aspirin. There is no current laboratory test that will measure the functional effect of aspirin and allow dose adjustment, but it is clearly important to avoid drug interactions, for example, nonsteroidal anti-inflammatory drugs, that can diminish the anti-platelet effectiveness of aspirin and other agents.

B. Other Anti-platelet Drugs

Clopidogrel is the alternative drug of choice, especially for patients who have side effects from aspirin. It has demonstrated efficacy in reducing the event rate for stroke and vascular death when compared with aspirin, and has been approved for the management of patients with cardiovascular, cerebrovascular, and peripheral vascular disease. Clopidogrel is also used in combination with aspirin in high-risk cardiovascular or cerebrovascular disease, and in angioplasty patients with implanted coronary artery stents.

Dipyridamole, another anti-platelet drug, has been used in conjunction with warfarin to prevent prosthetic heart valve embolization. It has also been used together with aspirin to provide a greater inhibition of platelet function. There is no clinical evidence, however, that the combination is better than aspirin alone in patients with atherosclerotic disease.

Abciximab has been approved for the treatment of patients with unstable angina destined for angioplasty and following angioplasty to prevent immediate reocclusion of dilated arteries. Multiple trials of ReoPro (EPILOG, EPISTENT, CAPTURE) in combination with heparin in patients undergoing angioplasty have shown significant reductions in reocclusion, myocardial infarction, and death at 30 days and 3 months. ReoPro has also been studied as an adjunct to thrombolytic therapy in patients with acute myocardial infarction. ReoPro used in combination with half-dose tissue-type plasminogen activator (t-PA; TIMI-14, SPEED) appears to be more effective than t-PA alone, achieving overall patency rates of 93%.

The peptide and peptidomimetic inhibitors **(eptifibatide, tirofiban)** show great promise in coronary artery disease patients. Trials of tirofiban and eptifibatide in angioplasty patients have shown improved outcomes, with decreased rates of reocclusion, myocardial infarction, and death at 30 days. When given in combination with heparin and aspirin (PRISM-PLUS, ESPRIT) to patients with unstable angina and non-ST elevation myocardial infarction, tirofiban therapy resulted in a 30%–40% reduction in rates of death, myocardial infarction, and recurrent ischemia. Moreover, since these agents have the advantage of being very short acting, they can be used as first-line therapy in unstable patients with angina who may require emergency angioplasty or coronary artery bypass grafting (CABG).

Therapeutic Guidelines

A. Aspirin

Aspirin in a starting dose of 325 mg, followed by a lower-dose regimen of 80–160 mg/d, is recommended as immediate treatment for acute chest pain (coronary artery disease), myocardial infarction, and thrombotic stroke. A daily dose of 81 mg/d (a baby aspirin) is recommended for maintenance therapy since it inhibits platelet function without impairing endothelial cell prostacyclin production. For the sake of convenience, an every-other-day 325-mg dose can be used with equal clinical effectiveness but does convey a 4- to 10-fold greater risk of gastrointestinal (GI) bleeding. Concurrent use of an anti-secretory agent (especially a proton pump inhibitor [PPI]) will reduce the risk of upper GI bleeding. Much higher doses (900 mg or more of aspirin daily) provide no greater inhibition of thromboxane metabolism and are associated with an even higher incidence of GI bleeding.

B. Clopidogrel

Trials of clopidogrel have used 75 mg once a day with a significant improvement in outcome in patients with coronary artery disease, stroke, or peripheral arterial disease. At this dose, the full effect is not seen for up to a week. If more immediate blockade is required, as with emergent angioplasty or an acute coronary event, a single clopidogrel loading dose of 300 mg may be given, followed by 75 mg/d for maintenance therapy. The combination of aspirin (325 mg) and clopidogrel (600 mg) given just before stent placement reduces poor vascular outcomes by 25%–30%. Once the stent is placed, low-dose aspirin should be continued for life, and clopidogrel probably for more than 1 year, but the exact duration for the latter is unknown. Clopidogrel, given in combination with aspirin, may be synergistic in the secondary prevention of cardiovascular events after myocardial infarction.

Clopidogrel resistance has been reported as a laboratory event (an inadequate decrease in platelet function despite appropriate dosing). Cytochrome CYP2C19 polymorphisms confer loss of clopidogrel function by preventing its conversion to the active thienopyrimidine metabolite. Indeed, there is some evidence that concomitant use of clopidogrel and PPIs, which generally decrease CYP2C19 activity, also leads to a slightly higher incidence of myocardial infarction. A definitive effect on clinical care needs confirmation, but an H2 blocker should be seriously considered over a PPI if clopidogrel is simultaneously prescribed.

C. Abciximab

The recommended dose of abciximab for angioplasty patients is 0.25 mg/kg given intravenously (IV) 10–60 minutes prior to the start of the procedure, followed by a continuous infusion of 0.125 μg/kg/min, up to a maximum dose of 10 μg/min, for at least 12 hours. Unstable angina patients should be maintained on a 10 μg/min infusion until angioplasty is performed. This should be accompanied by low-dose heparin (70 U/kg), adjusted to keep the activated clotting time (ACT) between 200 and 250 seconds in order to minimize bleeding complications. Special caution should be taken with patients who have received thrombolysis prior to angioplasty. If possible, abciximab treatment should be delayed for 12–18 hours until the thrombolytic effects have been largely reversed. When studied in combination with t-PA, the dose of both t-PA and heparin was reduced (t-PA: 15-mg bolus followed by a 35-mg infusion over 60 minutes; heparin: 60-U/kg bolus followed by a 7-U/kg constant infusion) to avoid excessive bleeding. Abciximab therapy is most effective in patients undergoing angioplasty or unstable angina with elevated troponin levels. It does not reduce 30-day mortality/myocardial infarction rates in patients with troponin-negative unstable angina.

The primary complication of abciximab therapy is a poorly understood, severe thrombocytopenia (10,000–50,000/μL) occurring within a few hours of receiving the drug in up to 1% of patients. In patients treated a second time, the incidence is much higher (4%–5%) and appears to be related to a drug-induced antibody. Platelet transfusion may be required to treat bleeding with this complication.

D. Tirofiban or Eptifibatide

Both tirofiban and eptifibatide are administered as a bolus followed by a continuous intravenous infusion. Effectiveness depends on the level of inhibition of platelet aggregation. The ESPRIT trial, which used a double bolus of eptifibatide, two 180-μg/kg doses 10 minutes apart, together with a continuous infusion of 2 μg/kg/min, achieved 85%–95% platelet inhibition. This dose is now recommended for angioplasty patients. Acute coronary event patients should receive only a single bolus and the identical infusion. Tirofiban is administered as a 0.4-μg/kg/min infusion for 30 minutes, followed by a continuous infusion of 0.1 μg/kg/min (the rate is halved for severe renal insufficiency). Both agents have very short half-lives. Once the infusion is discontinued, platelet aggregation returns to normal in 2–4 hours. Both tirofiban and eptifibatide also have been associated with an antibody-induced thrombocytopenia, but in a smaller number of cases, 0.1%–0.5% of treated patients.

E. Oral GPIIb/IIIa Inhibitors

Trials of the "first-generation" oral GPIIb/IIIa inhibitors (orbofiban, xemilofiban, sibrafiban, roxifiban) have yet to show a comparable benefit when compared with aspirin or the intravenous inhibitors. This may relate to an inability to achieve a constant blood level with oral dosing. In addition, thrombocytopenia is a common adverse reaction.

Laboratory Monitoring

No laboratory monitoring is absolutely required with aspirin or clopidogrel therapy, although several instruments are available to confirm that dosing is adequate for platelet inhibition; no studies have shown that the platelet function analysis (PFA), an in vitro bleeding time, correlates with clinical efficacy. Furthermore, other coagulation tests are not affected. ReoPro and the other newer platelet aggregation antagonists can be dose adjusted using mini-platelet aggregation studies if less than maximum inhibition is desired. However, clinical trials of these drugs have not tested the effectiveness of lower-dose regimens.

Adverse Effects

Low-dose aspirin therapy is not associated with an increased incidence of abnormal bleeding and does not pose a risk for the patient who requires an operative procedure. Patients taking aspirin who undergo coronary bypass surgery do not experience an increased amount of blood loss compared with aspirin-free patients and, in fact, there is evidence that continuing aspirin through the perioperative period is beneficial for coronary artery bypass patients. Similarly, clopidogrel therapy is not a contraindication to surgery. If the surgeon considers it important to reverse the aspirin effect prior to surgery, it is best accomplished by giving the patient a single intravenous injection of 0.3 μg/kg of desmopressin (DDAVP) just prior to surgery. Platelet transfusions will only be effective if the patient no longer has aspirin in their system, since the transfused platelets would be affected by circulating aspirin. If significant bleeding occurs with low-dose aspirin, the patient should be investigated for an accompanying platelet functional defect, especially type 1 von Willebrand disease (vWD; see Chapter 32).

Abciximab therapy in patients who are also receiving full-dose heparin is associated with a significant increase in both minor and major bleeding, most often bleeding at the femoral artery access site for cardiac procedures. Fortunately, intracranial hemorrhage is rare. Predictors of bleeding include heparin and abciximab dosage, small body size, larger sheath size, female sex, and advanced age. Bleeding may be controlled by using low-dose heparin, keeping the ACT between 200 and 250 seconds, or low-molecular-weight heparin (LMWH) without an apparent loss of effectiveness. Reduction in the dose of abciximab to lessen the aggregation defect as a way to reduce the bleeding complications has not been tested. Mild to severe thrombocytopenia can complicate abciximab therapy and require platelet transfusion. Since abciximab has a very long half-life and a demonstrable aggregation defect for up to 2–3 weeks, reversal can be difficult in the bleeding patient. If major bleeding does occur, both the abciximab and heparin should be discontinued, any obvious bleeding site such as the femoral access site should be controlled locally, and the patient should be given platelet transfusions and red blood cells as needed. Major surgery should be delayed for at least 12–24 hours after discontinuing abciximab. Better yet, if the need for an emergency CABG is anticipated, the patient should be treated with tirofiban or eptifibatide rather than abciximab to take advantage of the shorter duration of action (4–6 hours).

Platelet counts should be monitored since immediate, severe thrombocytopenia can occur with the initial exposure to abciximab. This is somehow related to the presence of naturally occurring IgG antibodies to platelet GPIIb/IIIa, which are reactive with abciximab-coated platelets. Caution must be exercised in interpreting automated platelet counts since ethylenediaminetetraacetic acid (EDTA)-pseudothrombocytopenia (see Chapter 31) has also been reported following abciximab; a blood smear should be examined to rule out platelet agglutination.

ORAL ANTICOAGULANTS (COUMARINS)

The coumarin compounds have been recognized for more than 50 years for their value in treating thromboembolic diseases. The 4-hydroxycoumarin derivative, warfarin sodium (Coumadin), is the preferred compound for clinical use.

Pharmacokinetics

Warfarin is a mixture of equal amounts of 2 active racemic isomers, the R and S forms. The drug is absorbed rapidly and completely, resulting in a peak plasma level in 90 minutes. It is then gradually cleared into liver cells, where it blocks vitamin K reductase enzymes, thereby depleting the cell of vitamin KH_2. The latter is an essential cofactor for the required (carboxylation of the vitamin K–dependent coagulation proteins: prothrombin; factors VII, IX, and X; protein C; and protein S (Figure 37–1). The R and S isomers are cleared by different pathways. The S isomer is oxidized and excreted in bile, whereas the R isomer is excreted in urine.

As highlighted in Figure 37–1, several factors will influence the effectiveness of warfarin therapy. Fluctuations in dietary intake and absorption of vitamin K will influence the dose response. Vitamin K is a fat-soluble vitamin and its absorption is impaired in conditions of fat malabsorption or with ingestion of drugs such as clofibrate and oral antibiotics. Liver functional status is also important; cirrhosis or passive congestion of the liver can increase sensitivity to warfarin by decreasing synthesis of the liver-dependent coagulation factors.

Several **drug interactions** can affect warfarin kinetics. The most important are those drugs (phenylbutazone, metronidazole, sulfa drugs, disulfiram, and amiodarone) that inhibit the clearance of the more active S isomer, since this significantly prolongs the prothrombin time (PT). Drugs that inhibit R isomer clearance (cimetidine and omeprazole) have a less pronounced effect on the PT. Other drugs that have been reported as potentiating the effect of warfarin include erythromycin, the anabolic steroids, phenytoin, quinidine, tamoxifen, isoniazid,

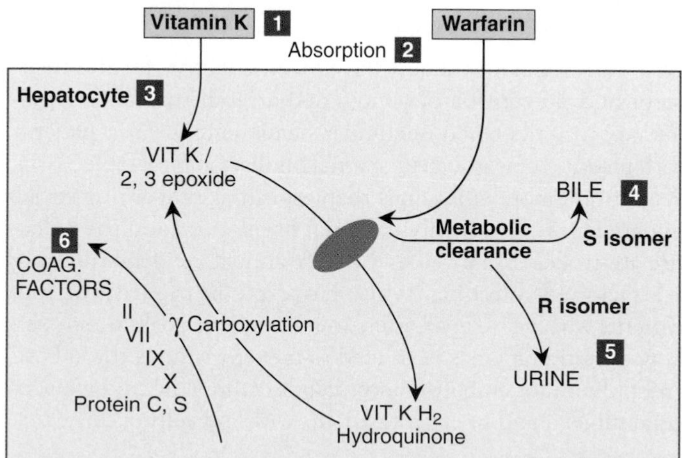

FIGURE 37–1. **Warfarin and vitamin K metabolism.** Warfarin blocks the normal reductase conversion of vitamin K epoxide to the hydroxyquinone (KH_2). This interferes with formation of the vitamin K–dependent factors—prothrombin (II); factors VII, IX, and X; and the anticoagulant proteins C and S. Therapeutic anticoagulation with oral doses of warfarin can be affected by multiple factors at several sites: (1) dietary content of vitamin K; (2) malabsorption of vitamin K; (3) liver function; (4) inhibition of S isomer clearance; (5) inhibition of R isomer clearance; and (6) coagulation-factor production (pregnancy, fever, hyperthyroidism).

ethacrynic acid, and ketoconazole. The mechanism involved is less clear.

Resistance to warfarin therapy due to drug interaction is usually caused by either reduced absorption (cholestyramine) or an increased rate of warfarin clearance (alcohol, barbiturates, rifampin, glutethimide, griseofulvin, and carbamazepine). Rarely, *VKORC1* mutations can cause extreme warfarin resistance, necessitating very high (>100 mg) weekly maintenance doses.

Genotyping for the enzymes responsible for warfarin metabolism may eventually become clinically useful for streamlining maintenance dosing. Commercial platforms are now available for rapid genotyping of the cytochrome P450, CYP2CP *2/*3, and the vitamin K epoxide reductase (*VKORC1*) isoforms. About 50% of individual variability in the INR is accounted for by these 2 polymorphisms, with the remainder dependent on body mass, age, and other demographics. Although genotyping for warfarin susceptibility is not yet FDA approved, it is possible that future algorithms with such testing will be implemented to be sure that patients who need lower maintenance dosing are not put at risk for high INR values. Based on studies to date, the only cost-effective genotyping strategy is in patients with non-valvular atrial fibrillation who are at high bleeding risk.

Age in general is an important **risk factor for bleeding** with oral anticoagulation. Although older patients generally require a lower warfarin dose to reach equivalent INR values, their dosing is more variable, resulting in wide swings in their INR. The latter may be related to diet and vitamin K intake or polypharmacy. Self-monitoring of INR values may help older patients as a guide to dose adjustments. Even so, the anticoagulated elderly patient clearly has a greater bleeding risk, especially intracranial, possibly because of age-related changes in vessel integrity.

Clinical Applications

Oral anticoagulant therapy has proven effective for the treatment and prevention of venous and arterial thrombosis, pulmonary thromboembolism, and systemic embolism in patients with prosthetic heart valves or atrial fibrillation (see Table 37–1). Warfarin is more efficacious than aspirin at preventing stroke in patients with non-valvular atrial fibrillation, and the reduction in stroke risk outweighs the 0.3% annual incidence of major (extracranial) bleeding. It also has a role in the treatment of patients with acute myocardial infarction and evolving strokes. Low-dose therapy has been used to prevent venous thrombosis and pulmonary embolism after major orthopedic and gynecologic surgery, and in cancer patients with indwelling catheters.

Therapeutic Guidelines

Full anticoagulation with warfarin takes at least 3–4 days. This period reflects the relatively long half-lives of factors II (prothrombin), IX, and X in circulation once synthesis is inhibited. Therefore, a patient who requires immediate anticoagulation should be given heparin. Warfarin therapy can be started simultaneously using a dose of 5–10 mg/d for the first 2 days, then reducing the dose appropriately for maintenance. Since it is impossible to accurately predict a patient's final maintenance requirement, which can range from 1–15 mg/d, a PT should be measured every 3–7 days (as an outpatient) to make appropriate adjustments in dosage. Only after the patient's response has stabilized should the frequency of the PT measurements be reduced. For patients who are stable on chronic therapy, the PT may be measured as infrequently as once a month.

In the non-urgent patient, oral anticoagulant therapy is best initiated by simply starting a daily maintenance dose of 5 mg. This dose schedule results in a smooth and balanced decline in factor levels (factors II, VII, and X, and protein C), avoiding the risk of increased thrombotic potential for the first 48 hours because of a rapid depletion of protein C. Only patients with a congenital deficiency in protein C or S are at significant risk of increased thrombosis, skin necrosis, or both if warfarin is initiated without heparin anticoagulation.

A. Maintenance Therapy

Maintenance therapy requires a well-educated patient, home/clinic monitoring of the INR, correlated measurements of the PT/INR by a reliable laboratory, and a recognized algorithm for adjusting the warfarin dose. The latter is most important if multiple care providers are interacting with the patient.

Recommended dose adjustments should be gradual, using modest daily changes planned over 1–2 weeks as follows for a target INR of 2–3:

- International normalized ratio (INR) <2: Increase the weekly dose by 5%–20%
- INR 3–3.5: Decrease weekly dose by 5%–15%
- INR 3.6–4: Withhold 0–1 day's dose and decrease weekly dose by 10%–15%
- INR >4: Withhold 1 day's dose and decrease weekly dose by 10%–20%

For very high INRs, 1 or 2 oral doses of vitamin K (2.5–5 mg) can be given, while continuing the warfarin therapy. This will speed the correction of the INR without completely reversing the patient's anticoagulation.

Recommended target ranges for anticoagulation are listed in Table 37–2. For most situations, an INR range of 2–3 is recommended. Higher-intensity anticoagulation has been reported to provide protection against recurrent myocardial infarction and stroke in patients following acute myocardial infarction. However, high-intensity regimens are associated with an increased incidence of bleeding complications. The same is true for patients receiving chronic anticoagulation to prevent embolism from mechanical heart valves. This situation has led to recommendations for less intense regimens, INRs of 1.5–2.5, and regimens that **combine lower-dose warfarin with low-dose aspirin**. The efficacy of these low-dose regimens appears to be comparable to that of the higher-dose approach in most instances, and bleeding complications are considerably less. Very low-dose warfarin, 1 mg/d, can significantly reduce the incidence of catheter-related thrombosis in cancer patients.

TABLE 37–2 • Target ranges for warfarin therapy

Condition	INR	Duration
Venous thrombosis		
Treatment	2.0–3.0	3–6 months
Prevention	1.5–2.5	Chronic
Atrial fibrillation		
Embolus prevention	2.0–3.0	Chronic
Myocardial infarction		
Embolus prevention postinfarction	2.0–3.0	2–3 months
Prevent reinfarction	3.0–4.5	Chronic
Mechanical heart valves		
Tissue valves	2.0–2.5	Chronic
Mechanical valves	3.0–4.0	Chronic
Arterial thrombosis		
Stroke prevention	2.0–4.0	Chronic

B. Management of Anticoagulated Patients during and after Surgery

The management of anticoagulated patients in the perioperative period depends on the reason for the warfarin therapy and the duration of anticoagulation. Without full-dose anticoagulation, patients with venous thromboembolism (VTE) run a risk of recurrence of greater than 1% per day in the first month following the event. Therefore, major surgery should be avoided when feasible for at least 1 month following a venous or arterial thromboembolism. If early surgery is required, the patient should probably receive heparin (either unfractionated or low molecular weight) perioperatively while the INR is less than 2—so-called bridging therapy. Unfractionated heparin has some advantage over LMWH. It can be discontinued 6–8 hours prior to surgery and restarted 12–18 hours later, minimizing the period of thromboembolic risk. Once-daily treatment with low-molecular-weight heparin (LMWH) is also an option for perioperative anticoagulation. If a patient cannot receive heparin because of the higher risk of bleeding, a vena caval filter should be considered.

The situation is very different for patients with a remote history of VTE without recurrence. These patients are at low risk of recurrent VTE in the perioperative period when oral anticoagulation is interrupted. They are best managed by simply discontinuing the daily warfarin dose 4–5 days before surgery and then restarting it as soon as possible following the operation. Because it takes 3–4 days for an INR in the range of 2–3 to fall below 1.5 and another 3 or more days to rise above 2.0, once the warfarin is restarted, the patient is subtherapeutic generally for only 4–8 days. If the INR has been maintained at levels above 3, the warfarin should be stopped 5–6 days earlier or a small subcutaneous dose of vitamin K (1 mg) can be given the day before surgery. Bridging anticoagulation with heparin is not warranted in low-risk patients because the bleeding risk with heparin ranges from 2%–4% in the postsurgical period and the case-fatality rate for a major bleed is about 8%–9%.

However, in patients at high risk for thromboembolism, bridging therapy with either unfractionated heparin or LMWH should be considered. Patients at increased risk of a perioperative VTE include those who are within 3 months of a venous or arterial thromboembolism; have a history of recurrent VTE, an inherited factor deficiency (antithrombin, factors C and S), or an underlying thrombogenic illness (metastatic cancer, diabetes, severe hypertension, congestive heart failure); or patients in whom cardioembolism is likely (mechanical heart valves and atrial fibrillation with valvular disease). Bridging therapy involves treating with heparin immediately before and after surgery to cover the gap in oral anticoagulation. Bridging studies of LMWH in mechanical heart valve patients have demonstrated a thromboembolism rate of less than 1% and major bleeding of about 3%, suggesting that bridging is safe in most surgeries. However, when a surgery is considered to be high risk for bleeding, the bleeding rate for heparin bridging can increase to as high as 6%. In this situation, it may be prudent to delay heparin in such patients for at least 24 hours postoperatively or withhold bridging anticoagulation completely.

C. Duration of Anticoagulation

How long to continue oral anticoagulation in patients with VTE is a topic of intense debate. Population studies have provided an overall estimate for the frequency of recurrent VTE, but it is important to evaluate each individual patient's risk.

Patients with VTE have an overall incidence of recurrent disease, once anticoagulation is discontinued, as high as 15% per year. However, when patients with malignancy, long-term immobilization, certain factor deficiencies, and thrombophilia are excluded, the incidence is much lower. Relatively healthy patients followed after a 6-month course of oral anticoagulation in one study had only a 1 in 200 patient-year chance of a fatal pulmonary embolism. Moreover, the case-fatality rate was 9% for recurrent VTE, exactly matching the case-fatality rate for anticoagulation-induced bleeding; long-term oral anticoagulation for VTE prevention carries about a 2% annual bleeding incidence.

Some studies suggest that treated VTE patients can be followed for recurrence risk on an individualized basis, for example, using the D-dimer. If the D-dimer result is prolonged (>500 ng/mL by enzyme-linked immunosorbent assay [ELISA]) 1 month after stopping anticoagulation for a first unprovoked VTE, those patients were at increased risk of VTE recurrence (9% annual rate) compared to those with a normal D-dimer (3.5% annual rate). Utilizing this approach may help in decision making with bleeding risk, but would require D-dimer cutoff values to be validated across multiple labs with different methods.

Another "personalized medicine" approach to optimizing the duration of anticoagulation for VTE is to determine thrombus resolution (vein recanalization) with serial venous ultrasonography. When compared to patients on fixed duration of therapy (>6 months), evidence for recanalization in one study was associated with a reduced incidence of recurrent VTE, permitting a shorter course of therapy in that subset. However, these data are too preliminary to justify changing clinical practice. Perhaps, in the future, measurements of vein recanalization and D-dimer levels, together with the age of the patient, bleeding risk, and complicating illness, can be incorporated in a decision-making algorithm that will help guide the duration of therapy.

Laboratory Monitoring

Although several laboratory tests can be used to monitor anticoagulation, the one-stage PT is the most popular. The test is quick and quite sensitive to reductions in the levels of prothrombin and factors VII and X. The PT is not significantly prolonged by heparin given in therapeutic amounts. Therefore, it can be used to monitor coumadin therapy without interrupting a continuous heparin infusion.

The sensitivity of the PT depends, however, on the type of thromboplastin used to initiate the reaction. Different commercial thromboplastins have different sensitivities, varying over a 2- to 3-fold range. This situation requires normalizing the prothrombin time ratio for different sensitivity thromboplastins (Figure 37–2). By knowing the relative sensitivity of a commercial thromboplastin, the **international sensitivity index (ISI)**, the nomogram in Figure 37–2 can be used to calculate the **international normalized ratio (INR)**. There is some evidence that the use of PT reagents with lower ISI values improves INR reporting by lowering its coefficient of variation by about two-thirds; for this reason, many manufacturers are moving to lower ISI reagents.

Traditionally, the PT has been measured on a venous blood sample by a local reference laboratory. However, instruments designed to do a PT on capillary whole blood, collected by finger stick, are now available for office use and patient self-testing. The CoaguChek, ProTime Monitor, and Avocet instruments have all been approved for home use. Care needs to be taken to standardize the instrument's results to those of the local laboratory to guarantee appropriate dosing. Success keeping any patient within a therapeutic range will also reflect the frequency of PT testing and the attention given to following up the patient. Many medical centers now offer an anticoagulation management service dedicated to tracking patients who receive warfarin or heparin. Studies suggest that these services do much better maintaining patients within an appropriate therapeutic range, with a significantly lower incidence of bleeding.

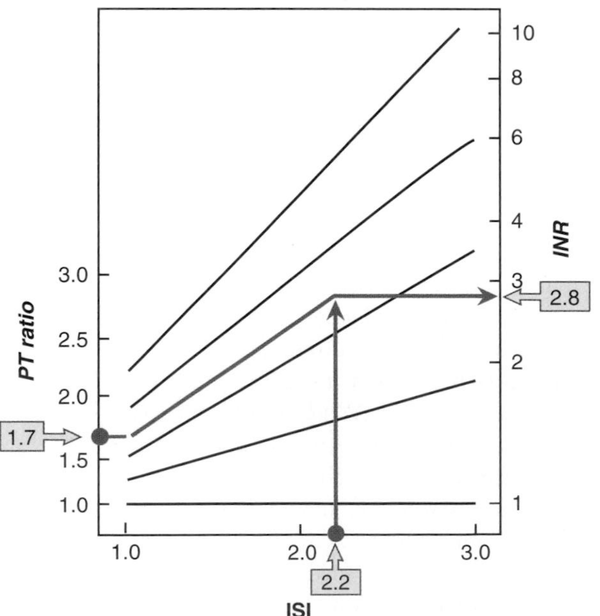

FIGURE 37–2. **Nomogram for determining the INR.** The prothrombin time (PT) must be corrected for the sensitivity of the thromboplastin reagent in use in the laboratory. By knowing the published sensitivity of the commercial thromboplastin (ISI), the nomogram is used to convert the measured PT ratio (patient's PT/control PT) to an INR. The figure shows the example of converting a PT ratio of 1.7 for a thromboplastin with an ISI of 2.2.

Adverse Events

A. Abnormal Bleeding

Abnormal bleeding is the principal adverse effect of oral anticoagulation. Risk factors that increase the likelihood of a bleed include advanced age; a preexisting medical condition, especially congestive heart failure or cancer, or bleeding diathesis; concomitant use of heparin or aspirin; and the intensity of the regimen. Generally, an INR below 3 should not by itself result in an abnormal bleed, while higher INRs are associated with a significant bleeding incidence of 20%–40% per year. The relative risk of bleeding can be, in part, predicted using the Blythe model, which uses various risk factors (age, recent stroke, cardiovascular disease, renal failure, diabetes mellitus) to derive a bleeding risk index. If a bleed occurs, the patient should be carefully worked up for an underlying medical condition. In the case of gastrointestinal bleeding, a full evaluation for ulcer disease or an occult neoplasm in the large bowel is required.

B. Contraindication of Warfarin during Pregnancy

Warfarin is **contraindicated during pregnancy**, especially during the first trimester. The drug freely crosses the placenta and can cause skin, bone, and central nervous system abnormalities in the fetus. Risk estimates for first trimester exposure are as high as 30%. Warfarin therapy at term will effectively anticoagulate the fetus with the possible risk of a significant fetal hemorrhage at delivery. If anticoagulation is required during pregnancy, heparin is a better alternative, especially the low-molecular-weight heparins (LMWH).

C. Reversal of Warfarin Anticoagulation

Warfarin anticoagulation can be reversed completely with vitamin K or transiently by the administration of fresh frozen plasma (FFP) to directly replace vitamin K–dependent coagulation factors. The latter should be reserved for emergency situations such as, for example, an anticoagulated patient who must undergo immediate surgery. To reverse an INR of 3 or greater in preparation for emergency surgery, the patient should receive 10–20 mL/kg of FFP (at least 1,000 mL) to increase levels of factors II, VII, IX, and X to at least 30% of normal. Vitamin K should also be given to correct factor production; otherwise, the PT will again rise as the infused factors, especially factor VII, which has a half-life of only 3–4 hours, are cleared.

CASE HISTORY • *Part 2*

A surgical procedure requires reversal of oral anticoagulation to guarantee adequate hemostasis during and after the operation. This does not generally apply, however, to low-dose (81 mg/d) aspirin therapy since, unlike high-dose antiplatelet drug therapy, it is not associated with increased perioperative bleeding.

The key to management of a patient on long-term warfarin therapy is to minimize the "unanticoagulated" interval and the associated risk for a thromboembolic event. Patients maintained at an INR of 2–3 can usually be managed by discontinuing their oral anticoagulant 4 days prior to their surgery to reach an INR below 1.5 on the day of surgery. This time interval will allow a return of depressed coagulation factors, in patients with normal liver function, to levels above 30%. If the patient has a higher chronic INR range (>3), then warfarin should be discontinued 5–6 days prior to the procedure.

If surgery is urgent, the time delay to "normalizing the INR" can be shortened by the administration of vitamin K or an infusion of fresh frozen plasma. However, while the INR may appear to rapidly shorten with vitamin K therapy, this is largely a result of a rapid return of factor VII, not factors IX, X, and II (prothrombin), which still require several days to recover. In addition, vitamin K therapy can make it extremely difficult to reinstitute warfarin therapy after surgery. Fresh frozen plasma must be given in volumes up to 1–1.5 L (one-third of the estimated plasma volume in a patient with an INR >2 and factor levels <5%) to reliably return the depressed factor levels to above 30%. This can be a major cardiovascular challenge and the effect will be short-lived since the half-life of factor VII is only 3–4 hours.

In this case, despite stopping her warfarin appropriately, the patient presented on the morning of surgery with only a partially corrected INR of 1.9. Since it was planned to restart warfarin as soon as possible following the surgery, she was not given vitamin K. Instead, she received 2 U of fresh frozen plasma just prior to the procedure; 1 hour after the infusion, the INR was 1.5.

Questions

- How should the patient be managed in the immediate postoperative period?
- When can her oral anticoagulation be restarted and how should it be accomplished?

When there is less urgency, vitamin K given orally will effectively reverse the warfarin effect within a few days. An INR greater than 4 can be brought into the therapeutic range within 24–48 hours by withholding the warfarin for that time and orally administering a single vitamin K dose of 2.5 mg. Several days of vitamin K therapy plus withdrawal of warfarin are required to completely reverse anticoagulation. Patients who have liver disease or have taken an overdose of warfarin can be resistant to therapy.

Vitamin K_1 (phytonadione) is the recommended preparation. It is available as 5-mg tablets, a liquid formulation containing 5–10 mg/mL for oral use, and a viscous liquid for injection (AquaMEPHYTON). A dose of 2.5–5 mg (2.5 mg if INR is between 6 and 10 or 5 mg if INR >10) of vitamin K_1 given orally is usually sufficient to decrease the INR to therapeutic levels of warfarin anticoagulation. Larger or multiple doses not only normalize the PT but also will make the patient resistant to reinstitution of warfarin therapy. Therefore, when a small dose of vitamin K is used to bring an elevated INR (>5) into the desired range of 2–4, warfarin need not be interrupted. With marked overdose or ingestion of rat poisons containing coumarin derivatives with extremely long half-lives, much larger and repeated doses of vitamin K will be required together with plasma infusions. Patients who have ingested rodenticides can require daily doses of 50–200 mg of vitamin K for months to counteract the coumarin effect.

UNFRACTIONATED HEPARIN

Unfractionated heparin is a heavily sulfated, complex polysaccharide that is naturally found in mast cell secretory granules. The commercial drug heparin is a mixture of glycosaminoglycan chain fragments of varying size (3,000–30,000 Da) extracted from bovine lung or porcine intestine. It is a highly effective anticoagulant for several clinical purposes.

Pharmacokinetics

Heparin acts by binding to and potentiating antithrombin 1,000-fold to inactivate circulating thrombin and activated factor X (Xa; Figure 37–3). Only the larger heparin molecules, those with at least 18 saccharide residues, are capable of inhibiting thrombin. Smaller heparin fragments have little effect on thrombin but do potently inhibit factor Xa. This difference in

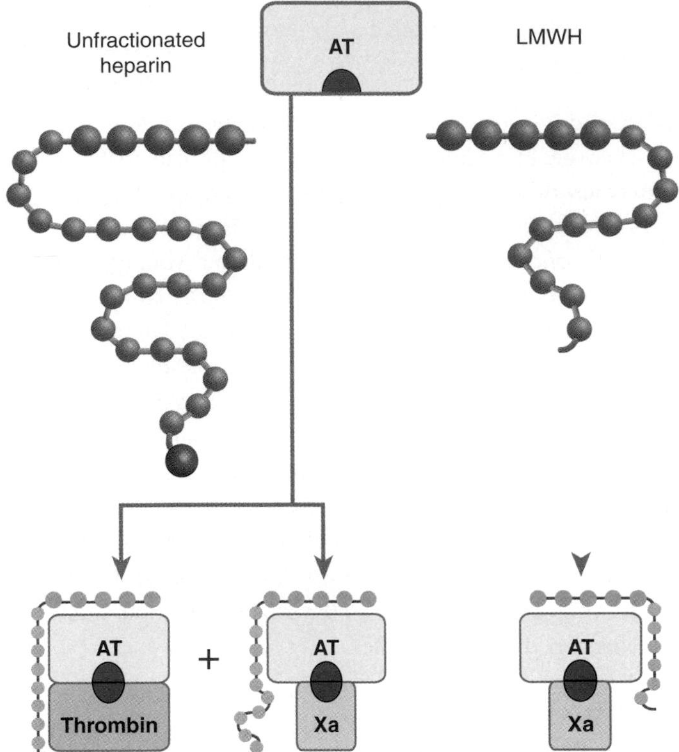

FIGURE 37–3. **Thrombin and factor Xa binding by unfractionated and low-molecular-weight heparin.** Both heparin types are capable of binding to antithrombin (AT) to catalyze the inactivation of factor Xa. Unfractionated heparin, because of its longer chain size, can also inactivate thrombin.

activity has been applied in the development of LMWH preparations. The heparin-antithrombin (AT) complex is more effective at blocking the activity of circulating thrombin than fibrin-bound thrombin; for the latter, direct thrombin inhibitors are required.

Heparin can only be administered by intravenous or subcutaneous injection. Given IV, its anticoagulant effect is immediate and easily monitored with the partial thromboplastin time (PTT). The dose response is not directly proportional to the dose administered. Clearance is biphasic, reflecting a rapid but saturable binding/uptake by plasma proteins, endothelial cells, macrophages, and hepatocytes, followed by a slower renal clearance phase. With increasing doses, the half-life of the drug in circulation lengthens significantly from 1 to several hours. Final degradation and elimination of heparin appears to involve endothelial cell and monocyte removal, hepatic metabolism, and renal clearance. Unlike the oral anticoagulants, the response to heparin is not affected by liver disease.

Heparin binding to plasma proteins can also reduce its anticoagulant activity. Since some of the plasma proteins responsible for heparin binding are acute phase reactants, ill patients can demonstrate heparin resistance. This is also seen in patients with pulmonary embolism or a large volume of thrombus. A significant decrease in AT levels secondary to liver or renal disease, or an inherited AT deficiency, will also interfere with the heparin response, since AT is required for its action.

TABLE 37–3 • Target ranges for heparin therapy

Recommended Dosage	PTT (times normal control)[a]
Venous thrombosis/pulmonary embolism	
Treatment: 5,000 U bolus, 1,000–1,500 U/h continuous infusion (28,000–40,000 U/24 h)	2.0–2.5
Prevention: 5,000 U SC 8–12 h	<1.5
Acute myocardial infarction	
With thrombolytic therapy: 5,000 U bolus, 1,000 U/h (to prevent rethrombosis): infusion (24,000/U/24 h)	1.5–2.5
Mural thrombus 8,000 U SC every 8 hours for prevention and to initiate warfarin	1.5–2.0
Unstable angina	
Treatment: 5,000 U bolus, 1,000 U/h continuous infusion (24,000 U/24 h)	1.5–2.5

[a]*Assumes PTT has been standardized against anti-Xa levels so that the therapeutic range for treating venous thrombosis is equivalent to an anti-Xa blood level of 0.3–0.7 U/mL.*

Clinical Applications

Heparin has been the traditional drug of choice whenever a patient requires immediate anticoagulation to treat or prevent venous or arterial thromboembolic disease (Table 37–3). It also has been used in the treatment of patients with unstable angina or acute myocardial infarction, and as adjunctive therapy following thrombolysis to prevent rethrombosis. Heparin has been the recommended agent for anticoagulation during pregnancy because it does not cross the placenta, and thus does not pose a risk to the fetus. However, because of the associated risk of bone loss with unfractionated heparin, LMWH is now recommended for pregnant women.

Heparin is routinely used to prevent intravascular clotting during extracorporeal circulation when patients undergo bypass surgery or hemodialysis. Low-dose heparin therapy can be used to prevent venous thromboembolism after orthopedic surgery and in patients for whom complete bed rest is required. Finally, heparin is a ubiquitous additive to intravenous fluids in order to prevent line clotting.

Therapeutic Guidelines

Heparin may be administered by continuous intravenous infusion or intermittent intravenous or subcutaneous injection. The intravenous route is preferred when immediate anticoagulation is desired, since the subcutaneous route is less dependable in time of onset and dose response. Intravenous heparinization should begin with a loading dose of 5,000 U (75 U/kg body weight) followed by a continuous infusion of 1,000–1,500 U per hour (28,000–40,000 U over the first 24 hours). An alternative approach is to use a weight-based nomogram where 80 U/kg is given as a loading dose, followed by a continuous infusion of

TABLE 37–4 • Heparin dose adjustment

PTT(s) (normal 27–35 s)	Start: 5,000-U bolus; 1,300 U/h continuous infusion
<50	Rebolus 5,000 U; increase infusion rate by 100 U/h
50–60	Increase infusion rate by 100 U/h
60–85	No change—60–85 s is therapeutic range
85–100	Decrease infusion rate 100 U/h
100–120	Stop infusion for 30 min, decrease rate 100 U/h
<120	Stop infusion for 60 min, decrease rate 200 U/h

18 U/kg per hour. Although overweight patients are more likely to achieve a therapeutic PTT within the first 24 hours by this approach, the PTT still needs to be closely monitored and the dose adjusted accordingly.

A. Dose Adjustment

For the first 48 hours, a PTT should be measured at 6- to 12-hour intervals and the rate of infusion adjusted to achieve a prolongation of between 1.8 and 2.5 times the normal PTT. Table 37–4 lists guidelines for dose adjustment according to the PTT measurement. The most common failure is achieving a therapeutic range within the first 12–24 hours. Therefore, close attention should be paid to the first few PTT measurements and the infusion rate adjusted appropriately. Regardless of the method used to dose adjust, weight-based nomogram or non-weight-based PTT-guided adjustment, only 50% of patients will reach the target range for the PTT by 24 hours. The rest will fall below or above the therapeutic range.

Dosing is more difficult when the drug is given IV or subcutaneously (SC) on an intermittent schedule. Intermittent dosing results in very high heparin levels immediately after injection, followed by a return of the PTT to near normal just prior to the next injection. To monitor therapy, the PTT should be obtained 1 hour prior to the next scheduled injection and the heparin dosage adjusted to keep the PTT at greater than 1.5 times normal. When a 12-hour schedule is used, there is a definite risk that the PTT will return to normal for some hours prior to the next treatment, thereby breaking the continuity of anticoagulation.

In general, patients receiving intermittent intravenous injections will require more heparin per 24 hours than those receiving continuous infusion (36,000 U versus 30,000 U per 24 hours on the average). Subcutaneous injection patients will also require higher 24-hour dosages of heparin. Moreover, they run the risk of erratic absorption from injection sites, which can lead to a loss of control, either too little or too great a PTT response.

B. Low-Dose Heparin and Other Therapies

Low-dose heparin, 5,000 U every 8 or 12 hours administered SC, will reduce the risk of venous thrombosis and pulmonary embolism in medical and surgical patients. The PTT is not prolonged and the risk of major bleeding is not increased, even when patients undergo major orthopedic surgical procedures. However, for the purpose of perioperative prophylaxis, LMWH or low-dose warfarin therapy (and now other anti-Xa and thrombin inhibitors) may be more effective. Full-dose heparin therapy can be safely given to cardiac patients as part of their treatment for an acute myocardial infarction and as an adjunct to thrombolytic therapy. Combination therapy with aspirin and/or clopidogrel is also safe and may be more effective in preventing coronary rethrombosis.

C. Addition of Warfarin for Chronic Anticoagulation

When chronic anticoagulation is indicated, warfarin therapy should be initiated at the same time the patient begins heparin. This approach should permit discontinuation of the heparin by the fourth to sixth day of warfarin therapy, once a therapeutic INR is achieved for 2 consecutive days. Delays in starting warfarin increase the risk of complications from heparin anticoagulation, whether abnormal bleeding or the development of heparin-induced thrombocytopenia (HIT)/thrombosis.

D. Treatment of Thromboembolic Disease during Pregnancy

One exception to the heparin/warfarin regimen is the treatment of thromboembolic disease during pregnancy, where LMWH, because of its lower risk of HIT and osteoporosis, is the drug of choice for both prophylaxis and treatment of women with symptomatic thromboembolic disease. For near-term management, patients may be switched to unfractionated heparin, 5,000–10,000 U SC twice a day, because of its shorter half-life. This also allows use of the PTT to monitor the level of anticoagulation during labor. Postpartum, women with symptomatic thromboembolic disease should receive at least 6–8 weeks of warfarin anticoagulation. Women with a history of an antiphospholipid antibody complicated by a thromboembolic event or previous miscarriage can be treated with LMWH or low-dose unfractionated heparin the first 34 weeks of gestation. This therapy is well tolerated and has been shown to increase the chance for a live birth.

Laboratory Monitoring

The **activated PTT** is the preferred laboratory test for monitoring heparin therapy. It is readily available in most hospital laboratories and will reflect heparin blood levels with considerable precision if well standardized. The reagents used in the PTT do influence the responsiveness of the test. Therefore, each laboratory should establish the therapeutic range in seconds for its own PTT method to correspond to an anti-Xa level of 0.3–0.7 U/mL.

Measurement of the **activated clotting time (ACT)** is used to monitor heparin therapy during extracorporeal circulation (bypass) and with cardiac procedures in the catheterization laboratory. For bypass, the issue is one of guaranteeing complete anticoagulation to prevent intravascular clotting, followed by full reversal of heparinization at the end of extracorporeal circulation. The major advantage of the ACT measurement, even though it is less precise, is that it can be performed in the operating room, avoiding the delay inherent in a laboratory PTT measurement. Recently, a direct measurement of heparin levels has been introduced using automated equipment.

Adverse Effects

A. Sudden, Severe Bleeding

The principal adverse effect of heparin is sudden, severe bleeding. Factors that increase the risk of hemorrhage include dose and route of administration, reduced levels of key coagulation proteins, thrombocytopenia, concomitant use of other anticoagulants or drugs that inhibit platelet function, and the presence of a medical or surgical illness that increases the risk of bleeding. As regards dosing, the incidence of major bleeding is proportionate to the cumulative daily dose of heparin and is also increased in those given intermittent intravenous or subcutaneous injections. When used in conjunction with thrombolytic therapy, marked hypofibrinogenemia increases the risk of spontaneous bleeding and hemorrhage with invasive procedures. Patients with renal failure or severe liver disease on heparin also have a greater risk of bleeding.

B. Heparin-Induced Thrombocytopenia and Platelet Thrombosis

HIT type II (immune-related) with thromboembolic complications is the other major adverse effect. When exposed to heparin for more than 5 days, patients can form IgG antibodies that are capable of binding the heparin-PF4 complex to the platelet surface, resulting in activation, aggregate formation, and the release of thrombogenic platelet microparticles, all leading to removal of platelets from circulation. An incidence of HIT of 10%–15% has been reported in patients who receive bovine heparin, whereas the incidence with porcine heparin is 4%–6%. Risk is in part related to the dose of heparin and the duration of therapy. Patients receiving full-dose heparin for more than 5 days are at greatest risk. Patients who are exposed to heparin on more than one occasion are also at increased risk and can exhibit an acute form of immune-related HIT with all of the manifestations of a drug reaction, including the sudden onset of dyspnea, shaking chills, diaphoresis, hypertension, and tachycardia. These patients are at extreme risk for a fatal thromboembolism if heparin is continued. See the full discussion of HIT presentation and treatment in Chapter 31.

HIT-induced platelet activation and thrombin generation can cause significant thrombosis and tissue damage, such as venous limb gangrene, and even death. The frequency of arterial or venous thrombosis in HIT patients depends on the clinical situation. While it may be no more than 1% in otherwise healthy patients, it can reach incidences of 40%–50% in postoperative patients with high levels of circulating thrombin after receiving heparin for more than 5 days. Therefore, the **platelet count** should be monitored as frequently as every other day when a patient is treated with heparin for longer than 5 days. Even a modest decrease in the platelet count (30%–50% reduction from baseline) can indicate the appearance of the pathologic heparin-PF4 antibody.

If there is a clinical suspicion of HIT because of an observed fall in the platelet count or a thrombotic or embolic event while on heparin, all heparin should be discontinued immediately, including heparin line flushes and all IV or SC dosing. This is true even when a laboratory assay for the HIT antibody is available. To continue heparinization while awaiting the test result runs the risk of a significant, even fatal thromboembolic event.

Because HIT itself is a hypercoagulable state, and because the responsible heparin is often being used in situations where anticoagulation is required (eg, coronary artery bypass surgery, presence of a deep venous thrombosis [DVT] or pulmonary embolus, dialysis), a direct thrombin inhibitor (DTI; eg, lepirudin or argatroban) should be started, using the PTT to monitor therapy. If long-term anticoagulation is necessary, oral anticoagulation with warfarin should be initiated when the platelet count has completely recovered and while the patient is still on a DTI, with at least a 2- to 3-day overlap once the PT has reached a therapeutic level (see Chapter 31).

C. Other Side Effects

Several less common but certainly serious side effects of heparin have been reported. These include hypersensitivity reactions, skin reactions, hypoaldosteronism with hyperkalemia, and osteoporosis. Long-term heparin therapy is associated with a 5%–7% loss in bone mass. LMWH is the best alternative. Urticaria, erythematous plaques, and even skin necrosis (the latter with HIT) can occur at the site of heparin injection.

D. Reversal of Heparin Anticoagulation

Heparin anticoagulation can be reversed by the intravenous infusion of protamine sulfate, a low-molecular-weight protein derived from fish sperm. One milligram of protamine neutralizes approximately 100 U of heparin. The treatment dose must be estimated according to the status of the heparin regimen and the predicted half-life of residual heparin in the patient. The calculated dose of protamine sulfate is then infused IV at a rate less than or equal to 5 mg per minute; a more rapid infusion can result in marked hypotension, dyspnea, bradycardia, and even anaphylaxis. In light of these side effects, it is best, if possible, to allow the heparin anticoagulant effect to naturally dissipate. This should occur within a matter of hours, unless very large amounts of heparin have been administered.

LOW-MOLECULAR-WEIGHT HEPARIN

Heparin molecules with fewer than 18 saccharides can be prepared chemically or enzymatically from natural heparin. Because of the smaller molecular size (average 5,000 Da), LMWH is less able to bind to antithrombin and thrombin simultaneously but does retain its ability to inhibit factor Xa (see Figure 37–3). LMWH does not inhibit platelet function or increase microvascular permeability to the same extent as heparin.

The smaller molecular size also affects the pharmacokinetics. LMWH has a lower binding affinity for endothelial cells and plasma proteins, including platelet factor 4, fibronectin, and vWF. This translates into a better dose-response relationship for therapeutically administered LMWH preparations. LMWH has a dose-independent plasma half-life that is 2–4 times longer than unfractionated heparin when given IV and 3–6 times longer when given SC at therapeutic doses, making it possible to administer LMWH on a less frequent schedule. Clinical trials of LMWH (enoxaparin) for the prevention of thrombosis during surgery have successfully used twice-a-day dosing regimens. Dalteparin, a longer-acting LMWH, can be administered once a day. The extremely reliable dose response to LMWH makes laboratory testing of the anti-Xa level unnecessary except in patients who weigh substantially more than 80 kg or have renal failure.

Clinical Applications

LMWH has now been studied in numerous randomized clinical trials aimed at the prevention and treatment of venous thrombosis in high-risk patients. In general, it appears to be a slightly more effective anticoagulant when compared with unfractionated heparin, while reducing the incidence of microvascular bleeding. Because of this, LMWH has become the preferred choice for prophylactic therapy for patients over age 40 who are undergoing a major surgical procedure, especially if they have a history of previous thromboembolic disease, a malignancy, a fracture, or spinal cord injury. Untreated, this group of patients has a 40%–80% incidence of deep venous thrombosis (DVT) and a 4%–10% risk for a pulmonary embolus (PE). LMWH prophylaxis reduces the risk of DVT by 75%–80%. In patients undergoing hip or knee surgery or long-bone fracture repair, LMWH reduces a 50% untreated incidence of DVT by 60%–70%. Treatment for 4–6 weeks post-surgery is recommended, since the risk of thromboembolism in hip arthroplasty patients extends well beyond the usual 7–10 days of standard prophylaxis. LMWH, specifically enoxaparin, has also been shown to be safer and more effective than warfarin in patients undergoing orthopedic surgery; those studies used thromboprophylaxis for 10–35 days following surgery, depending on relative VTE risk. Even in relatively minor procedures such as knee arthroscopy, the incidence of VTE is less with LMWH (for 7 days) treatment compared with local measures such as compression stockings.

Pregnancy clearly shows the safety profile of low-molecular-weight heparins, mostly from studies using enoxaparin, dalteparin, and nadroparin. The indications for LMWH in pregnancy include therapy for VTE, thromboprophylaxis for at-risk pregnancies, and prevention of recurrent fetal loss. For pregnant patients treated for VTE, there was a 1.15% VTE recurrence rate on LMWH therapy and a 0.5% incidence of arterial thrombosis, the latter occurring exclusively in lupus anticoagulant patients. For pregnant patients treated prophylactically or for previous fetal loss, the VTE incidence was 0.8%. Overall, pregnant patients on LMWH had a 2% rate of bleeding. In nearly 3,000 cases treated with LMWH, heparin-induced thrombocytopenia was not seen.

Patients with a complicated medical illness who are admitted to a hospital for at least 5 days can also benefit from low-dose LMWH (40 mg enoxaparin SC once a day) without an increase in bleeding complications. LMWH is comparable to or better than unfractionated heparin in unstable angina patients, but so far appears to provide no advantage over unfractionated heparin in angioplasty patients. Finally, LMWH may be the preferred anticoagulant for the initial treatment of patients with uncomplicated DVT or PE. It is more effective in preventing a subsequent embolus, while causing fewer bleeding complications. It also has the advantages of easier administration and a more reliable dose response. This makes laboratory testing unnecessary and opens the door to earlier discharge from the hospital or even treatment at home from day one in selected patients.

Overall, LMWH is a safe drug. It is somewhat more effective than unfractionated heparin, with a lower risk of significant bleeding. This reflects the reduced binding to platelets, vWF, and endothelial cells. The incidence of HIT and related thrombosis is also significantly lower with LMWH. However, because there is cross-reactivity, LMWH cannot be substituted for unfractionated heparin in known HIT patients. Unresolved issues include the risk of osteoporosis with long-term use and the poor effectiveness of protamine in reversing the LMWH anticoagulant effect. Protamine sulfate does not bind as well to low-molecular-weight fragments of heparin and will only neutralize the LMWH effect by about 10%.

Therapeutic Guidelines

In the United States, several LMWH preparations (enoxaparin, dalteparin, and ardeparin) have been approved for use in thrombosis prevention in surgery patients and in the treatment of thromboembolic disease (Table 37–5). Given in a dose of 30 mg

TABLE 37–5 • LMWH dose recommendations

Indication	Recommended Dose and Schedule
Prophylaxis	
General surgery	
Low risk	Enoxaparin 4,000 U before and then daily or dalteparin 2,000–3,000 U SC just before and then daily after surgery
High risk	Enoxaparin 3,000 U SC before and then bid or dalteparin 5,000 U SC before and then daily
Orthopedic surgery	Enoxaparin 3,000 U SC before and then bid or dalteparin 5,000 U SC before and then daily
Trauma/spinal injury	Enoxaparin 3,000 U SC bid
Immobility (bed rest secondary to medical illness: stroke, CHF, etc)	Enoxaparin 4,000 U SC or dalteparin 2,000–3,000 U SC daily
Treatment	
DVT or PE	Enoxaparin or dalteparin 100 U/kg SC bid
Unstable angina	Enoxaparin or dalteparin 100 U/kg SC bid

(3,000 anti-factor Xa IU) SC twice a day (40 mg once a day for general medical and surgical patients), enoxaparin is more effective than unfractionated heparin and has a lower incidence of bleeding complications. The longer-acting preparation, dalteparin (Fragmin), can be given once a day in doses of 2,500 or 5,000 U, depending on the severity of the surgery. Orthopedic surgery patients who receive LMWH prophylaxis for 4–10 days while in the hospital can be discharged off anticoagulants with little risk of subsequent symptomatic DVT or pulmonary embolism. Patients with an inherited thrombophilia or history of recurrent thrombotic disease may be maintained on warfarin following discharge to minimize the risk of late-occurring thromboembolism.

Full-dose LMWH, 1 mg/kg (100 U/kg) of enoxaparin given SC twice a day, is the best studied, and is therefore the preferred therapy in the treatment of DVT or PE. To guarantee effectiveness, dalteparin should also be given in a dose of 100 U/kg twice a day. LMWH can be used safely in patients with computed tomography (CT) scan–proven ischemic stroke to prevent paralysis/bed rest–induced thromboembolic disease. It can also be used in full dose for unstable angina with comparable efficacy to unfractionated heparin. LMWH can be used in the treatment of angioplasty patients to prevent restenosis, but holds no particular advantage over unfractionated heparin.

Cost-Effectiveness

LMWH is significantly more expensive than unfractionated heparin. For this reason alone, its use cannot be justified when unfractionated heparin is equally efficacious, as with low-dose prophylaxis in routine medical and surgical patients. However, a case can be made for LMWH as the more effective agent in orthopedic surgery patients and in the treatment of patients with venous thrombosis/thromboembolism. With orthopedic surgery, the lower incidence of postoperative thromboembolic disease provides a significant cost savings by preventing prolonged hospital stays for a complicating DVT or PE. In the treatment of the medical patient with venous thrombosis/thromboembolism or unstable angina, the elimination of the need for the heparin-infusion pump and laboratory testing (PTTs 2–4 times per day) makes the cost of unfractionated heparin and LMWH equivalent. An earlier discharge from the hospital, or even total treatment as an outpatient, makes LMWH the more cost-effective treatment strategy.

Adverse Effects

Just as with unfractionated heparin, the principal adverse effect of LMWH is bleeding. Although the risk at recommended dosages is somewhat less with LMWH, there is a dose relationship. Patients given more than 1 mg/kg twice a day have a higher incidence of bleeding. Renal failure patients are at special risk, since LMWH is primarily cleared through the kidney. In this situation, laboratory monitoring of anti-Xa activity is needed to adjust the LMWH dose. There have also been reports of spinal cord bleeds in patients receiving LMWH who have had epidural catheters placed. HIT can occur with any LMWH, albeit at a greatly reduced incidence compared with unfractionated heparin.

ANTI-Xa INHIBITORS

Fondaparinux (Arixtra) is a parenteral synthetic pentapolysaccharide that binds to antithrombin and specifically inhibits factor Xa. This FDA-approved drug holds the potential for replacing both unfractionated heparin and LMWH in the prevention and treatment of thromboembolic disease. After binding to and potentiating AT activity, fondaparinux can disengage to bind additional AT molecules. When used prophylactically in a dose of 2.5 mg SC once a day (half-life of 17 hours) for 3 weeks following knee, hip, or major abdominal surgery, it appears to be more effective than enoxaparin in preventing VTE, with a 3% incidence of bleeding complications. Some studies show a 50% decrease in VTE risk with fondaparinux compared with enoxaparin, and similar results have been noted with rivaroxaban, another Xa inhibitor approved in Canada and the European Union. Fondaparinux is usually started at least 6 hours following surgery. Once-daily subcutaneous fondaparinux (5–10 mg according to body weight) has been shown to be as effective as unfractionated heparin in the initial treatment of pulmonary embolus.

In acute coronary syndrome patients receiving VTE prophylaxis, fondaparinux at 2.5 mg SC once a day was as effective as enoxaparin but with lesser bleeding rates out to 30 days. Like enoxaparin, fondaparinux can be given without monitoring. Increased risk of bleeding is seen in patients weighing less than 110 lb, elderly people, and patients with renal dysfunction since fondaparinux is renally excreted like all of the anti-Xa inhibitors. **Parenteral idraparinux** has a very long half-life (80 hours) such that it is given as a weekly SC dose (2.5 mg) for VTE therapy. **Oral rivaroxaban**, with a half-life of 7 hours and given as a 10-mg dose once daily, appears to be at least as effective as enoxaparin for VTE prophylaxis after orthopedic surgery.

DIRECT THROMBIN INHIBITORS

Direct thrombin inhibitors (DTIs) have no plasma protein binding and thus do not require AT interaction in order to inhibit thrombin activity. DTIs are very effective at blocking thrombus growth, especially when thrombin is fibrin bound, a situation that is relatively resistant to heparin therapy. Heparin-induced thrombocytopenia is a major indication for DTI therapy because of the associated increase in fibrin-bound thrombin activity. In addition, because several of the new DTI drugs can be given orally, there is intense interest in their use for VTE prophylaxis.

Dabigatran is an orally absorbed DTI drug approved for use in Canada and the European Union. It is excreted renally and has a half-life of 17 hours. Given prophylactically at 150–220 mg once a day following orthopedic surgery, dabigatran was as effective as enoxaparin at preventing VTE. Another oral DTI, **ximelagatran**, was recalled because of hepatotoxicity.

Lepirudin (Refludan), a recombinant hirudin derived from yeast, is a highly specific direct inhibitor of thrombin, binding to thrombin without AT as a cofactor. It was initially studied in combination with t-PA in order to prevent the reocclusion of coronary arteries following successful thrombolysis. However, it did not appear to add significant value to the treatment outcome and there was a greater incidence of bleeding requiring transfusion. Lepirudin is FDA approved for the treatment of HIT. It is also at least as good as, if not better than, LMWH in the prevention of DVT in postoperative patients when given in a dose of 15 mg SC twice a day.

Lepirudin is considered by many to be the drug of choice for the treatment of HIT. It has no cross-reactivity with heparin and can be managed using the PTT to adjust the dose. After the clinician documents a baseline PTT in the normal range, the drug is administered IV in a bolus of 0.4 mg/kg over 15–20 seconds, followed by continuous infusion at a rate of approximately 0.15 mg/kg/h. The dose should then be adjusted to keep the PTT between 1.5 and 2.5 times normal. Renal failure patients will require a dose reduction of 30%–50%, since hirudin is primarily cleared through the kidney. If oral anticoagulation is initiated, the lepirudin dose should be reduced to keep the PTT at 1.5 times the control. The platelet count can show a rapid recovery, indicating a reversal of the HIT process of platelet activation and consumption.

Lepirudin is generally well tolerated. The most common adverse effect is bleeding, usually minor bleeding from puncture sites. However, blood loss sufficient to require transfusion is seen in up to 15% of patients. Lepirudin inhibition of thrombin is not reversible by any agents such as protamine. The half-life of lepirudin is approximately 90 minutes, although delayed clearances are seen in patients with renal disease. Unfortunately, lepirudin is associated with a 40%–75% incidence of antibody formation to the drug after 4 days of therapy; re-dosing lepirudin is therefore absolutely contraindicated since fatal anaphylaxis can occur.

Bivalirudin is a synthetic hirudin-like peptide that is cleaved by thrombin itself, thus producing a much more transient inhibition of thrombin. In fact, it has the shortest half-life of all the available direct thrombin inhibitors. It is largely metabolized in plasma, making it safer than hirudin for use in patients with either renal or hepatic failure. The dose response is also more predictable. This enhances its safety when used in situations like percutaneous transcoronary angioplasty (PTCA), where hirudin use has been associated with a greater incidence of bleeding complications. Bivalirudin is FDA approved as an alternative to unfractionated heparin for PTCA.

Desirudin, another short-acting hirudin derivative, is approved by the FDA for VTE prophylaxis following hip surgery. It shows promise for decreasing the incidence of venous thrombosis post–orthopedic surgery compared to both enoxaparin and unfractionated heparin.

Argatroban (Novastan), a substituted derivative of arginine, is a reversible inhibitor of both soluble and fibrin-bound thrombin. However, unlike lepirudin, it inhibits only the catalytic site of thrombin and lacks activity for the fibrinogen binding site. For this reason, it may have a somewhat lower efficacy than lepirudin, but argatroban is still effective (and FDA approved) for treatment of HIT. It is metabolized by the liver, and therefore has a greater safety margin in renal failure patients, but should be avoided in patients with liver disease. Like heparin, it is best administered as a continuous intravenous infusion (2.0 μg/kg per minute), titrated to achieve an activated PTT of 1.5–3 times baseline. Like lepirudin, argatroban prolongs the PT and INR, complicating the transition to oral anticoagulant therapy. Advantages of argatroban include its rapid reversibility—a half-life of 30 minutes—and unlike lepirudin, argatroban does not induce antibodies to itself, making it safe to use repeatedly if needed. It may, however, be associated with a higher incidence of major bleeding, especially in patients with HIT with thrombosis.

ANTICOAGULANTS IN DEVELOPMENT

A number of new agents are currently undergoing clinical trials. They include recombinant TFPI (tissue factor pathway inhibitor) and APC (activated protein C), NAPc2 (a nematode anticoagulant peptide), the thrombin mutant analogue PCA (protein C activator), and soluble thrombomodulin. PCA demonstrates the interesting property of comparable antithrombotic activity to both LMWH and APC, but unlike the latter agents, PCA does not increase bleeding in animal models.

THROMBOLYTIC DRUGS

Intravascular thrombi can be dissolved by thrombolytic drugs, such as streptokinase, urokinase, and t-PA. These agents are of greatest use in the treatment of patients with arterial thrombosis, including coronary, peripheral, and, less commonly, cerebral artery thrombosis.

Pharmacokinetics

Streptokinase binds to and activates plasminogen to form free plasmin. When given in doses of 250,000–1.5 million units IV, the active streptokinase-plasminogen complex is not inhibited by α_2-antiplasmin, and both fibrin and fibrinogen destruction occur. This situation continues as long as the drug is infused or for about 80 minutes after a single bolus dose. **Urokinase** is a serine protease that also lacks fibrin specificity. It is most often used as a continuous infusion by catheter to the site of a peripheral arterial thrombosis.

t-PA is also a serine protease. However, it is selective for plasminogen bound to fibrin clot, making it more clot specific. t-PA is naturally produced by endothelial cells to inhibit clot propagation. As a part of this natural cycle, only small amounts are released into circulation, and this quantity is rapidly inactivated by plasminogen activator inhibitor-1 (PAI-1) so as to prevent any effect on circulating plasminogen and fibrinogen. When **recombinant t-PA (rt-PA)** is administered to patients with coronary thrombosis, a loading dose is given, followed by a continuous infusion over 3–4 hours to a total of 100–150 mg of rt-PA. This situation results in plasma concentrations of t-PA that are several thousand times greater than physiologic levels. It is common, therefore, to see partial breakdown of circulating fibrinogen as well as clot lysis.

Clinical Applications

The principal application of the thrombolytic agents is to dissolve arterial thrombi to prevent irreversible organ damage. In the case of a thrombus or embolus in large arterial vessels, direct infusion of a lytic agent by catheter can result in effective clot lysis with little systemic fibrinogen destruction. With thrombosis of smaller arterial vessels, especially acute coronary artery occlusion, intravenous administration of either streptokinase or rt-PA can result in dissolution of the offending thrombus and return of blood flow. However, new clot formation may occur shortly after thrombolysis unless effective anticoagulation is maintained with heparin and anti-platelet drugs such as aspirin and clopidogrel.

Most patients with iliofemoral DVT will develop post-phlebitic syndrome with objective signs and symptoms of venous insufficiency, including skin thickening (nonpitting edema) and discoloration and, in some, nonhealing leg ulcers and venous claudication. Thrombolytic therapy for iliofemoral venous thrombosis has had variable success in decreasing the severity of post-phlebitic venous insufficiency. However, if and when clot lysis is complete, morbidity is reduced. Both catheter-directed urokinase therapy and venous t-PA have been used effectively. Thrombolytic drugs are also used to clear thrombosed intravenous catheters and in the treatment of life-threatening PE.

Adverse Effects

Thrombolytic agents not only dissolve intravascular clots but will also interfere with the normal coagulation sequence required for wound healing. Therefore, contraindications to thrombolytic therapy include recent surgery or an invasive procedure involving arterial puncture, a history of a previous cerebrovascular ischemic or hemorrhagic stroke, significant hypertension, recent gastrointestinal bleeding, or a history of a hemorrhagic diathesis. The incidence of complicating hemorrhage following intravenous streptokinase or rt-PA is directly related to the drug dosage or the concurrent use of heparin.

Some protocols in the treatment of coronary artery thrombosis have involved the administration of a **fixed dose of streptokinase or rt-PA** without regard for body size. It is not surprising, therefore, that women of lower body weight show a higher incidence of fibrinogen destruction and **complicating hemorrhage**. When thrombolytic agents are infused over many hours, as has been used for peripheral arterial or venous disease, fibrinogen destruction causing circulating levels to fall below 100 mg/dL with accompanying hemorrhage is much more common. Severe bleeding immediately following fibrinolytic therapy should be managed by discontinuing the heparin and administering cryoprecipitate if the measured fibrinogen level is less than 100 mg/dL. Finally, late-onset bleeding occurring hours or days after thrombolysis is invariably the result of concurrent heparin therapy, not the lytic agent.

Patients who have previously received streptokinase or have antistreptokinase antibodies resulting from a prior streptococcal infection are at risk of an adverse reaction to the drug. This includes an IgE-mediated acute allergic reaction and, on occasion, severe anaphylaxis. This is not true for rt-PA, which is a recombinant human protein. At the same time, the cost of rt-PA is far greater than that of streptokinase.

CASE HISTORY • *Part 3*

For most surgical procedures, anticoagulation can be safely instituted after 12–24 hours of demonstrated hemostasis. Some situations may temper that interval, including the nature of the operation, for example neurosurgery where bleeding into a closed space can be disastrous or when there is an ongoing difficulty with bleeding at the operative site.

In low-risk patients, warfarin therapy can be restarted with a daily dose of 5 mg until the INR is above 2.0. This patient is at somewhat greater risk due to her complicating illnesses (atrial fibrillation and a heart murmur), and therefore probably should be considered for bridging therapy with unfractionated heparin, starting 12–24 hours after surgery and continuing until the INR is in a therapeutic range for 1–2 days. She can then return to her maintenance warfarin dose. Cardiac ultrasound imaging to determine any valvular abnormality would assist in that decision. Instead of unfractionated heparin, some high-risk patients may be managed with a daily prophylactic dose of LMWH over the 3–5 days of reinstituting warfarin to establish a therapeutic INR. This may be especially useful for surgeries with increased thrombogenic potential, such as hip or knee replacement.

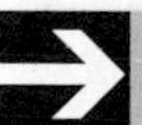

POINTS TO REMEMBER

Anti-platelet agents include aspirin, clopidogrel, the inhibitors of glycoprotein IIb/IIIa, and persantine. These drugs are efficacious in the treatment of arterial thromboembolism, especially when accompanied by abnormal vasculature, such as atherosclerosis.

Aspirin is the mainstay of arterial thrombosis treatment and prophylaxis; it is inexpensive and safe. Aspirin irreversibly inhibits the platelet cyclooxygenase pathway, blocking platelet release and aggregation. By itself or in combination with other anti-platelet agents or anticoagulants, it is used to treat and prevent coronary artery disease/myocardial infarction, transient ischemic attacks and completed stroke, and peripheral arterial disease.

Low-dose aspirin (81–162 mg per day) is as effective as higher doses and carries less risk of gastrointestinal bleeding. The addition of clopidogrel is suggested for patients with clinical resistance to aspirin (ongoing symptoms or signs of thromboembolism despite adequate aspirin treatment) and for patients following coronary angioplasty.

Clopidogrel is an ADP receptor blocker with similar indications for thrombotic therapy as aspirin. It is normally given in a daily dose of 75 mg. However, since its full effect is delayed for several days after initiating therapy, a loading dose of 300 mg should be given when more immediate activity is needed.

The parenteral and oral GPIIb/IIIa inhibitors (abciximab, eptifibatide, and tirofiban) are used for acute myocardial infarction and unstable angina. Intravenous abciximab allows for immediate onset and long-lasting effect, while the other oral inhibitors, because of their shorter half-life, can be used for patients who are likely to need angioplasty or bypass grafting. All of these inhibitors can produce thrombocytopenia as a side effect.

Anticoagulation therapy involves agents that decrease thrombin generation or block thrombin activity—coumarin compounds, heparins, anti-Xa agents, and direct thrombin inhibitors. These agents are key to prophylaxis against venous or cardiac/valvular thromboembolism and treating any and all types of acute arterial or venous thrombosis/embolic disease.

Oral anticoagulation is most often accomplished with warfarin, which decreases synthesis of active vitamin K–dependent factors II, VII, IX, and X, and also the natural anticoagulants, proteins C and S. The prothrombin time (PT) is used to monitor the effect of warfarin, although to adjust for variable reagent and instrument sensitivities, the PT is always reported with the accompanying INR (international normalized ratio).

Prophylaxis against recurrent venous thromboembolism (VTE) is a common indication for warfarin anticoagulation. Patients who have suffered a venous thrombosis should be anticoagulated for at least 6 months or longer, especially if the D-dimer remains elevated or the involved vein(s) fail to recanalize. Patients with recurrent VTE or inherent risk factors may require lifelong anticoagulation.

Unfractionated heparin is the drug of choice for immediate full anticoagulation when rapid reversibility is important. It acts by binding to antithrombin (AT) to inhibit thrombin activity. Because heparin also binds other proteins, its bioavailability may not be reliable, requiring frequent adjustments in dosing to maintain the PTT range.

Low-molecular-weight heparin, which primarily blocks factor Xa and not thrombin, is consistently bioavailable, allowing for weight-based once- or twice-daily administration without monitoring. The indications for LMWH are identical to that of unfractionated heparin, although its effect cannot be rapidly reversed.

The main complication of both unfractionated heparin and LMWH therapy is bleeding, although the incidence with LMWH is lower. Heparin-induced thrombocytopenia (HIT) is another potentially life-threatening complication. Frequent platelet counts are required to detect the appearance of the HIT antibody.

HIT is associated with a hypercoagulable state, which, in patients undergoing surgery, presents a very high risk for VTE and arterial thrombosis/embolism. In this situation, treatment with one of the direct thrombin inhibitors, lepirudin or other hirudin-based compounds, or argatroban, is indicated (see Chapter 31).

Thrombolysis can play an important role in managing arterial and large venous thromboembolic events, especially if life threatening. Streptokinase, urokinase, and t-PA have all been used successfully, but only t-PA is relatively fibrin specific, thereby reducing the risk of marked hypofibrinoginemia. Heparin is used concurrently to maintain anticoagulation.

The risk of bleeding with thrombolysis can be correlated with fibrinogen levels below 100 mg/dL. If bleeding occurs, heparin should be discontinued, and cryoprecipitate given. Contraindications to thrombolysis include hemorrhagic stroke, ongoing or recent gastrointestinal bleeding, and a history of bleeding disorder.

Newer anticoagulants include the anti-Xa agents—fondaparinux, the long-acting idraparinux, and the oral drug, rivaroxaban. These may be as effective as LMWH in treatment and prophylaxis of VTE and coronary arterial disease. Like LMWH, they do not require monitoring and appear to have a low bleeding incidence.

BIBLIOGRAPHY

Principles of Management

Anand S et al: Oral anticoagulant and anti-platelet therapy and peripheral arterial disease. N Engl J Med 2007;357:217.

Geerts WH et al: Prevention of venous thromboembolism: American College of Chest Physicians evidence-based clinical practice guidelines. Chest 2008;133:381S.

Palareti G et al: D-dimer testing to determine the duration of anticoagulation therapy. N Engl J Med 2006;355:1780.

Silverstein RL et al: Venous thrombosis in the elderly: more questions than answers. Blood 2007;110:3097.

Spyropoulos AC, Turpie AGG: Periopeative bridging interruption with heparin for the patient receiving long-term anticoagulation. Curr Opin Pulm Med 2005;11:373.

Verhovsek M et al: Systematic review: D-dimer to predict recurrent disease after stopping anticoagulation therapy for unprovoked venous thromboembolism. Ann Intern Med 2008;149:481.

Anti-platelet Drugs

Bhatt DL et al: ACCF/ACG/AHA 2008 expert consensus document on reducing the gastrointestinal risks of anti-platelet therapy and NSAID use: a report of the American College of Cardiology Foundation Task Force on Clinical Expert Consensus Documents. J Am Coll Cardiol 2008;52:1502.

Eisenstein EL et al: Clopidogrel use and long-term clinical outcomes after drug-eluting stent implantation. JAMA 2007;297:159.

Grines CL et al: Prevention of premature discontinuation of dual anti-platelet therapy in patients with coronary artery stents: a science advisory. J Am Coll Cardiol 2007;49:734.

Hulot JS et al: Cytochrome P450 2C19 loss-of-function polymorphism is a major determinant of clopidogrel responsiveness in healthy subjects. Blood 2006;108:2244.

Juurlink DN et al: A population-based study of the drug interaction between proton pump inhibitors and clopidogrel. CMAJ 2009;180:713.

Kastrati A et al: Abciximab in patients with acute coronary syndromes undergoing percutaenous coronary intervention after clopidogrel pretreatment: the ISAR-REACT 2 randomized trial. JAMA 2006;295:1531.

Mega JL et al: Cytochrome P-450 polymorphisms and response to clopidogrel. N Engl J Med 2009;360:354.

Patrono C et al: Low-dose aspirin for the prevention of atherothrombosis. N Engl J Med 2005;353:2373.

Patti G et al: Randomized trial of high loading dose of clopidogrel for reduction of periprocedural myocardial infarction in patients undergoing coronary intervention: results from the ARMYDA-2 study. Circulation 2005;111:2099.

Sabatine MS et al: Effect of clopidogrel pretreatment before percutaneous coronary intervention in patients with ST-elevation myocardial infarction treated with fibrinolytics: the PCI-CLARITY study. JAMA 2005;294:1224.

Simon T et al: Genetic determinants of response to clopidogrel and cardiovascular events. N Engl J Med 2009;360:363.

Steinhubl SR et al: Aspirin to prevent cardiovascular disease: the association of aspirin dose and clopidogrel with thrombosis and bleeding. Ann Intern Med 2009;150:379.

US Preventive Services Task Force: Aspirin for the prevention of cardiovascular disease: US Preventive Services Task Force recommendation statement. Ann Intern Med 2009;150:396.

Wolff T, Miller T, Ko S: Aspirin for the primary prevention of cardiovascular events: an update of the evidence for the US Preventive Services Task Force. Ann Intern Med 2009;150:405.

Oral Anticoagulants

Bodin L et al: Cytochrome P450 2C9 (*CYP2CP*) and vitamin K epoxide reductase (*VKORC1*) genotypes as determinanats of acenocoumarol senstivity. Blood 2005;106:135.

Douketis JD et al: The risk for fatal pulmonary embolism after discontinuing anticoagulant therapy for venous thromboembolism. Ann Intern Med 2007;147:766.

Eckman MH et al: Cost-effectiveness of using pharmacogenetic information in warfarin dosing for patients with nonvalvular atrial fibrillation. Ann Intern Med 2009;150:73.

Goldhaber SZ. Optimal duration of anticoagulation after venous thromboembolism: fixed and evidence-based, or flexible and personalized? Ann Intern Med 2009;150:644.

Hart RG, Pearce LA, Aguilar MI: Meta-analysis: antithrombotic therapy to prevent stroke in patients who have nonvalvular atrial fibrillation. Ann Intern Med 2007;146:857.

Olson JD et al: Laboratory reporting of the international normalized ratio: progress and problems. Arch Pathol Lab Med 2007;131:1641.

Prandoni P et al: Residual thrombosis on ultrasonography to guide the duration of anticoagulation in patients with deep venous thrombosis. Ann Intern Med 2009;150:577.

Sconce EA et al: The impact of *CYP2C9* and *VKORC1* genetic polymorphism and patient characteristics upon warfarin dose requirements: proposal for a new dosing regimen. Blood 2005;106:2329.

Heparin/LMWH

Camporese G et al: Low-molecular-weight heparin versus compression stockings for thrombprophylaxis after knee arthroscopy. Ann Intern Med 2008;149:73.

Greer IA, Nelson-Piercy C: Low-molecular-weight heparins for thromboprophylaxis and treatment of venous thromboembolism in pregnancy: a systematic review of safety and efficacy. Blood 2005;105:401.

Warkentin TE et al: Treatment and prevention of heparin-induced thrombocytopenia: American College of Chest Physicians evidence-based clinical practice guidelines. Chest 2008;133:340S.

Other Thrombin Inhibitors

Bauer KA: New anticoagulants. Curr Opin Hematol 2008;15:509.

DiNisio M, Middeldorp S, Buller HR: Direct thrombin inhibitors. N Engl J Med 2005;353:1028.

Eriksson BI et al: Oral dabigatran etexilate vs subcutaneous enoxaparin for the prevention of venous thromboembolism after total knee replacement: the RE-MODEL randomized trial. J Thromb Haemost 2007;5:2178.

Gruber A et al: Relative antithrombotic and antihemostatic effects of protein C activator versus low-molecular-weight heparin in primates. Blood 2007;109:3733.

Lassen MR et al: Rivaroxaban versus enoxaparin for thromboprophylaxis after total knee arthroplasty. N Engl J Med 2008;358:2776.

Thrombolytic Drugs

Iakovou I et al: Incidence, predictors, and outcome of thrombolysis after successful implantation of drug-eluting stents. JAMA 2005;293:2126.

SECTION IV
Transfusion Medicine

BLOOD COMPONENT THERAPY · 38

Blood transfusion became practical early in the twentieth century with the discovery of blood group antigens and methods for typing and matching donor to recipient. Subsequently, with the development of fortified anticoagulants to improve red blood cell preservation, the biocompatible plastic bag system that allows blood fractionation, and expanded testing to prevent disease transmission, modern concepts of blood component therapy gradually evolved. Transfusion practice is now a complex therapeutic discipline, requiring all the skills of a trained clinician. The transfusion of a blood component can never be taken lightly; it should only be given for a good reason after careful evaluation of the clinical situation.

Transfusions should always be targeted to the clinical problem, whether blood loss, anemia, or both; thrombocytopenia; or a coagulopathy. Only the most appropriate blood component(s) should be ordered and transfused (Table 38–1). It is also essential to take into account any special needs of the patient, for example, as in the immunosuppressed patient who should receive only irradiated products to avoid transfusion-associated graft-versus-host disease (TA-GVHD). Great care must be taken to prevent mistakes in matching donor product to recipient, and also in recognizing and treating transfusion reactions. All these items are the responsibility of the physicians and nurses involved in the patient's care.

WHOLE BLOOD

The practice of whole blood transfusion has largely been replaced by component therapy. However, some blood centers are able to offer whole blood or "modified" whole blood (whole blood minus the platelet component) for the treatment of large-volume blood loss. Its use can save time, cost less, and expose the recipient to fewer donors. In the patient with massive blood loss, transfusion of modified whole blood sustains coagulation factor levels in plasma, but platelets need to be replaced separately. There is increasing evidence that in the setting of massive hemorrhage or trauma, component transfusions that simulate the infusion of whole blood (ie, 1 U of plasma for each unit of red blood cells) leads to better outcome with regard to morbidity and mortality.

RED BLOOD CELLS

Transfusion of red blood cells is used to treat most anemia, regardless of cause, to improve oxygen delivery to tissues. A single unit of red blood cells contains all of the red blood cells from a 450-mL unit of whole blood (~200 mL of red blood cells) suspended in 130 mL of plasma/acid citrate dextrose (ACD) solution to give a hematocrit of about 60%. A red blood cell unit also contains sufficient white blood cells and platelets to induce alloimmunization to HLA antigens, and with storage, to increase levels of cytokines capable of producing a febrile transfusion reaction. For this reason, many blood banks and transfusion centers offer other red blood cell products including:

- **Leukodepleted red blood cells:** Red cell units can be passed through a microfiber filter to remove 99.9% of leukocytes, with a loss of 15%–20% of the red blood cells. This step reduces the risk of HLA alloimmunization, cytomegalovirus (CMV) transmission, and, if the cells are filtered prior to storage, cytokine-induced febrile reactions. This product should be considered for use in a patient with a history of recurrent febrile reactions, and is the preferred product for patients in need of long-term transfusion support (eg, hematopoietic

TABLE 38–1 • Blood components for transfusion

Red blood cells
Red blood cells
Leukodepleted red cells
Washed red cells
Irradiated red cells
Frozen (deglycerolized) red cells
CMV-negative red cells
Platelets
Pooled random donor platelets
Single donor pheresis platelets
HLA-matched single donor platelets
Coagulation factors
Fresh frozen plasma
Cryoprecipitate

malignancies, aplastic anemia, stem cell transplantation). In many centers, all of the red cell units available for transfusion are leukodepleted prior to storage.

- **Washed red blood cells:** These red cell units are prepared immediately before transfusion with repeated saline washes and a final suspension in saline. This procedure removes 99% of the original plasma. The primary indication for washed red cell units is to prevent adverse events during transfusion. In the past, patients with diseases such as paroxysmal nocturnal hemoglobinuria received washed units to prevent disease exacerbation from complement in the plasma fraction. With modern red cell production techniques, however, plasma makes up an extremely small fraction of a typical unit. However, for some conditions, such as patients with IgA-deficiency with anti-IgA antibodies, even a small amount of plasma can cause severe anaphylactic reactions. Thus, washed units may be used for these patients, and others with evidence of recurrent or severe allergic reactions to red cell transfusion. Over time, stored red cells also accumulate potassium in the supernatant plasma due to inhibition of the Na/K pump during cold storage. Therefore, washing of red cell units may also be appropriate to reduce or remove supernatant plasma for transfusions of infants or those patients at risk for hyperkalemia (eg, individuals with severe, dialysis-dependent renal disease).
- **Frozen (deglycerolized) red blood cells:** Like washed cells, cryopreserved red blood cells, once deglycerolized, are washed and suspended in saline for transfusion. Therefore, they can be used for the same indications as washed cells. The principal use of frozen red blood cells, however, is their long-term storage for the treatment of patients who are difficult to crossmatch because of rare blood types or the presence of alloantibodies to high-frequency red cell antigens.
- **Irradiated red blood cells:** This product is indicated for markedly immunocompromised patients (including those who receive myelosuppressive chemotherapy) in whom transfused lymphocytes might induce TA-GVHD. Red blood cells are exposed to a minimum dose of 2,500 cGy prior to transfusion. This treatment, while generally benign, will increase potassium levels in supernatant plasma. In addition, the "shelf-life" of an irradiated red cell unit is typically shortened because of the irradiation.
- **CMV-negative red blood cells:** This is a preferred product for CMV-negative recipients, especially those who are undergoing hematopoietic stem cell transplantation. Donors are typically tested for CMV based on the presence or absence of anti-CMV antibodies in their serum; those donors without IgM or IgG class antibodies are considered CMV negative. However, it should be noted that given the ubiquitous nature of CMV infection, most blood donor centers have very limited "CMV-safe" supplies. It has also been found that leukodepleted red cells are virtually equivalent to "CMV-safe" units with regard to virus transmission since the virus typically resides in white blood cells. Thus, most transfusion medicine specialists consider leukoreduced units to be equivalent to CMV-negative units for most indications.

Red Blood Cell Transfusion Therapy

A transfusion of red blood cells is not without risk, and therefore should only be performed when clearly indicated. Hospitals have strict transfusion guidelines that spell out when red cell transfusions are indicated—whether for blood loss related to a procedure, significant anemia (hemoglobin level <7–8 g/dL unless age, illness, or cardiopulmonary disease mandates a higher hemoglobin level), or ongoing hemorrhage. Red blood cells are used to improve oxygen delivery to tissues, not to treat hypovolemia (see Chapter 10). Although red blood cells do provide some volume expansion, actively bleeding patients will require further volume support with electrolyte, colloid, or plasma transfusions. Each unit of red blood cells given to an average-sized adult will increase the hemoglobin level by 1 g/dL (~3% hematocrit rise).

Patients can only receive transfusions with red blood cells of the same or a compatible ABO and Rh blood type. Furthermore, plasma antibodies to any one of several minor blood group antigens can make crossmatching difficult or even render the patient untransfusable. It is important, therefore, to have a basic understanding of the blood group antigen system.

A. Blood Group Antigens

Blood group antigens are inherited amino acid and carbohydrate moieties on the surface of the red blood cell that define the immune potential of the cell. When a person lacking an antigen receives antigen-positive blood, alloantibodies may form, resulting in a transfusion reaction with destruction of the transfused cells. Over 250 antigens, assigned to 23 blood groups, have been identified. However, only the ABO and Rh systems and a handful of so-called minor blood group antigens (Kell, Duffy, Kidd,

TABLE 38–2 • ABO and Rh phenotype frequencies (Caucasians)

Phenotype	Frequency (%)
O	43
A	44
B	9
AB	4
$Rh(D)^+$	85

and the MNSs systems) are of primary importance in transfusion practice. More extensive genotyping of minor blood group antigens is of value in tissue typing and the genetic localization of diseases whose genes are close to a blood group antigen locus.

1. ABO system—Historically, the naturally occurring isoagglutinins, anti-A and anti-B, were used to define the major blood types: A, B, AB, and O. The frequency of each blood type in Caucasian populations is listed in Table 38–2. Genetic analysis has since revealed many subgroups in the ABO system (A_2, A_8, cis AB, B_m, etc), which has helped to explain the variable expression of the A and B antigens.

To avoid a major adverse reaction, transfused blood must be type specific or type compatible. Type O patients have both anti-A and anti-B in their serum, and therefore must receive type O blood. Type B patients carry anti-A, and type A patients carry anti-B. Only type AB patients can accept red blood cells of any type without risk. Type O red blood cells, because they are antigenically silent, can be given to A, B, and AB patients in an emergency. Life-threatening hemolytic transfusion reactions are generally associated with transfusions of type A blood to type O recipients, especially those who carry a high-titer hemolytic anti-A alloantibody.

2. Rh system—The Rh blood group system includes 5 important antigens—D, C, c, E, and e, coded by 2 highly homologous genes on chromosome 1. The prevalence of Rh-negative (D-negative) people varies by race, from as high as 15% in Caucasians to less than 1% in Asians. D-negativity in Caucasians is most often due to a deletion of the entire *RHD* gene, setting the stage for a strong immune response upon exposure to the highly immunogenic D antigen with transfusion or pregnancy. Still, formation of anti-D is not a certainty; naive Rh-negative women come to term without sensitization by a D-positive fetus more often than not. Moreover, the risk of Rh immunization can be reduced to near zero by the administration of hyperimmune anti-D serum (Rh immune globulin) within 72 hours postpartum or following a mismatched transfusion. Much less commonly, hemolytic disease of the newborn can result from antibody formation to C, c, E, and e or a minor blood group antigen.

3. Kell system—The Kell antigens are coded by a gene on chromosome 7. Antibodies to the Kell blood group system (anti-K) have been associated with rapid destruction of Kell-positive red blood cells following transfusion, and an anemia of the newborn secondary to marrow suppression because of antibody interaction with erythropoietic precursors, not hemolysis. Outside of the ABO system, Kell is second only to D in terms of immunogenicity, that is, the ability to induce an alloantibody following transfusion or pregnancy.

4. Duffy system—The Duffy system consists of 2 polymorphic antigens—Fy^a and Fy^b, reflecting a single amino acid difference. Most African Americans (and 100% of West Africans) are Fy(a– b–), perhaps through natural selection, in as much as the Duffy antigen is an obligate receptor for *Plasmodium vivax* and *Plasmodium knowlesi*. Patients with this phenotype may form anti-Fy^a after transfusion but not anti-Fy^b because the Fy(a– b–) recessive gene still encodes normal amounts of Fy^b protein in nonhematopoietic tissues.

5. Other minor blood group antigens—Other minor blood group antigens of importance include the following:

- **The Kidd gene**, located on chromosome 18, codes for 2 antigens—Jk^a and Jk^b. Anti-Jk^a may cause severe immediate or delayed hemolysis after transfusion, as can anti-Jk^b to a lesser extent. Anti-Jk^a and -Jk^b are both dangerous antibodies because of their tendency to decrease to undetectable levels in between transfusions. In addition, both of these antibodies are often able to fix complement, indicating their propensity to mediate intravascular hemolysis. Thus, both anti-Jk^a and -Jk^b are common and potentially serious causes of delayed hemolytic transfusion reactions.
- **The Diego antigens**, Di^a and Di^b, have also been implicated as a cause of hemolytic disease of the newborn. Deficiency in band 3, which carries both the Diego and Wright antigens, has been associated with hereditary spherocytosis.
- **The MNSs system** is expressed on the red blood cell surface as 2 homologous proteins, glycophorin A (M and N antigens) and glycophorin B (S and s antigens). S and s antibodies have been associated with hemolysis, while M and N antibodies have not.
- **Lewis antigens** (Le^a and Le^b), **P antigen**, and **the Ii antigen** system are targets for IgM cold-reacting antibodies seen with cold agglutinin disease, Epstein-Barr virus and mycoplasma infections, and non-Hodgkin lymphomas. The rare P- or I-negative patient can form strong alloantibodies with transfusion.

B. Typing and Crossmatch

Each unit of donated blood is routinely typed prior to storage for both ABO and Rh (D) antigens. In addition, the plasma from the unit is tested for the presence of anti-A and anti-B and for other minor blood group antibodies using the **indirect antiglobulin test**. For the purpose of screening, this test uses a standard set of red blood cells, which express a full range of blood group antigens, to detect plasma IgG antibodies against minor blood group antigens. Approximately 0.5% of donated units will test positive. Even when present, these antibodies pose

TABLE 38–3 • Transmissible disease testing

Agent	Test
T. pallidum (syphilis)	Antibody
Hepatitis B (HBV)	HBsAg, anti-HBc (core antibody)
Hepatitis C (HCV)	Viral protein antibody, nucleic acid testing
CMV	Viral antibody (not routinely performed on all donations)
HIV-1 and -2	Viral antibodies, nucleic acid testing
HTLV-1 and -2	Viral antibody
West Nile virus	Nucleic acid testing
Trypanosomes	Antibody (not routinely performed on all donations)
Malaria	Antibody (EU and UK)
Babesiosis	Antibody (experimental, not routinely performed outside of the US)

little risk to the recipient, since the amount of donor plasma transfused with a unit of red blood cells is less than 20 mL. They do need to be recognized, however, when it comes to the preparation of platelets and fresh frozen plasma (FFP), where the amount of donor plasma transfused is considerably greater.

Donor blood is also tested for specific transmissible diseases (Table 38–3), and all components are quarantined until the test results are available. This approach, together with prescreening of all donors prior to phlebotomy, has made the blood supply extremely safe. For example, since the hepatitis C (HCV) enzyme immunoassay for viral antibody was introduced in 1990, the risk of HCV transmission in the United States has decreased from 1 in 500 to 1 in 100,000 U transfused, and with the advent of nucleic acid amplification testing (NAT, implemented as early as 1995 in some countries), the incidence of transfusion-transmitted HCV is now around 1 in 1 million. Because the window for onset of hepatitis B (HBV) infection and NAT detection is longer than for HCV, the risk for HBV red cell transmission is slightly higher, 3.6 per million in the United States. With NAT, the risk of HIV-1 and HIV-2 red cell transmission is 1 in 3 million and 1 in 15 million, respectively. To further reassure patients, some blood centers also routinely offer an **autologous blood service**, where patients can store their own blood in preparation for surgery. This further reduces, but certainly does not eliminate, the risk of disease transmission and transfusion reactions since errors can still occur because of mishandling of the blood at the time of transfusion.

Red blood cells can be stored for up to 42 days at 4°C. Most washed cells have to be used within 24 hours of preparation to guarantee sterility, although recent technological advancements have allowed for the preparation of thawed units, which "outdate" 2 weeks after their preparation. Prior to transfusion, the donor and the recipient must be matched for compatibility. This process includes selecting ABO and Rh type-specific blood, screening the recipient for serum antibodies, and performing a "major" crossmatch (testing donor cells against patient serum for ABO compatibility). This process is made much more difficult if the patient has a positive indirect antiglobulin test for minor blood group antibodies. In this situation, the antigen specificity of the antibodies must be identified to permit selection of donor units that lack the target antigen.

Compatibility testing can be both costly and time-consuming. This is especially true for the large amount of blood that must be selected and put aside each day in support of surgical procedures that may or may not require transfusion. There is also the issue of the time required for crossmatch when blood is needed urgently. These factors have led to a standard approach to ordering that addresses these logistical problems:

- **Fully crossmatched red blood cells:** Patients requiring an elective transfusion of red blood cells should receive fully crossmatched blood. This includes typing, screening for antibodies, and performing a major crossmatch of each unit. Depending on the workload in the blood bank and any underlying auto- or alloantibodies, several hours may be required before compatible blood will be available for transfusion.
- **Type and screen:** For surgical procedures where blood is only occasionally needed, it is common practice to determine the patient's ABO and Rh type and test the serum for red blood cell antibodies. If none are detected, type-specific blood is set aside but the major crossmatch is not performed. Then, if the patient requires transfusion, crossmatched red blood cells can be made available within 15 minutes, or if it is an emergency, the type-specific blood can be transfused and the crossmatch performed post facto to detect any mismatch.
- **Emergency crossmatch:** When blood is needed urgently, the blood bank can type and crossmatch red blood cells in 15–30 minutes, once a sample of the patient's blood is available. For patients who have already received transfusions, the blood bank usually has a sample on hand. If not, an extra delay can result. Antibody screening results will generally not be available prior to transfusion, but this poses almost no risk to the patient.
- **Uncrossmatched/type-specific red blood cells:** If a patient cannot wait the 15–30 minutes required to obtain crossmatched blood, ABO type-specific or, in a situation where the patient's blood type is unknown, type O-Rh(D) negative red blood cells can be transfused. When the supply of O-negative cells is exhausted, O-positive red blood cells can be substituted with little risk to the recipient; this practice should be done only if absolutely necessary in children and women of child-bearing age. The chance of a reaction to Rh-positive cells is very small; less than 0.5% of patients will be both Rh negative and have an anti-D antibody. A tube of the patient's blood should always be drawn prior to transfusion to avoid confusion and allow the blood bank to start crossmatching additional units. Since the supply of O-negative red blood cells is always limited, conversion of

the patient to type-specific or type-compatible, crossmatched blood should occur as soon as possible.

C. Administration

Red blood cells should never be administered without the informed consent of the patient. The risks involved and the alternatives to transfusion need to be explained, and the patient's consent needs to be documented. It is essential that any transfusion be taken very seriously. It is estimated that 1 in every 10,000–40,000 red blood cell transfusions given in the United States is ABO incompatible, not because of an error in crossmatching, but because of a clerical/management error. The most common errors are mislabeling of the patient's blood sample for typing and crossmatch, and failure to match the unit to be transfused with the right patient at the time of transfusion. Hospitals have written procedures for both sample collection and blood administration. If followed meticulously, these can go a long way toward eliminating transfusion errors.

The **rate of red blood cell administration** will vary with the clinical situation. When red blood cells are given electively to treat a chronic anemia, the first 25–50 mL of each unit should be administered slowly over 10–15 minutes, while closely monitoring the patient. If no immediate adverse reaction is observed, the rate can then be increased. The overall rate will vary depending on the patient's cardiovascular status, the number of units to be transfused, and the patient's tolerance. Signs of volume overload or the appearance of a transfusion reaction, such as fever and chills, will necessarily cut short the transfusion event. All red cell infusions must be completed within 4 hours of issue from the blood bank, but most transfusions last only 2–3 hours.

Red blood cells should never be diluted to decrease viscosity and improve the rate of infusion. The use of fortified anticoagulant solutions (Adsol, etc) for storage maintains the unit's hematocrit at about 60%, so infusion flow rates should not be a problem. If red blood cells are piggybacked to an existing indwelling catheter, only isotonic (0.9%) saline solution should be used in the main line; no medications or other infusions may be given via this route. Exposure to even small amounts of dextrose in water or hypotonic saline can result in clumping and hemolysis; lactated Ringer solutions can cause clot formation. When a higher rate of infusion is required, as with massive blood loss, a pressure bag or cuff can be used to speed delivery. However, flow will not significantly increase unless a large-bore catheter or needle (18 gauge or higher) is in place.

Warming is rarely necessary when red blood cells are given slowly. It is recommended, however, when multiple units are given at rates exceeding 50 mL per minute, when the patient has a high-titer cold agglutinin, or for a newborn receiving an exchange transfusion. Warming should always be done using an approved device designed specifically for blood warming. Never use a microwave to warm blood! Hypocalcemia secondary to citrate toxicity is rarely seen with red blood cell transfusions, even when multiple units are given in cases of massive blood loss. Citrate toxicity can be seen in adults undergoing apheresis procedures (due to the use of citrate as an anticoagulant) and newborns needing exchange transfusion.

Transfusion Complications and Adverse Reactions

Several adverse reactions can complicate a red blood cell transfusion (Table 38–4). Some are relatively frequent, such as febrile (cytokine-induced), non-hemolytic reactions; alloimmunization to HLA antigens; IgE-histamine–driven allergic reactions; and induction of minor blood group antibodies. Others are rare, but can be devastating. The most dreaded is an ABO-incompatible hemolytic transfusion reaction. The severity of reaction to an ABO-mismatched unit of red blood cells varies depending on the type of mismatch, with type A red blood cells administered to a type O patient expressing a high-titer anti-A antibody being the worst case scenario. The most severe reactions involve sudden intravascular hemolysis, which may go unrecognized until a large volume of cells has been infused. This reaction can result in acute renal failure or, when severe, even cardiovascular collapse and death.

The key to preventing a life-threatening reaction to transfusion is to closely monitor the patient during and after the transfusion. The **most frequent signs and symptoms** that accompany a hemolytic reaction include fever, chills, chest and low back pain,

TABLE 38–4 • Adverse effects of blood transfusion

Hemolytic reactions
ABO-incompatible, intravascular hemolysis
Non–ABO-incompatible, intravascular hemolysis
Delayed, extravascular hemolysis
Mechanical hemolysis of infused red cells
Febrile reactions
Septic (bacterially contaminated) reactions
Cytokine-induced fever
HLA alloimmunization reactions
Allergic reactions
Alloimmunization, decreased platelet survival
IgE-related histamine reactions
IgA-deficient anaphylaxis
Immunocompromised reactions
Transfusion-associated GVHD (TA-GVHD)
Transfusion-related immunomodulation (TRIM)
Infectious agent transmission
Bacterial or parasitic contamination (non-septic reaction)
Cytomegalovirus, West Nile virus
Viral hepatitis (B, C, other)
HIV and HTLV-I
Other adverse effects
Transfusion-related acute lung injury (TRALI)
Transfusion-associated circulatory overload (TACO)
Post-transfusion purpura (PTP)
Isolated hypotensive reactions
Iron overload

hypotension, and often a feeling of impending doom. The transfusion must be discontinued immediately and a venous blood sample drawn to look for intravascular hemolysis and to repeat the crossmatch. The further workup and management of the patient with intravascular hemolysis is discussed in Chapter 11.

A. Types of Reactions

Delayed hemolytic transfusion reactions are seen in patients who develop antibodies to one of the minor blood group antigens, most often to the Rh system (E or c), Kell, Fy^a, or Jk^a. Generally, this occurs in a patient who has already been immunized from a past pregnancy or transfusion, but whose antibody is below the limits of detection of a routine serum antibody screen. Typically, extravascular red blood cell hemolysis is clinically silent, other than a surprising fall in the hematocrit within a few days or even weeks. If this happens, a repeat of the serum antibody screen will usually detect the antibody. However, depending on the antibody class and specificity, moderate to severe intra- and extravascular reactions have been seen with minor blood group antigens.

Patients who have had multiple transfusions and patients receiving red blood cells that have been stored for long periods without leukodepletion often experience fever and/or chills, beginning, during, or several hours after the transfusion. This effect is not a hemolytic reaction. It is caused by cytokines released by contaminating leukocytes or alloantibodies to leukocyte and platelet HLA antigens. Transfusion with leukodepleted red blood cells, together with premedicating the patient with hydrocortisone, diphenhydramine, and/or acetaminophen, can greatly ameliorate this reaction. Patients who have had several febrile reactions to blood should receive only leukodepleted red blood cells, preferably cells leukodepleted at the time of donation, prior to storage.

Simple **allergic reactions** are common with transfusion. The incidence of hives and mild bronchospasm, perhaps related to IgE-related histamine response to infused plasma proteins, cytokines, or both, has been estimated to occur in 2%–10% of transfusions. **Atopic individuals** may be at greater risk. Treatment of affected patients with diphenhydramine, 25–50 mg orally or intravenously, usually ameliorates this reaction so that transfusion can be completed.

Transfusion-related acute lung injury (TRALI), a severe, sometimes fatal pulmonary reaction characterized by noncardiogenic pulmonary edema and hypotension, has been described in association with leukocyte or HLA-specific complement-activating antibodies in transfused platelets, plasma, or red cells. The passive transfer of these antibodies, which then react with the recipient's leukocytes, results in activation of neutrophils, adherence to pulmonary endothelial cells, microvascular pulmonary damage, and liberation of complement-derived anaphylatoxins. Most patients with TRALI present with tachypnea, dyspnea, and fever during or within 1–2 hours of transfusion; however, TRALI symptoms may manifest as late as 6 hours post-infusion. Signs include an increased A-aO_2 gradient, decreased breath sounds, and diffuse, bilateral infiltrates on chest films. Aggressive respiratory (and ventilatory) support with supplemental oxygen should be instituted as for any acute lung injury, but steroids and diuretics are of no benefit. The risk of TRALI is decreased by excluding multiparous women from donating blood, but this certainly affects the donor pool. In the United States and the United Kingdom, several efforts are under way to convert to an "all-male" plasma supply to reduce the risk and incidence of TRALI.

Red blood cell transfusions carry a special risk for the severely **immunocompromised patient**. Only irradiated red blood cells and, if the patient is CMV negative, CMV-negative or leukodepleted units should be used. Unirradiated red blood cells contain enough viable lymphocytes to cause TA-GVHD. Red blood cell transfusions are also believed to modulate the immune system. They have been used to induce tolerance in patients receiving renal transplants and may be associated with a higher incidence of postoperative infection and secondary cancers. Finally, although the risk of disease transmission is very small, **bacterial and viral infections secondary to transfusion** still can occur, the latter because of the variable window period between onset of viral infection (with transmissible risk) and earliest detection. The risk of infection for HBV, HCV, and human immunodeficiency virus (HIV) from well-screened, NAT-tested blood is less than 1 in 1.5 million units/components transfused.

IgA-deficient patients are very rare but are at considerable risk for a severe anaphylactic reaction if they have formed anti-IgA antibodies. Once identified, they should only receive a transfusion of washed or deglycerolized red blood cells. Any plasma component transfusion should be with product from an IgA-deficient donor.

Red Blood Cell Transfusion Alternatives

A. Autologous Blood Storage

Two to four units of blood can be collected from a normal-sized adult in the weeks prior to an elective surgical procedure and stored for use during surgery. Administration of erythropoietin can be used to facilitate the collection and maintain the patient's hematocrit as near normal as possible. The use of autologous blood can reduce, but certainly not eliminate, many of the risks of transfusion. The opportunity still exists for a clerical error or mistake in patient-unit identification. Bacterial contamination can also still occur. However, in situations where the blood supply is unreliable or the patient cannot be easily crossmatched, the use of autologous blood can be of value.

Autologous blood storage makes sense in a limited set of circumstances, primarily elective surgical procedures where transfusion of 2–4 U of red blood cells is predictable and sufficient. Orthopedic procedures such as total hip and major knee operations are one good example. Autologous blood storage is inappropriate in elective surgeries where blood loss is usually minimal (<1–2 U) or major procedures requiring more than 4 U. There is also the issue of whether, once collected, autologous blood should be returned to the patient regardless of the volume of blood lost. The patient owns the blood and since it cannot be given to another patient, many people think "why not?" This thinking has to be strongly discouraged. It not only violates the rules guiding transfusion practice but also runs the risk of unnecessary transfusion error, volume overload, and a supranormal postoperative hematocrit.

B. Red Blood Cell Salvage

Shed blood can be retrieved from the operative site and the red cells separated for perioperative transfusion. Red blood cell salvage has its greatest application in major surgical procedures, such as open-heart operations, where the site of blood loss is readily accessible. It can serve to reduce the need for allogeneic transfusion.

C. Erythropoietin Therapy

Besides increasing the amount of autologous blood that can be donated and stored, **perioperative erythropoietin therapy** can also reduce the need for transfusion. Erythropoietin will increase in vivo erythropoiesis preoperatively and postoperatively. When erythropoietin is given a week or more before, and continued for up to 10 days after major elective surgery, the immediate postoperative anemia is less and a 5%–6% rise in the hematocrit level can be seen by the tenth postoperative day (see Chapter 10). The number of units of red blood cells transfused is also reduced. Success, however, is very much dependent on the level of iron supply during treatment, so aggressive iron supplementation is essential.

D. Red Cell Substitutes

Red blood cell substitutes have been a dream for a long time. Perfluorocarbon emulsions and hemoglobin-based oxygen carriers have been studied for the past 50 years but have still not shown clear success and are often associated with many side effects. Third-generation compounds are still in the testing stage of development.

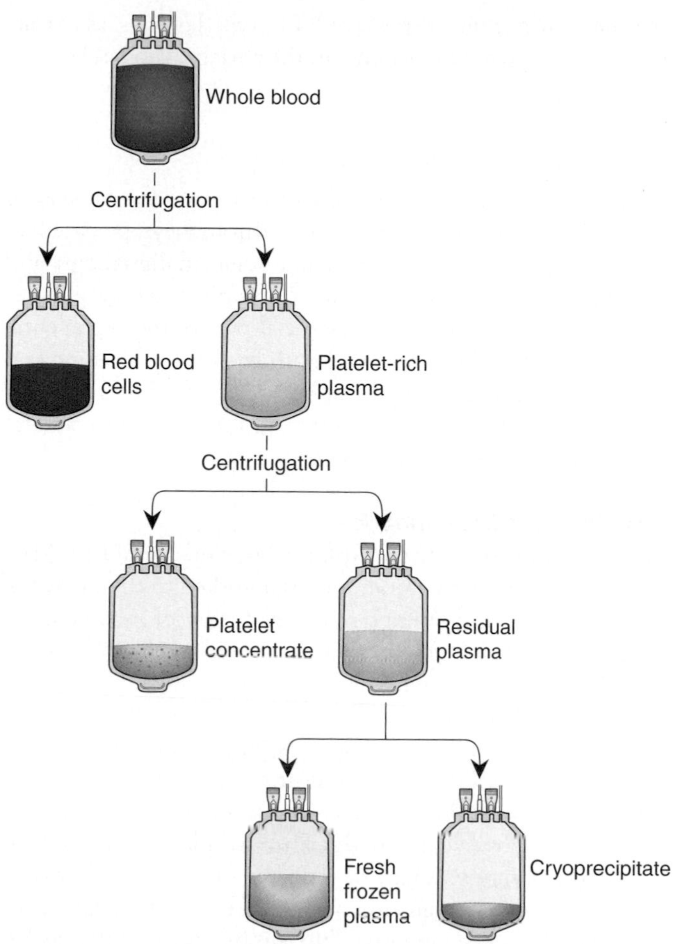

FIGURE 38–1. **Blood component preparation.** Diagram of the separation of whole blood into red blood cells, platelet concentrate, and FFP or cryoprecipitate, using the multibag system.

PLATELETS

Platelet concentrates can be prepared from individual units of donated blood **(random donor platelets)** or harvested from a single donor by cytapheresis **(apheresis, or single-donor platelets)**. In the United States, where blood is routinely collected using a multibag system (Figure 38–1), platelet rich plasma (PRP) is separated from red blood cells by centrifugation at a low G force. The PRP is then transferred to a smaller connected bag where, following a second spin at a higher G force to further concentrate the platelets, excess supernatant plasma is transferred to a third bag. About 50 mL of plasma/ACD solution is left behind. This method recovers about 60%–70% of the platelets from the original unit of blood, together with a portion of the leukocytes and a few red blood cells (<0.3 mL). Most platelet concentrates contain 10^8 or more leukocytes, which is enough to induce HLA alloimmunization and cause febrile transfusion reactions.

Random donor platelet concentrates can be stored for up to 5 days at 20°C–24°C. Although the normal survival of platelets in the circulation is 10 days, platelet recovery after transfusion is predictably reduced by 25% or more, mostly because of splenic sequestration. Between 4 and 6 U of random donor platelets are pooled to comprise a single platelet transfusion unit. When transfused into an average-sized adult, 6 U (a "6-pack") of random donor pooled platelets increase the platelet count by approximately 50,000/μL, usually enough to control any bleeding tendency. In patients with a qualitative platelet defect (eg, aspirin treatment), transfusion of platelets in an amount equivalent to 10%–20% of the circulating platelet count (1–2 pools) generally is sufficient to stop the bleeding.

Platelets in amounts equivalent to 6–10 pooled random donor units can be harvested from a single donor by cytapheresis, and many blood centers now employ plateletpheresis as their routine platelet production procedure. Each plateletpheresis unit has a volume of 200–500 mL and contains approximately 3×10^{11} platelets. Like random donor units, apheresis platelets can be stored for up to 5 days at 20°C–24°C. Single-donor apheresis platelet units are processed like platelets prepared from a unit of whole blood. They are ABO and Rh typed and tested for transmissible disease, and therefore are only available for transfusion once testing results are known, usually 24 hours after the draw. Most blood centers also provide single-donor apheresis platelets drawn from a registry of HLA-typed donors, as a strategy to improve platelet recovery in the patient who has become HLA alloimmunized.

Platelet Transfusion Therapy

The routine availability of platelet concentrates for transfusion has revolutionized the management of thrombocytopenia. Myeloablative chemotherapy for hematologic malignancies and bone marrow transplantation are 2 situations where platelet transfusions are an absolutely essential part of the therapeutic regimen. Platelet therapy is used both to prevent bleeding and to treat the patient with thrombocytopenia who is actively bleeding. Guidelines for platelet transfusions in various platelet disorders are discussed in Chapter 31.

A. Typing and Crossmatch

As with red blood cell transfusions, platelets should be ABO type-specific if possible. A-antigen is absorbed to the surface of platelets of type A patients, so a transfusion of incompatible platelets may result in a somewhat shortened survival. However, since this is a relatively minor issue, ABO-incompatible platelets can be given when the supply of type-specific platelets runs short, without risk to the patient. If large volumes of type-O donor plasma (>500 mL), containing anti-A and anti-B, are transfused to a type A, B, or AB patient, the direct antiglobulin test may turn positive and both transfused platelet and patient red blood cell survivals may be reduced. Reports of intravascular hemolysis due to high-titer anti-A and/or anti-B agglutinins in platelets have been reported, but this is a rare occurrence. Rh antigens are not present on the platelet surface, so the Rh type need not be considered. However, the small number of red blood cells present in platelet preparations from Rh-positive donors can induce anti-D antibody in an Rh-negative patient. This will not affect platelet survival and is only of consequence when the patient is of child-bearing age; in this circumstance, Rh-immune globulin is used to prevent alloimmunization and should be administered within 3 days of an Rh-mismatched transfusion.

Patients receiving transfusions of multiple units of platelets and other blood products are likely to become **"refractory,"** defined as a failure to achieve a respectable platelet count increment immediately following or within 1 hour of transfusion. Depending on the clinical illness, the cause may be multifactorial. Anti-platelet antibodies in the patient with idiopathic thrombocytopenic purpura or non-immune factors such as fever, sepsis, disseminated intravascular coagulation, and hypersplenism can all be responsible. However, alloimmunization to platelet and leukocyte HLA antigens also must be considered, especially for those patients who receive platelet and blood product transfusions over a long period, such as patients with hematologic malignancies or aplastic anemia. Pre-storage leukodepletion of platelet units is a major factor in reducing the risk of alloimmunization to HLA antigens.

To evaluate a patient for the possibility of platelet transfusion refractoriness due to HLA alloimmunization, patient serum is tested with platelets from multiple donors, usually an index pool drawn from the central donor institution representing a wide variety of HLA subsets. When there is evidence of reactivity, the patient is considered to be alloimmunized, usually to an HLA antigen, although such testing lacks specificity in identifying the target of a patient's antibody. However, if patients do test positive, several possibilities for transfusion exist. First, patients may receive "crossmatched" platelets, that is, platelets from a single donor that demonstrate no reactivity with their serum. In such a circumstance, the donor platelets lack target antigens and should circulate for a longer period of time post-infusion. Crossmatched platelets are a viable option for patients who demonstrate serological reactivity against a moderate number of donors in an index pool. If a patient's serum demonstrates reactivity against a high percentage of donors in an index pool, then the possibility of randomly finding crossmatch compatible units is low. In such cases, the patient should undergo HLA typing, which allows for the provision of HLA-matched platelets, typically drawn from an HLA-matched unrelated community donor(s). This approach often yields an improved post-transfusion recovery, confirming a significant component of alloimmunization. When crossmatched or HLA-matched platelets fail to induce an adequate post-transfusion platelet count increment, continued transfusion of random, non-matched donor platelets may be of clinical benefit, even though there is no apparent improvement in the platelet count.

B. Platelet Administration

Like red blood cells, platelets should be transfused using a standard filter set to exclude fibrin clots and debris. Microfiber filters are available to leukodeplete the platelet unit at the time of transfusion at the cost, however, of a 20%–25% loss of platelets. Leukodepletion also helps prevent CMV transmission and alloimmunization, whether random or apheresis platelets are used. Platelet units should be leukodepleted prior to storage to decrease cytokine production; this will reduce the severity of fever and chills in the sensitized patient. Moreover, sensitized patients should be premedicated and the platelets infused at a slower rate. Even in the face of severe fever and chills, platelet recovery may be respectable. Immunocompromised patients should receive irradiated platelets.

The effectiveness of a platelet transfusion can only be determined by its impact on the patient's platelet count and the control of ongoing hemorrhage (see Chapter 31). Measurement of the patient's platelet count at 1, 4, and 24 hours following transfusion can ideally be used to assess **recovery** (the incremental rise in the platelet count at 1 hour), and **survival** (the fall in the platelet count at 4 and 24 hours). This information is essential for planning subsequent platelet transfusions. The pattern of the response may also help identify the cause of apparent refractoriness (see discussion in Chapter 31).

C. Complications

All of the reactions previously listed for red cell components may be encountered during platelet infusion, and are treated accordingly. In addition, because platelets are stored at room temperature, the risk of bacterial contamination is significantly increased compared to other blood products. In fact, the rate of contamination of platelets is estimated to be as high as 0.1% of units transfused, although apheresis platelets generally pose a lower risk. Sepsis or high (>102°F/39°C) or persistent fever following transfusion should be reason to draw blood cultures and, if available, culture the remnant of the transfused unit. It is now a US Food and Drug Administration (FDA) requirement that all platelet units be tested for bacterial contamination prior to transfusion; this policy has decreased the rate of post-platelet transfusion sepsis.

COAGULATION FACTOR COMPONENTS

As an integral part of blood component therapy, blood centers prepare fresh frozen plasma (FFP) and cryoprecipitate as respective sources of coagulation factors at physiologic levels, and a concentrated product containing fibrinogen, von Willebrand factor (vWF), and factor XIII. FFP is most often used in patients with liver disease or those who require immediate reversal of warfarin anticoagulation. Both products are used for massive blood loss, where low factor and fibrinogen levels can result from dilution by the combination of colloid or electrolyte infusions, and large volume red cell transfusions. Low levels of coagulation factors, especially fibrinogen and the common pathway factors, can also result from the consumptive coagulopathy associated with trauma.

Fresh Frozen Plasma

FFP is harvested from donated whole blood as part of the preparation of platelet concentrates. Using a 3-bag system, the excess plasma/ACD solution left after the platelet concentrate centrifugation step (~200–250 mL) is transferred to the third bag, separated, and frozen within 8 hours of collection. FFP can then be stored for up to 1 year at -20°C. At the time of transfusion, it is thawed at 37°C, a process that takes 30–60 minutes. Once thawed, FFP should be transfused within 12 hours to guarantee adequate coagulation factor levels and sterility. FFP should be ABO compatible with the patient's red blood cells. Many blood centers also now provide a similar product known as plasma frozen within 24 hours of collection. As the name suggests, this product, unlike FFP, must be processed and frozen within 24 hours of initial collection. Plasma frozen within 24 hours is used because an 8-hour restriction often means that many whole blood donations cannot be used for FFP preparation. Thus, plasma frozen within 24 hours can help to alleviate or curb potential shortages of FFP. Studies have shown that the levels of coagulation factors in these products are virtually equivalent to FFP.

Plasma transfusion may be used in several clinical situations (Table 38–5). In all cases, FFP should be reserved for patients demonstrating coagulopathy by tests like the prothrombin time (PT) or partial thromboplastin time (PTT). A common misconception with FFP use is that the higher the PT/PTT, the larger the dose of plasma is needed. This is not necessarily the case. Like any pharmaceutical product, the dose of plasma depends primarily on the weight of the patient receiving transfusion. To sustain a baseline factor level of 25%–30% (ie, that which is necessary to maintain adequate coagulation function), a plasma dose of 10–15 mL/kg is often sufficient for most coagulopathic patients. In the setting of trauma, as a general rule, transfusions for massive blood loss should follow a 1:1:1 ratio of red cells:FFP:platelets as closely as possible; this ratio has resulted in improved hospital survival for combat injuries. Thus, a pool of platelets and 6 U of FFP should be transfused for every 6 U of red blood cells transfused, with additional FFP or platelets given according to the clinical situation (see Chapters 31 and 35).

TABLE 38–5 • Indications for coagulation factor replacement

Fresh frozen plasma
Massive blood loss/transfusion
Emergency reversal of warfarin therapy
Factor replacement in DIC
Treatment of hereditary coagulopathies (if purified factor unavailable)
Liver disease
Cryoprecipitate
Treatment of factor XIII deficiency
Fibrinogen replacement, particularly in DIC
Bleeding associated with uremia
Purified and recombinant factor preparations
von Willebrand disease
Inherited factor deficiencies

When FFP is used to treat a PT greater than twice the control value in an adult patient weighing 70 kg or more, an appropriate plasma dose of 4–6 U (~800–1,200 mL) must be given to achieve factor levels of greater than 30%. Each FFP unit increases coagulation factor levels by only 2%–3%. Thus, attempting correction of the PT may involve the transfusion of close to 1,500 mL of plasma/ACD solution, and unless the patient is actively bleeding, can result in volume overload and congestive heart failure. Certainly, subsequent FFP infusions may be limited by the large volumes required for an appreciable incremental impact on factor levels. In addition, any sustained benefit from transient FFP correction of the PT requires a normal level of coagulation factor production by the liver. Patients with severe liver disease will benefit only briefly, often for only a few hours, before the transfused coagulation factors, especially factor VII, decline and the PT rises once again. In this regard, it is also important to remember that the effects of plasma infusion induce only a temporary correction of coagulation tests. For instance, the duration of the correction of the PT following plasma infusion correlates with the half-life of factor VII, which is about 4–6 hours. Thus, the timing of plasma infusion is an extremely important aspect of FFP therapy. For the non-bleeding patient with a prolonged baseline PT who is receiving plasma transfusion to prevent complications from invasive procedures, the plasma should be infused as close as possible to the start time of the procedure. Provision of plasma more than 4–6 hours before the start of a procedure will only result in a return to a coagulopathic state at the time when the patient's procedure is to begin! One good strategy for prophylactic reversal of a prolonged PT prior to an invasive procedure is to infuse 1 U of FFP immediately before the procedure and 1 U during the procedure. In this way, the patient will attain maximal coagulation status precisely when it is most needed.

Like red cells and platelets, plasma can induce virtually all types of transfusion reactions. In fact, antibody-mediated reactions like TRALI are most common with plasma products because of the opportunity to encounter high-titered antibody (red cells and platelets have a much smaller plasma fraction). Allergic reactions are also quite common following plasma infusion. Finally, because of the large volumes sometimes necessary to replace coagulation factors in large patients or those with persistent, ongoing bleeding, plasma infusions may also commonly be associated with circulatory overload. Adverse events to plasma infusion are treated in the same way as those following transfusion of red cells or platelets, as discussed above.

Cryoprecipitate

Cryoprecipitate (cryo) is prepared by flash freezing fresh plasma and then thawing it at 4°C. This process leaves a residual precipitate, once the plasma/ACD supernatant is removed, of cryoproteins, including fibrinogen, fibronectin, vWF, and factors VIII and XIII. The procedure recovers 150–200 mg of fibrinogen and 80–100 U of factor VIII/vWF in 15 mL of residual plasma, a 10-fold concentration over FFP. Cryoprecipitate units can then be stored for up to 1 year at 4°C. The greatest advantage of cryo is its small volume—large amounts of fibrinogen can be replenished with only a few hundred milliliters of fluid. As with plasma infusions, cryoprecipitate is dosed by weight and is based, in part, on a patient's underlying fibrinogen levels. Since this calculation can be complicated and not easily performed in the acute setting, as a general rule, an adult patient with hypofibrinogenemia should receive a pool of 10 U of thawed cryo, which should be infused within 4 hours of pooling. Indications for cryoprecipitate therapy are listed in Table 38–5.

Each unit of cryoprecipitate will raise a patient's fibrinogen level by only 5–10 mg/dL. Thus, when it is used to treat hypofibrinogenemia (fibrinogen levels <100 mg/dL), a minumum of 10 U need to be pooled, which is sufficient to increase the circulating fibrinogen level in an average-sized adult by at least 100 mg/dL. Following transfusion, the fibrinogen level should be monitored and repeated infusions given to maintain levels above 100 mg/dL. The amount required will vary with the rate of fibrinogen consumption. Cryo can also be used as a low-volume therapy to replete factor XIII levels in the setting of congenital or acquired deficiencies. There is also growing evidence to suggest the use of cryo for bleeding associated with uremia. In this condition, circulating platelets do not function properly, often leading to microvascular oozing and bleeding. Although the mechanism of action of cryo in this setting remains unclear, it is theorized that the high levels of vWF attained post-infusion promote platelet adhesion and activation, helping to overcome acquired functional defects.

The treatment of von Willebrand disease (vWD) itself is often empirical and depends on the disease subtype. In the past, doses of cryoprecipitate ranged from 20–30 pooled units per day in an adult with severe type 1 or 3 disease to fewer than 10 U/d for those with mild disease (see Chapter 32). However, with the development of virally inactivated, intermediately purified factor VIII concentrates containing large amounts of vWF (eg, Humate-P), cryoprecipitate is no longer the product of choice in the treatment of vWD and should only be used for this indication if no virally inactivated factor VIII or vWF concentrates are readily available. Cryoprecipitate is also used in the operating room for the preparation of fibrin glue for topical surgical hemostasis.

Purified and Recombinant Factor Preparations

The treatment of the inherited coagulopathies has changed dramatically, first with the purification of individual factors from pooled plasma, then with viral inactivation methodology, and now with the synthesis of recombinant coagulation factors and growth factors, the latter including erythropoietin and now possibly useful thrombopoietin mimetics. Recombinant technology has opened the door to a highly sophisticated approach to the management of both bleeding disorders and some thrombotic pathologies. See Chapters 31, 33, 34, and 36 for a full discussion.

POINTS TO REMEMBER

Transfusions and the choice of the most appropriate blood component(s) should always be targeted to a specific clinical problem whether blood loss, thrombocytopenia, or coagulopathy.

Leukodepleted red blood cells are the units of choice for transfusion therapy for anemia, blood loss, or both. Frozen red blood cells are used for patients with rare blood types or alloantibodies to high frequency antigens.

Irradiated and CMV-negative/leukodepleted red cells are preferred for transplant and other immunocompromised patients. Washed red cells are reserved for rare patients who require removal of plasma to deplete IgA (IgA deficiency) or those at risk of hyperkalemia (dialysis dependence).

All blood products are tested for transmissible diseases, including viral hepatitis (HBV, HCV), HIV-1 and -2, and West Nile virus. Nucleic acid amplification testing (NAT) has greatly reduced the incidence of transfusion-transmitted viral infections. Testing of platelet units for bacterial contamination (because platelets are stored at room temperature for 5 days) has reduced the incidence of post-transfusion sepsis.

As a routine, patients should only receive ABO and Rh type-specific blood. In response to a "type and crossmatch" order from the physician, the blood bank determines the recipient's ABO and Rh type and screens for serum antibodies to minor blood group antigens. Selected units are then crossmatched (test of donor cells against patient serum for ABO compatibility). This procedure can take 30 minutes or more.

When patients require immediate red cell transfusion, uncrossmatched type O, Rh-negative, or ABO type-specific red cells can be used. FFP should also be type specific, but unless there is alloimmunization, platelet transfusions do not require typing.

Transfusion of incompatible (ABO mismatched) blood is most often the result of clerical and identification errors at the bedside, not a crossmatching error in the laboratory. Therefore, strict adherence to transfusion policies cannot be emphasized enough.

An ABO-mismatch hemolytic transfusion reaction (usually a unit of type A blood given to a type O patient) is characterized by fever, chills, chest and low back pain, and hypotension. If any of these signs are present, the transfusion must be discontinued immediately.

Other complications of transfusion include a delayed hemolytic transfusion reaction (due to a minor blood group incompatability), an IgE-driven allergic reaction, and TRALI, an infrequent but severe complication that must be aggressively treated with respiratory support.

Platelet transfusions are one of the mainstays of supportive care for thrombocytopenic patients receiving intensive chemotherapy where they are transfused prophylactically for severe thrombocytopenia and for any bleeding symptoms. Platelet transfusion is also indicated for bleeding caused by acquired (drug-induced) or congenital platelet dysfunction.

Platelet transfusions are given either as pools combined from 4–6 random single donors or as a cytapheresis unit prepared from 1 donor. Patients receiving chronic platelet transfusions have a high rate of alloimmunization, resulting in refractoriness to subsequent platelet transfusions. Platelet "crossmatching" for HLA-compatible platelets is used to improve platelet recovery in such patients.

Fresh frozen plasma (FFP) contains all of the coagulation factors at physiologic levels and is most often used to replace factors II, V, VII, X, and XI when there is liver disease or vitamin K deficiency induced by warfarin. Because of the short half-life of factor VII, correction of the PT is short-lived if these underlying abnormalities are not remedied.

Cryoprecipitate, an enriched product from plasma, has very high concentrations of fibrinogen, factor XIII, and vWF. Cryoprecipitate transfusion is used to treat bleeding associated with low fibrinogen levels, such as acquired with disseminated intravascular coagulation (DIC), and uremia, and congenital factor XIII deficiency.

BIBLIOGRAPHY

Borgman MA et al: The ratio of blood products transfused affects mortality in patients receiving massive transfusions at a combat support hospital. J Trauma 2007;763:805.

Kerkhoffs JLH et al: A multicenter randomized study of the efficacy of transfusions with platelets stored in platelet additive solution II versus plasma. Blood 2006;108:3210.

Marks PW: Thrombocytopenia and platelet transfusion. In: Simon TL, Snyder EL, Solheim BG, Powell CP, Strauss RG, Petrides M, eds: Rossi's Principles of Transfusion Medicine. Wiley Blackwell, 2009;199-210.

Pomper GJ: Febrile, allergic, and nonimmune transfusion reactions. In: Simon TL, Snyder EL, Solheim BG, Powell CP, Strauss RG, Petrides M, eds: Rossi's Principles of Transfusion Medicine. Wiley Blackwell, 2009;826-846.

Silliman CC, Ambruso DR, Boshkov LK: Transfusion-related acute lung injury. Blood 2005;105:2266.

Tormey CA, Snyder EL: Transfusion support for the oncology patient. In: Simon TL, Snyder EL, Solheim BG, Powell CP, Strauss RG, Petrides M, eds: Rossi's Principles of Transfusion Medicine. Wiley Blackwell, 2009;482-497.

INDEX

Note: Numbers followed by f and t denote figures and tables, respectively.

B

M

N

U